D0100325

MANUAL OF
CLINICAL LABORATORY
IMMUNOLOGY
THIRD EDITION

TALL
RB
46.5   Manual of clinical
.M36   laboratory immunology.
1986

Lake Tahoe Community College
Learning Resources Center
So. Lake Tahoe, CA   95702

MANUAL OF
CLINICAL LABORATORY
IMMUNOLOGY
THIRD EDITION

Editors:

Noel R. Rose

Department of Immunology and Infectious Diseases
The Johns Hopkins University School of Hygiene and Public Health
Baltimore, Maryland

Herman Friedman

Department of Medical Microbiology and Immunology
University of South Florida College of Medicine
Tampa, Florida

John L. Fahey

Department of Microbiology and Immunology
Center for Interdisciplinary Research in Immunology and Disease
UCLA School of Medicine
Los Angeles, California

LAKE TAHOE COMMUNITY COLLEGE
LIBRARY AND MEDIA SERVICES

American Society for Microbiology
Washington, D.C. 1986

Copyright © 1976, 1980, 1986
American Society for Microbiology
1913 I St., N.W.
Washington, DC 20006

Library of Congress Cataloging-in-Publication Data

Main entry under title:

Manual of clinical laboratory immunology.
    Rev. ed. of: Manual of clinical immunology. 2nd ed. 1980.
    Includes bibliographies and indexes.
    1. Immunodiagnosis—Handbooks, manuals, etc. 2. Immunology—
Handbooks, manuals, etc. I. Rose, Noel R. II. Friedman, Herman,
1931–   . III. Fahey, John L. IV. Manual of clinical immunology. [DNLM:
1. Immunological Technics. QY 25 M2942]
RB46.5.M36 1986   616.07′5   85–26675

ISBN 0-914826-66-2
ISBN 0-914826-70-0 (soft)

All Rights Reserved
Printed in the United States of America

Contents

Section A. GENERAL METHODOLOGY
Section Editor: Robert F. Ritchie

Section B. IMMUNOASSAY
Section Editor: Bruce S. Rabin

Section C. IMMUNOGLOBULINS AND B-CELL DISORDERS
Section Editor: Gerald M. Penn

Section D. COMPLEMENT AND IMMUNE COMPLEXES
Section Editor: Peter H. Schur

Section E. LYMPHOCYTE ENUMERATION
Section Editors: Noel L. Warner and John L. Fahey

Section F. CELLULAR COMPONENTS
Section Editor: Ross E. Rocklin

Section G. HOST RESPONSES TO BACTERIAL, MYCOTIC, AND PARASITIC DISEASES
Section Editor: Steven D. Douglas

Section H. VIRAL, RICKETTSIAL, AND CHLAMYDIAL IMMUNOLOGY
Section Editor: John L. Sever

Section I. IMMUNOHEMATOLOGY
Section Editor: Bruce C. Gilliland

Section J. ALLERGY
Section Editor: Reuben P. Siraganian

Section K. IMMUNODEFICIENCY
Section Editor: Evan M. Hersh

Section L. AUTOIMMUNE DISEASES
Section Editor: Eng M. Tan

Section M. TUMOR IMMUNOLOGY
Section Editor: Ronald B. Herberman

Section N. IMMUNOGENETICS AND TRANSPLANTATION IMMUNOLOGY
Section Editors: Edmond J. Yunis and Devendra P. Dubey

Section O. IMMUNOPATHOLOGY AND IMMUNOHISTOLOGY
Section Editor: David T. Rowlands, Jr.

Section P. LABORATORY MANAGEMENT AND ADMINISTRATION
Section Editor: Dan F. Palmer

Editorial Board

Steven D. Douglas   **Section G**
    The Children's Hospital of Philadelphia and Department of Pediatrics, University of
    Pennsylvania School of Medicine, Philadelphia, Pennsylvania 19104
Devendra P. Dubey   **Section N**
    Division of Immunogenetics, Dana-Farber Cancer Institute, Harvard Medical School,
    Boston, Massachusetts 02115
Bruce C. Gilliland   **Section I**
    Department of Medicine and Laboratory of Medicine, University of Washington,
    Seattle, Washington 98195, and Pacific Medical Center, Seattle, Washington 98144
Ronald B. Herberman   **Section M**
    Pittsburgh Cancer Institute, Pittsburgh, Pennsylvania 15213
Evan M. Hersh   **Section K**
    Department of Clinical Immunology and Biological Therapy, University of Texas
    System Cancer Center, M. D. Anderson Hospital and Tumor Institute, Houston, Texas
    77030
Dan F. Palmer   **Section P**
    Serology Training Unit, Centers for Disease Control, Atlanta, Georgia 30333
Gerald M. Penn   **Section C**
    Grant Medical Center and Department of Pathology, College of Medicine, The Ohio
    State University, Columbus, Ohio 43215
Bruce S. Rabin   **Section B**
    Department of Pathology, University of Pittsburgh, Pittsburgh, Pennsylvania 15261
Robert F. Ritchie   **Section A**
    Foundation for Blood Research, Scarborough, Maine 04074
Ross E. Rocklin   **Section F**
    Allergy Division, Department of Medicine, Tufts University Medical Center, New
    England Medical Center, Boston, Massachusetts 02111
David T. Rowlands, Jr.   **Section O**
    Department of Pathology, University of South Florida College of Medicine, Tampa,
    Florida 33612
Peter H. Schur   **Section D**
    Department of Rheumatology and Immunology, Brigham and Women's Hospital,
    Harvard Medical School, Boston, Massachusetts 02115
John L. Sever   **Section H**
    Infectious Disease Branch, National Institute of Neurological and Communicative
    Disorders and Stroke, Bethesda, Maryland 20892
Reuben P. Siraganian   **Section J**
    Clinical Immunology Section, Laboratory of Microbiology and Immunology, National
    Institute of Dental Research, Bethesda, Maryland 20892
Eng M. Tan   **Section L**
    Autoimmune Disease Center, Scripps Clinic and Research Foundation, La Jolla,
    California 92037
Noel L. Warner   **Section E**
    Becton Dickinson Immunocytometry Systems, Mountain View, California 90403
Edmond J. Yunis   **Section N**
    Division of Immunogenetics, Dana-Farber Cancer Institute, Harvard Medical School,
    Boston, Massachusetts 02115

Contributors

N. Franklin Adkinson, Jr.
The Johns Hopkins University School of Medicine at the Good Samaritan Hospital, Baltimore, Maryland 21239

C. R. Adolphson
Allergic Diseases Research Laboratory, Mayo Clinic, Rochester, Minnesota 55905

Vincent Agnello
Immunology Laboratory, Lahey Clinic Foundation, Burlington, Massachusetts 01805

M. Teresa Aguado
Department of Immunology, Research Institute of Scripps Clinic, La Jolla, California 92037

Aaron D. Alexander
Chicago College of Osteopathic Medicine, Chicago, Illinois 60615

Chester A. Alper
The Center for Blood Research, Boston, Massachusetts 02115

D. Bernard Amos
Division of Immunology, Duke University Medical Center, Durham, North Carolina 27710

Porter Anderson
The University of Rochester Medical Center, Rochester, New York 14642

Warren A. Andiman
Departments of Pediatrics and Epidemiology and Public Health, Yale University School of Medicine, New Haven, Connecticut 06510

Kenneth A. Ault
Hematology Division, Brigham and Women's Hospital, Boston, Massachusetts 02115

Henry A. Azar
Department of Pathology, University of South Florida College of Medicine, and Laboratory Service, James A. Haley Veterans' Hospital, Tampa, Florida 33612

Ajay Bakhshi
Metabolism Branch, National Cancer Institute, Bethesda, Maryland 20892

Stanley P. Ballou
Case Western Reserve University, Cleveland Metropolitan General Hospital, Cleveland, Ohio 44109

Robert C. Bast, Jr.
Duke University Medical Center, Durham, North Carolina 27710

Irene Batty
Wellcome Research Laboratories, Beckenham, Kent BR3 3BS, United Kingdom

Patrick G. Beatty
Fred Hutchinson Cancer Research Center, Puget Sound Blood Center, and Department of Medicine, Division of Oncology, University of Washington, Seattle, Washington 98104

Joseph A. Bellanti
Departments of Pediatrics and Microbiology and the International Center for Interdisciplinary Studies of Immunology, Georgetown University School of Medicine, Washington, D.C. 20007

Robert B. Belshe
Department of Medicine, Marshall University School of Medicine, Huntington, West Virginia 25701

Lee L. Berman
Department of Epidemiology and Public Health, Yale University School of Medicine, New Haven, Connecticut 06510

Wilma B. Bias
Division of Medical Genetics, Department of Medicine, The Johns Hopkins University School of Medicine, Baltimore, Maryland 21205

Dennis Bidwell
Nuffield Laboratories of Comparative Medicine, Institute of Zoology, Zoological Society of London, London NW1 4RY, England

Pierluigi E. Bigazzi
Department of Pathology, University of Connecticut Health Center, Farmington, Connecticut 06032

P. Andrew Biro
Dana-Farber Cancer Institute and Department of Pathology, Harvard Medical School, Boston, Massachusetts 02115

Francis L. Black
Department of Epidemiology and Public Health, Yale University School of Medicine, New Haven, Connecticut 06510

Larry Borish
Allergy Division, Department of Medicine, Tufts University School of Medicine, New England Medical Center, Boston, Massachusetts 02111

Robert Bortolussi
Infection and Immunology Research Laboratory, Izaak Walton Killam Hospital for Children, Halifax, Nova Scotia B3J 3G9, Canada

Lynda L. Bradford
Serology Section, California Department of Health Services, Berkeley, California 94704

Brenda L. Brandt
Department of Bacterial Diseases, Walter Reed Army Institute of Research, Washington, D.C. 20307

William E. Braun
Histocompatibility and Immunogenetics Laboratory, Department of Immunopathology, Cleveland Clinic Foundation, Cleveland, Ohio 44106

Robert R. Brubaker
Department of Microbiology and Public Health, Michigan State University, East Lansing, Michigan 48824

Philip A. Brunell
Department of Pediatrics, University of Texas Health Sciences Center, San Antonio, Texas 78284

C. Edward Buckley III
Departments of Medicine and Microbiology-Immunology, Duke University Medical Center, Durham, North Carolina 27710

C. Lynne Burek
Department of Immunology and Infectious Diseases, The Johns Hopkins University School of Hygiene and Public Health, Baltimore, Maryland 21205

Peter M. Burkholder
Veterans' Administration Medical Center and University of Michigan Medical School, Ann Arbor, Michigan 48105

Don G. Burstyn
Office of Biologics Research and Review, Center for Drugs and Biologics, Bethesda, Maryland 20892

C. B. Carpenter
Brigham and Women's Hospital, Boston, Massachusetts 02115

Philip B. Carter
Department of Microbiology, Pathology, and Parasitology, School of Veterinary Medicine, North Carolina State University, Raleigh, North Carolina 27606

Irene J. Check
Department of Pathology and Laboratory Medicine, Emory University, Atlanta, Georgia 30333

Max A. Chernesky
McMaster University Regional Virology Laboratory, St. Joseph's Hospital, Hamilton, Ontario, Canada L8N 4A6

T. Ming Chu
Diagnostic Immunology Research and Biochemistry Department, Roswell Park Memorial Institute, Buffalo, New York 14263

Laurence Corash
Department of Laboratory Medicine, University of California, San Francisco, California 94143

Jeffrey Cossman
Hematopathology Section, Laboratory of Pathology, National Cancer Institute, Bethesda, Maryland 20892

John P. Craig
Department of Microbiology and Immunology, SUNY Downstate Medical Center, Brooklyn, New York 11203

Marie C. Crookston
Department of Pathology, University of Toronto, and Department of Laboratory Hematology, Toronto General Hospital, Toronto, Ontario M5G 2C4, Canada

Richard M. Dauphinais
Department of Pathology and Laboratory Medicine, St. Francis Hospital and Medical Center, Hartford, Connecticut 06105

Sharad D. Deodhar
Department of Immunopathology, The Cleveland Clinic Foundation, Cleveland, Ohio 44106

Steven D. Douglas
The Children's Hospital of Philadelphia and Department of Pediatrics, University of Pennsylvania School of Medicine, Philadelphia, Pennsylvania 19104

Walter R. Dowdle
Centers for Disease Control, Atlanta, Georgia 30333

Gordon R. Dreesman
Southwest Foundation for Biomedical Research, San Antonio, Texas 78284

Devendra P. Dubey
Division of Immunogenetics, Dana-Farber Cancer Institute, Harvard Medical School, Boston, Massachusetts 02115

Christine S. Eisemann
Walter Reed Army Institute of Research, Washington, D.C. 20307

Carmen G. Espinoza
Department of Pathology, University of South Florida College of Medicine, and Laboratory Service, James A. Haley Veterans' Hospital, Tampa, Florida 33612

John L. Fahey
Department of Microbiology and Immunology, Center for Interdisciplinary Research in Immunology and Disease, UCLA School of Medicine, Los Angeles, California 90024

Anthony S. Fauci
National Institute of Allergy and Infectious Diseases, Bethesda, Maryland 20892

John C. Feeley
Division of Bacterial Diseases, Center for Infectious Diseases, Centers for Disease Control, Atlanta, Georgia 30333

Patricia Ferrieri
Departments of Laboratory Medicine/Pathology and Pediatrics and Clinical Microbiology Laboratory, University of Minnesota Medical School, Minneapolis, Minnesota 55455

Jordan N. Fink
Medical College of Wisconsin, Veterans' Administration Medical Center, Milwaukee, Wisconsin 53226

Thomas Folks
Laboratory of Immunoregulation, National Institute of Allergy and Infectious Diseases, Bethesda, Maryland 20892

Robert C. Foster
Atlantic Antibodies, Scarborough, Maine 04074

Janet M. Fowler
Department of Microbiology and Public Health, Michigan State University, East Lansing, Michigan 48824

Marvin J. Fritzler
Department of Medicine, Health Sciences Centre, Calgary, Alberta, Canada T2N 4N1

David A. Fuccillo
Microbiological Associates, Bethesda, Maryland 20816

Robert S. Galen
Department of Biochemistry, The Cleveland Clinic Foundation, Cleveland, Ohio 44106

J. Phillip Galvin
E. I. Du Pont de Nemours & Co., Inc., Glasgow Research Laboratory, Wilmington, Delaware 19898

M. R. Garovoy
University of California Medical Center, San Francisco, California 94143

Bruce C. Gilliland
Department of Medicine and Laboratory of Medicine, University of Washington, Seattle, Washington 98195, and Pacific Medical Center, Seattle, Washington 98144

Janis V. Giorgi
Human Immunobiology Group, Department of Microbiology and Immunology, UCLA School of Medicine, Los Angeles, California 90024

David Glass
Department of Rheumatology and Immunology, Brigham and Women's and Beth Israel Hospitals, and Department of Medicine, Harvard Medical School, Boston, Massachusetts 02115

G. J. Gleich
Allergic Diseases Research Laboratory, Mayo Clinic, Rochester, Minnesota 55905

John Godwin
Division of Hematology, The University of North Carolina at Chapel Hill, Chapel Hill, North Carolina 27514

Sidney H. Golub
Division of Surgical Oncology, UCLA School of Medicine, Los Angeles, California 90024

Sidney E. Grossberg
Department of Microbiology, Medical College of Wisconsin, Milwaukee, Wisconsin 53226

John A. Hansen
Puget Sound Blood Center, Fred Hutchinson Cancer Research Center, and Department of Medicine, Division of Oncology, University of Washington, Seattle, Washington 98104

John A. Hardin
Department of Internal Medicine, Yale University School of Medicine, New Haven, Connecticut 06510

Curtis Harris
Division of Infectious Diseases, Department of Pediatrics, Johns Hopkins University School of Medicine, Baltimore, Maryland 21205

Robert J. Hartzman
Naval Medical Research Institute, Bethesda, Maryland 20014

James C. D. Hengst
Allied Health and Scientific Products, Andover, Massachusetts 01810

Ronald B. Herberman
Pittsburgh Cancer Institute, Pittsburgh, Pennsylvania 15213

Kenneth L. Herrmann
Division of Viral Diseases, Center for Infectious Diseases, Centers for Disease Control, Atlanta, Georgia 30333

Evan M. Hersh
Department of Clinical Immunology and Biological Therapy, University of Texas System Cancer Center, M. D. Anderson Hospital and Tumor Institute, Houston, Texas 77030

John C. Hierholzer
Respiratory and Enteric Viruses Branch, Center for Infectious Diseases, Centers for Disease Control, Atlanta, Georgia 30333

F. Blaine Hollinger
Department of Medicine, Virology, and Epidemiology, Baylor College of Medicine, Houston, Texas 77030

H. W. Holy
Technical Consultants S.A., 1260 Nyon, Switzerland

Richard Hong
Department of Pediatrics, University of Wisconsin Clinical Science Center, Madison, Wisconsin 53792

William A. Hook
Clinical Immunology Section, Laboratory of Microbiology and Immunology, National Institute of Dental Research, Bethesda, Maryland 20892

Gail A. Hudson
Foundation for Blood Research, Scarborough, Maine 04074

Richard Insel
The University of Rochester Medical Center, Rochester, New York 14642

Thomas B. Issekutz
Infection and Immunology Research Laboratory, Izaak Walton Killam Hospital for Children, Halifax, Nova Scotia B3J 3G9, Canada

Anne L. Jackson
Becton Dickinson Immunocytometry Systems, Mountain View, California 94043

Deborah A. Jacobsen
Microbiology Research Laboratory, Mayo Clinic and Mayo Foundation, Rochester, Minnesota 55905

Elaine S. Jaffe
Hematopathology Section, Laboratory of Pathology, National Cancer Institute, Bethesda, Maryland 20892

Peter B. Jahrling
U.S. Army Medical Research Institute of Infectious Diseases, Fort Detrick, Frederick, Maryland 21701

Patricia Jameson
Department of Microbiology, Medical College of Wisconsin, Milwaukee, Wisconsin 53226

A. H. Johnson
Division of Immunologic Oncology, Lombardi Cancer Center, Georgetown University School of Medicine, Washington, D.C. 20007

Andrew Myron Johnson
Center for Blood Research, Boston, Massachusetts 02115

Irving G. Kagan
Parasitic Disease Consultants, Inc., Tucker, Georgia 30084

Leo Kaufman
Immunology Branch, Division of Mycotic Diseases, Center for Infectious Diseases, Centers for Disease Control, Atlanta, Georgia 30333

Douglas S. Kellogg
Sexually Transmitted Diseases Laboratory Program, Center for Infectious Diseases, Centers for Disease Control, Atlanta, Georgia 30333

Alan P. Kendal
Centers for Disease Control, Atlanta, Georgia 30333

George E. Kenny
Department of Pathobiology, University of Washington, Seattle, Washington 98195

Robert C. Knapp
Dana-Farber Cancer Institute, Boston, Massachusetts 02115

Richard B. Kohler
Indiana University Medical Center, Indianapolis, Indiana 46223

Stanley Korsmeyer
Metabolism Branch, National Cancer Institute, Bethesda, Maryland 20892

Irving Kushner
Case Western Reserve University, Cleveland Metropolitan General Hospital, Cleveland, Ohio 44109

Robert A. Kyle
Departments of Internal Medicine and Laboratory Medicine, Mayo Clinic and Mayo Foundation, and Mayo Medical School, Rochester, Minnesota 55905

Parviz Lalezari
Division of Immunohematology, Department of Medicine, Montefiore Medical Center, Albert Einstein College of Medicine, New York, New York 10467

H. Clifford Lane
Laboratory of Immunoregulation, National Institute of Allergy and Infectious Diseases, Bethesda, Maryland 20892

Paul H. Lange
Department of Urologic Surgery, University of Minnesota Medical School, Minneapolis, Minnesota 55455, and Urology Section, Veterans' Administration Medical Center, Minneapolis, Minnesota 55417

Jennifer Larsen
Division of Endocrinology and Metabolism, Department of Internal Medicine, University of Utah Medical Center, Salt Lake City, Utah 84132

Sandra A. Larsen
Treponema Research Branch, Centers for Disease Control, Atlanta, Georgia 30333

Thomas B. Ledue
Atlantic Antibodies, Scarborough, Maine 04074

Spencer H. S. Lee
Department of Microbiology, Faculty of Medicine, Dalhousie University, Halifax, Nova Scotia B3J 3G9, Canada

Maurice J. Lefford
Department of Immunology and Microbiology, School of Medicine, Wayne State University, Detroit, Michigan 48201

Flora Leister
Division of Infectious Diseases, Department of Pediatrics, Johns Hopkins University School of Medicine, Baltimore, Maryland 21205

Lawrence Levine
Department of Biochemistry, Brandeis University, Waltham, Massachusetts 02254

Joe B. Linker III
Department of Medicine, University of New Mexico, Albuquerque, New Mexico 87131

David Y. Liu
Department of Medicine, Harvard University Medical School, and Department of Rheumatology and Immunology, Brigham and Women's Hospital, Boston, Massachusetts 02111

Eufronio G. Maderazo
Medical Research Laboratory, Department of Medicine, Hartford Hospital, Hartford, Connecticut 06115, and Departments of Medicine and Pathology, University of Connecticut School of Medicine, Farmington, Connecticut 06032

James B. Mahony
McMaster University Regional Virology Laboratory, St. Joseph's Hospital, Hamilton, Ontario, Canada L8N 4A6

Annette E. Maluish
Program Resources, Inc., National Cancer Institute-Frederick Cancer Research Facility, Frederick, Maryland 21701

Charles R. Manclark
Office of Biologics Research and Review, Center for Drugs and Biologics, Bethesda, Maryland 20892

Peter W. A. Mansell
Department of Cancer Prevention, University of Texas System Cancer Center, M. D. Anderson Hospital and Tumor Institute, Houston, Texas 77030

Deborah Marcus
The Center for Blood Research, Boston, Massachusetts 02115

Joseph B. Margolick
Departments of Environmental Health Sciences and Immunology and Infectious Diseases, The Johns Hopkins University School of Hygiene and Public Health, Baltimore, Maryland 21205

Richard B. Markham
Departments of Medicine and Microbiology and Immunology, Washington University School of Medicine, and the Jewish Hospital of St. Louis, St. Louis, Missouri 63110

P. L. Masson
Unit of Experimental Medicine, International Institute of Cellular and Molecular Pathology, University of Louvain, B-1200 Brussels, Belgium

Robert J. Mayer
Dana-Farber Cancer Institute and Department of Medicine, Harvard Medical School, Boston, Massachusetts 02215

Bruce D. Meade
Office of Biologics Research and Review, Center for Drugs and Biologics, Bethesda, Maryland 20892

Virginia S. Mehl
Grant Medical Center and Department of Medical Microbiology and Immunology, College of Medicine, The Ohio State University, Columbus, Ohio 43215

Margaret E. Meyer
Department of Epidemiology and Preventive Medicine, School of Veterinary Medicine, University of California, Davis, California 95616

Eric M. Mickelson
Fred Hutchinson Cancer Research Center, Puget Sound Blood Center, and Department of Medicine, Division of Oncology, University of Washington, Seattle, Washington 98104

Malcolm S. Mitchell
University of Southern California School of Medicine, Los Angeles, California 90033

Thomas P. Monath
Division of Vector-Borne Viral Diseases, Center for Infectious Diseases, Centers for Disease Control, Fort Collins, Colorado 80522-2087

Alton C. Morgan, Jr.
NeoRx, Seattle, Washington 98119

Stephen A. Morse
Sexually Transmitted Diseases Laboratory Program, Center for Infectious Diseases, Centers for Disease Control, Atlanta, Georgia 30333

Maurice A. Mufson
Department of Medicine, Marshall University School of Medicine, Huntington, West Virginia 25701

C. Gwyneth Munn
Department of Clinical Immunology and Biological Therapy, University of Texas System Cancer Center, M. D. Anderson Hospital and Tumor Institute, Houston, Texas 77030

Nancy B. Murphy
Histocompatibility and Immunogenetics Laboratory, Department of Immunopathology, Cleveland Clinic Foundation, Cleveland, Ohio 44106

Betty Nakamoto
Division of Hematology, Department of Medicine, University of Washington, Seattle, Washington 98195

Robert M. Nakamura
Department of Pathology, Scripps Clinic and Research Foundation, La Jolla, California 92037

W. Stephen Nichols
Department of Pathology, Scripps Clinic and Research Foundation, and University of California, San Diego, La Jolla, California 92037

John F. Nitsche
Immutek Clinical Immunology Reference Laboratory, New Orleans, Louisiana 70115, and Tulane Medical Center, New Orleans, Louisiana 70112

Philip S. Norman
The Johns Hopkins University School of Medicine at the Good Samaritan Hospital, Baltimore, Maryland 21239

William D. Odell
Division of Endocrinology and Metabolism, Department of Internal Medicine, University of Utah Medical Center, Salt Lake City, Utah 84132

Herbert F. Oettgen
Human Cancer Immunology Laboratory, Memorial Sloan-Kettering Cancer Center, New York, New York 10021

Lloyd J. Old
Human Cancer Immunology Laboratory, Memorial Sloan-Kettering Cancer Center, New York, New York 10021

Ørjan Olsvik
Department of Microbiology and Immunology, Norwegian College of Veterinary Medicine, Oslo, Norway

Joseph V. Osterman
Naval Medical Research and Development Command, Bethesda, Maryland 20814

M. A. Palladino, Jr.
Genentech, Inc., South San Francisco, California 94080

Dan F. Palmer
Serology Training Unit, Centers for Disease Control, Atlanta, Georgia 30333

Thalia Papayannopoulou
Division of Hematology, Department of Medicine, University of Washington, Seattle, Washington 98195

Gerald M. Penn
Grant Medical Center and Department of Pathology, College of Medicine, The Ohio State University, Columbus, Ohio 43215

Stephen M. Peters
Department of Pediatrics and the International Center for Interdisciplinary Studies of Immunology, Georgetown University School of Medicine, Washington, D.C. 20007

Lawrence D. Petz
Department of Clinical and Experimental Immunology, City of Hope National Medical Center, Duarte, California 91010

A. C. Pier
Division of Microbiology and Veterinary Medicine, The University of Wyoming, Laramie, Wyoming 82071

Gerald B. Pier
Channing Laboratory, Department of Medicine, Brigham and Women's Hospital and Harvard Medical School, Boston, Massachusetts 02115

Margaret Piper
Department of Pathology and Laboratory Medicine, Emory University, Atlanta, Georgia 30333

Douglas Pohl
Immunology Laboratory, Lahey Clinic Foundation, Burlington, Massachusetts 01805

Bruce S. Rabin
Department of Pathology, University of Pittsburgh, Pittsburgh, Pennsylvania 15261

Francisco X. Real
Human Cancer Immunology Laboratory, Memorial Sloan-Kettering Cancer Center, New York, New York 10021

Errol Reiss
Immunology Branch, Division of Mycotic Diseases, Center for Infectious Diseases, Centers for Disease Control, Atlanta, Georgia 30333

Heinz Remold
Department of Medicine, Harvard University Medical School, and Department of Rheumatology and Immunology, Brigham and Women's Hospital, Boston, Massachusetts 02111

James M. Reuben
Department of Clinical Immunology and Biological Therapy and Department of Laboratory Medicine, University of Texas System Cancer Center, M. D. Anderson Hospital and Tumor Institute, Houston, Texas 77030

Margaret Rheinschmidt
Department of Laboratory Medicine, University of California, San Francisco, California 94143

John H. Rippey
St. Luke's Hospital Laboratory, Kansas City, Missouri 64111

Robert F. Ritchie
Foundation for Blood Research, Scarborough, Maine 04074

R. E. Ritts, Jr.
Microbiology Research Laboratory, Mayo Clinic and Mayo Foundation, Rochester, Minnesota 55905

Bruce A. Robbins
Department of Pathology, Scripps Clinic and Research Foundation, La Jolla, California 92037

Harold R. Roberts
Division of Hematology, Departments of Medicine and Pathology, Center for Thrombosis and Hemostasis, The University of North Carolina at Chapel Hill, Chapel Hill, North Carolina 27514

Ross E. Rocklin
Allergy Division, Department of Medicine, Tufts University School of Medicine, New England Medical Center, Boston, Massachusetts 02111

R. P. Channing Rodgers
Department of Laboratory Medicine, School of Medicine, University of California, San Francisco, California 94143, and Clinical Laboratory, Veterans' Administration Medical Center, San Francisco, California 94121

Paula J. Romano
Department of Surgery, Milton S. Hershey Medical Center, Pennsylvania State University, Hershey, Pennsylvania 17033

Noel R. Rose
Department of Immunology and Infectious Diseases, The Johns Hopkins University School of Hygiene and Public Health, Baltimore, Maryland 21205

Lanny J. Rosenwasser
Allergy Division, Department of Medicine, Tufts-New England Medical Center, Boston, Massachusetts 02111

Gordon D. Ross
University of North Carolina, Chapel Hill, North Carolina 27514

David T. Rowlands, Jr.
Department of Pathology, University of South Florida College of Medicine, Tampa, Florida 33612

Robert L. Rubin
Autoimmune Disease Center, Department of Basic and Clinical Research, Scripps Clinic and Research Foundation, La Jolla, California 92037

Shaun Ruddy
Division of Immunology and Connective Tissue Diseases, Department of Medicine, Medical College of Virginia, Virginia Commonwealth University, Richmond, Virginia 23298

R. Bradley Sack
Department of International Health, The Johns Hopkins University School of Hygiene and Public Health, Baltimore, Maryland 21205

Fred Sanfilippo
Department of Pathology, Duke University Medical Center, Durham, North Carolina 27710

Julius Schachter
Department of Laboratory Medicine, University of California, San Francisco, and San Francisco General Hospital, San Francisco, California 94110

Gerald Schiffman
Department of Microbiology and Immunology, Downstate Medical Center, State University of New York, Brooklyn, New York 11203

Nathalie J. Schmidt
Viral and Rickettsial Disease Laboratory, State of California Health Services, Berkeley, California 94704

Peter H. Schur
Department of Rheumatology and Immunology, Brigham and Women's Hospital, Harvard Medical School, Boston, Massachusetts 02115

John L. Sever
Infectious Disease Branch, National Institute of Neurological and Communicative Disorders and Stroke, Bethesda, Maryland 20892

M. R. Shalaby
Genentech, Inc., South San Francisco, California 94080

Michael J. Sheehy
American Red Cross and University of Wisconsin, Madison, Wisconsin 53792

Ziad M. Shehab
Department of Pediatrics, University of Arizona Health Sciences Center, Tucson, Arizona 85724

Isabel C. Shekarchi
Microbiological Associates, Bethesda, Maryland 20816

A. E. Sherrod
Department of Pathology, University of Southern California, Los Angeles, California 90033

Sidney Shulman
Sperm Antibody Laboratory, Metropolitan Hospital, New York, New York 10029

Ruth E. Siebenlist
Department of Microbiology, Medical College of Wisconsin, Milwaukee, Wisconsin 53226

Reuben P. Siraganian
Clinical Immunology Section, Laboratory of Microbiology and Immunology, National Institute of Dental Research, Bethesda, Maryland 20892

Alan R. Smerglia
Histocompatibility and Immunogenetics Laboratory, Department of Immunopathology, Cleveland Clinic Foundation, Cleveland, Ohio 44106

Merrill J. Snyder
Division of Infectious Diseases, University of Maryland School of Medicine, Baltimore, Maryland 21201

Frederick S. Southwick
Hematology-Oncology Unit, Massachusetts General Hospital, Boston, Massachusetts 02114

Glenn Steele
New England Deaconness Hospital, Dana-Farber Cancer Institute, and Department of Surgery, Harvard Medical School, Boston, Massachusetts 02215

James C. Sternberg
Diagnostic Systems Group, Beckman Instruments, Inc., Brea, California 92621

John A. Stewart
Division of Viral Diseases, Center for Infectious Diseases, Centers for Disease Control, Atlanta, Georgia 30333

Thomas P. Stossel
Hematology-Oncology Unit, Massachusetts General Hospital, Boston, Massachusetts 02114

Douglas M. Strong
Genetic Systems Corporation, Seattle, Washington 98121

Karen A. Sullivan
Histocompatibility and Immunogenetics Laboratory, Department of Medicine, Tulane University Medical School, New Orleans, Louisiana 70112

Arne Svejgaard
Tissue-Typing Laboratory, University Hospital (Rigshospitalet), DK-2200 Copenhagen N, Denmark

Eng M. Tan
Autoimmune Disease Center, Scripps Clinic and Research Foundation, La Jolla, California 92037

Gregory A. Tannock
Faculty of Medicine, Royal Newcastle Hospital, The University of Newcastle, Newcastle NSW 2300, Australia

Clive R. Taylor
Department of Pathology, University of Southern California, Los Angeles, California 90033

Jerry L. Taylor
Department of Microbiology, Medical College of Wisconsin, Milwaukee, Wisconsin 53226

Roger N. Taylor
Laboratory Program Office, Centers for Disease Control, Atlanta, Georgia 30333

Argyrios N. Theofilopoulos
Department of Immunology, Research Institute of Scripps Clinic, La Jolla, California 92037

E. Donnall Thomas
Fred Hutchinson Cancer Research Center and Department of Medicine, Division of Oncology, University of Washington, Seattle, Washington 98104

Peter Thomas
Mallory Gastrointestinal Research Laboratory, Boston City Hospital; Department of Medicine, Harvard Medical School; and Department of Pathology, Boston University School of Medicine, Boston, Massachusetts 02118

Carol Ann Toth
Immunology Laboratory, Lahey Clinic Foundation, Burlington, Massachusetts 01805

Edmund C. Tramont
Department of Bacterial Diseases, Walter Reed Army Institute of Research, Washington, D.C. 20307

Raymond R. Tubbs
Department of Pathology, The Cleveland Clinic Foundation, Cleveland, Ohio 44106

Rafael Valenzuela
Department of Immunopathology, The Cleveland Clinic Foundation, Cleveland, Ohio 44106

Robert L. Vessella
Department of Urologic Surgery, University of Minnesota Medical School, Minneapolis, Minnesota 55455, and Urology Section, Veterans' Administration Medical Center, Minneapolis, Minnesota 55417

Raphael Viscidi
Department of Medicine, The Johns Hopkins University School of Medicine, Baltimore, Maryland 21205

Alister Voller
Nuffield Laboratories of Comparative Medicine, Institute of Zoology, Zoological Society of London, London NW1 4RY, England

I. Kaye Wachsmuth
Division of Bacterial Diseases, Center for Infectious Diseases, Centers for Disease Control, Atlanta, Georgia 30333

Joseph L. Waner
Department of Pediatrics, University of Oklahoma Health Sciences Center, Oklahoma Children's Memorial Hospital, Oklahoma City, Oklahoma 73190

Peter A. Ward
Department of Pathology, University of Michigan Medical School, Ann Arbor, Michigan 48109-0010

Noel L. Warner
Becton Dickinson Immunocytometry Systems, Mountain View, California 94043

Marina L. Wasylyshyn
Division of Surgical Oncology, UCLA School of Medicine, Los Angeles, California 90024

Siok-Bi Wee
Department of Pediatrics, Johns Hopkins Hospital, Baltimore, Maryland 21205

Shelba D. Whaley
Diagnostic Immunology Training Section, Centers for Disease Control, Atlanta, Georgia 30333

L. Joseph Wheat
Indiana University Medical Center, Indianapolis, Indiana 46223

Arthur White
Indiana University Medical Center, Indianapolis, Indiana 46223

Hazel W. Wilkinson
Centers for Disease Control, Atlanta, Georgia 30333

Ralph C. Williams, Jr.
Department of Medicine, University of New Mexico, Albuquerque, New Mexico 87131

Merlin R. Wilson
Immutek Clinical Immunology Reference Laboratory, New Orleans, Louisiana 70115, and Louisiana State University Medical Center and Tulane Medical Center, New Orleans, Louisiana 70112

Robert J. Winchester
>Hospital for Joint Diseases, New York, New York 10003

Robert H. Yolken
>Division of Infectious Diseases, Department of Pediatrics, Johns Hopkins University School of Medicine, Baltimore, Maryland 21205

Charles R. Young
>Center for Vaccine Development, Division of Geographic Medicine, University of Maryland, Baltimore, Maryland 21201

J. W. Yunginger
>Allergic Diseases Research Laboratory, Mayo Clinic, Rochester, Minnesota 55905

Edmond J. Yunis
>Division of Immunogenetics, Dana-Farber Cancer Institute, Harvard Medical School, Boston, Massachusetts 02115

Ivan Yunis
>Division of Immunogenetics, Dana-Farber Cancer Institute, Harvard Medical School, Boston, Massachusetts 02115

Andrea A. Zachary
>Histocompatibility and Immunogenetics Laboratory, Department of Immunopathology, Cleveland Clinic Foundation, Cleveland, Ohio 44106

Norman Zamcheck
>Mallory Gastrointestinal Research Laboratory, Mallory Foundation, Boston City Hospital; Department of Medicine, Harvard Medical School; and Department of Pathology, Boston University School of Medicine, Boston, Massachusetts 02118

Wendell D. Zollinger
>Department of Bacterial Diseases, Walter Reed Army Institute of Research, Washington, D.C. 20307

Preface

This third edition of the *Manual of Clinical Laboratory Immunology*, like the first and second editions (entitled *Manual of Clinical Immunology*), represents a joint effort by members of the American Society for Microbiology (ASM) and the American Association of Immunologists to provide medical scientists and physicians interested in human immunology with a guide to the rapidly growing field of clinical laboratory immunology. The first edition of this manual developed as a natural extension of the *Manual of Clinical Microbiology*, which is now in its fourth edition as a highly successful publication of ASM. The first edition of the *Manual of Clinical Microbiology*, published in 1970, devoted approximately 100 pages to various serologic tests. As in many manuals of microbiology, immunology was considered only for the diagnosis of microbial infections by immunological means.

In 1975 a companion text to the *Manual of Clinical Microbiology* was conceived to deal exclusively with applications of immunology to detection and analysis of a wide variety of diseases, not only diseases induced by microorganisms. This *Manual of Clinical Immunology* would be devoted to methodologies which are used in the clinical laboratory for diagnosing infectious diseases as well as diseases of various other origins, such as autoimmunity, allergy, and cancer, and also to methods used in transplantation and transfusion immunology. Since the publication of the first edition of the manual in 1976, the acquisition of knowledge and the introduction of new and improved methods of clinical laboratory immunology have occurred rapidly. Developments such as immunoassays based upon enzyme-linked, radiolabeled, or fluorescein-labeled antibodies, as well as the newer hybridoma technologies and monoclonal antibodies, were included in a second edition of the *Manual of Clinical Immunology*, published in 1980. Subsequently, immunological methodology continued to grow at such a rapid pace that we believed that a revised and updated manual was needed in 1986.

The term "clinical immunology" is being utilized by physicians who diagnose and treat patients with immunological diseases. Therefore, we and the ASM Publications Board felt that the word "laboratory" should be included in the title of this manual, hence the revised title, *Manual of Clinical Laboratory Immunology*. As in the first and second editions, this manual deals almost exclusively with techniques and methods used in laboratory settings.

This manual is divided into sections, with distinguished immunologists serving as the editors of each section. The first section deals with the general methodology and contains chapters discussing the methods for antiserum preparation, characterization of such antisera, precipitin techniques, turbidity, nephelometry, particle immunoenhancement assays, complement fixation, and similar assays. A shortened immunoassay section discusses only the general principles of assays based upon enzymes, radioisotopes, and fluorescence, as we felt that detailed descriptions of each immunoassay are no longer necessary. The section on immunoglobulins and B-cell disorders describes methodologies for the detection of immunoglobulins, monoclonal gammopathies, and gene rearrangement. The section on complement and immune complexes contains chapters on the classical and alternative pathways, complement allotypes, and immune complexes.

A new section added to this edition details lymphocyte enumeration methods. Among them are the newer techniques of flow cytometry for identification of T- and B-lymphocyte subsets. The recommended (international) nomenclature for the clusters of differentiation (CD) with the lymphoid system is included in this section. The section on cellular components of the immune response system discusses not only delayed hypersensitivity testing by in vitro techniques but also one of the few in vivo techniques described in this manual, i.e., skin testing for delayed hypersensitivity, since this is such an important portion of the armamentarium of the clinical immunologist. Interleukins, lymphocyte-mediated cytotoxicity, natural killer cells, suppressor cells, and lymphocyte proliferation assays are also described in this section.

Several sections describe methods for the detection of infections caused by microorganisms, including bacteria, fungi, parasites, viruses, rickettsiae, and chlamydiae. The section on immunohematology describes blood grouping, immune drug-induced hemolysis, immunology of hemolytic diseases, and detection of hemoglobins. The section on allergy and allergic immunology includes a chapter on skin testing, as well as newer methods for measuring immunoglobulin E antibody, histamine release detection, and assessing arachidonic acid metabolism.

The section dealing with immunodeficiency describes congenital and acquired immunodeficiencies, including the acquired immune deficiency syndrome (AIDS). This section will serve as an important reference source for tests that specifically monitor individuals for virus-induced immunodeficiencies.

The section on autoimmunity describes immunofluorescence techniques and other tests for autoantibodies. The tumor immunology section has chapters dealing with methods for diagnosing lymphoid and mononuclear cell tumors, enzyme-linked immunoassays for tumor-associated antigens, and methods for monitoring of patients with different types of tumors.

The section on immunogenetic and transplantation immunity includes chapters dealing with various methods used in transplantation and immunogenetic laboratories.

A new section on immunopathology and immunohistology describes methods for demonstrating lymphocyte markers in solid tumors as well as immunohistochemical and immune electron microscopic techniques. The section on laboratory management and administration presents chapters discussing proficiency tests and organization of the clinical immunology laboratory.

As in the other editions of this manual, the methodologies described are presented in a manner understandable to students and to laboratory personnel in academic or community hospitals. Descriptions of laboratory tests are given in sufficient detail that a skilled technologist should be able to perform the procedures without referring to other manuals or books. Step-by-step methods are provided wherever possible. For areas in which a number of different techniques are available, the procedure(s) employed by the author(s) is described in detail. However, a brief discussion describing other methods is included, pointing out how and why these methods differ. All authors were instructed to keep the description of methods as brief as possible, but to describe the initial ingredients necessary for the test rather than indicating commercially available reagents or kits. When multiple sources are available, a list of different vendors or sources of reagents is provided. Whenever possible, those vendors or sources of reagents used by individual authors are described.

A difficult decision made by the Editorial Board for this edition of the manual was not to include an exhaustive listing of the literature of clinical laboratory immunology. Only in this way could the cost of the book be kept under control. We sincerely regret that due recognition cannot be given to the many colleagues who have made important contributions to the methodology of clinical immunology. However, because references and citations are used mainly for entry into the scientific literature, the chapters in this manual generally refer only to a few major articles or reviews.

We thank the Editorial Board of the manual, ASM, and the American Association of Immunologists, as well as the 250 authors, for the high quality of the chapters and for accepting the peer review procedure established for the manual. We are greatly indebted to all those who undertook the heavy commitment of time and effort. We are grateful to the staff of the ASM Publications Department (including Walter Peter, Susan Birch, Sara Joslyn, Marie Smith, and Ellie Tupper) for valuable assistance in the preparation of the manual and for extraordinary forebearance in publishing a volume which is eagerly awaited in this rapidly expanding field.

Noel R. Rose
Herman Friedman
John L. Fahey

Chapter 1

Section A. General Methodology

Introduction

ROBERT F. RITCHIE

Since the previous edition of this manual was published, great changes in laboratory methodology have occurred. Ironically, the improvements have spawned the desire for further improvements rather than generated comfort with what has become available. The problems thus generated fall into the following areas: (i) impatience with the speed of analysis, (ii) dissatisfaction with the precision and sensitivity of recent introductions, and (iii) concern that data generated by old methods, which may or may not have produced clinically specific information, can be assumed to correlate with newer methods. Compounding these concerns have been the promulgation of new regulations (i.e., diagnostic-related groups [DRGs]), cost containment programs, and reluctance on the part of laboratory workers to be laboratory experts and artists at the bench. The net result is that efforts, sometimes heroic and not always well directed, have been mounted by instrument manufacturers to produce the "perfect" instrument system which is, at the same time, extremely fast, precise, very inexpensive, fully automated, versatile, foolproof, etc. Descriptions of these exciting instruments in this volume would be of great interest to the readers, but unfortunately, these systems, several of which are already in existence, are understandably under tight security wraps. If these systems are viable, however, the 4th edition of this manual will be the most suitable forum for presentation of details about them.

The fixation of the laboratory and industry on the speed of analysis is often unwarranted. Manufacturers will at times exert tremendous efforts toward reducing the time for completion of an assay by a factor of 2 or shaving 5 to 10 min off the turnaround time, with the primary goal being to upstage the competition or at least satisfy the marketing department's distorted perception of user needs. The time required to complete an assay, particularly when automated devices are used, is of little consequence when most assays can be completed in an hour or less, with the remaining assays best managed by overnight processing. However, the buyer, already susceptible to nonscientific issues such as color, shape, color video terminals, etc., is now highly susceptible to the words "speed," "low cost," "state of the art," etc. In actual practice, the systems are little different from one another once the gaudy and occasionally misleading veneer of the sales pitch is removed. In a recent survey of several immunoassays, it was clearly shown that precision is no longer an issue, and the new methods all intercorrelated extremely well. They intercorrelate so well, in fact, that the decision to purchase one or another system falls on the nonscientific items, i.e., speed, cost, available automation, etc.

At first glance, the new devices seem to be ideal, offering great precision and speed, error detection, full and sophisticated automation, sample preparation, antigen excess checking, etc. The human cost, however, is that bench science, once the pride of the technologist, has been given over unwittingly to the data processing system and the instrument. Black-box technology is now available in most areas of the laboratory with the exception of some areas of cellular immunology. The consequence is that the need for highly trained technologists has rapidly diminished in the clinical laboratory except for establishments devoted to the development of new knowledge or for those still untouched by the new methodology. Even small laboratories in rural areas or in physicians' offices are to be profoundly affected. New devices have been created which are small, inexpensive, and capable of addressing a wide range of chemistries which they perform extremely well.

Furthermore, as a result of the fixation with labor-saving devices and the emphasis on error-free operation, black-box technology totally prevents manipulation of the reagents to be employed. Laboratorians must, usually against their will, use prepackaged materials as supplied by the manufacturer, for there can be no assurance that the results are valid if nonstandard reagents are used. Submerged in this approach is one very important and usually overlooked beneficial trade-off; if reagents optimized and prepackaged by a manufacturer are used, the user is freed of much of the responsibility for defective instruments or reagents by virtue of the software aborting analyses. Therefore, in exchange for potentially superior results, the operator has lost virtually all control and has been reduced to the status of a laboratory instrument custodian. One can easily visualize a new generation of instruments which, like new cars, inform the owner in a synthesized voice to refill the reservoirs, pat the optics chassis, and wipe the cuvette.

The future for the research laboratory does not look quite so Orwellian, at least at present. With the new instruments, laboratory developers are setting the stage for entirely new technology, from principles to instruments. One focus is subminiaturization, for which sample and reagent volumes are measured in microliters, reaction vessels are barely visible, and all materials are disposable. Power requirements are negligible, and self-contained pocket analyzers are already in development. The cycle is, nevertheless, repetitive. More and more analytical sophistication and facilities more widely disseminated in the community contrast with less need for highly trained and costly personnel and centralized facilities.

The natural evolution towards more sophisticated methods moved initially towards labeled immunoassays described elsewhere in this volume, but also towards highly advanced optical methods. Perhaps the major reason that the laboratory is changing so drastically is related to the electronics industry. Firms which create new devices have teams of engineers and computer and software specialists and only a sprinkling of biochemists spearheading the new science.

Turbidimetric and nephelometric analyses of soluble analytes such as proteins and haptens have largely replaced the gel techniques of the past. As a result, three new chapters have been added to this section, each written by an author deeply involved in the design and application of new instruments. Of the twelve chapters in section A, four cover space-age Model T's already in evolution for the future, and five cover techniques still requiring experts and manual dexterity.

It is likely that all future volumes of this manual will contain a section on manual immunochemical methods performed in gels. Simple and inexpensive, these methods can nonetheless be elegant and informative and can recover information not accessible by other means. In chapter 4, the focus is on nuances of the currently employed popular methods rather than on the more historical overview presented in the 2nd edition.

Immunoturbidimetric analyses of serum proteins are the oldest methods of observing antigen-antibody reactions, dating to the end of the last century. Instruments have continually evolved, from the first, introduced in the 1930s as a "photon reflectometer," to small, quite precise devices, and on to the present generation of rotary analyzers such as the Technicon RA-1000 and the Roche Cobas Bio and FARA, for which the coefficient of variation is now in the neighborhood of 3 to 6%, similar to standard chemistries performed colorimetrically. The author of chapter 5 has chosen one system as an example of up-to-date turbidimetric analysis.

Nephelometry, itself a method employed as early as 1907, rose to a high point of laboratory awareness with continuous-flow measurement of serum proteins by an endpoint method of analysis. This method, however, has been totally eclipsed by the rate nephelometric approach. The author of chapter 6, in fact a principle parent of the technique, reviews the subject and describes further applications.

In an effort to extend the sensitivity of protein and hapten analysis while at the same time reducing the size of the analytical sample, particles coated with antibody have been carefully evaluated. Chapter 7 describes successful approaches to extended sensitivity by the use of antibody-coated latex particles rather than soluble antisera and an even more advanced system in which a two-particle form of analysis is used. An elegant system with exquisite sensitivity, the particle immunoassay employs discrete analysis of dispersed versus aggregated particles and is described in chapter 8. If one considers that two separate antibody-coated particles can be brought together as a doublet by a dual event of antibody-antigen-antibody and that these discrete simple or compound particles can be measured individually at high speeds, perhaps sensitivity has reached close to the ultimate limit of measuring the number of individual antigen-antibody events.

Regardless of the advances being made in immunological methods, older techniques are often the spawning grounds for new ideas which advance the art. Current protocols are in transition from these stable and well understood if tedious manual tests to advanced methods achieving high speed, precision, and low cost. The older methods still warrant chapters in the 3rd edition. The agglutination assays (chapter 9), forerunners of the particle-enhanced assays described above, still play a major role in blood banking and infectious-disease serology and are still widely used because of their technical unsophistication, requiring virtually no expensive equipment. However, in view of the fact that many of these assays rely on biologically derived particles, e.g., erythrocytes and bacteria, they are somewhat subjective and have an inherent variability to which the user must be constantly alert. Since few of these assays are commercially available, in-house reagents are generally used, placing the burden of quality control on the clinical or research laboratory itself.

Closely related to the particle-enhanced assays are the complement fixation methods, which have largely resisted commercialization (chapter 10). Having long been a benchmark assay and a standard against which newer methods are compared has made complement fixation very resistant to displacement by high technology. The perception that complement fixation will be with us for many years as a reference method justifies its inclusion in this section.

Neutralization assays (chapter 11) are focused on those procedures which assess the abilities of an antitoxin to neutralize the infectivity or toxin production of a microorganism; to properly identify a putative organism, virus, or microbe; or to identify rises in anti-viral-antibody titers in paired sera from an infected person. Highly specific, these assays are nevertheless labor intensive and, in practice, are often used for retrospective confirmation of an illness suspected of being of unknown viral origin. Neutralization assays require scrupulous quality control, and as a consequence, the tests are used in large laboratories where the volume can justify the high costs.

Again, employing a living biological system, the cytolytic assays test the ability of an individual serum to react with a cell surface antigen or to detect a specific cell surface antigen with characterized antisera (chapter 12). Certain assays proceed only in the presence of complement, whereas others produce cytolysis without complement. As with assays described in chapters 10 and 11, the nature of the procedures so far precludes a contribution by sophisticated instruments. Quality control requirements are also stringent, but some advances in reproducibility have been made by using continuous cell lines with well-characterized surface antigens.

Finally, the hinge for all immunoassays must be recognized. Immunoassays can be no better than the antisera employed. Major improvements have been made in the quality of commercial antisera since the last edition of this manual. However, immunological reagents, both homegrown and commercial, still abound which are of poor titer, contain major contaminants, are not suited to the particular technology, or may not even be directed towards the antigen indicated on the label. Antiserum production and qualification remains largely a "black art," with most of the successful immunoassays achieved by simple trial and error (chapter 2). Chapter 3 describes a method which not only characterizes the concentration and avidity of antisera, but also precisely describes the performance of a given batch of antiserum in one or another of the precipitin methods. Extension to other technologies is implied.

Although the excitement of high technology draws the laboratory's attention and great strides are being made, there is always a price to be exacted. The price(s) relates to the inseparable problem of higher sensitivity being linked to the loss of specificity, with the latter being due to "noise," blurring the distinction between closely apposed numerical values, or similar clinical situations. The burden of minimizing the side effects of modern devices falls to the manufacturers of the electronic devices and incorporated microcomputers and eventually to the manufacturers of the immunochemical reagents. Ultimately, the re-

finements present the medical community with the need to translate the more precise data supplied to the laboratorian into improved patient care. The latter problem is perhaps the greatest challenge. Current budgetary restraints will allow only slow progress.

Undoubtedly, major advances in immunoanalysis will appear during the next 5 to 10 years, and the turmoil in the laboratory industry will not lessen as a result. We can speculate that new devices or methods employed in 1990 will be miniaturized, components will be prepackaged and the entire test module will be discarded, precision will be in the 2 to 4% range for the coefficient of variation, sensitivity will far exceed the clinical need, the devices may well be portable or even handheld in some cases and not require trained personnel, and multiple assays per sample will be commonplace. Costs will have fallen dramatically to meet the desire of physicians to control their laboratory testing in their own offices. Research versions of the instruments will appear somewhat later than the clinical models. Rather than being a pipe dream, prototypes for these advanced technologies already exist.

Chapter 2

Preparation of Polyclonal Antisera

ROBERT F. RITCHIE

With the ascendency of immunologic tests in virtually every field of biological science, one would expect the literature to be replete with in-depth studies of the theory and practice of polyclonal antibody production. Not surprisingly, however, this multimillion-dollar industry, built upon the successful production of superior antisera by many workers, has hidden its "secrets," which is understandable in light of its inability to achieve patent protection (9). The previous edition of this volume contains no section on the preparation of antisera, with only a few remarks on this subject in the introduction to section A. It was felt by the editors of the present edition that an effort should be made to set down in a logical fashion that which is widely recognized about the subject. Such a study could assist the novice in avoiding the many pitfalls by demystifying the subject and perhaps could give a perspective for those fortunate few who have made a usable immunologic reagent. Monoclonal antibody production, which is not significantly different from heteroclonal antibodies production in the traditional manner, is not addressed here.

GENERAL COMMENTS

See references 7, 17, and 19.

Despite erudite publications on this subject, antiserum production is still very much a "black art." Luck plays an inordinately large role, and even if a worker succeeds in producing a satisfactory product from an animal by whatever protocol, it is still advisable not to expect a repeat performance as a matter of course. Every worker who has devoted much effort to antiserum production can relate instances where success was achieved with only one of several animals. That animal may have produced antibody only once for a few days, with all subsequent efforts meeting failure in spite of strict adherence to what had been a successful protocol. These admonitions apply most to large animals such as the goat, horse, and donkey, whose lineage is basically that of a mongrel. Rabbits, guinea pigs, and even fowl have much narrower genetic makeups. It is only in purebred mice that the genetics of the immune response have allowed workers to achieve a degree of consistency and predictability in antiserum production. It is assumed that similar characteristics of consistency and homogeneity can be achieved for the production of immunogen.

CELLULAR RESPONSE

See reference 18.

The introduction into the host of a foreign substance capable of stimulating antibody production initiates a series of events which culminate in the entry into the circulation of immunoglobulin of different antibody classes, light-chain isotypes, and, depending on the number of epitopes on the immunogen, a variable number of idiotypic specificities. Large molecules, such as serum proteins, generate an enormous number of specificities—one from each clone stimulated—whereas only a single type is generated to synthetic polymeric materials due to a repetitive single epitope. It is this idiotypic diversity that contributes to the effective performance of an antiserum in the majority of modern immunoassays for complex molecules.

Upon the exposure of an animal to a foreign immunogen, a series of events occur. If the immunogen is cellular, microbial, or composed of complexes, the macrophage plays a key initial role. Even for soluble antigens, the emulsification with complete Freund adjuvant may reduce the molecules to relatively insoluble precipitates also requiring processing. Ingestion of the immunogen by the macrophage results in lysosomal enzymatic degradation to smaller fragments bearing the epitopic determinant of the original particle. The antigen is then transported to the surface of the macrophage, where it becomes accessible to the T lymphocyte. When presented in the context of Ia antigens, the T cell becomes activated. This activation is facilitated by macrophage secretion of interleukin-1 (IL-1), which in turn induces T-lymphocyte synthesis of interleukin-2 (IL-2), a T-cell growth factor (15). Stimulation of T-lymphocyte activation by macrophage-lymphocyte interaction leads to the secretion of many other immune mediators (lymphokines) which enhance B-lymphocyte function (3). The result is a coordinated immunologic response against the immunogen by macrophages, T lymphocytes, and B lymphocytes with the ultimate production of harvestable polyclonal antibody.

CELL-CELL INTERACTION

A requirement of T-cell activation involves interaction between the T lymphocyte and the macrophage in which the T cell recognizes antigen through a specific receptor on its surface along with Ia antigens on the surface of the macrophage encoded by the major histocompatibility complex. Recognition of foreign antigens by T lymphocytes cannot occur unless there is at least haploidentity at this Ia locus, i.e., the macrophage and lymphocyte derive from genetically related animals (11). Until recently, little was known of the T-lymphocyte antigen receptor; however, by utilizing nucleotide sequencing procedures of cDNA clones, the T-cell antigen receptor appears to be similar to immunoglobulin protein (20). This knowledge may soon lead investigators to further understanding of T-cell activation and its central role in immune modulation.

Cooperation between T and B cells is necessary for an antibody response; however, T-cell-independent antigens are capable of directly triggering B cells in the mouse. The proliferation of B lymphocytes is the rate-limiting factor dictating the concentration of antibody secreted by these activated plasma cells into the lymphatics and then the peripheral circulation (14). In the case of immunoglobulin G (IgG), which moves relatively freely through the vascular endothelium, the total mass of antibody present in an animal whose immune response to antigen has matured may be much larger than expected from the animal's blood volume. This fact can be capitalized upon by harvesting antiserum by plasmapheresis.

IMMUNOGEN

See references 4 and 5.

The initial step in antiserum production, the introduction of the immunogen, usually presents a variety of epitopes to the immunocompetent host. An epitope as it is described here is the minimum biochemical unit capable of stimulating an antibody response. In general, the larger molecules such as serum proteins or bacterial proteins contain many different epitopic sequences, each capable of evoking antibody production from a single clone of B cells. Some large molecules such as dextran or other polysaccharides produce much more homogeneous antibody specificity because of the highly repetitive nature of the immunogen. Generally speaking, immunogens that are composed of highly repetitive epitopes produce the best-precipitating antisera. At times, even monoclonal antibodies will precipitate when reacted with antigens of this type.

Proteins are the most commonly used immunogens. However, polysaccharides and oligosaccharides with a large degree of epitopic repetitiveness can be excellent stimulants of antibody production. Lipids and nucleic acids in combination with proteins can also be immunogenic in the intact animal.

Smaller molecules called haptens present fewer epitopes (sometimes only one) and so cannot evoke a satisfactory antibody response. Placing these limited epitopes close to a substance or carrier with significant immunogenicity through chemical linkage may induce different epitopic sequences, each capable of evoking antibodies specific for the carrier, the hapten-carrier bridge, and the hapten epitopes themselves. If the carrier is an alien protein such as keyhole limpet hemocyanin, antibodies to it do not contribute to any in vitro immunologic reaction. However, should there be a problem of cross-reactivity, adsorption with the carrier will remove all antibodies except those reactive with the hapten itself (10).

Haptens, in the form of drugs and steroids of low molecular weight, can be intensely immunogenic when coupled to the proper carrier protein (2). There is a lower limit to the molecular weight beyond which antibody cannot be induced easily. Molecules as small as 200 to 300 daltons can induce antibody. Some, when polymerized, will produce excellent antiserum, but, as a rule, once the molecular weight falls below 700 daltons the induction of antibody is increasingly difficult. Glycolipids, phospholipids, and carbohydrates can also induce antibody production (13).

If the problem is addressed from a different point of view, it can be seen that minor differences in epitopic structure may produce antibodies which will recognize two variants of a large immunogen (12). Proteins often express genetic polymorphism by differences in the hexose content attached to the protein backbone.

Conversely, antibody diversity may not be manifest even though chemical diversity is apparent in significant physicochemical or functional differences. For example, despite much effort, no antibody, either polyclonal or monoclonal, has been found to be able to distinguish between the phenotypes of alpha$_1$-antitrypsin in the human. The difference is due to a single hexose molecule.

Hemoglobin molecules differ in a variety of ways. Hemoglobin A2 differs from A in only 10 amino acids on one of the two chains; hemoglobin S differs in only a single amino acid on the β chain. The fact that some workers have produced precipitating polyclonal antibodies to hemoglobin S suggests that the physical difference plays a major role in this immunogenicity (8). These antibodies have been termed conformational.

If the immunogen bears epitopes which are, for the most part, common to several analytes, passive immunization or induction of tolerance in the animal before active immunization may be effective. An example is the production of antiserum to the IgG subclasses where each subclass differs from the other in only a few epitopes (16). The vast majority of the antibody is directed to the common portions of the molecules. By infusing the animal with large volumes of antiserum to the other subclasses, followed by the standard immunization with the desired immunogen, success has been achieved. Other examples are antisera to hemoglobins F and A2 and to the subtypes of haptoglobin. The procedure is demanding of staff, since sterile technique is required and not readily available in most animal holding facilities.

Immunogenicity is a term that, for the most part, lacks numerical descriptors. Workers experienced in producing a wide range of antisera recognize that some immunogens are exquisite in their ability to elicit antibodies while others often fail to elicit any response at all, let alone one which is satisfactory or usable. Alpha$_2$-macroglobulin, a high-molecular-weight protein, is one of the best inducers of antibody and will sometimes produce many milligrams of high-affinity antibody per milliliter within the first 3 weeks of immunization. Human myoglobin, on the other hand, often fails to produce any antibody, and only occasionally among the responders will there be an animal that produces an antibody of even modest potency.

A variety of maneuvers can be carried out to enhance immunogenicity; however, these can be risky. Some glycoproteins are relatively poor immunogens, and their effectiveness can be enhanced by desialidation with neuraminidase. An old method of enhancing immunogenicity was to precipitate the protein with alum, rendering it insoluble and presumably less mobile and thus less subject to excretion by the host. Denaturation, however, may sufficiently alter the immunogenicity so as to present the host animal with a material substantially different from the native molecule.

OTHER FACTORS AFFECTING ANTIBODY RESPONSE

Many species of animals have been used to produce antisera. Some are selected because they are easy to handle; some, because of the immunological or physical properties of the product; and some, because they do not possess a native substance antigenically similar to the proposed immunogen. In still others, the animal is chosen because it is phylogenetically and therefore antigenically very close to the species from which the immunogen is to be recovered; thus the animal will produce antibody to any of the minor differences. At present, most antisera are produced in the goat (followed by the rabbit). The goat is preferred because of its ease of handling and hardiness. Further, the size of the goat allows volume production from single animals if required. Although rabbits produce excellent precipitating antisera with superior physical properties, they present a significant increase in labor costs for volume production. Long-term maintenance of a producing rabbit is very labor intensive and therefore costly.

Commercial suppliers have occasionally used burros, donkeys, and other mid-size animals, but chiefly for promotional rather than scientific reasons, alleging that for a specific analyte a superior antiserum has been made. A better product may have been recovered, but unfortunately not because of the species.

Guinea pigs have been used to produce specific antibodies, e.g., human insulin. The principal reason is that guinea pig insulin is significantly different from human insulin, whereas goat and rabbit insulin are too similar to yield a satisfactory immune response.

Fowl, reptiles, and even fish have been immunized in the past in efforts to recover a special antiserum or to better understand the immune process. Fowl offer an advantage in that they produce antibodies which do not fix mammalian complement. Therefore, fowl antisera serve as useful blocking agents in the antibody-mediated complement-dependent cytotoxicity assay.

In the experimental animal the age of the host can influence the response. Young animals are more prone to develop tolerance to low doses of immunogen. The inevitable contaminants may therefore be less of a problem when an animal is started on its immunization schedule early in life. Young animals also are more easily paralyzed by large doses of antigen than are adults.

The size of the animal as a function of dose seems largely unrelated. A rabbit of 5 kg requires approximately the same dose of immunogen as a mature goat of 50 kg or a donkey of 200 kg. Mice also require disproportionately large doses of immunogen. The dose and rate of immunization are partially related to the host's body temperature; high temperatures require larger doses and more frequent administration, while cold-blooded animals will retain antigen for months without apparent effect until the body temperature rises to a critical level.

The route of immunization plays a major role in antiserum quality. Any route by which an immunogen can be introduced into the body for interaction with mononuclear cells will produce a response. The most commonly used routes are intramuscular, subcutaneous, and intradermal. Variations such as intrasplenic or intranodal injection have been employed with variable success. Injection into the popliteal space has been effective by placing small doses of antigen close to a large collection of immunocompetent cells. The use of footpad injection has fortunately fallen into disuse because of its cruelty, but it is basically the subcutaneous and intranodal routes combined.

Less frequently employed routes are immunogens directed through the skin via a blast of sterile nitrogen or in a solution of dimethyl sulfoxide which facilitates transport. Inhalation can be effective and gives rise to unexpected production of contaminating antibodies as a result of inhaling aerosols produced by human workers with upper respiratory tract infections. Ingestion can also be effective with some antigens: on a few occasions, the curiosity and appetite of our goats resulted in inadvertent immunization when plastic syringe, immunogen, and needle were all chewed and swallowed. Antibody was detected at the appropriate time.

The immunization schedule also affects the potency of an antiserum, playing an ill-defined yet important role. As a rule, immunogen is given to a naîve animal weekly for 3 weeks, followed by a month's rest and then a challenge. This schedule is often changed to multiple doses weekly until the titer is adequate. The protocol may produce low-potency antibody, but once a response is elicited careful attention is required to determine when the antibody concentration has reached a maximum and is therefore ready for harvesting.

Immunization dose is perhaps the most controversial part of the antibody production equation. The literature contains information suggesting doses over a 5-log range. The unfortunate fact is that extremely small doses will sometimes succeed with a given animal when larger doses fail and vice versa.

Long-term immunization can apparently increase the body burden of immunogen, resulting in deleterious effects controlled by a mechanism that is not well understood. Animals whose titer is falling may, in reality, be responding to excessive rather than to insufficient doses. The narrow range of optimal dosage is a relatively fine line, sharper for highly immunogenic materials than for those which do not stimulate good antibody production.

The two extremes of immunogen dosage play havoc with antibody response. Again, the frustrating feature is that no easily accessible parameter informs the worker in what part of the spectrum of response the animals are responding. At the low end, subliminal doses will not produce antibody and over time may actually inhibit production should the dosage reach levels that would ordinarily produce an excellent response. This phenomenon, known as tolerance, is probably active in all protocols involving immunogens that are "crude" or that have multiple epitopes of various densities.

At the other extreme, massive doses can result in the cessation of antibody synthesis, a condition termed immune paralysis. Depending on the route of immunization and on whether adjuvants are used, major swings in antibody concentration and quality may occur. Furthermore, other factors such as the health of the host play a role. Intercurrent infection can actually enhance immune responsiveness or, if severe, curtail antibody production. Most goat herds are infected with *Mycobacterium johnii*, which can sometimes be debilitating. However, infected and compromised animals may produce superior antisera. To enhance the host response to immunogen, a variety of materials called adjuvants have been used.

Adjuvants are agents which enhance antibody production by inducing an intense inflammatory response at the site of immunogen injection, bringing the necessary cellular components for the induction of antibody production (1). Several of the materials, such as complete Freund adjuvant and mineral oil, contain lipids. In the preparation of the immunogen, an emulsion of the aqueous and lipoid materials must be made. This may contribute to the slower release of material by its sequestration in insoluble lipid particles.

Protocols for the use of adjuvants vary considerably. Some workers use only complete adjuvants containing lipid and mycobacterial extracts. Others use only incomplete adjuvants. At times, a mixed protocol of complete and incomplete can also be effective. Even the addition of an intravenous boost can sometimes be salutary. Again, unfortunately, since there is as yet no means of clearly assessing the host's status, careful trial and error is the only approach. In the event that an animal fails to produce satisfactory antiserum, repeated and close monitoring is mandatory. A decision to increase or decrease the dosage or the frequency of injection is made based on the serial results. An experienced team will use every modality available.

ANTIBODY QUALITIES

During the course of immunization, specific antibody of the IgM and IgG classes can be found. The IgG antibody is preferred for several reasons: its concentration is highest and can reach 15 to 20 mg/ml, it is more stable to long-term storage, and it tolerates purification and isolation with minimal losses. IgM antibody presents serious problems in all of these areas.

Also, during immunization the avidity (the overall potency of an antiserum batch) changes as the animal's production matures (6). The avidity generally rises with time; however, overimmunization can result in a falling titer as the result of in vivo adsorption of highly active molecules by the injected immunogen. At times, only low-avidity antibody will remain. Close monitoring of antibody levels will show the fall immediately after immunization, and then the expected rise if the animal is on the proper protocol.

The purity or monospecificity of an antiserum is, as mentioned above, a function of the immunogen. As a rule, samples taken early in a program contain fewer and lower levels of contaminants and are therefore easier to render monospecific. Samples taken from animals years into a program have the highest level of contaminants, and the removal of these contaminants is much more difficult. Changes in the immunogen can prevent the "hardening" of the contaminant population. However, despite the extreme purity of an immunogen, with the exception of synthetic materials the antiserum will never be totally free of contaminants. Our experience extends to over 10,000 bleedings. The levels of contaminant antibodies may actually rise when any immunogen is used (and not only the specific target substance), further supporting the importance of using high-purity immunogen from the outset. If a serum shows no precipitin reactions in a properly balanced antigen-antibody gel system, substantial amounts can still be found if adsorption is carried out using columns of immobilized antigen. The eluate from such a column will contain surprising amounts and diversity of antibodies. It is a common observation that once a contaminant population becomes well established, it will remain throughout the life of the animal.

Perhaps the most frustrating feature of antiserum production to the novice and expert alike is that the immunogen, in its "pure" form, still elicits antibody whose specificity is either totally unwanted or cross-reactive with other molecular species; in other words, it is nonspecific. The old literature condemns using the goat as a source of antiserum because this animal produces so many nonspecific antibodies; in fact, however, it is basically this feature of sensitivity to small doses of immunogen that has made the goat the animal of choice for polyclonal antisera production. The problem lay in the size of the dose of immunogen given to the animal with each injection.

LITERATURE CITED

1. **Borek, F.** 1977. Adjuvants, p. 369–428. *In* M. Sela (ed.), The antigens, vol. 4. Academic Press, Inc., New York.
2. **Butler, V. P., Jr., and S. M. Beiser.** 1973. Antibodies to small molecules: biological and clinical applications. Adv. Immunol. **17**:255–310.
3. **Clayberger, C., R. H. DeKruyff, and H. Cantor.** 1985. T cell regulation of antibody responses: an I-A-specific autoreactive T cell collaborates with antigen-specific helper T cells to promote IgG responses. J. Immunol. **134**:691–694.
4. **Crumpton, M. J.** 1974. Protein antigens: the molecular basis of antigenicity and immunogenicity, p. 1–78. *In* M. Sela (ed.), The antigens, vol. 2. Academic Press, Inc., New York.
5. **de Weck, A. L.** 1974. Low molecular weight antigens, p. 141–248. *In* M. Sela (ed.), The antigens, vol. 2. Academic Press, Inc., New York.
6. **Donnenberg, A. D., G. J. Elfenbein, and G. W. Santos.** 1984. Secondary immunization with a protein antigen (tetanus toxoid) in man. Characterization of humoral and cell-mediated regulatory events. Scand. J. Immunol. **20**:279–289.
7. **Eisen, H. M. (ed.).** 1974. Immunology: an introduction to molecular and cellular principles of the immune response, p. 351–509. Harper & Row, Publishers, Inc., New York.
8. **Headings, V., S. Bhattacharya, S. Shukla, S. Anyaibe, L. Easton, A. Calvert, and R. Scott.** 1975. Identification of specific hemoglobins within individual erythrocytes. Blood **45**:263–271.
9. **Inglis, J. R.** 1983. Special feature on immunotechnology and industry: introduction. Immunol. Today **4**:125–139.
10. **Knight, G. J., P. Wylie, M. S. Holman, and J. E. Haddow.** 1985. Improved ^{125}I radioimmunoassay for cotinine by selective removal of bridge antibodies. Clin. Chem. **31**:118–121.
11. **Kurnick, J. T., P. Altevogt, J., Lindblom, O. Sjöberg, A. Danneus, and W. Wigzell.** 1980. Long term maintenance of HLA-D restricted T-cells specific for soluble antigens. Scand. J. Immunol. **11**:131–136.
12. **Lerner, R. A.** 1984. Antibodies of predetermined specificity in biology and medicine. Adv. Immunol. **36**:1–44.
13. **Marcus, D. M., and G. A. Schwarting.** 1976. Immunochemical properties of glycolipids and phospholipids. Adv. Immunol. **23**:203–240.
14. **Melchers, F., C. Corbel, and M. Leptin.** 1983. Requirements for B-cell stimulation, p. 669–682. *In* Y.

Yamamura and T. Tada (ed.), Progress in immunology, vol. 5. Academic Press, Inc., New York.

15. **Pike, B. L., A. Raubitschek, and G. J. V. Nossal.** 1984. Human interleukin-2 can promote the growth and differentiation of single hapten-specific B cells in the presence of specific antigen. Proc. Natl. Acad. Sci. U.S.A. **81:**7917–7921.

16. **Speigelberg, H. L., and W. O. Weigle.** 1968. The production of antisera to human γ G subclasses in rabbits using immunological unresponsiveness. J. Immunol. **101:**377–380.

17. **Steward, M. W.** 1984. Antibodies: their structure and function. Outline Series in Biology. Chapman & Hall, New York.

18. **van Furth, R.** 1983. The role of macrophages in the immune process. Birth Defects **19:**3–7.

19. **Wedgwood, R. J., F. S. Rosen, and N. W. Paul (ed.).** 1983. Primary immunodeficiency disease. March of Dimes Birth Defects Foundation, A. R. Liss, New York.

20. **Yanugi, Y., Y. Yoshikai, K. Loggett, S. P. Clark, I. Aleksander, and T. W. Mak.** 1984. A human T cell-specific cDNA clone encodes a protein having extensive homology to immunoglobulin chains. Nature (London) **308:**145–148.

Chapter 3

Characterization of Antisera

GAIL A. HUDSON

Understanding the quality of an antiserum is crucial in the development of a successful clinical immunoassay. Several characteristics contribute to antiserum quality.

Antibody concentration. Antibody concentration determines the extent to which antiserum must be diluted for use in an immunoassay. Since antiserum contains a mixture of serum components, the mass of a specific antibody cannot be measured directly. Instead, it must be indirectly represented by generating a functional immunoassay and measuring the milligrams of antigen that react with 1 ml of antiserum (antigen-binding capacity or titer). The term titer is also sometimes used to specify the extent to which antiserum must be diluted to perform optimally in a given assay.

Antibody reactivity. Antibody reactivity, also termed avidity, influences the slope of the standard curve, thereby affecting assay sensitivity and precision. Avidity results from a combination of such factors as binding strength (affinity), valency, precipitating ability, resistance to dissociating agents, and specificity. Because antiserum avidity varies independently of titer, both characteristics must be assessed in order to fully characterize a lot of antiserum.

Method. Because they are estimated indirectly from parameters within an immunoassay, antiserum characteristics are method dependent. For example, an antiserum that has a high avidity in radioimmunoassay, where binding affinity is critical, may have a relatively low avidity in nephelometry, where reactivity depends upon immunoprecipitation characteristics. Thus, it is important to define antiserum performance within the immunoassay system for which the antiserum is intended.

Other characteristics. Antiserum performance is affected by other, less well defined characteristics such as the ability of an antibody to produce a standard curve that has a wide dynamic range and differences in reactivity under various assay conditions (e.g., pH, temperature, ionic strength).

ASSESSMENT OF ANTISERUM FOR GEL TECHNIQUES

Radial immunodiffusion

Several procedures have been described for evaluating antiserum in standard and reverse radial immunodiffusion. In the Becker standard radial immunodiffusion procedure (2), various amounts of antigen diffuse radially from wells cut in a uniform layer of antibody-containing agar or agarose. After the reaction reaches equilibrium, the diameters of the precipitin rings are measured. The titer of the antiserum (the amount of antigen which reacts with 1 ml of antiserum) is calculated from the equation $T = (4V_{ag})/(P\pi hk_1)$, where T is the titer (milligrams of antigen bound per milliliter of antiserum), V_{ag} is the volume of antigen (microliters), P is the percentage of antiserum in the gel, h is the depth of the gel layer (millimeters), and k_1 is the slope of the line produced by plotting antigen concentration (milligrams per deciliter) versus the square of the diameter (millimeters) of the precipitin ring.

In the Reimer reverse radial immunodiffusion procedure (12), antiserum diffuses from wells cut into an antigen-containing gel, the diameter of the precipitin ring is measured, and an E value (equivalence value or titer) is calculated from the equation

$$E = \frac{t(D^2 - D_w^2)C_{ag}\pi}{4Q_{ab}}$$

where t is the gel thickness (millimeters), D and D_w are the diameters (millimeters) of the precipitin ring and of the well, respectively, C_{ag} is the concentration of antigen in the gel (micrograms per milliliter), and Q_{ab} is the volume of antiserum in the well (microliters).

As with all of the radial immunodiffusion procedures, both the Becker and the Reimer procedures assign numerical values to antiserum titer but do not measure antiserum avidity. No methods for defining antiserum avidity in diffusion-in-gel techniques have been published.

Electroimmunodiffusion

To determine antiserum titer, dilutions of test antiserum and of a standard antiserum solution are applied to wells and electrophoresed through an antigen-containing gel (reverse electroimmunodiffusion) (1). The mass of antibody in the test antiserum is calculated by comparing the peak heights of the unknown antiserum with those of the standards, whose antibody mass has been assigned by another immunoassay technique (unspecified).

Methods have been described for determining the avidity of affinity-purified antibody by either standard or reverse electroimmunodiffusion (4). The antisera are adjusted to equivalent protein concentrations (absorbance at 280 nm) and then electrophoresed through gels that have varying antigen concentrations. A plot of peak area (obtained by tracing on paper and weighing) versus antigen concentration gives a straight line whose slope indicates antiserum avidity. Different dilutions of the same antiserum give parallel lines, indicating that the slope of avidity versus antigen concentration is not affected by differing titers.

ASSESSMENT OF ANTISERUM FOR LIGHT-SCATTERING TECHNIQUES

Nephelometry

Until recently, antiserum for use in nephelometry was characterized by first making an arbitrary dilu-

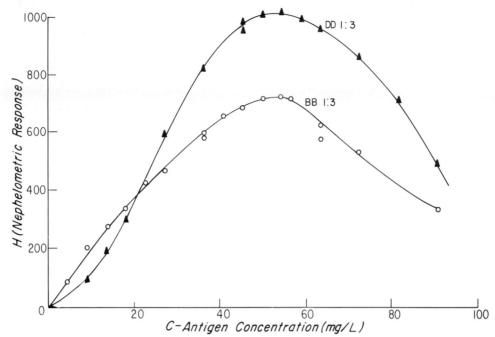

FIG. 1. Nephelometric standard curves for two anti-alpha$_1$-acid glycoprotein sera, each diluted threefold. Adapted with permission from Hudson et al. (8).

tion and then generating standard curves (plot of nephelometric response versus antigen concentration) (13). The slope of the curve within a defined antigen concentration range was compared with that of an acceptable homologous antiserum. Shortcomings to this approach are as follows. (i) Results are dependent upon the antigen range chosen. For example, Fig. 1 displays standard curves from two anti-alpha$_1$-acid glycoprotein sera (8), illustrating how antiserum BB gives a better response between 0 and 15 mg of antigen per liter, whereas antiserum DD gives a greater response in the range of 20 to 40 mg/liter. (ii) Measuring the slope of the standard curve produced by one antiserum dilution gives no indication of the slope that would be obtained with any other dilution, because no simple relationship exists between peak height and antiserum dilution. (iii) The slope of the standard curve represents a combination of titer and avidity, whereas separate assessments of these two parameters would be preferred.

Cambiaso et al. adopted the parameter C_{50}, defined as the antigen concentration giving a peak height equivalent to one-half of the maximum height of the standard curve, and designated it antigen-binding capacity (5). Gauldi et al. described antisera by two parameters, the peak height and the antigen concentration corresponding to the maximum point of the standard curve (7). Four antiserum pools were tested, but the relationship between the two parameters was not compared.

Hudson et al. devised an approach for characterizing antiserum that differentiates between titer and avidity and allows the optimum antiserum dilution to be predicted without trial and error (8). By using rate nephelometry, standard curves were generated from which two terms can be derived: H_{max}, the maximum nephelometric response, and C_{50}, the antigen concentration corresponding to one-half of H_{max} (Fig. 2).

Next, to determine how H_{max} and C_{50} vary with antiserum dilution, a series of standard curves was generated for several different dilutions of each antiserum (Fig. 3a). Plots of C_{50} versus antiserum concentration (reciprocal of dilution) yielded straight lines whose slopes (designated C_{coef}) indicate antiserum titer (Fig. 3b). Plots of H_{max} versus antiserum concentration produced second-order curves that were made linear by graphing the square root function (Fig. 3c). The slopes of these plots (designated $\sqrt{H_{coef}}$) represent antiserum avidity. Therefore, in rate nephelometry, doubling the antiserum concentration caused C_{50} to double and H_{max} to increase fourfold.

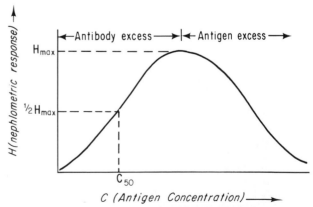

FIG. 2. Nephelometric standard curve. Maximum rate of change in light scatter is plotted as a function of antigen concentration. H_{max} is defined as the maximum nephelometric response attained. C_{50} is defined as the antigen concentration that corresponds to one-half of H_{max}. Reprinted with permission from Hudson et al. (8).

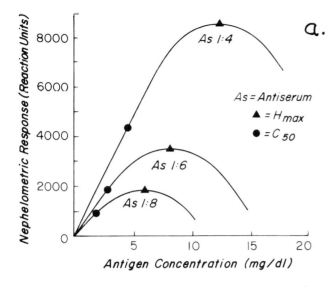

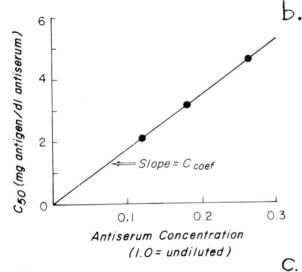

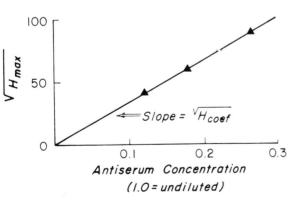

FIG. 3. Characterization of antiserum for use in nephelometric immunoassay. (a) Standard curves generated by using several different antiserum dilutions in a rate nephelometer. Two parameters, C_{50} and H_{max}, are determined. (b) Plot of C_{50} versus antiserum concentration. The slope is a measure of antiserum titer. (c) Plot of H_{max} versus antiserum concentration. The slope is a measure of antiserum avidity. Reprinted with permission from J. E. Haddow and R. F. Ritchie. Newer immunochemical techniques for the quantitation of specific proteins, p. 304. *In* R. A. Thompson (ed.), Recent advances in clinical immunology no. 2. Churchill Livingston, Edinburgh, 1980.

By understanding these generalized functions, it is possible to predict the characteristics of a standard curve that would result from any given dilution of antiserum, without testing the antiserum at several dilutions. Thirty-three lots of goat antiserum against the human proteins alpha$_1$-antitrypsin, alpha$_1$-acid glycoprotein, and immunoglobulin G were examined, and it was confirmed that these relationships held for all three analytes. Since it is not known what differences in antigen composition (e.g., size, charge, carbohydrate content) might affect these relationships, similar experiments will be required for other analytes before these generalized functions are adopted.

Turbidimetry

Singer et al. (14) used a combination of turbidimetry and the quantitative precipitin reaction of Kabat and Mayer (9) to determine antibody concentration. With a constant amount of antiserum, a standard curve was generated and the maximum response point was taken as the point of equivalence. The antibody concentration at the equivalence point was then estimated by the quantitative precipitin method (9).

ASSESSMENT OF ANTISERUM FOR LABEL IMMUNOASSAYS

Radioimmunoassay

In the Farr technique the antigen-binding capacity of an antiserum is measured by combining antiserum with excess labeled antigen, precipitating the immune complexes with 50% saturated ammonium sulfate, and measuring the amount of labeled antigen precipitated (10). The amount of antiserum that binds 33% of the label is calculated and then multiplied by 3 to give the antigen-binding capacity. Antiserum avidity is assessed by diluting the antiserum and antigen solutions 10-fold and determining the effect of dilution on the antigen-binding properties. Low-avidity antisera bind less antigen when diluted. In later modifications titers of antiserum were determined against a wide range of antigen concentrations, with avidity expressed as the slope of a regression plot of binding capacity versus antigen concentration.

The Scatchard plot was introduced for immunoassay by Berson and Yalow (3). First, the optimum antiserum titer is determined by combining various dilutions of antiserum with the amount of labeled antigen that is to be used in the assay. Titer is expressed as the reciprocal of the dilution that will bind 50% of the labeled antigen (Fig. 4a). Next, various amounts of unlabeled antigen compete with a fixed amount of labeled antigen for a limited number of antibody sites. The bound/free ratio is then plotted against the concentration of bound antigen, and the slope is equal to $-K$, where K is the equilibrium constant (affinity constant) for the reaction of antibody combining with antigen (Fig. 4b). Because antiserum contains a heterogeneous mixture of antibodies with various affinities, the plot seldom yields a straight line, and therefore the estimate of K is imprecise.

In the saturation method of Odell et al., portions of antibody are combined with various amounts of la-

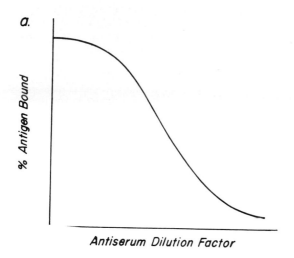

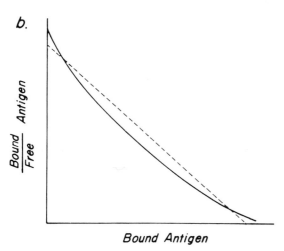

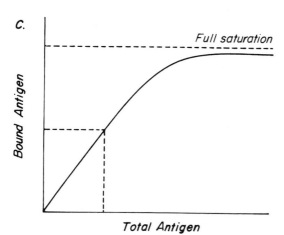

FIG. 4. Characterization of antisera for use in label immunoassays. (a) Screening for titer. The antiserum concentration which binds 50% of the antigen is chosen. (b) Scatchard plot for estimation of the average affinity constant, K. Since the line is not straight because of antibody heterogeneity, an average slope is calculated (- - -) which is equal to $-K$. (c) Saturation curve for estimation of average affinity constant, K. The concentration of free antigen at 50%saturation of antibody is equal to $1/K$. Reprinted with permission from G. Hudson, *in* M. Werner, ed., *CRC Handbook of Clinical Chemistry*, in press.

beled antigen, bound antigen is plotted versus total antigen, and the concentration of total antigen at 50% saturation is equal to $1/K$ (Fig. 4c) (11). The disadvantage of this method is that, in practice, the amount of bound antigen continues to increase, and a maximum is never really achieved. It is therefore necessary to estimate the saturation point, contributing to the imprecision of the technique.

Enzyme-linked immunosorbent assay

Most enzyme-antibody conjugates are characterized by measuring their reactivity against a single concentration of antigen under conditions used in an enzyme-linked immunosorbent assay (6). Several dilutions of antiserum are reacted with a fixed concentration (often 50 ng/ml) of immobilized antigen, the solid phase is washed and then reacted with substrate, and the absorbance is measured. The dilution of antiserum that produces an absorbance of 1.0 is referred to as the antiserum titer. Because absorbance is highly dependent upon assay conditions, these must be specified when the titer is reported.

LITERATURE CITED

1. **Axelsen, N. A., and P. J. Svendsen.** 1973. Reversed rocket immunoelectrophoresis. Scand. J. Immunol. **2**(Suppl. 1):155–157.
2. **Becker, W.** 1969. Determination of antisera titers using the single radial immunodiffusion method. Immunochemistry **6**:539–546.
3. **Berson, S. A., and R. S. Yalow.** 1959. Quantitative aspects of the reaction between insulin and insulin-binding antibody. J. Clin. Invest. **38**:1996.
4. **Birkmeyer, R. C., L. L. Keyes, and A. L. Tan-Wilson.** 1981. Determination of relative antigen-antibody affinities by quantitative immunoelectrophoresis. J. Immunol. Methods **44**:271–284.
5. **Cambiaso, C. L., P. L. Masson, J. P. Vaerman, and J. F. Heremans.** 1974. Automated nephelometric immunoassay (ANIA). I. Importance of antibody affinity. J. Immunol. Methods **5**:153–163.
6. **Engvall, E., and P. Perlmann.** 1971. Enzyme-linked immunosorbent assay (ELISA). Quantitative assay of immunoglobulin G. Immunochemistry **8**:871–874.
7. **Gauldi, J., P. Horsewood, and M. Koekkebaiker.** 1979. Nephelometric activity as a criterion of adequate antisera for use in immunofluorescence. Int. Arch. Allergy Appl. Immunol. **60**:186–194.
8. **Hudson, G. A., R. F. Ritchie, and J. E. Haddow.** 1981. Method for testing antiserum titer and avidity in nephelometric systems. Clin. Chem. **27**:1838–1844.
9. **Kabat, E. A., and M. M. Mayer.** 1961. Experimental immunochemistry, 2nd ed., p. 22–47. Charles C Thomas, Publisher, Springfield, Ill.
10. **Minden, P., R. T. Reid, and R. S. Farr.** 1967. Ammonium sulfate method to measure antigen-binding capacity, p. 13.1–13.22. *In* D. M. Weir (ed.), Handbook of experimental immunology. Blackwell Scientific Publications, London.
11. **Odell, W. D., G. Abraham, H. R. Raud, R. S. Swerdloff, and D. A. Fisher.** 1969. Influence of immunization procedures in the titer, affinity, and specificity of antisera to glycoproteins. Acta Endocrinol. Suppl. **140**:54.
12. **Reimer, C. B., D. J. Phillips, S. E. Maddison, and S. L. Shore.** 1970. Comparative evaluation of commercial precipitating antisera against human IgM and IgG. J. Lab. Clin. Med. **76**:949–960.
13. **Ritchie, R. F., and J. Stevens.** 1972. Qualifications for acceptable antiserum performance in the Automated

Immunoprecipitin System: a brief review of commercially available reagents, p. 9–14. *In* Advances in Automated Analysis, Technicon Symposia, 1971. Mediad Inc., Tarrytown, N.Y.

14. **Singer, J. M., J. Hengevels, S. C. Edberg, J. W. T. Lichtenbelt, and P. H. Wiersema.** 1977. Determination of antibody concentration using a stopped-flow turbidimetric technique. Immunol. Commun. **6:**517–535.

Chapter 4

Immunoprecipitation in Gels

ANDREW MYRON JOHNSON

Precipitation of antigen-antibody complexes from solution has been used since the 1920s for the quantification of antigens and antibodies. Reactions in gels were first utilized for immunochemical studies in the mid-1940s, when Oudin introduced one-dimensional, "simple" immunodiffusion in tubes containing agar gel. He demonstrated that a single antigen-antibody system gave a single precipitin band and that mixtures of systems in the same tube gave multiple, independent bands. With these observations, precipitin reactions became qualitative as well as quantitative. Gel methods have significantly higher sensitivity and greater resolving power than techniques with no support medium. In addition, the actual gels may be photographed and stored, since the insoluble immunoprecipitates formed at equivalence become trapped in the gel matrix.

Several modifications of Oudin's diffusion method have been developed subsequently, perhaps the most commonly used being double immunodiffusion and radial immunodiffusion (RID) for qualitative and quantitative studies, respectively. The combination of electrophoresis and, more recently, isoelectric focusing with simple diffusion and the utilization of electrical potential for the diffusion process itself have resulted in the introduction of a plethora of gel precipitin methods. A few of the more important of these methods are described in this chapter.

Immunodiffusion in gels is based on the same physicochemical principles as precipitin reactions in solution. The basic tenets of antigen or antibody excess and of equivalence are particularly important; indeed, the relative solubility of complexes with a significant excess of either reactant and the insolubility of these complexes near equivalence, or "optimal proportions," are critical to the visualization process, whether the gels are stained or not.

In the passive diffusion procedures (i.e., those in which electrical potential is not used to drive one or both reactants into the gel), rates of diffusion of the antigen and antibody affect both the rate of reaction and the location of precipitates within the gel matrix. Rates of diffusion are affected, in turn, by molecular size, temperature, gel viscosity and hydration, and interactions between matrix and reactants.

The passive immunodiffusion techniques share the major disadvantage of requiring several hours or even days before results are available. For quantification, they are relatively insensitive and labor intensive. At the same time, they are easy to learn and require no large or expensive equipment. The "active" procedures, those using electrophoresis, are faster and more sensitive but require more investment in training and equipment.

Of the passive procedures, double (Ouchterlony) immunodiffusion and RID are described in this chapter. In addition, electroimmunoassay (EIA; "rocket immunoelectrophoresis") and counterimmunoelectrophoresis (CIEP) of the active methods and immunoelectrophoresis (IEP) and immunofixation electrophoresis (IFE) of the combined methods are presented. Of these, double immunodiffusion and IFE are qualitative, IEP and CIEP are qualitative-semiquantitative, and the other methods are quantitative.

Support media

Passive immunodiffusion was originally performed in gels made from Noble agar, a mixture of polysaccharides obtained from algae. Agar contains a large number of impurities plus two major fractions. One of these fractions, agaropectin, contains large numbers of sulfate and carboxyl groups which interact with some proteins and which, in electrodiffusion methods, cause reverse buffer flow or electroendosmosis (EEO). Purified agarose, the other major fraction, is relatively free of these effects and is therefore preferable to agar for all of the techniques discussed here. Several grades of agarose are available commercially, characterized in part by the amount of EEO in each. High-EEO agarose is useful for most applications of CIEP, which require that immunoglobulins migrate cathodically. For most other procedures, medium- or low-EEO agarose is preferred.

Agarose also varies in other aspects, including gel strength and temperatures of solution and gelation. Many manufacturers give data for these qualities as well as for EEO. The routine use of high-quality agarose is recommended; for critical procedures, several lots should be tested, and a long-term supply of the chosen lot should be obtained. FMC Corp., Marine Colloids Div., Rockland, ME 04841, is perhaps the major supplier of high-quality, well-characterized agarose preparations.

Other support media may also be used for immunodiffusion, including, in particular, cellulose acetate membranes. Cellulose acetate is easier to use than agarose gels, but has the disadvantages of less clarity, reduced resolution with electrophoretic procedures, and the necessity for using surface application techniques. In contrast, sample wells can be molded or cut into gels. In general, sieving gels (starch and polyacrylamide, for example) are not recommended for immunodiffusion because of the prolonged times required for diffusion and the difficulty in washing out unprecipitated proteins if the gels are to be stained. These gels may be used, however, for IFE or immunoprinting (see below).

Buffers

See reference 4.

For passive (nonelectrophoretic) procedures, normal saline (0.15 M NaCl) may be used. However, phosphate-buffered saline with a neutral pH is recommended. For electrophoretic procedures, buffers with an alkaline pH (ca. 8.6) and low ionic strength are most commonly used. Several formulas have been recommended for various procedures; for general use, the following formulas, among others, work well.

Phosphate-buffered saline (for passive immunodiffusion)

Na$_2$HPO$_4$	13.88 g
NaH$_2$PO$_4$ · H$_2$O	2.43 g
NaCl	80.0 g

Add distilled water to make 1.0 liter. Dilute this solution 1 in 10 with distilled water for use.

Electrophoresis buffer. Mix the following in a 2-liter Erlenmeyer flask.

Diethyl barbituric acid	11.0 g
Sodium barbital	70.1 g

Add distilled water to make 1,400 ml.

Heat, with stirring, until all the salts have dissolved; cool to room temperature, and then adjust the pH to 8.6.

Dilute to 8 liters in a polyethylene carboy. (Alternatively, dilute to 2 liters, and then dilute 1 in 4 for use.)

Preparation of gels

Agarose gels with sample wells or troughs prepunched for the various procedures are available from several manufacturers. However, in-house preparation of gels is relatively simple and permits more flexibility. Agarose concentrations around 1% (wt/vol) generally work best, depending on the gel strength desired. As mentioned above, different grades of agarose are recommended for different procedures; some guidelines are given below in the descriptions of the specific procedures.

The agarose is weighed and placed in an Erlenmeyer flask or large test tube. The appropriate volume of saline or buffer (depending on the procedure) is added, and the agarose is dissolved by heating. This step may be done by placing the tube or flask into a boiling-water bath (or temperature block) or by heating it on a temperature-controlled surface at 100 to 110°C or on a simple hot plate. In the last two cases, the solution should be stirred (usually with a magnetic stirrer) or swirled frequently. Minimal boiling is permissible, but boiling over is likely to be a problem unless care is taken. Heating should continue until the solution is clear, i.e., there are no more undissolved agarose particles.

The solution may be used to pour gels immediately if antiserum is not to be added, or it may be kept covered at 60°C for up to 8 h. Agarose solutions may be kept at 4°C for a week or longer and then reheated as needed to melt the gel. Repeated heating results in evaporation and therefore concentration of the agarose and buffer salts; in addition, caramelization of the agarose may occur. Therefore, only a few careful reheatings are recommended. Alternatively, several gels may be poured at one time and kept at 4°C, well sealed to minimize evaporation.

For preparation of gels containing antiserum (e.g., for RID or EIA), the agarose solution must be cooled to approximately 50 to 52°C to prevent heat denaturation of the antibodies. It is recommended that the desired volumes of warm agarose solution and antiserum be pipetted into separate test tubes, brought to 52°C in a water bath (or temperature block), mixed, and inverted several times. The mixture can then be kept at 52°C until one is ready to pour the gel. To prevent premature gelling at the lower temperatures used for antiserum-containing gels, it is helpful to warm the gel-molding materials (glass, Mylar, U-frame) to 45 to 55°C in an oven or a stream of warm air. Excessively warm plates, however, will denature the antibodies.

In most cases, agarose-coated polyester (Mylar) backing is recommended for agarose gels to facilitate handling, staining, and preservation of the gels. This polyester is available in cut sheets of various sizes and in rolls from the Marine Colloids Div. of FMC as GelBond and from Serva Fine Biochemicals, Garden City Park, N.Y., as Gel-Fix. (If rolls are used, sheets should be cut to the desired size and left under a weight for a few days to reduce curling.) The backing should be applied to a clean glass plate to maintain absolute flatness. Be sure the hydrophilic (agarose-coated) surface is upward, away from the glass. If there is a question, apply a drop of water to each side; the drop will spread on the coated side but "bead" on the uncoated side. Spread a few drops of 10 to 20% glycerol on the glass plate, carefully apply the Mylar sheet with the uncoated side toward the glass, avoiding air bubbles, and then roll the surface with a photographic print roller to squeeze out excess moisture and to flatten the Mylar sheet. During this process, it is best to place the glass plate on an absorbent paper or cloth towel and to cover the Mylar with the protective paper with which it is sold, plus a second towel.

Any of several methods may be used to cast gels. In the simplest of these, the Mylar sheet (still on the glass plate) is laid on a perfectly level surface, and the appropriate volume of warm agarose solution is pipetted evenly onto the surface and allowed to spread. The backing and the solution should be warm enough to prevent too rapid gelation. For a gel 1 mm thick, the area of the backing is multiplied by 0.1 to obtain the volume of solution, in milliliters, which must be applied. For example, a 10- by 10-cm surface would require 10 × 10 × 0.1, or 10, ml of solution. Once gelation has occurred at room temperature, the gel should be covered with ordinary plastic kitchen wrap and placed in a refrigerator for at least 15 min before use.

Alternatively, a gel-molding frame may be used. This procedure results in more uniform gels but does require additional materials. The backing is prepared as described above, and then a spacer (usually a Plexiglas or Neoprene U-frame of the desired thickness) is applied to the Mylar surface, and a glass or Plexiglas plate (3 to 4 mm thick) of the same dimensions as the backing and frame is placed thereon. The unit is held together with large ("bulldog") paper clamps or similar clamps, such as those used for acrylamide gel frames. If antiserum-containing agarose is used, the frame should be warmed to 45 to 52°C before being filled; if the frame is too warm, the antibodies may be denatured. Agarose solution is carefully but rapidly pipetted into the mold from the open side. The agarose-filled mold is left upright until gelling is complete (15 to 20 min) and then placed in a refrigerator for at least 15 min before use. The frame is carefully pried open with a spatula, and the Mylar-backed gel is removed from the supporting glass plate. If the gel is not needed immediately, it may be completely covered with plastic wrap (air bubbles should be avoided) and kept at 4°C until use. Alternatively, the gel may be left in the frame with the top sealed with tape.

Gel knives, punches, and templates are available from many manufacturers, or they may be made from scalpel or Exacto blades; thin metal tubing, large hypodermic needles, or cork borers; and plastic sheets, respectively. In lieu of superimposed templates, the desired patterns may be drawn on paper or cardboard and placed under the Mylar-backed gel while the wells are cut or punched. The patterns used are dependent on the procedure; examples are described below.

Viewing gels after diffusion

If the concentrations of both antigen and antibody are high enough, precipitin lines may be seen immediately after diffusion. With the active (electrophoretic) methods, the lines may intensify if the gel is left at room temperature for several minutes after completion of the electrophoretic run. The unstained lines may also be photographed by diffused light, with either a commercial apparatus such as the Cordis camera or a simple box with indirect illumination.

For band intensification and gel preservation, the gels should be thoroughly washed to remove salts and unwanted proteins and stained. Cover the gel surface with a damp sheet of Whatman no. 1 filter paper; add several layers of paper towels or old newspapers, then a thick sheet of glass or plastic, and finally a 1- to 5-kg weight (a large bottle of reagent may be used). Press the gel for 15 to 30 min, and then soak it in 1 liter of phosphate-buffered saline for at least 2 h (preferably overnight). Alternatively, the gel may be repeatedly pressed and soaked in saline (three or four times, 30 to 45 min per soak). Press the gel again as described above. Dry the gel completely in an oven or a stream of warm air (e.g., from a hair dryer).

Any of the routine protein stain-destain systems may be used if staining is desired. Preference should be based upon desired sensitivity and photographic technique. Coomassie brilliant blue R250 is a good routine stain, either alone or in combination with crocein scarlet. The combined stain is available premixed from Polysciences, Inc., Warrington, PA 18976. If the gels are to be photographed and sensitivity is not a critical factor, amido black (alone or with nigrosin) is also an excellent stain.

The stain should be dissolved or suspended in a good fixative solution, particularly if the antigen molecules are small (less than 50,000 daltons) or if tight lattices are not formed. Some precipitates will redissolve slowly in standard methanol-acetic acid solutions; 10 to 20% trichloroacetic acid, 3% trichloroacetic acid plus 5% acetic acid, or 3.5% perchloric acid is a better fixative. Suspensions of 0.1% Coomassie blue G250 (versus R250) in 3.5% perchloric acid are excellent for staining immunofixation precipitates in acrylamide gels. For highest sensitivity, enhanced silver stains are recommended (9). With any staining system, high-quality reagents should be used.

The following stain solution may be used for fixation and staining at the same time. It should be discarded after one or two uses. (If gels are fixed beforehand, the solution may be used repeatedly.) The same solution without stain may be used for fixation.

Stain solution

Crocein scarlet (Eastman Kodak Co., Rochester, N.Y.) . . . . 250 mg*
Coomassie blue R250 (Sigma Chemical Co., St. Louis, Mo.). . . . . 15 mg
Trichloroacetic acid. . . . . 5 g
Glacial acetic acid . . . . 5 ml
*Optional

Add distilled water to make 100 ml.
Stir at 60°C until dissolved, filter, and store at room temperature in a closed bottle.
Leave the dried gel in the stain solution for 30 min. Destain in 0.5 to 1% acetic acid until the background is clear, rinse with water, and dry. Dried gels will keep for years at moderate temperature and humidity; for improved long-term storage, soak the gels for 30 min in 5 to 10% glycerol before drying them.

PASSIVE IMMUNODIFFUSION

Double (Ouchterlony) immunodiffusion

Although it is one of the older immunochemical techniques, double immunodiffusion remains one of the most versatile techniques for evaluating antigens and antibodies. The agarose (or agar) gel may be prepared with either electrophoresis buffer or phosphate-buffered saline, although the latter is preferred to minimize nonspecific precipitation of euglobulins (proteins relatively insoluble in low-ionic-strength solutions). The two reactants (antigen and antibody solutions) are applied via punched sample wells or a template applied onto the surface of the gel. Each reactant then diffuses radially outward, with concentration decreasing geometrically with increasing distance from the point of application. Where the antigen and antibody meet in optimal proportions, an insoluble precipitate will form. This precipitate may be viewed directly, or the gel may be washed to remove unprecipitated proteins and stained.

Procedure

1. Prepare the agarose solution (1% in phosphate-buffered saline), and pour the gel as described above. Gels may be formed in small petri dishes, on precoated microscope slides, or, preferably, on Mylar backing.

2. Using a drawn pattern under the gel or a template laid on top, punch wells in the desired pattern. Cut and aspirate the agarose plugs cleanly by using vacuum with a trap.

3. Place the prepared gel on a level surface. Fill the reactant wells with antiserum and antigen solutions as desired. Do not overfill. (Usually the antiserum is placed in the central well and different antigen solutions, or dilutions of a single solution, are placed in the outer six wells in a seven-well pattern [Fig. 1]. Any pattern may be used, however.)

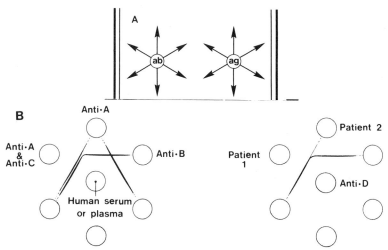

FIG. 1. Double (Ouchterlony) immunodiffusion. (A) Antigen (ag) and antibody (ab) are applied in wells cut into the agarose gel and diffuse radially toward each other. (B) Precipitin lines form where antigen meets its specific antibody in optimal proportions. These patterns are the common seven-well patterns; on the left, a complex antigen mixture is applied in the center well, and different antisera are applied in the peripheral wells. The curved line indicates complete identity of the reaction of anti-A in two wells with its corresponding antigen. B–anti-B and C–anti-C show patterns of nonidentity with A–anti-A. On the right, a single antiserum is used in the center well, and sera from two patients are used in the outer wells. The spur indicates that protein D in the serum of patient 1 has antigenic determinants not shared by D in serum from patient 2; i.e., this reaction is the reaction of partial identity.

4. Cover the gel with a tray containing a wet paper towel, or carefully place the gel in a humid chamber at room temperature.

5. Allow diffusion to proceed overnight or for as long as necessary for precipitin bands to form. (Larger proteins, longer diffusion distances, and lower temperatures will increase the required time.)

6. View or photograph the precipitin lines with indirect light; alternatively, wash and stain the gel as described above.

Irregular patterns may result from overfilling of wells, irregular well punching, or nonlevel incubation. Other potential problems include gel drying during diffusion because of exposure to dry air; overheating and denaturation of proteins; inadequate time for diffusion and resulting weakness of band intensity; bacterial or fungal contamination of gel solution, antigen, or antiserum, with resulting degradation; use of lipemic antigen or antiserum solutions, with intensive staining of the lipoproteins (if lipemic samples must be used, this problem may be reduced by adding 0.5% nonionic detergent, such as Triton X-100, to the wash solutions); and antigen or antibody excess. The last problem can be circumvented by trying several combinations of antigen and antibody dilutions.

RID

The gel preparation for RID is similar to that for double immunodiffusion, except that antiserum is added to the agarose solution before the gel is poured, as described above. Phosphate-buffered saline is again preferred. It is essential that monospecific antiserum with relatively high affinity be used. The use of immunoglobulin G (IgG) fractions of antiserum will produce clearer backgrounds. Table 1 gives volumes of antisera (IgG fractions) from Atlantic Antibodies,

Scarborough, ME 04074, for several proteins, with the sample dilutions indicated. Lower concentrations of antiserum may be used in most cases if the antigens are present at lower concentrations (e.g., in body fluids) or if higher dilutions of serum are used. Volumes indicated are for a gel 10 by 10 by 0.1 cm; change the volumes as necessary for other sizes of gels. RID is illustrated graphically in Fig. 2.

Procedure

1. Prepare a 1% agarose solution in phosphate-buffered saline.

2. Pipette 10 ml (for a gel 10 by 10 by 0.1 cm; adjust the volume as necessary) of warm agarose solution into a large test tube (15 to 25 ml). Place the tube in a water bath (or temperature block) at 52°C until the temperature has equilibrated (about 15 to 30 min, depending on the starting temperature of the agarose).

TABLE 1. Recommended antiserum and serum dilutions

| Analyte | RID | | EIA | |
	Sample[a]	Anti-serum[b]	Sample	Anti-serum
Prealbumin	1 + 10	0.5	1 + 10	0.15
Albumin	1 + 1,000	0.3	1 + 300	0.7
Alpha-1-antitrypsin	1 + 5	0.6	1 + 30	0.15
Alpha-2-macroglobulin	1 + 10	0.5	1 + 20	0.2
Haptoglobin	1 + 20	0.4	1 + 20	0.08
Transferrin	1 + 50	0.3	1 + 20	0.35
C3 complement	1 + 15	0.3	1 + 10	0.3
C4 complement	1 + 5	0.3	1 + 10	0.06
IgG	1 + 100	0.2	1 + 50	0.2
IgA	1 + 10	0.7	1 + 10	0.15
IgM	1 + 10	0.3	1 + 3	0.2

[a] Volume of serum or plasma plus volume of diluent.
[b] Microliters of IgG fraction of respective antisera (Atlantic Antibodies) per square centimeter of gel.

Diffusion of antigen from wells

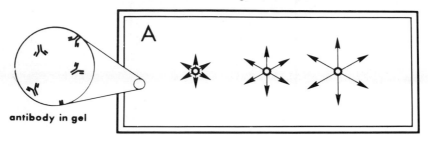

antibody in gel

Fixed-time assay

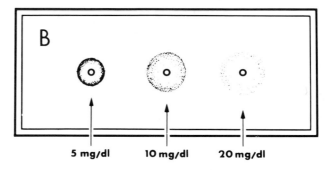

5 mg/dl   10 mg/dl   20 mg/dl

Endpoint assay

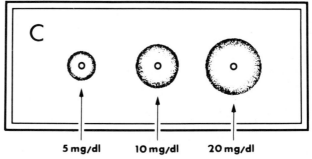

5 mg/dl   10 mg/dl   20 mg/dl

FIG. 2. RID. (A) Samples have been applied to wells in an agarose gel containing specific antibodies and allowed to diffuse. At the end of a specified time (B) or after completion of diffusion (C), the ring sizes are proportional to antigen concentration. Lower-concentration samples (e.g., 5 mg/dl in this case) reach completion earlier than higher-concentration ones (Fig. 3).

3. Pipette the desired volume of antiserum (Table 1) into a similar tube, and place the tube in the same water bath.

4. While these tubes are equilibrating, prepare the gel frame (or Mylar sheet on glass backing) as described above. If no frame is used, the backing must be on a perfectly level surface. In either case, it is best to warm the support to 45 to 50°C to prevent premature gelling. Do not overheat! (Temperatures over 56°C denature IgG.)

5. Pour or pipette the warm agarose into the test tube with the antiserum; cover this tube with Parafilm, and mix the contents by inverting the tube several times.

6. Either pour or pipette the warm agarose-antiserum mixture onto the backing, spreading the solution evenly over the surface. If a frame is used, pipette the mixture carefully but quickly into the frame, avoiding air bubbles.

7. Allow the agarose to cool at room temperature for 15 to 20 min and then at 4°C for an additional 15 to 20 min. (Gels which are well covered to prevent evaporational drying may be kept in the refrigerator for up to 1 week.)

8. Before use, cleanly punch 2.5- or 3-mm holes in the gel with a sharpened cork borer or a commercial or homemade punch. Aspirate the gel plugs and discard them. Holes should be at least as far apart in all dimensions as 1.5 to 2 times the maximum expected diameter of rings; this distance may be determined by trial, but as a starting point, 2 cm may be used. A template may be drawn and placed behind the gel backing, if desired.

9. Place the punched gel on a flat surface, and carefully pipette samples into the wells. The volumes for all standards and samples must be the same; precision of the assay increases directly in proportion

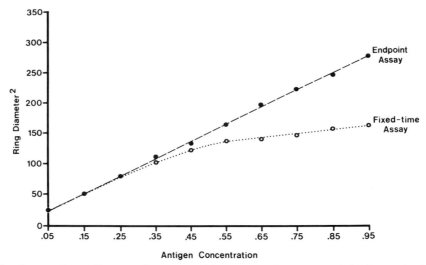

FIG. 3. RID graph. The two lines illustrate the improved linearity and precision of the longer (endpoint) type of assay. Concentrations of unknown samples may be interpolated graphically or arithmetically.

to the precision of measurement. Therefore, accurate micropipettes must be used. For the well size indicated (2.5 to 3 mm in diameter for a gel 1 mm thick), volumes should be not more than 5 μl. Wells must not be overfilled; reduce the volumes used or increase the well size as necessary.

10. Carefully place the loaded gel into a moist chamber. Diffusion will proceed faster in a 37°C chamber, but humidity must be more carefully maintained to prevent drying than is the case at room temperature. (Commercially prepared gels usually come in tightly sealed plastic containers. These gels should also be placed in humid chambers.)

11. The time required for diffusion depends in part on the size of the antigen being assayed. Diffusion of large molecules, such as IgM and alpha-2-macroglobulin, requires substantially longer than that of alpha-1-antitrypsin, for example. As discussed above, preliminary readings may be made after 12 to 24 h. Incubation should then be continued until ring size for the highest concentration standard has reached a plateau; measure again, and calculate final concentrations.

12. For the measurement of ring diameters, several reading devices are available from various manufacturers. A simple millimeter ruler may be used with a magnifying glass, however. Rings should be measured twice at right angles to compensate for irregular (noncircular) rings. The two measurements are then averaged (if the calculation is to be made as concentration versus square of ring diameter [d^2], the two values may simply be multiplied to give an estimated d^2).

13. Plot the standards as follows: on arithmetic graph paper, plot concentration on the y (vertical) axis and d^2 on the x axis; on semilogarithmic paper, plot concentration on the logarithmic axis and average diameter (not squared) on the arithmetic axis. Fit a smooth curve to the points, and then extrapolate concentrations of unknowns from the curve. An example of an RID graph is shown in Fig. 3.

Alternatively, ring areas may be determined by cutting out and weighing photographic images or by using a digitized planimeter such as the Zidas (Carl Zeiss, Inc., Thornwood, NY 10594). On arithmetic graph paper, plot area on the x axis and concentration on the y axis.

A computer or calculator may be used instead of graph paper to calculate a polynomial best-fit curve and to extrapolate unknowns with any of the above methods of measurement.

ACTIVE IMMUNODIFFUSION

CIEP

CIEP is related to double immunodiffusion in that antibody and antigen are diffused toward each other. However, in this case they are driven by an electric current rather than allowed to diffuse passively. As was mentioned previously, agarose with relatively high EEO (or agar) is used with a buffer system which will result in cathodic migration of the relevant antibodies and anodic migration of the antigen. For most proteins, standard barbital or Tris buffers at ca. pH 8.6 work well.

CIEP is commonly used as a qualitative procedure, especially in the rapid diagnosis of infectious diseases such as bacterial meningitis. If serial dilutions of antigen are applied, along with controls with known concentrations, the procedure becomes semiquantitative. The location of the precipitin line also gives an indication of concentration; higher antigen/antibody ratios result in a shift toward the antigen well and vice versa (Fig. 4).

Monospecific antiserum must be used for most purposes to prevent confusion. Antibodies with relatively high affinity and avidity are also recommended.

Procedure

1. Prepare agarose solution with electrophoresis buffer and high-EEO agarose (such as SeaKem HE or HEEO from FMC, depending on application). Pour a gel 1 mm thick of the desired dimensions, with Mylar backing.

2. With a template (either a metal or a plastic overlay template or a simple drawing behind the gel),

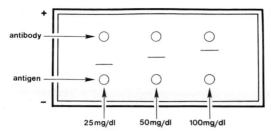

FIG. 4. CIEP. Samples containing antigen are applied in the cathodic wells, and specific antiserum is applied in the anodic wells. The two reactants are driven toward each other by an electrical potential. Precipitin lines form where the two reactants meet in optimal proportions. As shown, the procedure is semiquantitative if standards with known antigen concentrations are included.

punch parallel horizontal rows of 2.5- to 3-mm wells, as shown in Fig. 4. Multiple pairs of rows may be punched on the same gel, if it is wide enough. Be sure to align the anodic (antiserum) wells with the cathodic (antigen) wells in each pair of rows. Aspirate all agarose plugs from the wells.

3. Place the punched gel in the electrophoresis cell. Apply foam or filter paper wicks soaked in the electrode buffer to the anodic and cathodic edges of the gel, overlapping the agarose about 1 cm. The wicks must reach into the electrode buffer on each end.

4. With micropipettes, barely fill each of the anodic wells in each pair of rows with antiserum (for 2.5- to 3-mm wells in a gel 1 mm thick, 4- to 5-μl volumes should be used). Likewise, fill the cathodic wells of each pair with the control and test antigen solutions. Turn on the power supply (5 to 10 V/cm) for at least 1 h. (With this buffer-and-gel combination, a 10°C cooling plate, and a 10-cm gel distance between wicks, the current should be about 2 to 4 mA/cm of horizontal gel width.)

5. Turn off the power supply. Wait 15 to 30 min, and then remove the gel from the electrophoresis cell and examine it with indirect lighting for precipitin lines. Process the gel as described above for RID for staining and preservation.

EIA (rocket immunoelectrophoresis)

EIA was developed in the mid-1960s by Laurell as a rapid, precise method for quantification of plasma proteins (6). It is analogous to RID, except that an electrical potential is used to drive the antigen-containing solutions into the antibody-containing agarose gel. As is the case with CIEP, the time for diffusion is thereby reduced from several hours or days to a few hours. The resulting immunoprecipitates assume a triangular or "rocket" shape, with antigen concentrations directly proportional to the areas of the triangles or, more simply, to their heights.

The agarose-buffer system for EIA should result in a net migration of the antibodies as near zero as possible, unlike that in CIEP. The antigen may migrate anodically, cathodically, or both. Low- to low-medium-EEO agarose is used with the standard electrophoresis buffer for most purposes. Most plasma proteins migrate anodically in such a system; sample wells are therefore punched in a row near the cathodic

electrode wick. For proteins with cathodic migration, the wells should be at the anode; for bidirectional proteins, such as IgG and IgM, the wells should be near the center.

It is important to apply samples as quickly as possible, preferably with a low-voltage field across the gel during application. Otherwise, lateral diffusion may result in irregularly widened immunoprecipitates or even in mixing of antigens from adjacent wells. The low voltage should be maintained for several minutes while the antigen is migrating into the gel to minimize artifacts. Voltage is then raised and maintained for approximately twice the time required for the antigen to migrate the expected distance of the highest peak in the absence of antibody. For example, if a given electrophoretic system requires 2 h for ceruloplasmin to migrate 4 cm and if 4 cm is the expected height of the highest standard peak, the potential should be applied for 4 h.

At least three, and preferably five or six, standards should be run on each gel. These standards should bracket the entire range of concentrations to be assayed, since extrapolation beyond the standard range is fraught with error.

EIA is particularly useful for the assay of proteins in the "midrange," i.e., concentrations too low for precise assay by nephelometry or turbidimetry, but requiring extensive dilution for radioimmunoassay or similarly sensitive methods. These proteins include alpha-fetoprotein in amniotic fluid, immunoglobulins and complement components in urine and cerebrospinal fluid, antihemophilic factor antigen in plasma, and the like. Many clinical and research laboratories use this method for most plasma protein assays.

Procedure

1. Prepare a 1% agarose solution with electrophoresis buffer and low- or medium-EEO agarose.

2. Pipette 10 ml (for a gel 10 by 10 by 0.1 cm; adjust the volume as necessary) of the warm agarose solution into a large test tube (15 to 25 ml). Place the tube in a water bath (or temperature block) at 52°C until the temperature has equilibrated (15 to 30 min).

3. Pipette the desired volume of antiserum (Table 1) into a similar tube, and place the tube in the same water bath.

4. While these tubes are equilibrating, prepare the gel frame (or Mylar sheet on glass backing) as described above. If no frame is used, the backing must be on a perfectly level surface. In either case, it is best to warm the support to 45 to 50°C to prevent premature gelling. Do not overheat!

5. Pour or pipette the warm agarose into the test tube with the antiserum; cover this tube with Parafilm, and mix the contents by inverting the tube several times.

6. Either pour or pipette the agarose-antiserum mixture onto the backing, spreading the solution evenly over the surface. If a frame is used, pipette the mixture carefully but quickly into the frame, avoiding air bubbles.

7. Allow the agarose to cool at room temperature for 15 to 20 min and then at 4°C for an additional 15 to 20 min. (Gels which are well covered to prevent evaporational drying may be kept in the refrigerator for up to 1 week.)

8. Before use, cleanly punch 2.5- to 3-mm wells in the gel, and aspirate the plugs by using vacuum with

a trap. For most procedures, these wells should be in a single row 1 to 2 cm from the cathodic edge of the gel, with about 2 mm between wells. For proteins which migrate cathodically, wells should be at the anode; for IgG and IgM, wells should be near the center. If maximum peak heights are less than one-third the gel width, two parallel horizontal rows—one at the cathodic side and one just anodic to the center—may be used.

9. Place the punched gel on a flat surface, and carefully pipette samples into the wells. The volumes for all standards and samples must be the same; precision of the assay increases directly in proportion to the precision of measurement. Therefore, accurate micropipettes must be used. For the well size indicated (2.5 to 3 mm in diameter, gel 1 mm thick), volumes should be no more than 5 μl. Wells must not be overfilled; reduce the volumes used, or increase the well size as necessary.

10. Transfer the gel as quickly as possible to the electrophoretic apparatus, and apply electrode wicks. (If the setup permits, an electrical potential of 2 to 3 V/cm may be applied across the gel during sample application to the wells. This step minimizes passive diffusion of samples and results in better precision.)

11. Apply a potential of 2 to 5 V/cm for 15 to 20 min, and then increase the potential to 25 to 30 V/cm (depending on cooling efficiency of the electrophoresis cell). Maintain this potential for the time required to complete peaking (see discussion above). Alternatively, 5 to 10 V/cm may be applied overnight.

12. Turn off the power supply. Leave the gel in the cell for 15 to 30 min, and then remove and process the gel as described above for staining of RID gels.

13. Measure peak heights (from the middle of the sample wells to the tops of the peaks) to the nearest 0.1 mm.

14. Plot the standards on arithmetic graph paper, with peak heights on the x axis and concentrations on the y axis. Draw a smooth curve through the points, and then extrapolate unknown concentrations. Alternatively, a calculator or computer with a parabolic (quadratic) or cubic curve-fitting program may be used.

Careful attention to detail will usually result in sharp, triangular peaks which are easy to measure. Delay in sample application or in beginning electrophoresis will result in variable lateral diffusion and imprecision. Excessive electrical potential during the first few minutes will result in unequal migration in the gel and "diving" peaks which are difficult to measure. Excessively prolonged electrophoresis will result in buffer depletion and pH changes in the gel, with resulting dissolution of immunoprecipitates. Prolonged washing in water before staining may also result in loss of precipitates.

Two or, on occasions, three proteins may be assayed in the same gel, as long as the relevant antiserum concentrations are such that the peaks are of distinctly different heights. Examples include simultaneous assay of IgA and IgG or of transferrin and alpha-1-antitrypsin.

Variants of EIA

Fused rockets. The fused-rocket modification of the EIA is particularly useful in the characterization of protein fractions from preparative procedures such as column chromatography (8). Two rows of closely spaced sample wells are used, with sequential samples alternating in wells in the upper and lower rows. Antigenic identity of proteins in the fractions is indicated by fusion of the rockets, and relative concentrations are indicated by peak heights. Multispecific antisera, either mixtures of two or three monospecific sera or antiserum to whole human serum, are often used to detect contaminants in the preparations.

Crossed IEP. Crossed IEP is similar to fused rockets, except that the initial separation is performed by electrophoresis or isoelectric focusing (5). An actual strip of this initial separation is then applied to, or embedded in, a second gel containing antibodies. Electrophoresis is performed at right angles to the first separation. Rocket-shaped immunoprecipitates form wherever an antigen and specific antibodies to it are present in the gel. This technique may be used for quantification of several proteins at the same time (3). It is more often used in the detection of conversion products (particularly of complement components) and of complexes.

COMBINED (ACTIVE-PASSIVE) IMMUNODIFFUSION

IEP

IEP is a two-stage method in which an antigen mixture, such as plasma or serum, is separated by electrophoresis. Antiserum is then allowed to diffuse against the separated proteins at right angles to the separative migration. First introduced by Grabar and Williams in 1953, IEP has been used extensively since the development by Scheidegger of a microadaptation.

The initial separation may be performed in almost any solid or gel medium for electrophoresis; a trough parallel to the electrophoretic separation is subsequently filled with antiserum, which is allowed to diffuse against the antigens overnight. The procedure is illustrated in Fig. 5. The antiserum may be mono- or polyspecific; for identification of myeloma proteins (M-components), both types of serum are commonly used.

IEP is relatively insensitive to the antigen/antibody ratio. It is therefore the preferred method in many clinical laboratories for the detection of myeloma and Bence-Jones proteins. For the differentiation of minor differences in electrophoretic mobility, as with genetic variants of proteins or multiple bands with M-components, immunofixation electrophoresis (IFE; see below) gives far superior resolution. In general, IEP is an excellent method for detecting impurities in antigen or antibody preparations, although crossed IEP (see above) is more sensitive.

IEP has also been used in the past as a screening procedure for quantification of the major classes of immunoglobulins. As such, it is both qualitative and semiquantitative. Its usefulness in this regard has decreased with the advent of rapid, accurate quantitative methods such as immunonephelometry and turbidimetry. Agarose gel electrophoresis of serum is used along with these quantitative procedures to

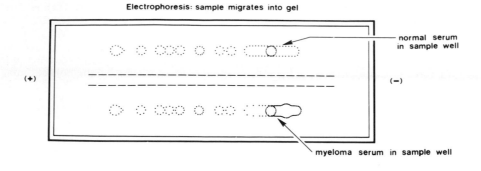

Electrophoresis: sample migrates into gel

normal serum
in sample well

(+)   (−)

myeloma serum in sample well

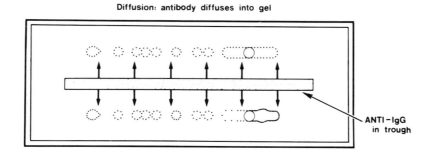

Diffusion: antibody diffuses into gel

ANTI−IgG
in trough

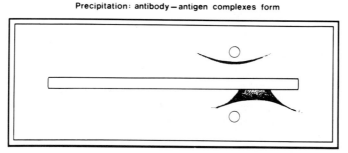

Precipitation: antibody−antigen complexes form

FIG. 5. IEP. Samples are applied to wells in agarose gels containing buffer, and electrophoresis is performed. The agarose in the central trough is removed, and antiserum (in this case, specific for IgG) is applied and allowed to diffuse overnight. Precipitin bands form where antigen and its specific antibody meet in optimal proportions.

screen for myeloma proteins and to confirm the quantitative assays. IFE, IEP, or both are then performed as required for positive identification of paraproteins.

Prepared gels and reagents for IEP are available from many commercial sources, including Corning Medical, Medfield, Mass., and Beckman Instruments, Inc., Brea, Calif. It is relatively easy to prepare gels in house, as explained below.

Procedure

1. Prepare a 1% solution of agarose (or 1.5% agar) in electrophoresis buffer.

2. Pour a gel 1 mm thick (without antiserum) as described above for CIEP. The width of the Mylar backing (and the resulting gel) is determined by the number of patterns to be run.

3. With an IEP template and matched cutter and punch, cut sample wells and antiserum troughs. Leave the gel strips in the antiserum troughs until electrophoresis is completed. Aspirate the gel plugs from the sample wells. (Sample wells should be near

the midpoint of the electrophoretic separation if agar or high-EEO agarose is used, but near the cathode for low- or medium-EEO agarose.)

4. Depending on the electrophoretic system in use, perform the following steps in the required order.

   a. Place the gel in the electrophoretic cell, and apply saturated electrode wicks, which must also contact the electrode solutions.

   b. Barely fill the antigen wells with the antigen solutions to be tested. Bromophenol blue may be used as a marker for electrophoretic migration.

5. Apply an electrical potential of 15 to 30 V/cm across the gel for the time required for the desired separation. If bromophenol blue is used, the second (albumin-bound) dye front may be used to ascertain completion of electrophoretic migration.

6. Remove the gel from the cell, and remove the gel strips in the antiserum troughs. Place the gel in a moist chamber or a tray containing wet paper towels. Barely fill the troughs with the appropriate antisera.

7. Allow the antisera to diffuse overnight or until precipitin arcs are visible. Examine the gels before or after staining, or both, as described above for double (Ouchterlony) immunodiffusion.

Prolonged diffusion will result in artifacts, especially at the anodic and cathodic ends of the run. Liquid-absorbed antisera may diffuse across the gel and form linear precipitates with antisera from adjacent troughs. Marked antibody excess may result in multiple, concentric arcs or Liesegang lines, which may be mistaken for multiple antigen reactivities. With IgG, these arcs or lines may be seen at one end of the overall precipitin arc if one subclass (particularly IgG4 anodically or IgG1 cathodically) is present at a very high concentration. Similar partial splitting of arcs may be seen with other proteins if there is catabolism or complexing with other substances.

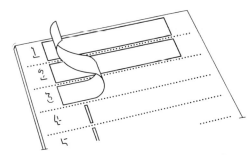

FIG. 6. Application of antiserum for IFE. After electrophoresis of samples in a thin-layer gel, cellulose acetate strips saturated with specific antisera are carefully applied over the gel (without air bubbles). Diffusion occurs in both directions between the gel and the strips; either or both may be washed in saline and stained for immunoprecipitates.

IFE

IFE was first described in its present format by Alper and Johnson (1) as a technique for the differentiation of genetic variants and catabolic products of proteins. It is similar to IEP except that antiserum is applied to the surface of the gel, rather than in a trough, after electrophoresis. Ritchie and Smith (7) suggested the application of antiserum via cellulose acetate or filter paper strips, thus permitting direct, side-by-side application of different antisera without cross-contamination. Arnaud et al. (2) subsequently demonstrated that the application strips themselves could be processed and stained, producing an "immunoprint."

The advantages of IFE include much more rapid diffusion (1 h compared with overnight), significantly higher resolution, and direct comparability to electrophoretic separations themselves. Increased resolution is particularly useful with oligoclonal banding, as seen with many IgA myelomas and with IgG patterns in cerebrospinal fluid of many patients with multiple sclerosis, central nervous system lupus erythematosus or syphilis, or subacute sclerosing panencephalitis. In most cases, the same gels (commercial or homemade) may be used for both screening electrophoresis and IFE.

IFE has the disadvantage, compared with IEP, of a much more restricted range of useful antigen/antibody ratios. Antigen excess results in broadened immunoprecipitates; with marked excess, "holes" appear in the centers of the patterns. This situation is usually less of a problem in identification of M-components than in genetic phenotyping and research applications, which require higher resolution. In addition, proteins with the same electrophoretic mobilities are less likely to be separated than is the case with IEP (for example, an M-component and free light chains with similar mobilities).

The initial separation may be made in cellulose acetate membranes or in most gel matrices. Resolution is generally better in gels, with agarose the preferred medium for routine use. Agarose gels may be prepared in the laboratory or purchased commercially; Corning Medical sells complete kits for immunofixation of myeloma proteins, including titered antisera.

Sieving gels, such as polyacrylamide and starch, may be used; however, diffusion and washing times must be extended severalfold. The immunoprint technique may be used to avoid this this extra time. Immunofixation may also be used after other gel separative procedures, such as isoelectric focusing.

Procedure

1. Perform electrophoretic separation by routine procedures. The protein of interest should be diluted to a concentration of approximately 5 to 50 mg/dl, depending on antiserum titer (for myeloma proteins, this titer may be estimated from a screening electrophoresis or determined by immunoassay). Do not fix the patterns chemically after electrophoresis!

2. Completely saturate a cellulose acetate strip, cut to the desired size, with diluted antiserum (Table 2). Drain the strip, and then blot quickly with a paper towel to remove excess antiserum.

3. Apply the strip(s) to the surface of the gel used for separation, being careful to avoid air bubbles under the strip(s) (Fig. 6).

4. Permit the antiserum to diffuse for 1 h in a moist chamber (or cover the gel with an inverted baking dish containing a paper towel).

5. Press, wash, and stain the gel as discussed above for RID.

TABLE 2. Suggested trial dilutions for IFE

Protein to be fixed	Sample[a]	Antiserum[b]
Alpha-1-antitrypsin	1 + 5	Neat, 1 + 1
C3 complement	1 + 4	Neat
C4 complement	Neat	Neat
Gc globulin	1 + 1	Neat
Properdin factor B	1 + 1	1 + 1
Transferrin	1 + 10	1 + 1, 1 + 2
IgG[c]	1 + 4, 1 + 5	Neat, 1 + 1
IgA[c]	1 + 1	Neat, 1 + 1
IgM[c]	Neat	Neat

[a] Volume of serum or plasma plus volume of diluent; urine and cerebrospinal fluid samples must be concentrated. Neat, Undiluted.

[b] Volume of IgG fraction or nephelometric-grade antiserum to respective protein (Atlantic Antibodies) plus volume of diluent.

[c] Myeloma proteins must be diluted to 20 to 100 mg/dl, final concentration. For identification of light chains, use neat antisera to kappa and lambda chains.

For identification of myeloma proteins, antisera specific for the heavy chains of the immunoglobulin classes and against kappa and lambda light chains may be applied on adjacent electrophoretic patterns of the same serum. Antisera specific for free light chains may also be used to detect the presence of these chains in serum or urine. For the detection of oligoclonal banding of IgG in cerebrospinal fluid, this fluid should be concentrated 50- to 100-fold before electrophoresis.

Illustrations were drawn by Thomas Jordan and are used with the permission of Atlantic Antibodies (A Charles River Company).

LITERATURE CITED

1. **Alper, C. A., and A. M. Johnson.** 1969. Immunofixation electrophoresis: a technique for the study of protein polymorphism. Vox Sang. **17:**445–452.
2. **Arnaud, P., G. B. Wilson, J. Koistinen, and H. H. Fudenberg.** 1977. Immunofixation after electrofocusing: improved method for specific detection of serum proteins with determination of isoelectric points. I. Immunofixation print technique for detection of alpha-1-protease inhibitor. J. Immunol. Methods **16:**221–231.
3. **Clarke, H. G. M., and T. Freeman.** 1968. Quantitative immunoelectrophoresis of human serum proteins. Clin. Sci. **35:**403–413.
4. **Clausen, J.** 1969. Immunochemical techniques for the identification and estimation of macromolecules, p. 404–572. *In* T. S. Work and E. Work (ed.), Laboratory techniques in biochemical and molecular biology. North-Holland Publishing Co., Amsterdam.
5. **Laurell, C.-B.** 1965. Antigen-antibody crossed electrophoresis. Anal. Biochem. **10:**358–361.
6. **Laurell, C.-B.** 1972. Electroimmuno assay. Scand. J. Clin. Lab. Invest. **29**(Suppl. 124)**:**21–37.
7. **Ritchie, R. F., and R. Smith.** 1976. Immunofixation. I. General principles and application to agarose gel electrophoresis. Clin. Chem. **22:**1735–1737.
8. **Svendsen, P. J.** 1973. Fused rocket immunoelectrophoresis, p. 69–70. *In* N. H. Axelsen, J. Krøll, and B. Weeke (ed.), A manual of quantitative immunoelectrophoresis. Universitetsforlaget, Oslo.
9. **Willoughby, E. W., and A. Lambert.** 1983. A sensitive silver stain for proteins in agarose gels. Anal. Biochem. **130:**353–358.

Chapter 5

Turbidimetry

ROBERT C. FOSTER AND THOMAS B. LEDUE

Clinical laboratories today are faced with demands for more tests of various kinds delivered at a lower cost. As a result, administrators and laboratorians look to automated instruments currently in place to perform both standard and exotic tests. New devices that perform a wide variety of tasks are an increasingly attractive alternative to less flexible dedicated machines. General-use spectrophotometers and clinical analyzers represent a resource in this regard. For example, many routine immunochemical assays for serum proteins are performed easily and competently on these instruments (16). In the previous edition of this manual, Buffone (2) described quasiequilibrium methods designed for nephelometric systems and adaptable to turbidimetric instruments. This chapter outlines the basic principles involved in turbidimetric immunoquantification and describes 12 fixed-time kinetic assays for serum proteins on a centrifugal analyzer (COBAS BIO with DENS 8326 data reduction package) by Roche. This article also serves as a practical guide for adapting these assays to other sophisticated chemistry analyzers.

THEORETICAL CONSIDERATIONS

Immune complexes formed in solution scatter light in proportion to their size, shape, and concentration. Under conditions of antibody excess, increasing amounts of antigen result in higher scatter. The inclusion of polymer enhancers such as polyethylene glycol (PEG) 8000 (formerly PEG-6000) in the reaction buffer significantly accelerates complex formation (7). Over the past 10 years, workers have exploited these phenomena in devising simple and accurate optical techniques to quantify plasma proteins in body fluids.

Various instruments measure different consequences of the interaction of light and particles in solution. Turbidimeters measure the reduction of incidence light due to reflection, absorption, or scatter. Readings are given in absorbance units (A) which reflect the ratio of incident to transmitted light ($A = 2 - \log_{10} T$, where T is percent turbidity). Nephelometers measure the amount of light scattered at a defined angle to the incident beam. Scattered light is measured against a dark background, amplified, and reported in arbitrary units. It might be concluded that nephelometric and turbidimetric measurements paint the same picture of immunochemical reactions. Instead, these measurements indicate that the total amount of light scattered is not equivalent to the amount of light absorbed. Immunocomplexes tend to scatter light forward, which makes the light indistinguishable from transmitted light for a turbidimeter (11). Large or concentrated complexes cause destructive interference patterns in light, reducing the scatter apparent to a nephelometer.

The question of which method offers better results is still debated. The theoretical and practical aspects of each approach have been reviewed (4, 8, 11, 12). It appears, however, that the ability of an instrument to provide accurate and precise results is less a function of the optical alignment than of instrument quality. It is meaningless to argue the advantages gained by detector placement if these advantages are lost to noisy electronics or poor cuvette design.

INSTRUMENT CONSIDERATIONS

Electro-optical system

Assay sensitivity depends on a specific signal that exceeds the variability of blank readings by 3 standard deviations. Most direct turbidimetric assays are performed at between 20 and 300 mA over a 0.5- to 1-cm light path. Within these specifications, the standard deviation of absorbance readings of a dilute suspension of inert particles (0.3-μm-diameter latex) should be less than 1.0 mA. In this case, an absorbance change of 3.0 mA is necessary to distinguish a change in antigen concentration from background noise.

Immune complexes between 35 and 100 nm in diameter result in the greatest change in absorbance of incident illumination in the near UV. Generally, illumination should be available between 290 and 410 nm with a half-band pass of less than 10 nm. Spectrophotometers that utilize diffraction grating monochromators are ideal. However, instruments that employ dichroic or interference filters also perform well.

The quality of reaction cuvettes or cells is extremely important but highly variable. A cuvette system should minimize variation between and within cells. Flow-through systems have the advantage of using the same cell for all measurements. Multicuvette systems use flat, highly polished optical windows that reduce stray or internally reflected light. Some cuvettes need only one optical surface, since the incident light travels parallel to the open axis of the cuvette. Disposable cuvettes attract dust and may contain plastic molding flakes. These particles present problems for turbidimetric assays that may not be evident in colorimetric applications.

The instrument's photodetector should view a narrow angle of light transmitted in line with the incident beam (0°). This setup reduces the effect of light scattered forward on the measurement of transmitted light. An instrument with a 3° acceptance angle, however, must have a more powerful (and expensive) light source than one that measures a 10° angle.

Mechanical systems

Pipetting limitations. Ideally, the pipetting station is incorporated into the analyzer unit. This arrangement eliminates errors associated with rotor handling and lessens demands on the operator. Sample pipettes should offer users a range of volumes between 2 and 50 µl in steps no greater than 2 µl. Imprecision within this range should show a coefficient of variation of less than 0.2%. Since most serum protein assays require sample dilution, the ability to automatically dilute samples or pipette small volumes (0.1 to 5 µl) is a distinct advantage. Reagent pipettes commonly deliver between 100 and 500 µl with an accuracy and precision of less than 1%. Many analyzers offer the addition of a second or third reagent via the sample or reagent pipette. With this arrangement, antiserum can be added to initiate a reaction after a sample blank has been taken or to test for antigen excess conditions.

Mixing and timing of measurements. The complete mixing of reactants must be accomplished rapidly and completely. This mixing eliminates localized concentrations of sample or antibody that can affect results. Centrifugal analyzers are ideal in this respect, since reactants are pipetted into separate chambers, spun into a reaction cell under centrifugal force, and mixed by changes in acceleration within 3 to 5 s of contact. Sample and control cuvettes are measured simultaneously within 1 s after reactant mixing. This measurement is often used as a combined blank for sample and reagent. The effects of centrifugal force, however, may cause the settling of large immune aggregates formed by concentrated reactants (8). Many clinical analyzers incubate reactants under no centrifugal force, and a few offer constant mixing as the reaction tray moves into various positions. In these systems, samples may be assayed undiluted with concentrated antibody. These instruments, however, mix samples and calibrators at different times and must rely on precise timing of equivalent readings. Furthermore, measurements usually cannot be taken within 15 s of reactant mixing, necessitating separate sample and reagent blanks.

Programming features

Blanking options. An instrument's ability to acquire sample and reagent blanks is an important consideration. Most chemistry analyzers offer one or both of the approaches depicted in Fig. 1 for the fixed-time kinetic assays described below (6).

The autoblank procedure calls for the mixing of diluted antibody and sample. An absorbance is recorded directly after mixing and serves as a combined sample-plus-antibody blank (A^0_{s+ab}). This reading is subtracted from the total absorbance of the reaction mixture after appropriate incubation (A^f_{s+ab}). Also subtracted is any change evident in the antibody reagent alone (dA_{ab}/dt). The net change in absorbance (dA_n/dt) is the corrected measure of specific precipitation. This blanking option offers a relatively short assay with good clinical performance.

The hold-blank procedure requires incubation of calibrators and samples in a buffer containing 4% polyethylene glycol (PEG). A sample blank absorbance (A^f_s) is recorded after sample incubation and before the introduction of concentrated antibody. A total reaction absorbance (A^f_{s+ab}) is taken after reaction incubation and corrected for the sample blank. A reagent blank (A^f_{ab}) is obtained by subtracting the absorbance of PEG-buffer alone (A^f_{PEG}) from that of

concentrated antibody incubated in PEG (A^f_{ab+PEG}). The reagent blank is also subtracted from A^f_{s+ab} to give an estimate of the net change in absorbance (dA_n/dt). This procedure is similar to that of quasiequilibrium methods outlined in the previous edition of this manual. Because of the accurate timing of readings offered by automated equipment, incubation times are considerably reduced. This blanking option does require, however, approximately twice the assay time as the autoblank method. Its advantage lies in the accuracy of the sample blank and the ability to include reaction signal that occurs during the mixing phase of the assay. The choice of blanking modes depends on the type of sample, quality of antibody reagent, and operational demands of individual laboratories.

Data reduction and analysis. The change in absorbance with respect to antigen concentration is characteristically nonlinear for immunoassays based on light scattering. Manual plotting has given way to sophisticated onboard curve-fitting options made possibly by powerful microprocessors. The four-parameter logit-log transformation used for many EMIT chemistries is adaptable to immunoquantifications. Also, simple second-order polynomial functions adequately describe precipitin curves within the range of most assays (2).

Antigen excess detection is important when immunoglobulins or acute-phase proteins are quantified. Abnormally high levels of target protein may exhaust the supply of available antibody. Ths situation results in small, slow-forming precipitates that give low absorbance signals. An instrument cannot distinguish these absorbances from equivalent signals formed when antibody is not limiting. Some instruments, however, can detect differences in reaction kinetics that flag antigen excess conditions (1, 8). This capability is advantageous, but not essential. Gross abnormalities in protein levels in serum are usually anticipated because of patient history or prior testing. An additional eightfold dilution of these samples confirms high levels. However, an assay should provide sufficient antibody to produce high signals from virtually all samples encountered.

SAMPLE AND REAGENT CONSIDERATIONS

Even a well-designed spectrophotometer is often held hostage by the limitations imposed by samples and reagents. In this section, reagent variability is outlined and assay performance is discussed in the light of these problems.

Samples

An underlying assumption of any immunoassay is that the dose responses for a given protein are the same in sample and calibration materials. Unfortunately, this assumption is not always the case. Highly lipemic samples are notorious for interfering with optical immunoassays. Chylomicrons and other large lipoproteins present high levels of nonspecific scatter. Also, hydrophobic macroglobulins, endogenous immune complexes, and monoclonal proteins may aggregate when they encounter conditions that significantly alter their native solubility. The inclusion of

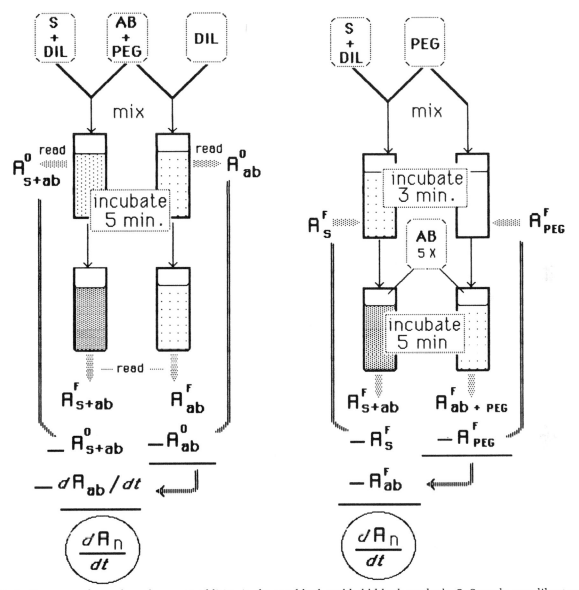

FIG. 1. Sequence of sample and reagent addition in the autoblank and hold-blank methods. S, Sample or calibrator; DIL, saline diluent; AB, antibody reagent; PEG, phosphate-buffered diluent containing 4% PEG 8000. Photometer readings and calculations are described in the text under blanking options.

PEG in the reaction solution favors this aggregation by reducing vibrational space and increasing protein-protein interactions. This nonspecific "signal" develops during the assay and is included in the total reaction absorbance. Generally, the higher the initial turbidity of the sample, the greater the change in the sample blank readings.

Dito (5) suggests that the use of dilute samples alleviates problems created by all but the most turbid samples. Very dilute samples, however, also reduce the degree of specific signal and compromise the assay. Pretreatment of turbid samples with various clearing agents has been reported to have some suc-

cess. This pretreatment introduces time-consuming sample manipulation that invites errors. Also, proteins associated with lipoproteins, such as C4, immunoglobulin A (IgA), and IgM, may be removed (14).

Automated instruments, with precise timing and blanking options, offer some hope for optical assays of turbid samples. Figures 2 and 3 compare results from turbid samples assayed at a 1:25 dilution for C4 (low-level protein). Samples were asayed by both the autoblank and hold-blank procedures and compared with results obtained by radial immunodiffusion. Protein values are significantly higher in the autoblank method than in the hold-blank procedure (Fig. 2). The

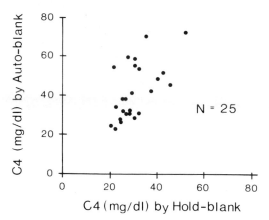

FIG. 2. Comparison of C4 values estimated in hyperlipemic samples by two turbidimetric blanking procedures.

radial immunodiffusion results indicate that the degree of overestimation is directly related to sample turbidity. Figure 3 depicts the exaggeration of C4 values as a function of the changes in sample blanks that occur over a 5-min assay. Note that preincubation of samples in PEG (hold-blank method) dramatically reduces, but does not eliminate, the effects of turbidity. The hold-blank procedure requires more reagent manipulation and assay time, but offers an advantage in assaying less-than-ideal samples for low-level proteins. The autoblank procedure yields excellent results when samples of normal turbidity are assayed. Both procedures are described in this article. Highly turbid samples, however, should not be assayed by direct photometric means.

Antisera

The antibody reagent presents additional problems. Antisera from virtually all commercial suppliers are

sufficiently monospecific to allow accurate assays of the major serum proteins. However, the variability found in antibody titer and avidity can alter assay results significantly. For example, low-avidity antibody is unsuitable for fixed-time turbidimetric assays because of slow complex formation and poor response at low antigen concentrations. Uncorrected variations in titer can change the shape of an assay's dose-response curve. The effects of these qualities on immunoassays are reviewed by Deverill and Reeves (3). Techniques for the characterization and monitoring of antisera are covered in chapter 3 of this manual and by Hudson et al. (9).

Optical clarity is as important in the antibody reagent as it is in other reactants. Most antisera, however, become turbid on dilution with PEG-buffer. Filtration removes much of this precipitation, but leaves small unfilterable complexes that contribute to the blank. The IgG fraction of a particular antiserum, however, shows very little turbidity when diluted in PEG. Figure 4 illustrates the signal-to-noise ratio at the low end of a transferrin assay with filtered and unfiltered reagents. The unfiltered IgG fraction provides a considerably lower blank than filtered serum. This difference has obvious benefits for assays that have low dose-response signals.

An antibody blank can also change during the assay. The addition of diluent to a working antibody mixture increases the solubility of unfilterable hydrophobic complexes and thus reduces the absorbance of the blank over time. The change in a reagent blank is directly related to the volume of diluent added. Figure 5 depicts the decrease in blank readings for two antibody reagents over 5 min. Note that the IgG fractionated material gives the lowest change in blank of all antibody preparations. The effects of a decreasing blank are reduced by minimizing the combined volume of sample and diluent. Also, both of the kinetic blanking methods described in the previous section include a measurement of a reagent blank. The change in this blank is subtracted from the total absorbance change for each sample.

Protein reference materials

The complexity, genetic variability, and instability of some serum proteins has frustrated efforts to estab-

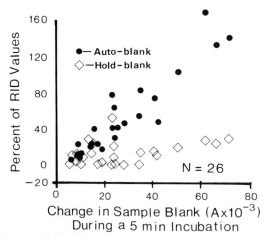

FIG. 3. Overestimation of C4 values plotted against the change in absorbance measured in sample blanks. C4 levels determined by hold-blank and autoblank methods are given as percentages of values indicated by radial immunodiffusion (RID). These percentages are plotted against the change in absorbance measured for each sample during a 5-min incubation in PEG-PBS buffer.

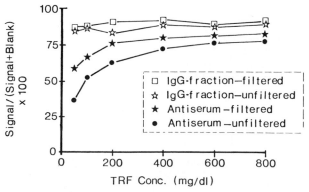

FIG. 4. Ratio of specific signal to total absorbance plotted against transferrin (TRF) concentration. Four antiserum preparations were used.

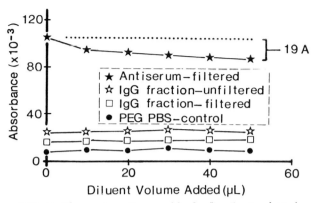

FIG. 5. Change in antiserum blank after 5 min plotted as a function of the volume of saline added to antibody reagent alone.

lish universally accepted standards. The World Health Organization distributes a lyophilized calibrator for 10 serum proteins which is based on a system of international units. Other commercial calibrators are based on various mass unit (weight-to-volume) standards. Often these standards disagree with one another. Recently the College of American Pathologists (CAP) released a secondary Reference Preparation for Serum Proteins (RPSP) that lists mass values for 12 proteins (13). These values were determined in an extensive collaborative study that estimated the mean of protein levels reported by laboratories using calibrators based on mass values. Many commercial suppliers now offer CAP-RPSP-based values for their calibrators to allow interlaboratory comparison of results.

We found that frozen (−20°C) samples of secondary reference calibrators from pooled serum provide stable results over a 2-year period for all proteins described herein. It is advisable to assay CAP-RPSP material (readily available) at intervals of 3 months to verify the stability of all calibrators and in-house controls.

Buffers

The composition of reaction buffers has been explored extensively over the past 10 years. Nonionic polymer enhancers speed the rate of complex formation by increasing the effective concentration of the reactants. The type and strength of buffering anion are also important considerations. The factors of pH and temperature, however, appear to have little effect over wide ranges. The effects of immunoenhancers and various ionic constituents of buffers are reviewed by Killingsworth (10) and Price et al. (12).

We recommend physiological saline as a diluent for samples, controls, and calibrators. Antibody is diluted with a 0.01 M phosphate-buffered saline (PBS) at pH 7.4 that includes 4% PEG 8000.

PERFORMANCE OF TURBIDIMETRIC ANALYSIS

We found a low-end assay limit for direct turbidimetric analysis of serum proteins at between 1 and 2 mg/dl. This limit corresponds to Buffone's (2) experi-

ence with nephelometric systems. Whicher et al. (16) reports that good spectrophotometers can detect 50 to 100 ng of target protein per cuvette with mild sample pretreatment. These methods are used to measure beta-1-glycoprotein and human placental lactogen in serum to 0.16 mg/dl with good precision.

The assays described here measure proteins that occur over a clinically important range of 10 to 8,000 mg/dl. The exceptions are C-reactive protein (CRP) in serum and albumin (ALB) and IgG in cerebrospinal fluid (CSF). With sample treatment, CRP can be measured to 0.4 mg/dl in processed calibration material. A more realistic low-level limit for serum samples, however, is 1 to 2 mg/dl. CSF samples need no manipulation because of low background absorption and scatter. IgG may be measured to 0.6 mg/dl in such samples.

In each assay listed in Table 1, values obtained for 98 patient samples agreed well with nephelometric determinations made on the Beckman Immunochemistry System. One exception was the haptoglobin assay that showed a significant underestimation of four samples with values above 200 mg/dl. Other high-level samples were unaffected. It is likely that these discrepancies are due to differences in light scattering exhibited among the phenotypic variants of the haptoglobin. Diluting these high-level samples to 50 to 100 mg/dl substantially reduced this underestimation.

General assay imprecision ran as high as 6.2% coefficient of variation between runs and as low as 1.3% within runs. As expected, the poorest precision occurred between runs of low-level proteins like C4.

PROCEDURES

Source of supplies

Buffer constituents. Buffer constituents are as follows: Sodium chloride (NaCl; no. S-9625; Sigma Chemical Co.); sodium azide (NaN$_3$; no. S-2002; Sigma); anhydrous dibasic sodium phosphate (Na$_2$HPO$_4$; no. S-0751; Sigma); anhydrous monobasic potassium phosphate (KH$_2$PO$_4$; no. P-5379; Sigma); PEG, molecular weight of 8,000 (PEG 8000; no. 15415-1; Kodak from American Scientific Supply).

Antisera and calibrators. The immunological reagents, calibrators, and controls for our work came from a single supplier, i.e., Atlantic Antibodies, Scarborough, Maine. Other manufacturers that offer similar high-quality reagents that are adaptable to the assays described here are Kallestad Laboratories Inc., Austin, Tex.; Tago Inc., Burlingame, Calif.; and Dako Corp., Santa Barbara, Calif. The IgG fractions of all antisera were used to ensure low reagent turbidity. A high-level (3×) calibrator was used to construct calibration curves. A normal-level (1×) preparation of pooled serum served as control material. The CAP-RPSP is available at a nominal cost through CAP, Skokie, Ill.

Instrumentation. A Roche COBAS BIO centrifugal analyzer was used to develop the assays described here. Most spectrophotometers that meet the requirements listed in the text can be used for these assays. In general, centrifugal analyzers excel. A review of selected equipment is given by Deverill and Reeves (4).

TABLE 1. Assay specifications and reagent dilutions for turbidimetric quantification of 12 serum proteins on a centrifugal analyzer

| Protein | Vol (μl) | | | Antiserum dilution for blanking method | | Approx calibration range (mg/dl) |
	Diluted sample	System diluent	Sample dilution	Auto	Hold	
Serum[a]						
ALB	7	20	1:800	1:75	1:15	670–11,000
AGP	12	15	1:25	1:50	1:10	18–140
AAT	12	15	1:25	1:25	1:5	20–320
A₂M	12	15	1:25	1:25	1:5	35–530
HPT	10	20	1:25	1:30	1:6	13–200
TRF	10	20	1:25	1:50	1:10	50–740
C3	13	25	1:25	1:50	1:10	20–320
C4	30	5	1:25	1:30	1:6	6–47[b]
IgG	4	25	1:25	1:50	1:10	150–2,500
IgA	8	20	1:25	1:20	1:4	27–435
IgM	20	5	1:25	1:30	1:6	15–245
CRP	25	5	1:5	1:10	1:4	1.5–12[b]
CSF						
ALB	2	25	Neat	1:75	NA[c]	2.7–43
IgG	25	25	Neat	1:75	NA	0.6–9.8

[a] AGP, α₁-Acid glycoprotein; AAT, α₁-antitrypsin; A₂M, α₂-macroglobulin; HPT, haptoglobin; TRF, transferrin.
[b] For assay of C4 and CRP, use five-point curve eliminating lowest point (6.25%).
[c] NA, Not applicable.

Miscellaneous. Miscellaneous necessary supplies are Gelman Acrodisc filters (no. 4192; 0.22-μm pore size) and latex suspension (0.3-μm particle size; no. LB-3; Sigma).

Preparation

Buffers. Use saline diluent for samples, calibrators, and controls. Dissolve 9 g of NaCl and 0.5 g NaN₃ in 950 ml of deionized water. Bring to 1 liter with water. For antiserum diluent (PEG-PBS), dissolve 1.15 g of NaHPO₄, 0.2 g of KH₂PO₄, 9 g of NaCl, 40 g of PEG, and 0.5 g of NaN₃ in 950 ml of deionized water. Bring to 1 liter with water, and adjust the pH with 1 M NaOH or 1 M HCl. Both reagents are stable for 1 year. Filter through a filter (0.45-μm pore size) before use.

Antisera. All assays described use antiserum IgG fractions diluted in PEG-PBS to the specifications listed in Table 1. Note that the autoblank and hold-blank procedures call for different antiserum dilutions. For best results, let the antiserum dilutions incubate for 30 min and then clarify them through a syringe filter (0.22-μm pore size). Working solutions of antiserum may be stored at 4°C for at least 2 weeks. Equilibrate these solutions to room temperature before use. Refilter the antibody if any cloudiness is apparent.

Calibrators. Prepare six calibrator levels (0.5 ml each) by dilution of the concentrated reference material with saline diluent. The neat calibrator represents the 100% curve point. Four serial dilutions create 50, 25, 12.5, and 6.25% curve points. Make a 75% curve level by mixing equal volumes of the 100 and 50% calibrators. Obtain the appropriate protein levels for the curve by multiplying the dilution percentages by the calibrator's value for assayed protein. Initial curve dilutions may be stored for 1 week at 4°C.

For most assays, dilute these stock curve levels and unknowns 1:25 (1 + 24) with saline. The assay for serum ALB, however, requires a 1:800 dilution of the stock curve and unknowns. Measuring CSF for IgG or ALB demands a 1:250 dilution of the stock curve, but no dilution of the unknowns. In this case, the values printed must be divided by 250 to correct for the dilution difference between curve and unknowns.

Prepare calibrators for the CRP assay with a concentrated CRP source at approximately 12 mg/dl. Use human serum deficient in CRP as a diluent. This calibration curve is then diluted 1:5 in PEG-PBS diluent and centrifuged at the same time as samples and controls.

Unknowns and controls. Fresh, fasting serum samples are preferred as unknowns and controls. For most of the assay proteins, these samples may be stored undiluted for 2 weeks at 4°C without significant degradation. Long-term storage should be at or below −20°C. Once thawed, a sample should be mixed well and assayed promptly. Handle controls in the same manner as unknowns.

Most assays listed here require a sample dilution of 1:25. This single sample dilution saves considerable time and reduces errors associated with sample manipulation. Serum samples assayed for ALB, however, are diluted 1:800 in saline. CSF is assayed without dilution. The assay for CRP in acute-phase sera requires that samples be diluted 1:5 in PEG-PBS, incubated for 30 min, and then centrifuged for 5 min at 15,000 × g to remove precipitates.

Instrument operation

The steps listed below describe programming of the Roche COBAS BIO and assume that the worker has a basic familiarity with the instrument. The analyzer parameters, however, may be applied to other instruments. Parameters common to all assays are listed in Table 1, and variable settings are given in Table 2.

TABLE 2. Instrument parameter settings for serum protein quantification on the Roche COBAS BIO

Parameter	Settings for blanking method[a]	
	Auto	Hold
1. Unit	8	8
2. Calculation factor	1,000	1,000
3. Standards 1 and 2		
4. Standards 3 and 4		
5. Standards 5 and 6		
6. Limit	0	0
7. Temp (°C)	25	25
8. Type of analysis	**7.5**	**7.6**
9. Wavelength (nm)	340	340
10. Sample vol (μl)	—[b]	—
11. Diluent vol (μl)	—	—
12. Reagent vol (μl)	**200**	**160**
13. Incubation time (s)	**0**	**180**
14. Start reagent vol (μl)	**0**	**40**
15. Time of first read (s)	1	1
16. Time interval (s)	300	300
17. No. of reads	2	2
18. Blanking mode	1	1
19. Printout mode	1	1

[a] Settings that differ between the blanking methods are printed in boldface.

[b] —, Sample and diluent volumes are listed in Table 1.

Instrument parameters for both autoblank and hold-blank procedures are listed in separate columns in each table.

1. Store parameters for each assay under a test number 20-40. Press ALPHA key and indicate a positive (+) reaction direction by entering 11. Label the assay with a three-letter code by using the appropriate numbers found in the systems function section of the operator's manual.

2. Enter the analysis type (7.5 or 7.6) under parameter 8, and return to the start of the parameter list.

3. Enter all parameters for a particular assay as they are given in Tables 1 and 2. Enter five or six calibrator concentrations in ascending order under parameter 3, i.e., standard 1. If five calibration points are used, enter a zero in position 6.

4. Place calibrator dilutions in the sample wheel in ascending order, starting with the lowest calibrator in position "CS."

5. Place antibody reagents in the reagent boat. For the autoblank method, place 20 ml of antibody solution in the primary reagent cavity. For the hold-blank method, place 20 ml of PEG-PBS diluent in the primary reagent cavity and 6 ml of antibody solution in the secondary reagent cavity.

6. Place a new cuvette rotor on the rotor housing, and secure the rotor with the plastic retaining ring. Close the cover and start the assay.

7. A list of curve parameters and sample values (in milligrams per deciliter) are printed after the run. To obtain a record of individual absorbances, change parameter 8 to analysis type 5, and change parameter 19 to printout mode 3. Depress the print button twice.

8. Calibration curve absorbances are automatically stored under the assigned test number. To use this curve for future runs, indicate printout mode 0 before initiating the assay.

Interpretation of results

Control and normal values will fall within the assay ranges listed in Table 2. The pattern of sample values, however, will most likely differ from published data because of a variety of population characteristics. The variability and interpretaion of serum protein values is reviewed extensively by Ritchie (15).

Each assay offers antibody excess conditions well above the assay range. Thus, samples with high protein levels create absorbances above the calibration curve and are flagged as "TOO HIGH." Further dilute these samples 1:4 and 1:8 with saline, and reassay. Values printed for samples with nonstandard dilutions must then be corrected to reflect the changed dilutions.

Antigen excess conditions may exist, however, when high levels of monoclonal proteins are present. This situation may result in readings that lie within the absorbance range of the calibration curve and cannot be distinguished from normal-level readings. Samples from patients with immunoproliferative disease should be assayed at additional dilutions of 1:100 and 1:200. A higher value for a more dilute sample indicates a high level of the analyte.

A relative antigen excess may occur with a polyclonal antibody to quantify an M component with restricted specificities. To get the most reliable estimate of a monoclonal protein, dilute the sample so that it is measured at the low end of the calibration curve. This dilution increases the relative concentration of antibodies specific for the common portion of the molecule.

For clear samples flagged as "TOO LOW," reassay them at a lower dilution, i.e., at 1:12.5. Lipemic samples, however, produce enough nonspecific precipitation to significantly bias results at this dilution.

LITERATURE CITED

1. **Anderson, R. J., and J. C. Sternberg.** 1978. A rate nephelometer for immunoprecipitin measurement of specific serum proteins, p. 409–468. *In* R. F. Ritchie (ed.), Automated immunoanalysis, part 2. Marcel Dekker, Inc., New York.

2. **Buffone, G. J.** 1980. Immunonephelometric and turbidimetric measurement of specific plasma proteins, p. 23–28. *In* N. R. Rose and H. Friedman (ed.), Manual of clinical immunology, 2nd ed. American Society for Microbiology, Washington, D.C.

3. **Deverill, I.** 1980. Kinetic measurements of the immunoprecipitin reaction using the centrifugal analyser, p. 109–124. *In* C. P. Price and K. Spencer (ed.), Centrifugal analysers in clinical chemistry. Praeger Publishers, London.

4. **Deverill, I., and W. G. Reeves.** 1980. Light scattering and absorption—developments in immunology. J. Immunol. Methods 38:191–204.

5. **Dito, W. R.** 1982. Quantification of serum proteins by centrifugal fast analyzer, p. 119–137. *In* S. E. Ritzmann (ed.), Physiology of immunoglobulins: diagnostic and clinical aspects. Alan R. Liss, Inc., New York.

6. **Eisenwiener, H. G., J. M. Kindbeiter, M. Keller, and K. Gutlin.** 1980. Photometry and the centrifugal analyser, p. 29–50. *In* C. P. Price and K. Spencer (ed.), Centrifugal analysers in clinical chemistry. Praeger Publishers, London.

7. **Hellsing, K.** 1978. Enhancing effects of nonionic polymers on immunochemical reactions, p. 67–112. *In* C. P. Price and K. Spencer (ed.), Centrifugal analysers in

clinical chemistry. Praeger Publishers, London.

8. **Hills, L. P., and T. O. Tiffany.** 1980. Comparison of turbidimetric and light-scattering measurements of immunoglobulins by use of a centrifugal analyzer with absorbance and fluorescence/light-scattering optics. Clin. Chem. **26:**1459–1466.

9. **Hudson, G. A., R. F. Ritchie, and J. E. Haddow.** 1981. Method for testing antiserum titer and avidity in nephelometric systems. Clin. Chem. **22:**1838–1844.

10. **Killingsworth, L. M.** 1978. Analytical variables for specific protein analysis, p. 113–137. *In* R. F. Ritchie (ed.), Automated immunoanalysis, part 1. Marcel Dekker, Inc., New York.

11. **Kusnetz, J., and H. P. Mansberg.** 1978. Optical consideration: nephelometry, p. 1–43. *In* R. F. Ritchie (ed.), Automated immunoanalysis, part 1. Marcel Dekker, Inc., New York.

12. **Price, C. P., K. Spencer, and J. Whicher.** 1983. Light scattering immunoassay of specific proteins: a review. Ann. Clin. Biochem. **20:**1–14.

13. **Reimer, C. B., J. Smith, T. W. Wells, R. M. Nakamura, P. W. Keitges, R. F. Ritchie, G. W. Williams, D. J. Hanson, and D. B. Dorsey.** 1982. Collaborative calibration of the U.S. National and the College of American Pathologists reference preparations for specific serum proteins. Am. J. Clin. Pathol. **77:**12–19.

14. **Ritchie, R. F.** 1975. Automated immunoprecipitin analysis of serum proteins, p. 376–425. *In* F. W. Putnam (ed.), The plasma proteins, vol. 2. Academic Press, Inc., New York.

15. **Ritchie, R. F.** 1979. Serum protein profile analysis and interpretation: some basic information, p. 227–242. *In* R. M. Nakamura, W. R. Dito, and E. S. Tucker III (ed.), Immunoassays in the clinical laboratory, vol. 3. Alan R. Liss, Inc., New York.

16. **Whicher, J. T., C. P. Price, and K. Spencer.** 1983. Immunonephelometric and immunoturbidimetric assays for proteins, p. 213–224. *In* J. W. Platz (ed.), CRC critical reviews in clinical laboratory sciences. CRC Press, Boca Raton, Fla.

Chapter 6

Rate Nephelometry

JAMES C. STERNBERG

Immunoprecipitation methods, based on quantitation of the precipitate formed when antigen-antibody reactions take place, provided one of the earliest tools for the study of immunochemical reactions.

The amount of precipitate developed at a fixed antibody concentration by variable amounts of antigen typically follows a parabolic curve, first described by Heidelberger and Kendall in 1935 (2). The ascending portion of the curve represents conditions with antibody in excess, and the amount of precipitate increases in proportion to the mass of antigen added. The level at which the addition of further antigen produces no increase in precipitation is the point of equivalence. A further increment in antigen mass will result in a decrease in the total precipitate developed. The descending limb of the curve defines the zone of antigen excess. There is, therefore, an ambiguity in the total mass of precipitate formed, since a single value of total mass developed can represent two distinct concentrations of antigen, i.e., one in the antibody excess zone and one in the antigen excess zone. This ambiguity presents the field of quantitative immunoassay with one of its most difficult problems.

The chemistry which leads to the configuration of the Heidelberger curve is generally well understood. Antibodies are typically divalent, whereas large molecular antigens such as proteins are multivalent. In the presence of a considerable excess of antibody, the predominant species present are excess free antibody and complexes of the form $Ag(Ab)_m$, where Ag is the antigen, Ab is the antibody, and m is the valence of the antigen. Larger complexes do not develop, since the antigenic sites are fully occupied by antibody molecules, and there is little probability of single antibody molecules bridging the gap between two antigens. Hence, little precipitate forms in extreme antibody excess.

When the concentration of antigen far exceeds the binding capacity of the amount of antibody present, soluble complexes of the form $(Ag)_2 Ab$, plus excess free antigen, predominate. The cross-linking of complexes required to produce precipitation is thus compromised and in extreme circumstances does not develop at all.

However, when the number of antibody combining sites closely approximates the number of antigen combining sites, extensive cross-linking occurs, permitting larger particles to develop. The condition called equivalence is the point at which maximal precipitate is formed.

The Heidelberger curve, from which it was possible to estimate antigen concentrations at a fixed antibody titer, was originally determined by weighing the precipitate or measuring its total protein content, usually after allowing the reaction mixture to stand overnight or longer at refrigerator temperature.

The process of radial immunodiffusion, in which the antigen diffuses outward into an antibody-containing gel, later provided a more convenient protein quantitation method. In this technique, a ring of precipitate, which provides visual evidence of equivalence, forms around the sample application point and moves radially outward until all antigen has been fixed into stable complexes. Protein concentration is evaluated simply by measuring the diameter of the arc; the entire determination requires 18 to 72 h to complete because of slow diffusion in the gel matrix.

Nephelometry, the measurement of scattered light, provides a convenient means of quantifying immunoprecipitation reactions. Light scattering occurs as a result of the elastic collisions of particles of all sizes with light quanta. The amount and nature of the scatter depend upon the size and shape of the particles, the wavelength of the light, and the refractive index of the medium.

Scatter for particles of different sizes is shown schematically in Fig. 1. Light traveling along the horizontal axis and striking a small particle leads to Rayleigh scatter, which is characterized by a symmetrical distribution of intensity such that the light scattered at any angle (theta) from the forward direction is equivalent to that scattered at an angle of 180° − theta. The forward and reverse scatters are equal. Scatter is minimal at 90° and is maximal at 0° (forward scatter) and 180° (back scatter).

With particles which have a dimension greater than 1/20 the wavelength of the light, the scatter develops asymmetry. The asymmetry (measured by the ratio of the light scattered at an angle, theta, to that scattered at 180° − theta) is unity for Rayleigh scatter, but becomes progressively greater than unity for angles (theta) < 90° as the particle size increases. This type of scatter is called Rayleigh-Debye scatter.

The sizes of several protein molecules relative to the wavelength of blue-to-green light (having a wavelength in air of 400 to 500 nm) are shown in Fig. 2. It can be seen that most protein molecules are much smaller than the wavelength of light and give only Rayleigh scatter. A molecular weight of about 3×10^6 is required to give a protein particle diameter of about 1/20 the wavelength of the light, and thus for the onset of Rayleigh-Debye scatter, but a molecular weight of 8×10^7 to 1×10^8 is required for significant Rayleigh-Debye scatter (as shown in recent work by George Wilson and co-workers at the University of Arizona; 7).

The direct antigen-antibody reaction initially forms small complexes which increase in size through cross-linking (Fig. 3, steps 1 and 2). These steps probably enable the molecular weight to reach only the onset of Rayleigh-Debye scatter (i.e., to reach about 3×10^6); at this size, however, most proteinaceous substances will begin to agglutinate by hydrophobic or charge-related interactions or both. Such interactions, which generally occur slowly in aqueous media, lead to

RAYLEIGH

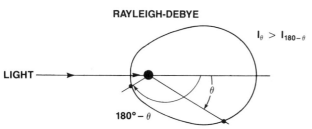

$$I_\theta = I_{180-\theta}$$

LIGHT

$180° - \theta$ θ

RAYLEIGH-DEBYE

$$I_\theta > I_{180-\theta}$$

LIGHT

$180° - \theta$ θ

FIG. 1. Angular distribution patterns for light scattered from small particles, showing Rayleigh scattering from particles having diameters less than 1/20 the wavelength of the light and Rayleigh-Debye scattering from somewhat larger particles.

1) $xAg + yAb \rightleftharpoons Ag_xAb_y$ (Rayleigh scatter)
   Immunochemical, primary

2) $n(Ag_xAb_y) \rightleftharpoons (Ag_xAb_y)_n$ (Rayleigh scatter if $nx < 10$)
   Immunochemical, secondary

3) $(Ag_xAb_y)_n + (Ag_xAb_y)_m \rightleftharpoons (Ag_xAb_y)_{n+m}$ (Rayleigh-Debye)
   Hydrophobic and charge-based, tertiary

FIG. 3. Primary, secondary, and tertiary steps in the buildup of immunochemical aggregates to produce light-scattering centers.

dimensions sufficient to produce significant scatter at visible wavelengths.

Many investigators recognized the applicability of light-scattering methods to the monitoring of immunochemical reactions to obtain quantitative information more rapidly than by earlier methods. Ritchie and co-workers (4) provided the basis for the Technicon Auto-Immuno-Precipitin System, a flow-through, fixed-time scatter instrument which served to considerably increase recognition of the usefulness of nephelometry. The work of Hellsing (3) on the enhancement of protein precipitation with polyethylene glycol suggested to others, including Buffone et al. (1) at the University of North Carolina, a group at Oak Ridge (10), and my laboratory (9), that it might be possible to make the immunoprecipitation measurements even more rapidly by using kinetic rather than endpoint methods.

The time course of the nephelometric signal in an immunoprecipitation reaction is shown in Fig. 4.

There is always some background of low-level Rayleigh scatter in the starting medium (Fig. 4A). This background scatter increases as the protein-containing sample is added. The subsequent addition of antiserum leads to a small increment in scatter, followed by scatter represented by a sigmoidal curve as the antigen-antibody reaction progresses and the hydrophobic and charge-based interactions between the resultant larger protein complexes provide observable scattering centers. Scatter is not a simple function of either size or concentration; both are changing during the course of the reaction, causing the curve showing scatter versus time to have a complex shape. In fact, no real endpoint is reached, since in the latter stages the larger particles agglomerate, reducing their number and decreasing the scatter signal. Very large particles tend to settle out from suspension, further decreasing the observed scatter.

The first derivative of the curve for scatter versus time (the rate curve) is the curve in Fig. 4B. Reaction conditions can be selected to cause the maximum of the rate curve (the steepest portion of the curve for

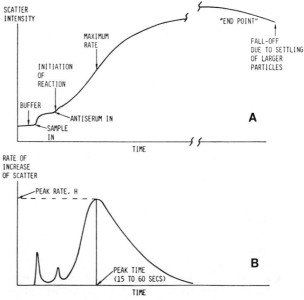

FIG. 4. Time course of the immunoprecipitation reaction. (A) Variation of intensity of scattered light versus time. (B) Rate of increase of scatter versus time.

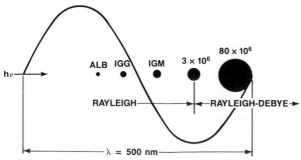

FIG. 2. Sizes of various serum proteins and aggregates of higher molecular weight in comparison to a wavelength of visible light.

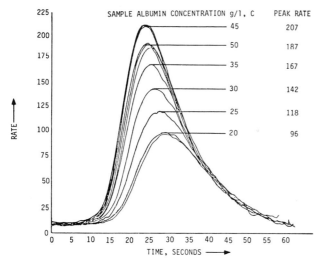

FIG. 5. Rate-versus-time curves for a series of antigen (albumin) concentrations at fixed antibody concentration. (The human serum samples were diluted 1:1,000 for measurement.)

scatter versus time) to occur a minute or less after injection of the triggering reagent. Such use of the rate of change of light scatter is called rate nephelometry.

In rate nephelometry, measurements are preferentially made in the antibody excess region, in which the maximum rate increases monotonically with the antigen concentration at a fixed antibody concentration. In antibody excess, the ratio of antibody to antigen concentration determines the stoichiometry of the complexes which initially form. These complexes then build up into immunochemical aggregates which reach the threshold of Rayleigh-Debye scattering size (about 3×10^6 daltons). Hydrophobic and charge-based interactions then take over to provide most of the observed scatter and rate signals.

In the antibody excess region, the peak rate increases and the time to peak rate decreases with increasing antigen concentration, up to the kinetic equivalence point. In Fig. 5, equivalence appears to lie between 35 and 50 g of albumin per liter. The peak rate then decreases with further increases in antigen concentration, just as the amount of precipitate obtained in the reaction represented by the Heidelberger curve decreases. A curve of maximum rate as a function of antigen concentration at fixed antibody concentration thus has the characteristics of a Heidelberger curve and can be regarded as a "kinetic Heidelberger curve."

The observed behavior is summarized in Fig. 6. The initial antigen concentration (x), antibody concentration (y), and antigen valency (m) are shown as indices with respect to the different regions of the kinetic Heidelberger curve. The steps cited are (1) the primary immunochemical formation of complexes, (2) the secondary immunochemical interlinking of complexes, and (3) the rapid buildup of scattering centers due to subsequent hydrophobic and charge-based interactions among the complexes. In the extreme cases of antibody and antigen excess, steps 2 and 3 cannot occur.

Kinetic Heidelberger curves are obtained by varying the amount of antigen at a fixed antibody concen-

tration. As the antibody concentration is increased, the kinetic equivalence point (the peak of the curve for maximum rate versus antigen concentration) moves to a higher antigen concentration, and the maximum amplitude of the curve increases, while the time to peak rate decreases. It thus becomes possible to design the reaction conditions to obtain satisfactory signal levels within suitable time intervals and therefore to provide a practical rate nephelometric system for immunochemical measurements.

The Beckman Immunochemistry System is an example of such a system. It provides continuous monitoring of both scatter and rate of change of scatter at a 70° forward angle in a stirred cylindrical reaction cell containing a lightly buffered phosphate-buffered saline–polyethylene glycol solution. The sample is introduced first, and the immunochemical reaction is then triggered by the introduction of the antiserum. The maximum rate of change of scatter due to the reaction is used by the instrument, in conjunction with a predetermined calibration curve, to measure the sample component of interest.

The stability of the shape of the calibration curve for a given lot of antiserum is excellent, making it possible to map out the curve shape for each lot, convert the curve into mathematical form, store the curve parameters on a machine-readable card, and reduce calibration for this complex curve shape to a single-point process. This approach has been shown to provide the basis for highly reliable serum protein determinations.

The double-valued nature of the kinetic Heidelberger curve requires a mechanism for ensuring that the measurements are made under antibody excess conditions or for alerting the user to possible antigen excess situations. A simple procedure has been devised whereby individual samples are checked for antigen excess by the addition of calibrator immediately after the normal measurement is made. A positive rate response obtained upon addition of the calibrator indicates that free antibody remains and that the previously measured value was created under antibody excess conditions. However, if antigen excess exists, the addition of calibrator produces no response, and the user is directed to repeat the measurement with a higher sample dilution.

The shape of the calibration curve and antigen excess check criteria are encoded as data on a ma-

Condition	In $Ag_x^{(m)} Ab_y^{(2)}$	Result
Extreme antibody excess	$\frac{y}{x} \geq m$	No steps (2), (3)
Antibody excess	$m > \frac{y}{x} > \frac{m}{2}$	Scatter ↑ as $\frac{y}{x}$ ↓
Equivalence	$\frac{y}{x} = \frac{m}{2}$	Maximum scatter
Antigen excess	$\frac{m}{2} > \frac{y}{x} > \frac{1}{2}$	Scatter ↓ as $\frac{y}{x}$ ↓
Extreme antigen excess	$\frac{y}{x} < \frac{1}{2}$	No steps (2), (3)

FIG. 6. Regions of the Heidelberger curve expressed in terms of the relative concentrations (x and y) of antigen (Ag) and antibody (Ab), respectively, present. The antibody has a valence of 2, and the antigen has a valence of m. Step numbers refer to the equations in Fig. 3.

chine-readable card supplied with each bottle of antiserum, thus eliminating the need for the operator to manually enter test parameters.

The rate nephelometric system has proven itself to be precise and accurate, as documented in the College of American Pathologists Laboratory Surveys (6). Those protein determinations most frequently requested of the clinical laboratory are conveniently measured by rate nephelometry. These tests include specific serum protein tests for immunoglobulin G (IgG), IgA, IgM, complements C3 and C4, properdin factor B, alpha-1-acid glycoprotein, albumin, alpha-1-antitrypsin, alpha-2-macroglobuin, haptoglobin, transferrin, and ceruloplasmin.

Two additional proteins of considerable clinical interest are C-reactive protein and rheumatoid factor. C-reactive protein, a useful index of inflammation, was little utilized in the United States before being made available by nephelometric methods. The analysis of rheumatoid factor represents an inverted system whereby antigen becomes the reagent for the measurement of human serum antibodies (in this case, IgM anti-IgG). The principles are identical to those of the antigen quantitation analyses described above and yield objective data considerably more precise than a highly subjective visual estimation of agglutination in a test tube or on a slide (6).

Small molecules, with a molecular weight of less than about 5,000, tend to be nonantigenic and are called haptens. These molecules can be conjugated to protein molecules to produce hapten-specific antibodies in animals. Since the haptens are generally only univalent, no cross-linking to produce precipitate occurs when the hapten is allowed to react with its antiserum.

The nephelometric measurement of haptens, therefore, requires a variant called nephelometric inhibition methods (5). A polyvalent hapten (or "developer antigen"), synthetically generated by conjugating several hapten molecules to a single protein molecule, will cross-link with antibody and can produce a precipitate. The presence of free, monovalent hapten, however, ties up antibody combining sites, decreasing the ability of the antibody to cross-link with any polyvalent hapten molecules present. The free hapten thus inhibits the nephelometric signal.

The rate nephelometric inhibition method has been applied to the measurement of several therapeutic drugs, and further methods are undergoing development at the present time. Rate nephelometric inhibition furnishes a rapid and convenient approach to the immunoassay of haptens with stable reagents.

Rate nephelometry has proven to be the method of choice for the measurement serum proteins, and commercially available tests include tests for IgG, IgA, IgM, C3, C4, C-reactive protein, haptoglobin, transferrin, albumin, alpha-1-antitrypsin, alpha-2-macroglobulin, alpha-1-acid glycoprotein, properdin factor B, ceruloplasmin, and rheumatoid factor. The performance of rate nephelometry in the measurement of therapeutic drugs has been generally good, but its precision for drugs has been significantly poorer than for proteins. Recent studies have identified the sources of the variation, and it now appears possible to make the performance of the method as precise for drugs as for proteins. Therapeutic drugs tested for by

rate nephelometry are phenytoin, phenobarbital, theophylline, gentamicin, tobramycin, primidone, lidocaine, quinidine, procainamide, NAPA, and carbamazepine.

In summary, although precipitation methods are not among the most sensitive, they are clearly among the most effective and convenient of the nonisotopic immunoassay techniques presently available. Rate nephelometry provides a rapid and reliable method, yet new studies suggest that its potential is even greater than has been appreciated.

Rate nephelometry also can be an extremely convenient research tool. We have found it valuable in general immunochemical studies and in the monitoring of labeling and purification processes involving proteins and other biological macromolecules. For this purpose, the instrument is provided with "manual mode" cards which may be selected to set up the appropriate instrument parameters for the sensitivity range required for the measurement. The instrument then reads out directly in rate or scatter units or both, which can be directed to a strip chart recorder providing a continuous record of the immunological reaction, facilitating selection by the user of the optimal conditions.

In labeling an antibody with an enzyme or fluorescent label, Sittampalam et al. (8) have shown that the residual titer of the labeled antibody after coupling is most conveniently measured by rate nephelometry; the residual enzyme activity after coupling can, of course, be monitored by its reaction with its substrate.

In column purifications with ion-exchange, exclusion, or affinity chromatography for protein separation, the elution of a protein of interest can be monitored virutally in real time by the use of rate nephelometry. If the eluted protein is an antibody, its direct reaction with its antigen can be observed; the elution of other proteins requires the use of their corresponding antisera for monitoring. Measurements are conveniently made down to eluted concentrations of 3 μg of the protein of interest per ml, and each measurement can be made within approximately 1 min of the elution of the protein fraction from the column. The isolation of desired fractions of haptens and labeled haptens can be monitored by nephelometric inhibition methods, with an antiserum to the hapten of interest in conjunction with a synthetic polyvalent hapten prepared by coupling multiple molecules of the hapten to a protein carrier molecule. The isolation of desired fractions of a hapten multiply conjugated to a protein can be monitored directly by using the antihapten antiserum as a reagent.

The sensitivity of rate nephelometry is also well suited to the rapid evaluation of monoclonal antibody titers in cell culture broths or in ascites fluid samples, provided that an antigen having multiple identical epitopes is available (if only a single epitope of a particular type is present on a macromolecular antigen, it is not possible for antibodies of a single clone directed against that epitope to lead to the buildup of cross-linked aggregates). For a hapten, it is necessary to use a conjugate bearing several (typically 5 to 20) molecules of the hapten bound to a protein carrier as the test antigen. Antibodies to bacterial, viral, or cell surface antigens can be monitored directly, provided that fairly clear suspensions of these species can be provided for testing.

The method is also applicable to the monitoring of other macromolecules, such as carbohydrates (with antisera or lectins as reagents) and nucleic acids. If the nucleic acids have been labeled, they can be monitored with antisera to the labels; single-stranded nucleic acids can be monitored with complementary DNA sequences which will hybridize to them.

LITERATURE CITED

1. **Buffone, G. J., J. Savory, and R. E. Cross.** 1974. Use of a laser-equipped centrifugal analyzer for kinetic measurement of serum IgG. Clin. Chem. **21:**1735–1746.
2. **Heidelberger, M., and F. E. Kendall.** 1935. A quantitative study and a theory of the reaction mechanism. J. Exp. Med. **61:**563–591.
3. **Hellsing, K.** 1972. Influence of polymer on the antigen-antibody reaction in a continuous flow system, p. 17. *In* J. D. Hamm (ed.), Automated immunoprecipitin reactions. Technicon Instruments Corp., Tarrytown, N.Y.
4. **Larson, C., P. Orenstein, and R. F. Ritchie.** 1971. An automated method for quantitation of proteins in body fluids, p. 101–104. *In* Advances in automated analysis. Technicon International Congress 1970, vol. 1, Clinical analysis. Futura Publishing Co., Mt. Kisco, N.Y.
5. **Riccomi, H., P. L. Masson, J. P. Vaerman, and J. F. Heremans.** 1972. An automated nephelometric inhibition immunoassay (NINIA) for haptens, p. 9–11. *In* J. D. Hamm (ed.), Automated immunoprecipitin reactions. Technicon Instruments Corp., Tarrytown, New York.
6. **Ritchie, R. F., and J. H. Rippey.** 1982. Performance on immunoglobulin G, IgA, and IgM tests in C.A.P. survey specimens. Am. J. Clin. Pathol. **78**(Suppl.)**:**644–650.
7. **Sittampalam, G., and G. S. Wilson.** 1984. Theory of light scattering measurements as applied to immunoprecipitin reactions. Anal. Chem. **56:**2176–2180.
8. **Sittampalam, G., G. S. Wilson, and J. M. Byers.** 1982. Characterization of antigen-enzyme conjugates: theoretical considerations for rate nephelometric assays of immunological reactions. Anal. Biochem. **122:**372–378.
9. **Sternberg, J. C.** 1977. A rate nephelometer for measuring specific proteins by immunoprecipitin reactions. Clin. Chem. **23:**1456–1464.
10. **Tiffany, T. O., J. M. Parella, W. F. Johnson, and C. A. Burtis.** 1974. Specific protein analysis by light-scatter measurement with a miniature centrifugal fast analyzer. Clin. Chem. **20:**1055–1061.

Chapter 7

Particle-Enhanced Immunoassays

J. PHILLIP GALVIN

The simplest type of immunoassay involves measurement of the agglutination of an antigen and its corresponding antibody as a function of the concentration of one of these components. As the immune complex of the antigens and antibodies grows in size, its light-scattering properties change, and the change can be monitored either visually or on a simple spectrophotometer or nephelometer. The sensitivity of these light-scattering immunoassays can be increased by attaching one of the reagents, for example, the antibody, to an inert support particle and then following the agglutination of the particle by the protein to be measured. Many types of support particles, including erythrocytes, clay, and polymer latex, have been used. This chapter will be devoted to the use of polystyrene latex particles and will describe their use both in kits to be used manually to give qualitative or semiquantitative results and also in automated instruments in which the particles can be the basis of methods comparable in sensitivity to enzyme immunoassays and radioimmunoassays (RIA).

PARTICLE REAGENT PREPARATION

The polystyrene latex particles are made by emulsion polymerization (1). The polymerization of the styrene monomer is carried out in an aqueous emulsion of the styrene monomer using surfactants such as sodium dodecyl sulfate or Aerosol OT. Potassium persulfate is the usual free radical initiator for the polymerization. The polymer is formed in the droplets of monomer-surfactant in the water. Particle size is most easily controlled by changing the concentration of the surfactant. For the manual kits based on visual observation of agglutination (see below), relatively large particles of 0.81-μm diameter have been used, but for the instrument-based methods of following the agglutination, much smaller particles are required for highest sensitivity (see Fig. 3), and particles of 0.1- to 0.2-μm diameter are preferred. If the particles are to be used with covalently attached protein, the surface of the particles must be modified to provide chemical groups capable of reacting with the protein. This modification is often done by preparing a seed emulsion of pure polystyrene particles and then continuing the polymerization with a mixture of monomers, styrene, and a modified styrene with the appropriate chemical substitution. This produces a "core-shell" structure with an inert polystyrene core and a chemically reactive copolymer shell containing groups such as epoxide, amino hydroxyl, and carboxyl. Proteins can be covalently linked to the particles by these various groups under simple reaction conditions. For example, amino groups of proteins can be linked to epoxides on the particles by being warmed to 50°C for 1 h at a pH of 8.

For many of the latex tests described in the literature, the particle reagents are prepared by simple adsorption of the protein onto the particle surface, followed by extensive washing or dialysis to remove unbound protein. However, most of the commercially available latex agglutination tests employ reagents in which the protein or antibody has been covalently attached to the particle by the technique described above. When making antibody particles, it is essential to retain immunoreactivity of the antibodies. Masson et al. have done considerable work on developing stable, reactive, covalently attached antibody particle reagents (6). They also have stressed the importance of using antibody fragments [Fab, Fab', F(ab')₂] as opposed to whole antibodies to overcome problems caused by nonspecific aggregation, and they have described procedures for making particles with the antibody fragments. Coating of particles with a protein such as human serum albumin (HSA) to cover the sites not occupied by the antibody or antigen also increases particle reagent specificity and stability (2). Particle reagents are usually stored in glycine-buffered saline.

PARTICLE-ENHANCED IMMUNOASSAY DESIGNS

All the various designs of particle-enhanced light-scattering immunoassays can be divided into two groups, i.e., direct agglutination and inhibition of agglutination (Fig. 1 and 2), regardless of the measurement technique. The direct particle agglutination assay can use either antigen- or antibody-coated particles. If a protein is to be measured, a particle reagent coated with the corresponding antibody is used. Conversely, if the test requires measurement of a specific antibody, particles coated with the corresponding antigen are used. In these direct assays the degree of agglutination increases with the concentration of the reagent being measured, and this increase is reflected by increased clumping with a manual kit or increased light-scattering signal with an instrumental model.

For increased sensitivity, and especially when the analyte is a hapten, agglutination inhibition immunoassays must be used (Fig. 2). It is usually preferable to make a protein-hapten conjugate and attach that to the particle rather than attach the hapten directly. The particle agglutination reaction can be inhibited by allowing the free hapten in the sample to compete with the hapten particle reagent for a limited number of antibodies. The reduction in the extent of agglutination of the particles is a measure of the concentration of the analyte in the sample. Alternatively, the antibody particles can be used and the concentration of the hapten in the sample can be measured by how much the hapten blocks binding sites on the particle and inhibits the particle agglutination by a hapten-protein conjugate. Finally, both the hapten conjugate or antigen and the antibody can be attached to particles, and again, the degree of inhibition of their

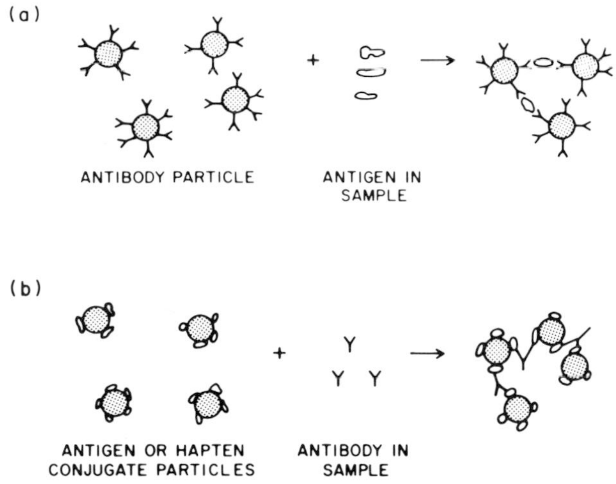

FIG. 1. Assay designs for particle agglutination immunoassays. (a) Antibody particles aggregated by the multivalent antigen in the sample. (b) Antigen particles are agglutinated by the corresponding antibodies in the sample. (From reference 3. Reproduced with permission of the College of American Pathologists, Skokie, Ill.)

agglutination will be a measure of the concentration of free hapten or antigen in the sample. All these assay designs are competitive-mode assays, and sensitivity is largely governed by the concentration and avidity of the antibody. In general, sensitivity is increased by decreasing antibody concentrations as long as an acceptable signal is maintained.

MANUAL KITS BASED ON LATEX AGGLUTINATION

Singer and Plotz (8) were the first to describe the use of latex particles for a diagnostic test, and they used the particles to follow changes in the titer of rheumatoid factor in patients' samples. This method is still in use today, and this technology is now the basis of many commercially available kits for a wide range of analytes. Many of the early reports of latex assay kits were based on reagents developed by the workers themselves. Now, however, kits are available commercially for the rapid identification of many microbial antigens without a culture step, for the detection of circulating antibodies, and for the measurement of drugs and even hormones, since particle immunoassay kits are the basis for pregnancy detection tests to be used in the home. Most of the kits are qualitative or semiquantitative, but some of the latest kits for therapeutic drug-monitoring give values of the drug concentration in narrow ranges of micrograms per milliliter by using serial dilution (4).

Many latex kits for the detection of bacterial antigens have been described for organisms such as *Haemophilus influenzae*, *Rickettsia* spp., group B streptococci, *Staphylococcus aureus*, *Neisseria meningitidis*, etc. In all of these methods, the latex particles are coated with the corresponding antibody and reacted with a sample (serum, urine, or cerebrospinal fluid) suspected of containing the bacteria. The test is performed on a slide, a series of test tubes, or a card provided by the kit manufacturer. The cards are often

preferred because of speed and ease of use and because it is easy to compare the results for the samples with those for the controls run directly on the same card. In running the test, a small volume (often 20 to 50 µl) of the samples and controls are placed in separate circles on the card, and a fixed amount of the well-shaken particle reagent suspension is added to each circle. The card is rotated on an electrical rotator at 100 rpm for 8 min and then read under a high-intensity lamp to determine the extent or absence of agglutination for each sample or control. The concentration or titer of the analyte in the sample can be estimated by comparison of its extent of agglutination with that of the controls. Often the test will involve a series of dilutions on the sample. Interference and nonspecific agglutination in particle-based assays for bacterial antigens have been ascribed to the presence of immunoglobulin M (IgM) antibodies in the sample (7). A pretreatment with protein A will remove these interfering antibodies, but not the bacterial antigens. Latex agglutination can identify organisms within a few minutes, and its sensitivity and specificity are comparable to those of staphylococcal coagglutination and better than those of counterimmunoelectrophoresis (9).

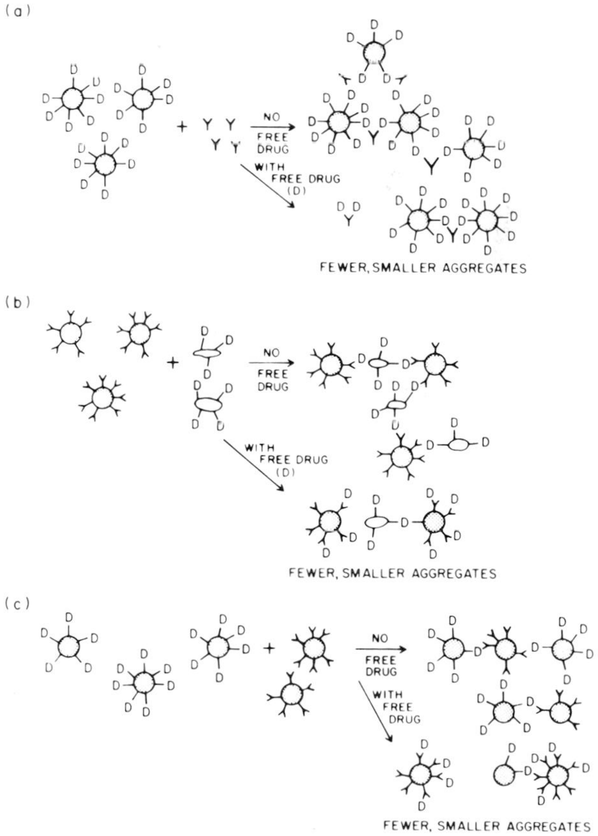

FIG. 2. Assay designs for particle-enhanced inhibition immunoassays. The examples are all drawn for a drug-monitoring immunoassay, but the same principles apply for other classes of analytes. (a) Inhibition of the agglutination of hapten particles. (b) Inhibition of the agglutination of antibody particles. (c) Dual-particle (antigen and antibody) inhibition immunoassay. (From reference 3. Reproduced with permission of the College of American Pathologists, Skokie, Ill.)

In serological tests in which antibody to a bacterial or viral protein is to be detected, the latex particles are coated with either cell surface or other antigen proteins from the bacteria or virus. Presence of the antibody is confirmed if the sample agglutinates the particles. Many of these tests are designed to detect IgM antibodies, and there is always the risk of nonspecific agglutination of the particles by other IgM antibodies in the sample. The titer of the antibody concentration in the patient can be estimated by serial dilution to find the level at which the particles are just agglutinated. This gives only a semiquantitative value for the level of, for instance, IgM in a patient with rheumatoid arthritis, but this value is useful for following changes over time or as a result of treatment.

In the Macro-Vue kits, manufactured by Hynson, Wescott & Dunning, the concentration of a therapeutic drug is measured by the inhibition method (Fig. 2). This system provides drug-coated latex particles and antisera and uses cards for running the assay. The patient sample is diluted to various concentrations according to the instructions of the manufacturer and each dilution and various controls are placed in separate wells. A standard amount of antibody is added to each well, and then the analyte-coated particles are added. After incubation on a rotator, inhibition of the agglutination at various dilutions of the patients' serum is compared with that of drug standards. In this way, the drug concentration can be estimated to within a few micrograms per milliliter and the kits are useful for monitoring the drug level in patients when instrumental methods are not available. Good correlation with RIA is claimed (4).

The inhibition reaction mode is also used in the many particle-based kits for the detection of pregnancy. β-Human chorionic gonadotropin (β-HCG) is covalently attached to the particle reagents. β-HCG appears in the urine of a pregnant woman very soon after she conceives. In the tests designed for home use, a urine sample is mixed with the particle reagent and antiserum. If β-HCG is present in the urine, it will react with the antibodies, and particle agglutination will not occur, whereas if β-HCG is absent, the particles will be flocculated. These tests can be very sensitive and, with a 90-min incubation, levels as low as 250 mIU of β-HCG per ml can be detected by these visual methods.

When these manual latex kits are used, it must be realized that their performance varies widely from manufacturer to manufacturer and also to some extent among different batches from the same manufacturer. Virtually all kits include positive and negative controls of the antigen or antibody to be measured, and the results are read for the performance of the test with the sample from the patient relative to that with the controls. Controls and particle reagents should not be used interchangeably from different kits.

INSTRUMENT-BASED PARTICLE-ENHANCED IMMUNOASSAYS

Although latex particle immunoassay kits are useful for the qualitative detection of various analytes without the need for expensive equipment, instrumental methods greatly increase the sensitivity achievable by this technology, as well as provide accurate quantita-

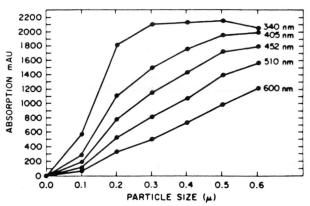

FIG. 3. Effect of particle size and wavelength on light scattering. The data were collected with different-sized polystyrene particles at various wavelengths. The greatest signal change is obtained with small particles measured at 340 nm. (From R. M. Nakamura, W. R. Dito, and E. S. Tucker, ed., *Clinical Laboratory Assays*, 1983. Reproduced with permission of the Masson Publishing Co., New York.)

tive data on the concentration of the analyte of interest. Usually the test can be performed in a much shorter time when an instrument is used. At least three measurement techniques have now been described in which particle-based immunoassays are capable of measuring analyte at levels as low as 1 ng/ml (7). These techniques are the particle-enhanced turbidimetric (PETINIA) (3), particle-counting (6), and Quasi-Elastic light-scattering immunoassay technologies (10).

The most important properties affecting the performance of a particle in an immunoassay are its size and refractive index. The optimum size will depend on the measurement technique. Thus, small particles will be preferred for a rate assay, whereas large particles will give a larger signal change in the endpoint mode. The relationship between particle size and the corresponding turbidimetric signal are shown as a function of both particle diameter and wavelength in Fig. 3. It can be seen that for highest sensitivity the measurement should be made at as low a wavelength as possible and that the latex particles should have as small a diameter as possible. Particle size also affects diffusion kinetics and, therefore, the rate of reaction. Light scattering also increases with the refractive index of the particle material.

Many direct agglutination immunoassays for a wide range of proteins and other analytes have been developed for use on spectrophotometers and other instruments (3). Gorman has coated particles with antibody to C-reactive protein and used them in a rate mode to measure the concentration of this acute-phase protein. Excellent correlation with the Beckman ICS rate nephelometric method was demonstrated, and the lowest level detected was about 10^{-9} M in the sample (Fig. 4). Leflar and Looney (5) have used the alternative procedure of antigen-coated particles to measure the concentration of the corresponding antibody. They used the streptolysin O-coated 0.14-μm polystyrene latex from Behring's Rapi-Tex ASO kit and used them in a method for measuring the antibody concentration on the Du Pont aca discrete clinical analyzer.

STANDARD CURVE

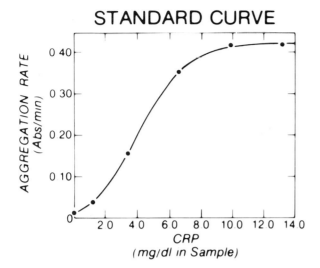

CORRELATION WITH RATE NEPHELOMETRY

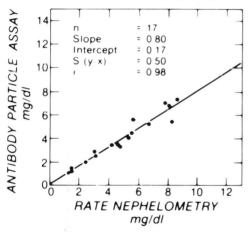

n	= 17
Slope	= 0 80
Intercept	= 0 17
S (y x)	= 0 50
r	= 0 98

FIG. 4. Particle-enhanced direct agglutination assay for C reactive protein (CRP). Standard curve and correlation with a nephelometric (nonparticle) method.

With an endpoint measurement, the detection limit was 100 IU/ml with 10% coefficient of variation at the 200 IU/ml medical decision level (Fig. 5). This assay principle can be used for many serological tests.

PETINIA technology has been used to monitor the concentration in serum of many drugs and proteins, including theophylline, gentamicin, tobramycin, and digoxin (3). In the theophylline method, the drug is covalently attached to the polystyrene particle with a short, polyamine linking molecule, and a monoclonal antitheophylline antibody is used to avoid the problem of cross-reactivity with caffeine that plagues most theophylline assays. As the concentration of theophylline in the patient sample increases, the rate of agglutination of the particle reagent is reduced. Both within-run and day-to-day precision are excellent, as is correlation with both high-pressure liquid chromatography and the Syva EMIT methods (Fig. 6).

The most sensitive particle-enhanced inhibition assay design involves using both antigen and antibody particles (Fig. 2). This approach has been used to develop a particle-based immunoassay for digoxin. This drug must be maintained at levels of 0.9 to 2.0 ng/ml of patient serum, and its use requires constant monitoring and the capability of reliably measuring drug levels below 1 ng/ml in the sample (3). The antibody particles are made from particles with a high refractive index and have a digoxin-HSA conjugate covalently attached. The antibody particles are first allowed to react with the sample. Ideally, there are only a few active antibody sites per particle, and if the sites react with digoxin from the sample, the antibody particle will not be able to agglutinate with the digoxin-HSA particles when they are added. With a sample fraction of 0.1, separation of 25 mA/min per ng/ml of digoxin was obtained, with a fair correlation with RIA.

DISCUSSION

There are many factors affecting the performance of particle-enhanced immunoassays used either as manual kits or as reagents on an automated instrument. With a properly maintained instrument, the test is likely to be run with a high level of reproducibility, but with manual kits it is essential that all important factors be controlled and performed identically every time for the results to be meaningful. These conditions include reagent concentration, incubation period and temperature, method of reading the tubes or cards, etc.

In the design or use of particle-based immunoassays all possible interactions both among the particles themselves and between the particles and other components must be considered. The assay milieu should maintain a stable dispersion of the particle reagents during storage but should then allow for rapid but specific agglutination to occur when the assay is initiated. Many workers report that glycine-based buffers provide the best storage medium. A "ballast" protein such as HSA or bovine serum albumin, added during particle reagent synthesis to block unoccupied sites on the particle, also improves reagent stability (2). A surfactant such as sodium dodecyl sulfate also is helpful in maintaining stable particle dispersions and in preventing nonspecific agglutination.

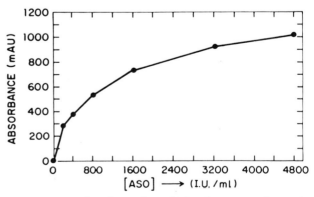

FIG. 5. Particle-enhanced agglutination assay for antistreptolysin O. Particles 0.14 μm in diameter are coated with streptolysin O. Measurement is at 340 nm (5). (From R. M. Nakamura, W. R. Dito, and E. S. Tucker, ed., *Clinical Laboratory Assays*, 1983. Reproduced with permission of the Masson Publishing Co., New York.)

STANDARD CURVE

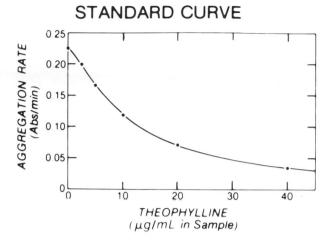

CORRELATION WITH EMIT·

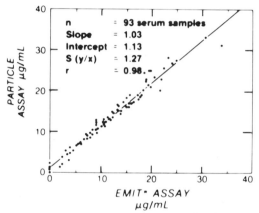

FIG. 6. PETINIA for theophylline. Results show the standard curve and the correlation of the PETINIA method with Syva's EMIT method.

The importance of polyethylene glycol in increasing the rate of reaction and sensitivity for non-particle agglutination immunoassays has been stressed by many workers. For particle-enhanced assays, the results are more complex. Polyethylene glycol certainly increases the sensitivity in some assays, but it can lead to self-aggregation, especially of antibody-coated particle reagents (6).

Two major sources of interference in latex-based immunoassays are the C1q component of the complement system and rheumatoid factor. The effect of C1q can be eliminated by heating the sample for 30 min at 56°C. Rheumatoid factor is an IgM antibody directed against the Fc portion of an IgG molecule. Thus, in any test using antibody-coated latex particles, there is always the risk of nonspecific agglutination by rheumatoid factor in the sample. The rheumatoid factor can be eliminated by digestion of the sample with dithiothreitol or mercaptoethanol. Another effective way of avoiding this source of interference is to use either F(ab')$_2$ or Fab' fragments instead of whole

antibody molecules when making the antibody particle reagent (6).

There are three major forces affecting the agglutination behavior of latex particles in an electrolyte (10). These forces are the van der Waals attraction, the Coulombic repulsion, and the antigen-antibody agglutination. The short-range van der Waals forces are independent of the pH and ionic strength. For stability, all particles in a suspension should carry the same electrical charge. Latex particles normally have a slight negative charge, and so the ionic environment must be adjusted to maintain this charge. However, the Coulombic repulsion must not be so strong as to prevent the antigen-antibody binding reaction. In most particle-based assays, the pH is usually between 6 and 9 and the ionic strength is adjusted so that nonspecific agglutination of the particles is just avoided. The suspensions of the latex particle reagents are increasingly unstable as the pH is lowered to less than 6.0. If the pH is below 4 or above 11, no specific immunoreactivity of the particles can be detected (2).

In summary, the particle-enhanced immunoassay is a very flexible and powerful technology which can be adapted to measure many different kinds of analytes with little or no expensive equipment. When the proper precautions are taken to avoid the various causes of nonspecific particle agglutination, it is capable of high sensitivity and specificity and in its ultimate form is comparable to enzyme immunoassay, fluorescence immunoassay, and RIA.

LITERATURE CITED

1. **Craig, A. R., W. A. Frey, C. C. Leflar, C. E. Looney, and M. A. Luddy.** 1984. Novel shell-core particles for automated turbidimetric immunoassays. Clin. Chem. **30:** 1489–1493.
2. **Dezelic, G., N. Dezelic, N. Muic, and B. Pende.** 1971. Latex agglutination in the human serum albumin-rabbit antiserum system. Eur. J. Biochem. **20:**553–557.
3. **Galvin, J. P.** 1984. Particle-enhanced immunoassays—a review, p. 17–30. *In* J. H. Rippey and R. M. Nakamura (ed.), Diagnostic immunology: technology assessment and quality assurance. College of American Pathologists, Skokie, Ill.
4. **Johnson, J. E., S. Crawford, and J. H. Jorgensen.** 1982. Evaluation of the Macro-Vue latex agglutination test for quantitation of gentamicin in human serum. J. Clin. Microbiol. **16:**299–302.
5. **Leflar, C. C., and C. E. Looney.** 1980. Scattering studies in immunoprecipitation methods. Clin. Chem. **26:**1074.
6. **Masson, P. L., C. L. Cambiasio, D. Collet-Cassart, C. C. M. Magnusson, C. B. Richards, and C. J. M. Sindic.** 1981. Particle counting immunoassay (PACIA). Methods Enzymol. **74:**106–139.
7. **Oxenhandler, R. W., E. H. Adelstein, and W. A. Rogers.** 1977. Rheumatoid factor: a cause of false positive histoplasmin latex agglutination. J. Clin. Microbiol. **5:**31–33.
8. **Singer, J. M., and R. M. Plotz.** 1956. The latex fixation test—applications to rheumatoid arthritis. Am. J. Med. **21:**888–892.
9. **Thirumoorthi, M. C., and A. S. Dajani.** 1979. Comparison of staphylococcal coagglutination, latex agglutination, and counterimmunoelectrophoresis for bacterial antigen detection. J. Clin. Microbiol. **9:**28–32.
10. **Von Schulthess, G. K., R. J. Cohen, N. Sakato, and G. B. Benedek.** 1976. Laser light-scattering spectroscopic immunoassay for mouse IgA. Immunochemistry **13:**955–962.

Chapter 8

Immunoassay by Particle Counting

P. L. MASSON AND H. W. HOLY

A newly introduced immunoassay to be used in a routine clinical laboratory should be nonisotopic. Of the many immunoassays currently available, the particle-counting immunoassay has the advantage of being completely automated for the quantification of both monovalent (hapten) and multivalent antigens over the range covered by radioimmunoassay (RIA). The particle-counting immunoassay is also suitable for the titration of antibodies and immune complexes. The analysis time of the instrument presently available (IMPACT, manufactured and sold by ACADE S.A., B-1200 Brussels, Belgium) (Fig. 1) is 50 min, with an assay rate of 60 samples per h. Table 1 lists the analytes which have been addressed. Although some 70 publications have described or made use of the particle-counting immunoassay, no publication details a manual method, largely because timing is so critical in all protocols. An extensive review of the method has been published (9).

PRINCIPLES OF THE ASSAY

Antigens are quantified by mixing a sample of serum, plasma, cerebrospinal fluid, or urine with antibody-coated latex particles of 0.8-μm diameter suspended in a suitable buffer. Sample antigen agglutinates some of the particles, so the number which remains dispersed decreases (Fig. 2). The antigen concentration is inversely proportional to the unagglutinated particle count (1, 3–5, 9).

Antibodies are analyzed similarly by using their agglutinating activity on the latex particles coated with antigen. The agglutinating activity of immunoglobulin G (IgG) antibodies can be reinforced by IgM rheumatoid factor (RF). The use of RF rather than an anti-immunoglobulin antiserum (Coombs reagent) has the advantage of not requiring a washing step to remove unbound immunoglobulins. Insolubilization of certain antigens, e.g., phospholipase A2, the allergen of honey-bee venom (7), and antigens from herpes simplex virus (10), can result in nonspecific binding of immunoglobulins without antibody activity. Such a cause of error can be avoided by the use of antibody-coated latex, which is agglutinated by the antigen. The antibody of interest is titrated by its inhibitory activity on the agglutination.

Immune complexes are measured by the agglutinating activity of RF (9) or mouse C1q (9) on latex particles coated with IgG. Immune complexes, which bind the agglutinator, decrease the agglutination of latex. Thus the concentration of immune complexes is proportional to the concentration of unagglutinated particles.

Latex coated with hapten molecules (Fig. 3) reacts with IgG antibodies against the hapten, whereupon the complex is agglutinated by introduced RF. When free hapten is present in the sample, the hapten also reacts with IgG antibodies and therefore inhibits agglutination, increasing the number of unagglutinated particles. The hapten concentration is proportional to the unagglutinated-particle count (2). When a monoclonal antibody is used, as in the commercial version of the triiodothyronine assay, RF can be replaced by an antiserum directed against the monoclonal antibody class.

A great deal of similarity exists in all methods, three of which are detailed in Fig. 4. The following interferences which frequently occur in latex agglutination have been overcome (9).

1. Agglutination by endogenous RF or the C1q component of complement. Only the F(ab')$_2$ of the IgG antibody is bound to latex; the interfering substances bind to the Fc region only.

2. Agglutination by protein-protein interaction. For each test, the pH and ionic strength of the reagents provided in kit form are carefully chosen to inhibit this interference. The publications describing each method detail the composition of the reaction media.

3. Agglutination by human antibodies to the animal immunoglobulin used for the assay. Serum of the animal providing the antisera is present in the diluents to absorb these antibodies.

4. Agglutination by human anti-F(ab')$_2$ antibodies. These antibodies are absorbed by the addition of aggregated F(ab')$_2$ of the animal providing the antisera to the reaction media.

5. Agglutination or inhibition by serum proteins. When the determinants of the antigen of interest resist pepsin digestion, samples are treated with pepsin to destroy interfering protein substances (8).

MATERIALS AND METHODS

Normal procedures for blood, urine, and cerebrospinal fluid collection should be used. Serum should be separated as soon as possible and then may be used directly. After being frozen and thawed, lipoproteins tend to precipitate, and this precipitation may interfere with particle counting. The lipids may be removed easily by mixing 2 volumes of the sample with 1 volume of Freon 113 (Serva, Heidelberg, Federal Republic of Germany) and then vortexing. A brief centrifugation (5 min at 5,000 rpm) will leave a clear supernatant suitable for the assay.

Reagents used for each assay have been well detailed in the literature (9). Those reagents commercially available are listed in Table 2. The manufacturers claim that all reagents which have not been opened are stable for 2 years and that reconstituted reagents are stable for 3 months at 4°C and for 2 weeks at room temperature (25°C).

To avoid interference from water or buffer containing dust or other particulated contaminants, all liquids are filtered with a 0.2-μm filter.

Most of the work has been done with carboxylated latex, obtained as a 100-g/liter suspension (Rhône-

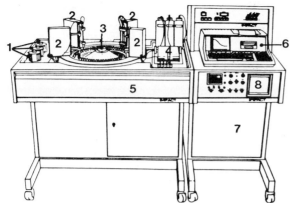

FIG. 1. IMPACT, an automated immunoassay by particle counting. 1, Three peristaltic metering pumps; 2, pipetting stations; 3, sampler tray; 4, large peristaltic pump; 5, optical particle counter; 6, computer; 7, electronic control unit.

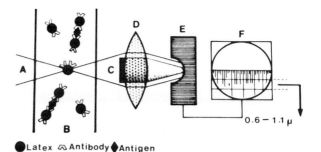

●Latex ⌢Antibody ◆Antigen

FIG. 2. Quantitation of antigens. A collimated beam of white light focused to a diameter of 7.5 μm passes through a flow cell (B) and impinges on a black spot (C). When a particle passes through this beam, light is diffracted past the black spot, collected by the lens (D), and focused onto the photomultiplier (E). The impulse from E, shown on the oscilloscope (F), is proportional to the size of the particle. Only the unagglutinated particles are electronically counted, thus separating bound from free. No physical separation is necessary. The IMPACT system is therefore a homogeneous assay.

TABLE 1. Immunoassays by particle counting

Analyte	Reference
Polyvalent antigen	
Alpha-fetoprotein[a]	3
C-reactive protein[a]	4
Ferritin[a]	5
Lactoferrin	
S-100 protein	10
Pregnancy-specific β₁ glycoprotein	4a
IgE	8
IgA	10
IgM	10
IgG and IgA subclasses	6
Thyroxine-binding globulin[a]	
Thyroglobulin	
Thyroid-stimulating hormone[a]	
Human placental lactogen[a]	
Human somatotropin	1
Capsular antigen of *H. influenzae* type b	
Capsular antigens of *Streptococcus pneumoniae* (83 serotypes)	
Antigen of *Streptococcus haemolyticus* type b	
Monovalent antigen[a]	
Thyroxine[a]	
Triiodothyronine[a]	
Digoxin	2
Antibodies	
RF	9
Anti-honey bee venom IgG (blocking) antibodies	7
Anti-*Brucella abortus* antibodies	
Specific IgE antibodies	8
Anti-myelin basic protein antibodies	9
Anti-thyroglobulin antibodies	
Anti-tetanus antibodies	
Antibodies against herpes simplex virus type 1	10
Immune complexes	
Detection with RF	9
Detection with mouse C1q	9

[a] Reagents commercially available.

Poulenc, Courbevoie, France), to which the antigen or the antibody in the form of F(ab')₂ fragments is coupled after carbodiimide activation of the particles.

The reaction medium often contains polymers which enhance the agglutination reaction, such as polyethylene glycol (molecular weight, 6,000) or Dextran T-500 (Pharmacia, Uppsala, Sweden) at the concentrations indicated in Table 3 and Fig. 4. As certain serum samples contain antibodies reacting with rabbit F(ab')₂, the reaction medium contains F(ab')₂ fragments to absorb these antibodies (1, 4). However, to be effective, the F(ab')₂ fragments have to originate from a pool of rabbit serum, because the anti-F(ab')₂ antibodies seem to react only with certain allotypic determinants. The fragments have to be used in an aggregated form, which can be obtained, for example, by treating them with glutaraldehyde. For the titration of IgG antibodies or for the assay of monovalent antigens such a digoxin (2) and thyroxin, RF is introduced as a diluted serum from a

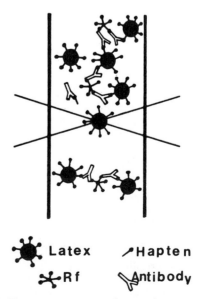

Latex   Hapten
Rf   Antibody

FIG. 3. Hapten assays. See the text for explanation.

Alpha-fetoprotein assay
1. 27 μl of serum + 108 μl of GBS → incubate for 5 min at room temperature
2. 27 μl of mixture from step 1 + 27 μl of GBS → incubate for 1 min at 37°C
3. 27 μl of additive GBS + aggregated rabbit F(ab')$_2$ → incubate for 1 min at 37°C
4. 27 μl of latex–anti-AFP → incubate for 30 min at 37°C
5. Go to step 6 below

Triiodothyronine assay
1. 90 μl of serum + 45 μl H$_2$O + 45 μl of pepsin → incubate for 5 min at room temperature (digestion)
2. 165 μl of Tris (2 M) quenching buffer → (pH 7.0) stop pepsin reaction 3 min at room temperature
3. 45 μl of mixture from step 2 + 27 μl of anti-T$_3$ (monoclonal) → incubate 1 min at 37°C
4. 27 μl of second antibody → incubate for 1 min at 37°C
5. 27 μl of latex-T$_3$ conjugate → incubate for 30 min at 37°C
6. Go to step 6 below

Thyroid-stimulating hormone
1. 45 μl of serum + 45 μl H$_2$O + 90 μl of pepsin → incubate for 5 min (pH 1.4) at room temperature
2. 145 μl of Tris (1 M) → (pH 7.4) stop pepsin reaction 3 min at room temperature
3. 45 μl of mixture from step 2 + Dextran (6%) in GBS → incubate for 1 min at 37°C
4. 27 μl of latex–thyroid-stimulating hormone antibody → incubate for 30 min at 37°C
5. Go to step 6 below

For all methods
6. 930 μl of GBS→ incubate for 2 min at 37°C
7. 20:1 dilution of GBS-Tween 20 → count the unagglutinated particles

FIG. 4. Assay procedures for automated particle-counting immunoassays of alpha-fetoprotein (AFP), triiodothyronine, and thyroid-stimulating hormone. GBS, Glycine-buffered saline.

TABLE 2. Tests and suppliers

Test[a]	Name of test and source of RIA kit	Correlation coefficient (r)	Regression equation[b]	Antigen excess (per liter)
T$_4$	Diagnostic Products Corp. Los Angeles, Calif.	0.96	$1.00x + 0.4$	
TSH	Diagnostic Products Corp. Los Angeles, Calif.	0.98	$1.42x - 0.23$	>200 mIU
IgE	PHADEBAS (modified) Pharmacia Uppsala, Sweden	0.99	$0.95x - 7.5$	>6,000 kIU
CRP	Nephelometric Disc 120 Travenol International Services, Inc. Brussels, Belgium	0.97	$1.04x - 9.3$	>940 mg
T$_3$	Gamma-Coat Clinical Assay Travenol International Services, Inc. Brussels, Belgium	0.93	$0.92x + 0.09$	
TBG	RIA-gnost Behring Marburg, Federal Republic of Germany	0.95	$0.95x + 0.126$	>320 mg
HPL	HPL-RIA bio Mérieux 1040 Brussels, Belgium	0.94	$0.86x + 0.08$	>16 mg
AFP	α-feto RIABEAD Abbott Laboratories, Diagnostics Div. North Chicago, Ill.	0.98	$1.08x + 0.06$	>1,300 kIU
Ferritin	Ferrizyme Abbott Laboratories, Diagnostics Div. North Chicago, Ill.	0.98	$1.09x + 2.3$	>2.6 mg

[a] T$_4$, Thyroxine; TSH, thyroid-stimulating hormone; CRP, C-reactive protein; T$_3$, triiodothyronine; TBG, thyroxine-binding globulin; HPL, human placental lactogen; AFP, alpha-fetoprotein.
[b] $y = a + bx$ and y = IMPACT.

TABLE 3. Standards and reagents for test kits

Test kit no.[a]	Vol of standard used (μl)	Composition (μl) of reagent and vol used; position on instrument[b]							
		Pepsin	H₂O	Diluent[c]	Quenching solution	Additive	Antiserum	Second antibody	Latex conjugate
T₄ IMP-05R	0, 10, 20, 40, 80, 160, 320 μg/liter (36)	5 mg/ml in 0.2 N HCl (90); P1	Particle >0.2 μm free (90); P2		0.2 M Tris and PEG 6000 (7% wt/vol) (250 μl); P3		Rabbit anti-T4 (27); P4	High-titer rheumatoid serum (27); P5	Albumin-T₄ covalently coupled (27); P6
TSH IMP-08R	0, 1, 2, 5, 10, 20, 50, 100 mU/liter (45)	5 mg/ml in 0.3 N HCl (90); P1	Particle >0.2 μm free (90); P2		1.6 M Tris buffer (271); P3	GBS + 6% Dextran (27); P5			Rabbit anti-TSH F(ab')₂ covalently coupled (27); P4
CRP IMP-06R	0, 1.5, 3, 6, 12, 20, 40, 80 mg/liter (27)			GBS[c] (2,000); P1 (180); P2 (180); P3					Rabbit anti-CRP F(ab')₂ covalently coupled (27); P4
IgE[d] IMP-10R	0, 10, 20, 50, 100, 200, 500, 1,000 kIU/liter (27)	5 mg/ml in 0.4 N HCl (72); P1	Particle >0.2 μm free (480); P1			Tris buffer, 2.0 M (27); P3	Rabbit anti-fragment F(c)″ of IgE (27); P4		Rabbit anti-IgE–F(c)″ F(ab')₂ covalently coupled (27); P6
TBG IMP-02R	0, 2, 5, 10, 20, 30, 40, 80 mg/liter (27)			GBS (2,180); P1 (45); P3					Rabbit anti-TBG F(ab')₂ covalently coupled (27); P4
T₃ IMP-04R	0, 0.4, 0.8, 1.6, 3, 6, 12 μg/liter (100)	5 mg/ml in 0.8 N HCl (45); P1	Particle >0.2 μm free (45); P2		2.0 M Tris buffer (112); P3		Mouse monoclonal anti-T3 (20); P4	Rabbit anti-mouse IgG (20); P5	Albumin-T₃ covalently coupled (20); P6
HPL IMP-04R	0, 0.25, 0.5, 1, 2, 4, 8, 16 mg/liter (27)			GBS (836); P1 (45); P2		Aggregated rabbit F(ab')₂ (27); P4			Rabbit anti-HPL F(ab')₂ covalently coupled (27); P6
AFP IMP-03R	0, 6.5, 13, 32.5, 54, 130, 325, 650 kIU/liter (27)			GBS (126); P1 (45); P2		Aggregated rabbit F(ab')₂ (27); P4			Rabbit anti-AFP F(ab')₂ covalently coupled (27); P6
Ferritin IMP-01R	0, 3.25, 6.5, 13, 32.5, 65, 130, 325 μg/liter (27)			GBS (126); P1 (45); P3		Aggregated rabbit F(ab')₂ (27); P4			Rabbit anti-ferritin F(ab')₂ covalently coupled (27); P6

[a] See Table 2, footnote a for explanation of abbreviations.
[b] See Fig. 3.
[c] GBS, Glycine-buffered saline.
[d] The manufacturers advise that a new formulation is being considered.

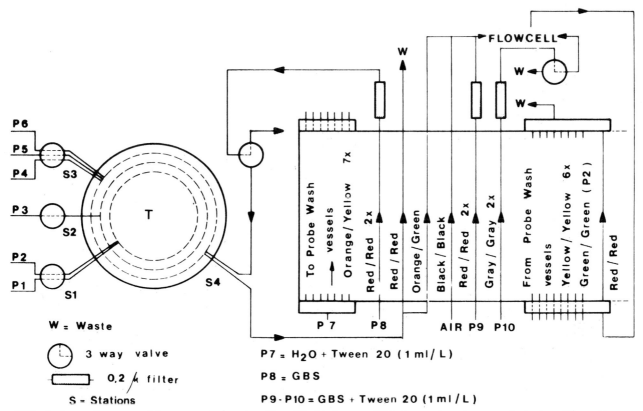

W = Waste

⌷ 3 way valve

▭ 0.2 μ filter

S = Stations

P7 = H₂O + Tween 20 (1 ml / L)

P8 = GBS

P9 - P10 = GBS + Tween 20 (1 ml / L)

FIG. 5. Operating steps of the automated system. Tray T holds 3 rows of 60 tubes each and moves clockwise with continuous vortex mixing, turning 1 position per min. The outer row of tubes is incubated at 37°C. S1 through S4 are pipetting stations (Fig. 6) capable of transferring sample from the inner to the middle tubes (S1) or the middle to the outer tubes (S2), or of simply adding reagents or buffer (S3), or of adding buffer and aspirating reacted mixture (S4). S1, S2, and S3 are fed by 4-channel peristaltic pumps which, when turning clockwise, aspirate sample and, when turning counterclockwise, discharge sample and diluent (Fig. 6). The amount of liquid handled depends on the tube size used and the number of turns commanded by the computer for the assay. According to Fig. 4, a typical assay for triiodothyronine is as follows: step 1 by S1 (P1, P2); step 2 by S2 (P3); steps 3, 4, and 5 by S3; and steps 6 and 7 by S4. Final dilution (20:1) is by the orange-green sample tube and P9. P10 is a reverse wash flow to clean the flow cell of particles between assays. It operates automatically.

rheumatoid patient that has a titer in the manual latex test of at least 1:500.

In the titration of specific IgE antibodies (8), radioallergosorbent test paper disks from Pharmacia can be used, but the sensitivity is such that a quarter of the disk is sufficient. After the antibodies are absorbed on the insolubilized allergen and appropriately washed, fragments of the IgE antibodies are recovered by digestion of the paper disk with pepsin. This digestion step proceeds in the incubating tray of the IMPACT instrument.

For the titration of immune complexes, all samples are treated first by dithiothreitol to inactivate endogenous IgM RF and then reoxidized with hydrogen peroxide or periodate to avoid inactivation of the added agglutinator (9). Reduction of the samples with dithiothreitol has also been found necessary for the assay of pregnancy-specific β₁ glycoprotein (SP1) (4a). In IMPACT, this treatment proceeds automatically in the incubation tray.

The operating steps of the automated system are illustrated in Fig. 5 and 6. The sequence of operations required for each assay and the data-handling algorithms are stored on cassette in a Hewlett Packard 85 computer, which is an integral part of the machine.

The operating steps may be summarized as follows.

1. Switch on the power.
2. Switch on the thermostat before the actual run.
3. Reconstitute the lyophilized latex conjugate (Table 3) with 6 ml of H₂O (the conjugate is stable for 3 to 4 months at 4°C).

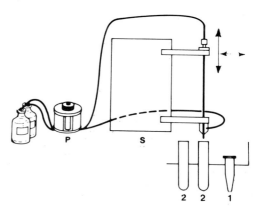

FIG. 6. Portion of automated system. P, Peristaltic metering pump; S, pipetting station; 1, sample tube; 2, reaction tubes; ↔, movement between 1 and 2 on computer command; ↕, movement up and down on computer command.

4. Reconstitute the lyophilized standards no. 1 through 8 with 1 ml of H_2O (sufficient for 10 to 15 standard curves). Other reagents should be ready for use (Table 3).

5. Load the central and outer rings (Fig. 5) with empty tubes.

6. Manually dispense approximately 100 μl of standards and samples into the tubes in the inner ring.

7. Secure the platten on the large peristaltic pump, and push the "22-Channel Pump" switch.

8. Place the appropriate pump tubes into reagent bottles (Fig. 5), and prime the metering pumps by pushing the appropriate switch.

9. Prime the reverse wash and diluent lines by pushing the "Reverse Flow" and "Diluent Valve" switches.

10. Load the program into the computer.

11. When the test list is shown on the computer screen, select the tests to be done by keying in the appropriate number.

12. Start the analysis by pushing the "GO" key on the computer.

RESULTS

Sensitivity for most assays is on the order of 0.1 to 1 ng/ml. In the case of the capsular antigen of *Haemophilus influenzae* type b, a meaningful agglutination has been observed at a concentration of 0.25 pg/ml. Increasing the concentration of particles or the antibody loading of latex increases the speed of the reaction but tends to decrease the sensitivity.

Particular attention has been paid to the latex coating and the preparation of the reaction medium to avoid nonspecific agglutination or inhibition and to obtain parallelism between samples and standards. Correlation coefficients calculated on a minimum of 100 results range from 0.93 to 0.99 for the assays of polyvalent and monovalent antigens (Table 2). The number of outliers between a particle-counting immunoassay and any RIA method is not greater than the number between two RIAs (1–5, 9).

Regarding precision, published data have been obtained in general on prototype instruments. Results obtained on the commercial version of the IMPACT instrument have recently been published for the assay of the pregnancy-specific β₁ glycoprotein. The interassay precision was assessed by using samples at three concentrations of SP1, i.e., 5, 35, and 245 ng/ml, and the assay was repeated each day for 15 days. The coefficients of variation were, respectively, 9.9, 9.2, and 9.8% (4a).

One possible weakness of direct methods such as agglutination and precipitation is the risk of antigen excess. An excess of agglutinator results in a decrease of agglutination. All reagents commercially available have been carefully checked for this possibility, and all inserts mention the concentration value at which a decrease of agglutination occurs (Table 2).

DISCUSSION

Latex agglutination has been used for about 30 years but was restricted to semiquantitative methods essentially for two reasons, i.e., the lack of a reliable instrument to measure the extent of the reaction and the multiple factors causing nonspecific agglutination or inhibition. Instrumental counting of particles has rendered latex agglutination not only more precise, but also at least 10 times more sensitive than when the agglutination is measured by turbidimetry or nephelometry and at least 1,000 times more sensitive than immunoprecipitation in gels. The interferences can be avoided as described by using various substances in the incubation medium and by removing the Fc fragment of the antibodies used to coat the latex.

With a suitable instrument to read agglutination and with reagents protecting the reaction from interfering factors, latex agglutination offers the advantages of rapidity and simplicity, as the principle rests on a direct reaction without any separation or washing steps as required for immunoprecipitation.

LITERATURE CITED

1. **Castracane, C. E., C. L. Cambiaso, L. A. Retegui, I. Gilbert, J. M. Ketelslegers, and P. L. Masson.** 1984. Particle counting immunoassay of human somatotropin. Clin. Chem. **30**:672–677.

2. **Collet-Cassart, D., C. G. M. Magnusson, C. L. Cambiaso, M. Lesne, and P. L. Masson.** 1981. Automated particle counting immunoassay for digoxin. Clin. Chem **27**:1205–1209.

3. **Collet-Cassart, D., C. G. M. Magnusson, J. G. Ratcliffe, C. L. Cambiaso, and P. L. Masson.** 1981. Automated particle counting immunoassay for alpha-fetoprotein. Clin. Chem. **27**:64–67.

4. **Collet-Cassart, D., J. C. Mareschal, C. J. M. Sindic, T. P. Tomasi, and P. L. Masson.** 1983. Automated particle counting immunoassay of C-reactive protein and its application to serum, cord serum and cerebrospinal fluid samples. Clin. Chem. **29**:1127–1131.

4a. **Fagnart, O. C., J. C. Mareschal, C. L. Cambiaso, and P. L. Masson.** 1985. Particle counting immunoassay (PACIA) of pregnancy-specific β₁-glycoprotein. A possible marker of various malignancies and Crohn's ileitis. Clin. Chem. **31**:397–401.

5. **Limet, J. N., D. Collet-Cassart, C. G. M. Magnusson, P. Sauvage, C. L. Cambiaso, and P. L. Masson.** 1982. Particle counting immunoassay (PACIA) of ferritin. J. Clin. Chem. Clin. Biochem. **20**:141–146.

6. **Magnusson, C. G. M., D. L. Delacroix, J. P. Vaerman, and P. L. Masson.** 1984. Typing of subclasses and light chains of human monoclonal immunoglobulins by particle counting immunoassay (PACIA). J. Immunol. Methods **69**:229–241.

7. **Magnusson, C. G. M., R. Djurup, B. Weeke, and P. L. Masson.** 1983. The use of particle counting immunoassay (PACIA) for the titration of specific antibodies: application to sera from honey-bee venom-desensitized patients. Int. Arch. Allergy Appl. Immunol. **71**:144–150.

8. **Magnusson, C. G. M., and P. L. Masson.** 1982. Particle counting immunoassay of immunoglobulin E antibodies after their elution from allergosorbents by pepsin: an alternative to the radioallergosorbent test. J. Allergy Clin. Immunol. **70**:326–336.

9. **Masson, P. L., C. L. Cambiaso, D. Collet-Cassart, C. G. M. Magnusson, C. B. Richards, and C. J. M. Sindic.** 1981. Particle-counting immunoassay (PACIA). Methods Enzymol. **74**:106–139.

10. **Sindic, C. J. M., M. P. Chalon, C. L. Cambiaso, E. C. Laterre, and P. L. Masson.** 1984. Inflammatory and immune reactions in the CSF of patients with herpetic encephalitis. Protides Biol. Fluids Proc. Colloq. **32**:179–182.

Chapter 9

Agglutination and Agglutination Inhibition Assays

W. STEPHEN NICHOLS AND ROBERT M. NAKAMURA

Agglutination reactions consist of the clumping of particulate matter such as cells or synthetic material by antibodies called agglutinins. The reaction takes place on the surface of particles, such as erythrocytes, bacteria, or latex, with antigen located to be available to specific binding sites on antibodies. Agglutination is an example of a secondary immune reaction, the primary event involving recognition of antigenic determinants by antibody. Secondary reactions manifest the binding event (Fig. 1) and include agglutination, flocculation, and precipitation. Tertiary reactions require physiologic manifestations of the binding event, such as phagocytosis, chemotaxis, and immune adherence.

Primary immunologic reaction is detected by such techniques as radioimmunoassay, enzyme immunochemistry, and fluorescence microscopy. Secondary reactions are often manifest by microscopic or gross visual observations. The first agglutination reactions involved bacterial agglutinins in experiments carried out by the early bacteriologists. This work led to the formulation of the idea of antibodies. The utility of this simple procedure—mixing antigen-laden particles with antibody—gave rise to the era of serodiagnosis in microbiology, advanced the understanding of the role of microorganisms in the cause of disease, and soon led to the discovery of the ABO blood groups. These same procedures find ubiquitous use in contemporary medicine. Practical use of agglutination procedures has expanded from the areas of infectious disease and immunohematology to the study of autoimmune disease, the endocrine assay, and other diverse areas. The classic techniques of direct agglutination have given rise to a variety of techniques involving coating of carrier particles with antigen (or antibody), either through passive adsorption processes or through covalent linkage of antigens to carrier via chemical manipulation.

PRINCIPLES OF AGGLUTINATION

Bordet proposed that agglutination takes place in two phases: (i) specific combination of antibody and antigen and (ii) visible aggregation of particles. Both phases are mediated by specific attraction between antibody and antigen. Particles such as erythrocytes and bacteria bear slight negative charges in suspension (the zeta potential) and repel each other, to an extent as hydrophobic colloids, so that the surface potential of these particles is such that specific cross-linkage of antigen-coated particles by a bridge of immunoglobulin G (IgG) antibody is at times prevented (8). Failure of particles to agglutinate after the primary reaction is called "incomplete" agglutination. The reduction of relative ionic strength of the test medium with protein or inorganic solute reduces distances among particles, allowing successful antibody bridging, formation of an extensive lattice of antigen-antibody complex, and agglutination.

Although charge is important in determining completeness of agglutination, it is evident that other effects play a role in the agglutination of particles by antibodies. Viscosity of the test medium also appears important to completion of agglutination, since the addition of low-charge polymerized molecules such as dextran also augments agglutination.

A chief disadvantage of the agglutination phenomenon is that the reaction is semiquantitative. Although agglutination may be carried out with standardized reagents and conditions, repeated results are only accurate to a fourfold difference in antibody titer. However, the fact that numerous systems lend themselves to agglutination reactions, the basic simplicity of agglutination systems developed to date, and the high sensitivity of agglutination-based reactions (Table 1; 5) encourage wide use of agglutination tests.

The successful application of agglutination reactions to antibody or antigen detection systems requires a stable particle, pure antigen, and specific antibody. Generally, use of the agglutination phenomenon also requires knowledge of the likelihood of completion of the reaction. IgM antibodies in the test medium usually aggregate particulate antigen based on the size of the IgM molecule, whereas IgG antibodies alone may fail to cause completion of the agglutination reaction. IgM is said to be 750 times more efficient than IgG in agglutination reactions.

It should also be remembered that the so-called prozone phenomenon may contribute to incomplete reaction in agglutination reactions, even where adequate titers of IgM antibodies exist in the test medium. The prozone phenomenon is produced by several factors. Serum of low dilution may fail to aggregate particles due to the coating of antigen sites with large numbers of individual antibodies, a situation which, under equilibrium conditions, decreases the number of complexes of cross-particle-linked antigen-antibody. Similarly, the amount of cross-linkage may also decrease with increasing antigen concentration. Moreover, the prozone phenomenon may be produced by alteration of proteins (heating) or through interference with the close approximation of particles, such as with excessive quantities of extraneous colloid material. In general, agglutination reactions may be read with the unaided eye, or a microscope or magnifying mirror may be used to increase sensitivity of detection of aggregates where agglutination is poor, partially completed, or near a prozone.

CLASSIFICATION OF AGGLUTINATION ASSAYS

Direct agglutination assay

The simple direct agglutination assay is the classic reaction involving clumping of cells or particulate

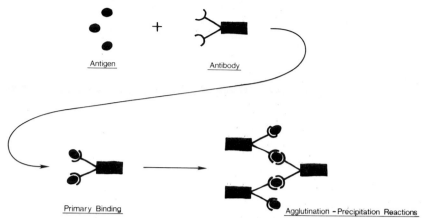

Antigen

Antibody

Primary Binding

Agglutination – Precipitation Reactions

FIG. 1. Secondary manifestations of antigen-antibody reaction.

antigen (Table 2). Reaction is brought about by specific antibody molecules with two or more receptors linking particles in suspension. Modifications of the test medium or of antigens close to the surface of erythrocytes may be necessary to demonstrate incomplete reactions. An example of an incomplete antibody is that encountered in the blood bank in testing for Rh blood group IgG antibody by direct hemagglutination (9). IgG antibody species may fail to agglutinate erythrocytes in saline or in dilutions of serum and saline. Modifying incomplete systems by any of several techniques allows detection of the incomplete reaction.

Incomplete antibodies may be demonstrated by using methods designed to decrease ionic strength or enhance fluid viscosity, or both, of the test medium (8). If test serum is enhanced with bovine serum albumin or with highly polymerized molecules such as dextran, polyvinylpyrrolidone, or Polybrene, charge and viscosity alterations of test media tend to reduce repulsive dielectric forces between cells with amplification of the sensitivity of agglutination reactions. Charge and viscosity modifications are generally brought about in the blood bank with 5 to 30% bovine albumin additive. Cells and bacteria are also rendered more agglutinable by enzyme treatment, presumably by increasing exposure of the surface antigen to antibody through removal of blocking

structures, perhaps through decrease in hydration or alteration of the surface charge, or through change in the configuration of external membrane components. Several enzymes have been investigated for these effects. These enzymes include bromelin, papain, and ficin. Procedures utilizing enzyme augmentation of agglutinins are now commonplace in blood banks in the workup of atypical antibodies in the Rh, Kidd, Lewis, and P systems, as examples. A one-stage enzyme test incorporates enzyme with serum and cells. Otherwise, erythrocytes may be pretreated with enzyme, washed, and subsequently tested with serum (two-stage test). Enzyme is normally used at a 0.5 to 1.0% concentration over a variable pH range. It must be remembered that enzyme may actually reduce agglutinability of certain systems such as the M and N erythrocyte antigens. Occasionally, nonspecific agglutination can occur in enzyme-treated systems. Low-ionic-strength salt solution is today employed as a convenient method of modifying incomplete agglutination reactions in the blood bank. Low-ionic-strength media supply fewer ions than does 0.85% saline, thus increasing association between cells and antibody. This treatment appears to reduce the total time for cell-cell interaction to occur, and hence the time of incubation may be shortened. The *Technical*

TABLE 1. Relative sensitivity of immunologic tests

Test	Minimum antibody (μg) N/ml detectable
Precipitation in liquid	20
Precipitation in gel	
Double diffusion (Ouchterlony).......	3–20
Radial diffusion (Mancini)	3–20
Immunoelectrophoresis	50–200
Agglutination	
Qualitative	0.05
Quantitative......................	0.02–0.1
Hemagglutination, indirect	0.001–0.01
Hemagglutination inhibition..........	0.001–0.01
Coombs test	0.01
Complement fixation.................	0.01–0.05
Fluorescent antibody	1.0
Particle-enhanced light scattering	0.001
Radioimmunoassay..................	0.001

TABLE 2. Agglutination techniques

Direct agglutination
  Classic (simple)
  Hydrophilic enrichment
  Enzyme augmentation
Indirect (passive) agglutination
  Antigen-coated particles
    Absorbed
    Covalently linked
  Antibody-coated particles (reverse passive)
Antiglobulin-mediated agglutination
  Coombs
    Direct
    Indirect
  Rose-Waaler
Agglutination
Particle-enhanced immunoassay
  PETINIA
  PACIA
  QUELS

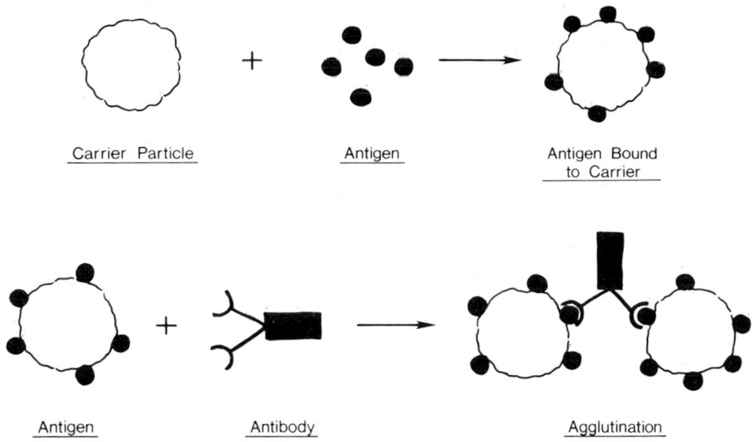

FIG. 2. Passive agglutination technique.

Manual of the American Association of Blood Banks serves as a general reference for blood bank techniques (7).

Indirect (passive) agglutination assay

The development of the technique of passive agglutination has had numerous ramifications in the laboratory (8). This versatile technique consists of agglutination of cells or particles coated with soluble antigen. Antibody may also be bound to particles, in a sense reversing the reaction (reverse passive agglutination) in this test. The cells or particles act as passive carriers of antigens or antibody in these assays (Fig. 2). Usually, antigen is physically adsorbed or covalently bound to the surface of particles. Human or animal erythrocytes may be used in developing erythrocyte indirect agglutination procedures (indirect or passive hemagglutination). One drawback of hemagglutination testing in general is the occasional presence of heterophile antibody in sera. Hence, serum samples for hemagglutination often require adsorption against uncoated erythrocytes for removal of nonspecific antibodies before the test.

Many proteins spontaneously adsorb to the surface of erythrocytes and are therefore convenient reagents for use in agglutination testing. Examples of such antigens include thyroglobulin, purified protein derivative, *Clostridium tetani* toxoid, *Corynebacterium diphtheria* toxin, human albumin, bovine serum albumin, and numerous hormones. Several other proteins adsorb relatively poorly to cells. Mild exposure of erythrocytes to tannic acid, trypsin, or other similar reagents increases the amount of cell-bound antigen, however. This technique provides for considerable versatility in hemagglutination testing. Proteins that fail to adsorb to erythrocytes or that undergo desorption from cells during attempts to carry out simple direct agglutination may be chemically linked to erythrocyte membranes through covalent bonding. One common procedure for chemical bonding of antigens to erythrocytes involves cross-linking with bisdiazobenzidine. This method has applications similar to those of the tanned-erythrocyte procedure. Other specialized methods of chemical bonding of antigen to cells include the use of metallic ions such as chromic chloride, 1-ethyl-3-(3-dimethylaminopropyl)-carbodiimide, and 1,3-difluoro-4,6-dinitrobenzene for antigen linkage to erythrocytes.

The development of indirect systems utilizing inert particles such as bentonite (potter's clay), latex (polystyrene polymer), collodion, and charcoal have considerably expanded the diagnostic capabilities of immunology laboratories in contemporary serodiagnosis (8). The carrier serves as an agglutinogen indicating specific interaction of antigen and antibody. It was first shown that latex-absorbed human gamma globulin underwent aggregation in the presence of serum rheumatoid factors, IgM antibodies to human immunoglobulin. Latex techniques have been extremely popular since that time, and rheumatoid factor is still detected by this method.

Latex spheres (0.81 μm) in suspension behave as inert colloid with a negative charge. Latex easily adsorbs protein and serves as a useful source of particulate antigen. Latex particles are sized, diluted, coated with antigen, and stored at 4°C until used. Coating of latex particles is carried out by passive means, although different proteins adsorb to different degrees. Optimal quantities of protein are used to sensitize particles, the highest concentration utilized yielding high-titer agglutination without nonspecific agglutination. Latex agglutination is still used today to detect rheumatoid factors (immunoglobulin-coated particles), as well as agglutinins to *Histoplasma capsulatum*, thyroglobulin, hormones, parasites such as *Trichinella sprialis*, and C-reactive protein. Antinuclear antibodies are occasionally identified with latex methodology in certain laboratories. Bentonite clay is a kind of aluminum silicate and is also used for adsorption of several types of proteins, including parasitic antigens, thyroglobulin, etc.

Antiglobulin-mediated assays

The most useful mode of detecting incomplete agglutinins was developed by Coombs et al., who used anti-immunoglobulin as a second antibody to directly cross-link incomplete agglutinins reacting with Rh and ABO blood cell antigens (Fig. 3). The antiglobulin reagent provides a bridge between antibodies hooked to adjacent erythrocytes and culminates in aggrega-

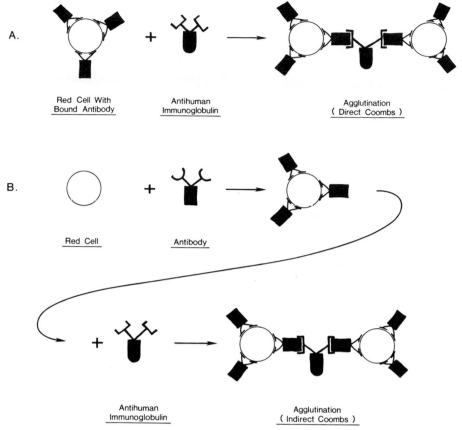

FIG. 3. Antiglobulin (Coombs) technique. (A) Direct test; (B) indirect test.

tion of cells or particles. The antiglobulin test is now commonly known as the Coombs test, and the most frequent application of the test today is still in the blood bank in the study of antigen-antibody systems, although the technique is also easily applied to several indirect hemagglutination tests.

The direct Coombs test predominantly utilizes antiglobulin to detect in vivo-sensitized erythrocytes. Anticomplement antibody may be employed in the Coombs test for detection of complement bound to sensitized cells. Patients with hemolytic disease which is secondary to either autoimmune antibody or antibody resulting from incompatible erythrocyte transfusion have erythrocytes that demonstrate positive Coombs testing. Coombs antiglobulin may be used at various dilutions to provide optimal conditions for agglutination, thereby increasing the sensitivity of the test.

Causes of autoimmune anemia include idiopathic etiology, such as cold agglutinin disease, lymphoproliferative disease, and hemolysis secondary to infection with any of several viruses or with *Mycoplasma pneumoniae*. The Coombs test is of great clinical use in delineating erythrocyte antibody sensitization in the sudden development of hemolytic anemia. Iatrogenic causes of hemolytic disease include infusion of incompatible blood units as well as antibody-mediated hemolysis secondary to sensitization with drugs.

The indirect Coombs test allows a search for free antibody in test sera. The indirect test is useful for screening sera for incomplete antibodies, as well as for the identification of problem antibodies with panels of erythrocyte antigens prepared from known erythrocyte donors. Serum is tested for the presence of incomplete antibodies by mixing cells of known antigenicity with donor serum and then washing the erythrocytes and combining the washed cells with Coombs antiglobulin reagent. Free serum antibody, if present, attaches to the cells and then demonstrates agglutination upon addition of the second antibody. Among the important achievements related to the Coombs technique, testing for Rh type and maternal sensitization to Rh(D)-positive fetuses has led to successful treatment of mother and fetus in prevention of Rh antibody-mediated hemolytic disease of the newborn (6).

In testing erythrocytes for antibody sensitization, it must be remembered that optimal reaction, and hence sensitivity of the agglutinating system, is dependent upon temperature. So-called cold and warm antibodies react best at approximately 4 and 37°C, respectively. The "cold" or "warm" nature of an antibody often influences the in vivo behavior of the antibody and the potential for hemolysis. Incomplete antibodies are often warm in their behavior.

The Rose-Waaler test is a specialized antiglobulin test with sheep erythrocytes sensitized with a subagglutinating dose of rabbit anti-sheep erythrocyte IgG. Rheumatoid factor combines with membrane-bound IgG and produces agglutination. At present, however, most tests for rheumatoid arthritis use latex particles.

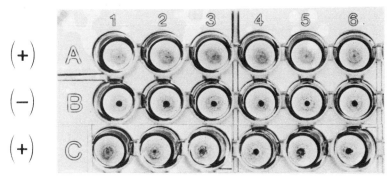

FIG. 4. Hemagglutination patterns observed in the microhemagglutination test for thyroid microsomal antibody. Row A, Positive agglutination pattern (wells 1 through 6); row B, negative pattern (wells 1 through 6); and row C, positive pattern (wells 1 through 3) and transition to negative pattern (wells 4 through 6).

DIAGNOSTIC USES OF AGGLUTINATION TESTS

Aside from the immunohematologic applications of agglutination reactions, numerous diagnostic procedures in the clinical laboratory utilize agglutination-based techniques. Many of these techniques are reviewed in depth in later chapters in this manual.

Some of the most useful tests involve agglutination of microorganisms for the immunologic diagnosis of infectious diseases such as salmonellosis, brucellosis, rickettsiosis, and several others. Early identification of initially high or rising titers of agglutinins to these organisms offers a powerful laboratory adjunct to clinical diagnosis.

The Widal test (8), designed in 1954, is exemplary of the applicability of agglutination reactions and is used primarily to identify antibody to various antigens incorporated in the *Salmonella* species, several of which are etiologic for dysentery. *Salmonella typhi* is the agent responsible for typhoid fever. In the Widal test, antibody screening is carried out against selected *Salmonella* species, usually those prevalent in a given geographic area. Test sera of several dilutions are incubated with killed organisms, with attention directed toward the possibility of the prozone phenomenon. Several different antigens exist among the members of bacterial species, so that antibodies against *Salmonella* species may be directed toward somatic, flagellar, or capsular antigens. A titer of somatic and flagellar antibodies equal to 1:80 or greater indicates an active infection. Lower titers are found among immunized individuals or in recent onset of infection.

Other organisms are also of great use in infectious disease surveillance with agglutination assays of serum antibody titers. These organisms include species of the genera *Brucella* (brucellosis), *Francisella* (tularemia), and *Bordetella* (pertussis).

The Weil-Felix test is also useful in the study of infectious disease and employs the so-called OX-2, OX-19, and OX-K strains of *Proteus vulgaris* to detect cross-reacting antibodies produced during rickettsial infections such as typhus and spotted fever. In the United States, Rocky Mountain spotted fever is caused by *Rickettsia rickettsii* after exposure to the tick vector. The Weil-Felix reaction is useful to screen suspected patients for high titers of *Proteus* agglutinins for presumptive diagnosis of spotted fever.

Several other agglutination tests are useful in diagnosing a wide variety of infectious diseases. As examples, indirect hemagglutination assays were once popular for the rapid detection of hepatitis B antigens. Differential adsorption of heterophile antibodies with agglutination of xenogeneic erythrocytes continues to be of use in the diagnosis of mononucleosis.

Several developments in the study of connective tissue and autoimmune diseases have demonstrated the usefulness of screening tests for specific tissue-directed antibodies. As an example, the tanned erythrocyte hemagglutination technique is used in recognizing antithyroid antibodies for the differential diagnosis of thyroid diseases. The method utilizes microtechnique involving a tray of small, round-bottomed wells substituting for test tubes. Serum is screened in several dilutions for antibody to thyroid antigens such as microsomal or thyroglobulin-related antigens. The results of the microtest are read with relative ease with a mirror or microscope. Agglutination of erythrocytes by antibody results in settling of a somewhat rigid matrix of aggregated cells diffusely spread over the bottom of microtest wells, whereas negative tests result in the settling of erythrocytes in a compact button at the base of the wells (Fig. 4). The finding of a high titer of antithyroid antibody is consistent with Hashimoto's autoimmune thyroiditis. A low (or negative) titer may suggest the possibility of the presence of other thyroid diseases such as hyperthyroidism or even thyroid carcinoma. Antinuclear antibodies of autoimmune nature are tested by using various nuclear antigens in similar hemagglutination tests. Saline-extractable antigens such as Sm and ribonuclear protein are conveniently linked to erythrocytes to screen for antibodies in lupus erythematosus and related diseases. Autoimmune antibodies are covered extensively in other chapters of this text.

Mixed agglutination technique is one of several recent ingenious applications of agglutination. Mixed agglutination is the formation of aggregates of two different particles (or cell types) with antibody reacting with similar antigenic determinants on both particles. The second particle acts as the indicator system. With this technique, cells or particles can be used to examine for the presence of antigenic determinants on the first particles. Solid tissue sections, for instance, may be tested for the presence of blood group antigens by exposing tissue sections to erythrocytes

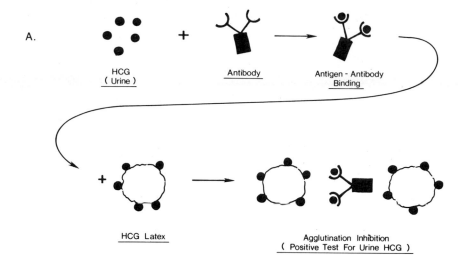

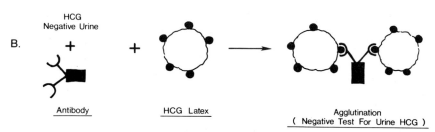

FIG. 5. Agglutination inhibition test for HCG. (A) Positive test; (B) negative test.

treated with anti-blood group (ABO) antibodies. An interesting "sandwich" reaction involving erythrocytes (E) sensitized with antierythrocyte antibody (A) and nonhemolyzing complement (C) has been developed to form a particle indicator system, the EAC. EACs are agglutinated in a form of the mixed cell reaction around B lymphocytes (EAC rosettes) by complement receptors residing on the B cells. B lymphocytes may be quantitated by enumerating EAC-rosetting lymphocytes. Another so-called rosetting technique exploits the human T lymphocyte-sheep erythrocyte (E) receptor. The performance of sheep erythrocyte mixed agglutination with T lymphocytes (E rosette formation) allows quantitation of T lymphocytes. These latter tests have been extremely helpful in differentiating hematologic neoplasms, although the tests are rapidly being replaced by other, more sensitive techniques.

Another useful non-antibody-mediated agglutination reaction in the blood bank and cellular immunology laboratory makes use of agglutinating substances called lectins (8). Usually derived from plants, lectins are molecules with specific carbohydrate receptors. Presently, a large array of lectins are available in blood banks for agglutination of erythrocytes through attachment to carbohydrate receptors such as A, B, and H antigens, thus providing an alternative method for the identification of blood group substances.

Agglutination inhibition

Inhibition of antigen-antibody reactions was first employed by K. Landsteiner. In agglutination inhibition reactions, assessment of specificity and titer of antibody is carried out based on competition between particulate and soluble antigens for antibody combining sites. In agglutination inhibition reactions, antibody and soluble antigen are ordinarily reacted together first. Antibody in the test medium reacts with the soluble antigen, subsequently inhibiting indirect agglutination of indicator particles or cells. An agglutination inhibition assay in current, popular use is the agglutination inhibition test for human chorionic gonadotropin (HCG). Testing for HCG in urine is a classic method for the laboratory confirmation of pregnancy. In the agglutination inhibition assay for HCG, reagent antibody is first reacted with test urine. The combination of HCG in urine with antibody prevents subsequent agglutination of reagent latex or erythrocytes sensitized with HCG (Fig. 5). A positive urine HCG test is consistent with pregnancy.

An important variation of agglutination inhibition reactions makes use of specific virus receptors on erythrocyte membranes. Influenza, rubella, and other viruses directly agglutinate erythrocytes. The inhibition of virus hemagglutination by specific serum antibody to virus is a particularly useful test in determining titers of antiviral antibody by microtiter methods. Testing women for antibodies to rubella virus by hemagglutination inhibition has been important in recognizing women at risk for development of the teratogenic effects of in utero rubella infection.

Particle-enhanced light-scattering immunoassays

A very simple method for increasing the sensitivity of immunoassays, such as the agglutination-based techniques, is to follow light scattering of the carrier particles. Three important techniques employing light scattering and agglutination have evolved. These techniques are capable of detecting levels of analytes to nanograms per milliliter, and, thus, they are comparable in sensitivity to radioimmunoassay.

The particle-enhanced immunoassays depend upon either light scattering (nephelometry) or light absorption (turbidimetry) measurements. Ordinarily, the study of antigen-antibody reactions by light scattering or absorption relates to the number of antigen-antibody complexes formed. Optimally, non-particle-based light-scattering immunoassays may be used to perform measurements of analytes in the 1 to 10 μg/ml range.

In the particle-enhanced light-scattering immunoassays, many types of support particles have been employed, including bacteria, erythrocytes, and metal sols. For the most part, polystyrene particles have been used in these assays. Either proteins or hapten molecules may be employed in coating inert particles.

Particle properties affecting these assays include size, concentration, shape, and refractive index. Basically, the rate of reaction depends upon the rate of diffusion of particles. Depending upon the nature of the analyte, agglutination and inhibition particle-enhanced immunoassays may be designed.

The most popular particle-enhanced immunoassays today include the particle-enhanced turbidimetric inhibition immunoassay (PETINIA), particle-counting immunoassays (PACIA), and particle-enhanced quasi-elastic light-scattering spectroscopy (QUELS).

PETINIA

Several different methods based on particulate reagents and turbidity measurements are available (3). Some of these methods employ drug-protein conjugates covalently bound to polystyrene latex particles (4). In the inhibition assay (PETINIA), the conjugate particle and free drug in the assayed sample compete for antidrug antibody. As the concentration of free drug is increased, less antibody is available for aggregation of the particles present in the reaction (inhibition of agglutination), and the turbidity measurement is altered in parallel.

PACIA

PACIAs involve measuring the numbers of particles present in an immunoassay system (2). In PACIA technique, the detection system is based on forward light scattering for sizing of particles flowing through an optical counting cell. Very large and very small particles are ignored by setting the threshold limits of the counting instrument; in this fashion, unagglutin-ated particles may be counted, while large particles are assumed to be aggregates of reacted particles.

To date, applications of PACIA have included measurements of several human serum proteins and drug haptens.

QUELS

In QUELS, a laser beam is employed to measure the mean diffusion constant ($\overline{D}$) of a particle suspension (3). This constant is inversely related to particle size. The QUELS procedures follow changes in $\overline{D}$ as a measurement of agglutination. QUELS has been described for measurement of HCG and luteinizing hormone.

Measurement methods based on light scattering for detection of agglutination of particles are sensitive and reproducible. Of the three methods, turbidimetry is easiest and may be run with standard laboratory spectrophotometric equipment.

The applications of agglutination techniques discussed in this chapter are but a few of the examples of this valuable technology. The agglutination tests show excellent sensitivity and specificity, comparing well with the versatility of other assays. Utility of agglutination methodology is likely to continue in the future.

QUALITY CONTROL

Sensitivity of agglutination tests varies with the antigen used, reagents, etc. (1). Definite differences exist among various commercial products. As with other kinds of immunologic tests, problems arise in agglutination testing due to the presence of cross-reacting and interfering antibodies in test sera. For example, *Brucella* antibodies cross-react with bacteria such as *Francisella*. Heterophile antibodies are particularly troublesome at times, and autoagglutination of particles or erythrocytes may occur in many tests. Control is therefore an absolute necessity in agglutination tests to ensure the quality of the results. Techniques must be standardized to achieve this end. Concentration of antigen, time, temperature, diluent, and the nature of carrier particles must always remain the same for a given test. McFarland standards may be used for opacity reference. Chemical techniques may be necessary for determining the amount of antigen used in tests. Standard reference materials are useful in obtaining consistent results over long periods of time.

Positive and negative control sera are indispensable in monitoring the quality and sensitivity of agglutination tests. Positive sera should be titered so that high and low or borderline reactivities are checked for each run of tests as well as for each new batch of reagents. An autoagglutination control should also be tested, and carrier particles should not react with sera without the presence of antigen. Finally, agglutination tests should be examined identically each time. The endpoint reaction should be standardized in individual laboratories.

LITERATURE CITED

1. **Batty, I.** 1977. Standards and quality control in clinical immunology, p. 219–236. *In* R. A. Thompson (ed.), Tech-

niques in clinical immunology. Blackwell Scientific Publications, Oxford.

2. **Boguslavski, R. C.** 1984. Immunoassays monitored by virus, particle, and metal labels, p. 211–219. *In* R. C. Boguslavski, E. T. Maggio, and R. M. Nakamura (ed.), Clinical immunochemistry: principles of methods and applications. Little, Brown & Co., Boston.

3. **Galvin, J. P.** 1983. Particle enhanced immunoassay—a review, p. 17–30. *In* J. H. Rippey and R. M. Nakamura (ed.), Diagnostic immunology: technology assessment and quality assurance. College of American Pathologists, Skokie, Ill.

4. **Hamil, P. A., J. C. Dickinson, W. A. Frey, J. E. Geltosky, and W. K. Miller.** 1982. Measurement of theophyllin on the DuPont automatic clinical analyzer. Clin. Chem. **28:**1611.

5. **Kwapinski, J. B. G.** 1972. Methodology of immunochemical and immunological research, p. 292. Wiley-Interscience, Inc., New York.

6. **Mohn, J. F., and R. M. Lambert.** 1973. Immunohematologic procedures, p. 71–106. *In* N. R. Rose and P. E. Bigazzi (ed.), Methods in immunodiagnosis. John Wiley & Sons, New York.

7. **Widmann, F. K. (ed.).** 1981. Technical manual, American Association of Blood Banks. J. B. Lippincott Co., Philadelphia.

8. **Williams, C. A., and M. M. Chase (ed.).** 1970. Methods in immunology and immunochemistry, vol. 3, p. 1–125. Academic Press, Inc., New York.

9. **Zmijewski, C. M.** 1978. Immunohematology, 3rd ed., p. 149–180. Appleton-Century-Crofts, New York.

Chapter 10

Complement Fixation Test

DAN F. PALMER AND SHELBA D. WHALEY

For a long time during the "serological era" now passing, the complement fixation test was considered the "emperor" of serodiagnostic assays, largely because it routinely made possible a degree of sensitivity not ordinarily achieved by other methods. In several serological areas, it was the reference test to which other methods were compared. Today, in spite of the recent development of procedures with much higher levels of sensitivity, it is still an important constituent of the viral, rickettsial, and fungal serologist's armamentarium.

When stripped to its bare essentials, the complement fixation test may be viewed as a sequence of two complement titrations: the first performed in the absence of a patient's serum specimen, and also in the absence of test antigen (in the procedure described in this chapter), and the second performed in the presence of these reactants. The difference, if any, between complement activities in the two titrations reflects the amount of complement "fixed" by the patient's antibody reacting with its homologous test antigen.

The procedure requires carefully predetermined concentrations of all components except the unknown immune reactant in the patient's specimen. All aspects of the test must be monitored by numerous controls because of the instability of complement, the biochemical and physical variation of erythrocytes, the immunochemical variation of hemolysin, and the narrow optimal range of diluent components. Of course, the reactions of these controls must be critically evaluated so that the validity of test results can be determined. This is especially important in the diagnostic test, because activity of complement in the presence of the patient's specimen and the test antigen is often enhanced or diminished nonspecifically by constituents of these materials.

The Centers for Disease Control in Atlanta, Ga., has established recommended minimal acceptable standards for hemolysin and complement used in the complement fixation test. Hemolysin should have a minimal optimal titer of 2,000, with no visible agglutination of erythrocytes in hemolysin titration reaction mixtures at hemolysin dilutions above 1:500. No microscopic agglutination should be evident in complement titration reaction mixtures with the dilution of hemolysin selected for sensitizing cells in the test. Complement should have a minimal hemolytic titer so that 0.4 ml of a dilution no more concentrated than 1:100 contains five 50% hemolytic units. Further, when complement is recommended for use in fungal, rickettsial, or viral complement fixation tests, it should be free from antibody against the test antigen when the complement is diluted no greater than 1:8.

All of the necessary controls, as well as the procedures for determining proper concentrations of test components, are described below. The test described is a standardized procedure developed in 1965 by the Centers for Disease Control (3, 4), and it adheres to sound theoretical principles. It is based on the 50% hemolytic unit of complement (CH_{50}) and the "plateau" method of hemolysin titration; it is described as a microtitration test for diagnostic serology.

MATERIALS REQUIRED

Reagents

Working barbital-buffered diluent (BBD)
    Gelatin-water solution
    Stock barbital solution, 5×
Sheep erythrocytes, 2.8% suspension
Hemolysin
Complement
Antigens
Reference sera, positive and negative
Sera from patients

Equipment

Centrifuge with tachometer and carriers for microtitration plates
Water baths, 37 and 56°C
pH meter
Suction apparatus
Centrifuge tubes, 10 and 50 ml
Test tubes, 13 by 100 mm
Microtitration diluters, droppers, and U-plates
Mechanical vibrator
Vortex mixer
Miscellaneous glassware

PREPARATION OF REAGENTS

Note. All chemicals used in this section should be reagent grade or the equivalent. Prepared reagents should be stored in a refrigerator at 4°C. When the test is performed, reagents should be kept in an ice bath to prevent degradation of complement activity.

Gelatin-water solution

1. Add 1 g of gelatin and approximately 300 ml of distilled water to a 1-liter Erlenmeyer flask.
2. Bring the mixture to a boil to dissolve the gelatin (do not boil excessively).
3. Allow the solution to cool, and add sufficient distilled water to bring the final total volume to 800 ml.

Note. Gelatin-water solution should not be used after 1 week of storage at 4°C.

Stock MgCl$_2$-CaCl$_2$ solution

1. Add 20.3 g of $MgCl_2 \cdot 6H_2O$ and 4.4 g of $CaCl_2 \cdot 2H_2O$ to a 100-ml volumetric flask.
2. Add distilled water to the flask to a total volume of 100 ml.
3. Mix by swirling. This makes a 1 M $MgCl_2$–0.3 M $CaCl_2$ solution.

Stock BBD

1. To a 2-liter volumetric flask add 1,500 ml of distilled water.
2. Add 83.0 g of NaCl and 10.19 g of sodium 5,5-diethylbarbiturate.
3. Mix the solution until the chemicals are completely dissolved.
4. Add 34.58 ml of 1 N HCl and mix by swirling.
5. Add 5.0 ml of stock $MgCl_2$-$CaCl_2$ solution.
6. Fill the flask to the 2-liter mark with distilled water and mix.
7. Check the pH as follows. Prepare a 1:5 dilution by adding 1 ml of the stock solution to 4 ml of distilled water, and check the pH. If the pH is below 7.3 or above 7.4, discard the stock solution and prepare a fresh solution.

Working BBD

Note. Working BBD must be made fresh daily.
1. Add 200 ml of stock BBD to a 1-liter flask.
2. Add 800 ml of gelatin-water and mix thoroughly (avoid excessive foaming).
3. Check the pH. If the pH is below 7.3 or above 7.4, discard the BBD and prepare a fresh solution.

STANDARDIZATION OF THE SHEEP ERYTHROCYTE SUSPENSION BY THE SPECTROPHOTOMETRIC METHOD

1. Filter preserved blood through two layers of sterile gauze into a 50-ml conical, graduated centrifuge tube (use only preserved blood which has aged 2 to 5 days).
2. Fill to the 50-ml mark with cold BBD.
3. Centrifuge at $600 \times g$ for 5 min.
4. Remove the supernatant fluid and leukocyte layer by suction.
5. Add cold BBD to fill the tube to the 50-ml mark.
6. Mix gently to resuspend the cells, and centrifuge at $600 \times g$ for 5 min.
7. Carefully remove the supernatant fluid and any remaining leukocytes by suction.
8. Repeat steps 5 through 7 two times for a total of three washes.
Note. Check the supernatant fluid after the second wash to determine if it is colorless. If not, the cells are too fragile and should be discarded. Obtain new blood and return to step 1.
9. Resuspend the cells in cold BBD and transfer the suspension to a graduated centrifuge tube.
10. Centrifuge at $600 \times g$ for 10 min.
11. Read and record the volume of packed cells.
12. Carefully remove the supernatant fluid without disturbing the cells.
13. Calculate the volume of BBD needed for a ca. 4% suspension by multiplying the volume of packed cells by 24.
14. Suspend the cells in the calculated volume of BBD.
15. Swirl gently to secure an even suspension.
16. Carefully pipette 1.0 ml of the ca. 4% suspension into a 25-ml volumetric flask.
17. Fill the flask to the 25-ml mark with cyanmethemoglobin reagent. (Cyanmethemoglobin reagent should be obtained commercially, mixed with 2,000 ml of distilled water, and stored at room temperature in the dark.)
18. Mix the solution well and allow it to stand for 20 min at room temperature.
19. Check the spectrophotometer if the standards were prepared on a previous day. Read the optical density of the 40 mg/100 ml standard and compare the reading with the previous reading for this standard. If the reading is not within 3% of the correct value, check the calibration of the spectrophotometer and, if necessary, prepare new standards and calculate a new target optical density (see Appendix for preparation of cyanmethemoglobin standards and calculation of the target optical density).
20. After 20 min, mix the solution and pour it into a cuvette.
21. Read the optical density of the solution against the reagent blank (0 mg/100 ml) at 540 nm. This value is the test optical density.
22. Calculate the final volume of the desired 2.8% suspension by using the following formula: final total volume = (optical density of test solution) × (original volume of test suspension − 1.0 ml)/(target optical density for a 2.8% suspension).

TITRATION OF THE HEMOLYSIN

Note. A hemolysin titration should be performed each time a new lot of cells or hemolysin is used.

Preparation of hemolysin dilutions

1. Reconstitute or otherwise prepare the hemolysin as instructed in the package insert. Note that 2.0 ml of 50% glycerol-treated hemolysin must be contained in a total of 100 ml to make a 1:100 dilution.
2. Store the 1:100 stock hemolysin dilution in a refrigerator at 4°C.
3. Add 9.0 ml of BBD and 1.0 ml of the 1:100 stock hemolysin dilution to a tube. Mix the solution well, using a Vortex mixer. This is the master 1:1,000 dilution.
4. Label tubes (15 by 125 mm) with the final hemolysin dilutions shown in Table 1.
5. Add the volumes of BBD shown in Table 1 to the respective tubes.
6. Add 1.0 ml of 1:1,000 hemolysin dilution to each tube. Mix the solutions well, using a Vortex mixer.

Preparation of a 1:400 dilution of complement

1. Prepare a 1:10 master dilution of complement by adding 0.1 ml of undiluted cold complement to 0.9 ml of cold BBD in a chilled glass test tube. Mix gently (avoid foaming).

TABLE 1. Preparation of hemolysin dilutions

Final hemolysin dilution	BBD (ml)	1:1,000 hemolysin dilution (ml)
1:1,500	0.5	1.0
1:2,000	1.0	1.0
1:2,500	1.5	1.0
1:3,000	2.0	1.0
1:4,000	3.0	1.0
1:8,000	7.0	1.0

2. Place the 1:10 dilution of complement in a refrigerator and allow it to stand for at least 20 min (complement diluted 1:10 must be kept cold and used within 1 day.)

3. Using a chilled tube, add 0.1 ml of 1:10 complement dilution to 3.9 ml of cold BBD for a 1:400 dilution.

4. Store the 1:400 complement dilution in an ice bath or in the refrigerator for at least 10 min before titrating. The solution must be used within 2 h.

Preparation of sensitized cells for hemolysin titration

1. Place seven tubes (15 by 125 mm) in a rack. Label the first tube 1:1,000, and label the remaining six tubes with the hemolysin dilutions shown in Table 1.

2. Add 1.0 ml of the standardized 2.8% cell suspension to each of the seven tubes.

3. Slowly add, with constant swirling, 1.0 ml of the 1:1,000 hemolysin dilution to the cell suspension in the 1:1,000 tube.

Note. To ensure proper sensitization, always add a hemolysin dilution to constantly swirling sheep cells.

4. For each of the six remaining tubes, mix the corresponding hemolysin dilution and add 1.0 ml to the sheep cells.

5. Shake the rack and incubate the seven tubes in a 37°C water bath for 15 min.

Setting up the hemolysin titration

1. Label seven tubes (13 by 100 mm) with the following hemolysin dilutions: 1:1,000, 1:1,500, 1:2,000, 1:2,500, 1:3,000, 1:4,000, and 1:8,000. Place the tubes in a test tube rack.

2. Add 0.4 ml of cold BBD to each tube.

3. When the 1:400 dilution of complement has been allowed to stand in a refrigerator for at least 10 min, add 0.4 ml of it to each of the seven tubes.

4. Add 0.2 ml of each of the sensitized cell suspensions to the appropriately labeled tube.

5. Mix each tube by shaking, or use a Vortex mixer set for gentle swirling.

6. Incubate the tubes in a 37°C water bath for 1 h; shake the tubes once after the first 30 min of incubation.

Determination of the optimal hemolysin dilution

1. Centrifuge the tubes at $600 \times g$ for 5 min.

2. Compare each tube with the color standards (see Appendix for the procedure for preparing color standards).

Note. Percent hemolysis is best estimated by reading the tubes against a white background illuminated by a daylight-type fluorescent light. If the tube matches a standard, read and record the percent hemolysis. If the tube does not match a standard, interpolate to the nearest 5% and record the reading.

3. Plot on ordinary arithmetic (linear) graph paper the percent hemolysis obtained with each dilution of hemolysin versus the dilution factor (Fig. 1).

4. Draw a line through the points plotted.

5. Examine the graph for a plateau, that is, the level at which increasing the amount of hemolysin produces no marked increase in percent hemolysis (Fig. 1).

Note. Commercial complement diluted 1:400 generally will yield 70 to 90% hemolysis on the plateau. With less active complement, it may be necessary to

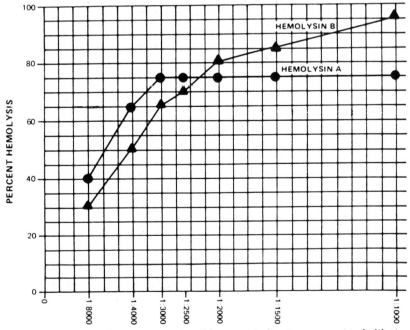

FIG. 1. Hemolysin titration examples, showing an acceptable curve indicating an optimal dilution of 1:2,500 (●) and an unacceptable curve (▲). The hemolysin dilution scale is prepared as follows. Let the left end of the scale be 0, and lay off a suitable length for the 1:1,000 dilution. Other dilutions are represented as fractions of this length. Thus, 1:1,500 = 2/3 of 1:1,000, 1:2,000 = 1/2 of 1:1,000, 1:2,500 = 2/5 of 1:1,000, 1:3,000 = 1/3 of 1:1,000, 1:4,000 = 1/4 of 1:1,000, and 1:8,000 = 1/8 of 1:1,000. Arithmetic graph paper 20 by 20 to the inch is most suitable, with a 6-in. horizontal distance used for the 1:1,000 dilution.

use a 1:300 dilution for the titration. With a very potent complement, it may be necessary to use a 1:500 dilution.

6. Read the second dilution on the plateau as the hemolysin dilution to be used for subsequent cell sensitization.

TITRATION OF THE COMPLEMENT

Note. Complement must be titrated each time an antigen titration or diagnostic test is performed.

Preparation of a 1:400 dilution of complement

Follow the instructions given above under Titration of the Hemolysin to prepare the 1:400 complement dilution.

Preparation of sensitized cells

1. Prepare a volume of the optimal hemolysin dilution slightly greater than half the volume of sensitized cell suspension needed.
2. Pipette a volume of the optimal hemolysin dilution into an equal volume of standardized 2.8% cell suspension, with rapid swirling.
3. Incubate the mixture for 15 min at 37°C in a water bath.

Setting up the complement titration

1. Label two sets of tubes (13 by 100 mm) 1 through 4 for performance of the titration in duplicate.
2. Add cold BBD in the amounts shown in Table 2 to both sets of tubes.
3. Add the 1:400 dilution of complement in the amounts shown in Table 2, and mix.
4. Add 0.2 ml of sensitized cells to each tube.
5. Shake the rack and incubate it in a 37°C water bath for 15 min.
6. After incubation for 15 min, remove the rack and resuspend unlysed cells.
7. Return the rack to the water bath for an additional 15 min to give a total of 30 min of incubation.

Reading the percent hemolysis

1. Centrifuge the tubes at $600 \times g$ for 5 min.
2. Compare each tube in the first set with the color standards. If the tube matches a standard, read and record the percent hemolysis. If the tube does not match a standard, interpolate to the nearest 5% and record the reading.
3. Read and record the percent hemolysis in the duplicate set.
4. Determine the average percent hemolysis for each pair of tubes containing the same volume of complement.

Determination of the volume of complement producing 50% hemolysis

1. Using the table in Fig. 2. read the $y/(100 - y)$ value for the average percent hemolysis of each pair of tubes.
2. Plot on log-log graph paper each volume of the 1:400 dilution of complement in milliliters against the corresponding $y/(100 - y)$ ratio value found in the table (Fig. 2).
3. Examine the graph to see whether two of the points fall on the left side of the vertical "1" line and two fall on the right (one point may fall on the vertical "1" line). If so, continue with step 4. If more than two points fall on the left side of the vertical "1" line, repeat the complement titration with a dilution of complement lower than 1:400 (i.e., 1:300). If more than two points fall on the right side, repeat the titration with a dilution of complement higher than 1:400 (i.e., 1:500).
4. Join the two points plotted for tubes 1 and 2, and find the midpoint of the line joining them.
5. Join the two points plotted for tubes 3 and 4, and find the midpoint of the line joining them.
6. Draw a line between the two midpoints.
7. Determine the slope of the line which joins the two midpoints, as follows. (i) From any point near the left end of the line joining the two midpoints, measure horizontally to a point 10 cm to the right. (ii) Measure the vertical distance in centimeters from that point upward to the line joining the two midpoints. (iii) Divide the vertical distance by 10 cm to obtain the slope. If the slope is 0.20 ± 10%, continue as described below. If the slope is not within ±10% of 0.20, repeat the complement titration.

Determination of the dilution of complement needed

1. From the intersection of the vertical "1" line with the line joining the two midpoints, draw a dotted horizontal line to the vertical axis on the left.
2. Read the volume in milliliters of the 1:400 dilution of complement (this volume contains 1 CH_{50}).
3. Determine the volume containing 5 CH_{50} by multiplying the volume containing 1 CH_{50} by 5 (5 CH_{50} in 0.4 ml is the concentration and volume required for performance of the antigen titration in tubes).
4. Calculate the dilution of complement necessary to obtain 5 CH_{50} in 0.4 ml:

$$\frac{\text{dilution of complement used in titration}}{\text{volume containing 5 } CH_{50}} = \frac{x}{0.4 \text{ ml}}$$

where x is the dilution of complement needed for 5 CH_{50}.

Example. The volume containing 5 CH_{50} at a 1:400 dilution is 1.3 ml (5 × 0.26 ml). The dilution of complement necessary to obtain 5 CH_{50} in 0.4 ml is calculated as follows:

$$\frac{400}{1.3} = \frac{x}{0.4}$$

The dilution of complement (x) is 1:123.

TABLE 2. Complement titration

Reagent	Vol (ml) in tube:			
	1	2	3	4
BBD	0.6	0.55	0.5	0.4
Complement, 1:400	0.2	0.25	0.3	0.4
Sensitized cells	0.2	0.2	0.2	0.2

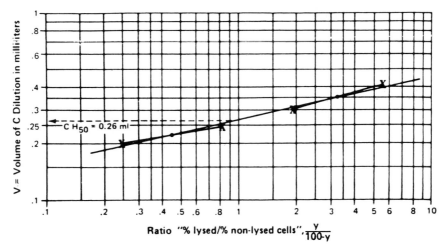

Table for conversion of "% lysed cells," y, to ratio "% lysed cells/% non-lysed cells." $\frac{y}{100-y}$

y	$\frac{y}{100-y}$	y	$\frac{y}{100-y}$	y	$\frac{y}{100-y}$
10	0.111	40	0.67	70	2.33
15	0.176	45	0.82	75	3.00
20	0.25	50	1.00	80	4.0
25	0.33	55	1.22	85	5.7
30	0.43	60	1.50	90	9.0
35	0.54	65	1.86		

Do not graph when "y" exceeds 90% nor when "y" is less than 10%.

FIG. 2. Titration of complement with a 1:400 dilution.

TITRATION OF THE ANTIGEN

Preparation of 1:8 reference antiserum and labeling of tubes

1. Prepare a 1:8 starting dilution of reference antiserum (6.3 ml of BBD plus 0.9 ml of antiserum), and inactivate the antiserum at 56°C for 30 min (the tubes should be covered).
2. Label six tubes for twofold master dilutions of antiserum, e.g., 1:16 through 1:512. (These dilutions of antiserum are examples only. In specific cases, a range of five or six dilutions, including two above and at least two below the known reference antiserum titer, must be used in the antigen titration.)
3. Label seven tubes for twofold test antigen dilutions, 1:2 through 1:128.
4. Label a tube for the known optimal dilution of reference antigen.
5. Label and arrange the tubes for the titration as shown in Table 3.

TABLE 3. Antigen titration example

Sample	% Hemolysis with:									
	Reference antiserum dilution							Complement control		
	1:8	1:16	1:32	1:64	1:128	1:256	1:512	5.0 CH$_{50}$	2.5 CH$_{50}$	1.25 CH$_{50}$
Test antigen[a]										
1:2	0	0	0	20	40	40	70	40	0	0
1:4	0	0	0	0	20	30	70	50	0	0
1:8	0	0	10	40	70	90	100	90	0	0
1:16	0	10	30	70	90	100	100	100	85	0
1:32	0	0	20	50	80	100	100	100	90	20
1:64	0	0	0	0	30[a]	80	100	100	100	50
1:128	0	10	20	40	70	100	100	100	100	50
Serum control	100	100	100	100	100	100	100	100	90	40
Reference antigen control	0	0	0	0	20	70	100	100	90	30
BBD								100	100	50

[a] The optimal test antigen dilution is 1:64, and the antigen is anticomplementary through the 1:8 dilution.

Preparation of further dilutions of reference antiserum

1. Add 3.0 ml of cold BBD to each of the six antiserum dilution tubes.
2. When the 1:8 dilution of antiserum has been inactivated for 30 min and cooled, prepare a 1:16 dilution by adding 3.0 ml of the 1:8 dilution to the BBD in the 1:16 tube; mix.
3. Prepare a 1:32 dilution by adding 3.0 ml of the 1:16 dilution to the BBD in the tube labeled 1:32; mix.
4. Continue preparing twofold master dilutions of antiserum until the 1:512 dilution has been prepared.

Preparation of test antigen dilutions and reference antigen dilution

1. Add 3.0 ml of cold BBD to each of the test antigen dilution tubes.
2. Prepare the starting dilution of 1:2 by adding 3.0 ml of undiluted test antigen to the BBD in the tube labeled 1:2.
3. Prepare further twofold dilutions of test antigen through 1:128 by adding 3.0 ml of the previous dilution of antigen to the BBD.
4. Prepare the known optimal dilution of reference antigen.

Setting up antigen titration

1. Add BBD in the volumes shown in Table 4 to the complement control tubes.
2. Add 0.2 ml of the starting reference serum dilution to each of the three complement-serum control tubes (Table 4).
3. For steps 3 through 7, refer to Table 3 to identify the tubes. Add 0.2 ml of each reference serum dilution to each appropriate test antigen dilution tube, serum control tube, and reference antigen tube.
4. Add 0.2 ml of each test antigen dilution to the seven test antigen dilution tubes and to each of the three complement-test antigen dilution control tubes.
5. Add 0.2 ml of reference antigen to each of the seven reference antigen tubes and to each of the three complement-reference antigen control tubes.

TABLE 4. Preparation of complement control tubes

Control tube and components	Vol (ml)		
	5 CH_{50}	2.5 CH_{50}	1.25 CH_{50}
Complement-diluent			
BBD	0.4	0.6	0.7
Complement	0.4	0.2	0.1
Complement-antigen[a]			
BBD	0.2	0.4	0.5
Antigen	0.2	0.2	0.2
Complement	0.4	0.2	0.1
Complement-serum[b]			
BBD	0.2	0.4	0.5
Serum	0.2	0.2	0.2
Complement	0.4	0.2	0.1

[a] Titrate each dilution of test antigen and the optimal dilution of reference antigen (include tissue antigen controls only when viral and rickettsial antigens are titrated).
[b] Use the starting dilution of reference serum employed in the antigen titration.

6. Add 0.2 ml of cold BBD (instead of antigen) to each of the seven serum control tubes.
7. Add 0.8 ml of BBD to a separate tube and label it cell control.
8. Shake the tubes and let them stand for 15 min at room temperature (22 to 25°C).

Preparation of complement for antigen titration

1. Prepare at least 40 ml of complement at the dilution determined in the complement titration, using a 1:10 dilution of complement prepared earlier.
2. Mix the diluted complement by swirling gently; avoid foaming.
3. Let the diluted complement stand for at least 20 min in an ice bath in a refrigerator.
4. When the complement has been in the refrigerator for at least 20 min, remove it, leaving it in the ice bath.
5. Add 0.4 ml of cold complement dilution (containing 5 CH_{50}) to each tube containing both serum and antigen and to each of the seven serum control tubes. (The cell control tube does not receive complement.)
6. Add the volumes of complement dilution (containing 5 CH_{50}) shown in Table 4 to the complement control tubes.
7. Shake all tubes and place them in a refrigerator for 17 to 18 h. On the following day, continue as described below.

Preparation of sensitized cells

1. Add 12 ml of standardized 2.8% cell suspension to a 50-ml Erlenmeyer flask.
2. Add 12 ml of optimal hemolysin dilution to the cells while swirling the flask rapidly.
3. Incubate the cells for 15 min in a 37°C water bath. While the cells are incubating, continue with steps 4 and 5.
4. Remove the test racks from the refrigerator and allow them to warm to room temperature.
5. Prepare color standards as indicated in the Appendix.
6. When the cells have been in the water bath for 15 min, remove them. Add 0.2 ml of sensitized cells to each tube in the antigen titration, and mix by shaking the racks.
7. Incubate the tubes in a 37°C water bath for 30 min.
8. Prepare record sheets for the titration.

Determination of optimal antigen dilution

1. Examine each tube for incomplete lysis. If a tube does not show complete lysis, centrifuge it at 600 × g for 5 min.
2. Read and record the percent hemolysis of the complement controls, using the color standards. Interpolate to the nearest 5%.
3. Compare the complement control readings with those in Table 5 to determine whether they are acceptable. If the control readings are not acceptable, disregard the test results.
4. Read and record the percent hemolysis of the remaining tubes.
5. Draw a line through the ca. 30% hemolysis endpoints of each antigen dilution. Interpolate where necessary (Table 3). The curve must not be drawn through any anticomplementary antigen dilution.

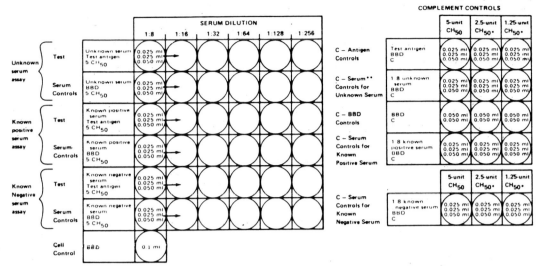

FIG. 3. Diagnostic test: micromethod. *, For 2.5-CH$_{50}$ controls, a 1:2 dilution of the complement (C) containing 5 CH$_{50}$ in 0.05 ml is used. For 1.25-CH$_{50}$ controls, a 1:4 dilution is used. **, Complement-serum controls can be omitted from the routine diagnostic test.

6. Select the dilution giving the greatest amount of fixation as the optimal antigen dilution (the dilution giving the highest titer with the specific antiserum). (i) If two antigen dilutions give identical fixation reactions within the optimal dilution curve, select the dilution which gives greater fixation to the right of the curve. (ii) If two antigen dilutions give identical fixation reactions, select the lower dilution, i.e., the more concentrated one. (iii) The titer of the test antigen with the reference antiserum must be within one twofold dilution of the titer obtained with the reference antigen and the reference antiserum. Note that the reference antiserum must react within one twofold dilution of its known titer when tested with the reference antigen.

Note. Antigens should not be anticomplementary at the dilution selected for use (the optimal dilution). Minimal acceptable titers for reference antisera and antigens have been established. See individual specifications for details (1, 2).

PERFORMANCE OF THE DIAGNOSTIC TEST (MICROMETHOD)

Preparation of 1:8 dilutions of sera

1. Label tubes (13 by 100 mm) for the 1:8 dilutions of unknown sera, known positive serum, and known negative serum.

TABLE 5. Acceptable[a] hemolysis for complement controls

Type of control	% Hemolysis		
	5 CH$_{50}$	2.5 CH$_{50}$	1.25 CH$_{50}$
Complement-BBD	100	90–100	40–75
Complement-antigen(s)	100	85–100	0–75
Complement-antiserum			
Patient	75–100		
Reference	100	90–100	0–75
Control	100	90–100	0–75

[a] Any result less than the range of hemolysis given is considered anticomplementary.

2. Add 0.7 ml of cold BBD to each tube, add 0.1 ml of each serum to its labeled tube, and mix.

3. Inactivate the serum dilutions for 30 min in a 56°C water bath. During this incubation period, label the plates.

Labeling plates for the diagnostic test

Label the rows of wells on plates for the diagnostic test as shown in Fig. 3 (each circle represents a well).

Preparation of twofold dilutions of sera in plates

1. When the 1:8 dilutions have been in the water bath for 30 min, remove them and allow them to cool to room temperature.

2. Use a 0.025-ml dropper to add 0.025 ml of cold BBD to each well which is to contain a serum dilution higher than 1:8.

3. Add 0.05 ml of the 1:8 dilution of unknown serum to the assay wells labeled 1:8 unknown serum.

4. Add 0.05 ml of the 1:8 dilution of known positive serum to the assay wells labeled 1:8 known positive serum.

5. Add 0.05 ml of the 1:8 dilution of known negative serum to the assay wells labeled 1:8 known negative serum.

6. Using 0.025-ml microdiluters, transfer 0.025-ml portions of the 1:8 dilutions to the wells labeled 1:16 dilution; twirl the microdiluters rapidly for 4 s to mix. Repeat this process through the 1:256 dilution of each serum.

Setting up the diagnostic test

1. Add 0.025 ml of the 1:8 dilution of unknown serum to each of the complement-serum controls for unknown serum (this step can be omitted from the routine diagnostic test).

2. Add 0.025 ml of the 1:8 dilution of known positive serum to each of the complement-serum controls for known positive serum.

3. Add 0.025 ml of the 1:8 dilution of known negative serum to each of the complement-serum controls for known negative serum.

Preparation of antigen dilutions (immediately before use)

1. Determine the volume of test antigen required by multiplying the number of wells receiving test antigen by 0.025 ml. Add a 0.5-ml excess for pipetting.

2. Prepare the test antigen at the optimal dilution determined during the antigen titration in tubes, using cold BBD; mix well with a Vortex mixer.

3. Add 0.025 ml of the optimal dilution of test antigen to each well in the test rows and to each well for the complement-antigen control.

4. Add 0.025 ml of cold BBD (instead of antigen) to each serum control well (the volumes in the wells of all assay rows must be equal).

5. Add BBD in the volumes shown in Fig. 3 to each complement control well, using an appropriate dropper pipette.

6. Place the plates on a mechanical vibrator and mix well.

Preparation of diluted complement for the micromethod

Note. Complement activity decreases as the final test volume becomes smaller (4). The dilution of complement containing 5 CH_{50} in 0.4 ml, determined in a complement titration performed in tubes in a total volume of 1.0 ml, can be used for the dilution of complement necessary to contain 5 CH_{50} in 0.05 ml in a total volume of 0.125 ml (micromethod), with the following modification: to achieve an acceptable range of percent hemolysis in the complement-BBD controls (Table 5), compensate for the loss of complement activity due to the reduction of test volume (micromethod) by subtracting 5 to 10 from the complement titer determined in tubes. For example, if a 1:120 complement dilution contains 5 CH_{50} in 0.4 ml, a less diluted complement (1:115 to 1:110) should contain 5 CH_{50} in 0.5 ml (micromethod).

1. Determine the volume of diluted complement required by multiplying the number of wells to contain 5 CH_{50} by 0.05 ml. Add several milliliters for pipetting and for preparation of the controls containing 2.5 and 1.25 CH_{50}.

2. Calculate the volumes of BBD and complement needed to prepare the required volume of complement at the dilution containing 5 CH_{50} in 0.05 ml.

3. Add the calculated volume of BBD to a small flask.

4. Add the calculated volume of complement dropwise to the BBD. (It is permissible to return to the 1:10 dilution of complement to make up this final dilution.)

5. Allow the diluted complement to stand in an ice bath or in the refrigerator for each least 20 min.

6. Prepare a 1:2 dilution of the diluted complement containing 5 CH_{50} in 0.05 ml. (i) Determine the volume of 1:2 dilution needed by multiplying the number of wells for the 2.5-CH_{50} controls by 0.05 ml. Add a 0.4-ml excess for pipetting. (ii) Calculate the volumes of BBD and complement needed to prepare the required volume of 1:2 dilution. (iii) Add diluted complement (containing 5 CH_{50} in 0.05 ml) dropwise to the calculated volume of cold BBD. (iv) Mix gently; avoid foaming.

7. Prepare the same volume of 1:4 dilution for the 1.25-CH_{50} controls.

Addition of complement to the test

1. Use a 0.05-ml dropper pipette to add 0.05 ml of diluted complement containing 5 CH_{50} to each assay well and to each 5-CH_{50} complement control well.

2. With a clean 0.05-ml dropper pipette, add 0.05 ml of the 1:2 dilution of complement to each 2.5-CH_{50} complement control well.

3. With another clean 0.05-ml dropper pipette, add 0.05 ml of the 1:4 dilution of complement to each 1.25-CH_{50} complement control well.

4. Using a mechanical vibrator, mix the contents of each plate after all complement has been added.

5. Stack the plates one on top of the other; place an empty plate on top of the stack as a cover.

6. Incubate the plates in a refrigerator at 4 to 6°C for 17 to 18 h. On the following day, continue as described below.

Preparation of sensitized cells

1. Determine the volume of sensitized cells needed for the test by multiplying the total number of wells in the test by 0.025 ml and adding at least 1.0 ml excess for pipetting.

2. Remove the standardized cell suspension from the refrigerator, and swirl it gently to secure an even suspension.

3. To a small flask, add a volume of standardized cells equal to half the volume of sensitized cells needed.

4. Add an equal volume of optimal hemolysin dilution to the standardized cells, with rapid swirling of the cells.

5. Incubate the cells in a 37°C water bath for 15 min.

6. Remove the test plates from the refrigerator.

7. Prepare 0, 30, 50, 70, 90, and 100% color standards (see Appendix).

8. Use a 0.025-ml dropper pipette to add 5 drops of each of the color standards listed in step 7 to the plate(s) containing the complement controls.

9. Add 0.025 ml of sensitized cells to each well except the color standard wells.

10. Seal each plate with transparent plastic tape.

11. Place the plates on a mechanical vibrator, and mix well to ensure an even suspension of the sensitized cells.

12. Incubate the plates in a 37°C water bath (by floating) for 30 min. A 37°C incubator may be used if necessary. Do not stack the plates.

Reading and recording test results

1. Centrifuge the plates for 3 min at 300 × *g*. If centrifuge carriers are not available, let the plates stand in a refrigerator for 2 to 3 h until the cells settle.

2. Read and record the complement controls by comparison with the color standards.

3. Compare the complement control readings with those in Table 5 to see whether they are acceptable. If the controls are not acceptable, disregard the test results and repeat the test. (If either BBD or complement-antigen controls are not acceptable, disregard all test results. If serum controls [1:8 dilution] on a single serum are unacceptable, the serum is anticomplementary and test results on this particular serum should be read with caution. If there is a definite difference between the anticomplement activity and the specific titer [i.e., anti-complement activity greater than fourfold less than specific titer], the serum may be reported as positive with the reservation that the titer is only approximate.)

4. If the complement control readings are acceptable, read and record the percent hemolysis in each well in the test.

Note. Each dilution of patient's serum yielding hemolysis of ≤30% is considered positive for antibody (with the restrictions stated above in parentheses).

APPENDIX

Preparation of Cyanmethemoglobin Standards and Calculation of the Target Optical Density (Absorbance)

Preparation of standards

1. Label five cuvettes for standards of 80, 60, 40, 20, and 0 mg/100 ml.
2. Add to the tubes the volumes of 80 mg/100 ml standard and cyanmethemoglobin reagent shown in Table 6.
3. Wrap five cork stoppers in Parafilm-M, and plug each cuvette.
4. Mix by inverting each cuvette.

Calculation of factor

1. Wipe each cuvette with a tissue to remove fingerprints; then read and record the optical density for each standard at 540 nm.
2. The sum of the cyanmethemoglobin concentrations of all the standards equals 200 mg per 100 ml.
3. Take the sum of the optical density readings of all the standards.
4. To calculate the factor, divide the sum of the concentrations by the sum of the optical density readings.

Calculation of target optical density

Use the factor to calculate the target optical density of the instrument for a 2.8% sheep erythrocyte suspen-

TABLE 6. Preparation of cyanmethemoglobin standards

Tube	Cyanmethemoglobin concn (mg/100 ml)	80 mg/100 ml standard (ml)	Cyanmethemoglobin reagent (ml)
1	80	4	0
2	60	3	1
3	40	2	2
4	20	1	3
5	0 (blank)	0	4

TABLE 7. Preparation of color standards

% Hemolysis	Hemoglobin solution (ml)	0.28% cell suspension (ml)
0	0.0	1.0
10	0.1	0.9
20	0.2	0.8
30	0.3	0.7
40	0.4	0.6
50	0.5	0.5
60	0.6	0.4
70	0.7	0.3
80	0.8	0.2
90	0.9	0.1
100	1.0	0.0

sion. Use the following formula: target optical density = (35.04 mg of cyanmethemoglobin per 100 ml)/factor

Preparation of Hemoglobin Color Standards

Preparation of hemoglobin solution

1. Use a 2.0-ml pipette to add 1.0 ml of a well-mixed 2.8% erythrocyte suspension to a test tube (15 by 125 mm).
2. Add 7.0 ml of distilled water, and shake the tube until all erythrocytes are lysed.
3. Add 2.0 ml of stock buffer solution to the tube.
4. Mix the hemoglobin solution thoroughly and set it aside until it is needed.

Preparation of 0.28% erythrocyte suspension

1. Remove the 2.8% erythrocyte suspension from the refrigerator, and shake the flask gently to secure an even suspension.
2. Use a 2.0-ml pipette to add 1.0 ml of the 2.8% suspension to a test tube (15 by 125 mm).
3. Add 9.0 ml of cold BBD to the tube with the 2.8% erythrocytes.
4. Mix the 0.28% erythrocyte suspension and set it aside.

Preparation of color standards

1. Label 11 tubes (13 by 100 mm) with the percentages of hemolysis shown in Table 7. Label the 0% standard with the date and time of preparation.
2. Use a 2.0-ml pipette to add hemoglobin solution in the amounts shown in Table 7.
3. Use a 2.0-ml pipette to add the 0.28% cell suspension in the amounts shown in Table 7.
4. Mix the standards by shaking the rack.
5. Centrifuge the tubes at $600 \times g$ for 5 min.
6. Remove the tubes from the centrifuge without agitation, and store them in a refrigerator at 4°C until they are needed.

LITERATURE CITED

1. **Centers for Disease Control.** 1975. Specifications and evaluation methods for immunological and microbiological reagents, vol. 1. Bacterial, fungal and parasitic. Centers for Disease Control, Atlanta, Ga.

2. **Centers for Disease Control.** 1975. Specifications and evaluation methods for immunological and microbiological reagents, vol. 2. Chlamydial, mycoplasmal and viral. Centers for Disease Control, Atlanta, Ga.

3. **Palmer, D. F.** 1981. A guide to the performance of the standardized diagnostic complement fixation method and adaptation to micro test. Centers for Disease Control, Atlanta, Ga.

4. **U.S. Public Health Service.** 1965. Standardized diagnostic complement fixation method and adaptation to micro test. U.S. Public Health Service Publ. 1228 (Public Health Monogr. 74).

Chapter 11

Neutralization Assays

STEPHEN M. PETERS AND JOSEPH A. BELLANTI

Neutralization refers to the loss of infectivity of a microorganism, e.g., a virus, or the loss of toxicity of a product of a microorganism, e.g., a toxin, after its interaction with specific antibody.

Toxin neutralization, the ability of specific antibody to neutralize toxin, forms one of the oldest of serological reactions. It can be demonstrated in vitro or in vivo. The serum to be tested is first added to a potent toxin in vitro and then injected into a living animal or cell culture system. The survival of the animal or the continued viability of a cell culture is used as an index of toxin neutralization and will occur when antibody (antitoxin) is present in the test serum. On certain occasions, when a toxin is mixed in vitro with its specific antiserum, visible precipitation or flocculation will occur because of toxin-antitoxin formation (9). The Schick test for the detection of antibody to diphtheria toxin and the Dick test for the detection of antibody to erythrogenic toxin of group A beta-hemolytic streptococcus are examples of in vivo toxin neutralization and are discussed in chapter 65.

The neutralization test is also employed for the measurement of antibody to a wide variety of viral agents and represents one of the most sensitive, specific, and clinically significant serological tests available. Shown in Table 1 is a list of serological procedures commonly employed for the detection of viruses or their products. The table indicates the use of neutralization tests in the context of other assays such as complement fixation and hemagglutination inhibition procedures. Virus-neutralizing antibody measured in this way correlates very well with protection and is the measurement commonly employed by several federal regulatory agencies in establishing the potency of many biological agents, e.g., diphtheria and tetanus toxins, and the measles antibody content in gamma globulin preparations.

CLINICAL INDICATIONS

Microbial toxins, by causing cell and tissue damage, are responsible to various degrees for the clinical manifestations of infection. The classic exotoxins of *Clostridium tetani*, *C. botulinum*, *Vibrio cholerae*, and *Corynebacterium diphtheriae* are elaborated proteins with enzyme activity. The prime defense of the host against exotoxins is through neutralization by specific antibody (antitoxin). This detoxification process leads to the production of toxin-antitoxin complexes that are usually removed by phagocytic degradation. However, under conditions of antigen excess, these complexes can be injurious to the host and lead to immunologically mediated disease, e.g., serum sickness.

Endotoxins, which are components of the cell wall of gram-negative bacteria, exhibit more generalized effects on the host. These effects include pyrogen release by polymorphonuclear leukocytes, resulting in fever; leukopenia caused by destruction of polymor-phonuclear leukocytes; and the initiation of the coagulation sequence, resulting in intravascular coagulation and sometimes shock. Although endotoxins evoke species-specific antibody, unlike exotoxins, there appears to be no neutralization of their toxic effect.

Neutralization tests for determining antitoxin levels are rarely performed in the diagnostic laboratory because of their complexity and the lack of clinical demand. Tests of neutralizing antibody for viruses, on the other hand, represent an important measurement of protective antibody and are commonly performed in diagnostic virology laboratories.

The virus neutralization test detects antibody which blocks the infectivity of a virus particle. Of the types of antibody produced, e.g., precipitating, complement fixing, and hemagglutination inhibition, the production of neutralizing antibody is the most specific antibody reaction against viruses. Because of this specificity, tests of virus neutralization are employed in two ways: (i) for the identification of putative agents isolated from the patient and (ii) for the determination of a specific viral illness by the rise in antibody titer observed in paired sera. Since neutralization antibody can persist for years, neutralization tests are also useful in serological epidemiology, where one is interested in knowing which viral agents have infected a given population in the past.

TOXIGENICITY TESTS FOR *CORYNEBACTERIUM DIPHTHERIAE*

The demonstration of toxin production is an essential prerequisite for the identification of *C. diphtheriae*. The toxigenicity tests may be performed by two methods, i.e., an in vitro agar plate technique and an in vivo guinea pig test. If the isolate is toxigenic and the species is confirmed by cultural, morphological, and biochemical characteristics, the toxin can then be screened by titration to determine its approximate potency so it can be used in the rabbit model for measuring diphtheria antitoxin in sera, as described below under Toxin Neutralization Tests.

In vitro test

At the Centers for Disease Control and many state health laboratories in the United States, a modification of the Elek method (2) is used. For this procedure, an autoclaved and cooled (48°C) basal medium, such as Difco Proteose Peptone agar (Difco Laboratories, Detroit, Mich.), is poured into a petri dish that contains a nonserous enrichment (Tween 80, glycerol, and Casamino Acids) and 1 ml of 0.3% potassium tellurite. The medium is then thoroughly mixed. Just before the agar hardens, a sterile filter paper strip (1.5 by 7 cm) which has been saturated in diphtheria antitoxin diluted to 100 U/ml is gently pressed into place on the agar surface with sterile forceps. To ensure a mois-

TABLE 1. Procedures for diagnosis of viral infections

| Virus | Identification of virus or its antigens | | | | Demonstration of antibody response | |
| | Recovery of virus | | Detection[a] | | | |
	Method[b]	Efficiency	Method	Efficiency	Method	Efficiency
Togaviruses[c]						
SLE, EEE, VEE, and WEE	TC	Good			CF, HI, SN	Good
Arenaviruses						
Lassa	TC	Good	IF	Good	IF, SN	Good
Lymphocytic choriomeningitis	Mice	Good			IF, SN	Good
Enteric viruses						
Coxsackievirus	TC, mice	Good			SN, CF	Good
Echovirus	TC, mice	Fair			SN	Good
Poliovirus	TC	Good			SN	Good
Rotavirus			IEM, ELISA	Good	IF, CF, ELISA	Good
Respiratory viruses						
Adenovirus	TC	Good	IF, EM	Fair	CF, SN, HI	Good
Coronavirus	OC, TC	Poor			CF, SN, III	Fair
Influenza	Eggs, TC	Good	IF	Good	HI, CF	Good
Mumps	TC	Good			CF, HI, SN	Good
Parainfluenza	TC	Good	IF	Good	CF, HI	Good
Respiratory syncytial	TC	Good	IF, ELISA	Good	CF, SN, ELISA	Good
Rhinovirus	TC	Good			SN	Good
Herpesviruses						
Herpes simplex 1 and 2	TC	Good	IF	Fair	SN, HI, ELISA	Good
Varicella-zoster	TC	Good	IF	Fair	SN, IF	Good
Cytomegalovirus	TC	Fair	EM	Low	CF, IF, ELISA	Good
Epstein-Barr	LC	Low	EM	Low	IF	Good
Exanthematous viruses						
Rubella	TC	Fair			HI, IF	Good
Rubeola	TC	Poor	IF	Fair	HI, CF, IF	Good
Variola-vaccinia	Eggs, TC	Good	EM, IF	Good	HI, CF	Fair
Hepatitis viruses						
Hepatitis A			IEM	Fair	ELISA, RIA	Good
Hepatitis B			RIA	Good	ELISA, RIA	Good

[a] By visualization or immunological technique.

[b] TC, Tissue culture; IF, immunofluorescence; EM, electron microscopy; IEM, immunoelectron microscopy; HI, hemagglutination inhibition; CF, complement fixation; SN, serum neutralization; RIA, radioimmunoassay; OC, organ culture; LC, lymphoma culture; ELISA, enzyme-linked immunosorbent assay.

[c] SLE, St. Louis encephalitis; EEE, Eastern equine encephalitis; VEE, Venezuelan equine encephalitis; WEE, Western equine encephalitis.

ture-free surface, the plate is then placed in a 37°C incubator to dry. Inoculation of the plate should be performed within 2 h after drying.

A loopful of the culture of suspected *C. diphtheriae* from growth on a slant of Loeffler or Pai medium or from suspicious colonies growing on tellurite plates is then streaked across the plate, perpendicular to the paper strip, in a single line. Five test cultures and positive and negative controls may be tested on a single plate without crowding, and each culture should be spaced about 1 cm from the preceding strip. The positive control culture is usually a stock strain of *C. diphtheriae* biotype intermedius.

The plate is incubated at 37°C for 1 to 3 days; toxigenic strains will show a positive reaction within 24 to 48 h after incubation. If toxin has been produced, it will have diffused into the medium and, at the regions of optimal proportions with the antitoxin, will have produced a thin white line of precipitate extending radially from the line of bacterial growth at an angle of approximately 45°C. If the strain is nontoxigenic, no lines of precipitation will occur. The lines are usually visible to the naked eye and can easily be read by transmitted light against a dark background. *C. diphtheriae* strains that are negative in vitro should be tested in an animal model.

In vivo test

The guinea pig test is carried out as follows.

1. Inoculate 12 ml of heart infusion broth with a suspected strain of *C. diphtheriae* which has been grown overnight on a Loeffler slant or on Pai medium.

2. Allow the broth to incubate at 37°C for 48 to 72 h. Turbidimetric measurements may be performed to ensure adequate growth, i.e., the attainment of a density of 3 on the McFarland turbidity standard. Heavy growth as judged by the naked eye is also sufficient.

3. Fill a 10-ml syringe fitted with a 22-gauge needle with the broth culture, which serves as the test inoculum.

4. Obtain two guinea pigs weighing approximately 300 g each. Shave or clip an area about 3 cm in diameter on the abdomen of each animal, and disinfect the area with 70% alcohol.

5. Inject one animal, which serves as the protected control, intraperitoneally with 250 U of diphtheria antitoxin.

6. After 1 to 2 h, inject both the control and the second guinea pig (unprotected) subcutaneously in the prepared area with 5 ml of the test inoculum.

7. If the strain is toxigenic, the unprotected guinea pig will die within 1 to 4 days or will have an area of

necrosis or inflammation at the injection site, and the protected guinea pig (receiving antitoxin) will not exhibit ill effects. If neither animal demonstrates an ill effect or shows any evidence of local necrosis, the suspected organism is nontoxigenic and may not be *C. diphtheriae*.

TOXIGENICITY TEST FOR *CLOSTRIDIUM TETANI*

To test for toxin production (3), inoculate two tubes of chopped meat medium with the organism after identification by cultural, morphological, and biochemical characteristics. Incubate both tubes at 35 to 37°C, one for 24 h and the other for 72 h, and test each tube separately for toxin production. Pipette 3 ml of culture supernatant into a 12-ml plastic centrifuge tube, and centrifuge at $12,350 \times g$ for 10 min. Fill a 1-ml syringe with 0.8 ml of the centrifuged culture fluid, and inoculate each of two 15- to 20-g mice intraperitoneally with 0.4 ml. The animals should be observed over a period of 1 week, although symptoms of flaccid paralysis followed by death usually occur in 2 to 4 days if toxin is being produced by the organism.

If the *Clostridium* culture fluid is toxic for the mice, animal protection tests with specific immune serum will confirm the identification of the organism. Neutralization of toxic culture fluid is usually accomplished by mixing 0.3 ml of specific *C. tetani* antitoxin, allowing the mixture to stand for 30 min at 37°C, and inoculating each of two mice intraperitoneally with 0.5 ml of the material.

TOXIN NEUTRALIZATION TESTS

Two highly specific types of in vivo tests of toxin neutralization are available, i.e., the rabbit intracutaneous test for detecting diphtheria antitoxin and the mouse toxin neutralization test for tetanus antitoxin determinations. For both of these tests, a preliminary procedure is to determine the appropriate test dose of the toxin sample employed by titrating it against a sample of standard antitoxin. Crude culture filtrates or partially purified preparations of diphtheria and tetanus toxins prepared in the laboratory are satisfactory for use in antitoxin titrations. Diphtheria and tetanus toxins are not available commercially; however, they may be obtained from pharmaceutical firms engaged in the manufacture of diphtheria and tetanus toxoids. On the other hand, International Standards of Diphtheria and Tetanus Antitoxin are available from the Bureau of Biologics, Food and Drug Administration, Rockville, Md.

Titration of diphtheria antitoxin in sera

The potency of an antitoxin is expressed in antibody units (AU). The appropriate test dose of diphtheria toxin is determined by titration against a standard antitoxin. In the method first described by Jensen (4), the dose of toxin is the Limes reacting dose (Lr)/20,000. The Lr is that amount of toxin which, when mixed with 1 AU of diphtheria antitoxin and injected intracutaneously, will stimulate a minimal area of redness. Therefore, the Lr/20,000 is that quan-

tity of toxin which will stimulate the same minimal area of redness in the presence of 1/20,000 AU. The general procedure, which is described in detail in chapter 65, requires that 0.5 ml of standard diphtheria antitoxin be added to serial dilutions of toxin which encompass the expected Lr/20,000 endpoint. The mixtures are incubated for 1 h at 37°C and then injected into the backs of rabbits in a randomized pattern. Three days after injection, the diameters of redness are measured in millimeters and plotted on graph paper against the log of the toxin. The interpretation of the test is that an erythema diameter of 8 mm represents the Lr/20,000.

After the determination of the Lr/20,000, diphtheria antitoxin levels in sera can be measured. Serial dilutions of inactivated sera are mixed with equal volumes of diphtheria toxin containing 20 Lr/20,000 per ml and injected into rabbits. The areas of erythema elicited by the toxin-serum mixtures are then averaged, and the antitoxin content of the serum is expressed as a range, i.e., the serum dilution which neutralizes the Lr/20,000.

Titration of tetanus antitoxin in sera

Titration of antitoxin in sera, which is the most sensitive system available to detect tetanus antitoxin, determines the neutralizing capacity of tetanus antibody to protect mice from death after a subcutaneous injection of tetanus toxin. The procedure is described in chapter 65 and follows the method of Barile et al. (1). As with diphtheria antitoxin, the tetanus toxin is initially titrated against a standard tetanus antitoxin to obtain the Limes toxin dose (L+)/1,000. The L+/1,000 is defined as that amount of tetanus toxin which, when mixed with 1/1,000 AU of antitoxin, causes the death of mice 96 h after subcutaneous injection. The L+/1,000 is obtained by mixing equal volumes of antitoxin containing 0.004 AU/ml with a narrow range of three- to fivefold dilutions of tetanus toxin. The mixtures are incubated for 1 to 3 h at 37°C and injected into the inguinal fold of panels of mice, which are then monitored for death during a 96-h period. The smallest dose of toxin which kills all of the mice is considered the appropriate L+/1,000 to use in the serum titration of the test sera.

In the determination of the antitoxin level in test sera, constant volumes of 10-fold dilutions of heat-inactivated serum are mixed with equal volumes of the L+/1,000 and incubated for 1 to 3 h at room temperature. Panels of mice are then injected subcutaneously in the inguinal fold and observed for 4 days. The serum titration endpoint (AU per milliliter) is routinely taken as that value between the dilution at which all animals die or survive.

VIRUS NEUTRALIZATION TEST

The high degree of immunological specificity of the antigen-antibody reaction permits the application of the virus neutralization test to two types of biological inquiries. The first type of inquiry is for determining the identity or antigenic relationship of a virus, and the second is for determining the level of antibody production after infection or immunization.

Identification of viruses in cell cultures

Upon receiving a patient specimen in the laboratory for virus isolation and identification, three types of culture cells (primary, semicontinuous, and continuous) are inoculated. These cells provide a wide range of virus susceptibility. They are as follows:

Primary cell culture
    Rhesus monkey kidney cells (RMK)
    African green monkey kidney cells (AGMK)
Semicontinuous
    Human embryonic lung fibroblasts (WI-38)
Continuous
    Human epidermoid carcinoma (HEp-2)

Depending upon availability and the virus isolate recovered, embryonated hen eggs and suckling mice are also employed for viral isolation.

During incubation the cell cultures are observed for viral cytopathic effect (CPE) and read on a scale of 1+ (25% with localized areas of cell alteration) to 4+ (almost complete cellular degeneration, with 75 to 100% CPE).

Identification of the virus isolate at a 50% tissue culture dose (TCD_{50}), which is determined by the Reed-Muench method (8), is performed against a composition of immune serum pools, including the A and B coxsackieviruses, echoviruses, and poliovirus types 1, 2, and 3. Antisera to other viruses, e.g., respiratory viruses, are employed in these situations.

Neutralization test for enteroviruses

Reagents
Human embryonic kidney cell cultures or monkey kidney cell cultures
Cell maintenance medium (minimal essential medium) supplemented with 2% inactivated fetal bovine serum, 100 U of penicillin per ml, 100 μg of streptomycin per ml, and 500 μg of neomycin per ml
Virus isolate from patient specimen, 100 TCD_{50}/0.2 ml
Lim–Benyesh-Melnick enterovirus immune serum pools (5–7), 20 AU/0.2 ml (Research Reagents Branch, National Institute of Allergy and Infectious Diseases, Bethesda, Md.).

Procedure
1. Prepare all eight serum pools to contain 20 AU/0.2 ml in minimal essential medium.
2. The unknown isolate should be diluted to contain 100 TCD_{50}/0.2 ml (see above).
3. Mix 0.2 ml of each serum pool with 0.2 ml of the diluted isolate.
4. Shake and incubate the virus-serum mixture at 37°C for 1 h.
5. Prepare two more 10-fold dilutions of the unknown isolate from the 100 TCD_{50} dilution.
6. Inoculate 0.2 ml of each virus-serum mixture into two primary kidney cell culture tubes.
7. Inoculate 0.2 ml of the three virus dilutions into two cell cultures. These are the virus controls. Include one uninoculated cell culture tube as a normal control.
8. Add 1.5 ml of the cell maintenance medium to all the inoculated tubes, the three virus controls, and one normal uninoculated kidney cell control.

9. Incubate the cultures at 37°C for 3 days, observing daily for neutralization of CPE. The virus controls indicate the TCD_{50} of virus used in the test.

Interpretation. The tubes containing the virus and its homologous immune serum will not show CPE, whereas those containing heterologous sera will show virus activity. The virus control tubes indicate the titer of the virus and prove that the dilution used in the test contained 100 TCD_{50} of the virus. The identity of the virus is confirmed by a neutralization test against the type-specific immune sera.

Measurements of neutralizing antibody in serum

The basic method for assaying the virus neutralizing activity of serum consists of mixing the serum with virus and incubating the mixture in a susceptible host system in which the presence of unneutralized virus may be detected. The level in serum of neutralizing antibody to a given viral agent can be determined by using a constant amount of virus and various concentrations of serum. This technique is more useful for demonstrating significant increases in antibody levels than in certain instances where constant amounts of serum are tested against various concentrations of virus. To establish a diagnosis, one must be able to show a significant rise in neutralizing antibody for a given virus between acute- and convalescent-phase serum specimens collected from the patient.

Assays in monolayer tube cultures
1. Inactivate the unknown serum (or known immune serum) at 56°C for 30 min to destroy heat-labile nonspecific virus-inhibitory substances.
2. Prepare fourfold serum dilutions (1:16, 1:64, 1:256, and 1:1,024) in the cell maintenance medium (minimal essential medium supplemented with 2% fetal bovine serum, 100 U of penicillin per ml, and 100 μg of streptomycin per ml).
3. Dilute the virus to contain 100 TCD_{50} in a volume of 0.1 ml of minimal essential medium (as described above under Identification of viruses in cell cultures).
4. Mix 0.1 ml of the serum dilutions with 0.1 ml of the test virus dilutions. The volume of serum-virus mixture prepared is dependent on the number of cell cultures to be inoculated.
5. Prepare a "virus control" by mixing a volume of test virus dilution with an equal volume of diluent (or known "normal" serum). Incubate this mixture under the same conditions as the serum-virus mixture. In the neutralizing-antibody assay, it is necessary to perform a concurrent titration of the virus to establish that the test dose actually contained approximately 100 TCD_{50}.
6. Incubate the serum-virus mixture for 1 h at room temperature.
7. Inoculate the mixture and virus controls in a volume of 0.2 ml into at least two monolayer tube cultures.
8. Incubate the inoculated cultures at 37°C and examine daily with a microscope for evidence of the ability of the serum to inhibit CPE of the virus.
9. In the constant virus-varied serum system, the antibody titer is expressed as the highest serum dilution which neutralizes the test dose of virus.

CONCLUDING REMARKS

Most clinical laboratories are not commonly called upon to perform tests of either diphtheria or tetanus toxin neutralization, primarily because specific therapy of patients with diphtheria or tetanus is begun at once and is based on clinical findings. Consequently, convalescence determinations are of little value in the diagnosis retrospectively and are generally used for epidemiological studies, i.e., where the history of absence of diphtheria vaccination shows clusters in certain socioeconomic populations. Although the rabbit intracutaneous test and the mouse neutralization test are extremely time consuming to perform, both assays have been shown to be very reliable and very precise in antibody measurement and methods of choice.

Virus neutralization tests, although simple in principle, are expensive in time and materials and may be difficult to interpret because of the variability in the titration endpoint and the possible nonspecificity of the neutralization. The technique of performing the test for neutralizing antibodies must be standardized for each viral agent within a laboratory to have valid comparisons of titers. Among the variables which must be considered are (i) the selection of the experimental animal, embryonated egg, or cell culture, (ii) the relative heat stability of the specific antibody and of possible interfering substances in serum, (iii) the use of one concentration of virus and various dilutions of serum, or vice versa, (iv) the temperature of the neutralizing mixture, and (v) the time at which CPE is read.

LITERATURE CITED

1. **Barile, M. F., M. C. Hardegree, and M. Pittman.** 1970. Immunization against neonatal tetanus in New Guinea. 3. The toxin neutralization test and the response of guinea pigs to the toxoids as used in the immunization schedules in New Guinea. Bull. W.H.O. **43:**453–459.
2. **Bickman, S. T., and W. L. Jones.** 1972. Problems in the use of the in vitro toxigenicity test for *Corynebacterium diphtheriae.* Am. J. Clin. Pathol. **57:**244–246.
3. **Dowell, V. R., and T. M. Hawkins.** 1979. Detection of clostridial toxins, toxin neutralization tests, and pathogenicity tests, p. 15–16. *In* Laboratory methods in anaerobic bacteriology. HEW publication no. 79-8272. Center for Disease Control, Atlanta.
4. **Jensen, C.** 1933. Die intrakutane kanin chen Methods zur Auswetung von diphtherie Toxin und Antitoxin. Acta Pathol. Microbiol. Scand., vol. 10, suppl. 14.
5. **Lim, K. A., and M. Benyesh-Melnick.** 1960. Typing of viruses by combinations of antiserum pools. Application to typing enteroviruses (coxsackie and echo). J. Immunol. **84:**309–317.
6. **Melnick, J. L., and B. Hampil.** 1970. WHO collaborative studies on enterovirus antisera, third report. Bull. W.H.O. **42:**847–863.
7. **Melnick, J. L., and B. Hampil.** 1973. WHO collaborative studies on enterovirus antisera, fourth report. Bull. W.H.O. **48:**381–396.
8. **Reed, L. J., and H. Muench.** 1938. A simple method of estimating fifty per cent endpoints. Am. J. Hyg. **27:**493–497.
9. **Zmijewski, C. M., and J. A. Bellanti.** 1985. Antigen-antibody interactions, p. 160–175. *In* J. A. Bellanti, Immunology III. The W. B. Saunders Co., Philadelphia.

Chapter 12

Cytolytic Assays for Soluble Antigens

PAULA J. ROMANO

In vitro assays which measure cytotoxicity can be divided into two general categories: (i) those which are independent of complement for a lytic effect and (ii) those which proceed only in the presence of complement. The first group of reactions comprises T-cell-mediated lysis, natural killing, and antibody-dependent cellular cytotoxicity (ADCC), whereas the latter group consists mainly of complement-dependent cytotoxicity with its many variations.

These clinical assays share several basic characteristics. All cytotoxic reactions proceed by virtue of an interaction with an antigen on the cell surface membrane. Specific recognition of this antigen must occur either by combination with antibody or through analogous recognition structures on other cells. Peripheral blood lymphocytes are generally used as target cells since they are easy to obtain. However, other cell types (e.g., derived from tumor tissue) are also used as target cells when the antigens under study are present on their surfaces. In many cases, continuous cell lines derived from the particular tissue are often preferred because of ease of procurement and standardization.

CELL SURFACE MEMBRANES

The cell surface membrane is a dynamic three-dimensional interface between the intracellular and extracellular environments of a cell. Besides maintaining the physical and metabolic integrity of the cell, this surface membrane is an elaborate sensory device capable of detecting environmental signals and translating them into internal signals which then induce, alter or regulate cellular activity. Since receipt and translation of signals are initially cell surface phenomena, these functions are dependent upon the existence of membrane-associated "receptors." Multiple receptor types can be identified on individual specialized cells. Moreover, separate receptors for different signals coexist on the same cell and communicate intracellularly through common chemical messengers (e.g., cyclic AMP).

Structural analysis

Functionally differentiated cells all have their own spectrum of surface receptors which demonstrate their potential diversity. Lymphoid cell differentiation begins in the primary lymphoid organs and continues in the peripheral tissues, bringing about distinctive changes of cell surface molecules which are recognized as markers of the various subpopulations of T and B cells. Some of these surface components which change with differentiation are actually antigenic (e.g., immunogenic or capable of eliciting an immune response in another individual). These surface antigens have been termed differentiation antigens, implying that changes in the life history of a cell are accompanied by concomitant changes in structures at the cell surface. Many of these differentiation antigens are alloantigens (i.e., antigens which differ among members of the same species). Other cell surface molecules, not normally immunogenic, serve as distinct binding sites for physiological or structural components, or both, and generally are referred to as lymphocyte surface receptors.

Functional analysis

The way in which the cell membrane performs its function of signal recognition is not completely understood; however, several key elements are necessary. The first component involved is the receptor itself, which functions as a discriminator for detecting particular specific regulatory signals. Receptors thus serve for the selective recognition of extracellular signals and for the subsequent initiation of a message across the membrane and into the cytoplasm or nucleus. Second, also present is some type of intervening component which translates this binding activity of the receptor into the appropriate membrane signal. The third element involved is the effector or amplifier component, which is responsible for actually communicating altered cell surface activity into the cell interior. Although the structural diversity of cell surface receptors is predictable from specialization of cell function and the variety of regulatory signals, there is no a priori reason for diversity of effector mechanisms. In fact, different cell types (obviously having different receptors) employ only a few common response mechanisms, which reflect some general properties inherent in membrane structure and function. Lymphocyte responses to receptor binding generally fall into three categories, i.e., proliferation, cytotoxic responses, and production of lymphokines. This chapter will concentrate on in vitro assays which measure cytotoxicity.

COMPLEMENT-INDEPENDENT CYTOLYTIC ASSAYS

Cell-mediated target cell destruction can be effected by several different types of leukocytes: cytotoxic T lymphocytes (CTL), natural killer (NK) cells, and killer (K) cells that lyse antibody-coated target cells. The interrelationships between the lymphoid cytotoxic cells are not clear and may overlap to some degree.

Cytotoxicity is one major type of reaction by which lymphocytes can respond to antigen recognition. The lytic response consists of three phases: establishment of contact between cytotoxic cells and target cells (subsequent to cell surface receptor binding), development of cytotoxic activity, and death of the target cells. T-cell-mediated cytotoxicity is antigen specific, as only cells bearing the original sensitizing antigens are killed efficiently. This recognition of target cell antigens by CTL is probably an active phenomenon, as it can be abolished by metabolic inhibitors or low temperature. Contact between target and CTL cells causes metabolic changes associated with secretory activity. Moreover, cytotoxicity is unidirectional: a cytotoxic cell is capable of sequentially lysing several targets and therefore is not destroyed by the lytic process (2). The exact mechanism of cell lysis is still unclear, but the release of lytic enzymes or other toxic products has been suggested. In the human, the subset of T lymphocytes to which this activity is attributed can be identified with monoclonal antibodies, such as the OKT8 and Leu 2 reagents.

In addition to cytotoxic T effector cells, two additional sets of lymphocytes have the capacity for lytic activity, i.e., K cells and NK cells. The lineage of these cells, whether of T- or B-cell origin, is still uncertain; consequently, they have been difficult to characterize. The cytotoxic reaction mediated by K cells is termed ADCC. Lymphocytes from nonimmune donors are incubated with target cells in the presence of antibody specific for the target cells. K cells have receptors for immunoglobulin G antibodies which actually mediate the ADCC reaction. This phenomenon differs from T-cell-mediated killing in two respects: (i) the effector lymphocytes bind to the antibody of the antibody-target cell complex rather than to the target cell itself, and (ii) the cytotoxic effector cells are not specifically sensitized. NK cell activity is based on the fact that unsensitized lymphocytes from normal individuals are spontaneously cytotoxic for a variety of target cells. Antibody is not involved in this reaction, nor is the thymus required for development of NK cells. It has been suggested that the NK system is a possible surveillance mechanism to protect the individual against tumors and that it may complement T-cell-mediated killing in its biological role. The cytotoxic assay systems outlined here are all based on the release of chromium-51 (^{51}Cr) from prelabeled target cells as described below for cytotoxic T cells.

CTL

Sensitized lymphocytes may directly participate in cell-mediated immune responses by killing cells with the relevant surface antigens (e.g., cells infected with the sensitizing viruses and certain tumor cells) in the absence of antibody or complement or both. The cell-mediated lympholysis assay was perfected by in vitro studies of tumor allograft immunity (CTL cell phenomenon) in inbred mice (7). This cell-mediated lympholysis technique measures the release of radio-active label from donor target or tumor cells incubated in the presence of sensitized lymphocytes. These cells from immune animals (CTL cells) are incubated with ^{51}Cr-labeled target cells in various ratios of CTL to target cells. The mixtures are centrifuged, and the amount of radioactivity released into the supernatant is taken as an index of target cell damage brought about by the CTL cells. Utilizing this cell-mediated lympholysis assay in certain murine lymphocyte-target cell systems, as much as 70% of the radioactivity can be found in the supernatant after a 1-h incubation, with a ratio of 100 lymphocytes per target cell. Ample evidence exists that the CTL cells are a segment of the thymus-derived population of lymphocytes. Conse-

quently, this type of cell lysis is considered T-cell-mediated cytotoxicity.

CTL do not require additional immune factors to exert lytic activity, as each cell possesses surface receptors for antigen which confer specificity. Recent discoveries elucidating the structure and function of this T-cell receptor show that it recognizes foreign antigen only in conjunction with a histocompatibility molecule.

The generation of CTL requires exposure to the sensitizing antigen, usually through blood transfusion or transplantation. Hence, CTL have been implicated as playing a significant role in graft rejection. In addition, they may have a positive effect in viral infection by lysing those cells which contain virtually encoded cell surface components.

Alterations or abnormalities in cell-mediated immunity occur in a broad spectrum of diseases and in varying degrees of severity. The most pronounced disorders include the congenital syndromes of thymic hypoplasia and severe combined immunodeficiency. Acquired disorders include neoplasms such as Hodgkin's disease in which deficiency in cellular immunity appears integrally related to the disease process and parallels the clinical course. Acquired cellular immunodeficiency may also result from immunosuppressive therapy such as that used for posttransplant patients. In addition, deviations from the normal responses occur in certain infections such as leprosy and mycobacterial and viral diseases, as well as sarcoidosis and certain autoimmune diseases.

NK cells

A fact clearly emerging from all studies of cellular cytotoxicity is that it is not possible to investigate specific cytotoxic responses of patients or sensitized donors without taking into account the existence of another mechanism of cytotoxicity which is nonspecific, but nevertheless increasingly important, i.e., natural killing. Natural killing is based on the fact that unsensitized lymphocytes from normal individuals are spontaneously cytotoxic for a variety of target cells (8). The human NK cell has been identified as an Fc-receptor-bearing lymphocyte with no surface immunoglobulin. Most of the cytotoxicity of human NK cells is nonspecific in that target cells are lysed according to their susceptibility to lysis and to the cytotoxic efficiency of the effector cells from a particular donor. Interferon has a role in natural killing in vitro. However, many target cells that do not produce detectable amounts of interferon are, nevertheless, lysed by human lymphocytes. The existence of high NK-cell activity in nude and neonatally thymectomized mice provides an explanation for the resistance to tumors in these animals. Moreover, patients with X-linked agammaglobulinemia, a primary immunodeficiency with a total lack of B cells and circulating antibodies, have normal NK-cell activity (4). In addition, immunogenetic factors affect NK-cell function, as normal individuals show different (Fig. 1), though consistent, levels of NK-cell activity (unpublished data). Although the relevance of NK cells to disease states or to normal immunoregulatory functions is still unclear, there are accumulating data to suggest that these cells may play a role in immune

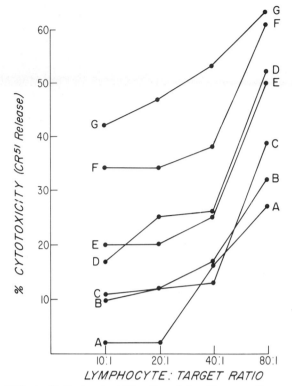

FIG. 1. Variation in NK cell activity. Target cells were K562 lymphoid cell line. Effector cells were Ficoll-Hypaque-purified lymphocytes from seven normal human donors (A through G) tested simultaneously for their spontaneous cytotoxic activity (NK) against K562 cells in the same assay.

surveillance against primary tumors or those arising from carcinogenic agents such as viruses, chemicals, or irradiation (3). The ^{51}Cr release assay is also used to monitor NK-cell activity.

ADCC

Another in vitro model of the interrelationship between antibody and immune cells has been described, wherein antibody enhances cellular cytotoxicity. For some years, it has been known that lymphoid cells from nonimmune animals may attack and lyse target cells coated with specific anti-target cell antibody. Several studies have shown that an antibody having this activity can be of the immunoglobulin G class and that effector cells are thymus-independent lymphocytes, bearing receptors for the Fc portion of immunoglobulin on their surface (1). This phenomenon differs from T-cell-mediated cytotoxicity in two respects: (i) lymphocytes bind to the antibody of the antibody-target cell complex, rather than to the target itself, and (ii) the effector cells do not have to come from specifically immunized animals. These cell-mediated lympholysis reactions, which involve specific anti-target cell antibody or lymphocyte-dependent antibody, have been studied primarily in heteroimmune situations, but there is also evidence for the presence of lymphocyte-dependent antibody activity in multiparous women (10), transplantation immunity (9), autoimmunity (5), and tumor systems (6).

Different methods have been used to determine the presence of lymphocyte-dependent antibody activity; however, all the methods are designed to expose target cells to serum with the putative antibody, in the absence of complement, and then to determine the extent of target cell destruction after the addition of normal lymphocytes. ^{51}Cr release is the most widely used technique for detection of this type of antibody.

COMPLEMENT-DEPENDENT CYTOTOXICITY

If antibodies directed against the surface of cells are able to fix complement, a cytotoxic reaction will occur. The combination of specific cytotoxic antibody and cell surface antigen, in the presence of complement, will result in lysis of the antigen-carrying target cell as monitored by dye exclusion from live cells or release of the isotope ^{51}Cr from labeled target cells. Clinically, this experimental approach can be used either to detect the production of specific antibody by assaying against cells known to have the respective antigen (e.g., tumor-specific antibody versus tumor cell antigen) or to detect the presence of a particular antigen on cells in question by testing them with sera (xenogenic, allogenic, or autologous) known to contain antibody directed against the antigen (e.g., cells from tumor patient versus xenogeneic antitumor sera).

Because blood samples from patients are generally obtained in small amounts and also because it is wise to freeze any remaining cells or sera for further retesting, the microcytotoxicity assay has particular appeal. This assay, originally developed for histocompatibility testing, can be adapted for other uses. The microliter quantities needed of both cells and sera, along with the rapidity and reproducibility of this technique, make it very popular. However, other methods, e.g., ^{51}Cr release by target cells in the presence of antibody and complement, have also gained wide acceptance, especially if they are simultaneously used in one of the non-complement-mediated tests described above.

TECHNIQUES

General Techniques

Lymphocyte purification

Heparinized (20 U/ml) peripheral blood is diluted 1:3 with phosphate-buffered saline (PBS) and then layered over a cushion of 3 ml of 9% Ficoll–33.9% Hypaque in a tube (16 by 125 mm). These gradients are centrifuged for 20 min at 1,100 × g. Cells are removed from the interface with a 9-in. (ca. 23-cm) Pasteur pipette, with care being taken to remove little, if any, of the Ficoll-Hypaque. These cells are then washed two times with PBS and once with medium and then suspended in medium and counted. (Additional purification steps to remove monocytes or to obtain enriched populations of T and B lymphocytes may also be employed if necessary).

^{51}Cr labeling technique

The ^{51}Cr labeling technique is based on the observation that radiolabeled sodium chromate (^{51}Cr), after diffusion through the cell membrane as chromate ion,

TABLE 1. ^{51}Cr labeling for 1-ml final volume of preparation

Type of cell	^{51}Cr (μCi)	Incubation time (h)
Freshly isolated	300	2
Cultured	100–300	1

is retained in the cytoplasm for a relatively prolonged period of time. Therefore, ^{51}Cr release from a labeled target cell into the supernatant fluid does not occur unless the cell membrane is sufficiently damaged to allow the efflux of intracellular molecules. Moreover, since the released ^{51}Cr is no longer the chromate anion and is not reutilized by either lymphoid or target cell multiplication, the only parameter measured is lysis of target cells.

Media. Most enriched media are suitable for the ^{51}Cr labeling technique. Ca^{2+} and Mg^{2+} ions are essential both for the participation of complement and for the steps leading to cell-mediated lysis. Hence, Eagle minimal essential medium, medium 199, and McCoy medium are all acceptable.

Serum. Fetal calf serum (FCS) is generally used for most in vitro assays. However, occasional experimental procedures will more closely resemble in vivo conditions when autologous serum is used. This modification in technique is best resolved in a preliminary pilot experiment. The medium is generally supplemented with heat-inactivated 10% serum by volume.

Cell concentration. Cells to be used as targets can be labeled in any quantity which is easy to manipulate, usually no less than 3×10^6 and up to a maximum of 10×10^6 cells. Although a total of 10^6 cells will generally provide more than enough targets, it is wise to label an excess amount to compensate for differential fragility and cell loss during washing steps.

Labeling technique. The half-life of ^{51}Cr is 27 days; hence, it is imperative to compensate for radioactive decay. Moreover, freshly isolated cells generally take longer to incorporate the radioactive label than do cultured cells (Table 1). Cells to be used as targets are dispensed into conical tubes. When only a small number (3×10^6 to 5×10^6) are available, the cells are more easily handled in a smaller tube (15 ml, conical), whereas larger numbers of cells can be adequately manipulated in a 50-ml tube. Cells are washed in medium with serum by centrifugation at $800 \times g$ for 10 min at room temperature. The supernatant is removed, the appropriate amount of radioisotope is added, and the volume is made up to 1 ml with medium with serum. The test tube containing cells is placed in a beaker in a 37°C water bath, with occasional mixing for the given incubation period. The uptake of ^{51}Cr is terminated by filling the test tube with cold medium (with serum) and washing at 4°C for 10 min at $800 \times g$. This procedure is repeated three times (four or five times for a 15-ml tube) to completely eliminate free ^{51}Cr, as the residual isotope will contribute to high background control counts per minute during the assay. Finally, the cells are counted and suspended at the working concentration. Target cells are then kept at 4°C until dispensed into the microtiter plate wells. If expense is an important consideration, it is advisable to run a pilot study with as little as 2% serum. The type of medium for washing can also be varied, e.g., Hanks balanced salt solution (HBSS) or PBS, thus reserving the enriched medium for the assay itself.

Culture vessel. Round-bottom microtiter plates (0.25-ml capacity; Linbro) are now widely used in most ^{51}Cr release assays; however, the test can also be performed in plastic (but not glass) test tubes (12 by 75 mm).

Effector cell concentration. Various ratios of effector to target cells should be used in each experiment to establish the linearity of the lytic response. Doubling dilutions are easiest to manipulate, beginning with 80:1, 40:1, 20:1, 10:1, etc.

Test Procedures

Antibody-dependent, complement-mediated test

National Institutes of Health modified technique

1. Dispense 1 μl of appropriate serum into each well of a Falcon microtest plate (no. 3034) with a Hamilton syringe (no. 705).

2. Dispense 1 μl of cells (2.0×10^6 to 2.5×10^6 cells per ml) into microtest plate wells with a Hamilton syringe.

3. Incubate at room temperature for 30 min.

4. Contents of the wells are then washed by adding 10 μl of HBSS to each well with a Hamilton syringe (no. 750). Allow the cells to settle for 10 min.

5. The excess fluid is then removed by inverting the plate with a quick snap of the wrist ("flick") over a large waste container.

6. A 5-μl volume of rabbit complement with titers for optimum dilution previously determined is added to each well with a Hamilton syringe (no. 725).

7. Incubate for 1 h at room temperature.

8. After incubation, flick the plates again (as in step 5).

9. A 10-μl volume of 0.3% trypan blue (in EDTA) is then added to each well, cells are permitted to settle again for 10 min, and the plate is flicked to remove excess dye, thus allowing better visualization of cells.

10. A 20-μl volume of HBSS is added to each well. Cells are allowed to resettle for 10 min before being read on an inverted phase microscope. The microtest plates may be held overnight by applying 2 drops of 37% formaldehyde to the filter paper strips for preservation of the cells and then refrigerating them at 4°C.

^{51}Cr release

1. Serum (10 μl) and cells (10 μl; 10^6 cells per ml) are added to wells of a microtiter plate (Linbro no. 76-013-05) or plastic tubes (12 by 75 mm) with a Hamilton syringe (no. 705).

2. Incubate for 30 min at room temperature.

3. The contents of the wells (or tubes) are then washed by adding HBSS (100 μl to each well or 1 ml to each tube) with a Hamilton syringe (no. 1005). Plates (or tubes) are then centrifuged for 10 min at 250 $\times g$, and the supernatant is removed.

4. Rabbit complement (10 μl, with titers for optimum dilution previously determined) is then added to each well (or tube) and allowed to incubate for 1 h at room temperature.

5. The reaction is stopped at the end of the incubation period by the addition of 200 μl of cold HBSS or PBS to each well (or 1 ml to each tube).

GENERAL SCHEMA

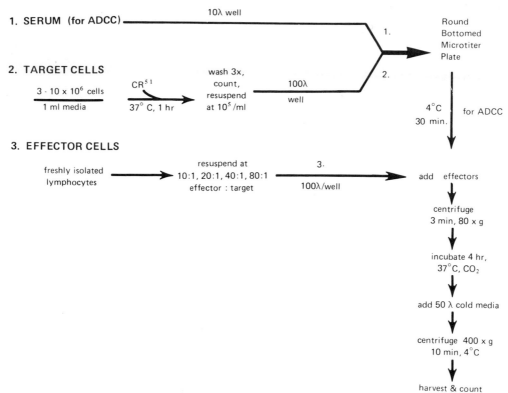

FIG. 2. General experimental design for complement-independent ^{51}Cr release assays (ADCC, CTL cell, NK cell), with tissue-cultured cells and microtiter plates.

6. The plates (or tubes) are immediately centrifuged for 10 min at 900 × g at 4°C.

7. A 100-µl volume of supernatant is carefully removed with an Eppendorf disposable pipette, placed in Biovials, and counted in a Beckman automatic gamma counter.

8. Maximum ^{51}Cr release control is set up with 100 µl of 1% Triton X-100 added to 10 µl of cells and counted.

9. The amount of ^{51}Cr released in the experimental wells is divided by the maximum release and expressed as the percentage of maximum release.

ADCC

Sera. All sera used in ADCC are decomplemented by heat inactivation at 56°C for 30 min and stored frozen in small samples at −70°C. The dilution of antiserum should be determined by prior titration. Normal human serum or FCS should be used as diluent to keep the total serum concentrations constant in all samples.

Cells. Lymphocytes for use as target or effector cells are prepared by the technique described above. Effector cells must not be treated with Tris NH$_4$Cl to remove erythrocytes. This treatment abolishes killing ability.

Assay. See Fig. 2 for a general schema of the assay.

1. With a Hamilton syringe, add 10 µl of serum or serum dilution to each well of a microtiter plate.

2. Add 10 µl of ^{51}Cr-labeled target cells (10^4 cells per well) in the same manner.

3. Incubate for 30 min at 4°C.

4. With a Hamilton syringe, add 100 µl of the effector cells at various effector and target ratios (10:1 to 100:1).

5. Centrifuge at room temperature for 3 min at 80 × g to facilitate cell contact, and then incubate for 4 h at 37°C in a humidified CO$_2$ incubator.

6. Add 50 µl of cold medium or PBS to stop the reaction.

7. Centrifuge at 400 × g for 10 min at 4°C.

8. With an Eppendorf pipette, carefully remove 50 µl of the supernatant from the side of each well and transfer it to a Biovial.

9. Count for ^{51}Cr release in a Beckman automatic gamma counter.

Controls

1. Place triplicate samples of 10 µl of target cells in 100 µl of 1% Triton X-100 detergent and count for a maximum release of ^{51}Cr.

2. Set up each plate of a multiplate experiment as shown in Table 2.

Calculation: % Specific lysis = (cpm experimental − cpm spontaneous release)/(cpm maximum − cpm spontaneous release) × 100, where each figure represents the mean of triplicate samples.

T-cell killing

Medium. Use RPM1 1640 supplemented with L-glutamine and 10% heat-inactivated FCS.

TABLE 2. Contents of control plates in ADCC assay with 10 μl of target cells

Control no.	Antibody (10 μl)	Effector (100 μl)
1[a]	Medium	Medium
2[a]	Serum	Medium
3[b]	Medium	Cells

[a] Necessary to determine that the antibody is not cytotoxic.

[b] Used as a spontaneous release in the calculation of results.

Target cells. ^{51}Cr-labeled target cells are suspended in medium with 10% FCS at a concentration of 10^5 cells per ml and kept at 4°C until they are ready to be dispensed, as ^{51}Cr is released spontaneously from most cells at a rate of 2 to 4%/h at room temperature.

Effector cells. Lymphocytes to be tested for CTL-cell function are suspended in medium with 10% FCS at a concentration of 8×10^6 cells per ml. Various ratios of effector to target cells are used (depending on the quantity of cells available for testing), preferably in doubling dilutions of 80:1, 40:1, 20:1, and 10:1. When a more precise evaluation of the lymphocyte subpopulation involved in killing is desired, T cells can be used as effector cells in this assay after their separation according to methods described elsewhere in this manual.

Assay. Effector cells (100 μl) are dispensed into microtiter plate wells (triplicate samples for each effector/target cell ratio), and then 100 μl of target cells (10^4 cells per well) is added. Plates are centrifuged for 3 min at $80 \times g$ to facilitate cell contact and then placed in a humidified CO_2 incubator at 37°C. Time course of killing must be empirically established for each antigen system, although 4 to 6 h of incubation is generally sufficient to observe target cell lysis, which is significantly increased over background.

Controls. For maximum release, place triplicate samples (100 μl each) of target cells with 100 μl of 1% Triton X-100 detergent. For spontaneous release, place triplicate samples of 100 μl of target cells with 100 μl of medium with 10% FCS.

Calculation: % Specific release = (cpm experimental − cpm spontaneous release)/(cpm maximum − cpm spontaneous release) × 100

NK cells

Assay. The methodology for detection of NK cells is essentially similar to the T-cell killer assay, with the exception that the cytotoxicity detected is natural, not derived from a sensitization process.

LITERATURE CITED

1. **Bach, J.** 1982. Transplantation immunity and cytotoxicity phenomena, p. 399–429. *In* J. Bach (ed.), Immunology, 2nd ed. John Wiley & Sons, Inc., New York.
2. **Berke, G.** 1983. Cytotoxic-T-lymphocytes—how do they function? Immunol. Rev. **72:**1–42.
3. **Herberman, R., T. Timonen, C. Reynolds, and J. Ortaldo.** 1980. Characteristics of NK cells, p. 89–104. *In* R. Herberman (ed.), Natural cell-mediated immunity against tumors. Academic Press, Inc., New York.
4. **Koren, H. S., D. B. Amos, and R. H. Buckley.** 1978. Natural killing in immunodeficient patients. J. Immunol. **120:**796–799.
5. **Kumagai, S., A. Steinberg, and I. Green.** 1981. Antibodies to T cells in patients with human systemic lupus erythematosus mediated ADCC against human T cells. J. Clin. Invest. **67:**605–614.
6. **Lamon, E. W., H. M. Skurzak, E. Klein, and H. Wigzell.** 1973. *In vitro* cytotoxicity by a nonthymus-processed lymphocyte population with specificity for a virally determined tumor cell surface antigen. J. Exp. Med. **136:**1072–1079.
7. **Nabholz, M., and H. MacDonald.** 1983. Cytolytic T lymphocytes. Annu. Rev. Immunol. **1:**273–306.
8. **Ortaldo, J., and R. Herberman.** 1984. Heterogeneity of natural killer cells. Annu. Rev. Immunol. **2:**359–394.
9. **Ting, A., and P. I. Terasaki.** 1975. Lymphocyte-dependent antibody crossmatching for transplant patients. Lancet i:304.
10. **Trinchieri, G., M. DeMarchi, W. Mayr, M. Sevi, and R. Ceppellini.** 1973. Lymphocyte-antibody lymphocytolytic interaction (LALI) with special emphasis on HLA. Transplant. Proc. **5:**1631–1649.

Chapter 13

Section B. Immunoassay

Introduction

BRUCE S. RABIN

The previous two editions of the *Manual of Clinical Immunology* have presented information regarding a number of tests which can be performed by ligand assays. The first chapter of this section will summarize relevant information for each of the assays previously presented. The other chapters in this section will present general principles of ligand assays with an emphasis on data processing, troubleshooting, the enzyme-linked immunosorbent assay technique, and new types of ligand procedures.

Monoclonal antibodies are being used more frequently in ligand assays and have made dramatic changes in both the specificity and sensitivity of these procedures. Ligand assays are now commonly used in immunology, chemistry, hematology, and microbiology laboratories. Ligand assays have even entered into the over-the-counter market with the availability of pregnancy tests to be used at home. There is every reason to believe that clinical laboratories will continue to adopt ligand assays rapidly and that these tests will introduce cost savings and more rapid turnaround time in the clinical laboratory.

Chapter 14

Summary of Immunoassay Test Procedures

BRUCE S. RABIN

For each of the following immunoassay tests, the indications for the use of each procedure, normal results, and pertinent comments are provided. The number of the page on which the test appears in either previous edition of this manual is given in parentheses with the name of each test.

Antibody to acetylcholine receptor (2nd ed., p. 386)

Indications. To assist in the diagnosis of myasthenia gravis.

Normal. Negative.

Comments. Antibodies to the acetylcholine receptor are present in approximately 90% of patients with myasthenia gravis. The assay can be used to distinguish myasthenic patients from patients whose neuromuscular transmission is impaired by genetic defects which do not involve such antibodies. The assay can also be used to monitor immunosuppressive or other therapy in myasthenic patients.

The absolute value of antibody does not correlate closely with disease severity.

Antibody to LSP (liver-specific lipoprotein) (2nd ed., p. 413)

Indications. There is a close relationship between antibody to LSP and piecemeal necrosis of periportal hepatocytes on liver biopsy.

Normal. Negative.

Comments. The test may prove to be of value in allowing a noninvasive assessment of the intensity of periportal inflammation, particularly during follow-up of patients receiving immunosuppressive drug therapy for chronic active hepatitis. In the assessment of asymptomatic carriers of hepatitis B serum antigen, up to 10% of such individuals may have unsuspected chronic active hepatitis detectable by a positive test for antibody to LSP.

Antibody to thyroglobulin (2nd ed., p. 403)

Indications. Useful for detecting the presence of autoimmune thyroid disease (chronic lymphocytic thyroiditis, Graves' disease, primary hyperthyroidism).

Normal. Negative.

Comments. There is a high degree of correlation between positive radioimmunoassay results for antithyroglobulin antibodies and one of the autoimmune thyroid disorders.

Antiglomerular basement membrane antibody (2nd ed., p. 376)

Indications. To identify and follow patients with antiglomerular basement membrane antibody disease.

Normal. Negative.

Comments. Patients with Goodpasteur's disease represent approximately two-thirds of all patients with this antibody. However, rapidly progressive as well as milder forms of glomerulonephritis alone are present in another one-third. An occasional disease confined to the lung is encountered.

Cyclic nucleotides (2nd ed., p. 409)

Indications. Cyclic nucleotides may play a role in the differentiation of lymphocytes and the regulation of lymphocyte function.

Normal. Levels for various tissue are dependent upon extraction methods and assay procedures. Thus, basal and stimulated levels must be interpreted by each laboratory.

Comments. Cellular levels of cyclic nucleotides may be altered by cell surface receptors being bound by either their substrate or an antibody to the receptor. Cyclic nucleotides are involved in the functional activity of T and B lymphocytes, the activation of macrophages, neutrophil chemotaxis, phagocytic enzyme secretion, lymphokine release, and lymphocyte-mediated killing of foreign cells.

Estradiol (1st ed., p. 239)

Indications. The most potent of the estrogens. Measurement may be useful in the establishment of the endocrine status of women in whom menstruation fails to take place after discontinuation of oral contraceptive tablets.

Normal. Values are low at the beginning of the menstrual cycle. In between it exhibits two peaks, one at midcycle just before rupture of the follicle and another at the midpoint of the luteal phase. In the pre-ovulatory period, it is <50 pg/ml. The high point may be 150 to 500 pg/ml.

Comments. Women who show consistently low estradiol levels with high levels of FSH (follicle-stimulating hormone) in the blood may suffer from primary ovarian failure. Low levels of both estradiol and FSH reflect a pituitary or hypothalamic cause for amenorrhea.

Gastrin (1st ed., p. 182)

Indications. To detect increased serum gastrin levels in patients with Zollinger-Ellison syndrome.

Normal. Range of 20 to 160 pg/ml.

Comments. Fasting serum gastrin levels may be increased with pernicious anemia and other forms of atrophic gastritis with gastric atrophy, including patients with carcinoma of the stomach with decreased or absent gastric secretion. Patients with renal failure and massive resection of the small intestine may have increased gastrin levels.

HCG (Human chorionic gonadotropin) and PL (placental lactogen) (1st ed., p. 213)

Indications. HCG levels can be used for the diagnosis of normal or ectopic pregnancy and in the evaluation of abortion, trophoblastic tumors, testicular tumors, and ectopic production by nontrophoblastic tumors. The primary indication for the determination of PL is to suggest the presence of fetal-placental growth retardation during the third trimester of pregnancy.

Normal. HCG levels in various conditions are as follows.

(i) Normal pregnancy. Values vary in relation to the number of days or weeks after the last normal menstrual period.

(ii) Ectopic pregnancy. Usually in the range of 150 to 800 mIU/ml, but may be lower.

(iii) Evaluation of threatened abortion. During the first trimester, plasma levels below normal range are associated with abortion.

(iv) Evaluation of trophoblastic tumors. Usually over 5×10^3 mIU/ml and as high as 6×10^6 mIU/ml.

(v) Evaluation of testicular tumors. Values can be used as a tumor marker to follow response to chemotherapy. Measurement of HCG provides a rational basis for deciding when to begin and when to stop chemotherapy in patients with HCG-producing diseases.

Placental lactogen is usually below 4 µg/ml.

Comments. A variety of assay procedures with varying sensitivities are available to detect HCG. The sensitivity of each procedure can be evaluated by reading the package inserts which come with each test. PL is markedly decreased in association with hydatidiform mole and choriocarcinoma. The combination of high HCG and low PL may have diagnostic value. Some nontrophoblastic tumors are associated with increased PL.

HGH (Human growth hormone) (1st ed., p. 197)

Indications. For evaluation of short stature possibly due to isolated HGH hyposecretion, deficiency in association with other anterior pituitary deficits, and hypersecretion by a pituitary tumor resulting in gigantism or acromegaly.

Normal. Basal level of <3 ng/ml.

Comments. To evaluate HGH secretion, either inhibition or provocation tests are used. An adequate response implies a functionally normal hypothalamic pituitary growth hormone axis, but an inadequate response does not by itself differentiate between primary hypothalamic and primary pituitary disease.

Insulin (1st ed., p. 172)

Indications. To distinguish insulinoma from other causes of hypoglycemia.

Normal. Levels of <30 µU/ml in nondiabetic individuals of normal weight after an overnight fast.

Comments. The preferable method of diagnosing an insulinoma is with a fasting insulin suppression test. A diagnosis of insulinoma should alert the physician to the possibility of the presence of other endocrine adenomas.

LH/FSH (Luteinizing hormone/follicle-stimulating hormone) (1st ed., p. 206)

Indications. Can be used in the diagnosis of polycystic ovary syndrome, psychogenic amenorrhea, pituitary tumors, and ectopic tumor production. Follow-up of patients with choriocarcinoma and hydatidiform mole.

Normal. LH values are <15 mIU/ml for adult males and between 30 and 200 mIU/ml in postmenopausal females. In menstruating females, levels are related to the timing of the sample within the menstrual cycle, as there is a midcycle peak.

FSH values are up to 15 mIU/ml for adult males and 200 mIU/ml for postmenopausal females. Menstruating females have a midcycle peak.

Comments. Measurement of LH and FSH is valuable in the assessment of hypothalamic and pituitary function. Usually a single determination is sufficient to distinguish between primary and secondary gonadal failure in the adult. A provocative testing using clomiphene may be required for adequate assessment of hypothalamic or pituitary reserve.

Plasma cortisol and urinary free cortisol (1st ed., p. 231)

Indications. To provide an estimate of the rate of secretion of cortisol by the adrenal cortex to establish whether the patient has significant hypo- or hypercorticism.

Normal. Cortisol is secreted intermittently by the adrenal gland under episodic stimuli from the pituitary. Cortisol secretion is nearly 0 between 11 p.m. and 12 midnight. Between 2 and 8 a.m. there are about six short bursts of cortisol secretion. Two more bursts of secretion occur later in the morning or early afternoon. Afterwards, the plasma concentration decreases steadily until it reaches the nadir previously described late at night. Serum assays are most useful in evaluating responses to adrenal stimulation or suppression tests. Urinary free cortisol correlates with the concentration of the free plasma fraction and, therefore, with cortisol-mediated function in target tissues.

Comments. Secretion of cortisol by the adrenal cortex occurs in response to ACTH (adrenocorticotropin), to diurnal rhythm, and to stress. Measurements of plasma and urinary free cortisol are indicated whenever Cushing syndrome or adrenal cortical insufficiency, organic or functional, primary or secondary, is suspected. Because of the circadian rhythm, no single determination, either in plasma or in urine, is likely to be of much clinical significance.

Progesterone (1st ed., p. 242)

Indications. Useful for investigations of the occurrence of ovulation, the induction of ovulation by therapeutic means, ovulatory and anovulatory dysfunctional bleeding, corpus luteum insufficiency during short luteal phases, problems of fertility, and suppression of progesterone levels during the luteal phase by oral contraceptives.

Normal. Levels are <1 ng/ml during the pre-ovulatory phase and reach a peak of 10 to 20 ng/ml approximately 4 to 6 days after the luteinizing hormone surge.

Comments. Progesterone is partially responsible for cyclic changes in the endometrium which are necessary for attachment and growth of an embryo.

Prostaglandin (2nd ed., p. 406)

Indications. To measure a variety of physiological regulatory products

Normal. Less than 500 pg/ml.

Comments. Prostaglandins have clinical usefulness in that they can be used for determination of pregnancy in the first trimester. Specific reasons to quantitate levels of prostaglandins in serum or tissue are still lacking. Intensive research is being done in this field, and prostaglandin assays should be considered of research interest only.

Renin (1st ed., p. 190)

Indications. Of diagnostic value in various disease states.

Normal. Highly variable. Related to posture and sodium intake.

Comments. About 15% of patients with central hypertension have excessive renin which is secondary to lesions in the kidney or its vascular supply. This leads to increased aldosterone production and subsequent changes in sodium and potassium excretion. Renin-secreting tumors are extremely rare. Malignant hypertension is associated with an elevated plasma renin.

Testosterone (1st ed., p. 248)

Indications. Testosterone is responsible for all of the androgenic changes associated with sexual development, including growth spurt, increased muscle mass, increase in penis size, sexual hair, prostatic growth, and deepening of the voice.

Normal. Testosterone concentrations in healthy individuals are 1.5 to 11.4 pg/ml for menstruating females and 56 to 240 pg/ml for males.

Comments. Serum testosterone levels are relatively constant. In young men, there is a circadian pattern of testosterone secretion with the highest levels occurring at about the time of wakening.

Thyroid-stimulating antibodies (2nd ed., p. 391)

Indications. There are a variety of assays to detect antibodies which may be present in patients with diffusely hyperplastic thyroid glands.

Normal. Negative.

Comments. Due to the variety of antibodies which may be involved with thyroid stimulation, a textbook of endocrinology should be consulted.

T4 (Thyroxine), T3 (triiodothyronine), and TSH (thyroid-stimulating hormone) (1st ed., p. 222)

Indications. These tests are valuable in diagnosing and following the course of disease in patients with hyper- or hypothyroidism.

Normal. Due to the necessity for evaluating the patient's history and physical findings in addition to interpreting the various thyroid function tests, it is recommended that an endocrinology textbook be referred to for the evaluation of the laboratory procedures used to diagnose thyroid function.

Chapter 15

Data Processing of Immunoassay Results

R. P. CHANNING RODGERS

This chapter has three goals: to outline the features of a good automated assay data reduction package, to provide assistance in selecting among the computer programs which are currently available, and to present a glossary of key terms pertaining to assay data reduction and quality control.

NECESSITY OF AUTOMATED DATA REDUCTION

The manual computation of assay results is a salutary exercise which every assayist should undertake at least once. Detailed instructions have been provided elsewhere (11). A proper evaluation of assay results includes not just the creation of a calibration curve and interpolation of test results to obtain concentration estimates, but evaluation of assay error and the performance of quality assurance tests. By the end of such an experience, the assayist will better appreciate that a thorough evaluation of assay results on a routine basis is only practical if done by computer. The error and quality assurance computations are particularly demanding and are generally omitted when data reduction is performed manually. In practice, good quality control requires the use of automated data reduction.

The two goals of a thorough assay analysis are to extract an estimate of the analyte concentration in the unknowns and to estimate the amount of error present in the assay process. This error can be subdivided into two components, i.e., that due to systematic error and that due to random error. The random error (imprecision) can be estimated in the form of a confidence interval about the analyte concentration estimate. This interval allows the formal statistical comparison of assay results. For example, a clinician can decide to what extent the difference between two drug or hormone levels is due to random error inherent in the assay process as opposed to a genuine change in concentration. Most assay quality assurance tests are designed to detect either a change in the imprecision or a shift in the amount of bias error. Routine quality control tests indicate that a problem exists and may require that assay results be discarded. They are not designed to specifically indicate the source of the problem, which requires additional (chemical) testing and application of the assayist's insight.

FEATURES OF AN IDEAL ASSAY DATA REDUCTION PACKAGE

Figure 1 summarizes the sequence of events occurring in a sound assay data reduction program. To avoid redundancy, definitions of technical terms (which appear in the glossary below) are not provided in the main text. The reader may want to review this glossary before proceeding.

Three forms of incoming information are provided by calibrators (or standards), test specimens (or unknowns, to use assay jargon), and quality control specimens. Calibrators are assumed to contain known amounts of analyte. There are numerous types of calibrators, discussion of which is beyond the scope of this presentation (see reference 11). Test specimens are presented to the assay as singleton samples, in replicate, or in multiple different dilutions. There are numerous types of quality control specimens; the most common type, often referred to as a quality control pool sample, is a sample drawn from a pool of material held in long-term storage which is analyzed in each assay run.

Because the use of quality control pool specimens can substantially increase the cost of performing an assay, there have been attempts to limit the number required. A formal cost effectiveness analysis of this problem has demonstrated the complexity inherent in the attempt to determine an optimal number of quality control tubes (12). The best established (arbitrary) guidelines advise that three quality control pools be used (representing low, medium, and high analyte concentrations) and that these pools be placed in groups throughout the assay to enable the worker to detect temporal drift.

All samples are processed by the same analytical method, the final result of which is a response for each sample. When replicate data are available, the random error present in the response can be computed, and a response-error relationship can be determined. If quality control and unknown samples require treatment different from what the calibrators require (such as a preliminary purification step), the response-error relationships for calibrator, unknown, or quality control data may differ.

The responses obtained from the calibrators are used to create a calibration curve. The responses from the unknowns and quality control samples are interpolated through this curve to obtain analyte concentration estimates. The response-error relationships and calibration curve together yield information required to compute an imprecision profile, which completely characterizes the performance of the assay with respect to random error. As with the response-error relationship, the imprecision profiles for calibrators, unknowns, or quality control data may not be identical. The imprecision computations allow the assignment of confidence intervals for the analyte concentration estimates obtained for unknown and quality control samples. Various specialized quality control procedures can be carried out to help pinpoint the origin of a problem indicated by the general tests. These procedures include tests for temporal drift, the presence of cross-reacting species, and interference from other binding substances.

As the only test specimens analyzed in different assay batches, the quality control samples are the

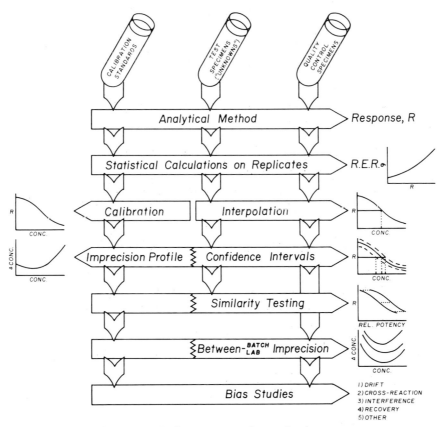

FIG. 1. Comprehensive assay data reduction system.

chief source of information concerning between-assay variability. A between-assay imprecision profile can be constructed and will lie above the within-batch profile described above, as it includes within-batch error as well as the additional sources of variability that appear between different batches.

If the laboratory participates in a good external quality control program, between-laboratory variability may also be computed. This variability could be summarized in a between-laboratory imprecision profile, which would lie above the between-batch profile.

COMPUTATIONAL METHODS

Obviously, any program attempting to perform the above calculations is worthless if it does them incorrectly. Valid computational methods must be employed at each step. This brief discussion is not intended to provide instructions for writing an assay program. Indeed, creation of a valid program is technically demanding and should be undertaken only by a team experienced in assay methodology, assay biostatistics, numerical methods, and sound programming practice. The goal of this presentation is to provide criteria for judging the quality of available programs.

Underlying every major assay data reduction program is a fundamental but rarely mentioned assumption that the assay response follows a normal (Gaussian) error distribution, which allows the use of parametric statistical methods. This assumption limits the choice of a response function to one which fulfills this criterion.

The enormous outpouring of literature dealing with the choice of a calibration curve-fitting equation has been summarized elsewhere (10, 13). Empirically minded workers may be attracted to the use of spline and related methods which mimic manual curve fitting, but the statistical shortcomings of these methods have prompted Finney to label their advantages "illusory" (6). At the opposite extreme, theoretically inclined assayists may be drawn to the use of complex formulas based on chemical models. These formulas are inescapably oversimplified representations of the complexities of assay systems and have some of the same statistical drawbacks as the spline family.

What is required is a formula which is sufficiently flexible in form to accommodate most assays in use, straightforward to computationally fit the data, easy to interpret geometrically, and containing as small a number of parameters as possible, allowing statistical tests to be performed on the results. The only formula in common use which fulfills these criteria is the four-parameter logistic equation, a generalization of the widely used logit-log method. This equation is appropriate for assays which yield response (y) data resembling a symmetric sigmoid when plotted with a logarithmic x (analyte concentration) axis, as follows:

$$y = \frac{a - d}{a + (x/c)^b} + d$$

where a and d represent the upper and lower asymptotes of the curve, respectively, c is the analyte concentration corresponding to the inflection point of the curve (where the response is midway between a and d), and b is the negative of the slope of the curve when plotted with logit-log coordinates. Most traditional radioimmunoassays employing bound, labeled ligand or the bound-to-total ratio as response are well represented by this formula. It has been equally successful with newer nonisotopic methods. For the unusual assay method which cannot be represented by the strictly symmetrical sigmoid shape of this formula, a fifth parameter may be added.

This formula should be fitted to calibration data by using iteratively reweighted nonlinear least-squares methods. Weighting is required because the error in response is not uniform over the range of assay results. The weights employed should not be arbitrarily defined as in some programs, nor based on the assay data in the current batch, which almost always are insufficient in number to allow good statistical estimates to be made. Weights should be determined from the accumulated data of (generally 10 to 30) previous assay batches, as embodied in a pooled response-error relationship. This relationship can be approximated by many simple equations, perhaps the most successful being the power function put forth by Finney (5): $E = a_0 \cdot y^J$. Here, E represents the variance in response, and y is the response. The value of a_0 is determined for each assay batch, and the value of J tends to remain roughly constant between runs of the same assay method. This model also has the advantage of being readily interpretable. If $J = 0$, variance is constant; if $J = 1$, the variance is directly proportional to y; and if $J = 2$, the coefficient of variation is constant. In radioimmunoassays examined to date, J tends to take on a value slightly larger than one.

Quality of fit may be judged by analysis of variance methods, even though these analyses will be approximations in the instance of a nonlinear model. Another useful tool for assessing systematic lack of fit is the examination of a plot of weighted residuals. With an appropriate model, these should vary randomly from batch to batch. If there is a shape to this plot which is consistently reproducible across batches, the curve-fitting model may be inappropriate for the assay under consideration.

Rigorously computed confidence intervals will contain contributions from three sources of uncertainty, i.e., uncertainty in the calibration curve response data, uncertainty in the location of the equation fitted to it (attributable to uncertainty concerning the ability of the curve-fitting model to actually represent the calibration curve), and uncertainty in the test response data being interpolated through the calibration curve. Given the mathematical complexities inherent in error computations for an algebraically nonlinear system, the confidence limits are almost always computed by making some simplifying assumptions, such as neglecting all but the term for the uncertainty in the test value being interpolated (which assumes that the calibration curve location is known exactly) and assuming that the calibration curve can be approximated by a straight line in the region around a given response.

Although calibration, interpolation, and confidence limit calculation make up the bulk of routine assay computations, some pre- and postprocessing are also required. The incoming data should be checked to screen out obvious nonsense, such as that which might arise with the misordering of data. Gross outliers should be indicated, although rejection of any outlier at any point in the assay should require human intervention, as automatic systems are too prone to abuse. If quality control or test specimens are subjected to a preliminary purification step, corrections must be made for the amount of analyte lost in this procedure. When multiple dilutions of a test preparation are assayed, a program should be able to compute a single properly weighted average analyte concentration estimate and to check for similarity (parallelism) with the calibration curve to look for statistical evidence against the fundamental assumption that test preparations and calibrators behave identically.

Given the technical complexities of assay computations and the different assumptions which can be made, it is not surprising that current implementations yield differing results. Two studies have suggested that differences in data-processing methods may account for a significant portion of between-assay variability. One of these reports demonstrated that different implementations of the same calibration curve-fitting model (the logit-log method) yielded significantly different results (7, 8). These findings suggest three things, i.e., that data-processing errors should not be dismissed as a negligible component of analytical error, that there is much more to developing a data reduction package than simply specifying a curve-fitting model, and that insufficient attention has been paid to the standardization of assay reduction software.

SELECTING A PROGRAM

In the selection of a program, a number of questions must be asked. Most importantly, is the program based on a sound statistical approach which has been correctly implemented, as discussed above? Does the program work on equipment already in hand, or must new hardware be purchased? How easily are the raw data entered? (Automated transfer is desirable to reduce clerical error and save time.) Is the program well documented and easy to use? How well are the results presented? Does the program interact well with preexisting software such as that used for report generation and data archiving? How expensive is the program? How much local computer expertise is required to install and maintain it? How good is the external support for maintenance and training?

Assay data reduction packages fall into two basic categories according to their source, i.e., commercial and public sector. Commercial programs are generally accompanied by better instructions for installation and use, but they rarely document the numerical methods they employ. Some of these packages are quite expensive. Sometimes they are sold as an adjunct to a piece of measuring equipment or to encourage the purchase of a manufacturer's assay supplies. Not a single commercial program reviewed by this author embodies the methods of the ideal program outlined earlier, and some programs are extremely crude from a statistical viewpoint. One example is offered by a program which provides numerous calibration curve-fitting models and numerous different weighting schemes, but offers no way to determine which combination of these models and schemes may be statistically valid. This same program offers no confidence limit computations.

Public-sector programs (those developed by academic and public health institutions) tend to be superior regarding statistical completeness and rigor, but they are often accompanied by poor documentation and may require some on-site computer expertise to install and operate. Some of these programs require licensing fees, but most are freely obtainable. Whereas most commercial programs are tied to a particular piece of computing hardware, the public-sector programs tend not to be. A difficulty which accompanies this freedom is that machine-specific functions such as the graphical display of results, automated transfer of raw assay data, report generation, and archiving of assay results may be rudimentary.

Examples of computationally sound public-sector programs are the FORTRAN and BASIC programs of Rodbard and his colleagues (4), the FORTRAN program of Raab and McKenzie (9), the World Health Organization Apple BASIC program (3), and the International Atomic Energy Agency HP-41C program (2). The Rodbard and Raab programs are best suited for use on medium to large computers. The program of the International Atomic Energy Agency runs on a small hand-held computer. It is statistically sophisticated, but because it is comparatively slow and requires manual data entry, it is probably best suited for use when assays are infrequent, assay batch size is small, or financial constraints are placed on the purchase of hardware.

Rodbard and his co-workers (10) have also developed numerous ancillary programs which may be applied to assay quality control, assay design optimization, and ligand binding studies. There are a number of programs for microcomputers such as the Apple and IBM PC which are claimed to be adaptations of the work of Rodbard (available from the source cited in reference 4). Potential users should be careful to verify the fidelity of these adaptations before putting them to routine use.

CONCLUSIONS

Assay data reduction and quality control are innately intertwined processes. The computations required are tedious and hence error prone, mandating the use of automated methods. Construction of a statistically sound assay data reduction program is a complex undertaking; it is preferable to select and use a preexisting program. Currently available commercial programs are either difficult to evaluate properly due to proprietary secrecy or computationally deficient. The noncommercial programs recommended above are statistically sound but may lack certain practical features required by laboratories which offer routine service and may require effort to install, use, and maintain.

GLOSSARY

Here I offer a glossary of basic terms. The terms are consistent with those offered by the International Federation of Clinical Chemists (1), except for definitions of bias and accuracy, for which the IFCC definitions depart from well-established usage.

Accuracy: the degree to which an analyte concentration estimate corresponds to the true value, rarely knowable absolutely. Inaccuracy is caused by a combination of random and bias errors.

Algebraic linearity: refers to a form of algebraic equation in which the parameters of interest appear only to the first power. This category excludes equations in which parameters are taken to powers other than one or appear as exponents, in denominators, or inside special functions such as trigonometric functions. This term is not to be confused with geometric linearity. An example of an equation which is algebraically linear in its parameters $(a_0, a_1 \ldots a_n)$ is the nth order polynomial $y = a_0 + a_1 \cdot x + a_2 \cdot x^2 + \ldots + a_n \cdot x^n$, of which the straight line is a special case (n set to 1), but which includes a large number of nongeometrically linear forms. An example of an algebraic equation which is nonlinear in its parameters is the four-parameter logistic equation discussed above.

Analysis of variance (ANOVA): a statistical method which allows the overall variation in experimental results to be broken down into components originating from distinct causes. In assay, this method may be applied to an analysis of the quality of fit of a calibration curve equation, comparing the deviations of the curve from the data to the random scatter in the data. It is also highly useful in between-batch and between-laboratory quality control.

Analyte: the substance to be measured

Analyte concentration estimate: the concentration of analyte in a test specimen which is estimated by the assay procedure. Also sometimes known as dose, a term from the earlier biological assay field.

Analytical method: the physical and chemical manipulations to which calibrators and test specimens are subjected to produce their corresponding assay response values

Analytical sensitivity: a vague term generally associated with the ability to detect small concentrations, but in fact used with multiple meanings, thus provoking immense needless debate. The IFCC recommends using some mathematically defined term such as the lower detection limit (see below). This term is analogous to but not to be confused with diagnostic sensitivity.

Analytical specificity: a vague term associated with the ability to detect analyte as opposed to nonanalyte. The use of cross-reaction profiles is preferable. The term is analogous to but not to be confused with diagnostic specificity.

Batch: a single processing session in which a set of specimens is subjected to the assay analytical method

Between-batch random error: the random error which accrues in an assay system, including within-assay random error and the additional sources of random error which are observed when comparing results obtained from repeated analysis of the same specimen in different batches of the same assay method

Between-laboratory random error: the random error which is observed in measurements of the same specimen in different laboratories, including within-assay error, between-batch random error, and the additional sources of random error which are observed when comparing such results

Bias: systematic error. Causes include a decay in the performance of the final detection device, specimen misidentification, decay of calibrators or test specimens, nonidentity of the chemical behavior of calibrators and test specimens (as with cross-reaction and interference), and other causes.

Calibration curve: the plotted or mathematically describable relationship between the response and the analyte concentration

Calibrator: a known concentration of the analyte, used in creating the calibration curve. Also known as a standard. There are multiple varieties (reference, relative, others).

Confidence interval: the analyte concentration range contained within a set of confidence limits

Confidence limits: statistically defined limits about an analyte concentration estimate, which reflect the random error inherent in the result. For example, 95% limits define a region within which, 95% of the time, the true estimate (in the absence of bias error) would be expected to fall (were the measurement with the accompanying computation of confidence limits to be repeated many times).

Continuous response assay: an assay in which the response varies over a continuous range of values or over a discrete range which is so large as to be well approximated by a continuous range, as in radio-immunoassay

Cross-reaction: the reaction with the specific assay binding substance of some chemical entity other than the analyte in such a way as to falsify the measured amount of analyte

Cross-reaction profile: a plot of the bias error in the estimated concentration of analyte as a function of the concentration of a specified cross-reacting species at a given fixed concentration of analyte

Cumulative sum chart: a variety of quality control chart. The cumulative sum of deviations (from the expected value) of some quality control parameter is plotted. Various statistical tests are available to determine if the plotted points indicate a quality control problem.

Drift: a temporal shift in bias of assay results. Drift may sometimes be detected by placing quality control pool specimens at regular intervals in the assay batch.

Imprecision profile: a plot of imprecision (generally expressed as the width of a confidence limit of some specified level of certainty and a given level of replication of calibrators and unknowns) versus analyte concentration. This profile is also known as a precision profile.

Interference: used in many different ways in clinical chemistry. For example, this term is used to refer to the bias error in a spectrophotometer reading produced by the absorption of a given frequency of light by substances other than the one of primary interest. In a ligand assay, the term usually refers to the presence of something which can mimic the chemical behavior of the binder, producing bias error. As an example, the presence of thyroid-binding globulin could interfere with the assay of thyroid hormone.

Interpolation: the process of reading the response for an unknown through the calibration curve to obtain an analyte concentration estimate

Least squares (method of): a procedure for fitting a mathematical function to data in which the sum of the second powers of the vertical distances between the function and the data points is minimized. This meth-

od can be broken down into linear least squares and nonlinear least squares depending on whether the equation being fitted is algebraically linear or not. Linear fitting may be done by rather rapid noniterative computational procedures. If the error (in the vertical direction) in the original data is Gaussian, estimates for the random error inherent in the parameter estimates can be computed. These estimates will follow Gaussian distributions and therefore will be interpretable in probabilistic terms. If the nonlinear least-squares method is employed, an iterative (stepwise) method of solution must be used, and rigorous probabilistic interpretation of the parameter estimates is risky.

Lower detection limit (LDL): the (statistically defined) lowest concentration which is distinguishable from the lowest calibrator concentration (generally zero). This limit should be reported along with its associated level of statistical confidence. It is also referred to as the minimum detection limit, minimum detectable dose, or lower detection limit, among other expressions.

Outlier: defined in two senses; (i) a member of a replicate set which lies far from the other members of the set, presumably due to some extraordinary error; (ii) the mean of a replicate set for a calibrator which lies far from the calibration curve location suggested by the other calibrators, again presumably due to some extraordinary error

Parallelism testing: the process of determining whether the curve which can be drawn from the responses obtained from multiple dilutions of a test specimen can be superimposed upon the calibration curve by a simple multiplicative rescaling of the x axis of the test curve; also referred to as similarity testing, which is perhaps more appropriate, as "parallelism testing" derives from the early days of biological assay, when straight-line calibration relationships were employed

Pooled response-error relationship: a response-error relationship which is obtained by pooling information from a number of consecutive assay batches (generally 10 to 30) to achieve better estimates of the expected error than would be possible with the limited information available in a single batch

Power function: plot for a specified quality control test of the probability of rejection of an assay result as a function of the amount of error present (either bias or random)

Precision: a qualitative term concerned with the reproducibility of a result and hence with its random error. The IFCC has recommended the avoidance of this term, preferring the use of some precisely defined mathematical expression of random error, such as a set of confidence limits with its associated level of statistical significance.

Quality control chart: a plot of some assay performance parameter, most often the measurement obtained for a quality control pool, plotted chronologically on a flow chart. Statistical tests may be performed to ascertain if deviations from the average result would be so rare (if attributed to the usual amount of random error of the assay) as to represent a possible quality control problem. This chart is also known as a Shewhart chart, after the man who invented it (for use in industrial quality control), and a Levey-

Jennings chart, after the authors who introduced Shewhart's idea to the clinical pathology community.

Quality control (QC) pool: a large collection of analyte-containing material which is stored to preserve it over a long period of time. Samples are taken and analyzed (with each assay batch in earlier assays but with decreasing frequency in some newer commercial assays) to assist in detecting exceptional error (particularly useful for bias).

Quantal response assay: an assay in which the response is some value which varies over a discrete range of values (example: 1, 2, 3, ... *n*) rather than over a continuous range. An example is the type of biological assay in which a small number of animals are employed and the response is the proportion of animals killed by a given dose of analyte. This assay requires statistical methods not discussed in this chapter.

Random error: error arising from chance occurrences rather than systematic causes. Important sources in practice include pipetting, timing, counting, and detection errors. See also: precision, imprecision, sensitivity, lower detection limit, confidence limits.

Recovery: the amount of added analyte detected when a known amount of calibrator is added to a test preparation which has been previously assayed. Significant deviations from 100% suggest the presence of bias error.

Replicate: a repeated analysis of a calibrator, quality control specimen, or unknown, as when a specimen is said to be run in duplicate, triplicate, ... *n*-plicate. Such analysis is the only source of information about random errors.

Residual: the vertical distance between a data point (in assay, this is often the mean of replicates obtained for a given calibrator concentration) and the mathematical equation fitted to it. If the residual is properly weighted for the amount of data it represents and for its variance, it is referred to as a studentized residual.

Response: some mathematical function of the final measurement taken from the assay analytical method

Response-error relationship: a plot of the error in the selected response versus the response

Run: assay jargon for the process of analyzing a single assay batch

Standard deviation: a measure of the random error inherent in a set of measurements of the same quantity (equal to the square root of the variance). Although the standard deviation may be computed for any given set of numbers, it is interpretable in strict probabilistic terms only if the data are drawn randomly from a Gaussian population.

Test specimen: a sample, generally a biological fluid, a portion of which is presented to the assay process to determine the concentration of analyte present

Unknown: assay jargon for the test specimen

Upper detection limit (UDL): the (statistically defined) highest concentration which is distinguishable from the highest calibrator concentration; should be reported along with its associated level of statistical confidence

Valid analytical range: the range between the upper and lower detection limits

Variance: a measure of the random error inherent in a set of measurements of the same quantity, equal to the second power of the standard deviation

Weighting: the use of some estimate of random error in the process of regression to take into account the relative error of the data being fitted. The final fit will pay more attention to data of higher precision than to data of lower precision. In assay work, the inverse of the variance (estimated from a pooled response-error relationship) should be employed.

Within-assay random error: the random error observed in assay results analyzed in a single batch

LITERATURE CITED

1. **Buttner, H., R. Borth, J. H. Boutwell, and P. M. G. Broughton.** 1976. Provisional recommendations on quality control in clinical chemistry (International Federation of Clinical Chemistry, Committee on Standards). Clin. Chem. **22**:532–540.

2. **Dudley, R. A.** 1982. Radioimmunoassay (RIA) data processing on programmable calculators: an IAEA project, p. 411–421. *In* Radioimmunoassay and related procedures in medicine. International Atomic Energy Agency, Vienna.

3. **Edwards, P. R., and R. P. Ekins.** 1982. Development of a microcomputer radioimmunoassay (RIA) data-processing program for distribution by the World Health Organization, p. 423–442. *In* Radioimmunoassay and related procedures in medicine. International Atomic Energy Agency, Vienna.

4. **Faden, V. B., J. C. Huston, P. J. Munson, and D. Rodbard.** 1980. RIAPROG. Logit-log radioimmunoassay data processing. Biomedical Computing Technology Information Center, Nashville, Tenn.

5. **Finney, D. J.** 1976. Radioligand assay. Biometrics **32**:721–740.

6. **Finney, D. J.** 1983. Software requirements for statistical analysis of immunoassays, p. 597–607. *In* W. M. Hunter and J. E. T. Corrie, (ed.), Immunoassays for clinical chemistry. Churchill Livingstone, Edinburgh.

7. **Jeffcoate, S. L., and R. E. G. Das.** 1977. Interlaboratory comparison of radioimmunoassay results. Ann. Clin. Biochem. **14**:258–260.

8. **Pegg, P. J., and E. M. Miner.** 1982. The effect of data reduction technic on ligand assay proficiency survey results. Am. J. Clin. Pathol. **77**:334–337.

9. **Raab, G. M., and I. G. M. McKenzie.** 1982. A modular computer program for processing immunoassay data. *In* D. W. Wilson, S. J. Gaskell, and K. Kemp (ed.), Quality control in clinical endocrinology. Proceedings of the 8th Tenovus Workshop. Alpha Omega Publishers, Inc., Cardiff, Wales.

10. **Rodbard, D.** 1978. Data processing for radioimmunoassays: an overview, p. 477–494. *In* S. J. Natelson, A. J. Pesce, and A. A. Dietz (ed.), Clinical immunochemistry: chemical and cellular bases and applications in disease, vol. 3. American Association for Clinical Chemistry, Washington, D.C.

11. **Rodgers, R. P. C.** 1981. Quality control and data analysis in binder-ligand assay. Scientific Newsletters, Inc., Anaheim, Calif.

12. **Rodgers, R. P. C.** 1984. A formal model for the cost-effectiveness of assay quality control procedures, p. 51–62. *In* A. Albertini, R. P. Ekins, and R. S. Galen (ed.), Cost/benefit and predictive value of radioimmunoassay, vol. 18. Proceedings of the International Symposium on Cost and Benefit of Radioimmunoassay, Milan, Italy, 15–16 May 1984. Elsevier Science Publishers, Amsterdam.

13. **Rodgers, R. P. C.** 1984. Data analysis and quality control assays: a practical primer, p. 253–308. *In* W. R. Butt (ed.), Practical immunoassay. The state of the art. Marcel Dekker, Inc., New York.

Chapter 16

Solving and Preventing Problems in Ligand Assay

RICHARD M. DAUPHINAIS

Radioimmunoassay (RIA) heralded the clinical application of ligand assay methodology 25 years ago with the measurement of peptide hormones. The introduction of RIA made feasible the analysis of large numbers of specimens at a level of sensitivity and specificity previously attained only by the tedious processing of individual samples preliminary to biological or chemical analysis. In more recent years, the application of nonisotopic methods has contributed further to progress in ligand assay technology, sharing with RIA the same analytical principle and the same antisera, standards, and quality control materials. Even the procedural steps, including separation techniques, are essentially the same for both methods, the only fundamental difference being the labeled antigen employed. Together with RIA, these techniques have been considered superior to alternative procedures that are subject to various chemical or biological interferences.

As a microanalytical technique, however, ligand assay is not without pitfalls of its own. For example, the measurements of serum cobalamin (vitamin B_{12}) and folate by radioassay were considered natural replacements for the older microbiological methods employing *Euglena* or *Lactobacillus* species because of the latter methods' laborious and lengthy techniques and the problems of drug interference. In 1978, however, radioassay methods were demonstrated to miss 10 to 20% of patients with proven pernicious anemia, due to the nonspecificity of the commercial intrinsic-factor binding agents used (7). It was found that virtually all intrinsic-factor preparations available were contaminated, in some cases up to 100%, with "R protein" that bound not only cobalamin, but also certain metabolically inactive analogs. Correction of this problem by the use of "purified" intrinsic factor, intrinsic factor plus blocking agents to R protein, or binders other than intrinsic factor helped to allay the skepticism of clinicians and laboratorians toward the new measurements. Some companies, however, continued to market the old kits. In addition, further uncertainty and confusion appeared with changes in new or existing vitamin B_{12}-folate methods such as combined measurements, boil versus no-boil methods of protein denaturation, erythrocyte folate determinations, source of standards, solid-phase supports, separation techniques, modification of normal ranges, use of indeterminant ranges, and clinical criteria for "normals," to name a few. Although assays for vitamin B_{12} and folic acid may represent an extreme example, searching for a reliable method can be an exhausting process.

When a commercial manufacturer asked us to evaluate a new, combined vitamin B_{12}-folate method by correlating it with our existing kit method, we found this approach was not valid. The validity of our reference method, as it pertained to the patient's clinical condition, was questionable in several of the results. Of 52 consecutive patients considered normal by our reference method, 49 failed to meet our criteria of normal based on their clinical history or hematological picture. We therefore reestablished our vitamin B_{12}-folate reference ranges and investigated four different kits in the process. Almost all of our ranges differed significantly from those of the manufacturer (Table 1). The kit we were asked to evaluate (Kit B) never reached the market. Our existing method (Kit A) was dropped. A third kit (Kit C) was one of four changes made by a single manufacturer in the course of 1 year (something to consider when establishing your own reference ranges). Over 10% of our serum and erythrocyte folate values were rejected because of recent vitamin intake or ingestion of food. My own serum folate was elevated (28 ng/ml), apparently from having had the breakfast cereal "Total" the day blood was drawn ("100% Minimum Daily Requirement . . .?").

Establishing an in-house reference range is generally recommended for any procedure, especially when ranges supplied by manufacturers for a "normal" population may be based on inadequate criteria (e.g., "apparently normal individuals," "apparently healthy adults undergoing routine physical examination," etc.). Establishing such an in-house range is not always without problems, however. Manufacturers may be reluctant to supply sufficient kits for this purpose, either free or at a nominal charge. A small laboratory may have limited resources and may have to accumulate "normals" by using the same lot of reagents and instrumentation. The reference range may not reflect the population of patients tested. For example, most laboratory normal ranges are established on a relatively young group (laboratory technologists, staff volunteers, etc.) with an average age around 30. Most vitamin B_{12}-folate-deficient patients are older, with an average age in the 60s. Moreover, the level of vitamin B_{12} is age dependent and normally lower in older individuals. It may also be necessary to evaluate "abnormal" populations, since an overlap or indeterminant range often exists between deficiency and normal. Once an adequate population is sampled, confirmation of the reference range should be done by nonparametric statistical methods.

It is clear that accuracy, both analytical and clinical, must remain a primary goal for those who perform ligand assays. Analytical accuracy, i.e., how well a specified analyte is quantified, is the primary responsibility of the laboratory. Clinical accuracy invokes consideration of the validity of the test as an indicator of a particular clinical condition. The laboratory can monitor the latter component of accuracy only through effective interaction with the clinical staff or other source of reliable clinical input.

How does the well-informed laboratorian design assays best to detect and prevent the reporting of inaccurate values? The answer to the question is

TABLE 1. Comparison of determined and commercial reference ranges of four commercial kits for vitamin B_{12}, serum, and erythrocyte folate

Analyte and kit	n^a	Reference range	
		Determined[b]	Commercial (kit insert)
Vitamin B_{12} (pg/ml)			
Kit: A	103	168–792	260–1,030
B	98	172–806	276–1,254
C	97	163–1,135	171–953
D	90	183–996	242–1,241
Serum folate (ng/ml)			
Kit: A	92	2.9–18.7	1.9–14.0
B	87	2.7–9.8	1.6–12.9
C	87	3.4–13.3	2.6–18.8
D	80	2.4–21.3	2.8–21.8
Erythrocyte folate (ng/ml)			
Kit: A	93	178–853	120–674
B	89	126–513	122–380
C	88	225–705	160–650
D	99	171–816	179–777

[a] In-house "normal" controls.
[b] ±2 standard deviations of the geometric mean.

complex, since the laboratorian relies heavily upon the efficacy, facilities, and quality control of the manufacturer of analytical raw materials. The quality of reagents available can be controlled by the user only to a very limited degree. However, the procedures, facilities, and personnel involved in the collection and storage of specimens for analysis, the storage and preparation of reagents for assays, the design and conduct of the analysis, and the collection, treatment, and interpretation of data are all under the specific control of the laboratory. Knowledge of problems that may be encountered in ligand assay is prerequisite to reliable performance to minimize the production of spurious results. It is the goal of this chapter to create an awareness of problems that may occur with this methodology and to point out the means and practices at the disposal of the laboratory for the prevention, detection, and, where possible, resolution of these problems.

COLLECTION OF SPECIMENS

Inappropriate collection and handling of specimens can be the cause of inaccurate results obtained for patient specimens. In general, it is recommended that serum or plasma be separated from cellular components as soon as possible. Cell-free, nonhemolyzed specimens should be apportioned in duplicate or triplicate and stored under the best conditions to maintain chemical stability (see below) until they can be analyzed. Several ligands show no significant detrimental effect after delayed separation of serum from clot, but the changes are variable and their magnitude will increase with longer contact times. Some substances, such as adrenocorticotropin and folate, degrade more rapidly than others at room temperature, and these analytes should be processed without delay. Adrenocorticotropin is adsorbed strongly on glass, a process which can be minimized by using plastic

tubes for sample collection as well as for all steps of the analytical procedure. The hormone is rapidly destroyed by proteolytic enzymes in the blood. The use of enzyme inhibitors such as mercaptoethanol or Trasylol (aprotinin) and of low temperatures during storage, extraction, and assay of samples will protect the concentration of the hormone. Prior extraction of samples eliminates proteolytic enzymes and may be recommended even when a very specific antibody is used. No significant loss of the hormone is seen either before or after extraction when it is stored at −70°C.

Hemolysis should always be avoided in specimen collection. Although some assays are unaffected, others, such as serum folate determination, will be completely invalidated by marked hemolysis. In liquid scintillation analysis, hemolysis and bilirubin may cause significant quenching.

Lipemia of serum in general or high levels of triglycerides, cholesterol, or both in particular may produce erroneous results in some assays by interfering with antigen binding, even when antibodies are linked to a solid support. Lipemia may also affect homogeneous enzyme immunoassays (EIAs) utilizing malate dehydrogenase activity by inhibiting the enzyme. Measurements of triglycerides and cholesterol will not help predict this effect. The only way to validly estimate the degree of lipid interference is by a comparison of results before and after clearance of the lipids from the patient's serum. Clarification should be by ultracentrifugation, not by dilution. No appreciable loss of ligand should occur with ultracentrifugation. Otherwise, the use of lipemic samples in ligand assays should be avoided.

The collection of specimens for assay of vitamin B_{12} and folate requires special considerations. These analytes may deteriorate on exposure to strong light. Specimens for erythrocyte folate assays should be collected in tubes containing ca. 1.5 ng of EDTA per ml, and a hematocrit should be performed on the sample of whole blood. Ascorbic acid, added to stabilize folate samples, should not be used in vitamin B_{12} samples because apparently it destroys B_{12}.

Anticoagulants added to specimens in appropriate concentrations to preserve certain analytes may play havoc with the assay of other analytes, frequently by interfering with binding or precipitation of the antigen-antibody complex. Thus, EDTA, by chelating Ca^{2+} in plasma samples, can beneficially inactivate complement and prevent its inhibitory effect on precipitation in double-antibody procedures. Excessive concentrations of EDTA or heparin, however, may themselves inhibit the precipitation step. In addition, heparin also appears to have a modest vitamin B_{12}-binding capacity. The lithium salt of heparin may also stimulate a sharp increase in the release of B_{12}-binding proteins by granulocytes, which can interfere with the B_{12} assay. Heparin, either from the specimen tube or from heparinized patients, may interfere in the assay for carcinoembryonic antigen. Heparin should also be avoided in the collection of renin samples, since it appears to inhibit the action of renin on its substrate. Heparin can also interfere with the charge on ion-exchange resins used as binding or separating agents in ligand assays. Inhibition of the uptake of free ligand in an RIA system results in more counts in the bound fraction and lower values for the sample.

Specimens for serum hepatitis analysis may be drawn in heparin-containing tubes without apparent effect on the results. However, serum samples from patients on heparin therapy, particularly renal dialysis, may occasionally contain fragments of fibrin. Fibrin tends to coat the polystyrene beads used in solid-phase hepatitis testing and trap radiolabeled antibody on the beads, producing false high (positive) counts. Fibrin coating of the beads with resultant trapping of labeled antibody may also occur in some neutralization tests. To avoid inaccuracy due to known or suspected presence of fibrin, incubate the patient's original serum specimen at 40 to 45°C for 30 min, centrifuge it at $1,200 \times g$ to precipitate any fibrin, and repeat the assay. Other radioligand assays employing polystyrene beads may be similarly affected by fibrin fragments.

Certain other analytes require particular attention in specimen collection. Samples drawn for ligand assay of prostatic acid phosphatase should not be acidified as for the conventional enzyme analysis. Because of diurnal variation, the time of collection of cortisol specimens should be noted; sequential levels must be collected at the same time each day. Digoxin samples should be drawn at least 5 to 6 h after the last oral maintenance dose of the glycoside, preferably 24 h later and just before the next dose. Initial studies suggest that samples for antibody testing of anti-intrinsic factor should not be drawn until 48 h after a B_{12} injection. Monitorial levels of antibiotics, such as gentamicin or tobramycin, should include "trough" concentrations, the residual levels in serum just before the next dose, particularly in patients with renal impairment. Prolactin levels exhibit circadian rhythm, but generally stabilize between 10 a.m. and noon. Therefore, it is best to draw blood for assay of the hormone during that interval. Care should be taken in drawing the sample, since any undue stress during venipuncture may be associated with a sudden, increased output of prolactin. Occasional analytes, e.g., prostaglandins, are difficult to measure accurately because of their extreme susceptibility to a number of variables related to the collection and processing of blood samples and require very special care in their handling.

The proper collection of renin specimens is essential to ensure accuracy of results. They should be drawn in tubes containing EDTA to give a final concentration of 1 ng/ml. Time of day and the activity, salt intake, and specific medications of the patient should be defined. If samples are taken from different anatomical sites, these sites also should be indicated. Other details of the recommended method of handling specimens are controversial. Most methods have required drawing samples in prechilled syringes or Vacutainer tubes and maintaining them on ice during processing, either for immediate assay or for storage in a freeezer. In recent years, investigators have emphasized that cryoactivation of "prorenin" elevates measured total plasma renin activity. As a result, newer methods advocate performing the test at room temperature, thus eliminating the need to chill samples during collection. However, we have found that keeping specimens on ice during processing maintains relatively stable renin activity, as evinced through repetition of

analysis. If the samples are not to be assayed immediately, they are stored in a freezer, preferably at −40°C. (We have some evidence of angiotension I generation at freezer temperatures above −20°C.) Ideally, renin specimens should be handled promptly, i.e., within 30 min of collection, before significant changes occur at room or refrigeration temperatures.

The use of salivary samples to estimate circulating free levels of drugs or hormones in plasma may be affected by salivary protein concentration. The analysis of saliva may be limited to molecules not strongly bound to plasma proteins. Some drugs such as aminoglycoside antibiotics do not appear in saliva to any significant extent, presumably due to their extremely low lipid solubility. Immunoassays of these materials in saliva can play no part in routine monitoring of antibacterial therapy.

A final precaution concerns radioactive contamination in samples. Such radioactivity may remain with the bound labeled antigen, leading to an underestimation of analyte in the test sample. In charcoal techniques, radioiodinated (^{125}I) human serum albumin from blood volume studies will be counted with the bound complex. This is not a problem in techniques using solid-phase or double-antibody (without accelerator) separation of bound from free antigen. Serum contamination may also occur from two isotopes commonly used in scanning procedures, i.e., technetium (^{99m}Tc) and gallium (^{67}Ga), the gamma energies of which are close to that of cobalt (^{57}Co). ^{67}Ga is protein bound and clears slowly, with 5% of its radioactivity remaining after 48 h. It may still be a problem 2 weeks later. ^{99m}Tc is mostly protein bound but has a shorter half-life and is cleared fairly rapidly, with 3 to 4% of its radioactivity remaining after 24 h. Radioactivity may still be a problem 1 day after administration, but usually not after that. Suspected radioactive contamination of a specimen can be confirmed by counting the original serum or plasma sample. Resultant assay errors may possibly be circumvented by repeating the assay of the sample with a duplicate prepared in the usual way, but omitting the assay tracer. The difference in counts represents true assay radioactivity.

STORAGE OF REAGENTS AND TEST SPECIMENS

The physical state and temperature of individual ligand assay reagents and specimens awaiting analysis must be chosen to preserve maximal stability during short- and long-term storage. Many serum analytes are actually stable for several hours or days at room temperature. Insulin is unstable at room temperature and requires refrigeration or freezing. Gastrin is unstable at room temperature and refrigeration and somewhat unstable at freezing, and it is best stored deep frozen (−70°C). The stability of erythrocyte folate in nonhemolyzed whole-blood samples is largely a function of temperature and may be maintained for at least 3 days refrigerated (4°C) without any added preservatives. Mailing of samples, however, should be avoided.

The manufacturer or source of a purchased reagent chemical should be able to advise on storage of the chemical in the dry or liquid state before use, storage temperature, need for desiccation, and expected duration of stability. Generally, technical specialists available for consultation by telephone will be able to answer specific questions about product storage. In commercial kits, the package insert is required to contain this information. Storage of reagent components prepared or purchased by the user poses additional questions of preserving chemical stability, answers to which may require researching the literature to find what approaches have been taken successfully by others.

Recommended storage temperatures will often require refrigeration or freezing of all or part of assay kits. It is preferable to use metal containers and adequate spacing of stored materials. Moreover, the requirement of freezing temperatures for preservation of more labile chemicals should indicate the use of a non-self-defrosting type of freezer whose cooling capacity is checked regularly. Ideally, a thermometer with a recording device should be placed in each piece of cooling equipment used for storage and checked regularly. In addition, installation of an electronic alarm to signal temperatures that are too high can prevent the laboratory from using reagents or analyzing specimens that may have been subject to damaging storage conditions.

Some commercial kits are designed for one-time use immediately after reconstitution or thawing of reagents. However, anticipated repetitious use of the same reagent would generally be an indication for storing it in numerous separate vessels, each containing the volume required for one use. Large volumes of working solutions should be stored in well-washed, very well rinsed borosilicate glass containers with glass or plastic stoppers.

The radiolabeled analyte is the assay reagent probably most susceptible to alteration or damage during storage. That is because radioactive, biological, and immunochemical properties all represent a possible target of alteration. The bond joining the radioactive atom to the ligand may be labile. Thus, molecules with covalently bonded radioiodide are susceptible to deiodination, and tritium can exchange with other hydrogens in the molecule or in the solvent. The radioactive atom may also induce molecular rearrangement of the ligand that would affect its immunochemical or binding properties; hence, association-dissociation characteristics of the antigen-antibody or ligand-binder complex may be altered. For these reasons, the labeled ligand must not be used beyond the shelf life recommended by the kit manufacturer, regardless of the half-life of the radionuclide.

Any possible deleterious effects a vessel surface might have upon its contents would be most pronounced during storage, when contact between the surface and the contained material is lengthy. Containers employed for storage of patient specimens and reagents should be of adequate quality and composition. Recommendations of the manufacturer of the radioassay kit or component should be followed closely. A first concern is that constituents of or materials adherent to container surfaces might leach into the stored specimen or reagent. These substances would include ions, detergent residue, silicon excess, plasticizers, etc. Second, adsorption of solutes to container surfaces could alter the concentration of analyte in stored specimens or the potency of standards or binding proteins. Third, chemical reactions catalyzed by reactive groups on the glass or plastic surface might alter the analyte or otherwise interfere with the assay of the stored specimen or use of the reagent. These hazards may be minimized by appropriate siliconization of glass tubes, inclusion of an inert protein (e.g., bovine serum albumin or gelatin) in the buffer solution to coat tubes preferentially, or use of plastic tubes of particularly nonporous composition.

PREPARATION OF REAGENTS AND SAMPLES FOR ASSAY

Preparation of reagent solutions requires volumetric delivery equipment of great precision and accuracy in the range of volumes for which each piece is employed. For mixing large-volume solutions, glass volumetric pipettes of high-quality manufacture seem to be safe choices for use with glass volumetric flasks. Smaller volumes are delivered most accurately by positive-displacement dispensers. The technique for use of any piece of volumetric equipment is as important as the quality of the equipment in that lack of skill in or knowledge of its use can completely obviate satisfactory performance of measurements. Uniform procedures and techniques should be practiced by all technicians who participate in performing a test day after day.

A variety of manual and semiautomated pipetting devices are available that are capable of delivering microliter volumes of fluids at a coefficient of variation of about 1%, a desirable limit, although these claims refer to aqueous fluids only, not the more viscous serum samples. The temperature of the pipette, especially that of semiautomated pipettes, should be the same as the solution being pipetted to avoid errors in reproducibility and accuracy. Prerinsing the pipette tip also diminishes errors in replication. Even with optimal use and care, pipetters are subject to wear, contamination, and deterioration due to age. In addition, faulty disposable tips can produce inaccurate measurements. Volumetric delivery apparatus should be calibrated regularly with verification of accuracy and reproducibility of volumes as part of a routine quality control program.

In mixing solutions whose concentrations must be critically controlled, such as standard or reference solutions, consistent temperatures are extremely important. These may be more difficult to achieve at certain times of the year when room temperatures may fluctuate widely. A recommended method of circumventing this problem is to handle all standard solutions, patient samples, and diluents at ice-water temperature. Cooled to 4°C, all solutions will have volumes measured with the same small degree of error (using apparatus calibrated for 20°C delivery). Since all solutions (i.e., standards, specimens, and controls) will be subject to the same error, any resulting inaccuracy would be minor compared to the uncontrolled error incurred from fluctuation of temperatures. Day-to-day inconsistencies in solution preparation thus are diminished.

The preparation of reagents occasionally requires the use of a balance for weighing buffer salts, assay standard, etc. The accuracy of the balance claimed by the manufacturer must be within the range of accuracy demanded by the weighing intended and the analytical method employed.

Ultimately, the preparation of reagents results in solutions. The user laboratory will usually have to add at least a solvent, often water, to premeasured buffer salts. The water employed as the reagent solvent (and also for at least the final rinses of any glassware used to contain assay reagents or specimens) should be free from any detectable microbiological contaminants. It must be of maximal chemical purity, devoid of metal ions, macromolecules, and pyrogens. Commercially bottled sterile water intended for use in intravenous injections has been used to prepare reagents and may be microbiologically sterile, but it contains many chemical impurities (revealed by high-pressure liquid chromatography [HPLC]) which may potentially interfere with or inhibit chemical and microbiological determinators. To achieve the desired degree of purity, a laboratory might have to install facilities to distill, deionize, and decontaminate its water. Such facilities themselves require cleaning and maintenance. Resin beds used for deionization will in time develop microbiological contamination, as will rubber or plastic tubing used in conjunction with water delivery systems. Filters of small pore size installed distal to a contaminated resin bed will prevent spread of the contaminating growth of microorganisms but will not remove pyrogens, their metabolic by-products. Rubber and plastic tubing may leach out some of their monomeric components over a period of time.

Salts and other ancillary reagents used in buffers that must be furnished by the user laboratory should be of the highest analytical reagent quality. The most commonly used buffers in RIA are Tris, phosphate-buffered saline, and barbital. Binding characteristics of reagents used with these buffers may differ due to variations of light sensitivity; i.e., phosphate-buffered saline systems are essentially insensitive, barbital is somewhat sensitive, and Tris is very sensitive to light. Therefore, UV light or bright sunlight should be excluded during assay procedures utilizing Tris buffer systems.

Reagents should be mixed effectively and thoroughly, but not destructively. Thus, stirring, either mechanical or manual, will usually be preferable to shaking. Blending small volumes in a Vortex mixer, particularly when solutions contain protein, can induce denaturation; mixing by gently withdrawing and expelling the liquid a number of times is preferable. Certain flocculent materials or lyophilized proteins seem to be dissolved most effectively when allowed to remain immersed in the delivered solvent (or floating on top of it) until the passage of time induces dispersal or wetting, followed by dissolution. In certain cases, gentle stirring at elevated temperatures may be helpful.

Final pH adjustments of solutions are best performed as short a time before the solutions are needed as possible. The pH meter should be reliably accurate and properly calibrated during use by a technician familiar with its operation.

Care should also be taken in the dilution of serum samples since dilution represents that assay condition that will most disturb protein-ligand equilibrium in the sample. The concentration of free hormone, for example, will alter after the addition of binding reagents to the extent of the binding properties (affinity and binding capacity) of the endogenous carrier proteins.

DESIGN AND CONDUCT OF LIGAND ASSAYS

As indispensable as ligand assay has become as a laboratory technique, there is potential for a variety of methodological problems. Some of these problems relate to nonspecific interferences such as medications, serum proteins, or radioactivity previously administered. Technical errors may also occur with any of the procedural steps, but in some cases are unique to the type of ligand assay system used. These errors are discussed in the context and sequence in which they may be encountered in the laboratory.

Calibrator, standard or reference material

The calibrator (standard) curve usually is derived from activity bound in the presence of standards at five or six concentrations. The curve should circumscribe the normal range, with sufficient overlap of areas above and below normal to provide clinically relevant data. The main problems relating to standards are miscalibration (e.g., incorrect dilution) and stability of stored solutions of standards. The ultimate accuracy of values determined in the assay is irrevocably dependent upon the accuracy of the concentrations assigned to the standards or calibrators. If these concentrations are incorrect, the values of patient specimens interpolated from the curve will be inaccurate. If standard solutions have been overdiluted or for any other reason are less potent than the concentrations indicated on the standard curve, the concentrations of test specimens evaluated from the curve will be inaccurately elevated. Conversely, underdilution of standards, or any factor causing the standards to be more potent than indicated on the curve, will result in inaccurately depressed values. Calibration of kit standards in terms of international standards or reference preparations would largely resolve calibration problems.

Problems with inappropriate measurements are frequently seen in assays operated down to their detection limits, i.e., for substances which are secreted intermittently or below a measurable threshold (e.g., human growth hormone) or which are readily measurable in patients in one clinical state (e.g., thyroid-stimulating hormone [TSH] in hypothyroids) but not in another (e.g., TSH in hyperthyroids) (5). A correct assessment would be to state the value as "less than" a threshold level of a kit rather than reporting an absolute value based on an unrealistically wide working range. The best evaluation of a threshold level is in an analyte-free human serum sample, where the analyte is lacking due to normal physiology or a diseased state, rather than having been physically or chemically removed, e.g., by charcoal adsorption or immunosorption.

Critically important to the preparation of accurate standards and patient specimens, as well as to the dilution of controls, is the selection and effective operation of volumetric dilution equipment, as discussed above. Final dilution of standards and calibrators should be made immediately before use in the assay. When possible, it is preferable not to prepare the assay standards by serial dilution because a small error in the dilution of any single standard is necessarily amplified in all subsequent dilutions. Standards should be determined at least in duplicate as a matter of good practice. If the variability of results obtained for standards and samples is so great that the distinction among responses of standards at different concentrations is unclear, the use of a larger number of replicates should be considered. Standard solutions, patient specimens, and controls all should be at the same temperature when delivered into assay tubes.

Antiserum or binding protein

High-affinity antisera should be used for ligand assay measurements to avoid excessive escape of bound tracer during the various reaction steps. Variations in antibody affinity may be minimized by keeping all manually controlled steps (e.g., length of incubation, centrifugation) the same for each tube or assay.

Final dilution of the binding-protein solution is best made just before use in an assay since this solution is generally more stable when maintained in the concentrated form. If special care is taken to perform dilutions with consistent accuracy through proper use of well-designed volumetric dilution and mixing equipment, interassay variation will be minimized. However, an assay will not necessarily produce unusable values because of slightly incorrect dilution of the binding-protein solution. For example, in an RIA, slight overdilution of the antibody would cause the higher-concentration standards, controls, and test specimens to be determined somewhat less precisely, just as slight underdilution would result in less confident determination in the low-concentration range. (The converse relationship would obtain in an immunoradiometric assay, i.e., radiolabeled binding protein.)

The most important considerations in handling the binding-protein solution are that precisely the same volume of binder be delivered to each assay tube (except to those that measure nonspecific binding) and that homogeneity of the solution be maintained by appropriate mixing during the period of delivery to tubes. Vigorous mixing should be avoided so as not to risk denaturation of the binder protein.

Labeled ligand

The labeled ligand represents the major difference among ligand assay methods, and although many alternatives to radioactive tracers have been proposed, no single all-purpose label has been identified that is without drawbacks of its own. The most common labels other than radioactive labels are enzymatic, fluorescent, and chemiluminescent. Which method is used is largely related to the advantages and disadvantages of each and to the preference of the user. Nonisotopic methods have become popular by eliminating the problems of handling and disposing of radioactive materials. Many research laboratories, however, prefer to use radioactive labels because of

their small size, resulting in less steric hindrance to the reaction of antigen with antibody than occurs with the much larger nonisotopic labels. Other factors relate to stability, available instrumentation, and practicability.

The labeled ligand usually requires refrigeration as a ready-to-use liquid reagent but may be supplied as a dry solid. Reconstitution, as well as final dilution of a concentrated tracer, should take place shortly before the tracer is to be used in the assay. Radiolabeled ligands degrade more readily in aqueous solutions. Their deterioration will contribute to a loss of assay sensitivity among other things, producing an inability to detect small amounts of analytes.

As with the binding-protein solution, slight differences in concentration or specific activity in the tubes from one performance of the assay to the next usually will not influence the overall analytical accuracy. However, gross errors in dilution of the labeled ligand will destroy the analytical usefulness of the assay. The most important consideration in handling the labeled ligands is that exactly the same volume of homogeneous solution be delivered to each tube within a given assay.

Separation of bound from free labeled ligand

The precision and accuracy of a ligand assay are directly related to the efficiency of the chemical or physical agent and the equipment employed to separate bound from free ligand. Incomplete removal of the free fraction from the bound complex adds significantly to the imprecision of the test by raising the determined level of nonspecific binding (see below). Consequently, the sensitivity of the system suffers as the minimum detectable concentration of analyte is raised.

The optimal concentration of separating agent relative to that of ligand-binder complex and the conditions for incubation should be determined for the assay system by either the user laboratory or the reagent kit manufacturer (and confirmed by the user) before institution of the test. Reagents commonly used for separation include chemical or biological agents, such as anti-gamma globulin, polyethylene glycol, ammonium sulfate, and *Staphylococcus aureus* protein A, and physical agents, such as charcoal, silica, or resin. Slight differences in preparation of the separation reagent may reduce the accuracy of the assay. For example, solutions made from a new lot of reagent or suspensions given inadequate time for mixing before or during use may perform less efficiently.

In double-antibody separation methods utilizing anti-gamma globulin, the rate of reaction between first and second antibodies is relatively rapid, but formation of a precipitate is a more protracted process. Incubation times for these procedures are generally overnight, and one should be wary of so-called "shortened" assays until they have been thoroughly examined. Ways of speeding up these assays include increasing the concentration of second antibody (which increases the use of an already-expensive reagent), or the use of an "accelerator" such as polyethylene glycol, which has to be added in the right concentration to avoid nonspecific precipitation of the ligand being measured. Patient sera with elevated globulin content may be associated with increased nonspecific binding in polyethylene glycol separation, which would not be seen in a straightforward double-antibody procedure, a clinically important effect when ligand concentrations are low (1).

Some steroid assays utilizing brief incubation intervals may exhibit prominent cross-reaction with closely related steroids. The ability of antisera to distinguish between these interfering substances depends more on their dissociation rate with the antibody than their association rate. By prolonging the incubation period, the more rapidly dissociating steroids are replaced with the more slowly dissociating specific analyte which reaches maximum by incubating until equilibrium conditions are reached.

Immobilization of antibody to a solid phase improves the simplicity and efficiency of separation but may result in low recovery of antibody activity, reducing assay sensitivity. Particulate solid preparations require constant suspension to minimize incubation times but may be partially counterbalanced by increasing the viscosity of the incubation medium or using magnetized particles and a magnetic field.

The use of physical agents such as charcoal requires continuous mixing for adequate suspension before addition to reaction tubes. Magnetic stirrers, therefore, are convenient, but tend to generate heat, and temperature changes affect adsorption rates onto charcoal, which already suffers from relatively poor selectivity. Prolonged contact of reaction mixtures with charcoal should be avoided, and the tubes should be decanted as soon as possible after centrifugation. Double-antibody techniques also require prompt decanting, but the pellet is extremely frail and may be lost if not handled gently. Polyethylene glycol methods pack a more solid pellet and minimize this problem.

If aspiration of the supernatant is performed, the vacuum system should be connected to a trap to avoid contamination of a central vacuum outlet, particularly with radioactive systems. Splashing of aspirated material through a water faucet outlet should also be avoided to prevent aerosol formation and scattering of droplets.

Centrifugation is an integral part of the separation step of many ligand assays. If centrifugal force and temperature are not properly maintained, separation may be incomplete, resulting in partial loss of precipitate during decantation or aspiration of the supernatant. Inconsistency would appear from run to run. Invalid assays may result. Adequate relative centrifugal force (g value) delivered to the assay tubes results from different rotor speeds in different instruments. The required number of revolutions per minute for separation in a given assay system is calculated from the radius measured from the center of the rotor to each horizontal tube bottom in the carrier and obviously will vary from one centrifuge to the next. Even with maintenance of constant rotor speed during centrifugation, in certain equipment the relative force delivered to each tube may differ according to its position in the carrier. Extending the time of centrifugation usually will compensate for this defect in instrument design, but prolonged centrifugation should be avoided to prevent escape of tracer from the bound complex or resolubilization of double-antibody complexes.

Detection of centrifuge malfunction often is difficult because, once initial settings of force and temperature are made, variation during the instrument's automatic operation may go unnoticed. It is good practice to watch the speed indicator while the rotor accelerates to the prescribed speed and to check the indicator during operation. Nonrefrigerated centrifuges will build up heat within the spinning chamber, which might cause partial denaturation or, at least, influence the integrity or precipitation of the ligand-binder complex.

After separation of the free from bound ligand by centrifugation, the supernatant phase must be removed with as little cross-contamination as possible. One usually finds that either decantation or aspiration will yield the most satisfactory results in a given assay system, provided that the technician performing the separation is skilled and well practiced. At this point in the procedure, it is possible for carelessness or lack of skill to destroy the consistency and accuracy of the assay for the reasons cited above.

Nonspecific binding and interference

Ideally, ligand assays involve only one variable, i.e., the concentration of specific analyte, but a variety of other factors can interfere with its measurement. In a ligand assay system, the labeled species itself or fragments thereof may bind to reagents in the reaction mixture other than the specific binder and be separated with the specific-protein-bound fraction. Significant activity may bind to the wall of the reaction tube. The physical separation of bound from free ligand results in a certain amount of residual supernatant liquid trapped in the precipitate. These factors add to the background "noise" of the test system.

In radioligand assay systems, regardless of the origin of background radioactivity counted with the bound fraction (whether due to real or apparent binding), many assays require monitoring of the nonspecific component at each performance of the test. This monitoring is usually accomplished by delivering to duplicate tubes the radioactive ligand and nonreactant reagents but omitting the specific binding protein and standard material. In RIA systems with binder immobilized to a solid material, it is usually not possible for the user to add the separating agent—glass or plastic beads, paper disks, coated tubes, etc.—without the antibody attached. In such a case, the nonspecific binding of the system can be estimated by delivering a 100- to 1,000-fold molar excess of nonradioactive ligand to a complete reaction mixture of reagents. The excess nonradioactive species should displace all specifically bound radioactivity.

The justification for subtracting the measured nonspecific binding of an assay system from the counts obtained for each tube, including standards, controls, and test specimens, is that the nonspecific component represents a very small percentage of the total binding activity. It is further presupposed that the assay binding agent constitutes the only binding activity in the system. If either of these assumptions is invalid, as with the presence of an anomalous binding substance (e.g., an autoantibody), totally inaccurate values for the sample may result (3). In patients with thyroid disease, for example, one may see high concentrations of autoantibodies to thyroid hormones, although these high concentrations are rare, but even low concentrations, which are more common, will cause spuriously high or low ligand assay results depending on how the hormone-antibody complex is separated. A test specimen can generally be checked for the presence of anomalous binding activity in an assay by adding the serum sample to all the usual reagents but omitting the assay binding protein. The incubation, separation, and quantitation are carried out as usual. If the resultant binding markedly exceeds the nonspecific binding of the system measured as described above, it may signal the presence of factors that prevent accurate analysis by routine means. Identification of such a specimen indicates the need to extract the analyte from or otherwise neutralize that interference.

Enzymes are particularly sensitive to their physical environment, and their activity is greatly affected by a number of parameters, some of which are unique to EIAs, e.g., substrate depletion, build-up of product inhibitors, high levels of endogenous enzyme, etc. (2). The more universal factors of temperature, pH, ionic strength, and protein composition also affect these systems, as they affect any other.

A number of different enzymes have been used successfully as labels, each enzyme with certain advantages and disadvantages. All of the chromogens for horseradish peroxidase are unstable to various degrees, requiring preparation immediately before use. Mutagenic and carcinogenic properties of some of these chromogens have been reported, and they should be handled with care. Sodium azide, a commonly used bacteriostatic agent, is a potent inhibitor of horseradish peroxidase activity. EDTA and phosphate, commonly used in plasma, are both inhibitory to alkaline phosphatase. EIA should not be used with plasma as a general rule. "Hook effects" are more often seen with solid-phase EIAs than with RIA, although the level at which a hook effect occurs will vary with different kits.

The avidin-biotin system has found use in some EIAs, in which it serves to chemically amplify the antibody-antigen reaction to facilitate its measurement using an enzyme label. Biotin is a vitamin which binds with an unusually high affinity (10^{15} M^{-1}) to the protein avidin. If the assay system utilizing avidin-biotin is not properly constructed, a variety of problems may ensue with its use, e.g., in reagent additions where binding takes place at a very rapid rate, and pipetting intervals will be more significant for one reagent addition than for another (D. Senn, personal communication).

Problems with fluorescence immunoassays include light scattering by samples containing high concentrations of lipids or other large complexes, resulting in summation of fluorescent signal. Bilirubin acts as an endogenous fluorophore and, together with hemoglobin, may absorb part of either the excitation or the emission beam. Quenching effects may be seen with temperature increases, low pH, changes in polarity, the presence of trace oxidizing agents or dissolved oxygen, and nonspecific binding to serum proteins (albumin). The light source should avoid even small variations in light intensity, since the intensity of fluorescence is directly proportional to the intensity of incident light. Better instruments, including lasers, can overcome this problem by utilizing the ratio of emitted light to incident light ("ratio recording") on which to base their measurements. In this case, the ratio stays the same even if the incident light varies.

Chemiluminescence, the chemical production of light, typically requires the oxidative excitation of luminol, in alkali, in the presence of a catalyst. A liquid scintillation detector can be modified as a luminometer, but use of strongly light-absorbing or fluorescent solutes may interfere with measurements since total light emitted from a sample will be collected, regardless of scattering. The color of the emitted light is often strongly dependent on pH. If a solid-phase system is used but not washed properly, serum components (i.e., adenine or pyridine nucleotides or certain enzymes) may react directly in the chemiluminescent reaction. Bioluminescence, a special form of chemiluminescence found in biological systems, frequently employs the catalytic protein luciferase, which is sensitive to thiol reagents and inhibited by volatile anesthetics, riboflavin, cyanide, and certain heavy metals. High concentrations of salts and buffers also inhibit the enzyme, but this inhibition can be overcome by dilution and accounted for by constant addition calibration. Luciferase is temperature dependent, with an optimum at 25 to 28°C.

Fluorometric assays for plasma cortisol have a marked positive bias (overestimation). Competitive protein-binding methods, which incorporate a solvent extraction stage, result in underestimation, presumably due to incomplete recovery of steroid. By replacing these earlier methods with the more specific immunoassays, the accuracy of the new measurements was considered superior and appropriate to provide clinically useful values on which treatment of patients could reliably be based. However, even immunoassay methods for cortisol may suffer from problems with specificity. Patients undergoing dynamic studies (i.e., metyrapone inhibition) will frequently demonstrate paradoxically elevated cortisol levels which, by HPLC, are found to be due to elevated levels of 11-deoxycortisol, the precursor to cortisol, and possibly to other interfering steroids (6). Some institutions now prefer to measure cortisol only by HPLC to ensure accuracy.

Alterations in serum proteins have been incriminated in a variety of behavior patterns in ligand assay analysis. Methods supposedly measuring unbound analog for free thyroxin (T4) may actually measure the albumin-bound hormone fraction and be influenced by the level of albumin in the serum (10). Interpretation of free-T4 values should be done with caution in patients with abnormal concentrations of serum albumin, e.g., those with nonthyroid severe illness. In conditions associated with low or absent albumin (hereditary analbuminemia) or abnormal albumin binding of analog tracer (familial dysalbuminemic hyperthyroxinemia), false low or false high levels of free T4, respectively, may be obtained. In some solid-phase assays, albumin may even inhibit binding of labeled T4 to the immobilized T4 antibody, giving false high results. If a patient is on heparin therapy, moreover, the concentration of nonesterified fatty acids is increased due to the release of lipoprotein lipase from the vascular endothelium, and, like thyroxine, nonesterified fatty acids will bind strongly to albumin, displacing residual labeled T4, the concentration of which increases in the specific bound fraction, resulting in apparently lower values for free T4. In general, thyroid function tests should be deferred to the convalescent phase of major illness, and blood should not be collected while the patient is receiving heparin (8).

Abnormal immunoglobulin (myeloma) paraproteins may affect homogeneous EIAs for serum thyroxine and other ligands. Interference is created by turbidity of the paraproteins in the reaction mixture, resulting in increased absorbance and marked underestimation of hormone concentration.

Heterophilic antibodies may interfere with a number of ligand assays, especially when the ligand in question is close to its detection limits. Heterophilic antibodies in the sera of healthy people may be due to drinking uncooked cow's milk (anti-bovine antibodies), to immunization with a vaccine obtained from bacterial culture on a medium enriched with homogenate of rabbit lung (anti-rabbit antibodies), and to receiving anti-human thymocyte serum (anti-rabbit antibodies). Interference by anti-rabbit antibodies in an immunoradiometric TSH assay has been reported as high as 20% in some special groups. Of patients in Sweden with elevated TSH values, 5% are estimated to have anti-rabbit antibodies. Sera with heterophilic anti-sheep antibodies have reportedly interfered with an alpha-fetoprotein immunoradiometric sandwich technique in which both sides of the sandwich used sheep antibodies. The cause was assumed to be ingestion of raw cow's milk, resulting in the production of anti-bovine antibodies which markedly cross-reacted with ovine (sheep) immunoglobulins (4). These problems may be resolved by including nonimmune serum from the animal in question (producing the antibodies) to the assay reaction mixture. The heterophilic antibodies present will be neutralized, preventing distortion of the assay.

A digoxin-like immunoreactive substance is present in premature and full-term infants not on digoxin therapy and cross-reacts in various degrees with different digoxin ligand assay kits (9). The nature and significance of this substance are unclear but may be sufficient to compromise the usefulness of a measured value for digoxin in the clinical management of newborns requiring digoxin treatment. Concentrations of digoxin-like immunoreactive substance apparently peak 4 to 6 days after birth, with highest concentrations occurring in the babies with lowest birth weights. Digoxin measurements on newborns should be interpreted carefully.

Drugs and their metabolites that are structurally related to substances measured by ligand assay represent a potential source of interference which should be considered in evaluating results inconsistent with clinical conditions. For example, danazol, a drug structurally related to testosterone and commonly used to treat endometriosis and benign breast disease, will competitively displace testosterone (and cortisol) from plasma proteins and inhibit production of testosterone-binding globulin and thyroxine-binding globulin. It interferes with the immunoassay of testos-

terone in some systems and affects thyroid function tests by its suppression of pituitary function.

Several different ligand assay techniques are also available for therapeutic drug monitoring. Generally, these methods show good agreement among themselves and with highly specific methods such as gas-liquid chromatography or HPLC. In patients with renal disease, however, there may be an accumulation of drug metabolites (and possibly other substances) that will cross-react with the therapeutic drug-monitoring immunoassays that may not be readily appreciated. It is recommended that, in uremic patients, these assays be validated by the laboratories (or manufacturers) against a reference method such as HPLC.

CONTROLS

Most laboratories now depend on commercially prepared kit reagents to perform the various clinical ligand assays available. However, large differences have occurred in the past for some insulin and thyroid-related RIA kits, due to lot-to-lot changes or variation in standard concentration assigned to individual kits. While short-term in-laboratory analytical variation is largely under the control of individual laboratories, long-term variation is largely related to changes in kit components. This fact emphasizes the importance of establishing international reference standards for ligand assay kits commercially available in different countries. In the meantime, one should look for the best analytic reagents for each analyte of interest.

The first and sometimes only means at the disposal of the laboratory for monitoring its own accuracy and detecting inaccuracy is the routine analysis of commercially prepared "controls," i.e., solutions containing one or more analytes in a serum or simulated serum diluent. The advantages of using commercially prepared controls are several. The commercial manufacturer has facilities to ensure consistent, accurate concentrations, chemical stability, and a long-lasting supply of the preparation that are almost certain to exceed the analogous facilities of even the best user laboratory. The commercial concern probably will have wide distribution of the product and, therefore, a broad-based consensus of quantitative results obtained with kits of various manufacturers. These data usually are furnished in the literature that accompanies the control preparation. Thus, the absolute values obtained by widely dispersed laboratories using the same or different analytical reagents will be available for comparison.

The user laboratory should monitor the reproducibility of the control values determined in successive repetitions of the assay to derive its own interassay variation for the control preparation. Each assay should contain control samples whose analyte content corresponds to normal and above- and below-normal results that might actually be obtained in the assay of clinical specimens. It is of practical value to monitor the consistency of analysis at points associated with medical decisions. One should avoid using commercial controls which do not contain an appropriate concentration of analyte at the decision level, e.g., ferritin (decision level, ±10 µg/liter). If a commercial kit supplies its own "in-kit" controls at these critical levels, it would be preferable to use them in the absence of suitable commercial preparations.

There are several important applications of the routine analysis of controls. Initially, the similarity of the laboratory's mean result for the control to the consensus value provides some degree of confidence in its performance of the test compared with that of other groups. Day-to-day consistency of control values provides an index of reproducibility of test results. On the other hand, a sudden departure from the laboratory's mean values for controls may signal an inaccurate performance of the test and, depending on the degree of disparity of values, might indicate that results obtained for specimens from patients should not be reported until the results are repeated and confirmed. Finally, careful examination of the pattern of control values obtained over a period of time may reveal a subtle drift of the assay results due, for example, to gradual deterioration of a reagent.

The control specimens should be positioned at intervals throughout the assay, with each control at more than one position, if possible. The latter strategy aids in detecting a "position effect," that is, disparate progress of the binding reaction or separation step(s) or both at different positions in the assay. For example, it might be seen that samples analyzed at the end of the assay are evaluated consistently higher (or lower) than the same samples appearing earlier in the test sequence. Identification of a position effect might logically lead first to verifying the calibration of the thermostat on incubation equipment and the accuracy of laboratory timers. If an incubation has proceeded at less than the prescribed temperature or for too short a time, the reaction may not have reached completion throughout the set of assay samples. Frequent checks of both timing and thermostatic equipment should be part of the laboratory's preventative maintenance program.

Eliminating inaccuracy due to a position effect may be accomplished by careful examination of each of the component reactions of the assay to discover which may have been timed so critically that even a slight difference in the treatment of samples nearer the beginning from the treatment of those at the end of the test has resulted in higher (or lower) values. If a critical reaction step(s) is identified, appropriate modification of the procedure for handling or dispensing reagents or of the duration or temperature of incubation or limitation of the number of tubes processed in a single performance of the assay probably will solve the problem.

When a source of suitable controls for an assay is located, it is wise to purchase a supply of the preparation that will last at least several months. One may then dissolve a portion of the material, using the very best quantitative chemical technique, dispense it into suitable containers in volumes corresponding to that consumed at each performance of the assay, and store it under conditions that ensure greatest chemical stability. If no commercial source of a control preparation for a particular ligand assay can be located, an effort should be made to purchase the purified chemical and prepare an in-house control.

In addition to the external control discussed above, it is useful to repeat the determination of actual test specimens from the preceding assay, such as one sample selected from each of the normal and abnormally high and low ranges. This practice furnishes random confirmation of the result obtained on the specimens selected. Also, it has been our experience that the repetition of actual test samples might detect a problem that routine repetition of the commercial control does not. One cannot say whether this is referable to the presence of some stabilizer or preservative in the commercial preparation or perhaps to the absence of some undefined constituent of normal serum. Through objective evaluation of the results obtained for control preparations and test specimens repeated from the previous run, results of an assay may be judged reliable, unreliable, or partially acceptable. The last is illustrated by the finding that values for repeated samples may agree with values previously obtained in some parts of the analytical range but not in others. In such a case, the laboratory could consider reporting results on test specimens that fell in the assay's reliable range but withholding values in the questionable range.

GENERAL REMARKS

Problems detected in an assay may be dramatic—such as no standard curve, all tubes binding at background or nonspecific level, all the controls elevated (or reduced), etc.—or they may be mild and gradual in onset—such as values determined for controls drifting higher (or lower) over a period of weeks, rising incidence of patient samples falling in abnormal ranges, apparent decline of maximum radioactivity bound to antibody, and so forth. Although the strategy invoked to solve the former type of problem differs superficially from that used to investigate the latter, in both cases identification of the cause of the problem is of secondary importance to resumption of accurate testing. Therefore, it may be desirable to substitute an entire, new set of reagents immediately while an orderly examination of the possible causes for assay failure takes place without pressure due to an accumulation of test requests.

The most valuable resource of the ligand assay laboratory is its technical staff. Notwithstanding the quality of chemical reagents and equipment and the sophistication of automated instrumentation, it is the technician who intelligently uses these elements to perform and analyze assays. Appropriate training in quantitative chemical technique and education in the principles of methodologies practiced combine to prepare a competent technologist. But it is the motivated, attentive assistant who will detect errors, irregularities, and unusual results, solve dilemmas, and otherwise provide the support essential to the conduct of a thoroughly reliable ligand assay program.

I express appreciation to Mary Zern for her invaluable assistance in preparing this chapter.

LITERATURE CITED

1. **Bolton, A. E.** 1981. Radioimmunoassay, p. 69–83. *In* A. Voller, A. Bartlett, and D. Bidwell (ed.), Immunoassays for the 80s. University Park Press, Baltimore.
2. **Carter, J. H.** 1984. Enzyme immunoassays: practical aspects of their methodology. J. Clin. Immunoassay **7:**64–72.

3. **Clayton-Hopkins, J. A., G. C. Schussler, A. H. Rule, R. A. DeLellis, and M. N. Lassman.** 1978. Binding of triiodothyronine (T3) to circulating autoantibody in a euthyroid woman. Endocrinology **102**(Suppl.):118.

4. **Hunter, W. M., and P. S. Budd.** 1980. Circulating antibodies to ovine and bovine immunoglobulin in healthy subjects: a hazard for immunoassays. Lancet **ii:**1136.

5. **Hunter, W. M., I. McKenzie, and R. R. A. Bacon.** 1981. External quality assessment schemes for immunoassays, p. 155–168. *In* A. Voller, A. Bartlett, and D. Bidwell (ed.), Immunoassays for the 80s. University Park Press, Baltimore.

6. **Jezyk, P. D., and R. M. Dauphinais.** 1983. Cortisol specificity by immunoassay and HPLC before and after metyrapone. J. Clin. Immunoassay **6:**296–301.

7. **Kolhouse, J. F., H. Kondo, N. C. Allen, E. Podell, and R. H. Allen.** 1978. Cobalamin analogues are present in human plasma and can mask cobalamin deficiency because current radioisotopic dilution assays are not specific for true cobalamin. N. Engl. J. Med. **299:**785–793.

8. **Mardell, R., and T. R. Gamlen.** 1982. Discrepant results for free thyroxin by radioimmunoassay and dialysis procedures explained (letter). Clin. Chem. **28:**1989.

9. **Pudek, M. R., D. W. Seccombe, B. E. Jacobson, and M. F. Whitfield.** 1983. Seven different digoxin immunoassay kits compared with respect to interference by digoxin-like immunoreactive substance in serum from premature and full-term infants. Clin. Chem. **29:**1972–1979.

10. **Stockigt, J., V. Stevens, E. L. White, and J. W. Barlow.** 1983. "Unbound analog" radioimmunoassays for free thyroxine measure the albumin-bound hormone fraction. Clin. Chem. **29:**1408–1410.

Chapter 17

Enzyme-Linked Immunosorbent Assay

ALISTER VOLLER AND DENNIS BIDWELL

Enzyme immunoassays, based on enzyme-labeled immunoreactants, especially antibodies, are playing an increasingly important role in the diagnostic laboratory. Although radioimmunoassay has been much longer established, it is now largely confined to the endocrinological laboratory. The short shelf life of the isotopes used for labeling (usually I^{125}) and the administrative inconveniences based on legislation (due to possible health risks) have restricted the further expansion of radioimmunoassays. In microbiology, immunofluorescence is still widely used for the measurement of antibodies and increasingly, with monoclonal antibodies, for the specific detection of organisms in clinical samples. However, the necessity for well-trained staff and the subjective nature of immunofluorescence limit its use. In contrast, the enzyme-linked immunosorbent assay (ELISA) (2) has long-lived reagents, is free from limiting legislation, and is adaptable to simple tests and to sophisticated automation. In addition, its variety of detection systems, which range from visual to photometric with colored, fluorescent, or luminescent substrates, have all contributed to the dramatic expansion of ELISA procedures and applications over the last few years.

Enzyme immunoassays can be subdivided into two main groups, i.e., homogeneous immunoassays, in which the enzyme activity is altered during the immunological reaction of the labeled reagent (see chapter 19), and heterogeneous immunoassays, in which the enzyme activity of the labeled immunoreagent is not affected by the participation of that immunoreagent in an immunological reaction. Of necessity, in the heterogeneous assays there must be a step to separate the reacted from the unreacted labeled reagent.

Despite the attractions of the homogeneous assays, it is the heterogeneous enzyme immunoassays, particularly the ELISA, which have attracted most attention. In this chapter the discussion will be restricted to the ELISA.

The ELISA is based on the premise that one immunoreagent can be immobilized on the carrier surface while retaining its activity and the reciprocal immunoreagent can be linked to an enzyme in such a manner that both the enzymic reactivity and the immunoreactivity of this conjugate are retained. The choice and preparation of the immunoreagent-sensitized solid phase and the enzyme conjugates deserve detailed consideration, and these factors will be considered after the general assay designs.

ASSAYS FOR ANTIBODY

Indirect method

A. The indirect method has been widely used for the measurement of antibody in virtually all human and animal infections. The particular attraction is that only single conjugates (e.g., enzyme-labeled anti-human globulin) are needed to measure antibody in any species. Immunoglobulin class-specific conjugate (e.g., enzyme-labeled anti-human immunoglobulin A [IgA]) also permits immunoglobulin class-specific antibody assessments.

The procedure of the indirect method is as follows.

1. Wells of plastic microplates are sensitized by passive absorption with the relevant antigen. The plates are then washed, and they can be stored (dry) if required.

2. The test samples (usually serum) at one dilution are incubated in the sensitized wells, and any antibody in the serum reacts with the immobilized antigen. A subsequent washing removes all unreacted serum components.

3. Enzyme-labeled anti-human immunoglobulin conjugate is added and incubated in the wells, and this conjugate reacts with the antibody captured by the solid phase-immobilized antigen in step 2. After incubation, excess unreacted conjugate is washed away.

4. The enzyme substrate, in solution, is incubated with the solid phase. The rate of degradation of the substrate, usually indicated by the color intensity of the substrate solution, is proportional to the antibody concentration in the test sample used in step 2.

5. The reaction is stopped, and the color intensity is estimated visually or photometrically. Kinetic measurements on the substrate breakdown can be made. In this case, the reaction need not be stopped.

Solid phase-antigen→test sample (antibody)→anti-species immunoglobulin-enzyme→substrate (color)

A variety of modifications can be made to the basic indirect method, and a few of these modifications are described below.

B. The indirect method as described above is suitable only when a pure or reasonably purified antigen is available. If that is not the case, then the solid phase can be coated with specific antibody, followed by the crude antigen, and then after it is washed, the usual indirect method is performed. In this modification it is essential that the antibody used to sensitize the solid phase not react with the enzyme-labeled antiglobulin.

Solid phase-antibody→impure antigen→test sample (antibody)→anti-species immunoglobulin-enzyme→substrate (color)

C. In step 3 of the example above, unlabeled antiglobulin can replace the conjugate, and this step is followed, after the antiglobulin is washed, by an extra step in which an enzyme-labeled antiglobulin conjugate reactive with the first antiglobulin is used.

Solid phase-antigen→test sample (antibody[1])→Anti-species[1] immunoglobulin→anti-species[2] immunoglobulin-enzyme→substrate (color)

D. Enzyme-labeled protein A can be used instead of the anti-species immunoglobulin conjugate. This method will of course be effective in the detection of antibody only in those species (e.g., humans, rabbit, etc.) whose immunoglobulin reacts with protein A.

Solid phase-antigen→test sample (antibody)→protein A-enzyme→substrate (color)

Sandwich method

In the sandwich method, the solid phase is coated with antigen, and then the test sample (for antibody) is added, followed by enzyme-labeled antigen and finally substrate. This method has been successfully used to detect anti-hepatitis b surface antigen.

Solid phase-antigen→test sample (antibody)→antigen-enzyme→substrate (color)

IgM antibody assays

Although the indirect method is good for the detection of total antibody and IgG antibody, it is not always so effective for IgM antibody assay. There are particular problems in the assay of IgM; e.g., false-positives occur due to the simultaneous presence of IgG antibody and IgM anti-IgG (rheumatoid factor), which will react with the enzyme-labeled anti-IgM conjugate. False-negatives can also occur if there is a vast excess of IgG antibody, often of a higher affinity, which competes for the limited amount of immobilized antigen, thus reducing the availability of antigen for reaction with the IgM antibody. These problems can be overcome to some extent by preadsorption of the test sera with particles sensitized with either anti-IgG or heat-aggregated IgG to remove the IgG antibody and rheumatoid factor, respectively. An alternative is to carry out an IgM antibody class capture ELISA as follows.
1. The solid phase is coated with antibody to IgM.
2. Test sera are incubated with the anti-IgM solid phase (any IgM in the sample is captured).
3. Enzyme-labeled antigen (or unlabeled antigen, followed by enzyme-labeled specific antibody) is then incubated.
4. Enzyme substrate is added.
In this method an immunoseparation of IgM is achieved during the ELISA procedure. This method has been particularly effective for hepatitis A IgM antibody detection, and since in that test infected feces are used as the antigen, it is clear that purified antigen is not necessary.

Solid phase-anti-IgM→

sample IgM ⟨ ↗antigen →antibody-enzyme→substrate (color)
↘antigen-enzyme→substrate (color)

ASSAYS FOR ANTIGENS

Sandwich method

A. Again, the immunometric or sandwich method with excess labeled antibody is the most popular procedure. The basic sandwich method is illustrated below and can be summarized as follows.

1. Specific antibody (or immunoglobulin-containing antibody) is bound to the solid phase.
2. Test sample, being assayed for antigen, is incubated with the solid phase and then washed.
3. Enzyme-labeled specific-antibody conjugate is incubated with the solid phase and then washed to remove unreacted conjugate.
4. Enzyme substrate solution is added, and the rate of its degradation is proportional to the antigen concentration in the test sample.

Solid phase-antibody→sample (antigen)→antibody-enzyme→substrate (color)

Note. This sandwich method can also be used to measure antibodies. In step 2 a reference amount of antigen is tested alone in one well, and in another well it is mixed with the test sample thought to contain antibody. If antibody is present, it will reduce the amount of antigen which can react with the solid phase, and so less conjugate will be fixed, and less substrate will be degraded. The difference in substrate degradation between antigen alone and antigen plus sample is proportional to the antibody content in the test sample. This method is appropriate when purified antigen is unavailable but materials with known antigen content are available.
Again, a variety of modifications are possible, and these can be advantageous in particular situations.

B. The plate coating can be a monoclonal antibody with one specificity for the antigen, and the conjugate can be made by enzyme labeling a monoclonal antibody that reacts with a different site on the antigen. The major advantage of this approach is that it permits steps 2 and 3 of the regular sandwich method to be combined, the sample and conjugate being incubated at the same time. This approach also eliminates one washing and allows assay time to be reduced.

Solid phase-monoclonal antibody[1]→sample (antigen) + monoclonal antibody[2]-enzyme→substrate (color)

C. If the plate-coating antibody is of one species (e.g., sheep) and unlabeled antibody in step 3 is from a second species (e.g., rabbit), then an extra step, 3a, can be introduced in which an enzyme-labeled anti-species immunoglobulin (e.g., enzyme-labeled anti-rabbit immunoglobulin) is used.

Solid phase-antibody[1]→sample (antigen)→antibody[2]→anti-immunoglobulin[2]-enzyme→substrate (color)

Although this procedure involves an extra step, it means that only one antispecies reagent is needed (e.g., antirabbit), and this reagent can be used with antisera of any specificity made in that species. This procedure can be especially valuable if only low-titered antisera are available and if a wide variety of antigens are to be detected.

D. The plate coating can be made with a F(ab)² fragment of the antiserum. The sample is then added, followed by unlabeled antisera as described above in C, but then enzyme-labeled protein A conjugate can be used in place of the enzyme-labeled anti-species immunoglobulin. In this case we have a "universal conjugate" suitable for use with most antisera.

Solid phase-F(ab)^2→sample (antigen)→antibody→ protein A-enzyme→substrate (color)

E. Attempts have been made to increase sensitivity of the ELISA by using biotin-avidin systems. The sandwich method can be performed in the usual way up to and including sample incubation. This step is followed by the addition of biotin-labeled antibody, which is followed by the addition of avidin-labeled enzyme.

Solid phase-antibody→sample (antigen)→antigen-biotin→enzyme-avidin→substrate (color)

Alternatively, the same procedure can be carried out with biotin-labeled antibody and enzyme, with unlabeled avidin to connect them.

Solid phase-antibody→sample (antigen)→antibody-biotin→avidin→enzyme-biotin→substrate (color)

HAPTEN ASSAYS

There are particular problems associated with the small size of haptens which prohibit the usual sandwich method and make the inhibition approach more suitable. One well-documented system is based on the inhibition principle as follows.

A. Two conjugates of the hapten are made, a different carrier being used in each substance (e.g., keyhole limpet hemocyanin, bovine serum albumin [BSA], or thyroglobulin). One of these conjugates is used to raise an antiserum, which is enzyme labeled. The other carrier hapten is used to coat the solid phase.

1. Solid phase is coated with carrier hapten (e.g., keyhole limpet hemocyanin-hapten).

2. Sample being assessed for hapten added to antibody made against the other carrier-hapten (e.g., anti-BSA-hapten) is incubated in solid phase which, after incubation, is washed.

3. Enzyme-labeled anti-species immunoglobulin is added, incubated, and washed.

At the same time, a reference test is set up in which a sample free of the hapten is used. The difference in absorbance values between the test with the reference sample and that with the test sample reflects the hapten level in the test sample.

Solid phase-carrier protein-hapten→sample (hapten + antibody)→antiglobulin-enzyme→

substrate ⤳ sample hapten positive (no color)
      ↘ sample hapten negative (color)

B. Alternatively, a classical type of competitive assay can be performed. However, this assay is less commonly employed because of the potential problems encountered in enzyme labeling different haptens.

Solid phase-carrier-antibody→hapten-enzyme + sample (hapten)→substrate

↗ sample hapten positive (no color)
↘ sample hapten negative (color)

The above examples are not comprehensive and are just a few of the various approaches which can be used in ELISA, but they serve to illustrate the permutations which make these tests so suitable for measuring virtually all diseases of humans, animals, and plants. Those interested in the applications should consult one of the comprehensive reviews (1, 4–6).

PRACTICAL NOTES

All ELISA tests are complex, multicomponent systems, and if they are to be precise and sensitive, careful selection of the components and test parameters must be made. In this section the assay components will be dealt with individually in the sequence in which they are used in the test.

Solid phase

Either antigen or antibody is attached to a solid-phase support to allow for the easy separation of reacted and unreacted reagents. In the vast majority of ELISA systems, the solid phase consists of plastic materials molded in the form of tubes, paddles, beads, disks, and particularly microplates. The microplates have been readily accepted, especially in the infectious disease laboratory, since they permit batch processing and this facilitates reagent additions and washing. Coated beads are convenient when only a few tests are being done, but they are less suitable for testing large numbers of samples.

The plastics used for the solid phase are very relevant to the performance of the test. Since the immunoreagents are usually passively adsorbed onto the surface of the solid phase, the amount taken up and the reproducibility of the uptake are critical. Different plastics have quite distinct uptake characteristics; e.g., polystyrene takes up much less protein than does polyvinyl chloride, and thus polystyrene might be used where a low coating level is acceptable and where nonspecific uptake from the sample (e.g, serum) is to be minimized. In contrast, when a high coating level is to be achieved (e.g., with antibody for antigen detection tests), then polyvinyl chloride would be the better choice. In addition to variations in the composition of the plastic, the production method can also influence the characteristics of the plastic. In particular, there can be variations between wells in different positions on the microplates. The better manufacturers have minimized this problem, but users should still carry out pilot studies with their own immunoreagent and the candidate plastic solid-phase materials.

The coating of the solid phase will be influenced not only by the solid phase itself, but also by the purity and concentration of the immunoreagent, by the diluent, and by the time and temperature used for the coating. Again, preliminary trial and error coatings with any particular coating material are recommended; however, the following observations can be used as a general guide. Aqueous diluents at neutral or alkaline pH (especially carbonate or phosphate buffers) have been used successfully for most proteins. Purified proteins can usually be used at a concentration of 1 to 10 μg/ml in such buffers and with overnight incubation at refrigerator temperatures (approximately 4 to 8°C). With some plastics, e.g., polyvinyl chloride, the uptake can be very rapid and is virtually complete within 1 h at room temperature.

Some materials (e.g., haptens) cannot be directly adsorbed onto the plastic surfaces, and it is then necessary to link them to a carrier protein (e.g., BSA) and then to adsorb the carrier hapten to the plastic.

The purity of the coating immunoreagent is of the greatest importance, since any heterologous material will compete for available space on the plastic. Plates coated with the immunoglobulin fraction of an antiserum may give adequate results in sandwich antigen detection assays, but the sensitivity will always be improved when specific antibody separated by affinity chromatography is used. Antibody used for coating in such assays must have an affinity that permits adequate sensitivity and a steep dose-response curve over the appropriate analyte range. For antibody assays, the antigen must of course have the right spectrum of reactivity, but, in addition, for ELISA it must be free of extraneous material so that adequate amounts of the antigen can be immobilized. Affinity-purified antigens give the best results, and it is becoming more practicable to prepare these with the aid of monoclonal antibodies. Antigen-coated plates are best evaluated first with positive and negative reference sera and then with a panel of representative samples. Some sera react with the tissues from which antigens have been isolated (e.g., cell culture). In such instances control "antigen" must be prepared from the uninfected tissue, and all samples must be tested against that antigen as well as against the specific antigen. The result of this nonspecific reaction must be subtracted from the microbial antigen result to permit estimation of the antigen-specific reaction.

One advantage of ELISA is that the coated solid phase has long-term stability. This stability is best achieved by washing the coated solid phase after the coating process and then postcoating with an irrelevant protein (e.g., BSA), drying it (37°C or below), and storing the coated solid phase in an impervious material (e.g., foil package) with desiccant at refrigerator temperatures. Microplates stored in this way can remain completely reactive for up to at least 5 years. Stability, however, must not be assumed; several workers have found that some monoclonal antibodies, but not all, can lose activity on the solid phase even within weeks or months.

There are numerous reports in the literature on bonding of the immunoreagent to plastic by means of various chemicals such as glutaraldehyde, by complexing the immunoreagent with urea, or by lowering the pH. Our experience has been that these methods may result in higher absorbance values but that both controls and positives increase proportionally; i.e., there is no improvement in signal-to-noise ratios. Covalent bonding can be carried out by cyanogen bromide treatment of cellulose, Sepharose, polyacrylamide, and other solid phases, but these matrixes are much less convenient for the separation washing steps.

Sample

It is important that the analyte be measured over the concentration range in which the ELISA has steep dose-response characteristics. In practice this usually means diluting the sample. It is possible to alter components of the test, e.g., antigen concentration and conjugate dilution, so that one serum dilution can be used for testing antibodies in a variety of diseases. The major reason for high nonspecific reactivity is sample components that stick directly to the coated plastic surface. To prevent this, a wetting agent (e.g., Tween 20) must often be used, and in some systems it is also necessary to include additional "blocking" materials in the sample diluent. Most people have used BSA in this context, but it may be appropriate to use other materials, e.g., uninfected cell culture fluid of the same source as that used to produce a viral antigen or "nonimmune" immunoglobulin of the same species that was used to raise the antisera for conjugates. When sera are being tested for immunoglobulin class-specific antibodies, especially IgM, there can be false-negatives due to competition between antibodies in the different immunoglobulin classes and there can be false-positives (IgM) where IgG antibody is present with rheumatoid factor (IgM anti-IgG). These problems can be minimized either by pretreatment of the test sera to remove rheumatoid factor (e.g., by aggregated immunoglobulin) and IgG (by protein A or by anti-IgG solid phase) or by prior separation of the serum component, or the capture assay system described above can be used.

Conjugate

As mentioned above, the conjugate is almost always antibody linked to enzyme, and there are three main variables, i.e., the antibody, the enzyme, and the method used to link them together. Ideally the antibody used should be of a high affinity and as purified as possible. However, in practice it is found that the immunoglobulin fraction of a polyclonal antiserum is often adequate, although better results are obtained with affinity-purified antibody or with monoclonal antibody. There is now a wide choice of inexpensive enzymes available with appropriate substrates.

For general purposes, horseradish peroxidase is a good choice. The enzyme is cheap and readily available in a purified form, it can be conjugated by several methods, and there is a good variety of chromogenic substrates available. In some situations (e.g., when the antigen itself has peroxidase activity), alkaline phosphatase is a good alternative, and β-galactosidase is now becoming more popular since it is convenient to use with fluorogenic substrates. Urease, penicillinase, and glucose oxidase can also be used as labels.

Initially, most enzyme antibody conjugates were prepared with glutaraldehyde as a cross-linking reagent. Subsequently the periodate method has largely replaced the glutaraldehyde method, especially for peroxidase conjugation. The periodate method has been found very satisfactory by many workers, but others favor maleimide and the new bifunctional reagents such as N-succinimidyl-3-(2-pyridyldithio) propionate (SPDP) for conjugates. The linkage procedure should produce a good yield of conjugate which has maximal immunological and enzymic activity and which is stable. All of these methods achieve these objectives.

Substrates

For most purposes, the chromogenic substrates are suitable. These are initially colorless and on degradation produce a colored, soluble product. For peroxidase, *ortho*-phenylenediamine (OPD) is most commonly used. This substance produces a strong-yellow product, and when the enzyme reaction is stopped by acid, the color conveniently changes to orange-brown. This peroxidase substrate, along with many others, is light sensitive and this characteristic, coupled with fears (probably exaggerated) over its safeness, has led to the use of alternatives such as 5-aminosalicylic acid, 2,2-azino-di-(3-ethyl-benzthiazoline sulfonic acid-6) diammonium salt (ABTS), and 3,3′, 5,5′-tetramethylbenzidine (TMB) to be employed. It is very convenient if the substrate can be provided in the form of tablets, and this is possible with OPD (and the buffer can be included in the tablet). Similarly, tablets of 4-nitrophenyl phosphate are suitable for use with alkaline phosphatase conjugates. Fluorescent substrate products are increasingly popular because they can be detected at very low levels. Methyl umbelliferyl phosphate and methyl umbelliferyl galactoside are suitable for alkaline phosphatase and β-galactosidase conjugates, respectively.

It is usual to permit substrate incubation for a given time (e.g., 30 min) and then to stop the enzyme reaction by means of acid, alkali, etc., and to measure the absorbance of the solution of the substrate product. This is easily done in one of the many ELISA readers now available, but an alternative is to make kinetic measurements during the substrate incubation.

Quality control

In the past it was often asserted that the ELISA was less precise than radioimmunoassay. This was probably due to the fact that well-established radioimmunoassay systems, often commercially produced, were being compared with enzyme immunoassays of laboratory origin made by workers with little understanding of quality control. It is now being appreciated that ELISA can give high precision only if care is taken to standardize all components. In particular, attention must be paid to the solid phase, whose properties can vary according to composition and manufacture, and variations can occur both between manufacturers and in different production batches. In addition, in the multitest formats (e.g., microplate), variation can even occur between different well positions in the format. Careful initial selection of materials and pilot test monitoring on new batches of solid-phase materials are essential. The second main area of variation is in the conjugates. This variability can often be related to the antibody; i.e., different animals or different hybridomas, even though reactive against the same epitope, can vary greatly. The conjugation method can also influence the conjugate performance, as can diluents used and storage conditions. Only by trial-and-error pilot studies on actual reference samples and then by vigorous adherence to the conditions established can accurate results be generated.

APPENDIX 1
Preparation of Enzyme-Labeled Antibody Conjugates

For further information, see reference 3.

Immunoglobulin preparation

The material for labeling may be prepared by salt fractionation or, preferably, by affinity chromatography.

Ammonium sulfate precipitation

Add 2.0 ml of serum to 2.0 ml of phosphate-buffered saline (PBS). Stir the mixture at room temperature, and slowly add 4.0 ml of saturated ammonium sulfate (pH 7.0). After 45 min, centrifuge the mixture at 3,000 rpm for 20 min, and discard the supernatant fluid. Suspend the deposit in half-saturated ammonium sulfate and centrifuge again. Discard the supernatant fluid, wash the pellet with half-saturated ammonium sulfate, and centrifuge. Finally, suspend the pellet in about 2.0 ml of saline and dialyze it extensively against saline (three times, against 2 liters of saline each time) at 4°C. Determine the protein concentration by reading the absorbance at 280 nm. Store frozen until used.

Affinity chromatography

The objective of affinity chromatography is to separate the specific antibodies from the antisera. This is done on cyanogen bromide-activated Sepharose 4B (CNBr4B). A suitable grade of CNBr4B is obtainable from Pharmacia Fine Chemicals, Inc., Sweden.

Preparation of the column is as follows.

1. Weigh 1 g of dry CNBr4B, and measure 200 ml of 1 mM HCl. Add a little of the HCl to the CNBr4B to permit swelling, and then transfer to a sintered glass filter and slowly wash through with the remainder of the HCl, taking about 15 min. Carry out one final wash in a flask with the coupling buffer (8.4 g/liter of 0.1 M NaHCO$_3$ [pH 8.3] plus 29.2 g/liter of 0.5 M NaCl). This procedure will provide 3.5 ml of swollen gel.

2. Dissolve 10 mg of antigen in a small volume (10.0 ml) of coupling buffer, and mix with the swollen gel suspension (3.5 ml) (using an end-over-end mixer, not a magnetic stirrer) for 2 h at room temperature or overnight at 4°C.

3. Wash away excess protein, and block the remaining active groups on the CNBr4B by first washing with 20 ml of coupling buffer and then adding 20 ml of 1 M glycine buffer (pH 8) and leaving for 2 h at room temperature.

4. Pack the gel into a column and wash with 10 ml of coupling buffer and then with 10 ml of glycine hydrochloride (pH 2.4) buffer. Repeat this procedure five times to remove any unadsorbed protein. Finally, wash the column through with 20 ml of PBS (pH 7.4) containing 0.02% sodium azide.

5. Dialyze 2 ml of the antiserum from which antibody is to be purified against PBS (0.1 M, pH 7.4) overnight at 4°C, and then add slowly to the affinity column prepared as described above. Pass excess PBS (0.1 M, pH 7.4) through the column at about 10 ml/h. Collect 2-ml fractions and determine absorbance at

280 nm. Those samples with absorbance at 280-nm represent the nonantibody proteins which are not required. When no further protein is being eluted, add glycine hydrochloride buffer (pH 2.4) plus 0.5 M NaCl (requires approximately 50 ml) to elute the bound antibody. Collect 2-ml fractions in tubes containing 0.1 ml of 3 M Tris hydrochloride (pH 7.4). Monitor absorbance at 280 nm, and pool all protein-containing fractions. These represent the specific antibody. Store at −20°C until required.

Protein A

It may not be necessary or possible to separate the specific antibody, but an IgG fraction may be acceptable. In this case protein A (a suitable purified grade is obtainable from Sigma Chemical Co.) instead of the antigen can be coupled to the CNBr4B column, and the procedure outlined above can be followed. This IgG fraction will have substantially fewer contaminants than that produced by salt fractionation and is preferable for ELISA conjugates.

Preparation of F(ab)^2

It may be necessary to use F(ab)^2 fragments either for coating the solid phase (e.g., when a protein A or anti-Fc conjugate is used) or in conjugates. The F(ab)^2 fragment can be prepared from the immunoglobulin fractions or specific antibody separated from the antisera as described above.

1. Make up 25 mg of the immunoglobulin to 2 ml in saline, and dialyze against 0.1 M acetate buffer (pH 4.0) overnight at 4°C. The dialysate should have a pH of 4.0.
2. Add 1 mg of pepsin (a suitable grade is obtainable from Sigma) and incubate overnight at 37°C. Maintain at pH 4.0 by the addition of dilute acetic acid or alkali.
3. Centrifuge at 3,000 × g for 15 min to remove any precipitate. Dialyze the supernatant against 0.1 M sodium borate buffer (pH 8.0) overnight at 4°C (2 liters).
4. Apply the supernatant containing the digested immunoglobulin fragments to a 2.0- by 45-cm column of Ultrogel AcA44 (LKB Instruments, Inc.) equilibrated with 0.1 M sodium borate buffer (pH 8.0). Elute F(ab)^2 fragments by the addition of 0.1 M sodium borate buffer (pH 8.0). Collect 1-ml fractions, monitor absorbance at 280 nm, and pool the F(ab)^2-containing fractions. Store frozen until used.

Conjugation methods

Horseradish peroxidase is used in all the examples given below. However, a number of alternative enzymes are listed in Appendix 3.

Periodate method

1. Dissolve 4 mg of peroxidase (Reinheitszahl [RZ] 3.0 for at least 200 U/mg of protein) in 1.0 ml of H$_2$O. Add 0.2 ml of freshly made up 0.1 M NaIO$_4$. Stir 20 min at room temperature (color should change from gold to green; if it does not, new periodate is needed).

2. Dialyze against 1 mM sodium acetate buffer (pH 4.4) overnight at 4°C.
3. Add 8 mg of immunoglobulin in 1 ml of saline to the enzyme, and immediately add 15 µl of 1 M carbonate buffer (pH 9.5). Stir 2 h at room temperature.
4. Add 0.1 ml of fresh sodium borohydride solution (4 mg/ml in H$_2$O). Allow to stand 2 h at 4°C. Dialyze overnight against PBS at 4°C. Store at 4°C until purified as described below.

One-step glutaraldehyde method

1. Add 2 mg of immunoglobulin in 0.5 ml of PBS to 5 mg of enzyme. Dialyze against PBS overnight at 4°C.
2. Make the volume up to 1.25 ml with PBS. Add 10 µl of 25% glutaraldehyde solution. Mix well. Leave at room temperature for 2 h. Dialyze against PBS overnight at 4°C with two changes of 2 liters of PBS at 4°C.
3. Dilute the conjugate to 4.0 ml with PBS buffer, and store at 4°C until purified.

Two-step glutaraldehyde method

1. Dissolve 10 mg of enzyme in 0.2 ml of 0.1 M phosphate buffer (pH 6.8) containing 1.25% glutaraldehyde. Leave the mixture overnight at room temperature.
2. Dialyze the mixture against normal saline (or pass it down a Sephadex G25 column) to remove free glutaraldehyde. Adjust the volume by concentration or dilution to 1 ml in normal saline. This solution is the activated enzyme.
3. Mix 1 ml of the solution containing 5 mg of immunoglobulin with 1 ml of the activated enzyme solution and 0.1 ml of carbonate-bicarbonate 1 M buffer (pH 9.5). Allow the mixture to stand at 4°C for 24 h.
4. Add 0.1 ml of 0.2 M lysine solution, and keep the mixture at room temperature for 2 h. Dialyze the mixture against PBS (pH 7.2) overnight at 4°C. Store at 4°C until purified as described below.

SPDP

SPDP is obtainable from Pharmacia.

1. Add 12 mg of SPDP to 1 ml of ethanol. Dissolve by warming to 45 to 50°C for a few seconds. Mix. Repeat until dissolved. This is the SPDP solution.
2. In a beaker, add 12.5 µl of SPDP solution to 2 ml of immunoglobulin solution (1 mg/ml in PBS). Leave at room temperature for 30 min. As the antibody is being processed, slowly add 350 µl of SPDP solution, with stirring, to 3 ml of enzyme solution (4 mg/ml in PBS). Leave at room temperature for 30 min.
3. Remove excess SPDP by filtration on a 10-ml column of Sephadex G25 with PBS. Collect the immunoglobulin-containing fractions and pool (easily done by monitoring at 280 nm). Also, remove excess SPDP from the enzyme by filtration on a 10-ml Sephadex G25 column with PBS. Collect the brown fractions and pool. Add 8 mg of dithiothreitol per ml collected, mix, and allow to stand 20 min at room temperature. Again filter on a 10-ml Sephadex G25 column. Pool the colored fractions.

4. Mix the enzyme fraction from step 3 with the immunoglobulin fraction from step 3. Leave overnight at room temperature.

5. Pass the mixture down a Sephadex G25 column. Collect fractions that absorb at both 280 and 405 nm. Pool and store at 4°C.

Avidin-biotin

A suitable grade of biotin (biotinyl-N-hydroxysuccinimide) is obtainable from Calbiochem-Behring Corp. A suitable grade of avidin is obtainable from Sigma.

Biotin labeling of immunoglobulin is performed as follows.

1. Make up immunoglobulin to 10 mg/ml in 0.1 M $NaHCO_3$. Add 100 μl of 0.1 M biotin dissolved in distilled dimethyl formamide (34 mg/ml). Allow to react at room temperature for 60 min. Dialyze overnight at 4°C against several changes of PBS.

2. Centrifuge at 5,000 × g for 15 min. Mix the supernatant with an equal volume of glycerol, and store at −20°C.

Avidin labeling of peroxidase is achieved by the two-step glutaraldehyde method (see above) with 5 mg of peroxidase and 2.5 mg of avidin.

Purification of conjugates

The objective of the purification of conjugates is to improve the conjugates by removing free enzyme might lead to higher nonspecific reactions. Unconjugated antibody may also be removed, as it can reduce conjugate reactivity.

The free enzyme may be removed by salt precipitation or by gel filtration.

Salt precipitation

After dialysis, the conjugate is mixed with an equal volume of saturated ammonium sulfate. The precipitate contains the conjugated antibody, and the free enzyme is in the supernatant, which is discarded. The details of the precipitation, washing, centrifugation, and dialysis are as given above in the description of the ammonium sulfate precipitation of immunoglobulin from serum.

Gel filtration

A column of Sephadex G25 (e.g., PD 10, Pharmacia) is washed with the buffer which was used to dialyze the conjugate. The conjugate is added to the column in that buffer and is eluted with the same buffer. Fractions of the effluent are collected, and absorbance at 280 nm is determined to indicate the immunoglobulin and at 405 nm to indicate the enzyme. Those fractions with high absorbance at both wavelengths are pooled. They represent the conjugated immunoglobulin.

Unconjugated immunoglobulin can be removed from the conjugates, although this is not usually essential. This procedure can be done by column separation using Ultrogel AcA44 (LKB). Alternatively, peroxidase conjugates can be purified from unlabeled immunoglobulin on concanavalin A-Sepharose columns (Pharmacia). The conjugate will bind to the lectin, whereas the free immunoglobulin will pass through. Enzyme-labeled immunoglobulins can then be eluted by the addition of α-methyl-D-mannoside.

Storage of conjugates

When prepared and purified as described above, the conjugates should be stabilized by the addition of BSA to a final concentration of 1%. For long-term storage, the undiluted conjugates can then be mixed with an equal volume of glycerol and stored at −20°C. They will not freeze at this temperature, and samples can be removed by micropipettes as required while the bulk is retained at −20°C.

If the conjugates are to be stored at higher temperatures, a preservative is required. Merthiolate (0.01%) is suitable for peroxidase, and sodium azide (0.02%) can be used with most other enzymes (but not with peroxidase, as some permanent inhibition of peroxidase occurs).

It is preferable to store the stock conjugates in a concentrated form. At the time of use, the conjugates can be diluted in a suitable diluent, e.g., PBS-Tween. It may be necessary to add additional protein to the diluent to reduce nonspecific binding. BSA (5 to 10%) or nonimmune immunoglobulin from the same species as that used to prepare the antisera is a suitable additive.

APPENDIX 2
Materials Found to be Satisfactory in ELISA

Solid-phase carrier

1. Disposable polystyrene microtitration plates, types M129A or B (Dynatech Laboratories, Inc.). These plates are useful for indirect tests since nonspecific adsorption during test procedures is low. (They are also available as 8- or 12-well strips.)

2. Disposable polyvinyl chloride microtitration plates, type M29 (Dynatech). These plates are especially suitable for antigen detection assays since they can be coated with higher levels of antibody.

3. Polystyrene beads for coating can be obtained from Precision Ball Bearing Co.

Coating buffer

Carbonate-bicarbonate buffer (pH 9.6) consists of 1.59 g of Na_2CO_3, 2.93 g of $NaHCO_3$, and 0.2 g of NaN_3 made up to 1 liter with distilled water. Store at 4°C for not more than 2 weeks. If the coating is not satisfactory in this buffer, then an alternative at a lower pH (e.g., PBS or Tris) should be tried. Some monoclonal antibodies in particular may coat better in these other buffers.

PBS

PBS consists of 8 g of NaCl, 0.2 g of KH_2PO_4, 2.9 g of $Na_2HPO_4 \cdot 12H_2O$, and 0.2 g of KCl in 1 liter of distilled water. The pH is 7.4. Store at 4°C.

PBS-Tween

Mix as described above for PBS, with 0.5 ml of Tween 20 per liter.

Enzymes and substrates

The highly purified grades of enzymes and substrates are obtainable from Sigma and other leading manufacturers.

Peroxidase conjugates (substrates)

1. OPD

OPD (40 mg) is dissolved in 100 ml of 0.1 M citrate phosphate buffer (pH 5.0). (Tablets containing OPD plus buffer are obtainable from Pitman Moore, Inc.)

The substrate solution is made up just before use, and 40 μl of 30% H_2O_2 is added. The substrate is light sensitive and must be shielded from strong light. After incubation at room temperature for up to 30 min, the reaction is stopped by the addition of 1 N H_2SO_4 or 2.5 N HCl. This step causes a further color change from yellow to orange-brown. Any dilution of strong samples should be made in buffer containing the correct proportion of acid. Absorbance of OPD is read at 492 nm.

2. TMB

Dissolve 10 mg of TMB in 1.0 ml of dimethylsulfoxide. Add TMB-dimethylsulfoxide dropwise with mixing to 100 ml of 0.1 M sodium acetate-citric acid buffer (pH 6.0). Add 20 μl of 30% hydrogen peroxide. Use immediately. A pale-blue color is produced which, on stopping with 2 M H_2SO_4, changes to bright yellow. The absorbance is read at 450 nm.

3. ABTS

Dissolve 10 mg of ABTS in 100 ml of citric phosphate buffer (pH 5.0; 24.0 ml of 0.1 M citric acid plus 26 ml of 0.2 M Na_2HPO_4 made up to 100 ml with distilled water). Add 20 μl of 30% hydrogen peroxide and use immediately. This substrate produces a green color. The absorbance is read at 405 nm.

4. 5-Aminosalicylic acid

Dissolve 100 mg of recrystallized 5-aminosalicylic acid in 100 ml of 0.01 M sodium phosphate buffer (pH 6.0) containing 1 mM EDTA. Immediately before use, add 20 μl of 30% hydrogen peroxide. Stop the reaction with 1 M NaOH. This substrate produces a brown color. The absorbance is read at 450 nm.

5. 3-(p-Hydroxyphenyl)propionic acid

3-(p-Hydroxyphenyl)propionic acid can be used to generate a fluorescent product. Add 0.25 g of the recrystallized acid to 50 ml of 0.1 M sodium phosphate buffer (pH 8.0). When dissolved, add 20 μl of 30% hydrogen peroxide. Use immediately. Incubate in the usual way, and then measure fluorescence at 320 nm excitation and 405 nm emission.

6. 3,3'-Diaminobenzidine

3,3'-Diaminobenzidine (DAB) produces an insoluble product and is suitable for use with dipsticks, immunoblot, ELISA techniques, etc.

Dissolve 3 mg of DAB in 10.0 ml of 10 mM phosphate buffer (pH 6.8) containing 0.01 M EDTA. Add 3 μl of 30% hydrogen peroxide. Filter before use, incubate as usual, and wash reacted material to remove excess substrate. The insoluble brown product can be observed visually.

7. 4-Chloro-1-naphthol

4-Chloro-1-naphthol (4C1N) produces an insoluble product and is an alternative to DAB.

Dissolve 30 mg of 4C1N in 10 ml of methanol (can be stored at 4°C in a dark bottle for 14 days). For use, to 10.0 ml of triethanolamine-buffered saline (pH 7.5; see below), add 2 ml of 4C1N solution and 5 μl of 30% hydrogen peroxide. Use immediately. This substrate produces an insoluble blue product.

Triethanolamine-buffered saline (pH 7.5) is made up of the following:

NaCl	7.5 g
Triethanolamine	2.8 ml
1 M HCl	17.0 ml
$MgCl_2 \cdot 6H_2O$	0.1 g
$CaCl_2 \cdot 2H_2O$	0.02 g

Make up to 1 liter with distilled water.

Alkaline phosphatase conjugates

A suitable grade of enzyme should have a specific activity of about 1,000 U/mg of protein.

Alkaline phosphatase is a good alternative to peroxidase although rather more expensive. It is often used when the antigen or sample contains excessive amounts of peroxidase activity, which precludes the use of peroxidase.

The following substrates are suitable.

1. p-Nitrophenyl phosphate

Tablets of p-nitrophenyl phosphate (5 mg) are obtainable from Sigma. These should be stored below 0°C in the dark. Immediately before use, dissolve one 5-mg tablet per 5 ml of diethanolamine buffer which has already been warmed to room temperature.

Diethanolamine buffer contains 97 ml of diethanolamine, 800 ml of distilled water, 0.2 g of sodium azide, and 100 mg of $MgCl_2 \cdot 6H_2O$. HCl (1 M) is added to bring the pH to 9.8, and then distilled water is added to 1 liter. Store at 4°C in the dark. The substrate reaction can be allowed to proceed for up to 24 h, although it is usually stopped within 30 min. The reaction is stopped by the addition of 50 μl of 3 M NaOH to each well. The substrate produces a soluble yellow product, the absorbance of which can be read at 405 nm.

2. Methyl umbelliferyl phosphate

Methyl umbelliferyl phosphate produces a fluorescent product.

Dissolve 3.5 mg of *n*-methyl umbelliferyl phosphate in absolute alcohol. Add to diethanolamine buffer (see above) to give a final concentration of 0.025 mg/ml.

The substrate solution is used immediately and is incubated in the usual way. Fluorescence is measured in a fluorimeter with excitation at 360 nm and emission at 440 nm. It can also be observed visually under a UV lamp. The reaction can be monitored kinetically or it can be read after a given time (e.g., after 20 to 30 min). It is not necessary to stop the reaction.

3. Fast red

Fast red produces an insoluble product and is used for the same purposes as the peroxidase substrates producing colored products.

Dissolve 40 mg of naphthol As-Mx (5-chloro-2-toluidinediazonium chloride hemizine chloride) phosphate sodium salt in 100 ml of 0.2 M Tris hydrochloride buffer (pH 8.0). Dissolve 25 mg of fast red TR (3-hydroxy-2-naphthoic acid, 2,4,-dimethylanilide phosphate) salt in 5 ml of distilled water. Mix an equal volume of each solution, filter, and use immediately. The product is red. Wash to remove excess substrate.

β-Galactosidase conjugates

β-Galactosidase is often the enzyme chosen for ELISA tests with fluorescent endpoints, although it can also be used with colored substrates.

1. *ortho* Nitrophenyl-β-D-galactosidase

ortho-Nitrophenyl-β-D-galactosidase (ONPG) produces a colored soluble product.

Prepare a stock solution of ONPG by dissolving 90 mg of ONPG in 10.0 ml of PBS (heat to 50°C to dissolve). This solution will keep for several days when stored at room temperature in the dark. Dilute the stock solution 1:10 in PBS (pH 7.5) containing 10 mM $MgCl_2$ and 0.1 M 2-mercaptoethanol. Stop the reaction with 1 M Na_2CO_3. The absorbance of the yellow product is read at 410 nm.

2. Methyl umbelliferyl galactoside:

Methyl umbelliferyl galactoside produces a fluorescent product.

Dissolve 300 μg/ml of 4-methyl umbelliferyl β-D-galactopyranoside in 0.1 M Tris citrate buffer (pH 8.5) containing 1% BSA, 0.001 M $MgSO_4$, and 0.0002 M $MnSO_4$. Incubate in the usual way for up to 24 h. Fluorescence can be determined kinetically or read after a given time without stopping the reaction. Fluorescence is determined with excitation at 360 nm and emission at 440 nm.

Glucose oxidase conjugates

Glucose oxidase conjugates represent alternatives to peroxidase conjugates. Suitable substrates are as follows.

1. Glucose-OPD

Dissolve 1 g of D-glucose in 100 ml of citric acid-phosphate buffer (pH 5.0) containing 40 mg of OPD (see above) and 100 U of peroxidase (RZ = 3.0). Stop the reaction with 2.5 N HCl. This substrate produces a soluble orange product. The absorbance should be read at 490 nm.

2. Glucose-nitroblue tetrazolium

Dissolve 150 mg of D-glucose in 10 ml of 0.1 M phosphate buffer (pH 7.2). Add 5 mg of nitroblue tetrazolium and 1 mg of phenazine methosulfate. Filter and use at once. This substrate produces an insoluble blue product and can be used for the same purposes as the other insoluble products described above.

3. Glucose-DAB

Dissolve 1 g of D-glucose in 100 ml of 0.1 M phosphate buffer (pH 6.8). When dissolved, add 5 mg of DAB tetrahydrochloride and 100 U of peroxidase (RZ = 3.0). Filter before use. This procedure produces an insoluble brown product.

Urease conjugates

Urease conjugates are often used when a visual test is required.

Dissolve 8 mg of bromocresol purple in 1.48 ml of 0.01 M NaOH. Make the volume up to 100 ml with fresh distilled water. Add 100 mg of urea and then add EDTA to a final concentration of 0.2 mM. Adjust the pH of the solution with 1 mM HCl to pH 5.0. A soluble product is produced with a marked color change from yellow to blue as the pH changes.

APPENDIX 3
Indirect Microplate ELISA

Determination of working strengths of antiglobulin conjugates

It is necessary to determine the approximate potency of antiglobulin conjugates, but it is not always possible to do this in a new system where the antigen activity is unknown and reference sera may not be available. In such situations a measure of the relative potency of new conjugates, which can be a rough guide to their working dilution, can be carried out on plates coated with the appropriate immunoglobulin, as described below.

1. Human IgG is diluted to 100 ng/ml in coating buffer (see Appendix 2). A 100-μl volume of this solution is added to each well of a polystyrene microtiter plate (see Appendix 2), and the plate is covered and put into a humid chamber at 4°C for 18 h. The contents of the wells are then shaken out, and the wells are refilled with PBS-Tween and allowed to stand for 2 or 3 min. This washing procedure is repeated twice more.
2. Dilutions of the conjugate to be tested are made in PBS-Tween, and 100 μl of each dilution is added to duplicate wells. The plate is covered and incubated for 1 h at room temperature. The washing procedure is repeated.

TABLE 1. Results of sample test for antibody detection by ELISA[a]

Serum	Absorbance value at antigen dilution of:					
	1:50	1:100	1:200	1:400	1:800	1:1,600
Strongly positive	1.2	1.04	0.84	0.68	0.42	0.29
Weakly positive	0.64	0.41	0.3	0.22	0.19	0.09
Negative	0.23	0.13	0.08	0.06	0.05	0.06
PBS-Tween	0.09	0.02	0.02	0.02	0.04	0.02

[a] The highest dilution of antigen giving a value of 0.8 after 20 min of substrate incubation with the strongly positive serum and under 0.1 with the negative serum is used in all subsequent tests. In the example shown, the antigen is used at a dilution of 1:200. Results are expressed as absorbance at 492 nm.

3. A 100-μl amount of the enzyme substrate (see Appendix 2) is added to each well. After 20 min at room temperature (about 23°C), the reaction in all wells is stopped by the addition of 50 μl of stopping solution (see Appendix 2). The absorbance of the contents of each well is then read in a spectrophotometer with a microcuvette (see Appendix 2).

The conjugate dilution giving an absorbance value of about 0.8 with the immunoglobulin solution at 100 ng/ml is then further assessed as described below.

An indirect microplate ELISA (see below) is then carried out with conjugate dilutions close to that determined as described above. The antigen will be that which is to be used in subsequent clinical assays. A positive reference serum and a negative reference serum are tested with a series of conjugate dilutions. The conjugate dilution that yields a high positive value (e.g., 0.8) and a low negative value (e.g., <0.1) in about 20 min of substrate incubation time is used for all subsequent tests.

Checkerboard titration to determine optimal antigen coating level for indirect microplate ELISA for assay of antibody

1. Serially dilute antigen in coating buffer. Add 100 μl of each dilution to a vertical row of wells in a microplate. Cover, and put in a humid chamber at 4°C for 18 h. Wash the plates as described above.
2. Three reference sera, i.e., a strong positive, a weak positive, and a known negative, are diluted 1:100 in PBS-Tween. Add 100 μl of each dilution to a horizontal row of wells in the plate. To one more row add PBS-Tween. Incubate for 1 h at room temperature in a humid chamber. Wash the plate.
3. Dilute enzyme-labeled antiglobulin conjugate to working dilution in PBS-Tween. Add 100 μl to all test wells in the microplate. Incubate at room temperature for 1 h. Wash the plate.
4. Add 100 μl of substrate solution to all test wells. Incubate at room temperature (in the dark if necessary) for 20 min.
5. Add 50 μl of stopping solution to each test well. Observe the color change and measure the absorbance spectrophotometrically at the appropriate wavelength. The results of such a checkerboard are given in Table 1.

Indirect microplate ELISA

1. Dilute the antigen to working dilution in coating buffer as determined above. Coat all wells with 100 μl

of the antigen solution for 18 h at 4°C. Wash the plates. (After being washed, plates can be stored dry at 4°C.)
2. Add 100 μl of each test serum diluted 1:100 in PBS-Tween to duplicate wells. Include at least two wells with positive and negative reference sera on each plate. Incubate for 1 h at room temperature. Wash the plate.
3. Add 100 μl of the working dilution of the conjugate to each well. Incubate for 1 h at room temperature. Wash the plate.
4. Add 100 μl of substrate to all wells. Incubate for 20 min at room temperature.
5. Add 50 μl of stopping solution to each well, and read the absorbance in a spectrophotometer.

Interpretation of results

Day-to-day variations in test conditions make it essential to correct all values of test samples to the reference positive sample as follows: correct sample value = (measured absorbance of sample × 0.8)/ absorbance of reference positive sample.

The results can be reported as follows.
1. As positive or negative. A threshold cutoff point is determined on the basis of the highest values obtained on a group of negative samples. Values above the cutoff are considered positive.
2. As ratios of sample values to the mean value of a group of negative samples. Ratios above two or three times the mean negative value are usually considered positive.

It is also possible to express the results as endpoint titers, but this involves making serial dilutions of the test sample.

APPENDIX 4
Sandwich ELISA for Measurement of Proteins

Checkerboard titration to find the working dilutions of the reagents

1. The immunoglobulin fraction of the antisera, or purified antibody, to the protein under test is diluted in coating buffer to give 10, 1, and 0.1 μg of protein per ml. Add 100 μl of each dilution to three vertical columns of wells in a microplate (usually polyvinyl chloride). Keep the plates in a humid chamber for 18 h at 4°C, and then wash with PBS-Tween in the usual way.
2. Add 100 μl of the strongly positive antigen solution to one horizontal row of wells, and add the weakly positive and the negative reference samples to other horizontal rows of wells. Incubate for 1 h at room temperature, and wash with PBS-Tween in the usual way.

TABLE 2. Checkerboard for determination of working dilution of reagents in the sandwich ELISA for protein[a]

Coating and conjugate dilution in PBS-Tween	Absorbance value of reference antigen samples		
	Strongly positive (25 ng/ml)	Weakly positive (1.5 ng/ml)	Negative
10 μg/ml			
1:1,000	1.17	0.15	0.09
1:5,000	0.46	0.03	0
1:25,000	0.12	0	0
1 μg/ml			
1:1,000	>2	0.25	0.10
1:5,000	0.91	0.12	0.01
1:25,000	0.25	0.01	0
0.1 μg/ml			
1:1,000	0.42	0.13	0.13
1:5,000	0.11	0.03	0.02
1:25,000	0.03	0	0

[a] The coating antibody could be used at 1 μg/ml and the conjugate at a 1:5,000 dilution. For the sake of economy, further titration of the coating antibody and conjugate could be made around those levels.

3. Dilute the conjugate in PBS-Tween. Three dilutions are usually adequate, e.g., 1:1,000, 1:5,000, and 1:25,000. Add 100 μl of each conjugate dilution to one vertical row of the plate coated with each level of antibody (Table 2). Incubate for 1 h at room temperature. Wash in the usual way.

4. Add 100 μl of substrate solution. Incubate for 20 min at room temperature, and then add 50 μl of stopping solution. Determine the color change in a spectrophotometer.

From the results, working dilutions for the reagents can be found. Further checkerboard titrations with closer dilutions can be carried out to economize on reagents. Once established, reagent dilutions and test conditions must not be changed.

In the example given, quantitative measurements are not necessary. In this case, only sample with values significantly above the negative control (e.g., 0.10) are considered positive. For quantitative assays a standard curve has to be established with reference samples. In many instances the test specimen may have to be diluted so that it can be read off the standard curve.

LITERATURE CITED

1. **Avrameas, S., P. Druet, R. Masseyeff, and G. Feldmann.** 1983. Immunoenzymatic techniques, p. 1–410. Elsevier Science Publishers, Amsterdam.
2. **Engvall, E., and P. Perlmann.** 1972. ELISA. III. Quantitation of specific antibodies by enzyme linked immunoglobulin in antigen coated tubes. J. Immunol. **109:** 129–135.
3. **Ishikawa, E., M. Imagawa, S. Hashida, S. Yoshitake, Y. Hamaguchi, and T. Ueno.** 1983. Enzyme labeling of antibodies and their fragments for enzyme immunoassay and immunohistochemical staining. J. Immunoassay **4:**209–327.
4. **Talwar, G. P.** 1983. Non-isotopic immunoassays and their applications, p. 1–436. Vikas Publishing House, New Delhi.
5. **Voller, A., and D. E. Bidwell.** 1980. The enzyme linked immunosorbent assay (ELISA). A review of recent developments with abstracts of microplate applications, p. 1–126. MicroSystems Ltd., Guernsey, Channel Islands.
6. **Voller, A., D. E. Bidwell, and A. Bartlett.** 1979. The enzyme linked immunosorbent assay (ELISA): a guide with abstracts of microplate applications, p. 1-125. Flowline Press, Guernsey, Channel Islands.

Chapter 18

General Principles of Radioimmunoassay

JENNIFER LARSEN AND WILLIAM D. ODELL

The technique of radioimmunoassay (RIA) is based on antibody recognition of the substance to be quantified (analyte). The technique is used in either competitive or excess-reagent conditions. Under competitive conditions a purified radiolabeled form of the analyte (label) competes with unlabeled analyte for binding to limited amounts of antibody. In the excess-reagent or sandwich technique the antibody is usually labeled and is used in excess concentration. Analyte is measured when bound to the radiolabeled antibody. In both forms of immunoassay, a method of separating bound label (to either analyte or antibody) from label not bound (free) is required. The competitive assay will be primarily discussed here. In this brief review, we will cover general principles, antibody production and selection, radiolabeling techniques, and separation methods.

The competitive RIA has several components to be discussed; each has its own characteristics and properties. Each component must be individually characterized in detail and these characteristics must be thoroughly understood before the assembled assay can be effectively used. "Troubleshooting" assays that do not perform optimally also require detailed knowledge of these component characteristics. RIA techniques are used extensively to quantify small concentrations of peptide, protein, and steroid hormones, antibodies to a variety of antigens, drugs, and chemicals, carbohydrates, and lipopolysaccharides.

Due to space constraints, this is not meant to be a comprehensive review of the subject. For further reading about specific techniques or problems of RIA techniques not covered in this chapter, the reader should consult one of the many texts dealing with the topic in greater detail.

GENERAL PRINCIPLES

The RIA involves recognition of antigenic determinants which have molecular weights of 600 to 800. However, analytes with smaller molecular weights can be quantified; the antibody is generated against a conjugated form of the analyte, and the antigenic site includes the analyte plus a portion of the carrier or conjugated protein. For a larger analyte (e.g., proteins) many antigenic sites exist and many different RIAs for the same analyte can be developed. If the analyte is a protein hormone which is metabolized during its circulation in the body, the antigenic portion may be biologically inactive. For example, some parathormone RIAs react with the carboxy-terminal portion of the protein. Fragments containing this determinant circulate in blood but are not biologically active. In renal failure these metabolized hormones accumulate in the blood due to decreased clearance and inaccurately reflect parathormone secretion. Under the same conditions, biologically active amino-terminal fragments circulate in much smaller quantities.

ANTIBODY

The antibody used may be part of a polyclonal antiserum prepared by in vivo immunization or may be a monoclonal antibody produced in vitro. Commonly, antibodies are produced by the immunization of animals with purified analyte. A variety of animals have been used for this purpose. Larger-molecular-weight (over about 6,000) peptides or proteins are mixed with complete Freund adjuvant and injected subcutaneously or intracutaneously into the desired animal. The adjuvant assures slow absorption of the antigen and both stimulates and facilitates antigen phagocytosis by macrophages which subsequently transmit the information to immunocompetent cells, which produce the antibody. Small substances with molecular weights less than 6,000, such as peptides, steroids, thyronines, and drugs, are covalently conjugated to carrier proteins, as they are otherwise not immunogenic. Examples of carrier proteins are albumin and thyroglobulin. Serum from the injected animal is then harvested at assigned intervals to test for antibody titer and, when found to be adequate, is further characterized as below.

Antisera are now frequently being produced in vitro by cell lines representing nonsecretory myeloma cells fused with lymphoid cells from hyperimmunized animals. These cells produce antibodies that can be harvested and characterized for use in assay procedures much like antibodies harvested from live animals. Once a cell line has been developed to produce a specific antibody, a pool of homogeneous (monoclonal) antibody with known affinity and specificity can be produced more easily and rapidly than by animal injection. Thus, extensive research is presently being performed to improve this methodology to make it readily applicable for a wider variety of assays.

Titer

Titer is the dilution of antiserum used in the assay, selected to bind 30 to 50% of the label. It is determined by incubating serial dilutions of antiserum with a small amount (trace) of label (Fig. 1). (Trace is defined as equal to or smaller than the smallest amount of analyte to be determined.) The dilution or titer used may vary, depending on the nature of the assay. Usual titers range from $1:10^5$ to $1:10^6$ or more. The terms "initial" and "final" titer refer to the titer added to the assay tube and the titer in the completed assay tube, respectively. For example, 100 μl of an antiserum with an initial titer of $1:10^5$ added to an assay tube with a total volume of 1 ml (1,000 μl) represents a 1:10 dilution, giving a final titer or

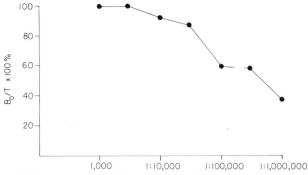

FIG. 1. First antibody dilution in an RIA for human growth hormone. Notice that as the dilution of the first antibody (in this case, rabbit anti-human growth hormone) increases, specific binding (B_0/t) decreases.

dilution of $1:10^6$. For communication purposes, final titer is preferable since assay volumes often differ.

Specificity

Specificity refers to the degree with which the antibody recognition of its antigen or analyte is unique. It is usually determined by setting up a dilution of the analyte to be measured and a wide range of dilutions of potentially cross-reacting analytes under assay conditions. In some instances a purification step can separate cross-reacting antigens before assay, permitting use of a less specific assay.

Affinity

Affinity is defined as the avidity or "tightness" of binding between an antibody and the analyte. It may be numerically represented by the affinity constant (K_a). K_a values for antisera in an optimal RIA usually range between 10^{-9} and 10^{-12} mol/liter. Affinity is related to the sensitivity possible in the final assembled assay system. As will be discussed, precision of the assay and separation method also affect sensitivity. The affinity may be estimated by using the Scatchard plot or the Woolf plot (Fig. 2). For most immunoassay data the Woolf plot has a statistical advantage for more accurate estimates of the number of antibody molecules and the dissociation constant (K_d). For a more detailed discussion, see Keightley and Cressie (7).

LABELED ANALYTE

Importance of the radiolabeled analyte

The use of a high-quality radiolabel improves both sensitivity and precision of the assay by producing a more uniform population of radiolabeled analytes with maximal affinity for the antibody binding site. Although several radioisotopes may be used, ^{125}I is most commonly used to label peptides, proteins, and thyronines, and ^3H is used most often for steroids. ^{125}I can also be conjugated to steroids to be used in RIA.

For substances such as drugs which exist in blood in much larger concentrations than hormones, longer-

life isotopes such as ^{14}C may be used. However, the very low counting rates seen with small concentrations generally preclude the use of ^{14}C for hormone RIA. ^3H-steroids, usually containing 2 to 6 tritiums per molecule, are generally available in high-quality form from commercial sources. The degree of purity should be ascertained. ^{125}I-peptides are often prepared by the researcher, and special consideration of preparation, purification, and storage is warranted.

Labeling peptide or protein analytes

As previously indicated, ^{125}I is most commonly used for radioiodinating peptide or protein hormones. This isotope has a half-life of 60 days and is a "soft" gamma emitter. The latter property makes shielding of radiation effects easier. ^{131}I has been used, but its shorter half-life (8 days) and "hard" gamma emission make it a lesser choice. For labeling peptides, ^3H and ^{14}C are less attractive because of very long half-lives, markedly decreased disintegrations per minute, and the fact that they are beta emitters. For routine assay use when sensitivity is not a problem, 10,000 to 25,000 cpm is generally used in each assay tube (~0.01 μCi per tube) and the mass of label is approximately equal to the smallest amount of analyte to be quantified. Where maximal sensitivity is required (e.g., ACTH [adenocorticotropin] and calcitonin RIA) and a sufficiently high-affinity antiserum is available, the label is reduced further in mass to 1 to 2 pg. (The starting assay B/F or B/B_0 is also often reduced. This is discussed later.) With usual specific activities, counting rates for such assays may be only 1,000 to 2,000 cpm, and under research laboratory conditions, very adequate assays may be run. In clinical laboratories and in commercial RIA kits, low counting rates are considered a negative selling point, and sensitivity is often sacrificed to achieve a level of 10,000 to 20,000 cpm.

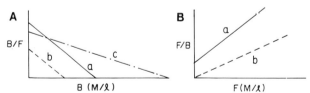

FIG. 2. Scatchard and Woolf plots. B, Analyte or hormone bound to antibody (both radiolabeled and unlabeled), expressed in moles per liter; F, unbound label (free). (A) Scatchard plot of antigen-antibody binding where line a represents one population of antibodies. Slope of line a equals $1/K_a$, and the x intercept is equal to the total number of available binding sites. Line b represents another antibody population with identical K_a (identical slope) but a smaller number of total binding sites. Line c has a greater x intercept, thus a larger number of binding sites, and a greater slope, thus a smaller K_a. (B) Woolf plot, another statistical representation of antigen-antibody binding. In this case F/B is plotted against F (as moles per liter). The slope of the line is equal to 1/number of total binding sites, and the x intercept is equal to $-K_a$. Thus line b has a greater x intercept, representing a smaller K_a than line a. Line b has a smaller slope, representing a greater number of total binding sites than line a.

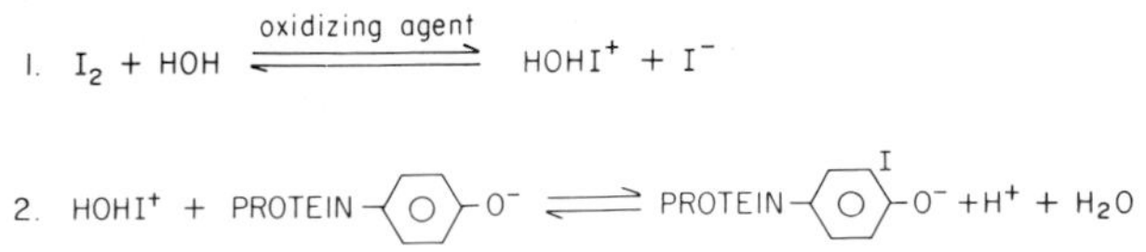

1. $I_2 + HOH \xrightleftharpoons{\text{oxidizing agent}} HOHI^+ + I^-$

2. $HOHI^+ + PROTEIN\text{-}\langle O \rangle\text{-}O^- \rightleftharpoons PROTEIN\text{-}\langle \overset{I}{O} \rangle\text{-}O^- + H^+ + H_2O$

FIG. 3. The iodination reaction.

Radiolabeling: the chemical reaction

The technique used is important to provide adequate combination of ^{125}I with the protein or peptide to be labeled and to minimize damage to the peptide or hormone (primarily through oxidation). Iodine can be introduced into tyrosyl residues via a reaction which produces a cationic iodinium (I^+) ion from iodide (I^-), available from the commercially available $Na^{125}I$, through oxidation. This active form interacts with the charged phenolic hydroxyl moiety on the tyrosyl residue of a protein or peptide (see Fig. 3).

Several methods exist to obtain the active iodinium form. Although many authors favor one method over another, it is our experience that as long as the iodination method is optimized any of the methods can be used successfully even for labile peptides. Lactoperoxidase and chloramine-T (8) methods are the most widely used.

Regardless of which method is used, the first step is to lower the pH of commercially available $Na^{125}I$ to 7.0, since it is usually provided at high pH. Iodination occurs optimally at this lower pH. Once oxidation has occurred, it should be stopped quickly to prevent hormone damage by adding a reducing agent (5 α-metabisulfite) or excess nonhormonal protein (albumin).

If chloramine-T is selected as the oxidizing agent, it is worth noting that past methods have tended to use an excess of chloramine-T which may result in damage of the hormone. Sample protocols for three commonly used methods are given in Tables 1 through 3. Because of space limitations we limit our discussion to the chloramine-T and lactoperoxidase methods. Other methods which the interested reader can con-

sult for greater details are given in references 4, 5, and 8.

Purification of radiolabeled hormone

Once the peptide or protein has been radioiodinated, it is essential to separate damaged peptide, high-quality label, and free ^{125}I. A number of procedures have been used for purification, including chromatoelectrophoresis, acrylamide gel electrophoresis, starch gel electrophoresis, ion-exchange chromatography, concanavalin A chromatography, and immunocolumn chromatography. We currently prefer ion-exchange chromatography for small noncarbohydrate peptides (6), concanavalin A chromatography for glycoprotein hormones (LH, FSH, TSH, hCG [luteinizing hormone, follicle-stimulating hormone, thyroid-stimulating hormone, human chorionic gonadotropin]) (9), and Sephadex column chromatography for non-carbohydrate-containing proteins over 5,000 molecular weight. At the time of writing, early reports of use of high-pressure liquid chromatography for purification of peptides and proteins are appearing. This newer method may prove highly useful.

Small peptides (under 5,000 molecular weight). By use of a carboxymethyl-Sephadex, SP-Sephadex, or quaternary aminoethyl-Sephadex column (Pharmacia Fine Chemicals, Inc.), carbohydrate-free small peptides may be purified by ion-exchange chromatography. We have used this technique for preparation of radioiodinated GnRH (gonadotropin-releasing hormone), calcitonin, parathormone, endorphin, vaso-

---

TABLE 1. Chloramine-T iodination sample protocol

1. In a small plastic vial (Brinkmann) to be used as the reaction vessel, add the following ingredients in the order given:
   a. 20 μl of 0.05 M phosphate–0.15 M NaCl buffer (pH 7.4) containing 1 to 2 μg of the protein to be radioiodinated
   b. 50 μl of 0.5 M phosphate buffer (pH 7.5)
   c. 1 mCi of carrier-free, high-specific-activity $Na^{125}I$ (about 2.5 μl)
   d. 5 μl of 0.15 M NaCl–0.05 M phosphate buffer (pH 7.4) containing 2.5 μg of chloramine-T (to be prepared fresh before use by combining 5 mg of preweighed chloramine-T in 10 ml of buffer and mixing for 15 to 40 s just before adding to the reaction vessel)
2. Stop the reaction after 30 s by adding 300 μl of 1% bovine serum albumin or 10 μl of sodium metabisulfite (5 μg).
3. Rapidly transfer contents of reaction vessel to the column selected for purification, washing the vessel several times with volumes of 1% bovine serum albumin.

TABLE 2. Lactoperoxidase-hydrogen peroxide method

1. Add the following reagents in order at room temperature to the reaction vessel (glass tube, 10 by 75 mm):
   a. 2 to 5 μg of the protein to be radioiodinated in 5 μl of 0.01 M phosphate–0.15 M NaCl buffer (pH 7.4)
   b. 50 μg of lactoperoxidase in 10 μl of 0.1 M sodium acetate (pH 5.6)
   c. 1 mCi of carrier-free $Na^{125}I$
   d. 25 μl of 0.4 M sodium acetate buffer (pH 5.6)
2. The reaction is initiated and maintained by 100 to 200 μg of hydrogen peroxide at 10-min intervals, usually for a total of 30 min. Occasionally, smaller amounts of hydrogen peroxide may be used for hydrogen-sensitive proteins (such as hCG).

TABLE 3. Lactoperoxidase-glucose oxidase sample protocol

1. Add all reagents in the order listed to reaction vessel at room temperature (*except* glucose oxidase, which should be kept at 4°C until added):
   a. 15 μl of 0.01 M phosphate–0.15 M NaCl buffer (pH 7.5)
   b. 2 to 5 μg of the protein to be iodinated
   c. 1 mCi of ^{125}I
   d. 50 μg of lactoperoxidase in 10 μl of 0.1 M sodium acetate (pH 5.6)
   e. 5 μl of glucose oxidase
   f. 25 μl of 0.1% glucose
2. Mix reaction by finger-flicking the vessel for 1.5 min.
3. Add 0.5 ml of 0.01 M phosphate buffer (pH 7.5).
4. Transfer entire contents to separation-purification column.

pressin, oxytocin, ACTH, and β-MSH (β-melanocyte-stimulating hormone). With cation-exchange chromatography, one should use a pH one unit below the estimated pK_a, and with anion-exchange one pH unit above the estimated pK_a should be used. A column (0.9 by 12 cm) is prepared at 10°C and packed by gravity. Under the most simple conditions, the iodinated reaction mixture is placed on the column, and initially a shallow linear osmolar gradient is applied at 40 to 50 ml/hr. Fractions of 2 to 3 ml are collected. Free iodine and albumin will be eluted first, followed by peptides and, much later, unlabeled and monoiodinated damaged proteins. From these data one can select or derive a two-step elution buffer gradient to elute first the free iodide (low osmolality), followed by a higher osmolality buffer to elute the noniodinated and iodinated undamaged material (300 to 400 ml later). Elution tubes are checked for maximal immunoreactivity with excess antiserum, and all tubes containing 90 to 100% immunoactivity are pooled.

Glycoproteins. Concanavalin A (Pharmacia Fine Chemicals, Inc.) column chromatography, used to purify labeled hormones, results in fractions with over 90 to 95% immunoreactivity for all four glycoproteins of many animal species. It is prepared as a column (8.5 by 40 mm) at room temperature, washed with 1% bovine serum albumin in phosphate-buffered saline (0.01 M phosphate–0.15 M NaCl; pH 7.4). The iodination mixture is added to the top of the column and then washed with phosphate-buffered saline until collected fractions reach a stable plateau of radioactivity. The column-bound glycoprotein is then eluted by 50 ml of methyl-α-D-glucopyranoside (0.2 M) in phosphate buffer solution, and all fractions are collected in 3-ml volumes in tubes containing 50 μl of 1% bovine serum albumin in phosphate buffer to prevent adsorption of label to glass. Excess antibody (1,000× greater concentration than that used in a usual assay) can be incubated with diluted samples from each eluate tube to determine optimal fractions to be used for assay. This will result in rapid binding to estimate immunoreactivity quickly (2 to 4 h at room temperature with polyethylene glycol or 24 h at 4°C with second antibody).

Larger nonglycoproteins. Larger-molecular-weight, noncarbohydrate proteins can be purified by use of long (1 by 100 cm) Sephadex column chromatography or with starch gel or acrylamide gel electrophoresis. We commonly employ Sephadex columns. As with the previously discussed purification methods, the immunoreactivity of the organic peak is assessed with excess antiserum.

Assessment of quality

Quality is routinely assessed by determination of each of the following: (i) immunoreactivity at a working dilution under assay conditions; (ii) immunoreactivity in the presence of excess antibody; (iii) nonspecific binding (binding in absence of antibody); and (iv) specific activity. Specific activity is a measure of the efficiency of the radiolabeling procedure. It can be estimated by using the mass of the peptide used for iodination and the disintegrations per minute of ^{125}I used for radioiodination, multiplied by the estimated efficiency of organification (radioactivity in the free

iodide peak compared with that of the labeled hormone peak). A more accurate measurement of specific activity is to compare the bound versus free values (B/F) of a standard curve with known amounts of standard with the B/F values of varying amounts (counts per minute) of labeled hormone. Equating comparable B/F points on the two curves can allow a comparison of counts per minute per microgram that can be readily converted to microcuries per microgram or to disintegrations per minute per micromole.

REFERENCE MATERIAL OR STANDARD

Assay results are given in terms of some reference or standard material. For steroids or thyronines where highly pure material is available with ease, results are given in terms of mass of the hormone. Even for these hormones, the assayist should verify the purity of the reference preparation. For peptide or protein hormones, results are often stated in terms of a national or international reference preparation. Since supplies of such standards or reference materials are often limited, a second standard characterized and assigned a potency in the individual laboratory is often developed and used. Such laboratory standards should be quantified in direct comparison with the international standard in multiple independent assays at different times, and a mean potency should be assigned. In our laboratory we perform 10 such independent assays before assigning a potency to our laboratory standard. Several facts are worth considering before developing or using a reference material for protein hormones. (i) Circulating proteins exist in several forms: polymorphology. (ii) Preparations purified from pituitary or other gland sources may well be different from circulating forms. (iii) Species differences exist, making it highly desirable to select a reference source from the same species as the one the assay will be used to measure. (iv) Protein hormones, especially in purified form, are unstable; thus, small samples, snap frozen and stored, may slowly lose biological and immunological potency over several months.

The World Health Organization and other agencies preparing international standards carefully assess stability and store freeze-dried materials in inert gas-filled and sealed ampoules to prevent or delay potency loss. Extreme caution in selection of preparation and storage conditions in the assay lab is urged.

SEPARATION METHOD

General

In our opinion, the separation method introduces the greatest source of error in the RIA procedure. This method distinguishes the antibody-bound analyte from the free analyte. No perfect method exists; each has its own individual limitations which may be preferable in one circumstance over another. The methods used include chromatoelectrophoresis, gel filtration, immunoprecipitation, chemical separation, adsorbent techniques, solid-phase separation, and polymerized antibodies. These methods predominantly depend on a size difference between free analyte versus analyte bound to antibody. Larger-molecular-weight substances, e.g., viruses, may be separated more easily by solid-phase techniques or special sandwich assay procedures, in which the size difference between bound and free portions is less important to separation.

Chromatoelectrophoresis is historically important as the first method used by Yalow and Berson (10). It is seldom used now as it is more time-consuming than other methods and impractical for large numbers of samples. Immunoprecipitation, chemical separation, and adsorption techniques are used most frequently, so they will be discussed in greater detail.

Immunoprecipitation

The immunoprecipitation method is known as double-antibody precipitation because it involves the use of a "first" antibody (the antisera described previously) and a less-specific "second" antibody, an anti-gamma globulin, which is directed against the first antibody. Typically, the first antibody (e.g., rabbit anti-human TSH) is permitted to react with analyte and reach equilibrium. The second antibody (e.g., goat anti-rabbit immunoglobulin) is added to permit precipitation of the immunoglobulin complex. The tubes are then centrifuged, and the supernatant is discarded by decanting or aspirating. The precipitate represents the heavier antigen-antibody complexes (bound antigen), and the counts per minute is determined.

Although it is not commonly appreciated, even this seemingly simple technique has multiple sources of imprecision and "misclassification" (i.e., errors in assigning bound as free or vice versa). For example, since first antibodies are usually used in very great dilutions (e.g., $1:10^6$), reaction with second antibody would take many days to reach equilibrium. Thus, carrier immunoglobulin (e.g., normal rabbit serum) is added to increase total immunoglobulin concentrations. The time required for the second antibody separation method to reach completion varies with immunoglobulin concentration, temperature, and osmolality and pH of buffers. The time to reach completion may be further hastened by addition of a chemical separation technique (e.g., polyethylene glycol) to the immunological separation method (3). The optimal amount of second antibody to be added varies with the amount of immunoglobulin present. Rigorous assessment of the optimal amount of second antibody required must be made under the individual assay conditions for every batch or lot of second antibody used. Commonly, commercial kits (for cost reasons) employ an amount of second antibody close to the inflection point on a second-antibody titration curve. Because of this, small errors in pipetting second antibody result in misclassification of bound and free hormone. The serious assayist or researcher should select an amount of second antibody on the upper plateau or flat maximal-response portion of the dose-response curve. In this region, pipetting errors in second antibody have little effect on assay precision. Once optimized, specific assay conditions should be held rigidly constant to ensure reproducibility of results.

Chemical separation

The chemical separation method also depends on differences in solubility of immune complexes (bound) and free analyte. Many chemicals have been used for separation, including ethanol, sodium sulfite, ammonium sulfate, and trichloroacetic acid. The most widely used is polyethylene glycol (Carbowax) (3), which can be prepared in a variety of concentrations and either used alone or in combination with a second antibody for fast turn-around time in RIA. It can be used with a variety of hormones, but is particularly useful for thyronine and steroid assays. As discussed for double-antibody separation, careful dose-response curves should be constructed with serially varying concentrations of polyethylene glycol versus amount bound, and a concentration should be chosen that maximizes specific binding while minimizing nonspecific binding.

Adsorbent techniques

Adsorbent techniques employ differential surface binding between free and the larger bound analyte. Larger molecules bind less well than smaller ones. The adsorbent technique is capable of separating a small free analyte from a large bound one. It will not work for large-molecular-weight analytes. With this technique the precipitate optimally contains the free fraction, which is discarded. The supernatant contains the soluble bound portion, which is decanted and assessed for radioactivity. The concentration of both electrolytes and proteins can greatly affect this method by interfering with surface adsorption. Examples of materials used as adsorbents include talc, silica, resins, staphylococcal protein A, and cellulose. Charcoal coated with dextran is the most widely used adsorbent (1), particularly in steroid assay systems. The concentration of both charcoal and dextran should be optimized for each particular assay. It is important to emphasize that dextran coating is employed only to make the charcoal more sticky to insure a formed pellet. Dextran does not create a molecular sieve to assist in molecular discrimination (1). The easiest technique is to prepare the dextran-coated charcoal as a suspension in buffer and, while stirring it continuously, to pipette a fixed volume of suspension to each assay tube.

CONCLUSION

RIA techniques have been important to our ability to measure extremely small amounts of proteins and hormones in body fluids. Advances in these techniques have largely been responsible for the great strides made in the last 10 to 15 years in endocrinology research as well as in many other fields. However, much research is still being done to improve the convenience, turn-around time, reliability, sensitivity, and reproducibility of the RIA, as well as to broaden its scope of applicability.

LITERATURE CITED

1. **Binoux, M. A., and W. D. Odell.** 1973. Use of dextran coated charcoal to separate antibody-bound from free hormone: a critique. J. Clin. Endocrinol. Metab. **36:**303–310.
2. **Bolton, A. E., and W. M. Hunter.** 1973. The labeling of proteins to high specific radioactivities by conjugation to a ^{125}I-containing acylating agent. Biochem. J. **133:** 529–539.
3. **Desbuquois, B., and G. D. Aurbach.** 1971. Use of polyeth-

ylene glycol to separate free and antibody-bound peptide hormones in radioimmunoassays. J. Clin. Endocrinol. Metab. **33:**732–738.

4. **Donabedian, R. K., R. A. Levine, and D. Seligson.** 1972. Microelectrolytic iodination of polypeptide hormones for radioimmunoassay. Clin. Chem. Acta **36:**517–520.

5. **Fraker, P. J., and J. C. Speck.** 1978. Protein and cell membrane iodinations with a sparingly soluble chloramide, 1,3,4,6-tetrachloro-3a,6a-diphenylglycoluril. Biochem. Biophys. Res. Commun. **80:**849–857.

6. **Heber, D., W. D. Odell, H. Schedewie, and A. R. Wolfsen.** 1978. Improved iodination of peptides for radioimmunoassay and membrane radioreceptor assay. Clin. Chem. **24:**796–799.

7. **Keightley, D. D., and N. A. C. Cressie.** 1980. The Woolf plot is more reliable than the Scatchard plot in analysing data from hormone receptor assays. J. Steroid. Biochem. **13:**1317–1323.

8. **Odell, W. D., and D. Heber.** 1980. Radioiodination of peptides and proteins for radioimmunoassays or radioreceptor assays, p. 329–338. *In* N. R. Rose and H. Friedman (ed.), Manual of clinical immunology, 3rd ed. American Society for Microbiology, Washington, D.C.

9. **Patritti Laborde, N., Y. Yoshimoto, A. R. Wolfsen, and W. D. Odell.** 1979. Improved method of purifying some radiolabeled glycopeptide hormones. Clin. Chem. **25:** 163–165.

10. **Yalow, R. S., and S. A. Berson.** 1961. Immunological specificity of human insulin: application to immunoassay of insulin. J. Clin. Invest. **40:**2190–2198.

Chapter 19

Analytical Fluid-Phase Fluorescence Immunoassays

ROBERT M. NAKAMURA AND BRUCE A. ROBBINS

Fluorescence immunoassay (FIA) procedures are currently widely used in many clinical laboratories for the detection and quantitation of drugs, hormones, proteins, and peptides in biological fluids (7, 11, 12). These FIA procedures are rapid, sensitive, and adaptable to automation and have been recommended as alternatives to radioimmunoassays and enzyme immunoassays.

Most fluorophores or fluorescent compounds are organic compounds with a ring structure. When the compound absorbs light, there is an excitation of electrons, which oscillate in resonance. With the absorption of light of shorter wavelength, the energy can be emitted in the form of light of longer wavelength, with a short time lapse between absorption and emission of light. The approximate time interval between absorption of energy and emission of fluorescence is less than 10^{-9} s with use of the standard labels such as fluorescein isothiocyanate (10).

Fluorescence, phosphorescence, and delayed fluorescence are types of photoluminescence in which molecules are excited by interaction with photons of electromagnetic radiation (10, 11). In fluorescence, the release of light energy is immediate or from the singlet state (antiparallel electron spin) and has lifetimes in the range of 0.1 to several hundred nanoseconds. In phosphorescence, there is a delayed release of energy from the triplet state (parallel electron spin). The phenomenon of delayed fluorescence results from the two intersystem crossings, first from the singlet to the triplet state and then from the triplet to the singlet state.

The sensitivity of early FIA procedures was impeded by many factors, including the high background fluorescence of biological fluid samples such as serum. Advances have been made in instrumentation and immunochemical reagents such that certain analytes may be detected at a concentration of 10^{-15} M.

In the quest for specific FIAs which have the sensitivity of radioimmunoassays, special instrumentation which allows kinetic measurements of the antigen-antibody reactions to minimize interference with background fluorescence has been developed. A new technique involves the use of a time-resolved fluorometer (15, 17, 21). In this method, a fast light pulse excites the label, and the fluorescence is measured after a certain time has elapsed from the moment of excitation to reduce nonspecific background fluorescence and increase the sensitivity of the assay. Various fluorescent probes such as pyrenebutyric acid, with a decay time of 100 ns, or chelates of europium, with a decay time of microseconds, have been used (17, 21).

This chapter will be limited to analytical fluid-phase FIA and will not include those FIAs involving cells and flow cytometry. The various FIAs may be classified as follows: (i) heterogeneous or homogeneous; (ii) ligand or antibody labeled; (iii) competitive or noncompetitive; (iv) solid phase or non-solid phase.

HETEROGENEOUS FIA

The heterogeneous FIA involves a separation step for the labeled-unlabeled reagent. This step eliminates many of the problems associated with sample background fluorescence. Most of the commercially available assays utilize a solid-phase antigen or antibody system. The assay can be developed either as a competitive or noncompetitive type.

For the solid-phase FIA, there are four commonly employed methods.

(i) Indirect method (Fig. 1). Specific antibody in the sample binds to a solid-phase antigen. The matrix is washed and reacted with fluorescence-labeled antibody. After a second wash, the fluorescence is quantitated.

(ii) Competitive method (Fig. 2). Labeled and unlabeled analytes compete for a limited number of antibody sites immobilized on a solid matrix. The matrix is washed, and the bound fluorescence is quantitated.

(iii) Sandwich method (Fig. 3). The analyte antigen reacts with matrix-bound antibody. The solid-phase matrix is washed and reacted with fluorescence-labeled antibody. After a second wash, the fluorescence is quantitated. This method is not readily adaptable for the assay of haptens.

(iv) Fluoroimmunometric method. The analyte reacts with labeled antibody in solution. Residual labeled antibody binds to excess solid-phase bound antigen. The solid-phase matrix is washed, and the fluorescence is quantitated. In contrast to the sandwich method, this method can be used for the assay of both haptens and complex proteins.

Solid-phase FIAs have been developed for the serologic assay of antibodies to rubella, nuclear antigen, toxoplasmosis, and many other viral antigens (11, 12). With the use of a dedicated instrument, the solid-phase FIA has the advantage of excellent precision when compared with manual methods using subjective endpoint detection.

FIA methods have been developed for serum protein, haptens, and hormones such as cortisol, progesterone, and thyroxine (5–7).

HOMOGENEOUS FIA

By definition, homogeneous FIAs do not require the separation of bound and free unknowns. The homogeneous FIAs have the following features. (i) With standard instrumentation, the assay sensitivity is limited near 10^{-10} M of analyte. (ii) Special instrumentation is required to achieve an assay with high sensitivity. (iii) Impurities in the sample can increase with background interference. (iv) Relatively pure immunochemical reagents are required.

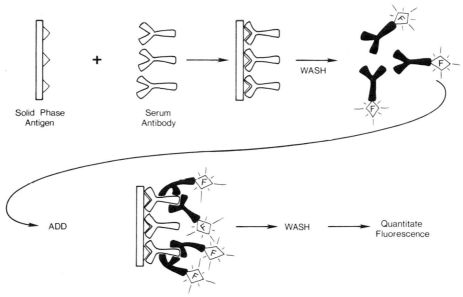

FIG. 1. Indirect method of solid-phase FIA. This assay is a heterogeneous method for the detection of specific antibody in serum.

HOMOGENEOUS ASSAYS BY FLUORESCENCE ENHANCEMENT OR QUENCHING

The fluorescence intensity of a fluorescent label of the analyte conjugate can undergo fluorescence quenching or enhancement subsequent to immunologic reaction of the labeled analyte (13, 14, 16).

In the fluorescence quenching method, the binding of a chromophoric hapten by antibody causes a marked decrease of antibody tryptophan fluorescence (14). Smith (16) has described an enhancement fluoroimmunoassay of thyroxine (T-4). A fluorescent derivative of T-4, when bound to anti-T-4 serum, demonstrated a three- to fourfold enhancement of fluorescence. The assay involves a short incubation step after the mixing of the sample, labeled T-4, and specific antiserum, with subsequent measurement of the fluorescence enhancement (Fig. 4). An Aminco-Bowman fluorometer was used to measure the degree

of fluorescence. Fluorescein–T-4 conjugate is not an efficient fluorophore since there is intramolecular quenching of the fluorescein fluorophore by the iodine atoms of the iodothyronine portion of the T-4 molecule. Such iodine-containing molecules are efficient quenchers of fluorescence. However, when specific antibody binds to T-4, there is enhancement of fluorescence. This enhancement is best explained in terms of inhibition of quenching when the iodothyronine moiety becomes interlocked with the combining site of the specific anti-T-4 antibody.

A major disadvantage of this method is the variability of levels of intrinsic serum fluorescence in the patient samples. The assay procedure would require either a reliable technique to remove background interference of the intrinsic serum fluorescence or a special instrumentation to increase the sensitivity and specificity of the assay. With the use of a conventional fluorometer, the technique as published is less sensi-

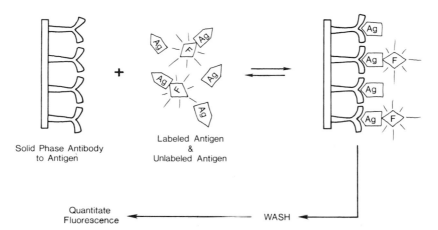

FIG. 2. Competitive solid-phase FIA for antigen (Ag). This assay is a competitive heterogeneous FIA for the detection of antigens. It is useful for detection of haptens or drugs.

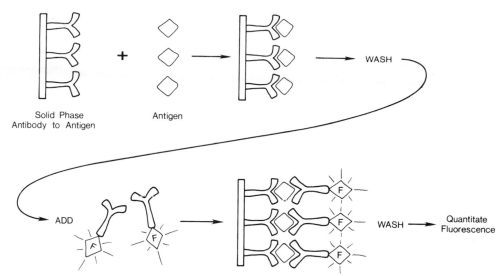

FIG. 3. Sandwich FIA for antigen. This noncompetitive FIA is useful for the detection of a polyvalent antigen.

tive than standard radioimmunoassay methods for T-4; however, removal of the variable background serum sample fluorescence would allow sufficient sensitivity to measure total T-4 levels in clinical patients.

Homogeneous fluorescence excitation transfer immunoassay

The fluorescence excitation transfer method has been applied to the analysis of morphine, a morphine-albumin conjugate, and human immunoglobulin G (IgG). This immunoassay employs two labels (20). Fluorescein is employed as the acceptor or quencher. Fluorescein isothiocyanate has a maximum emission of 525 nm, and tetramethyl or tetraethyl rhodamine has a strong absorption peak at 525 nm. Therefore, when fluorescein isiothiocyanate-labeled antigen and rhodamine-labeled antibody bind, there is a quenching of fluorescein isiothiocyanate fluorescence when the two labels are within 5 to 10 nm of each other.

There are two variants of the method. In the first, the antigen is labeled with fluorescein and the antibody is labeled with rhodamine. This method may be referred to as the direct antigen-labeling method. With fluorescein and rhodamine as the fluorescer and quencher, respectively, the average distance between them must be sufficient to permit dipole-dipole coupled excitation energy transfer within the antigen-antibody complex. In the assay procedure for quantitation of antigen in unknown samples, the unlabeled antigen would compete for the rhodamine-labeled antibody and reduce available binding sites, with a resultant decrease in fluorescence quenching.

The second method is similar to the first except that the antigen is labeled indirectly by employing a fluorescein-labeled antibody or Fab antibody fragment. This method is useful for the assay of antigen with multivalent antigenic determinants. Separate portions of specific antibody of Fab antibody fragments are labeled with fluorescein and rhodamine, respec-

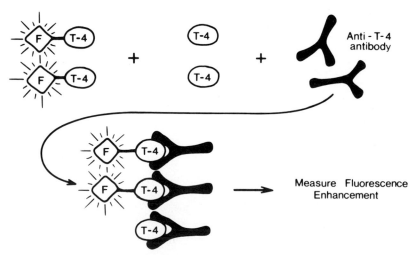

FIG. 4. Fluorescence enhancement immunoassay for T-4. When specific antibody binds to fluorescein-labeled T-4, there is a three- to fourfold enhancement of fluorescence.

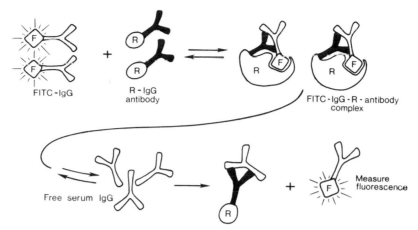

FIG. 5. Direct antigen-labeled fluorescence excitation transfer immunoassay. Fluorescein isothiocyanate (FITC)-labeled IgG and free IgG compete for the specific rhodamine (R)-labeled anti-IgG. The fluorescein-labeled IgG is quenched by increasing the amounts of rhodamine-labeled anti-IgG.

tively. The admixture of differently labeled fluorescein-tagged antibody or Fab antibody fragments and rhodamine-labeled antibody would reduce the intensity of the fluorescer by adjusting the ratio and amount of donor and acceptor so that they react in close proximity to permit energy transfer.

A disadvantage of the indirect labeling method is that immunochemically purified antibodies are required to avoid excessive fluorescence background due to nonspecific fluorescer-labeled proteins. These assays have potential sensitivity to the 100-pmol range (20). The advantages over heterogeneous assays include speed, avoidance of the separation step, and stability of the reagents.

Direct antigen-labeled fluorescence excitation transfer immunoassay

The direct antigen-labeling technique was studied in the assay of morphine. The addition of increasing amounts of rhodamine-labeled antimorphine to a fixed concentration of morphine-fluorescein will produce decreases in fluorescence intensity which will approach a minimum value with excess antibody. A maximum quenching of 72% was observed with an

excess of specific antibody labeled with 15 molecules of rhodamine. In the studies by Ullman et al. (20), the fluorescence measurements were made with a Perkin-Elmer MPF-2A spectrofluorometer equipped with Baird-Atomic B-4 and B-5 fluorescein filters (The Perkin-Elmer Corp., Norwalk, Conn.). The excitation light was at 470 nm, and the emission maximum was found near 520 nm. The direct antigen-labeling method has been applied to assays for human IgG with the use of fluorescein-labeled IgG and rabbit anti-human IgG labeled with rhodamine (Fig. 5).

Indirect antigen-labeled fluorescence excitation transfer immunoassay

The indirect antigen-labeling assay method is useful for antigens with multiple determinants and requires an immunochemically purified preparation of fluorescein-labeled antibody or Fab antibody fragments. The assay has been applied to a hapten such as morphine by employing morphine-albumin conjugates (albumin-M30) which have 30 molecules of morphine bound to 1 molecule of albumin (20). The assay was sensitive for albumin-M30 and codeine to a level of 1 nmol.

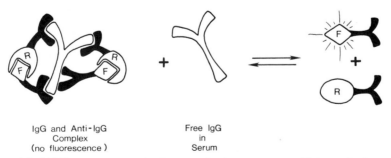

FIG. 6. Indirect antigen-labeled fluorescence excitation transfer immunoassay. This method is useful for the assay of a protein antigen such as IgG with multiple antigenic determinants. The procedure requires an immunochemically purified preparation of fluorescein-labeled antibody. The admixture of fluorescein- and rhodamine (R)-labeled antibodies in the proper ratio will reduce the intensity of the fluorescer. The addition of unlabeled antigen will change the balance of the antigen and antibody-labeled complex, and the degree of fluorescence in the free solution is directly proportional to the unlabeled antigen concentration.

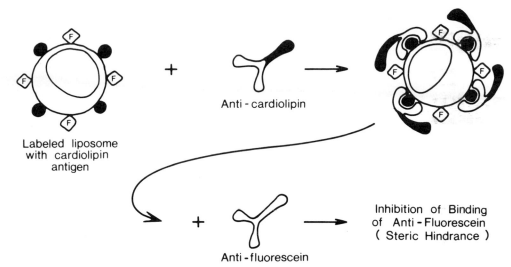

FIG. 7. Fluorescent protection assay for anticardiolipin antibody. The fluorescein-labeled antigen is reacted with the anticardiolipin antibody (analyte). The antibody-labeled antigen complex in turn will sterically inhibit the reaction of the fluorescein-labeled antigen with antifluorescein antibody. The antifluorescein antibody, when reacted with fluorescein, will quench the fluorescence. The anticardiolipin antibody level is directly related to the degree of fluorescence observed.

Similarly, an indirect assay was developed for human IgG with separate portions of two immunochemically purified antibodies to human IgG, one labeled with fluorescein and the other labeled with rhodamine (Fig. 6). The assay employed a 1:7 molar ratio of Ab-F4.3/Ab-R10 in reaction with human IgG, and 40% maximum quenching of fluorescein was observed. The sensitivity of the assay for human IgG was less than 100 pmol.

Antigen-labeled fluorescence protection or indirect quenching assay

In the indirect quenching technique, the antigen is labeled with fluorescein, and the antigen-specific antibody will sterically inhibit the reaction of the antibody specific for fluorescein. The specific antibody to fluorescein will quench the fluorescence of fluorescein after binding to the fluorophore. The specific anti-

fluorescein may be coupled to dextran or complexed with antibodies to the antifluorescein to increase the size and decrease the ability to interact with the fluorescein coupled to the surface of the antigen within a small space. The procedure may be used to assay for antibody to the antigen or the antigen concentration in a homogeneous system. Ullman used the technique for assay of T-4 levels in serum and also as a test for anticardiolipin antibody, similar to a serologic screening test for syphilis (19). Liposomes with the cardiolipin antigen are labeled with fluorescein. When the fluorescein-labeled antigen is first reacted with anticardiolipin antigen, antibody-labeled antigen complex in turn will inhibit the reaction of the fluorescein-labeled antigen with antifluorescein antibody by steric hindrance. The cardiolipin antigen concentration measured is directly related to the degree of fluorescence observed in the reaction (Fig. 7).

The assay for T-4 involves fluorescein-labeled T-4

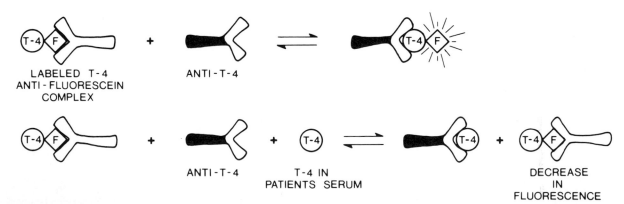

FIG. 8. Antigen-labeled fluorescence protection assay for T4. Fluorescein-labeled T4 is complexed with low-affinity antifluorescein antibody which decreases the fluorescence of fluorescein. When anti-T4 is added, the anti-T4 reacts with the fluorescein-labeled T4 and pulls it away from the specific antifluorescein antibody. The T4 in the assay sample will bind to the anti-T4 antibody, and the level of T4 is correlated with the decrease in fluorescence.

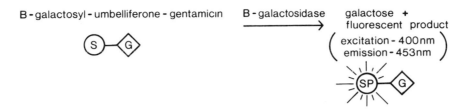

FIG. 9. Hapten-substrate conjugate in homogeneous FIA. The cleavage of the substrate (S) conjugate by the enzyme β-galactosidase will cause the release of galacton (G) and a fluorescent substrate product (SP).

complexed with low-affinity antifluorescein antibody, which decreases the fluorescence of fluorescein (Fig. 8). When anti-T-4 is added, it reacts with the fluorescein-labeled T-4 and pulls it away from the specific antifluorescein antibody, with a resulting increase in fluorescence. In the assay of serum samples with high concentrations of T-4, the anti-T-4 will react with the T-4, and the fluorescence will be decreased since antifluorescein will remain complexed to the labeled T-4. The assay shows very little interference with background serum proteins. It is feasible to measure T-4 levels in clinical samples in a sensitive and reproducible fashion.

Nargessi et al. (13) have developed similar indirect quenching fluorescence immunoassays for human serum albumin, human IgG, and human placental lactogen.

Homogeneous substrate-labeled FIAs

The substrate-labeled assay has been adapted to measure gentamicin (4) and tobramycin (3). In the gentamicin assay, gentamicin is coupled to β-galactosylumbelliferone to form a nonfluorescent substrate.

The free β-galactosylumbelliferone–gentamicin conjugate will react with the enzyme β-galactosidase to form a fluorescent product (Fig. 9). However, when the β-galactosylumbelliferone–gentamicin is combined with specific antibody, the linking of specific antibody by steric hindrance will not allow cleavage of the conjugate-antibody complex by β-galactosidase (Fig. 10). The procedure does not require a separation step and is a sensitive homogeneous assay. The rate of production of fluorescence was proportional to the gentamicin concentration, and the fluorescence assay yielded values which compared with a radioimmunoassay for gentamicin in clinical serum samples. The fluorescence assay requires 1 μl of serum and can easily detect levels of gentamicin of less than 1 μg/ml. The assay procedure is completed in 2 to 3 min, and the fluorescence rate reaction is measured with an Aminco-Bowman spectrophotofluorometer equipped with temperature control for the sample compartment.

The principle of a homogeneous substrate-labeled FIA was used to detect specific binding proteins (2). For example, biotin was coupled directly to umbelliferone through an ester bond. Hydrolysis of

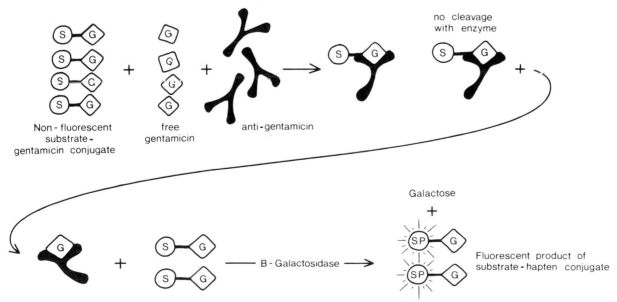

FIG. 10. Homogeneous substrate (S)-labeled FIA for gentamicin (G). Gentamicin is coupled to the substrate, and the complex forms a nonfluorescent substrate. The substrate can be cleaved by the enzyme β-galactosidase to form a fluorescent product (SP). However, when the substrate complexed with gentamicin is allowed to react with specific antigentamicin antibody, there is no cleavage with β-galactosidase. By this procedure one can assay for free gentamicin in serum, and the concentration will correlate with the amount of fluorescent product liberated by the enzyme reaction.

Chapter 20

Section C. Immunoglobulins and B-Cell Disorders

Introduction

GERALD M. PENN

Disorders of the B-cell system, either alone or in conjunction with defects of other cell systems, are currently the most common ailments to confront today's clinical laboratory immunologist. The expressions of the B cells, immunoglobulins, are usually altered qualitatively or quantitatively by these disease processes. In many instances these alterations are highly specific for a group of diseases, while in other cases they are nonspecific changes and only suggest a diagnosis. Section C will concentrate on those procedures which are utilized in the clinical immunology laboratory predominantly for the identification or assessment of B cells. Other procedures which evaluate B cells as well as other compartments of the immune system will be discussed in the appropriate sections of this manual. In addition, this section will emphasize those diseases for which the procedures discussed are essential for their diagnosis. For the most part, these diseases are the monoclonal gammopathies or immunoproliferative diseases. The B-cell lymphomas/leukemias, B-cell immune deficiencies, and autoimmune diseases are discussed in other sections of this volume.

In chapter 21, Virginia Mehl and I discuss the nomenclature and structure of the immunoglobulins and describe two procedures for their evaluation, namely, immunoelectrophoresis (IEP) and immunofixation electrophoresis (IFE). The main emphasis of this chapter is the interpretation of patterns generated in these assays by the use of commercial reagents and supplies (kits).

Irene Check and Margaret Piper co-authored chapter 22, entitled "Quantitation of Immunoglobulins." They describe three procedures for the measurement of immunoglobulin concentration: rate nephelometry, radial immunodiffusion, and enzyme-linked immunosorbent assay. The first two of these procedures employ commercial reagents and supplies, whereas the third method uses a procedure developed within Check and Piper's laboratory. An essential ingredient of this chapter is their excellent coverage of the pitfalls encountered in each procedure.

The third chapter of this section, chapter 23 authored by Robert Kyle, summarizes and integrates the information of the previous two chapters. He describes in-house procedures for IEP and IFE and demonstrates the use of other laboratory and clinical data for the diagnosis of multiple myeloma and other monoclonal gammopathies.

The fourth and final chapter of section C (chapter 24) was prepared by Jeffrey Cossman, Ajay Bakhshi, and Stanley Korsmeyer. They describe a procedure for detecting immunoglobulin gene rearrangement and hence demonstrating monoclonality of the B cell.

This type of procedure is useful when a serum, urine, or cell surface immunoglobin anomaly is not produced by a lymphoproliferative process. Section C would not be complete without a look at tomorrow's clinical laboratory technology.

Although the primary goal and objective of this section is to describe those procedures which are used to evaluate B cells, a secondary purpose is to discuss reasons for establishing these procedures in the laboratory and for formulating the criteria for performance of each procedure. It is obvious that admission screening by serum protein electrophoresis or the performance of IEP and IFE on all sera from patients with anemia or pulmonary infections would lead to an ineffective utilization of financial resources. It is also apparent that a 62-year-old patient with hypercalcemia and proteinuria, admitted for anemia of unknown etiology, should have additional laboratory testing beyond a urinalysis, complete blood count, and general biochemical profile. The former case is an example of laboratory overutilization, while the lack of additional testing in the second example is an underutilization of laboratory resources. Although underutilization appears to reduce laboratory expenses, the increase in length of stay due to delay in diagnosis actually increases the overall laboratory as well as hospital expenses. It is generally accepted that a good indicator of optimal laboratory utilization is minimal average test cost per individual diagnosis or disease-related group. Thus, the clinical immunology laboratorian must understand the effect of introducing a new procedure on the above ratio. The laboratorian should also recognize the benefits of establishing criteria for the performance of these procedures in regard to preventing over and underutilization.

An algorithm our laboratory has used to prevent over- and underutilization is illustrated in Fig. 1. The suggested clinical criteria are listed as a guide for the clinicians. Upon receiving a request for serum IEP, a screening immunochemical evaluation (ICE) profile is performed. The ICE profile consists of serum protein electrophoresis and quantitation of immunoglobulin G, A, and M and kappa and lambda light chains. These procedures are not as labor intensive as IEP or IFE and are excellent screening procedures to prevent overutilization of the other two more costly assays.

Laboratory criteria are also established to minimize underutilization of the above tests. If any of these criteria are met, protein electrophoresis assay is performed on serum, urine, or both. When a monoclonal protein is detected, the ICE profile and other laboratory procedures are initiated automatically. The essential factors of this algorithm which lead to cost effectiveness are cooperative medical staff, readily

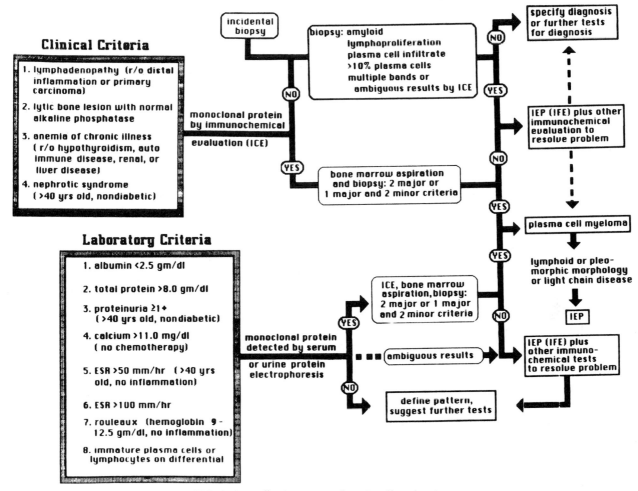

FIG. 1. Cost-effective approach to B-cell evaluation.

available clinical information, and fast turnaround time of the ICE profile and the protein electrophoresis. The use of similar algorithms or strategies has been shown to generate immense cost savings for the laboratory and hospital.

LITERATURE CITED

1. Sher, P. P., J. F. Caldas, G. W. Cole, G. M. Penn, B. E. Statland, P. Vincent, and H. Weitzman (ed.). 1984. Economic challenges to the clinical laboratory. Part 2: Trends in utilization. Technicon Instruments Corp., Tarrytown, N.Y.

Chapter 21

Electrophoretic and Immunochemical Characterization of Immunoglobulins

VIRGINIA S. MEHL AND GERALD M. PENN

The characterization of the immunoglobulins in a clinical specimen such as serum, urine, or cerebrospinal fluid (CSF) is performed in an attempt to answer several clinically relevant questions. (i) Does an immunoglobulin anomaly exist? (ii) Is this anomaly polyclonal or monoclonal? (iii) Is the anomaly indicative of a specific benign or malignant process?

The complete characterization of immunoglobulins often requires several different laboratory assays. A single method that will permit the identification of all immunoglobulin abnormalities does not exist. Zone electrophoresis and immunoelectrophoresis (IEP) are the most common techniques used to evaluate immunoglobulins; however, immunofixation electrophoresis (IFE) may also be extremely helpful. The quantitation of kappa and lambda light chains by rate nephelometry in conjunction with immunoglobulin quantitation and zone electrophoresis is currently being introduced as an alternative method for the identification and characterization of immunoglobulins in serum and urine. In this chapter these four methods will be extensively discussed in terms of their clinical indications, advantages, and disadvantages.

STRUCTURAL AND FUNCTIONAL CHARACTERISTICS OF IMMUNOGLOBULINS

Immunoglobulins comprise 20% of serum proteins and represent that component of serum which confers immunity. Immunoglobulins were originally termed gamma globulins as a result of their typical electrophoretic migration on zone electrophoresis. It is now recognized, however, that immunoglobulins may also migrate in the alpha-2 and beta regions. This diverse electrophoretic mobility reflects a variation in the carbohydrate and amino acid content of immunoglobulins. Immunoglobulins also demonstrate great functional diversity in their specificity of antigen binding and their biological activities.

Although heterogenous, all immunoglobulins have the basic structure shown in Fig. 1. This basic structural unit consists of two heavy chains (molecular weight, 55,000) and two light chains (molecular weight, 22,500) joined by interchain disulfide bonds. The first ca. 110 amino acids on the N-terminal end of both the heavy and light chains are termed the variable region and represent the site of antigen binding. The remaining portion of the heavy and light chains is termed the constant region. Amino acid sequencing studies of the variable regions have demonstrated that they have considerable variation in amino acid sequence and are primarily responsible for the heterogeneity of serum immunoglobulins. A certain degree of homology has been demonstrated in the variable regions, with hypervariable or "hot" spots identified at specific amino acid locations. These hypervariable regions appear to contribute directly to the antigen-binding site and produce the idiotypic antigens found on all immunoglobulins. The genetic mechanism responsible for the generation of these hypervariable regions will not be discussed here. For further information, see reference 7.

The constant region, as the name implies, demonstrates relatively little variation in amino acid sequence between members of the same class or type. Located on the C-terminal end of the polypeptide chain, the constant regions contain approximately 110 amino acids on the light chains and 330 amino acids on the heavy chains. Based on antigenic and structural characteristics of the constant regions, two types of light chains and five types of heavy chains have been described. The light-chain types are termed kappa and lambda. Lambda light chains have been further divided into four subtypes based on two amino acid differences. The heavy-chain types are designated gamma, alpha, mu, delta, and epsilon. These heavy-chain types correspond with the five immunoglobulin classes, i.e., immunoglobulin G (IgG), IgA, IgM, IgD, and IgE. IgG and IgA are further divided into subclasses based on a few amino acid differences. The constant portion of the heavy chains is responsible for the distinct and varied biological characteristics associated with the nine classes and subclasses of immunoglobulins. Also varied among classes and subclasses are the location and number of interchain disulfide bonds. The biological and chemical characteristics of the immunoglobulins are presented in Table 1.

Immunoglobulins from all five classes are composed of the basic structural unit described above. Two identical heavy chains and two identical light chains are joined by disulfide bonds. Both types of light chains are found in each class of immunoglobulin, but never on the same molecule. In serum and other body fluids, IgG, IgD, and IgE exist as monomers consisting of a single four-polypeptide unit. Serum IgM, in contrast, is present as a pentamer with five structural units joined by a small glycoprotein termed the J chain. IgA, which also utilizes the J chain to aid in polymerization, is usually observed in secretory fluids as a dimer with an attached secretory component. Serum IgA, which exists predominantly as a monomer, may polymerize further to contain two, three, four, or five of the basic structural units.

The heavy and light chains present in immunoglobulin molecules do not exist as linear polypeptides but have loops produced by intrachain disulfide bonds. The loops contain approximately 110 amino acids and are termed domains. Light chains contain two domains designated V_L and C_L. Heavy chains contain domains V_H, C_H1, C_H2, and C_H3. An additional domain, designated C_H4, is found on mu and epsilon

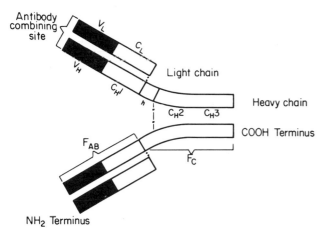

FIG. 1. Immunoglobulin structure, showing fragments resulting from papain digestion. Used by permission from reference 4.

heavy chains. Each domain has been shown to be associated with specific biological functions.

The hinge region is located on the heavy chain between the C_H1 and C_H2 domains. This region consists of approximately 20 amino acids and is rich in the amino acid proline. The hinge region is responsible for the flexibility of the immunoglobulin molecule.

Immunoglobulins can be digested into distinct, well-characterized fragments by certain enzymes. The study of these various fragments was invaluable in determining the biological function and structure of immunoglobulins. The hinge region is the site of action of the enzyme papain. Papain digestion results in the production of three fragments, i.e., two identical Fab fragments and an Fc fragment. The Fab fragment contains the entire light chain and the V_H and C_H1 domains of the heavy chain. This fragment retains the ability to bind to an antigenic determinant; however, it does not possess the biological activities associated with an intact immunoglobulin. The Fd fragment represents that portion of the heavy

chain that is not included in the Fc fragment. The Fc fragment, which contains the heavy chain domains C_H2 and C_H3, does not bind antigen; however, it does contain the class antigenic determinants and also biological activity.

Pepsin attacks the heavy chain on either side of the C_H2 domain, resulting in the production of the $F(ab')_2$ fragment and also two Fc' fragments. The Fc' fragment consists only of the C_H3 domain. The $F(ab')_2$ fragment contains both Fab fragments and the hinge region. The $F(ab')_2$ fragment not only can bind antigens, but as a result of its bivalent nature can cross-link and subsequently precipitate antigens.

MONOCLONAL IMMUNOGLOBULINS

Immunoglobulins present in normal human serum demonstrate an electrophoretic heterogeneity that results partially from class and subclass differences but is mainly due to the great diversity of variable regions seen on the heavy and light chains that compose serum immunoglobulins. Each specific antibody with its unique amino acid sequence is the product of a single clone of plasma cells. All immunoglobulins produced by a given clone of plasma cells have identical amino acid sequences; consequently they are of the same class, subclass, light-chain type, and idiotype. The idiotypic antigens are due to the hypervariable regions of the V_H and V_L areas. A clone of plasma cells represents the proliferation of a mature B cell after antigen stimulation. Excessive proliferation of any given plasma cell clone is normally prevented by the vast array of immune regulatory systems that are active during an immune response.

In multiple myeloma, solitary plasmacytoma, and certain other malignancies of B-cell origin (immunocytomas), a single clone of plasma cells proliferates in an uncontrolled fashion. These malignant plasma cells may produce a large number of identical immunoglobulins that demonstrate a restricted or limited electrophoretic mobility (Fig. 2). The immunoglobulin produced by a single clone of plasma cells are termed monoclonal immunoglobulins. Structural-

TABLE 1. Characteristics of immunoglobulin classes

Class	Heavy-chain type	No. of subclasses	Molecular formula	Mol wt	Sedimentation coefficient	% Carbohydrate	Mean serum concn	Biological half-life (days)	Biological functions
IgG	Gamma	4	H_2L_2	150,000	7	4	1,200 mg/dl	23	Crosses placenta; activates complement by classical pathway
IgA	Alpha	2	$(H_2L_2)_n$ $n = 1–5$	170,000	7, 10, 14	9	235 mg/dl	6	Secretory antibody; activates complement by alternate pathway
IgM	Mu	1	$(H_2L_2)_n$ $n = 5$	900,000	19	15	150 mg/dl	5	Distribution limited to intravascular space; activates complement by classical pathway
IgD	Delta	1	H_2L_2	185,000	7	18	5 mg/dl	2.8	Cytotrophic antibody for lymphocytes
IgE	Epsilon	1	H_2L_2	200,000	8	18	20 IU/ml	1.5	Cytotrophic for mast cells; immediate hypersensitivity

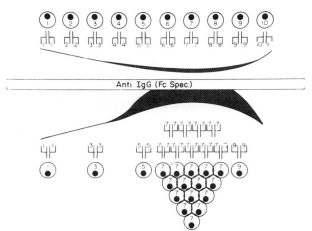

FIG. 2. Polyclonal and monoclonal plasma cell proliferation. Used by permission from reference 4.

ly, these monoclonal immunoglobulins are usually not abnormal. In fact, most of the current information on the structure of immunoglobulins was obtained by the study of monoclonal proteins isolated from the sera of patients with multiple myeloma. The abnormality of monoclonal immunoglobulins resides in their abundant homogeneity.

PRINCIPLES OF ELECTROPHORESIS

Electrophoresis may be defined as the movement of a charged particle within a solvent when that solution is placed in an electrical field. Electrophoresis is an extremely effective method of separating macromolecules for the characterization of components within a mixture or the isolation of macromolecules from a mixture. Electrophoresis can therefore serve as an analytical or a preparative procedure.

In zone electrophoresis, a small quantity of solution is placed on a buffer-saturated support medium. When an electrical potential is applied to the buffer, macromolecules in solution will migrate. The rate of migration is determined by the energy of the electrical field, the resistance of the support medium, and the net charge of the macromolecule at a given voltage; the larger the net charge, the greater the velocity of migration.

In the clinical laboratory, zone electrophoresis is currently used to separate the components of not only serum, but also CSF, urine, and other body fluids. Five major protein bands are seen on most routine serum protein electrophoretic patterns. These bands include albumin and alpha-1, alpha-2, beta, and gamma globulins. If high-resolution electrophoresis is performed, as many as 15 separate bands can be identified in normal serum samples.

PRINCIPLES OF IEP

The identification of serum protein components can usually be achieved by the use of two procedures, IEP and IFE. In IEP, serum proteins are first separated based on their electrical charge. Antiserum is then placed in a trough that runs parallel to the protein migration, and the separated proteins are precipitat-

ed by an immunodiffusion reaction. The precipitin arc location of a specific serum protein is determined not only by its electrophoretic mobility, but also by its serum concentration, diffusion characteristics, and the potency of the antiserum. By combining zone electrophoresis with immunoprecipitation, IEP permits an identification and characterization of serum protein components that would not be possible by zone electrophoresis or immunodiffusion alone. The clinical indications and interpretation of serum IEP patterns will be discussed in more detail later in this chapter. See reference 4 for a comprehensive discussion of IEP interpretation.

PRINCIPLES OF IFE

In addition to IEP, IFE may be used to identify and characterize serum proteins. IFE, similarly to IEP, combines zone electrophoresis with immunoprecipitation. In IFE, serum samples are first separated by electrophoresis on a buffer-saturated support medium. After electrophoresis, the medium is overlaid with antiserum reactive with the specific serum protein to be evaluated. If the antigen and antibody are present in the proper concentrations (near or in the equivalence zone), an immunoprecipitin band is formed. The monospecific antiserum "fixes" the specific serum protein. Nonprecipitated serum proteins and antiserum are removed by washing the medium in a saline solution, and the immunoprecipitin is stained for proper visualization. As will be discussed below, IFE is a valuable tool in the identification of "occult" paraproteins. See reference 5 for an extensive discussion of IFE.

CLINICAL INDICATIONS FOR THE EVALUATION OF IMMUNOGLOBULINS BY PROTEIN ELECTROPHORESIS

The possibility of an immunoglobulin anomaly is suggested by certain abnormal laboratory results. When any of the following abnormalities are observed, especially in a patient over 40 years old, electrophoresis of the serum, urine, or CSF should be considered: increased sedimentation rate, presence of rouleaux on peripheral blood smear, immature plasma cells on peripheral blood smear, elevated total serum protein concentration, proteinuria, hypercalcemia with normal alkaline phosphatase, and increased CSF protein without evidence of active inflammation.

There are also certain clinical signs that indicate the need for serum and urine electrophoresis and IEP. These signs in an older individual alert the physician to the possibility of a malignancy that may include a monoclonal gammopathy in its clinical presentation. These signs include chronic normochromic normocytic anemia of unknown etiology, nephrotic syndrome in the nondiabetic older patient, osteolytic lesions, and lymphadenopathy.

The malignant diseases associated with a serum monoclonal gammopathy include multiple myeloma, B-cell lymphoma (including Waldenström's macroglobulinemia), heavy-chain disease, and amyloidosis. Monoclonal proteins may also be present in the serum of a patient without a detectable immunoproliferative process. Transient minor monoclonal gammopathies are often seen during an infection or in association with hypergammaglobulinemia. It is important to distinguish these minor M proteins of the IgG class from the minor IgM monoclonal proteins often associated with a malignant lymphoma.

Electrophoresis of a clinical specimen can also indicate numerous clinical conditions other than monoclonal gammopathies. The procedure in these cases is not diagnostic; however, specific electrophoretic patterns in various body fluids are associated with different clinical entities. Protein electrophoresis can therefore aid in the development of a differential diagnosis. A diffuse polyclonal increase in serum immunoglobulins may occur in connection with an inflammatory process, chronic liver disease, infection, and connective tissue disease. In a patient with proteinuria, electrophoresis of the urine can determine if the elevated urinary protein is Bence Jones protein associated with multiple myeloma or if the patient has nonspecific proteinuria, possibly due to the nephrotic syndrome. Electrophoresis of CSF can also aid in the diagnosis of multiple sclerosis (MS).

Electrophoresis of serum or urine samples may be performed on a variety of support media, the most common being cellulose acetate and agarose gel. Normal serum produces a typical five-band electrophoretic pattern on these standard electrophoretic support media. High-resolution electrophoresis systems are also available from several commercial suppliers. These systems may resolve as many as 15 bands in a normal serum sample. They permit the detection of minor monoclonal bands, especially monoclonal light chains that are often obscured in standard electrophoresis. High-resolution agarose gel electrophoresis is also extremely valuable in the detection of oligoclonal bands in CSF. Many individuals feel that the additional bands seen on high-resolution electrophoresis are more confusing than helpful and do not contribute significantly to patient care. The unit cost per assay is also considerably more for high-resolution electrophoresis. The decision to use a high-resolution or a standard electrophoresis system should be based on the preference of the individual interpreting the electrophoretic patterns. An important fact to be remembered, however, is that regardless of the electrophoresis system employed, a normal serum protein electrophoretic pattern may occur in conjunction with a malignant monoclonal gammopathy. The monoclonal protein may be hidden in the beta globulins, e.g., in light-chain disease or monoclonal proteins of the IgD class. A normal serum protein electrophoretic pattern is also common with heavy-chain disease.

CLINICAL INDICATIONS FOR THE EVALUATION OF IMMUNOGLOBULINS BY IEP AND IFE

Serum or urine IEP or IFE is essential for the definitive diagnosis of multiple myeloma, macroglobulinemia, or heavy-chain disease. (For a complete discussion of the clinical staging of multiple myeloma, see reference 1.) IEP or IFE is also indicated if a monoclonal spike or immunoglobulin anomaly is seen on a serum protein electrophoresis performed for other clinical reasons.

Characterization of immunoglobulin anomalies by IEP and IFE includes differentiation of monoclonal from polyclonal anomalies, identification of monoclonal immunoglobulin fragments, and a semiquantitative estimation of the immunoglobulin concentrations. IEP and IFE are limited by the fact that they are only as sensitive as the antisera used. The clinical laboratory should always test a commercial antiserum against a series of known monoclonal proteins, including Bence Jones proteins. The laboratory should also have several different antisera available. A paraprotein in a serum or urine sample may fail to react or give an aberrant reaction with a particular antiserum.

IEP is routinely used in our laboratory for characterization of immunoglobulin anomalies. When compared with IFE, IEP utilized considerably less antiserum and technician time. Both procedures readily permit identification of the heavy- and light-chain type of most monoclonal proteins; however, IEP is superior for the evaluation of multiple paraproteins with similar electrophoretic mobilities and for the characterization of immunoglobulin fragments. IEP does have certain limitations. A minor monoclonal protein is often missed if other serum immunoglobulins are at normal or elevated levels. In addition, the light-chain type of an IgM monoclonal protein cannot usually be identified by IEP unless the patient's serum is first reduced or a cuglobulin precipitation is performed.

In those circumstances in which IEP yields inconclusive results, we use IFE to characterize the paraprotein. IFE readily identifies the light-chain type of IgM monoclonal proteins and is extremely valuable in the identification of minor monoclonal proteins. IFE is also considerably easier to interpret than is IEP. The accurate interpretation of infrequently encountered IEP patterns often requires considerable experience. The IFE procedure we currently employ utilizes agarose gel slides produced by Worthington Diagnostics (Freehold, N.J.) and requires an overnight incubation. IFE kits have recently become available from several commercial suppliers, including Beckman Instruments, Inc. (Brea, Calif.) and Helena Laboratories (Beaumont, Tex.). In our limited experience with the Paragon IFE system from Beckman, we found that the procedure required the same amount of technician time as IEP and had the advantage of same-day results.

USE OF RATE NEPHELOMETRY FOR THE DETECTION AND CHARACTERIZATION OF SERUM IMMUNOGLOBULIN ANOMALIES

IEP or IFE (or both) is currently used by most laboratories to identify immunoglobulin abnormalities in serum and urine. In many cases, this same information could be obtained by rate nephelometry. If a single monoclonal spike is seen on serum electrophoresis, the class and light-chain type of this paraprotein can usually be determined by measuring the serum level of IgG, IgA, IgM, and kappa and lambda light chains. Difficulties may be encountered when serum levels of IgG, IgA, and IgM are normal and when multiple monoclonal bands are seen on serum electrophoresis. Problems may also occur with light-chain disease and IgD or IgE monoclonal proteins. IEP or IFE (or both) is required for the identification of these immunoglobulin abnormalities.

Rate nephelometry can also be used for the differentiation of monoclonal and polyclonal increases in serum immunoglobulins. This distinction can be difficult to make by serum electrophoresis alone. Monoclonal proteins of the IgM and IgA class often polymerize and do not produce a sharp monoclonal spike. Calculation of the kappa/lambda ratio in the serum sample can rapidly distinguish monoclonal and polyclonal hypergammaglobulinemia.

In addition to monoclonal gammopathies, an abnormal kappa/lambda ratio may also be encountered in patients with immunoglobulin deficiencies and autoimmune diseases. A thorough review of other laboratory data and the clinical history is indicated when these problematic patients are encountered. The use of rate nephelometry to detect or characterize monoclonal proteins requires considerably more evaluation in a clinical setting; however, it may represent an extremely cost-effective way of evaluating immunoglobulin anomalies. We currently use the Beckman rate nephelometer with Kallestad reagents (antisera) for this type of immunochemical assessment (see chapter 22 for definitive details of the procedure).

For additional information on the kappa/lambda ratio, see references 3 and 6.

INTERPRETATION OF SERUM ELECTROPHORESIS AND IEP PATTERNS

Examples of the use of electrophoresis, IEP, IFE, and rate nephelometry to characterize serum immunoglobulin anomalies are demonstrated in Fig. 3 through 7. The majority of patients with multiple myeloma have serum immunoglobulin anomalies similar to that shown in Fig. 3. A single monoclonal protein is present that is easily detected by serum electrophoresis and readily characterized by rate nephelometry. The serum samples presented in Fig. 4 through 7 require more extensive procedures for accurate characterization of the serum immunoglobulin anomalies.

Figure 3A demonstrates the serum electrophoretic patterns obtained with normal control serum and serum from a patient with multiple myeloma. The patient's serum electrophoretic pattern shows a large monoclonal spike (arrow). A monoclonal protein of the IgG class is strongly suspected due to the location of this restriction at the more cathodal segment of the gamma region. Serum electrophoresis also demonstrated a sharp reduction in the other immunoglobulins and the near absence of C3. This was a sample that was mailed to the laboratory, and the breakdown of the third component of complement during transport is not uncommon.

In the majority of sera that contain a single large monoclonal band on serum electrophoresis, the class and light-chain type of this paraprotein can be identified by the measurement of the serum levels of IgG, IgA, IgM, kappa and lambda light chains, and the kappa/lambda ratio. The following are the serum protein quantitations obtained with the sample shown in Fig. 3A: IgG, 5,380 mg/dl; IgA, 10.5 mg/dl; IgM, 13.3 mg/dl; kappa chain, 106 mg/dl; lambda

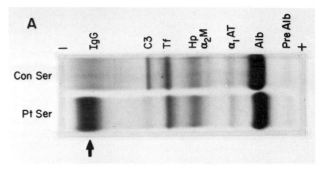

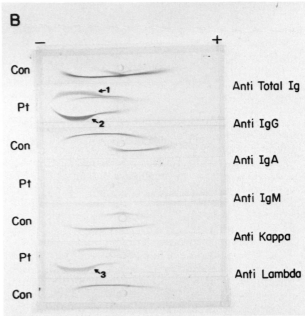

FIG. 3. Electrophoresis and IEP of a serum sample containing an IgG lambda monoclonal protein. Serum electrophoresis (A) detects a large monoclonal spike in the gamma region (arrow) and a near absence of C3. Serum IEP (B) detects a bowing of the precipitin arc with anti-total immunoglobulin (Ig) serum (arrow 1), anti-IgG serum (arrow 2), and anti-lambda serum (arrow 3). Con, Control; Pt, patient; Ser, serum; Tf, transferrin; Hp, haptoglobin; α_2M, α_2-macroglobulin; α_1AT, α_1-antitrypsin; Alb, albumin.

chain, 6,480 mg/dl; and kappa/lambda ratio, 0.016. These results identify the paraprotein as an IgG lambda. A polyclonal decrease in IgA and IgM is also apparent. Normal adult ranges for serum immunoglobulins were previously established at the following levels: IgG, 565 to 1,765 mg/dl; IgA, 85 to 385 mg/dl; IgM, 45 to 245 mg/dl; kappa chain, 510 to 1,300 mg/dl; lambda chain, 250 to 720 mg/dl; and kappa/lambda ratio, 1.3 to 2.7. The light chains are measured in milligram-per-deciliter equivalents of IgG.

The serum IEP shown in Fig. 3B confirms the presence of an IgG lambda monoclonal protein. A large bowing of the major IgG precipitin arc is seen when the patient's serum reacts with anti-total immunoglobulin (arrow 1). The same bowing is seen with anti-IgG serum and anti-lambda serum (arrows 2 and 3, respectively). This IEP pattern is indicative of an IgG lambda monoclonal protein. Precipitin lines are not easily observed when the patient's serum reacts

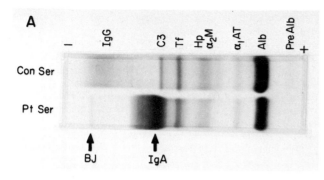

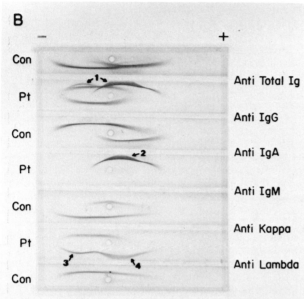

FIG. 4. Electrophoresis and IEP of a serum sample containing an IgA lambda monoclonal protein and monoclonal lambda light chains. Serum electrophoresis (A) detects a large monoclonal spike (arrow IgA) and a second minor restriction (arrow BJ). Serum IEP (B) detects a double bowing of the precipitin arc (arrow 1) with anti-total immunoglobulin. The major precipitin arc (IgA lambda) corresponds with those produced with anti-IgA (arrow 2) and anti-lambda (arrow 4). The slower small arc of the anti-total immunoglobulin reaction (lambda BJ) is duplicated only by the anti-lambda serum (arrow 3). For abbreviations, see the legend to Fig. 3.

with anti-IgA and anti-IgM, indicating a large decrease in the serum levels of these immunoglobulins.

The serum electrophoretic pattern in Fig. 4A demonstrates a large restriction in the beta-gamma region (arrow IgA). In comparison to the monoclonal spike seen in Fig. 3A, the M protein in Fig. 4A is a much faster-migrating monoclonal protein, and the band appears considerably broader or wider. These two characteristics suggest an IgA monoclonal protein. IgA often polymerizes, resulting in a broad rather than a sharp monoclonal band on serum electrophoresis. A second band is identified by arrow BJ. This minor band may represent Bence Jones protein or a second minor monoclonal protein.

The following are serum protein quantitations determined by rate nephelometry for the sample in Fig. 4A: IgG, 293 mg/dl; IgA, 7,260 mg/dl; IgM, 14.7 mg/dl;

kappa chain, 146 mg/dl; lambda chain, 2,062 mg/dl; and kappa/lambda ratio, 0.07. These results identify the major monoclonal bands as an IgA lambda monoclonal protein; however, these values are of little assistance in identifying the second protein band seen on serum electrophoresis. IEP or IFE is required for a definitive evaluation of the serum. An alternative approach, sufficient for clinical use, is the performance of urine electrophoresis to demonstrate a large band with the same electrophoretic mobility as the slower serum band, identifying it as a probable Bence Jones protein.

The IEP pattern produced by this patient's serum is shown in Fig. 4B. A double bowing of the precipitin arc is seen with anti-total immunoglobulin (arrow 1). The reactions of anti-IgA (arrow 2) and anti-lambda (arrow 4) identify the major restriction as an IgA lambda monoclonal protein. The slower small arc of the anti-total immunoglobulin reaction is duplicated

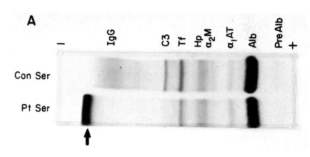

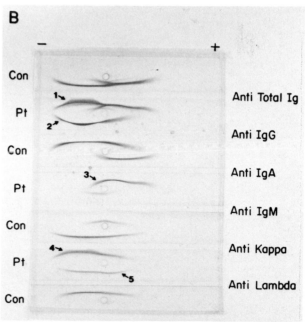

FIG. 5. Electrophoresis and IEP of a serum sample containing a diclonal monoclonal gammopathy composed of a major IgG kappa and a minor IgA lambda monoclonal protein. Serum electrophoresis (A) detects a single monoclonal spike in the gamma region (arrow). Serum IEP (B) demonstrates a major bowing of the precipitin arc with anti-total immunoglobulin (arrow 1), anti-IgG (arrow 2), and anti-kappa (arrow 4). A minor bowing of the precipitin arc is produced with anti-IgA (arrow 3) and anti-lambda (arrow 5). For abbreviations, see the legend to Fig. 3.

by the anti-lambda serum (arrow 3), signifying probable monoclonal lambda light chains. This small arc corresponds with the minor slow-migrating band seen on serum electrophoresis. The definitive identification of Bence Jones protein is based on the reaction of the

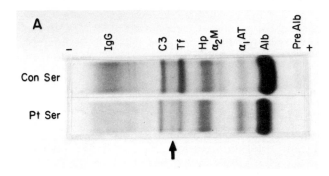

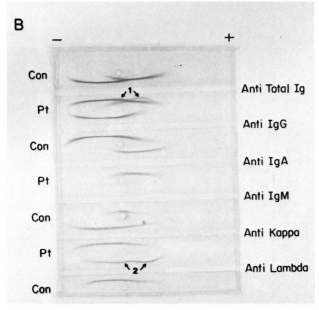

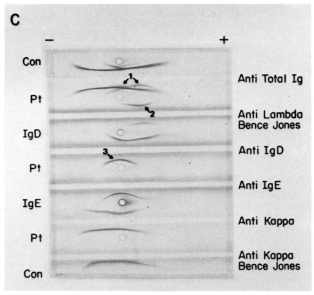

protein with free light-chain-specific antiserum or the use of urine electrophoresis to demonstrate in the urine a major band with the same electrophoretic mobility as the serum component. A precipitin arc is not seen with the patient's serum and anti-IgM, and the arc produced with anti-IgG is considerably reduced when compared with the control. These findings indicate a polyclonal decrease in IgG and IgM, which agrees with the serum immunoglobulin quantitations obtained by rate nephelometry.

The serum electrophoretic pattern shown in Fig. 5A illustrates a single large monoclonal band in the gamma region. The remainder of the immunoglobulins in the gamma region appear reduced, suggesting a polyclonal decrease in the other serum immunoglobulins. C3 is also decreased. Serum protein quantitations were as follows: IgG, 2,630 mg/dl, IgA, 320 mg/dl; IgM, 71.9 mg/dl; kappa chain, 1,770 mg/dl; lambda chain, 263 mg/dl; and kappa/lambda ratio, 6.7. Inspection of these data indicates an IgG kappa monoclonal protein.

Examination of the IEP pattern (Fig. 5B) confirms the presence of an IgG kappa monoclonal protein. Bowing of the major precipitin arc is observed when the patient's serum reacts with the anti-total immunoglobulin, anti-IgG, and anti-kappa sera (arrows 1, 2, and 4, respectively). The serum sample presented in this figure appears very similar to that of Fig. 3. On close examination of the pattern, however, a second minor monoclonal protein is observed. The second smaller precipitin arc is seen with anti-IgA and anti-lambda (arrows 3 and 5, respectively). This IEP pattern is consistent with a diclonal gammopathy composed of an IgG kappa and a minor IgA lambda monoclonal protein. The minor monoclonal protein was not suspected from the serum electrophoretic pattern or serum immunoglobulin quantitations. However, the clinical value of detecting the second minor component is questionable. This example demonstrates the difficulties that may be encountered with the complete identification and characterization of serum protein anomalies.

The serum electrophoretic pattern demonstrated in Fig. 6A shows only a possible band (arrow) located between transferrin and C3. When a minor monoclonal band is seen on serum protein electrophoresis, this protein usually cannot be identified by the results of serum immunoglobulin quantitation. The following are the serum immunoglobulin levels obtained for this patient: IgG, 851 mg/dl; IgA, 151 mg/dl: IgM, 42.9

FIG. 6. Electrophoresis and IEP of a serum sample containing an IgD lambda monoclonal protein and lambda Bence Jones protein. Serum electrophoresis (A) detects a minor monoclonal band (arrow) in the beta-gamma region. Serum IEP (B) demonstrates a double bowing of the precipitin arc with anti-total immunoglobulin (arrow 1) and anti-lambda (arrow 2). A corresponding heavy-chain reaction is not observed with anti-IgG, anti-IgA, or anti-IgM; however, the slower small arc of the anti-total immunoglobulin reaction is duplicated by the anti-IgD serum (C, arrow 3). The faster-migrating arc of the anti-total immunoglobulin reaction corresponds with a precipitin arc produced with anti-lambda Bence Jones (C, arrow 2). For abbreviations, see the legend to Fig. 3.

mg/dl; kappa chain, 631 mg/dl; lambda chain, 700 mg/dl; and kappa/lambda ratio, 0.9. The kappa/lambda ratio is reduced, but the serum levels of

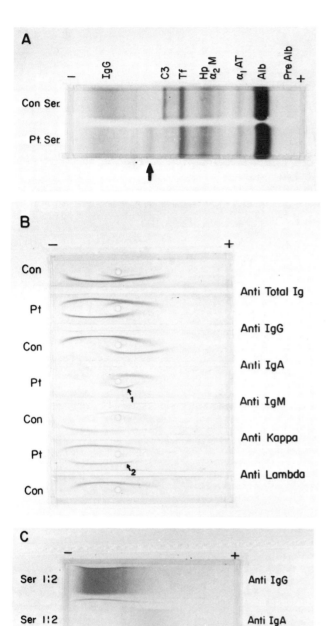

IgG, IgA, and IgM appear normal. Inspection of these data suggests the presence of lambda Bence Jones protein. Serum IEP is obviously required to verify the suspected lambda Bence Jones protein in this patient's serum.

The serum IEP pattern shown in Fig. 6B demonstrates a double precipitin arc (arrow 1) produced with the anti-total immunoglobulin serum. The anti-lambda serum shows a similar reaction (arrow 2). A heavy-chain reaction is not seen. This IEP pattern suggests light-chain disease or, less likely, a monoclonal protein of the IgD or IgE class. Two lambda precipitin arcs favor the IgD possibility, however, since most IgD monoclonal proteins are IgD lambda and are associated with lambda Bence Jones protein in the serum. To complete the characterization of this monoclonal protein, the patient's serum was tested by IEP with anti-total immunoglobulin, anti-lambda Bence Jones, anti-IgD, anti-IgE, anti-kappa, and anti-kappa Bence Jones sera. The resulting IEP pattern (Fig. 6C) demonstrates that the patient's serum contains not only lambda Bence Jones protein (arrow 2), but also an IgD lambda monoclonal protein (arrow 3). Anti-lambda Bence Jones serum binds to an epitope that is hidden in the intact immunoglobulins, and consequently the antiserum will not precipitate an intact immunoglobulin.

The serum electrophoretic pattern shown in Fig. 7A shows a minor monoclonal band in the beta-gamma region (arrow). There are C3 breakdown products anodal to transferrin, and the C3 band is absent. The following are the serum immunoglobulin levels: IgG, 689 mg/dl; IgA, 89.2 mg/dl; IgM, 146 mg/dl; kappa chain, 590 mg/dl; lambda chain, 377 mg/dl; and kappa/lambda ratio, 1.56. These serum immunoglobulin quantitations are of no assistance in the identification of the minor restriction seen on electrophoresis. Serum IEP (Fig. 7B) demonstrates an abnormal IgM arc (arrow 1). The quantity of this M protein is insufficient for the light-chain type to be definitively identified by IEP; however, a small, intense precipitin arc (arrow 2) is seen in the lambda precipitin line, suggesting an IgM lambda monoclonal protein. The inability to identify the light-chain type is very common with IgM monoclonal proteins. As a result of their pentamer structure, they diffuse at a much slower rate than monomeric IgG and IgA. The anti-light-chain sera are neutralized by the polyclonal IgG and IgA before the arrival of the IgM.

The light-chain type of an IgM monoclonal protein can be readily identified by IFE. IFE identified this minor monoclonal protein as an IgM lambda protein (Fig. 7C). The band seen on serum electrophoresis was precipitated by anti-IgM and anti-lambda sera.

FIG. 7. Electrophoresis and IEP of a serum sample containing a minor IgM lambda monoclonal protein. Serum electrophoresis (A) detects a minor monoclonal band in the beta-gamma region (arrow) and a sharply decreased C3. Serum IEP (B) detects a bowing of the precipitin arc with anti-IgM (arrow 1) and an increased intensity with anti-lambda (arrow 2). IFE (C) detects a monoclonal band with anti-IgM and anti-lambda. For abbreviations, see the legend to Fig. 3.

CHARACTERIZATION OF IMMUNOGLOBULINS IN URINE

Electrophoresis and IEP are extremely valuable in identifying immunoglobulin anomalies present in urine samples. When proteinuria is demonstrated by urinalysis, it is important to distinguish between proteinuria due to renal disease and Bence Jones proteinuria that may occur with multiple myeloma or other immunoproliferative diseases. Electrophoresis of a concentrated urine sample is indicated to resolve this clinical question. The prerenal proteinuria pattern most commonly caused by multiple myeloma typically produces an electrophoretic pattern with a band in the beta or fast-gamma region. This band produced by Bence Jones protein should always be identified by IEP. Identification and quantitation of the Bence Jones protein from a 24-h urine sample is extremely important in the clinical evaluation of multiple myeloma. If Bence Jones proteins are present in a urine sample, their excretion rate is directly proportional to the size of the tumor burden and can be used to monitor the effectiveness of therapy.

Figure 8A shows a urine electrophoretic pattern consistent with the interpretation of Bence Jones proteinuria. A single monoclonal band is seen in the urine gamma region that is not observed in the serum pattern. This band is identified as lambda Bence Jones protein by IEP (Fig. 8B). IEP demonstrates a bowed precipitin arc produced with the anti-total immunoglobulin serum (arrow 1) and duplicated with the anti-lambda serum (arrow 2). This IEP pattern identifies the protein as lambda Bence Jones. A careful evaluation of this urine IEP also reveals polyclonal light chains and a trace amount of polyclonal IgG.

CHARACTERIZATION OF IMMUNOGLOBULINS IN CSF

The diagnosis of MS is based on the clinical presentation; however, three distinct laboratory results are currently used to aid in this diagnosis. These results are an IgG index above 0.7, oligoclonal bands on CSF electrophoresis, and a CSF myelin basic protein level of >4 ng/ml.

The IgG index and the presence of oligoclonal bands in CSF are direct reflections of local production of immunoglobulin in CSF and have a high predictive value in the diagnosis of MS. The clinical indications for ordering an IgG index and electrophoresis of CSF include an unexplained increase in CSF total protein or the presence of MS in differential diagnosis.

To calculate the IgG index, serum and CSF levels of IgG and albumin are first measured by rate nephelometry or another suitable method. These values are then compared by the following formula:

$$\text{IgG index} = \frac{\text{CSF IgG/serum IgG}}{\text{CSF albumin/serum albumin}}$$

By comparing the concentrations of albumin in serum and CSF, the IgG index accounts for an increased CSF total protein resulting from permeability changes in the blood-brain barrier. The use of serum IgG within the equation corrects for an elevated CSF IgG due to hypergammaglobulinemia or monoclonal gammopathies. The normal range for the IgG index is 0.4

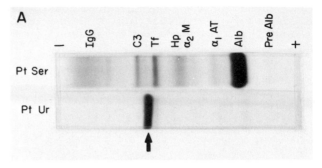

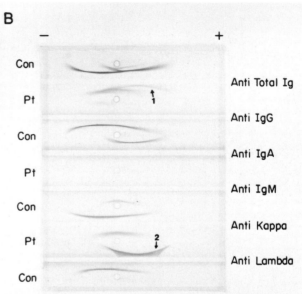

FIG. 8. Electrophoresis and IEP of a urine sample containing lambda Bence Jones protein. Urine electrophoresis (A) detects a monoclonal band in the beta region (arrow). Urine IEP (B) detects a bowing of the precipitin arc with anti-total immunoglobulin (arrow 1) and anti-lambda (arrow 2). For abbreviations, see the legend to Fig. 3.

to 0.53. We consider a value above 0.7 as a significant elevation and indicative of local production of immunoglobulins within the CSF.

Oligoclonal means "a few" clones (in contrast to one or many). The term oligoclonal bands refers to the multiple bands detected in the gamma region on CSF agarose gel electrophoresis. These bands result from the expansion of a limited number of plasma cell clones within the central nervous system and require high-resolution agarose gel electrophoresis or its equivalent for detection. CSF oligoclonal bands may also result from serum paraproteins; consequently, it is extremely important to compare the serum electrophoretic pattern with the CSF pattern.

Oligoclonal bands are often absent during the early stage of MS; however, once they appear, they remain in the CSF electrophoretic pattern and are characteristic for that patient. Oligoclonal bands are detectable in the CSF of 90% of patients with MS; however, oligoclonal bands are not pathognomonic for MS. They may be present in the CSF of patients with central nervous system lupus erythematosus, subacute sclerosing panencephalitis, neurosyphilis, or

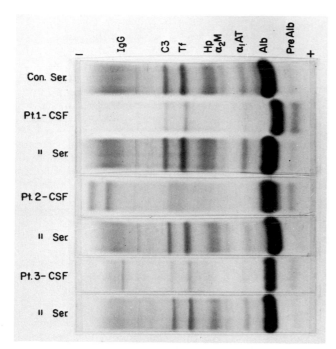

FIG. 9. Electrophoresis of serum and CSF. The CSF electrophoretic pattern of patient 1 was normal. Electrophoresis detects oligoclonal bands in CSF from patients 2 and 3. For abbreviations, see the legend to Fig. 3.

bacterial or viral meningitis. Oligoclonal bands are also not a good prognostic indicator. The intensity or number of these bands does not correlate with remission or exacerbation.

Figure 9 demonstrates CSF electrophoretic patterns. Patient 1 has a normal CSF electrophoretic pattern. A prominent prealbumin band is present, and the albumin as well as the CSF transferrin variant (Tau) band is readily seen. Tau, the CSF transferrin variant, is a carbohydrate-deficient protein with a slightly slower electrophoretic mobility than serum transferrin. Additional serum proteins that may be detected on CSF electrophoresis include alpha-1 antitrypsin, C3, and polyclonal IgG. The alpha-2 macroglobulins are noticeably absent with normal CSF. Oligoclonal bands are detected in the CSF electrophoretic patterns of patients 2 and 3. Note that two prominent oligoclonal bands are present in the CSF from patient 2. The CSF from patient 3 contains one major and four minor bands.

See reference 2 for additional information on the use of the IgG index, oligoclonal bands, and myelin basic protein in the diagnosis of MS.

IEP REAGENTS

Reagents needed for IEP include IEP films, IEP buffer, control serum, antisera, tracking dye, NaCl, glacial acetic acid, 95% ethanol, and Coomassie brilliant blue.

IEP reagent preparation and handling

IEP films (Kallestad Laboratories, Inc., Austin, Tex.). IEP films are packaged in a plastic box (two films per box) within a sealed shipping bag. Store the films in an unopened shipping bag at 20°C. If a single film is needed, remove the film from the box. Return the plastic box containing the unused film to the shipping bag, add several drops of tap water to the shipping bag, and reseal the bag with tape.

IEP barbital buffer (Kallestad Laboratories). IEP barbital buffer contains 0.027 M barbital, 0.023 M sodium acetate, and 0.015 M sodium azide (pH 8.6). It is packaged in vials containing 8.36 g of dry reagents. Store the vials at 20°C.

Dissolve the contents of the vials in a 1,000-ml volumetric flask. After reconstitution, store IEP buffer at 2 to 4°C. IEP buffer may also be stored at room temperature for a maximum of 2 weeks in the electrophoresis chamber.

If the polarity of the electrophoresis chamber is reversed after each use, the IEP buffer may be used four times.

Quantitrol (Kallestad Laboratories). Quantitrol is used for the human serum control. It is packaged in lyophilized form and stored at 2 to 8°C.

Reconstitute each vial of lyophilized Quantitrol with 0.5 ml of distilled water. Reconstituted Quantitrol is stable at 2 to 8°C for 28 days.

Tracking dye (Kallestad Laboratories). Tracking dye contains 0.4% bromphenol blue and is packaged in 0.5-ml vials. Store tracking dye at room temperature.

Specific antisera (Kallestad Laboratories). The following specific antisera are routinely used in serum IEP: anti-total human immunoglobulin, anti-human IgG, anti-human IgA, anti-human IgM, anti-human kappa chain, and anti-human lambda chain. Store the antisera at 2 to 8°C.

IEP stain. Add 5.0 g of Coomassie brilliant blue R (Sigma Chemical Co., St. Louis, Mo.) to a 1,000-ml volumetric flask. Add 450 ml of 95% ethanol, 450 ml of distilled water, and 100 ml of glacial acetic acid, and mix well. Let the mixture stand overnight at room temperature, and then filter through Whatman no. 5 filter paper.

Store the mixture at room temperature in a closed container. Discard the stain when a visible floating precipitate forms.

Destaining solution. To a 1,000-ml volumetric flask, add 450 ml of 95% ethanol, 450 ml of distilled water, and 100 ml of glacial acetic acid. The solution should be mixed well. Destaining solution is stored at room temperature.

Physiological saline. Mix 8.5 g of NaCl with 1,000 ml of distilled water in a 1,000-ml volumetric flask. Store the mixture at room temperature.

IEP EQUIPMENT AND PROCEDURE

IEP equipment and supplies

Electrophoresis chamber with power supply
Hamilton syringe
Polyethylene tubing
MLA pipette, 50 μl
Disposable MLA pipette tips
Volumetric flasks, 1,000 ml
Beakers, 1,000 ml
Magnetic stirrers
Stir bars

Whatman 3-mm chromatography paper
Glass plates (12 by 12 by 1 in. [ca. 30 by 30 by 2.5 cm])
Two 1-kg weights
Staining dishes

IEP procedure

1. Pour approximately 1 liter of buffer into the electrophoresis chamber. Tip the chamber so that the buffer level is equal on both sides.

2. Carefully remove the IEP film from the plastic box and shake it to remove any excess moisture from the wells and troughs.

3. Place the IEP film on a black sheet of paper. This will aid in visualizing the wells and troughs. Record the film identification number on the worksheet.

4. Attach approximately 5 in. (13 cm) of polyethylene tubing to a Hamilton syringe.

5. The IEP film contains wells numbered 1 through 7. Using the Hamilton syringe with the polyethylene tubing, carefully add 1 μl of the control serum to wells 1, 3, 5, and 7.

6. Remove the portion of the polyethylene tubing contaminated with the control serum by cutting off approximately 1 in. (2.5 cm). Add patient's serum to wells 2, 4, and 6.

7. Again cut off the contaminated portion of the polyethylene tubing. Using the Hamilton syringe and polyethylene tubing, add tracking dye to well 1.

Note. Extreme care must be exercised when adding control and patient sera to the wells. If a drop of serum lands on the agar, the IEP pattern will be distorted and the IEP film must be discarded.

8. Carefully place the IEP film on the bridge of the electrophoresis chamber. The agar side is up with the right or positive edge toward the anode. The edges of the IEP film are placed in the buffer by use of gauze pads or chromatographic paper moistened with buffer. If two gels are to be run simultaneously, care must be taken to ensure that the gels are not touching each other or the ends of the electrophoresis chamber.

9. Place the lid on electrophoresis chamber, connect leads to the power supply, and turn the power supply on. Adjust the voltage of the power supply to 125 V.

10. When the albumin-tracking dye complex has migrated 35 mm as indicated on the film, the electrophoresis is completed. Turn off the power supply and disconnect the leads. Carefully remove the IEP film and return it to the plastic shipping box.

11. Place the IEP film on a flat surface. Add 50 μl of the appropriate antisera to each trough with a 50-μl MLA pipette, as follows: trough A, anti-total immunoglobulin; trough B, anti-IgG; trough C, anti-IgA; trough D, anti-IgM; trough E, anti-kappa chain; and trough F, anti-lambda chain. Gently tilt the IEP film after the addition of each antiserum to ensure the equal distribution of antiserum throughout the entire trough.

12. Incubate the IEP film in the plastic shipping box for 18 to 20 h at room temperature. During the incubation period, the interior of the plastic shipping box should be kept moistened.

13. After the incubation, press the IEP film for 1 h, as follows. Place the film on a paper towel, and cover it with a damp piece of chromatography paper. Be sure no air bubbles are present. Add several layers of newspaper, followed by a glass plate (12 by 12 by 0.5 in.). Place two 1-kg weights on top of the glass.

14. Wash the film in physiological saline for 60 min with constant stirring. Two to four films may be washed in a 1,000-ml beaker.

15. Change the saline and wash for another 60 min.

16. Press the IEP film again as described in step 13.

17. Dry the film at room temperature or by use of hot air until no wet agar is seen.

18. Stain with Coomassie brilliant blue for 5 min.

19. Decolorize by gently agitating the IEP film in the destaining solution for approximately 20 min. Transfer the film to fresh destaining solution, and decolorize until the background is clear.

20. After decolorization, air dry the IEP film.

IFE REAGENTS

Reagents needed for IFE include Panagel slides, electrophoresis buffer, specific antisera, Coomassie brilliant blue, NaCl, glacial acetic acid, and ethanol.

IFE reagent preparation and handling

Panagel slides (Worthington Diagnostics, Freehold, N.J.). Store Panagel slides at room temperature, and keep them in the sealed plastic packing pouch until ready for use.

Panagel electrophoresis buffer (Worthington Diagnostics). Panagel electrophoresis buffer is a sodium barbital buffer (pH 8.6). Dry reagents are shipped in a sealed packet that is stored at room temperature before reconstitution.

Dilute the contents of the package in 1,000 ml of distilled water. Mix thoroughly until all dry reagents have dissolved. Store at room temperature.

Electrophoresis buffer may be used for two successive electrophoretic runs if the polarity of the Panagel electrophoresis chamber is reversed.

Specific antisera (Kallestad Laboratories). The following specific antisera are routinely used in IFE: anti-human IgG, anti-human IgA, anti-human IgM, anti-human kappa chain, anti-human lambda chain, anti-human CRP, anti-human free kappa chain, and anti-human free lambda chain. Antisera are stored at 2 to 8°C.

Coomassie brilliant blue stain. See IEP reagent preparation and handling, above.

Destaining solution. See IEP reagent preparation and handling, above.

Physiological saline. See IEP reagent preparation and handling, above.

IFE EQUIPMENT AND PROCEDURE

IFE equipment and supplies

Panagel migration unit (Worthington Diagnostics) (unit includes electrophoresis chamber, power supply, and cooling block)
Vented drying oven (Worthington Diagnostics)
Stopwatch
Panagel application blotter strips (Worthington Diagnostics)
Sepraphore III cellulose-polyacetate electrophoresis strips (1 by 6 in. [ca. 2.5 by 15 cm]) (Fisher Scientific Co., Cincinnati, Ohio).
MLA pipette, 10 μl

Disposable MLA pipette tips
Volumetric flasks, 1,000 ml
Beakers, 1,000 ml
Moist chamber
Mechanical stirrer
Stir bar
Whatman 3-mm chromatograph paper
Glass plates (12 by 12 by 1 in.)
Two 1-kg weights
Staining dishes

IFE procedure

1. Permit the serum sample to come to room temperature.

2. Prepare dilutions of patient's and control sera with Panagel electrophoresis buffer. The choice of serum dilutions should be determined by the size of the monoclonal band in the original serum high-resolution electrophoresis. Extreme care must be taken in choosing the appropriate serum dilutions. The incorrect choice of serum dilutions may result in either inability to detect a minor monoclonal protein or a prozone effect. For the detection and characterization of minor monoclonal proteins, the following serum dilutions are routinely used in our laboratory: IgG, 1:5; IgA, 1:2; IgM, 1:2; kappa chain, 1:5; lambda chain, 1:5. When an attempt is made to detect serum proteins other than immunoglobulins, serum is routinely diluted 1:1.

3. Add 500 ml of Panagel electrophoresis buffer to each side of the electrophoresis chamber.

4. Remove a Panagel slide from the sealed plastic pouch. Remove and discard the styrofoam insert.

5. Carefully remove the blue application mask and wipe it dry with gauze. Remove and discard the inner white sheet.

6. Cover the entire gel surface with a piece of chromatography blotting paper. Remove the paper after 15 s and repeat the blotting procedure with a fresh piece of chromatography paper.

7. Gently blot application points with a Panagel application blotter strip. After 15 s, carefully remove the blotter strip.

8. Carefully place the application mask on the gel. The mask must be properly aligned. Gently rub the mask with gauze pads to eliminate trapped air bubbles.

9. Using a 10-μl MLA pipette, apply 10 μl of serum dilutions at 15-s intervals. Let the serum absorb into the gel for 7 min. Application slits should not be allowed to dry.

10. Remove serum dilutions at 15-s intervals by carefully blotting the application slit with a Panagel application blotter strip.

11. Gently remove the blue application mask and discard it.

12. Invert the Panagel cooling block on the counter top, and remove excess moisture from the interior surface with a gauze pad. When the cooling block is not in use, it should be stored at 0 to 8°C. The cooling block may be used for three consecutive runs before it requires recooling. The cooling block is recooled by a 12-h incubation at 0 to 8°C.

13. The anode side of the cooling block is the side with the rubber gasket. Insert the agarose gel in the cooling block with the high-numbered side under the rubber gasket.

14. Carefully place the cooling block in the electrophoresis chamber. Electrophorese for 40 min at 200 V.

15. After electrophoresis, remove the agarose film and place it in a moist chamber. We routinely use an IEP plastic box for a moist chamber.

16. Soak Sepraphore III strips with the appropriate antisera, as follows. Place antiserum in a test tube (12 by 75 mm). Using forceps, carefully place a Sepraphore III strip in the test tube. Tilt the test tube and moisten the entire strip with antiserum. Then, using forceps, carefully remove the Sepraphore III strip from the test tube. Excess antiserum is removed by gently touching the end of the strip to the test tube.

17. Place the Sepraphore III strips on the surface of the agarose at the location of the protein of interest. Using the blunt end of the forceps, remove any air bubbles under the strips.

18. Incubate agarose film in the moist chamber for 2 h at room temperature.

19. After the incubation period, remove the Sepraphore III strips and press the agarose film for 30 min, as follows. Place the film over a paper towel on a flat surface. Moisten a piece of chromatography paper, and place it over the agarose film. Be sure no air bubbles are present. Add several levels of newspaper, and then place a glass plate (12 by 12 by 1 in.) on the newspaper, followed by two 1-kg weights.

20. Transfer the agarose film to a staining dish containing physiological saline, and rinse for 12 to 15 h. During the rinsing phase, the saline should be changed at least once and should be constantly agitated by a mechanical stirrer.

21. After overnight rinsing, press the agarose gel as described in step 19 for 30 min.

22. Dry the film at room temperature or in a vented air oven.

23. Stain the film by immersion in Coomassie brilliant blue stain for 5 min.

24. Decolorize the film in destaining solution for 15 min or until the background is clear.

25. After decolorization, air dry the agarose film.

LITERATURE CITED

1. **Durie, B. G. M., and S. E. Salmon.** 1975. A clinical staging system for multiple myeloma. Correlation of measured myeloma cell mass with presenting clinical features, response to treatment, and survival. Cancer **36**:842–854.

2. **Gerson, B. S., R. Cohen, I. M. Gerson, and G. H. Guest.** 1981. Myelin basic protein, oligoclonal bands, and IgG in cerebrospinal fluid as indicators of multiple sclerosis. Clin. Chem. **27**:1974–1977.

3. **Mason, D. Y.** 1975. Measurement of kappa/lambda light chain ratios by haemagglutination techniques. J. Immunol. Methods **6**:273–282.

4. **Penn, G. M., and J. Batya.** 1978. Interpretation of immunoelectrophoretic patterns. American Society of Clinical Pathologists, Chicago.

5. **Ritchie, R. F., and R. Smith.** 1976. Immunofixation. III. Application to the study of monoclonal proteins. Clin. Chem. **22**:1982–1985.

6. **Skvaril F., A. Morell, and S. Barandun.** 1982. Imbalances of kappa/lambda ratio of immunoglobulins, p. 21–35. *In* S. E. Ritzman (ed.), Protein abnormalities, vol. 2. Pathology of immunoglobulins: diagnostic and clinical aspects. Alan R. Liss, Inc., New York.

7. **Wall, R., and M. Kuehl.** 1983. Biosynthesis and regulation of immunoglobulins. Annu. Rev. Immunol. **1**:393–422.

Chapter 22

Quantitation of Immunoglobulins

IRENE J. CHECK AND MARGARET PIPER

Clinical indications for immunoglobulin quantitation

The spectrum of abnormalities in serum immunoglobulin concentrations is broad. Abnormal concentrations range from a virtual absence of one or more of the three major classes (immunoglobulin G [IgG], IgA, and IgM) to polyclonal increases in one or more immunoglobulins. IgA deficiency is the most common selective immunoglobulin defect. Polyclonal increases in immunoglobulins are commonly seen in chronic inflammation; for example, IgA is increased in association with chronic liver disease. In most cases, quantitation of immunoglobulins is performed because the patient is clinically suspected to have an immunoglobulin deficiency or a monoclonal immunoglobulin.

Patients with monoclonal immunoglobulins include those with multiple myeloma, but monoclonal immunoglobulins also occur in other B-cell malignancies such as non-Hodgkin's lymphoma and chronic lymphocytic leukemia and in benign monoclonal gammopathy. In rare cases, these paraproteins may be of the IgD or IgE class, and IgD or IgE quantitation would be indicated (IgE quantitation is covered in another chapter in this book). Immunoglobulin quantitation may be used in conjunction with immunoelectrophoresis or immunofixation (see chapter 21) to identify a monoclonal immunoglobulin (paraprotein) and to measure the extent of suppression of the normal immunoglobulins. The clinical course of the disease can be monitored by measuring the concentration of the paraprotein. Although this is usually accomplished by densitometric quantitation of serum protein electrophoretic patterns, immunoglobulin quantitation is preferable in some cases. These cases may include patients with extremely high concentrations of paraprotein and those whose paraprotein band is not clearly separable from other, normal serum proteins.

Immunoglobulin quantitation may also be ordered to follow up the finding of an abnormal ratio of albumin to gamma globulin in a screening serum chemistry profile or an abnormal pattern on serum protein electrophoresis. Selective deficiencies of one or more subclasses of IgG and IgA have been documented. There are four major subclasses of IgG and two of IgA, and decreased serum levels of each subclass can occur despite normal total immunoglobulin concentrations. Such subclass deficiencies have been associated with a myriad of disorders, including increased susceptibility to infections (11). The diagnostic application of immunoglobulin subclass quantitation has been hampered by the lack of standardized assays for these immunoglobulins, largely due to the difficulty in producing potent specific antisera. The production of monoclonal antibodies to immunoglobulin subclasses and the effort by the World Health Organization (WHO) to standardize the reagents should improve this situation in the next few years (12).

There are also diagnostic indications for the quantitation of immunoglobulins in body fluids other than serum (7). Parallel measurements of serum and cerebrospinal fluid IgG and albumin concentrations are used to calculate the permeability of the blood-cerebrospinal fluid barrier and to detect increased IgG synthesis within the central nervous system. These tests, together with high-resolution agarose gel electrophoresis to look for oligoclonal bands, are helpful in the work-up of patients with multiple sclerosis and other inflammatory neurological disorders. The quantitation of IgA in saliva is used to determine if children with recurrent upper respiratory tract infections are able to produce secretory IgA. The quantitation of IgG in serum and urine of patients with the nephrotic syndrome, when compared with the relative concentrations of other serum proteins of various molecular sizes, can be used to determine the type of glomerular damage (selective versus nonselective proteinuria). Quantitation of immunoglobulins in synovial fluids may be included in the work-up of patients with collagen vascular diseases. Finally, the measurement of immunoglobulin concentrations in tissue culture fluids may be included, for example, as part of the evaluation of the cellular basis for hypogammaglobulinemia (16).

Selecting a method for immunoglobulin quantitation

The work load and the nature of the immunoglobulin disorders evaluated will vary depending on whether the laboratory serves a primary-care or tertiary-referral patient population, the relative numbers of pediatric and adult patients, and the extent to which the laboratory participates in clinical research projects. In selecting a method for immunoglobulin quantitation, the first considerations should be the precision of the method (within-day, day-to-day, and interlaboratory coefficients of variation [CVs]) and its accuracy (standardization relative to the WHO International Reference Preparation for serum proteins). The ease of the assay, cost per test, turnaround time, and equipment expense relative to the work load will determine which method is best for the individual laboratory. All of the methods which are available to quantitate immunoglobulins utilize specific antibodies to the antigens (IgG, IgA, or IgM) and can be classified into two major categories: those involving measurement of the physical properties of the immune complexes formed between the antigen and the antiserum (turbidimetry, light scattering, precipitation in gel) and those in which the amount of labeled antibody bound to the antigen is measured (labels can include enzymes, fluorescent compounds, and radioisotopes). Within each category, there are numerous techniques. A thorough discussion of their relative merits with numerous primary references was written by Normansell (10). We recommend selecting a com-

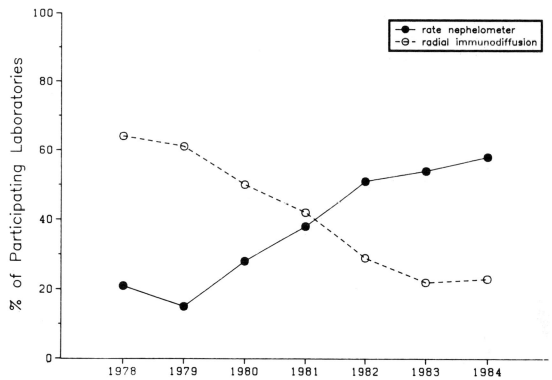

FIG. 1. Trends in laboratory use of rate nephelometry and RID to quantitate IgA, based on CAP proficiency surveys.

mercially available kit. These kits provide reference sera with the expected ranges of the analytes, facilitating quality control of the assays. In addition, it is impractical and time-consuming for an individual laboratory to standardize all of the variables so that the precision of the assays is comparable to that of the best commercial kits. A review of the College of American Pathologists (CAP) special diagnostic immunology surveys (3) for 1978 through 1984 provides data obtained from the 627 (in 1978) to over 1,000 (in 1983) clinical laboratories subscribing to these proficiency surveys. For the immunoglobulin quantitation section of the survey, the CAP sends each laboratory four unknown specimens each year. The laboratory quantitates IgG, IgA, and IgM in each sample by its routine method and returns the results, together with information about the method used, to the CAP. The data are compiled, and the mean, standard deviation, and CV for each test are summarized for each method. A useful feature of the report is the fact that the results obtained by using the reagents or instruments of each vendor are listed, provided that the kit or instrument was used by 20 or more laboratories.

Figure 1 shows the changing trends in use of the two most commonly used methods, rate nephelometry and radial immunodiffusion (RID). Of 915 laboratories participating in one of the IgA surveys in 1984, 58% used rate nephelometry, 11% used one of the Mancini technique (endpoint) (9) RID kits, and 12% used one of the Fahey-McKelvey technique (timed diffusion) (5) RID kits (see the section on RID below). The remaining 19% were distributed among turbidimetric, electroimmunodiffusion (rocket immunoelectrophoresis), radioimmunoassay, immunofluorescence, and other nephelometric and RID techniques.

This analysis yields a "field-tested" estimate of the precision of each method for a side-by-side comparison. In one specimen containing an approximately normal concentration of IgG (654 ± 96 mg/dl, tested by 687 laboratories in 1979), the CV ranged from 3.9% for 129 laboratories using rate nephelometry to 41.2% for 20 laboratories using one of the RID procedures. In one specimen assayed for IgA (107 ± 22 mg/dl, tested by 639 laboratories in 1978), the CV ranged from 4.9% for 52 laboratories using rate nephelometry to 29.2% for 82 laboratories using endpoint laser nephelometry. Although these are extreme examples, two- to threefold differences in CVs among methods are seen in almost every survey. A proficiency testing summary analysis prepared by the Centers for Disease Control in 1984 found that approximately 54% of 386 participating laboratories used nephelometry and 41% used RID to assay IgA (2). The RID results in general showed greater variability than the nephelometry results, but the results were not separated by manufacturer. Data about the performance of instruments or kits in the CAP surveys can be useful when the laboratory is considering a new procedure.

In this chapter, we describe the details of three procedures: rate nephelometry, RID, and solid-phase enzyme-linked immunosorbent assay (ELISA). Rate (kinetic) nephelometry is an excellent automated method for measuring serum immunoglobulins as well as several other serum proteins. The technique has been in routine laboratory use for several years and yields precise results rapidly. Because it requires a major investment in the instrument or a commitment to purchase a large volume of reagents (reagent rental plans), it is not appropriate for many laboratories with a small work load. Careful use of RID

TABLE 1. Normal ranges for concentrations of human immunoglobulins in serum

Method	n	Concn (mg/dl)[a]		
		IgG	IgA	IgM
Rate nephelometry[b]	120	994 (639–1,349)	171 (70–312)	156 (56–352)
RID[c]	199–303	1,047 (564–1,765)	177 (85–385)	126 (45–250)

[a] Means and 95% ranges are shown.
[b] Beckman ICS reagent test kits.
[c] Kallestad Endoplate test kit.

techniques can provide acceptable results within 24 h in the smaller laboratory. Finally, we describe our ELISA for IgG because it provides the nanogram sensitivity required for quantitating immunoglobulins in cell culture fluids and can be adapted to quantitate immunoglobulin subclasses by modifying the antibodies used.

Commercial methods for immunoglobulin quantitation by other techniques include solid-phase fluorescence immunoassays (FIAX 400 System from International Diagnostic Technology, Inc., Santa Clara, Calif.; Particle Concentration Fluorescence Immunoassay from Pandex Laboratories, Inc., Mundelein, Ill.) and turbidimetric methods using fast (centrifugal) analyzers (COBAS-BIO from Roche Diagnostic Systems, Nutley, N.J.; Mutilstat III F/LS from Instrumentation Laboratory Inc., Lexington, Mass.; ENCORE Special Chemistry Systems from Baker Instrument Corp., Allentown, Pa.) or the Du Pont Automated Chemistry Analyzer (Du Pont Co., Wilmington, Del.). These methods require sophisticated instruments which perform a variety of other chemical assays and would not be purchased solely for immunoglobulin quantitation.

Finally, although quantitation of kappa and lambda light chains in serum is not usually included in immunoglobulin measurements, the ratio of kappa to lambda light chains is sometimes measured as a screening test for abnormalities in serum immunoglobulins. Detection of an abnormal ratio of kappa to lambda light chains may signal the presence of a monoclonal immunoglobulin (15), which is presumably confirmed by the appropriate immunoelectrophoretic or immunofixation analysis. Unfortunately, this technique may miss low levels of monoclonal immunoglobulins which are readily visible on serum protein electrophoresis, especially on high-resolution agarose gels. The finding of a "normal" kappa-to-lambda ratio may mislead the clinician.

STANDARDIZATION

Results obtained with different reagents and in different laboratories can be standardized by relating the results to a common calibrator. WHO has prepared reference standards for serum immunoglobulin quantitation which are expressed in international units. The Centers for Disease Control and CAP collaborated to provide the CAP Reference Preparation for Serum Proteins (RPSP) which is calibrated, both in international units and in milligrams per deciliter, to the U.S. National Reference Preparation for Human Serum Proteins (13), which in turn is traceable to the WHO standard for serum immunoglobulins.

The U.S. National Reference Preparation for Human Serum Proteins (catalog no. IS1644) may be obtained free of charge by writing to the Director, Biological Products Division, Center for Infectious Diseases, Centers for Disease Control, Atlanta, Ga. Only one vial per year per individual, or ten vials per year per manufacturer of related reagents, is allowed in order to preserve an adequate supply of the standard. The CAP RPSP may be purchased without restriction from the College of American Pathologists, Skokie, Ill. Many commercial firms now standardize their reagents to these materials, and in fact several firms were involved in the calibration of the standards. When possible, the use of RPSP-standardized reagents is desirable.

NORMAL IMMUNOGLOBULIN LEVELS

Normal ranges for human serum immunoglobulins vary with age, sex, race, and a variety of environmental factors. A review of this topic was published by Maddison and Reimer (8). The normal values should be determined by each laboratory with as many individuals as possible, taking care that the demography of the group of normal individuals is comparable to that of the patient population. Table 1 shows the normal ranges stated in the package inserts for the two commercial methods described in this chapter. Normal ranges for children differ significantly with age (1).

ANTISERA

The antisera used should be monospecific and give a linear response over the required range, which is usually at least 20 to 200% of normal mean values. Additional requirements vary according to the assay. Nephelometry, for example, requires a higher-affinity antibody than does RID, and the sera must be free of turbidity. The antiserum must react with all of the phenotypes of the antigen. Sera with a highly abnormal immunoglobulin subclass distribution, or sera containing paraproteins of a rare allotype or of a subclass which is normally low, may yield variable results relative to the standard curves obtained with different antisera.

Because the sera of some persons contain antibodies to ruminant proteins, "back reactions," in which the patient serum reacts with, for example, the goat antiserum to human IgA, may obscure a condition of selective IgA deficiency. The use of rabbit antiserum to quantitate this protein will minimize the problem. In other patients, the presence of rheumatoid factors which react with the antiserum to IgG can alter the apparent concentration of IgG. Antisera calibrated for microprocessor-controlled rate nephelometry are currently available from two sources (see below). Separate antisera for RID assays are not required since these are incorporated into the commercially available plates. The antisera for the ELISA are listed in that section below.

The IgG fraction of the antiserum is preferable because nonspecific protein absorption which increases the background values in many assays is minimized. Unwanted reactions, for example, anti-light chain reactivity in an antiserum used to quantitate IgG, should be removed by using solid-phase immunoabsorbents. Commercial suppliers of antisera supply documentation of the specificity of the antisera, usually demonstrated by immunoelectrophoresis. However, in using the antiserum for a more sensitive procedure, such as ELISA, the investigator must verify that the specificity is retained under the more stringent test conditions. The development of monoclonal antibodies might allow the standardization of antisera among laboratories. Many monclonal antibodies do not precipitate because antigens with repeated determinants are required for lattice formation. This problem can be overcome by utilizing mixtures of monoclonal antibodies against different determinants (4). Monoclonal antibodies can react well, however, in direct binding (as compared with precipitation) assays. They are also uniquely suited for detecting minor antigenic determinants, such as some of the subclass- or allotype-specific determinants. For detecting total IgG, on the other hand, each monoclonal antibody must react with a determinant present on all four subclasses. Proceed with caution when using poorly characterized monoclonal antibodies in clinical assays. Regardless of whether monoclonal antibodies are prepared in a research or an industrial laboratory, pitfalls such as inappropriate allotypic reactivity or nonreactivity with rare allotypes must be avoided. In some cases, this can only be done by testing large numbers of sera or monoclonal immunoglobulins from patients with widely disparate genetic backgrounds.

RATE NEPHELOMETRY

Principle

Soluble immune complexes formed by the reaction of antibody with antigen in a dilute solution will scatter incident light of the appropriate wavelength. If the concentration of antibody is held constant, the amount of complex formed depends directly on the concentration of antigen in the mixture, provided that the antibody is in excess. The addition of polyethylene glycol enhances the formation of the immune complexes under dilute conditions so that accurate results are obtained rapidly. These principles are applied in endpoint laser nephelometers (Diagnostic Div., Cooper Biomedical, Malvern, Pa. [formerly Hyland Laboratories, Inc., Costa Mesa, Calif.]; Calbiochem-Behring, La Jolla, Calif.). These instruments measure the maximum scatter in an antigen-antibody reaction mixture; the antigen concentration in an unknown sample is calculated from a dose-response curve gen-

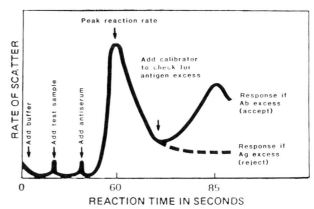

FIG. 2. Sequence of events during an automated nephelometric reaction. Buffer and test sample are added to the flow cell, and the background level of light scatter is zeroed. Antibody is added, the rate of scatter is electronically monitored, and the peak rate is determined. Samples with reaction rates above a certain threshold (see Fig. 5) are tested for antigen excess by injecting additional calibrator serum. A reaction mixture in antibody excess will produce a second rate signal, while one in antigen excess will not. In the latter case, the instrument will automatically test the next higher dilution. (Modified from the Beckman ICS operator's manual; used by permission.)

erated with reference sera containing known concentrations of immunoglobulins.

Since the amount of light scatter also depends on the relative size of the complexes, the relationship between the amount of scatter and time after addition of antiserum to an antigen solution is sigmoidal. Very early in the reaction (less than 5 s), the immune complexes are too small to scatter light. Once a threshold is exceeded, the scatter increases directly with time. As the reactants are used up, the rate of increase in scatter decreases and the scatter approaches the maximum value. The inflection point of the rate curve gives the peak rate of complex formation and is proportional to the antigen concentration, provided that all other conditions are constant and the solution is in antibody excess (Fig. 2).

The kinetic or rate nephelometer from Beckman Instruments, Inc. (Fullerton, Calif.) focuses a high-intensity light on the center of a cuvette or flow cell in which immune complexes are being formed and continuously monitors the light scattered by the complexes. Forward-scattered 450- to 550-nm light, collected at an angle of 70°, is filtered, imaged onto a photomultiplier tube, and converted into an electrical signal which is fed into a microprocesser. The rate constants and characteristics of the antigen dose-response curve are entered into the instrument for a particular batch of antiserum. The instrument is calibrated with a single dilution of calibrator serum. A reading of the background light scatter of the test sample is taken, antiserum is added, and a microprocessor interprets a signal that pipetting has occurred, determines the peak rate of scatter formation, and solves a cubic equation to calculate the antigen concentration. The result is obtained in 10 to 40 s with an effective concentration range of as low as 1.1 to as high as 21,600 mg/dl, depending on the antibody.

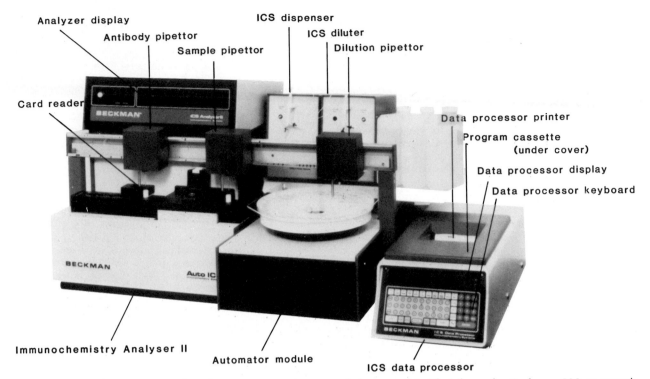

FIG. 3. Principal components of Beckman automated rate nephelometer. (Modified from the Beckman ICS operator's manual; used by permission.)

Equipment

The following procedure is designed for the Automated Immunochemistry System (Auto ICS) manufactured by Beckman. The Auto ICS consists of three major components: the Immunochemistry Analyzer II, which is a rate nephelometer equipped with a quartz-iodide lamp; an automated pipettor-dilutor module; and a microcomputer-data processor (Fig. 3). The analyzer may be separated from the other components and used manually (see below).

The microcomputer is the interface between the optical system of the analyzer and the data processor, as well as an integral part of the electronic system controlling the sequence of operation. The microcomputer is programmed for each antibody and calibrator by inserting accompanying cards into the analyzer card reader. These cards contain the necessary information for converting light scatter units to specific protein concentrations. The microcomputer also directs the analyzer and data processor displays, which provide instructions to the operator, describe operations in progress, and show the results. The automator module consists of pipettor "cars" mounted on a track, a 40-position turntable for patient samples and dilutions, a fixed-ratio diluter, and a fixed-volume dispenser. Racks to hold special dilutions of calibrator serum used in checking reactions for antigen excess and racks for buffer, diluent, and waste bottles are also provided.

The following supplies are also required.

Flow cell-related items
Reference cuvette for adjusting scatter
Disposable flow cells (changed daily)
Teflon-coated stir bars

Sample-handling items
Conical sample cups (0.5 ml) for patient and control sera
Sample cups (2.0 ml) for antigen excess calibrator dilution
Dilution cups segments for serum dilutions (each segment contains five groups of four cups)
Pipette tips for pipette and dilution modules (automatic mode)
Pipettes and pipette tips (42 and 100 μl) (manual mode)
Disposable transfer pipettes for adding specimens to sample cups

Other materials
Reagent bottle covers which prevent evaporation but allow pipette tips to enter
Paper for the printer
Cassette tape containing protein mode program

Reagents

The reagents listed below are available in pretested ready-to-use form. At present there are two suppliers of antisera for the Auto ICS, Kallestad Laboratories (Austin, Tex.) and Beckman. Kallestad reagents are calibrated with the CAP RPSP and are frequently less expensive than those from Beckman. They performed comparably to the Beckman reagents in the 1983 and 1984 CAP surveys. The user must weigh these factors against the increased difficulty in solving technical problems. We have found that using an instrument manufactured by one firm and purchasing reagents from a competing firm increases the time needed to solve technical problems, since the laboratory must first determine whether a problem is due to the reagent or instrument malfunction and then deal with technical representatives from both firms.

> Buffer, nephelometric grade (2 liters; store at room temperature); added to flow cell before sample and antibody injections; contains polyethylene glycol to enhance immune complex formation
>
> Diluent, nephelometric grade (2 liters; store at room temperature); used to dilute calibrator, control, and test samples
>
> Reagent kits for measurement of IgG, IgA, and IgM; each kit contains one vial of prediluted antiserum (goat) and calibration serum with attached program cards (store at 4°C); the same calibration serum is used for each antiserum
>
> Normal control serum (store at 4°C) with preassayed mean values for IgG, IgA, and IgM

Sample

Serum, collected after centrifugation of a clotted fasting blood specimen, is preferred. Centrifuged or filtered clear specimens of cerebrospinal fluid, urine, and other body fluids can also be analyzed. Store the specimen at 2 to 8°C overnight or at −20°C for longer periods of time. Hemolyzed or icteric specimens do not interfere with the assay, although the appearance should be noted when reporting the results. Specimens that are grossly lipemic or which are otherwise turbid may produce excessively high scatter signals; in this case, the microcomputer will stop the analysis and display the message "EXCESS SCATTER" or "UNSTABLE SAMPLE." Dilute the sample or centrifuge it to remove the interfering material, and rerun.

Quantitation of patient sera

Although the Auto ICS is microprocessor controlled, it has many components which must be properly set up, aligned, and monitored. Initially, at least one operator should be trained by the manufacturer's representative and should write a protocol specifying the details of the procedure for the particular laboratory. Before operating the Auto ICS, each operator should thoroughly read the operator's manual and the laboratory protocol and be instructed by an operator thoroughly familiar with the system.

Overview. The reagent rack can hold up to six different antisera. Although anti-IgG, anti-IgA, and anti-IgM are relevant here, the laboratory could include assays for C3, C4, haptoglobin, transferrin, or other serum proteins in the same run. The sample turntable has a capacity for 40 samples, including patient, calibrator, and control sera. The instrument is programmed to assay one to six proteins per specimen (depending on the antisera used); the specified proteins may differ for each specimen, but all of the assays are performed before moving on to the next sample.

Preparing to operate the instrument. This complex instrument requires numerous daily maintenance checks before beginning the run. The operator's manual provides a log sheet (Fig. 4) to record each of the following tasks as they are performed.

To begin, check the scatter signal and adjust it, if necessary, to 120 ± 20 scatter units. Replace the flow cell and stir bar, the pipettor module tips, and the cups

for the calibrator dilution used to check for antigen excess. Check the pinch valve and peristaltic valve tubing for leaks and crimps. Check that the data processor printer has an adequate paper supply. Inspect the levels of the diluent and buffer bottles to ensure an adequate supply for the run, and empty the waste bottle.

Bring the antisera and the calibrator and control sera to room temperature. Check and record the lot numbers and expiration dates, and make sure that the amounts of all sera and antisera are sufficient for the run. Place the antiserum bottles in the reagent rack, and replace their stoppers with reagent covers. These covers prevent evaporation while allowing the pipettor tips to enter the bottles.

Programming the analyzer. Immunoglobulin quantitation is performed with the protein mode program, one of several modes of programming the instrument. Load this program into the microcomputer memory by inserting the appropriate cassette. Select the protein mode, and enter the date, operator's name, and any comments by using the keyboard on the data processor unit. Insert the program cards attached to the antiserum and calibrator bottles into the analyzer card reader. Follow the sequence (antiserum 1, antiserum 2, . . . antiserum 6, calibrator 1, etc.) indicated on the data processor or analyzer display. The rack position of each antiserum, the characteristics of its dose-response curve, and the concentrations of IgG, IgA, and IgM in the calibrator serum are entered automatically via the program cards.

Loading samples onto the turntable. Place a clean, 0.5-ml conical sample cup for the calibrator serum in the position directed by the data processor display, and add a minimum of 350 µl of calibrator. Add sample cups for the controls and for each patient specimen into the outer ring of the turntable, label the cups, and dispense at least 250 µl of each sample. Place a sufficient number of dilution segments next to the sample cups in the turntable. For each sample, enter the specimen identification number (turntable position), the proteins to be assayed (antiserum bottle position number), and the starting dilution to be used with each antiserum if different from that automatically predetermined (see below). Keep in mind that such an alteration of the starting dilution may well require manual antigen excess checks.

Automated run. Start the run. The Auto ICS calibrates the system for each antiserum, prepares fixed dilutions of each sample (1:6 [B], 1:36 [C], 1:216 [D], 1:1,296 [E]), and adds 600 µl of buffer to the flow cell. The pipettor delivers 42 µl of the appropriate sample dilution to the reaction cell, takes a base-line reading of the light scatter, adds 42 µl of antiserum, and measures the rate of increase in the light scatter (Fig. 2). The microprocessor calculates the concentration of the analyte (IgG, IgA, or IgM) and prints the result. For each analyte, the analyzer automatically selects a starting specimen dilution (IgG, dilution D; IgA and IgM, dilution C) (Fig. 5). If the rate of complex formation is outside the measuring range (linear dose-response relationship), the next higher or lower dilution is assayed automatically. In the upper portion of the measuring range, the instrument checks for antigen excess by adding additional antigen (calibrator serum). The result is valid if the reaction mixture is in

AUTO ICS MONTHLY MAINTENANCE LOG

Month _____   Year _____   Auto ICS Serial # _____

DAILY MAINTENANCE	1	2	3	4	5	6	7	8	9	10	11	12	13	14	15	16	17	18	19	20	21	22	23	24	25	26	27	28	29	30	31
Read and Record Zero Scatter, 0000 ± 15, Procedure A																															
Read and Record Scatter Reference 120 ± 20, Procedure A																															
Replace Flow Cell and Stirrer; Twist to Seat																															
Replace Antibody Tip, Procedure B																															
Replace Sample Tip, Procedure B																															
Check Printer Paper																															
Check Ribbon																															
Check Reagent Levels																															
Check System for Leaks																															
WEEKLY MAINTENANCE																															
Wash Sample Tray and Cover																															
Inspect Pinch Valve Tubing, Procedure C																															

MONTHLY MAINTENANCE

	Date	Initials		Date	Initials
Replace Diluter Tip, Procedure D	____	____	Clean Printhead Track with Alcohol and Lubricate, Procedure H	____	____
Clean Pipettor Track Procedure E	____	____	Inspect Septum for Wear and Leakage	____	____
Replace Air Filter, Procedure F	____	____	Clean Cassette Tape Reader Assembly Head, Procedure I	____	____
Flush System with Distilled Water, Procedure G	____	____	Verify Pipettor Module Alignment, Procedure J	____	____

FIG. 4. Worksheet for the maintenance procedures for the Beckman rate nephelometer. (Modified from the Beckman ICS operator's manual; used by permission.)

antibody excess and additional immune complexes are formed (Fig. 2). If not, the next dilution is assayed either until the condition of antibody excess is met or until three sequential dilutions are tested. Using the

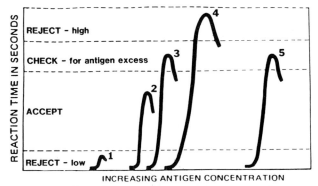

FIG. 5. Effect of antigen concentration on reaction rate. The nephelometer data processor is programmed to detect reaction rates that are below or above the range for each antibody (curves 1 and 4). Such samples are automatically retested at the next lower (more concentrated) or higher dilution. Reaction rates in the "check" range could represent reactions in either antibody excess (curve 3) or antigen excess (curve 5) and are tested for antigen excess (see Fig. 2). Samples whose reaction rates fall in the "accept" range are not tested further. (Modified from the Beckman ICS operator's manual; used by permission.)

standard cassette for the protein mode, the system must be recalibrated after analysis of 40 samples. If a run contains fewer than 40 samples, the user may add new samples and assay them with the antibodies already programmed and calibrated for up to 1 h after completing the first run. A recently updated version of this program allows for processing of more than 40 samples without recalibration and for addition and calibration of new antisera while retaining calibration of previously added antisera. It retains calibration for up to 24 h.

STAT run. The STAT mode allows the user to operate the instrument manually. It can be used to interrupt an automated run after calibration or to perform assays without entering the automated protein mode. Calibration, dilutions, and analysis are all performed manually. STAT measurements are not restricted to antibodies programmed in the automated run, but they must coincide with the cassette tape program currently loaded in the tape reader. This mode is also used when the concentration of the analyte is below the measuring range of an automated run. Results may be obtained either by assaying the undiluted specimen or by adding more than 42 μl of sample to the flow cell.

Quantitation of immunoglobulins in body fluids other than serum

Measurements of immunoglobulins in cerebrospinal fluid, saliva, urine, or joint fluid can be made in the automated or manual mode, provided that the specimens are clear and not too viscous. In most cases, the analyte concentration will be much lower than in normal serum, so the assays should start with a more concentrated dilution of the specimen. For example, to measure IgG in cerebrospinal fluid (normal range, 0.5 to 6.1 mg/dl), start with the B dilution intead of the D dilution normally used to measure serum IgG. Adjust the dilutions of other fluids similarly, based on the expected range of protein concentrations. The principal pitfall is the possibility of missing a condition of antigen excess, since the instrument detects an abnormal rate of immune complex formation based on parameters established for serum. This can be avoided by verifying that the immunoglobulin result is reasonable when compared with the total protein concentration and the electrophoretic pattern (see below) or by running the sample a second time, starting at the D dilution. A condition of antigen excess can be checked manually.

General considerations. Because this nephelometric method is a rate analysis, it is subject to any conditions which might affect the rate of immune complex formation, even if they do not affect the final equilibrium. These conditions include the order of addition of reagents, the temperature, and the efficiency of mixing in the cuvette. Care must be taken to keep running conditions as constant as possible. This is facilitated, in part, by the fact that much of the logic of the assay is programmed into the instrument and operator error is minimized. In addition, standardized reagents are readily purchased, although errors in manufacture or calibration do occur.

Control sera. Control sera with immunoglobulin values in the physiologic range are available from the manufacturers of nephelometric-grade antisera. In addition, we recommend the use of two in-house serum pools, one containing elevated (1 to 2 times the upper limit of normal) and one containing abnormally low (15 to 20% of normal) quantities of IgG, IgA, and IgM. The laboratory can save appropriate patient sera, pool them, and freeze them in 0.3-ml aliquots at −70°C. Alternatively, one can dilute and similarly store a pool of normal control serum for the low pool and a pool of calibrator serum spiked with sera containing monoclonal immunoglobulins for the high pool.

Place a control sample at the beginning of each run to check the calibration procedure. Recalibrate the system if the result is outside of a range of 2 standard deviations of the stated mean. Each automated run should include a normal control and a "low-pool" sample; large runs should also include a "high-pool" sample. These controls should be spaced evenly among the patient samples. Mean values and ranges for each pool should be established over time. The low pool ensures the quality of abnormally low results and can aid in troubleshooting. Subtle problems in calibration, instrument operation, or reagent quality may be detected sooner at low immunoglobulin values. A high pool checks the quality of abnormally high immunoglobulin values (e.g., paraproteins). Results of low and high pools should be evaluated together with normal control results to monitor reproducibility over time.

Abnormal values. We strongly recommend performing serum protein electrophoresis in parallel with immunoglobulin quantitation. The appearance of the gamma globulin region on the electrophoretic membrane will identify patients with paraprotein bands and those with hypo- or hypergammaglobulinemia. The nephelometric immunoglobulin values should be comparable. The most common cause for a discrepancy is the presence of an undetected condition of antigen excess in the assayed serum dilution.

Abnormally low values present special problems. If a serum sample is below the range on the B dilution, test the neat serum in duplicate with the STAT mode. First check for nonspecific protein interference by adding 42 μl of undiluted serum to the flow cell. Simulate antibody injection by inserting an empty pipette tip, and observe the display. If a peak reaction rate is found, the specimen cannot be assayed undiluted. Repeat the assay with a 1:2 or 1:3 dilution of the serum, and correct the result by the appropriate dilution factor. If a specimen is expected to have a low value of the analyte (e.g., IgG in cerebrospinal fluid), program the automated mode to begin at a lower dilution and check by rerunning the sample at the automatically programmed dilution.

High concentrations of monoclonal immunoglobulins may present an abnormal spectrum of antigenic determinants to the antiserum, resulting in less than optimal rates of scatter formation. Retesting the sample at the next higher dilution frequently yields quantitative results that are more in line with densitometric scan data.

Record keeping. A daily log of reagent lot numbers and control values is essential. Reviewed regularly, it can help detect trends and changes in the performance of the Auto ICS and provides a quick reference for troubleshooting problems. Notes on performance problems and corrective action taken are also invaluable for long-term operation and maintenance.

Troubleshooting

The Auto ICS analyzer, automater, and data processor are equipped with a number of aids for troubleshooting. Detailed in an extensive section in the operator's manual are simulated sample tests and tests of isolated components of the Auto ICS which may be performed to aid in identifying a problem. These problems can be mechanical or they may relate to reagents or signaling errors between different modules. In all cases, experience, attention to detail, and a healthy dose of common sense are extremely important.

It is not possible to consider here all problems that may be encountered. The reader is referred to the operator's manual for a complete discussion. In our experience, however, the problems encountered most often were signaled by out-of-range controls, results which made no sense, unusual calibration results, or a comment from the data processor (e.g., "calibrator out of range"). The reasons for these problems vary from forgetting disposable items (e.g., special calibrator dilution cups, dilution segments) and running out of reagents during the run to errors in alignment, tubing problems (e.g., crimps, leaks), or improper diluter and dispenser calibration. In extreme cases, circuit boards or modules have been replaced. Careful attention to specimen pipetting, dilution, and dis-

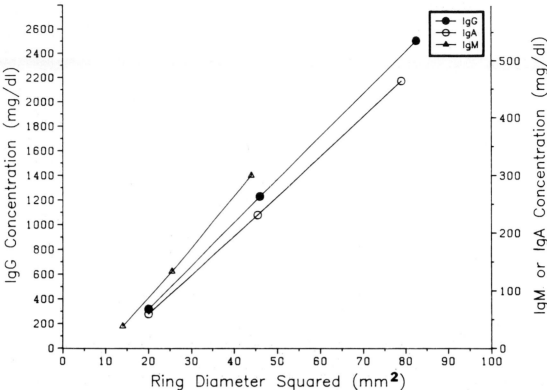

FIG. 6. Sample graph of reference serum values for endpoint RID assays to quantitate IgG, IgA, and IgM.

pensing when repeating a faulty run often helps to identify sources of error. In all cases, a log of problems and corrective action taken is invaluable for future troubleshooting and identification of repeated problems.

Maintenance

Timely and consistent maintenance is an important aspect of success with nephelometry. The manufacturer sponsors workshops where one or more technologists can learn detailed procedures. The daily, weekly, and monthly maintenance schedule illustrated in Fig. 4, with procedures specified in the operator's manual, should be observed. Quarterly maintenance procedures include replacing all peristaltic pump tubing and the flow cell septum, lubricating syringes, and lubricating and calibrating the diluter and dispenser.

RID

Principle

The method of RID to quantitate immunoglobulins was made possible when the relationship between antigen concentration and the diameter of the precipitin ring formed when antigen diffuses into an antibody-containing gel was described in 1965. Mancini et al. (9) showed that at equivalence (or endpoint) the relationship between the antigen concentration and the squares of the ring diameters is linear (endpoint method) (Fig. 6). Fahey and McKelvey (5) found that the ring diameters could also be measured before equivalence, when a linear relationship exists be-

tween the log of the antigen concentration and the ring diameter (timed-diffusion method) (Fig. 7).

In either method, equal volumes of reference sera and test samples are added to wells in an agarose gel containing a monospecific antiserum. Timed diffusion gives results in 18 ± 0.5 h, but the measured precipitin rings are dependent on time and temperature; these factors affect the rate of formation of the precipitin ring, which continues to grow until equivalence. The endpoint method requires 48 h (72 h for IgM), and the resulting precipitin rings are independent of variations in time and diffusion rate but are affected by marked changes in temperature. CAP survey data show no significant differences in the performance of the two methods as evaluated by CVs. Both methods are highly dependent on the molecular size of the antigen because this affects the diffusion coefficient and therefore the diameter of the precipitin ring.

RID is relatively simple to perform and requires little or no investment in capital equipment. The time required to obtain results, particularly if repeated tests are necessary, and the strong dependence on antigen size are its major limitations. The CVs of immunoglobulin measurements average 2 to 3 times those obtained with rate nephelometry.

Equipment

This procedure is written for the Kallestad RID Endoplate Immunoglobulin Test Kit. The kit can be used for either endpoint or timed-diffusion determinations. This procedure describes the timed-diffusion method. Required for the assay but not provided in the kit are the following items.

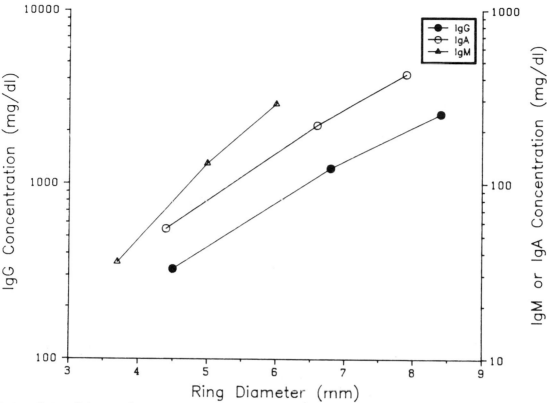

FIG. 7. Sample graph (two-cycle semilogarithmic) of reference serum values for timed RID assays to quantitate IgG, IgA, and IgM.

Volumetric pipette capable of dispensing 5 μl (calibrate regularly)

Pipette tips

Saline, 0.85%

Reticle or viewer capable of accurately measuring precipitin rings to 0.1 mm

Two-cycle semilogarithmic graph paper

Other commerical sources for immunoglobulin quantitation by RID include Calbiochem-Behring, Cooper Biomedical, ICL Scientific (Fountain Valley, Calif.), and Meloy Laboratories, Inc. (Richmond, Va). RID plates designed for the timed-diffusion method usually contain less antibody than those intended for the endpoint method in order to produce measurable rings in a shorter time. Timed-diffusion plates cannot be used for the endpoint method unless this is specifically stated by the manufacturer.

Reagents

The Kallestad Endoplate Immunoglobulin Test Kit consists of the following.

1. Buffered agarose-antiserum plates (Endoplate) preserved with 0.1% sodium azide (store at 2 to 8°C in a zip lock bag; stable to expiration date). Kits for various immunoglobulin ranges are available. The following are approximate ranges (in milligrams per deciliter) for reference sera: regular range, 350 to 2,400 for IgG, 50 to 400 for IgA, 50 to 350 for IgM, and 1 to 8 for IgD; low range, 20 to 350 for IgG, 4 to 60 for IgA, and 5 to 50 for IgM; ultralow range, 1 to 24 for IgG.

2. Human reference sera containing high (no. 1), medium (no. 2), and low (no. 3) concentrations of IgG, IgA, and IgM, whose values are calibrated against the CAP RPSP (see section on standardization, above). These sera are used to generate the dose-response curves for the assay. The approximate concentrations (in milligrams per deciliter) of IgG, IgA, and IgM, respectively, are 2,500, 400, and 300 in reference 1; 1,000, 200, and 125 in reference 2; and 400, 60, and 30 in reference 3. The actual concentrations vary among different lots. Reference sera are preserved with 0.1% sodium azide (store at 2 to 8°C).

Not included in the kit but recommended for use with each assay is a control serum (such as Quantitrol from Kallestad Laboratories) or an in-house-prepared pooled human serum control.

Sample

Samples are the same as for the nephelometric procedure.

Quantitation of immunoglobulins in patient sera

1. Bring all agarose plates, reference sera, and control sera to room temperature before use.

2. Remove the plate from the zip lock bag and inspect the wells. If they are moist, allow the uncovered plate to remain at room temperature until the moisture has evaporated.

3. Mix all patient and control samples thoroughly by inverting them several times.

4. Apply 5 µl of reference sera 1, 2, and 3 to each of three wells, using the volumetric pipette. Apply 5 µl of control serum to a fourth well and 5 µl of each patient specimen to the remaining wells. If additional plates are required, use the same lot number and include at least one reference or control serum per plate. See below (quality control) for conditions under which a single reference serum determination may be used in place of the three-point dose-response curve.

5. Carefully replace the lid and place the plate in the zip lock bag. Seal the bag and incubate it at room temperature (23 ± 2°C) on a level surface for 18 h.

6. Using the viewer, measure the ring diameters to the nearest 0.1 mm. Measure the samples in the same order that they were applied, taking approximately as much time between samples as it took to apply them.

7. Construct a standard curve by plotting the concentration of each reference serum on the logarithmic scale against the precipitin ring diameter on the linear scale. Connect the adjacent points.

8. Determine the control and patient sample concentrations by locating the ring diameter on the standard curve and reading the concentration on the logarithmic scale. Samples outside the concentration range defined by the low reference serum must be reassayed on "low-level" plates. Samples whose ring diameters are greater than that of the high reference serum must be diluted and reassayed (see below).

Quality control

Each RID kit contains a report which gives expected mean ring diameters and a range of 2 standard deviations for each reference serum and for the Quantitrol control serum. Accept the assays if the ring diameters of all reference sera and the control serum fall within these ranges. If an in-house control is used, establish a mean and range of 2 standard deviations for the ring diameter. Repeat assays which do not meet these criteria.

The manufacturer suggests that a single-point validation of the reference curve may be used for all runs performed by the endpoint method within 6 to 8 weeks with a single lot number of plates and provided that certain criteria are met. All three references and a control serum are run the first time the plates are used, and a standard curve is drawn. The control value must fall within the expected concentration range, and the x intercept (diameter-squared axis) on the Endoplates must be 11 ± 3 mm^2 for regular and low-level plates or 18 ± 3 mm^2 for ultralow-level plates. Later assays using the same lot number of plates and references may be validated by running only the highest reference. If the ring diameter is within 0.2 mm of the original ring diameter, controls and patient sample values may be read from the original curve. If not, the entire curve should be run again, together with the patient and control sera.

Patient samples with results which are higher than reference 1 must be diluted in saline and reassayed to obtain a value which falls within the reference range. Multiply the obtained concentration by the dilution factor for the final result. Patient samples with values lower than reference 3 must be reassayed on low-level plates.

Sources of error

Errors in RID results may be caused by distortion of the wells, improper filling of the wells, incorrect or inconsistent measurement of the diameter of the precipitin rings, variation in the conditions of incubation, or the presence of abnormal immunoglobulin molecules. Wells may be distorted by improper sample application. To prevent this, hold the pipette so that the tip is vertical and does not touch or nick the edges of the wells. Other causes of error include partial dehydration of the plates due to improper sealing and storage, failure to remove excess moisture from the wells before applying the sample, and introduction of bubbles into the wells. The precipitin rings must be measured as objectively as possible. The consistency of the measurements can be improved if all persons performing the assays compare and agree on their criteria for measurement.

The timed-diffusion method is especially sensitive to changes in temperature and incubation time. Consistent results depend on incubation times of 18 ± 0.5 h at a temperature of $23 \pm 2°C$. A shorter incubation time or a lower temperature will increase the slope of the reference curve and result in decreased sensitivity of the assay. If plates that are standardized for both methods are used, some authors suggest reporting preliminary results based on the timed-diffusion method and reading the final results by the endpoint method. In practice, this is cumbersome.

Abnormal molecules or aggregates of immunoglobulins cannot be measured accurately by RID because their diffusion coefficients differ from those of the standards. In gamma heavy-chain disease, for example, the paraprotein molecule is smaller than the molecules of the IgG standards, and the paraprotein concentration will appear high. With IgM paraproteins, monomeric forms are frequently present, again resulting in falsely high values. Immunoglobulin aggregation, which is especially likely with IgA, IgM, or IgG3 paraproteins or in sera with rheumatoid factor, may result in falsely low values.

ELISA FOR HUMAN IgG

Principle

Numerous protocols have been developed for solid-phase ELISAs, and many of them are described in detail by Saunders (14) and by Normansell (10). The procedure described here is a sandwich configuration in which insolubilized antibody to human IgG is used to "capture" the antigen (IgG). The captured antigen is reacted with a biotinylated second antibody to human IgG which is then detected by its binding to a complex of biotin-avidin-horseradish peroxidase (6). The amount of bound complex is quantitated by reaction of the enzyme with a chromogenic substrate. The resultant color is measured spectrophotometrically and is proportional to the antigen concentration. A dose-response curve for IgG is generated by using the CAP RPSP.

The peroxidase is conjugated to avidin, a 68,000-molecular-weight glycoprotein with a high affinity (10^{15} M^{-1}) for the small-molecular-weight vitamin biotin. Because this affinity is much higher than that of antibody for most antigens, the binding of avidin to biotin is essentially irreversible. Avidin has four binding sites for biotin, and most proteins can be conjugated with several biotin molecules.

Microtiter plates form the solid phase. The first antibody is covalently coupled to a bovine serum albumin (BSA) layer adsorbed onto the plate. This minimizes denaturation of the antibody due to hydrophobic interactions with the polystyrene plates. The procedure can be modified to quantitate IgG subclasses by substituting murine monoclonal antibodies of the appropriate specificity (12) for the biotinylated antibody to human IgG. A third antibody, biotinylated anti-mouse IgG, is then added, and the reaction with the biotin-avidin-enzyme complex occurs as described above. Reference sera for immunoglobulin subclass quantitation are not currently available, although a WHO committee is working on this problem. In the meantime, most laboratories standardize these assays by using purified paraproteins of the appropriate subclass.

Equipment and supplies

Automated microtiter plate reader (Titertek Multiscan filter photometer with vertical light path; Flow Laboratories, McLean, Va.)

Automated microtiter plate washer (Titertek Multiwash; Flow Laboratories)

Vibrator mixer, platform style (Arthur H. Thomas Co., Philadelphia, Pa.)

Microtiter plates (polystyrene, 96 well, flat bottom; Linbro, Flow Laboratories)

Pipettes: air displacement variable-volume pipettes (Rainin Instruments, Brighton, Mass.); Titertek Multichannel 12-channel pipettes (Flow Laboratories); positive-displacement pipettes with accuracy of ±1% of dispensed volume (Scientific Manufacturing Industries, Emeryville, Calif.)

Reagents

Phosphate-buffered saline (PBS) (pH 7.3) with 0.02% BSA fraction V (Sigma Chemical Co., St. Louis, Mo.) (PBS-BSA)

PBS with 0.05% Tween 20 (Sigma) (PBS-Tween)

Glutaraldehyde, 200 mg/dl in PBS, with pH adjusted to 7.0

ortho-Phenylenediamine substrate solution: 3.5 mM hydrogen peroxide–2.3 mM ortho-phenylenediamine–50 mM citrate–100 mM phosphate (pH 5), prepared 15 to 30 min before use

2.5 N sulfuric acid

Solid-phase (capture) antiserum: anti-human IgG made in goats (Cappel Laboratories, West Chester, Pa.), specific for heavy and light chains (cross-reacts with IgA and IgM), diluted 1:500 in PBS-BSA

Vectastain ABC kit (human IgG) (Vector Laboratories, Inc., Burlingame, Calif.) (contains avidin DH, biotinylated horseradish peroxidase H, affinity-purified biotinylated anti-human IgG [prepared in goats]): dilute biotin-conjugated goat anti-human IgG serum 1:500 by adding 20 µl to 10 ml of PBS; prepare avidin-biotin complex (ABC) reagent by diluting the avidin solution in PBS (pH

7.5) containing 0.1% Tween 20 (2 drops to 10 ml of buffer), and then add 2 drops of biotinylated horseradish peroxidase H, mix, and allow to stand for 30 min before use

Reference serum for standard curve: CAP RPSP (when reconstituted according to instructions, this contains 818 mg of IgG per dl)

Control sera: pooled normal human serum or one of the commercial controls available for use with nephelometric or RID procedures as described above

Preparation of anti-human-IgG-coated microtiter plates

1. Add 20 µg of BSA in 0.1 ml of water to each well, and dry at 37°C. Wash the plates five times with PBS-Tween, using the automated plate washer.

2. Add 0.1 ml of diluted glutaraldehyde and incubate for 30 min at room temperature. Wash the plates five times with water, and allow them to air dry at 37°C. These plates can be stored at room temperature for 3 months.

3. Add 0.1 ml of goat anti-human IgG (1:500) to each well. Incubate at 37°C overnight. Wash five times with PBS-Tween.

4. Add to each well 0.1 ml of BSA (50 mg/dl), incubate for 1 h at 37°C, and wash again five times.

Quantitation of IgG in serum or other fluids

1. For the standard curve, prepare the following dilutions of RPSP in PBS-BSA, using positive-displacement pipettes: 1:50,000, 1:100,000, 1:200,000, 1:400,000, 1:800,000, and 1:1,600,000.

2. Add 0.1 ml of each RPSP dilution (in duplicate) to wells of the anti-IgG-coated plate. Add 0.1 ml of PBS-BSA to four additonal wells for the negative control. Add 0.1 ml of the test specimens (in duplicate) to the remaining wells of the plate. If testing cell culture fluid, use undiluted and 1:3 dilutions; if testing biological fluids other than serum, adjust the dilutions according to the estimated concentration of IgG. Incubate for 2 h at 37°C, and wash five times in PBS-Tween.

3. Add 0.1 ml of biotinylated goat anti-human IgG (1:500 dilution) to each well. Incubate for 1 h at 37°C, and wash five times with PBS-Tween.

4. Add 0.1 ml of ABC reagent (1:100) to each well. Prepare the ABC reagent according to package directions; after incubating the mixture for 30 min at room temperature, dilute it 1:2 in PBS, add it to the plate, and incubate for 30 min at 37°C. Wash the plate five times with PBS-Tween.

5. Add 0.1 ml of ortho-phenylenediamine solution to each well. Incubate for 5 min at room temperature in a water bath by placing the microtiter plate in a shallow tray of water on the platform vibrator. Add 0.1 ml of 2.5 N sulfuric acid to stop the reaction.

6. Measure absorbance at 492 nm with the Titertek Multiscan microtiter plate reader.

7. Plot the mean absorbance values versus the concentration of IgG in the RPSP standard on linear graph paper (Fig. 8). Interpolate the concentration of IgG in test samples by using absorbance values in the linear portion of the dose-response curve. If the pho-

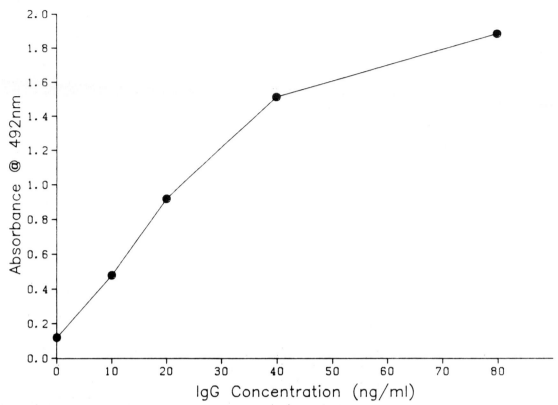

FIG. 8. Dose-response curve for quantitation of IgG by ELISA. The microtiter plate solid-phase ELISA utilizing biotin-avidin-horseradish peroxidase reagents is described in the text. Various dilutions of the CAP RPSP yield the different concentrations of antigen.

tometer output is sent directly to a microcomputer, these plots and calculations can also be performed automatically. If the absorbance readings are above the linear portion of the curve, repeat the assay with more dilute samples.

Sources of error

The major sources of error include nonspecific binding of the antigen to the solid phase and cross-reaction of the second antibody with the capture antibody. Appropriate blanks will identify these problems. Nonspecific antigen binding is minimized by treating the plates with BSA after conjugating them with the first antibody and by washing the plates thoroughly at each step. Interactions of the first and second antibodies are minimized if both are made in the same animal species, e.g., goat. The washing steps are critical. Careful monitoring to ensure adequate vacuum pressure during washing is particularly helpful. Due to the sensitivity of these assays, small errors in pipetting are readily magnified.

Optimal concentrations of each antibody must be determined, and the linear range for antigen measurement must be established. The final enzymatic reaction is affected by variations in time, temperature, and concentration of the reactants. Care should be taken to standardize these factors. Preservatives and oxidative or reducing agents may inactivate the peroxidase. The substrate used here is also unstable in light.

We thank Christine Papadea for providing details of the ELISA procedure which she developed, Devery Howerton for reviewing the nephelometer and RID procedures, Mary Beth Kidd for preparing the illustrations, and Joyce Brents for typing the manuscript.

LITERATURE CITED

1. **Cejka, J., D. W. Mood, and C. S. Kim.** 1974. Immunoglobulin concentrations in sera of normal children: quantitation against an international reference preparation. Clin. Chem. **20**:656–659.
2. **Centers for Disease Control.** 1983. Proficiency testing summary analysis. Immunochemistry 1983 II. Centers for Disease Control, Atlanta, Ga.
3. **College of American Pathologists.** 1978–1984. Special diagnostic immunology survey. College of American Pathologists, Skokie, Ill.
4. **Deverill, I., R. Jefferis, N. R. Ling, and W. G. Reeves.** 1981. Monoclonal antibodies to human IgG: reaction characteristics in the centrifugal analyzer. Clin. Chem. **27**:2044–2047.
5. **Fahey, J. L., and E. M. McKelvey.** 1965. Quantitative determination of serum immunoglobulins in antibody-agar plates. J. Immunol. **94**:84–90.
6. **Guesdon, J.-L., T. Ternynck, and S. Avrameas.** 1979. The use of avidin-biotin interaction in immunoenzymatic techniques. J. Histochem. Cytochem. **27**:1131–1139.
7. **Killingsworth, L. M.** 1982. Clinical applications of protein determinations in biological fluids other than blood. Clin. Chem. **28**:1093–1102.
8. **Maddison, S. E., and C. B. Reimer.** 1976. Normative values of serum immunoglobulins by single radial immunodiffusion: a review. Clin. Chem. **22**:594–601.

9. **Mancini, G., A. O. Carbonara, and J. F. Heremans.** 1965. Immunochemical quantitation of antigens by single radial immunodiffusion. Immunochemistry **2**:235–254.
10. **Normansell, D. E.** 1982. Quantitation of serum immunoglobulins. Crit. Rev. Clin. Lab. Sci. **17**:103–170.
11. **Oxelius, V.-A.** 1984. Immunoglobulin G subclasses and human diseases. Am. J. Med. **76**(Suppl. 3A):1–5.
12. **Reimer, C. B., D. J. Phillips, C. H. Aloisio, D. D. Moore, G. G. Galland, T. W. Wells, C. M. Black, and J. S. McDougal.** 1984. Evaluation of thirty-one mouse monoclonal antibodies to human IgG epitopes. Hybridoma **3**:263–275.
13. **Reimer, C. B., S. J. Smith, T. W. Wells, R. M. Nakamura, P. W. Keitges, R. F. Ritchie, G. W. Williams, D. J. Hanson, and D. B. Dorsey.** 1982. Collaborative calibration of the U.S. National and the College of American Pathologists reference preparations for specific serum proteins. Am. J. Clin. Pathol. **77**:12–19.
14. **Saunders, G. C.** 1979. The art of solid-phase immunoassay including selected protocols, p. 100–118. *In* R. M. Nakamura, W. R. Dito, and E. S. Tucker III (ed.), Immunoassays in the clinical laboratory. Alan R. Liss, Inc., New York.
15. **Skvaril, F., A. Morrell, and S. Barandum.** 1982. Imbalances of kappa/lambda ratios of immunoglobulins, p. 21–36. *In* S. E. Ritzmann (ed.), Protein abnormalities, vol. 2. Pathology of immunoglobulins: diagnostic and clinical aspects. Alan R. Liss, Inc., New York.
16. **Waldman, T. A., and S. Broder.** 1982. Polyclonal B-cell activators in the study of the regulation of immunoglobulin synthesis in the human system. Adv. Immunol. **32**:1–63.

Chapter 23

Classification and Diagnosis of Monoclonal Gammopathies

ROBERT A. KYLE

The monoclonal gammopathies are a group of disorders characterized by the proliferation of a single clone of plasma cells that produce a homogeneous monoclonal (M) protein. Each monoclonal protein consists of two heavy polypeptide chains of the same class and subclass and two light polypeptide chains of the same type. In contrast, an increase in polyclonal immunoglobulins consists of one or more heavy-chain classes and both light-chain types.

The different types of monoclonal immunoglobulins are designated by capital letters that correspond to the class of their heavy chains, which are designated by Greek letters: γ in immunoglobulin G (IgG), α in IgA, μ in IgM, δ in IgD, and ϵ in IgE. Their subclasses are IgG1, IgG2, IgG3, and IgG4, or IgA1 and IgA2, and their light-chain types are kappa (κ) and lambda (λ).

The monoclonal gammopathies may be classified as follows:

I. Malignant monoclonal gammopathies
  A. Multiple myeloma (IgG, IgA, IgD, IgE, and free light chains)
    1. Overt multiple myeloma
    2. Smoldering multiple myeloma
    3. Plasma cell leukemia
    4. Nonsecretory myeloma
  B. Plasmacytoma
    1. Solitary plasmacytoma of bone
    2. Extramedullary plasmacytoma, solitary and multiple
  C. Malignant lymphoproliferative diseases
    1. Waldenström's macroglobulinemia or primary macroglobulinemia (IgM)
    2. Malignant lymphoma
  D. Heavy-chain diseases (HCD)
    1. γ HCD
    2. α HCD
    3. μ HCD
    4. δ HCD
  E. Amyloidosis
    1. Primary
    2. With myeloma
    (Secondary, localized, and familial amyloidoses have no monoclonal protein)
II. Monoclonal gammopathies of undetermined significance
  A. Benign (IgG, IgA, IgD, IgM, and, rarely, free light chains)
  B. Associated with neoplasms of cell types not known to produce monoclonal proteins
  C. Biclonal gammopathies

MONOCLONAL PROTEINS

Relation to normal immunoglobulins

Although monoclonal proteins have long been considered abnormal, studies during the past several years have strongly suggested that they are only excessive quantities of normal immunoglobulins. The striking feature of monoclonal proteins that led investigators to consider them abnormal is their homogeneity. Whereas normal IgG in human serum is electrophoretically heterogeneous and is distributed from the α_2 to the slow γ regions, IgG monoclonal proteins are localized in their electrophoretic migration.

Kunkel (4) showed that each heavy-chain subclass and light-chain type in monoclonal proteins has its counterpart among normal immunoglobulins and among antibodies. After the discovery of the two types of light chains (κ and λ) in myeloma proteins in a ratio of approximately 2:1, these same light chains were detected in essentially the same ratio among normal immunoglobulins. Similarly, the IgG and IgA subclasses and IgD class were discovered among myeloma proteins and then found as normal serum components. These identifications have gradually weakened the belief that the monoclonal proteins of multiple myeloma and macroglobulinemia are abnormal and have suggested that they represent the overproduction of a normal product by a clone of abnormally functioning cells. However, many of the heavy chains found in the heavy-chain diseases show significant deletions of amino acids: they are abnormal immunoglobulins.

Even the antigenic determinants ("idiotypic specificities" or "individual antigenic specificities") that are associated with the binding sites were believed to be associated uniquely with myeloma proteins but have been shown to occur among antibodies. Conversely, studies of highly purified antibodies have revealed a homogeneity approaching that seen in monoclonal proteins. In some instances, after primary immunization with a carbohydrate antigen, monoclonal immunoglobulins consisting of a single light-chain type and a single IgG heavy-chain subclass have been seen.

The possibility expressed by Kunkel (4) that myeloma proteins are individual antibodies and are products of the individual plasma cells arising from a single clone of malignant cells has been supported by their antigen-combining activity. Monoclonal antibody activity in humans has been associated with cold agglutinin disease as well as with a wide variety of bacterial antigens including streptolysin O, staphylococcal protein, *Klebsiella* polysaccharides, and *Brucella* organisms. It is almost certain that more monoclonal human proteins will be found to have antibody activity. It has been postulated that all myeloma proteins may have such activity. The generation of antibody diversity has been discussed recently by Rose (8).

In this view, as illustrated in Fig. 1, the normal assortment of IgG molecules comprises minute

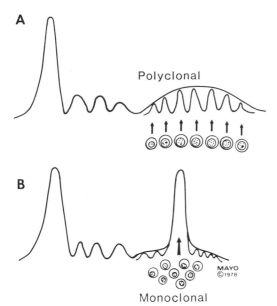

FIG. 1. Polyclonal and monoclonal electrophoretic patterns. Anode and albumin are on the left; cathode is on the right. (A) Broad outline comprising small peaks of many different homogeneous proteins that have been produced by many different plasma cell clones (polyclonal). (Each protein is represented here in normal amount, related by arrow to its peak.) (B) Tall, narrow peak of homogeneous protein (single heavy-chain class and subclass and single light-chain type), which is the excessive output of a single clone (monoclonal). (From R. A. Kyle and P. R. Greipp. 1978. The laboratory investigation of monoclonal gammopathies. Mayo Clin. Proc. **53:**719–739. By permission.)

amounts of homogeneous proteins from many diverse single clones of plasma cells, and so is polyclonal. If a single clone escapes the normal controls over its multiplication, it reproduces excessively and synthesizes an excess of protein with a single heavy-chain class and subclass and light-chain type. This monoclonal protein often is associated with a neoplastic process. Support for the one-cell, one-immunoglobulin concept comes from the studies of the cellular localization of these proteins. Experiments performed with antisera to light chains have shown that nearly all individual plasma cells contain κ or λ light chains but not both.

Patterns of overproduction

Normally, plasma cells produce heavy chains and a slight excess of light chains that spill over into the urine. In IgG myeloma, about 75% of patients have an excess of light chains that may be excreted into the urine (Bence Jones proteinuria) or catabolized. This small excess of light-chain production could be due to an imbalance in translation or transcription within the clone or to a possible suppression of heavy-chain synthesis in the clone. In other instances, no heavy chain is produced by the plasma cell, and only excessive quantities of light chains are detected (light-chain disease). Finally, a small proportion of myeloma cells do not secrete either heavy or light chains in detectable amounts because of a simple failure of synthesis or a blocking of secretion; these cells are called

nonsecretory. In heavy-chain disease, portions of the heavy chains of IgG, IgA, IgM, or IgD are present in serum or urine.

LABORATORY METHODS FOR THE STUDY OF MONOCLONAL PROTEINS

Analysis of the serum or urine for monoclonal proteins requires a sensitive, rapid, and dependable screening method to detect a monoclonal protein and a specific assay to identify it according to its heavy-chain class and light-chain type. Electrophoresis on cellulose acetate membrane is satisfactory for screening. (Agarose is more sensitive than cellulose acetate in detecting small monoclonal bands. See Immunoelectrophoresis for identification, below, for a discussion of the principles and a description of the specific methods involved.) After that, immunoelectrophoresis or immunofixation, or both, should be employed to confirm the presence of a monoclonal protein and to distinguish the immunoglobulin class and light-chain type of which it is made.

Analysis of serum for monoclonal proteins

Serum protein electrophoresis should be done in all cases in which multiple myeloma, macroglobulinemia, or amyloidosis is suspected. In addition, the test is indicated in any case of unexplained weakness or fatigue, anemia, elevation of the erythrocyte sedimentation rate, back pain, osteoporosis, or osteolytic lesions or fracture, immunoglobulin deficiency, hypercalcemia, Bence Jones proteinuria, renal insufficiency, or recurrent infections. Serum protein electrophoresis also should be performed in peripheral neuropathy, carpal tunnel syndrome, refractory congestive heart failure, nephrotic syndrome, orthostatic hypotension, or malabsorption, because a localized band or spike is strongly suggestive of primary amyloidosis. Electrophoresis on cellulose acetate membranes is an excellent screening test because it can be done easily and rapidly.

The use of cellulose acetate electrophoresis also has its disadvantages. The strip must be examined so that a minor band is not missed. Despite the sensitivity of electrophoresis on cellulose acetate, a small quantity of monoclonal protein may be obscured in the β or γ band and may escape notice. A band on the cellulose membrane, though somewhat discrete, may be fuzzy, making differentiation between a monoclonal and a polyclonal peak difficult. Monoclonal light chains (Bence Jones proteinemia) usually are not detected by this type of electrophoretic procedure.

Interpretation of results

The first peak at the anodal (positive) end of the serum electrophoretic pattern is albumin, and the next peak is α_1-globulin, which contains α_1-antitrypsin, α_1-lipoprotein, and α_1-acid glycoprotein (orosomucoid). The third peak, α_2-globulin, is composed mainly of α_2-macroglobulin, α_2-lipoprotein, haptoglobin, ceruloplasmin, and erythropoietin. The major components of the β-globulin peak are β-lipoprotein, transferrin, plasminogen, the third component of complement, and hemopexin.

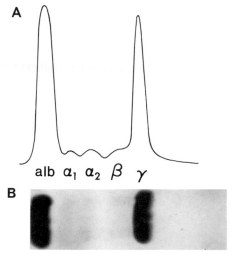

FIG. 2. (A) Monoclonal pattern of serum protein as traced by densitometer after electrophoresis on cellulose acetate (anode on left): tall, narrow-based peak of γ mobility. (B) Monoclonal pattern from electrophoresis of serum on cellulose acetate (anode on left): dense, localized band representing monoclonal protein at right. (From R. A. Kyle and P. R. Greipp. 1978. The laboratory investigation of monoclonal gammopathies. Mayo Clin. Proc. **53**:719–739. By permission.)

Fibrinogen (in plasma) appears as a discrete band between the β and γ peaks. Therefore, the specimen should be examined for a clot when a small localized band is seen in this region. The presence of a clot suggests that the plasma has converted to serum after the electrophoresis has been done. If no clot is seen, thrombin should be added to the sample; add 30 μl of bovine thrombin (1,000 U/dl) to 100 μl of the sample. Prompt development of a clot indicates the presence of fibrinogen. If the β-γ band can no longer be detected when electrophoresis is repeated, the presence of fibrinogen is proved. Fibrinogen may be detected also by immunodiffusion (Ouchterlony) by utilizing fibrinogen antisera. Fibrinogen may be present because the sample has not clotted sufficiently or if the patient has received heparin, i.e., the sample is actually plasma rather than serum. If no evidence of fibrinogen is found, immunoelectrophoresis should be done because the β-γ band might represent a small monoclonal protein.

Immunoglobulins (IgG, IgA, IgM, IgD, and IgE) make up the γ component, but it must be emphasized that they are also found in the β-γ and β regions and that IgG extends to the α_2-globulin region. Thus, an IgG monoclonal protein may range from the slow γ region to the α_2-globulin region.

A decrease in albumin and increases in α_1- and α_2-globulins, and occasionally in γ-globulin, are non-specific features of inflammatory processes (tissue inflammation and destruction) such as infection or metastatic malignancy. Broad-based γ-globulin peaks or wide bands with fuzzy borders blending into the background are seen in chronic infections, connective-tissue diseases, and liver disease and sometimes in apparently normal persons.

Hypogammaglobulinemia (<0.6 g/dl) is characterized by a definite decrease in the γ component, and the diagnosis should be confirmed by quantitative determination of the immunoglobulin levels. Hypogammaglobulinemia may be congenital (such as in Bruton's sex-linked or "Swiss-type" combined deficiency) or acquired (idiopathic or related to nephrotic syndrome, multiple myeloma, amyloidosis, chronic lymphocytic leukemia, lymphoma, or treatment with corticosteroids). The presence of a normal or modest increase in the β band associated with a decrease in the γ band raises the possibility of multiple myeloma or amyloidosis. In this situation, proteinuria of the Bence Jones type is often present, and immunoelectrophoresis or immunofixation of the serum and urine is necessary. Hypogammaglobulinemia is seen in about 15% of patients with multiple myeloma and in approximately 30% of patients with primary systemic amyloidosis.

A large decrease in the α_1-globulin component is usually due to a congenital deficiency of α_1-antitrypsin and may be associated with recurrent pulmonary infections and chronic obstructive pulmonary disease.

After electrophoresis, a monoclonal protein (having a single heavy-chain class and single light-chain type) usually appears as a narrow peak (like a church spire) in the γ, β, or α_2 region of the densitometer tracing or as a dense, discrete band on the cellulose membrane (Fig. 2). In contrast, an excess of polyclonal immunoglobulins (having one or more heavy-chain types with both κ and λ light chains) makes a broad-based peak or broad band (Fig. 3) and usually is limited to the γ region. In 1 to 2% of sera, there is an additional monoclonal protein of a different immunoglobulin class or light-chain type; this situation is designated biclonal gammopathy (5).

A tall, narrow, homogeneous peak or a discrete band is most suggestive of monoclonal gammopathy of undetermined significance, multiple myeloma, or Waldenström's macroglobulinemia, but monoclonal peaks may also occur in amyloidosis and in lymphoma.

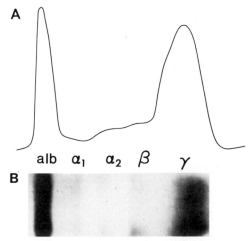

FIG. 3. (A) Polyclonal pattern from densitometer tracing after paper electrophoresis of serum (anode on left): broad-based peak of γ mobility. (B) Polyclonal pattern from electrophoresis of serum on cellulose acetate (anode on left): band at right is broad, and advancing and trailing edges both are diffuse. (From R. A. Kyle and P. R. Greipp. 1978. The laboratory investigation of monoclonal gammopathies. Mayo Clin. Proc. **53**:719–739. By permission.)

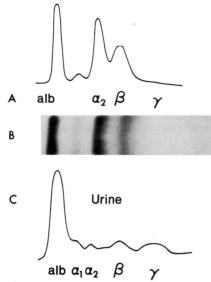

FIG. 4. Nephrotic syndrome. (A) Serum electrophoretic pattern (densitometer tracing; anode on left) showing decreased albumin (narrow peak), increased α_2 and β peaks, and hypogammaglobulinemia. (B) Cellulose acetate pattern (anode on left). (C) Urine electrophoretic pattern (anode on left); most of the protein is albumin. (From R. A. Kyle and P. R. Greipp. 1978. The laboratory investigation of monoclonal gammopathies. Mayo Clin. Proc. **53**:719–739. By permission.)

Other shapes may misleadingly suggest a monoclonal protein in the serum. For example, a large, broad peak in the α_2-globulin area may represent free hemoglobin-haptoglobin complexes resulting from hemolysis. The serum is often pink and suggests the possibility of hemolysis. Another serum sample should be obtained from the patient. Large amounts of transferrin in patients with iron deficiency anemia may produce a localized band in the β region. The point of application of the specimen in the cathodal area is also suggestive of a monoclonal protein. Usually, this can be recognized when the two faint lines of the applicator are visible.

Certain other conditions have distinctive electrophoretic patterns. The nephrotic syndrome produces a serum pattern featuring decreased albumin and γ-globulin and increased α_2- and β-globulins (Fig.4A and B). The increased α_2- and β-globulins may produce a pattern that looks like a monoclonal peak of rapid mobility, and this might be mistaken for a myeloma protein. The urinary pattern, however, consists mainly of albumin (Fig. 4C). Chronic infections, connective-tissue diseases, and chronic liver diseases may be characterized by large, broad-based polyclonal patterns. This is particularly true in chronic active hepatitis, where the γ component may be 4 or 5 g/dl or more. This large γ band may be confused with that seen in multiple myeloma or macroglobulinemia. Occasionally, lymphoproliferative processes may have a large polyclonal increase in immunoglobulins.

However, a monoclonal protein may appear as a rather broad band on the cellulose acetate membrane or a broad peak in the densitometer tracing and can be mistaken for a polyclonal increase in immunoglob-

ulins. Presumably, this is due to aggregates or polymers, and immunoelectrophoresis or immunofixation is required for identification.

It must be emphasized that a patient can have a monoclonal protein when the total protein concentration, β- and γ-globulin levels (Table 1), and quantitative immunoglobulin values are all within normal limits. A small monoclonal peak may be concealed among the β or γ components and therefore be missed. The cellulose acetate pattern and densitometer tracing may appear to be normal even though a monoclonal protein is present. A monoclonal light chain (Bence Jones proteinemia) is rarely seen on the cellulose acetate tracing. In some cases of IgD myeloma, the monoclonal protein has a small peak or is not evident at all. Often the monoclonal protein is not apparent in the heavy-chain diseases. In fact, the serum protein electrophoretic pattern is normal in half the cases of α heavy-chain disease, and an unimpressive broad band in the α_2 or β region is the only electrophoretic abnormality. The characteristic sharp band or peak, which is suggestive of a monoclonal protein, is not seen. In μ heavy-chain disease, the electrophoretic pattern is normal except for hypogammaglobulinemia, and a dense band is uncommon. In γ heavy-chain disease, there usually is a localized band in the β-γ region, but often the band is broad, appears heterogeneous, and is more suggestive of a polyclonal than a monoclonal protein. Thus, a normal value for the components of the electrophoretic pattern or a normal-appearing or nonspecific pattern may still contain a monoclonal protein, and, consequently, the use of immunoelectrophoresis or immunofixation is crucial for confirmation.

Immunoelectrophoresis for identification

Immunoelectrophoresis is necessary for the identification of a monoclonal protein and for the determination of its heavy-chain class and light-chain type. It should be performed in all cases in which a sharp peak or band is found in the cellulose acetate tracing or when myeloma, macroglobulinemia, amyloidosis, or a related disorder is suspected. Immunoelectrophoresis is particularly helpful in determining whether a solitary plasmacytoma is localized. After tumoricidal radiation therapy, the monoclonal protein should disappear. Its persistence suggests disseminated myeloma. Immunoelectrophoresis is essential in the differentiation of a monoclonal from a polyclonal increase in immunoglobulins. Monospecific antisera must be used to determine whether the increase of a heavy-chain class is associated with an increase of either κ or

TABLE 1. Serum protein electrophoresis: normal values (180 cases)

Fraction	Normal values (g/dl)[a]
Total protein	6.3–7.9
Albumin	3.1–4.3
α_1-Globulin	0.1–0.3
α_2-Globulin	0.6–1.0
β-Globulin	0.7–1.4
γ-Globulin	0.7–1.6

[a] The 2.5 to 97.5 percentile.

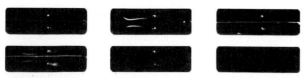

FIG. 5. Immunoelectrophoretic patterns in myeloma. Anode is on the left; cathode is on the right. Trough of each slide contains monospecific antiserum: (upper row) antisera to IgA(α) in first trough, to IgG(γ) in second, and to IgM(μ) in third; (lower row) antisera to κ in first and to λ in second (no sample in third position). The serum from the first patient, placed in the top well of each slide, has produced thickening and bowing of the IgG arc and a similar change in the λ arc, results that indicate the presence of IgG(λ) monoclonal protein. The serum from the second patient, placed in the bottom well of each slide, has produced thickening and asymmetry of the IgA arc and a similar change in the κ arc; so IgA(κ) monoclonal protein is present. (From R. A. Kyle and P. R. Greipp. 1978. The laboratory investigation of monoclonal gammopathies. Mayo Clin. Proc. **53:**719–739. By permission.)

λ light chains when the excess protein is monoclonal or with an increase in both light-chain types when the excess protein is polyclonal. Polyclonal increases of immunoglobulins are usually associated with an inflammatory process, and a monoclonal protein is usually associated with a neoplastic or potentially neoplastic proliferation of B lymphocytes.

In immunoelectrophoresis, the serum specimen is placed in wells on microscope slides covered with 1% agar or agarose. The serum from one patient is placed in each upper well, and the serum of a second patient or a normal sample is placed in each lower well. Electrophoresis separates the various proteins. Then a trough is cut into the agar—between the wells and parallel to the line of migration of the components—and each trough is filled with a monospecific antiserum. Proteins from the electrophoresed sample (antigen) and from the antisera (antibody) are then allowed to diffuse toward each other and to form precipitin lines or arcs where the antigen and the antibody meet (Fig. 5). Use of monospecific antisera is essential in order to determine whether the increase of a heavy-chain class is associated with an increase of either κ or λ light chains (monoclonal protein) or an increase in both light-chain types.

Reagents for immunoelectrophoresis

Barbital buffer consists of 184.80 g of barbital sodium and 33.12 g of barbital (must be dissolved in hot distilled water). These reagents are placed in a 5-liter volumetric container and diluted to 18 liters with distilled water. The buffer (pH 8.6, 0.05 M) is stored at 4°C until use.

Agar (1%) is prepared as follows: mix 4 g of agar with 400 ml of barbital buffer, heat to dissolve, and add 9 drops of 1% thimerosal (Merthiolate).

Procedure for immunoelectrophoresis

Six glass microscope slides are placed in a plastic slide holder. The electrophoresis chamber (LKB Multiphor electrophoresis system; LKB Instruments,

Inc., Rockville, Md.) will hold three slide holders, so six serum samples can be run at one time.

1. Place six clean microscope slides in the slide holder, and put the slide holder on a previously leveled table.

2. Apply several drops of warm agar (1% Noble agar in barbital buffer) to the microscope slides to make a seal between the slides and at both ends of the row of slides to prevent excess loss of agar.

3. After allowing the agar seal to cool, apply a total of 10 ml of warm agar to one row of three slides.

4. Add 10 ml of warm agar to the second row of three slides.

5. Allow the slides to cool at 4°C in a humidity chamber until needed. They should be chilled for at least 0.5 h before use.

6. Record the name and number of the patient whose serum will be placed in the wells. This is easily done by stamping an outline of the six troughs on a sheet 21.5 by 28 cm, where the arcs can be drawn and results of interpretation can be recorded.

7. Punch the well-trough pattern, using an LKB die with a 1-mm trough and a diffusion distance of 5.1 mm from the trough.

8. Remove the agar from the wells only with gentle suction.

9. Fill the wells with serum using Fisher capillary tubes (Fisher Scientific Co., Pittsburgh, Pa.). The top wells of five slides in the holder are filled with the same patient's serum, and the bottom well of each slide is filled with the serum or urine of a different patient.

10. Add a small quantity of indicator dye (amido black-nigrosin in acetic acid) to the patient's serum in the first slide.

11. Fill the wells of two more slide holders with the sera of four additional patients, and place the three slide holders in the electrophoresis chamber. Be certain that the wicks are in good contact with the agar on all three slide holders. Set the voltage at 180, which produces approximately 40 mA.

12. The current is applied continuously until the indicator dye has migrated 15 to 20 mm. This takes approximately 1 h.

13. Shut the current off and take the slide holders from the electrophoresis chamber.

14. With suction, remove the agar gently from the troughs.

15. Fill the troughs with monospecific antisera to IgG, IgA, IgM, κ, and λ.

16. Store the slide holders in a humidity chamber at room temperature for 24 h.

17. Observe the immunoelectrophoretic patterns in a view box. The abnormal patterns can be photographed using a 35-mm camera with a macromatic lens and black-and-white film. The negatives are stored in plastic.

Interpretation of results

Potent antiserum to whole human serum produces more than 30 precipitin arcs and causes difficulty in interpretation. Therefore, monospecific antisera to IgG, IgA, IgM, IgD, and IgE as well as to κ and λ light chains should be used. In addition to their monospecificity, the antisera must be potent. It is most impor-

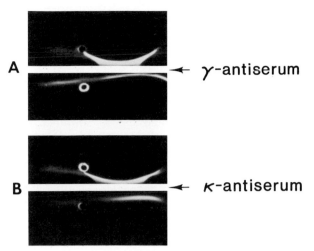

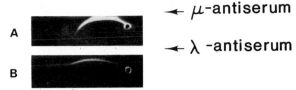

FIG. 6. Immunoelectrophoretic patterns obtained in myeloma. Anode is on the left; cathode is on the right. (A) Antiserum to IgG(γ) shows a thickened arc from a patient's serum in the top well; for comparison, a normal arc from normal serum is in the bottom well. (B) Antiserum to κ chains shows a thickened arc that is similar to the IgG arc (top well); for comparison, note the normal arc from normal serum (bottom well). Thus, the patient's serum contains IgG(κ). (From R. A. Kyle and P. R. Greipp. 1978. The laboratory investigation of monoclonal gammopathies. Mayo Clin. Proc. **53**:719–739. By permission.)

FIG. 7. Immunoelectrophoretic patterns in macroglobulinemia. Anode is on the left; cathode is on the right. (A) With antiserum to IgM(μ), the IgM arc is thickened and bowed. (B) With antiserum to λ, bowing of the arc corresponds to the IgM arc; this indicates the IgM(λ) monoclonal protein (macroglobulinemia). (From R. A. Kyle and P. R. Greipp. 1978. The laboratory investigation of monoclonal gammopathies. Mayo Clin. Proc. **53**:719–739. By permission.)

tant for each laboratory to test its antisera. For example, to ascertain the specificity and strength of IgG(γ) antiserum, it should be run against known IgA(κ), IgA(λ), IgM(κ), and IgM(λ) monoclonal sera; against several known IgG(κ) and IgG(λ) monoclonal sera; and against serum and urine containing monoclonal κ or λ light chains. It is always useful to have antisera from various sources available when typing monoclonal proteins because the antigenic determinants of some monoclonal proteins are so limited that they will not be recognized by all antisera.

In multiple myeloma, monospecific antisera to IgG, IgA, IgD, IgE, or κ or λ produce a localized thickening or bowing of a heavy-chain arc and similar thickening or bowing of a light-chain arc. The alterations in the heavy-chain and light-chain arcs should be about the same distance from the well. Occasionally, a thickened arc appears to be cut off abruptly near the trough. This appearance may be due to antigen excess and precipitation of the arc in the trough or to formation of a soluble antigen-antibody complex. In this situation, immunoelectrophoresis should be repeated with serum diluted 1:5 or 1:10. Most precipitin arcs form within 24 h. If diffusion is allowed to continue more than 24 h, the arcs become diffuse and exaggerated so that interpretation is difficult. The presence of an additional light-chain arc (double bowing) without a similar bowing of a heavy-chain arc indicates a free monoclonal light chain (Bence Jones proteinemia).

The immunoelectrophoretic pattern of an IgG(κ) monoclonal protein is shown in Fig. 6. In immunoelectrophoresis of an IgG protein, the abnormality in the precipitin arc may occur anywhere from the slow γ to the α₂ region. Polyclonal increase of a specific immunoglobulin often produces a rather localized thickening of the heavy chain, but there is no corresponding localized thickness of a single light chain because both the κ and λ light chains are increased. One must find a localized increase of one (and only one) light-chain arc before diagnosing the presence of a monoclonal protein.

In Waldenström's macroglobulinemia, IgM antiserum and κ or λ produce a dense localized arc (Fig. 7). Sometimes the monoclonal IgM protein does not show an accompanying light-chain abnormality, and thus misleadingly suggests μ heavy-chain disease. Immunofixation is helpful in this situation (Fig. 8). The addition of a reducing agent, such as dithiothreitol, to the serum usually makes IgM(κ) or IgM(λ) monoclonal protein identifiable (Fig. 9). Monoclonal IgM proteins may appear to be an application artifact on the cellulose acetate membrane. However, this supposed artifact may represent an IgM(κ) or IgM(λ) protein.

The serum protein electrophoretic pattern of a monoclonal protein may be relatively broad-based, a finding that suggests a polyclonal increase in immunoglobulins. As shown in Fig. 10, immunoelectrophoresis with monospecific antisera reveals impressive thickening and bowing of the IgA arc and a similar thickening and bowing with κ antisera; this appearance indicates a monoclonal IgA(κ) protein. The tendency of IgA monoclonal protein to produce polymers

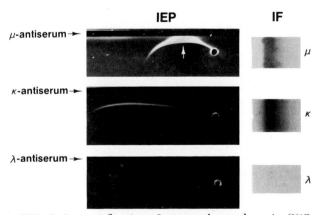

FIG. 8. Immunofixation. Immunoelectrophoresis (IEP; anode on left) shows a pronounced thickening of the arc with μ (IgM) antiserum but no similar changes with κ or λ antiserum. Immunofixation (IF) shows a dense, localized band with μ antiserum and a dense, localized κ band, indicating monoclonal IgM(κ) protein.

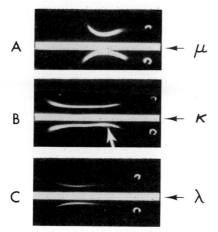

FIG. 9. Top well of each slide contains patient's serum (anode on left); bottom wells contain the same patient's serum exposed to dithiothreitol. (A) μ antiserum in trough: localized IgM arc. (B) κ antiserum in trough. Note the bowing of the κ arc in the bottom portion of the slide and the normal κ arc in the top portion. (C) λ antiserum: normal arcs. This patient has a monoclonal IgM(κ) protein. (From R. A. Kyle and P. R. Greipp. 1978. The laboratory investigation of monoclonal gammopathies. Mayo Clin. Proc. **53**:719–739. By permission.)

may be the reason for the broadness of the peak. Some patients with Waldenström's macroglobulinemia have had cellulose acetate tracings with a dense but broad band which appeared to be a polyclonal increase but which actually represented a monoclonal IgM protein. The monoclonal protein may precipitate near the application well (euglobulin) and produce no diagnostic arcs. Repetition with a lower-ionic-strength buffer or the addition of a reducing agent

may resolve the problem. Immunofixation may also be useful. IgM and IgG proteins are most frequently involved.

It must be emphasized that the densitometer tracing of a monoclonal protein may show a small peak, or the monoclonal protein may be concealed in the normal β band or γ area and may not be discovered until immunoelectrophoresis is done (Fig. 11). The cellulose acetate strip should also be examined, even when the β- or γ-globulin values are within normal limits, because small monoclonal proteins may be present. Normality of immunoglobulin values does not exclude a small monoclonal protein, particularly with IgG, since a small monoclonal protein may account for most of the quantitative IgG level, though it still is within normal limits. IgD myeloma frequently produces only a small peak or band, and it may not be very discrete. The α and μ heavy-chain-disease sera never show a dense band or sharp peak on electrophoresis and can be detected only with immunoelectrophoresis; γ heavy-chain disease often produces a broad band on electrophoresis, and the diagnosis can easily be missed. Hence immunoelectrophoresis or immunofixation is necessary for the diagnosis of these diseases.

Pitfalls of immunoelectrophoresis

The agar must be free from bubbles and other impurities because they will produce distortions in the precipitin arcs. The agar must be of uniform depth throughout the plate because unequal depth can cause aberrations of the arcs. Drying or freezing of the agar plates will prevent satisfactory electrophoresis and

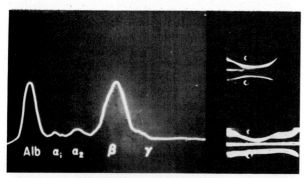

FIG. 10. Results of electrophoresis and immunoelectrophoresis of serum from patient with multiple myeloma (anode on left). (Left) Serum electrophoretic pattern on paper with a rather broad β peak that appears to be polyclonal. (Upper right) Result of immunoelectrophoresis of patient's serum (top well) and normal serum (bottom well), with IgA(α) antiserum in center trough; note the thickened and bowed IgA arc. (Lower right) Result of immunoelectrophoresis, showing reaction to κ-chain antiserum: prominent arc from patient's serum (top well) and elongated arc without localized thickening from normal serum (bottom well). These results confirm the presence of monoclonal IgA(κ) protein. (Modified from R. A. Kyle, R. C. Bieger, and G. J. Gleich. 1970. Diagnosis of syndromes associated with hyperglobulinemia. Med. Clin. North Am. **54**:917–938. By permission of W. B. Saunders Co.)

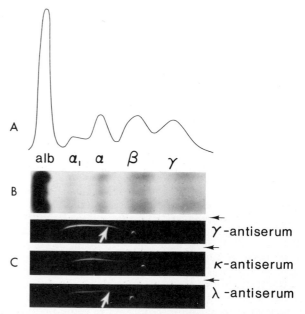

FIG. 11. Results from analyses of serum sample containing monoclonal protein. (A and B) Electrophoresis produced normal patterns in densitometer tracing and on cellulose acetate (anode on left). (C) Immunoelectrophoresis (anode on left) produced localized bowing of IgG(γ) and λ arcs, indicating IgG(λ) protein. (From R. A. Kyle and P. R. Greipp. 1978. The laboratory investigation of monoclonal gammopathies. Mayo Clin. Proc. **53**:719–739. By permission.)

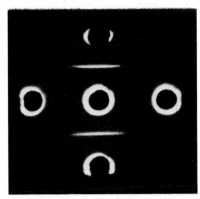

FIG. 12. Immunodiffusion with antiserum to IgD in central well and sera of two patients with IgD myeloma in the top and bottom wells. Dense precipitin bands confirm the presence of IgD protein. (From R. A. Kyle, R. C. Bieger, and G. J. Gleich. 1970. Diagnosis of syndromes associated with hyperglobulinemia. Med. Clin. North Am. **54:**917–938. By permission of W. B. Saunders Co.)

diffusion of the samples in the agar. In cutting and removing the agar from the wells and troughs, great care must be taken to avoid any irregularities or splitting of the agar, because this will allow the antiserum to produce bowing or asymmetry of the arcs, which is suggestive of a monoclonal protein. The agar should not be pulled away from the microscope slide because antisera can run under the agar. During electrophoresis, the wicks must maintain a good contact between the slide holder with the microscope slides and the buffer, or electrophoresis of the serum will be irregular. The inadvertent dropping of sera or antisera on the agar slide will produce new arcs or artifactual distortion of the arcs and make interpretation very difficult.

Immunodiffusion (Ouchterlony) for screening

All sera should be screened for the possibility of IgD or IgE monoclonal proteins. This screening is absolutely essential when bowing of the κ or λ arcs is seen without an accompanying abnormality of the IgG, IgA, or IgM arc. It is economical to screen the sera of all our patients by Ouchterlony immunodiffusion, using antisera to IgD and IgE against each patient's serum. The central well is filled with a monospecific IgD or IgE antiserum, and each surrounding well is filled with undiluted serum from each patient. Dense precipitin lines form if the patient has an increased concentration of IgD or IgE (Fig. 12). All sera forming a precipitin line are then studied further by immunoelectrophoresis with monospecific antisera to IgD, IgE, κ, and λ. Since most sera produce no reaction on immunodiffusion, immunoelectrophoresis is not necessary.

Since four to six sera can be screened with 7 or 8 μl of IgD or IgE antiserum by immunodiffusion, but 60 μl of antiserum is needed to perform immunoelectrophoresis on two sera, prior screening by immunodiffusion saves a significant amount of antisera.

Method (Ouchterlony)

1. Coat the microscope slides with 1% agar, as described above for immunoelectrophoresis, except

that the agar is dissolved in 0.01 M potassium phosphate (pH 7.4) and 0.15 M sodium chloride.

2. Punch wells as shown in Fig. 12. A die that makes six or eight wells around the central well, rather than four, may be used.

3. Fill the central well with IgD or IgE monospecific antisera. Fill one of the peripheral wells with the serum of a patient with known IgD or IgE myeloma as a control. Place the sera to be tested in the other wells. Place slides in the humidity chamber at room temperature for 24 h. Read the lines and photograph them, as for immunoelectrophoresis.

Immunofixation for identification

Immunofixation is useful when results of immunoelectrophoresis are equivocal. The appropriately diluted serum or urine sample is placed in a small trough in 1% agarose. Electrophoresis is performed, and, immediately afterward, monospecific antisera are placed over the electrophoresed protein. Excess protein is removed by washing in saline, and bands corresponding to an antigen-antibody complex remain. This is stained and read (Fig. 13).

Immunofixation is helpful when one suspects a monoclonal protein and finds only bowing of a single heavy chain or a single light chain on immunoelectrophoresis, especially in cases of monoclonal IgM protein in which the bowing of the light chain is not apparent on immunoelectrophoresis. Immunofixation is also useful in detecting a small monoclonal protein in the presence of normal background immunoglobulins or a polyclonal increase in immunoglobulins. It is particularly advantageous in treated myeloma or macroglobulinemia when looking for a small monoclonal serum protein after the band has disappeared on electrophoresis; in suspected amyloidosis, for the detection of small monoclonal immunoglobulin or monoclonal light chain; or in apparently solitary plasmacytoma or extramedullary plasmacytoma after treatment with radiation. It is also helpful in the recognition of a biclonal gammopathy (Fig. 14). Immunofixation is more sensitive than immunoelectrophoresis in detecting a monoclonal protein in the urine, especially in recognizing a monoclonal heavy-chain fragment in the urine of patients with myeloma or amyloidosis (Fig. 15).

Despite the advantages of immunofixation, immunoelectrophoresis is recommended as the initial procedure because it is technically easier and the results generally are satisfactory. In addition, interpretation of immunofixation may be misleading, and one can overdiagnose or underdiagnose monoclonal

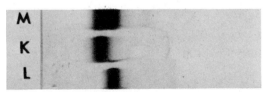

FIG. 13. Serum immunofixation. Two discrete IgM bands are seen in the top portion. One band corresponds to κ (middle portion), and the other, to λ (lower portion). The patient has a biclonal gammopathy [IgM(κ) and IgM(λ)].

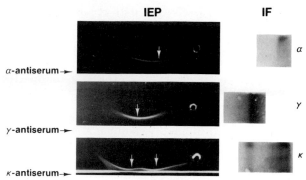

FIG. 14. (Left) Serum immunoelectrophoresis (IEP; anode to left) shows bowing of IgA and IgG arcs corresponding to double bowing of κ. This patient has a biclonal gammopathy [IgA(κ) and IgG(κ)]. (Right) Serum immunofixation (IF) shows a localized IgA(α) band in the top position corresponding to the κ band in the lower position. The localized IgG(γ) band in the middle position corresponds to the similar κ band in the lower position.

proteins because the dilution of the serum or urine specimen is crucial.

Reagents for immunofixation

The barbital buffer is the same as for serum immunoelectrophoresis. Agarose (1%) in barbital buffer is used. The gels are stained with 0.05% amido black and 0.05% nigrosin in 2 liters of 5% acetic acid.

Procedure for immunofixation

1. The dilutions of the serum are based on the size and type of the monoclonal protein. IgG is diluted with Veronal buffer to 0.10 g/dl, IgA to 0.13 g/dl, and IgM to 0.15 g/dl. IgD and IgE are not diluted.

2. An LKB Multiphor basic unit is used. The cooling system should be turned on 30 min before electrophoresis is started. The preparation should be kept at 4 to 10°C. The buffer tanks are filled with barbital buffer.

3. Pour warm (60°C) 1% agarose solution on the hydrophilic side of a gel bond film (25.4 by 12.7 cm; Bio-Products, Rockland, Maine). Approximately 30 ml of agarose will produce a 1-mm layer. The surface must be level because uneven levels of agarose will

distort the bands. The agarose should be poured at least 1 h before use and stored in a humidity chamber at 4°C.

4. Cut a narrow strip of Whatman filter paper no. 1, and place the smooth side of the paper on the gel where the sample is to be applied. Be sure no bubbles are present. After the paper has been evenly applied, carefully peel it off. Apply the sample application foil on top of the gel. The edges of the slits should protrude face down. Avoid bubbles between the foil and the gel.

5. Add 10 μl of amido black-nigrosin in acetic acid to the diluted serum sample, and mix. Apply 5 μl of diluted sample over each slit. Do not touch the gel surface with the tip of the pipette. Carefully peel off the foil when the diluted sample has been completely absorbed (in approximately 5 min).

6. Immediately after application of the sample, position the gel plate on the cooling plate with a layer of barbital buffer under the plate. Avoid trapping air bubbles between the gel and the cooling plate. Eight layers of Whatman filter paper no. 1 are used as wicks. Place heavy glass bars on top of the wicks to ensure good contact on the gels. Electrophoresis is carried out at 130 mA or 300 V with the cooling system between 4 and 10°C. Electrophoresis is terminated when the dye has migrated 3.5 to 4 cm (in approximately 20 min).

7. Soak the cellulose acetate strips (1 by 4 cm) in the appropriate monospecific antisera and apply them to the gel surface immediately after the plate has been removed from the electrophoresis chamber. Care must be taken to keep air bubbles from being trapped beneath the strips. Place the gel in the humidity chamber for 0.5 h at room temperature, and then remove and discard the cellulose strips.

8. Place Whatman filter paper no. 1 soaked in 0.15 N saline directly over the entire gel film. Overlay the filter paper with 5 to 10 dry paper towels. Weights (5 to 10 lb; approximately 2 to 5 kg) should be placed on the towels for at least 10 min. Carefully remove the paper towels and Whatman filter paper and wash the gel in 500 to 1,000 ml of saline for 2 h.

9. Place Whatman filter paper no. 3 over the entire film and dry with forced air in an oven at 56°C. The film is then stained with amido black-nigrosin stain for 2 to 5 min. The film is then destained in multiple changes of tap water with the agarose side facing down and dried as described above.

Interpretation of results

A sharp, well-defined band of a single heavy-chain class and light-chain type is seen in monoclonal gammopathy, while broad, diffuse, heavily stained bands with heavy- and light-chain antisera are characteristic of a polyclonal gammopathy. Interpretation is sometimes difficult because overdilution of a serum sample will result in loss of the monoclonal band. However, inadequate dilution of a specimen may obscure the recognition of a small monoclonal heavy or light chain in a sample with a normal background of immunoglobulins. In addition, underdilution may produce a dense polyclonal band which may be misinterpreted as a monoclonal protein. Consequently, technical and interpretive expertise is necessary for the proper diagnosis.

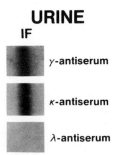

FIG. 15. Urine immunofixation. The localized IgG(γ) band in the top position corresponds to the localized κ band in the middle position. This patient has an IgG(κ) monoclonal fragment in urine.

Two-dimensional gel electrophoresis

Two-dimensional gel electrophoresis is a powerful technique for protein separation and is occasionally useful in the diagnosis of monoclonal gammopathies. The technique of two-dimensional gel electrophoresis separates heavy and light chains on the basis of their electrical charges and molecular sizes. Identification of γ, μ, and α heavy chains is readily established, but less than 80% of κ chains and λ chains can be identified correctly. In this high-resolution technique, a sample containing the protein mixture is subjected to isoelectric focusing in cylindric tube gels, followed by electrophoresis using slab gel-sodium dodecyl sulfate (SDS). A serum sample is mixed with an SDS dissociation buffer and reduced with 2-mercaptoethanol. Isoelectric focusing is done in a gradient of pH 4 to 10 established in cylindric tube gels of 3.5% acrylamide. The gels also contain 9 M urea and 2% Nonidet P-40. After 10,000 V · h of focusing, the gels are removed from the glass tubes and equilibrated with a buffer containing SDS and bromphenol blue. The isoelectric focusing gel is fused to the top of the SDS-polyacrylamide gel electrophoresis slab gel. Electrophoresis proceeds in a 10-place tank at 600 mA (approximately 150 to 250 V) until the dye has migrated within 1 cm from the end of the gel. The gel is stained with Coomassie blue or silver stain.

Two-dimensional gel electrophoresis is useful in identifying a small monoclonal protein when results with immunoelectrophoresis and immunofixation have been equivocal. It is also useful in identifying a second protein component in patients with biclonal gammopathies as well as identifying γ, μ, or α heavy-chain disease. If the serum protein is very small, immunoprecipitates can be made from the patient's serum and from control sera, using antisera to the appropriate immunoglobulin types. Two-dimensional gel analysis of these immunoprecipitates often reveals the monoclonal protein (10).

Quantitation of immunoglobulins

Quantitation is more useful than immunoelectrophoresis in the detection of hypogammaglobulinemia. In many laboratories, quantitation is performed by radioimmunodiffusion (1). In this method, antiserum to the specific immunoglobulin (IgG, IgA, IgM, or IgD) is mixed with agar and layered on a plate. Known concentrations of a specific immunoglobulin and the unknown serum are placed in wells. The size of the precipitin zone is proportional to the antigen in the test serum, so the precipitin zone surrounding each well is measured and compared with the known standards. (See chapter 22 for further discussion.)

In cases of macroglobulinemia, the high concentration of IgM may produce soluble, invisible complexes, leaving the appearance of no immunoglobulin. Low-molecular-weight (7S) IgM produces a spuriously elevated IgM value because its rate of diffusion is greater than that of the 19S IgM used as a standard. Similarly, polymeric IgA will produce spuriously low values because the standards consist of 7S IgA.

If a large number of quantitative tests for immunoglobulins are performed, an automated immunoprecipitin system is practical. In this system, the degree of turbidity produced by antigen-antibody interaction is measured by nephelometry in the near-UV region. Since the method is not affected by the molecular size of the antigen (as is radioimmunodiffusion), the nephelometric technique measures 7S IgM accurately.

Serum viscometry

Serum viscometry should be done in every case with more than 3 g of IgM monoclonal protein per dl or more than 4.0 g of IgA or IgG protein per dl and in any case of oronasal bleeding, blurred vision, or neurologic symptoms suggesting a hyperviscosity syndrome. The Ostwald-100 viscometer is a satisfactory instrument for this purpose. Distilled water and serum, separately, are made to flow through a capillary tube, and the quotient of the flow duration (serum/water) is the viscosity value (normal, <1.6). The Wells Brookfield viscometer (Brookfield Engineering Laboratories, Stoughton, Mass.) is preferred because it is more accurate, requires less serum (about 1.0 ml), and can perform at different shear rates and at different temperatures. In addition, determinations can be made much more rapidly, especially if the viscosity of the serum sample is high. In a series of 100 samples from normal blood bank donors, 95% had a value of 1.8 cP or less at a shear rate of 23/s (6 rpm). Symptoms of hyperviscosity are rare unless the value is greater than 4 cP. Some patients with a value of 10 cP or more do not have symptoms of hyperviscosity.

Sia test

The Sia test for euglobulins is performed by adding a drop of serum to a tube of distilled water. A positive result is the formation of a precipitate or flocculant as the serum is diluted by the water. This test has been recommended for the diagnosis of macroglobulinemia, but many false-positive and some false-negative reactions are seen. In addition, positive reactions may be seen with IgG and IgA monoclonal proteins. The Sia test is largely of historic interest, and it is not recommended.

Cryoglobulins

The serum should be evaluated for the presence of cryoglobulins. Cryoglobulins are proteins that precipitate when cooled and dissolve when heated (Fig. 16).

Fresh, centrifuged serum (5 ml) kept at 37°C is placed in a graduated centrifuge tube and incubated at 1°C (in an ice bath in a refrigerator or cold room) for 7 days. If a precipitate or gel is seen, the tube is centrifuged at 2,000 rpm (750 × g) for 30 min at 1°C, and the cryocrit is read. The supernatant is removed, and the precipitate is washed three times in 1 ml of normal saline at 4°C. Then 1 ml of saline is added to the precipitate, and the precipitate is placed in a 37°C water bath for 30 min. Immunoelectrophoresis is performed on the cryoprecipitate with monospecific antisera to IgG, IgA, IgM, κ, and λ.

Cryoglobulins may be classified as follows: type I (monoclonal—IgG, IgM, IgA, or, rarely, monoclonal light chains); type II (mixed—two or more immunoglobulins, of which one is monoclonal); and type III

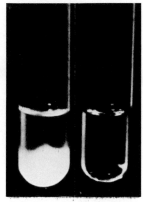

FIG. 16. Cryoglobulinemia. (Left) Precipitate formed on exposure to 1°C. (Right) Disappearance of precipitate when heated to 37°C. (From R. A. Kyle and P. R. Greipp. 1978. The laboratory investigation of monoclonal gammopathies. Mayo Clin. Proc. **53**:719–739. By permission.)

(polyclonal—in which no monoclonal protein is found).

In most cases, monoclonal cryoglobulins are IgM or IgG, but IgA and Bence Jones cryoglobulins have been reported. Surprisingly, many patients with large amounts of cryoglobulin are completely asymptomatic, whereas others with small monoclonal cryoglobulins in the range of 1 to 2 g/dl have pain, purpura, Raynaud's phenomenon, cyanosis, and even ulceration and sloughing of skin and subcutaneous tissues on exposure to the cold. The temperature at which the cryoglobulin precipitates is much more important than the amount of protein. Some patients have had serious problems because of the precipitation of proteins at room temperature. In contrast, others have had no symptoms upon exposure to cold despite having 4 to 5 g of a monoclonal IgG or IgM cryoprotein precipitating at 4°C.

Cryoglobulinemia may produce a spurious elevation of the leukocyte count on the model S Coulter Counter. This is due to particles formed by combination of the cryoglobulin and fibrinogen.

Most commonly, mixed cryoglobulins (type II) consist of IgM-IgG; but IgG-IgG and IgA-IgG combinations have also been reported. Usually, the quantity of mixed cryoglobulin is less than 0.2 g/dl and may not reach maximal amounts for 7 days. The serum protein electrophoretic pattern indicates normality or diffuse hypergammaglobulinemia. Patients with mixed cryoglobulinemia frequently have vasculitis, glomerulonephritis, or lymphoproliferative or chronic infectious processes. Hepatic dysfunction and serologic evidence of previous infection with hepatitis B virus were common in some series (2). In a review of renal findings in 44 cases of essential mixed cryoglobulinemia, Tarantino et al. (9) reported nephrotic syndrome in 8 patients and acute renal failure in 2 others. Proteinuria or hematuria, or both, were found in 28 patients.

Pyroglobulins

Pyroglobulins precipitate when heated to 56°C and do not dissolve when cooled. They are usually discovered when serum is inactivated for the Venereal Disease Research Laboratory test. Pyroglobulins resemble Bence Jones protein in that both precipitate when heated to 60°C, but the two can be distinguished easily by immunoelectrophoresis with appropriate antisera. In most cases, pyroglobulinemia is associated with multiple myeloma, but it may also occur in macroglobulinemia, lymphoproliferative syndromes, and other neoplastic diseases. Pyroglobulins are usually of the IgG class but IgM and IgA pyroglobulins have been seen.

ANALYSIS OF URINE FOR MONOCLONAL PROTEINS

When patients who have gammopathies are studied, analysis of urine is essential. The use of sulfosalicylic acid, or Exton's test, is best for the detection of protein. Sulfosalicylic acid detects albumin and globulin as well as Bence Jones protein, polypeptides, and proteases. False-positive reactions may be induced by penicillin or its derivatives, tolbutamide metabolites, sulfisoxazole metabolites, and certain organic roentgenographic contrast media.

Dipstick tests are used in many laboratories to screen for protein. The dipstick is impregnated with a buffered indicator dye that binds to protein in the urine and produces a color change proportional to the amount of protein bound to it. However, the dipsticks are often insensitive to Bence Jones protein and should not be used when a possibility of Bence Jones proteinuria exists.

Almost from the time of the discovery of the unique thermal properties of urinary light chains, screening tests for their detection have been in use. All have shortcomings, but the heat test of Putnam et al. (7) is the simplest and is generally satisfactory. In this test, 4 ml of centrifuged urine is mixed with 1 ml of 2 M acetate buffer (pH 4.9) and heated at 56°C in an incubation bath for 15 min. The formation of a precipitate that disappears after 3 min in a 100°C bath but reappears with cooling indicates the presence of Bence Jones protein.

Most, but not all, monoclonal light chains in the urine precipitate at 40 to 60°C, dissolve at 100°C, and reprecipitate on cooling at 40 to 60°C. Occasionally, the result of the heat test is positive even though the patient's urine reveals no sharp peak or localized globulin band on electrophoresis and no evidence of a monoclonal light chain on immunoelectrophoresis. Such urine usually produces a broad-based γ band and normal-appearing κ and λ arcs. Presumably, the positive result of the test is due to an excess of polyclonal light chains. Such false-positive results occur most often in cases of renal insufficiency, connective-tissue disease, or malignant disease. However, the results of the Bence Jones heat test have been negative in some cases in which urinary electrophoresis has shown a dense globulin band or spike and immunoelectrophoresis has demonstrated a monoclonal light chain. It is obvious that the heat test for Bence Jones protein has many shortcomings and can be used only as a rough screening procedure. The recognition of Bence Jones proteinuria depends on the demonstration of a monoclonal light chain by electrophoresis and immunoelectrophoresis or immunofixation of an adequately concentrated urine specimen.

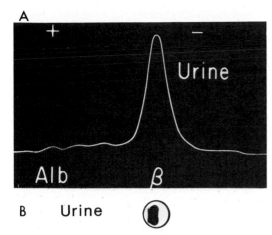

FIG. 17. Results of electrophoresis of urine from a patient with monoclonal protein. (A) Densitometer tracing: tall, narrow-based monoclonal peak of β mobility. (B) Cellulose acetate electrophoretic pattern; the dense band of β mobility represents monoclonal light chain. (From R. A. Kyle and P. R. Greipp. 1978. The laboratory investigation of monoclonal gammopathies. Mayo Clin. Proc. **53**:719–739. By permission.)

Determination of total protein

Coomassie brilliant blue dye combines with proteins in urine to form a dye-protein complex. The amount of color present is proportional to the quantity of protein in the specimen and is measured at 610 nm in a microcentrifugal analyzer (MCA III). Appropriate standards and controls are necessary.

Electrophoresis

In all patients with a monoclonal serum protein, electrophoresis, as well as immunoelectrophoresis, of urine should be performed. Additionally, both tests should be done in all instances of multiple myeloma, Waldenström's macroglobulinemia, amyloidosis, monoclonal gammopathy of undetermined significance, heavy-chain diseases, or suspicion of these entities. Immunoelectrophoresis of urine should also be done in evaluation of older patients with an "idiopathic" nephrotic syndrome.

First, a 24-h collection of urine must be made for the determination of the total amount of protein excreted per day. This is most important when following the course of a patient with a monoclonal light chain in the urine because the amount of protein correlates directly with the size of the plasma cell burden. An aliquot of the 24-h urine specimen must first be concentrated to approximately 3 g/dl (Minicon-B15 concentrator; Amicon Corp., Lexington, Mass.). Rarely, one specimen may be contaminated by another because of a leak in the concentrator.

A 5-ml amount of urine that has been centrifuged for 10 min at 2,000 rpm (750 × g) is added to the concentrator, and when the volume has decreased, 3 to 5 ml more of centrifuged urine is added. The volume of urine is reduced to 0.05 ml (×200) whenever possible. Allow urine to concentrate for 3 h. The urine concentrate is placed on the cellulose polyacetate

membrane with a Drummond Microdispenser and applicator (just as with serum). The number of applications depends on the protein concentration of the urine: one of 6.5 g/dl or more, two of 4.0 to 6.5 g/dl, three of 2.0 to 4.0 g/dl, four of 1.0 to 2.0 g/dl, and five of concentrations less than 1 g/dl.

A urinary monoclonal protein appears as a dense, localized band on the cellulose acetate strip or a tall, narrow, homogeneous peak on the densitometer tracing (Fig. 17). Generally, a monoclonal protein in urine produces a wider band than a monoclonal protein in serum, so immunoelectrophoresis must be done. Occasionally, two discrete globulin bands may be seen in the cellulose acetate tracing of the urine. These bands may be a monoclonal light chain plus a monoclonal immunoglobulin fragment from the serum, or they may be monomers and dimers of the monoclonal light chain (Fig. 18). Therefore, immunoelectrophoresis with the appropriate heavy- and light-chain antisera is necessary. Rarely, two monoclonal light chains (κ and λ) have been noted in the urine.

A polyclonal increase of light chains is seen as a very broad band extending through most of the γ region; it

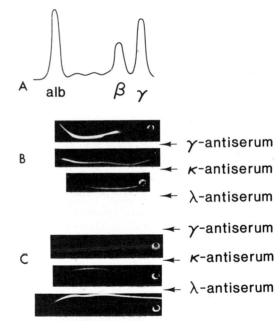

FIG. 18. (A) Densitometer tracing (anode on left) of urine showing albumin, β, and γ peaks. This pattern may represent either monoclonal immunoglobulin plus free monoclonal light chains or monomers and dimers of monoclonal light chain. (B) Immunoelectrophoresis of concentrated urine (anode on left) shows a dense IgG(γ) arc (top), double bowing of the κ arc corresponding to the IgG(γ) arc and one other κ arc representing free monoclonal κ chains (middle), and a small amount of polyclonal λ chains (bottom). This pattern is indicative of IgG(κ) monoclonal protein plus free monoclonal κ chains in urine. (C) Immunoelectrophoresis of urine (anode on left) of another patient with β and γ peaks in the electrophoretic pattern. IgG(γ) (top) shows no arc, antiserum to κ (middle) shows normal-appearing κ arc, and antiserum to λ (bottom) shows dense, doubly bowed λ arc overwhelming antiserum. This pattern is consistent with monomers and dimers of monoclonal λ light chain. (From R. A. Kyle and P. R. Greipp. 1978. The laboratory investigation of monoclonal gammopathies. Mayo Clin. Proc. **53**:719–739. By permission.)

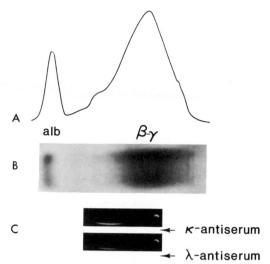

FIG. 19. Urine with polyclonal increase of light chains. (A) Densitometer tracing after electrophoresis (anode on left). Note broad-based β-γ peak. (B) Electrophoretic pattern on cellulose acetate (anode on left): small albumin band and broad β-γ band, with advancing and trailing edges that are diffuse and fading into background. (C) Immunoelectrophoresis (anode on left) with κ and λ antisera showing both arcs, which appear to be normal and represent a polyclonal increase of light chains. (From R. A. Kyle and P. R. Greipp. 1978. The laboratory investigation of monoclonal gammopathies. Mayo Clin. Proc. **53**:719–739. By permission.)

has fuzzy, indistinct cathodal and anodal borders. The densitometer tracing is broad-based, and immunoelectrophoresis shows both κ and λ arcs (Fig. 19).

In the nephrotic syndrome, a large albumin band and small α_1, α_2, β, and γ bands can be seen in the urine electrophoretic pattern.

Immunoelectrophoresis for identification

Immunoelectrophoresis establishes the presence or absence of light chains and determines whether they are monoclonal or polyclonal.

The concentrated urine specimen is placed in a well on a microscope slide covered with 1% agar or agarose and is subjected to electrophoresis to separate the various components. A trough is cut into the agar—parallel to the line of migration of the components—and is filled with specific antiserum. Proteins from the sample that has undergone electrophoresis (antigen) and from the antiserum (antibody) are then allowed to diffuse toward each other and to form precipitin lines or arcs along the line of contact between antigen and antibody. (This can be done on the sixth microscope slide in each slide holder.)

Immunoelectrophoresis should be performed on the urine of any patient with suspected monoclonal gammopathy, even if the sulfosalicylic acid test is negative for protein. It is not unusual for the urine osmolality to be normal or elevated and for the reaction for protein to be negative, yet immunoelectrophoresis of concentrated urine reveals a small localized globulin band and immunoelectrophoresis demonstrates a monoclonal light chain. Immunoelectrophoresis with monospecific antisera should be performed on the urine of every adult who develops the nephrotic syn-

drome with no evident cause. In a number of cases in which electrophoresis of urine showed a large amount of albumin and insignificant amounts of globulin, the urine also contained a monoclonal light chain. Most of these patients had primary systemic amyloidosis, although some had multiple myeloma or light-chain deposition disease. A monoclonal light chain in the urine is sometimes the first clue that the nephrotic syndrome is due to amyloidosis or related disorders.

Immunoelectrophoresis of concentrated urine is performed with antisera to κ and λ and the appropriate heavy chain. It should be done in all cases in which there is a sharp peak or band in the globulin region of the cellulose acetate tracing, in all cases with a monoclonal protein in the serum, and in all cases in which myeloma, macroglobulinemia, amyloidosis, or a related disorder is known or suspected.

If electrophoresis of the urine reveals a localized globulin spike but immunoelectrophoresis with κ and λ antisera does not demonstrate a monoclonal light chain, the presence of γ heavy-chain disease should be suspected. Immunoelectrophoresis should then be done with antisera to IgG (γ heavy chains) (Fig. 20).

Theoretically, it would be best to use antisera that recognize only free κ or λ immunoglobulins rather than light-chain antisera that recognize light chains that are either free or in an intact immunoglobulin. However, such antisera are not readily available, and most are either nonspecific or not potent enough. In addition, some patients have a heavy- and light-chain

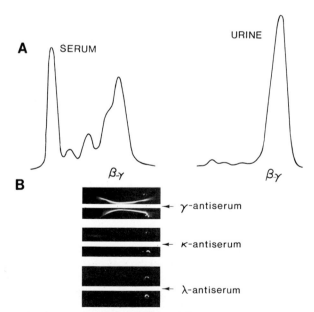

FIG. 20. Heavy-chain disease. (A) Densitometer tracings (anode on left) for serum (note tall peak of β-γ mobility) and urine (note tall β-γ peak). (B) Immunoelectrophoresis (anode on left). The top well in each slide contains serum, and the bottom well contains concentrated urine. With γ antiserum, a dense, thickened, asymmetric arc is seen in both serum and urine. With κ antiserum a faint, fuzzy arc is seen in serum and no arc is seen in urine, and with λ antiserum there is a faint, fuzzy λ arc in serum and none in urine. This patient has monoclonal γ chain in serum and urine (γ heavy-chain disease). (From R. A. Kyle and P. R. Greipp. 1978. The laboratory investigation of monoclonal gammopathies. Mayo Clin. Proc. **53**:719–739. By permission.)

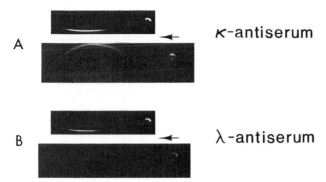

A   κ-antiserum

B   λ-antiserum

FIG. 21. Immunoelectrophoresis of urine (anode on left). (A) The urine in the top well shows a normal arc, and the urine in the bottom well reveals a bowed κ arc. (B) The urine in the top well reveals a normal λ arc, and the urine in the bottom well shows no λ arc. The patient whose urine is in the top wells of both slides has a polyclonal increase in light chains, whereas the urine of the patient in bottom wells has monoclonal κ protein. (From R. A. Kyle and P. R. Greipp. 1978. The laboratory investigation of monoclonal gammopathies. Mayo Clin. Proc. **53:**719–739. By permission.)

fragment that free κ or λ antisera would not recognize in the urine. Consequently, κ and λ antisera that are monospecific and potent and that recognize both free and combined light chains should be used.

A monoclonal protein forms an arc with κ or λ antisera that is bowed locally or restricted, whereas a polyclonal increase of light chains causes elongation and fuzziness of both κ and λ arcs (Fig. 21). In cases of renal insufficiency, faint, fuzzy, elongated κ and λ arcs are often seen, but if there is an underlying multiple myeloma or amyloidosis, an additional bowed or restricted arc with either κ or λ antisera may also be seen. Because of the arc configurations, there is usually little difficulty in distinguishing monoclonal from polyclonal light chains in the urine.

Occasionally, a thickened monoclonal arc appears as if cut off abruptly near the trough. This phenomenon may result from antigen excess or from formation of a soluble antigen-antibody complex. Consequently, immunoelectrophoresis should then be repeated with unconcentrated urine. Sometimes the monoclonal light-chain content of the urine is so high that the unconcentrated urine must be diluted to make an arc visible.

Immunofixation

Immunofixation may be helpful in detecting monoclonal Bence Jones proteins. Various concentrations of urine are electrophoresed on agarose gel, and the gel is overlaid with monospecific antisera. Formation of a localized band indicates the presence of a monoclonal protein. This technique is more sensitive than immunoelectrophoresis. Immunofixation is most helpful when a monoclonal light chain occurs in the presence of a polyclonal increase in light chains. It is also useful in detecting monoclonal heavy-chain fragments in the urine.

The need for collection of a 24-h urine specimen cannot be overemphasized. This allows one to measure the amount of the monoclonal protein excreted in the urine, which is a reliable indication of the effect of

chemotherapy (6) or evidence of progression of the disease and is also very useful in following the course of a patient who has amyloidosis and the nephrotic syndrome.

For demonstrating a monoclonal protein in the urine, electrophoresis and immunoelectrophoresis or immunofixation of an adequately concentrated specimen are the methods of choice.

Immunodiffusion

Urine studied by immunoelectrophoresis may be examined initially by immunodiffusion utilizing κ and λ light-chain antisera and a neat (unconcentrated) urine specimen as well as a concentrated urine specimen. A dense precipitin band confirms the presence of protein of that type (Fig. 22). Again, the concentrated urine may overwhelm the antisera without forming a band. Consequently, a faint band suggests the possibility of a monoclonal protein, and immunoelectrophoresis should be done with a more concentrated urine specimen to determine whether the band on immunodiffusion represents a monoclonal increase of light chain or merely polyclonal light chains. Immunodiffusion is more sensitive than immunoelectrophoresis and is a useful screening test, but it reacts to both monoclonal and polyclonal light chains; therefore immunoelectrophoresis or immunofixation must always be performed to prove that the protein detected is monoclonal.

DIFFERENTIATION OF MGUS FROM MULTIPLE MYELOMA AND MACROGLOBULINEMIA

The term monoclonal gammopathy of undetermined significance (MGUS) denotes the presence of a monoclonal protein in persons without evidence of multiple myeloma, macroglobulinemia, amyloidosis, or other related diseases. The term benign monoclonal gammopathy is misleading because it is not known at the time of diagnosis whether a monoclonal protein will remain stable and benign or will develop into symptomatic multiple myeloma, macroglobulinemia, or amyloidosis.

Persons with MGUS usually have (i) less than 3.0 g of the monoclonal protein per dl in the serum and none or small amounts of Bence Jones proteinuria, (ii)

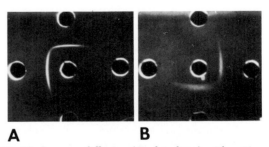

A   B

FIG. 22. Immunodiffusion (Ouchterlony) with antisera to κ (A) and λ (B) in the center of each slide. The top well and the left well show a κ band and no λ band in urine. The wells on the bottom and the right show a dense λ band and no κ band. (From R. A. Kyle and P. R. Greipp. 1978. The laboratory investigation of monoclonal gammopathies. Mayo Clin. Proc. **53:**719–739. By permission.)

fewer than 5% plasma cells in the bone marrow aspirate, and (iii) no anemia, hypercalcemia, renal insufficiency, or osteolytic lesions (unless caused by other disease). The only basis for deciding that the condition is benign is the absence of an increase of the monoclonal protein and absence of immunoproliferative disease during long-term follow-up. Differentiation of MGUS from myeloma or macroglobulinemia is fraught with difficulty at the time of recognition of the monoclonal protein. Help may be derived from the size of the serum monoclonal protein, levels of normal polyclonal or background immunoglobulin, presence and amount of Bence Jones proteinuria, number of plasma cells in the bone marrow, presence of osteolytic lesions, plasma cell-labeling index, serum β_2-microglobulin level, presence of J chains in plasma cells, and presence of monoclonal idiotypic peripheral blood lymphocytes.

The serum level of the monoclonal protein is often helpful. A monoclonal protein level of 3 g/dl or more usually indicates overt multiple myeloma or macroglobulinemia, but some exceptions, such as smoldering myeloma, do exist.

Levels of immunoglobulin classes that are not associated with the monoclonal protein (normal polyclonal or background immunoglobulins) have been suggested as being helpful in differentiating benign from malignant monoclonal gammopathies. Although reduction in normal polyclonal immunoglobulins is usual in multiple myeloma, a reduction of uninvolved immunoglobulins has been found in some patients whose monoclonal protein has followed a benign course for many years. Consequently, levels of uninvolved immunoglobulins are not a reliable differentiating feature.

The association of Bence Jones proteinuria with a serum monoclonal protein usually indicates a neoplastic process. My colleagues and I have seen many patients with a monoclonal gammopathy and a small monoclonal light chain in the urine that has remained stable for many years. We have also seen several patients with Bence Jones proteinuria (>0.8 g/day) for more than 10 years without development of multiple myeloma or amyloidosis.

The presence of more than 5% plasma cells in the bone marrow is suggestive of myeloma; but in some patients who have a more pronounced plasmacytosis, the process has remained stable for long periods. Conversely, single bone marrow specimens from patients with overt myeloma may have fewer than 5% plasma cells because the distribution of malignant cells may be spotty. Although plasma cells show morphologic atypia in multiple myeloma, these features also may appear with MGUS and smoldering multiple myeloma. Most observers agree that an atypical plasma cell does not indicate multiple myeloma. Experience has shown that plasma cell nucleolar size, grade, and asynchrony are of limited use in differentiating benign monoclonal gammopathy from multiple myeloma. The presence of increased numbers of lymphocytes, plasmacytoid lymphocytes, and plasma cells is suggestive of macroglobulinemia rather than a benign process.

The presence of osteolytic lesions is suggestive of multiple myeloma, but metastatic carcinoma may produce lytic lesions and plasmacytosis. My colleagues and I have seen several patients with a serum monoclonal protein, plasmacytosis, and lytic lesions secondary to a metastatic carcinoma.

A bone marrow plasma cell-labeling index, obtained by high-speed autoradiography, determines the percentage of plasma cells actively synthesizing DNA and is helpful in differentiating patients with overt multiple myeloma from those with benign monoclonal gammopathy or smoldering multiple myeloma (3). In 43 cases of benign monoclonal gammopathy and 9 of smoldering multiple myeloma, the patients' physicians had requested bone marrow examinations because of the possibility of multiple myeloma. The [^{3}H]thymidine-labeling index values determined in these 52 cases were compared with those in 23 cases of overt multiple myeloma. The plasma cell-labeling index correctly classified 62 (83%) of the 75 cases, and a linear discriminate function combining the labeling index and percentage of plasma cells improved the accuracy to 92% (69 of 75 cases). Occasionally, the plasma cell-labeling index is normal in patients with multiple myeloma.

Serum β_2-microglobulin levels may be helpful in differentiating benign monoclonal gammopathies from multiple myeloma in some instances. The β_2-microglobulin levels correspond to the monoclonal protein values: both decrease with chemotherapy but increase with relapse. However, the β_2-microglobulin level is similar in patients with low tumor cell mass (stage I or II myeloma) and MGUS and therefore is of limited value.

The presence of J chains in plasma cells may help to differentiate benign from malignant monoclonal gammopathies. In patients with multiple myeloma, J chains are present in more than 60% of the IgG-containing plasma cells, whereas in patients with benign monoclonal gammopathy, the J chains are in a minority of their plasma cells. Patients with Waldenström's macroglobulinemia also have cytoplasmic J chains. Both false-positive and false-negative findings occur, so this is not a reliable finding in differentiating benign from malignant disease.

T-lymphocyte populations have been studied in benign and malignant monoclonal gammopathies. In general, OKT4+ T cells are reduced in patients with multiple myeloma or Waldenström's macroglobulinemia and are normal in patients with benign monoclonal gammopathy. However, overlap exists, so this is not a reliable differentiating feature. The mixed lymphocyte reaction in patients with benign and malignant gammopathies is not significantly different from that in normal controls and does not help in differentiation. Increased numbers of monoclonal idiotype-bearing peripheral blood lymphocytes have been detected in multiple myeloma, but fewer have been detected in benign monoclonal gammopathy. Again, there is considerable overlap between benign and malignant disease. Increased numbers of immunoglobulin-secreting cells in the peripheral blood are characteristic of overt multiple myeloma, but such cells also have been noted in benign monoclonal gammopathy.

Other tests and criteria—including the presence or absence of chromosomal abnormalities, ABO blood group profiles, phytohemagglutinin stimulation of lymphocytes, and delayed skin hypersensitivity studies—have not proved to be adequate for differentiating benign monoclonal gammopathy from multiple myeloma. The content of plasma cell acid phosphatase is elevated in multiple myeloma, in contrast to benign monoclonal gammopathy, but overlap occurs.

In my experience involving patients with MGUS, the initial hemoglobin level, size of the serum monoclonal protein, number of plasma cells in the bone marrow, and levels of normal immunoglobulins do not differ significantly from those found in patients whose conditions progressed to multiple myeloma or amyloidosis or in patients whose conditions remained stable. Analysis of age, sex, presence of organomegaly, presence of small amounts of monoclonal light chain in the urine, serum albumin, and IgG subclass did not help to distinguish initially between patients with MGUS and those in whom multiple myeloma or macroglobulinemia developed.

The most reliable means of distinguishing a benign course from a malignant course is the serial measurement of the monoclonal protein. If the serum monoclonal protein is less than 2.0 g/dl, electrophoresis should be repeated 6 months after its discovery; if the concentration has not increased, electrophoresis should be repeated annually thereafter. If the monoclonal protein is 2.0 g/dl or more and there is no evidence of myeloma or macroglobulinemia after appropriate laboratory tests, electrophoresis should be repeated 3 months after the recognition of the monoclonal protein. If electrophoresis shows stability, it should be repeated in 6 months and if there is still no progression, electrophoresis should be performed every 6 to 12 months thereafter depending on the clinical findings. If the monoclonal protein increases more than 0.5 g/dl, immunoelectrophoresis of a 24-h urine specimen and a hemoglobin determination should be done. Determination of serum calcium and creatinine levels, as well as bone marrow and roentgenographic examinations, should be considered. If a monoclonal protein is present in the urine, the patient should be followed up more closely. It should be emphasized that serum protein electrophoresis, rather than quantitation of immunoglobulins, is recommended for follow-up because the former is more reproducible and less expensive.

The clinician must continue the periodic reexamination of patients with MGUS to determine whether the disorder is benign or is the initial manifestation of multiple myeloma, systemic amyloidosis, macroglobulinemia, or other malignant lymphoproliferative disorders.

This work was supported in part by Public Health Service research grant CA-16835 from the National Institutes of Health and by the Toor Myeloma Research Fund.

LITERATURE CITED

1. Fahey, J. L., and E. M. McKelvey. 1965. Quantitative determination of serum immunoglobulins in antibody-agar plates. J. Immunol. 94:84–90.
2. Gorevic, P. D., H. J. Kassab, Y. Levo, R. Kohn, M. Meltzer, P. Prose, and E. C. Franklin. 1980. Mixed cryoglobulinemia: clinical aspects and long-term follow-up of 40 patients. Am. J. Med. 69:287–308.
3. Greipp, P. R., and R. A. Kyle. 1983. Clinical, morphological, and cell kinetic differences among multiple myeloma, monoclonal gammopathy of undetermined significance, and smoldering multiple myeloma. Blood 62:166–171.
4. Kunkel, H. G. 1968. The "abnormality" of myeloma proteins. Cancer Res. 28:1351–1353.
5. Kyle, R. A., R. A. Robinson, and J. A. Katzmann. 1981. The clinical aspects of biclonal gammopathies: review of 57 cases. Am. J. Med. 71:999–1008.
6. McLaughlin, P., and R. Alexanian. 1982. Myeloma protein kinetics following chemotherapy. Blood 60:851–855.
7. Putnam, F. W., C. W. Easley, L. T. Lynn, A. E. Ritchie, and R. A. Phelps. 1959. The heat precipitation of Bence-Jones proteins. I. Optimum conditions. Arch. Biochem. Biophys. 83:115–130.
8. Rose, D. R. 1982. The generation of antibody diversity. Am. J. Hematol. 13:91–99.
9. Tarantino, A., A. De Vecchi, G. Montagnino, E. Imbasciati, M. J. Mihatsch, H. U. Zollinger, G. Barbiano Di Belgiojoso, G. Busnach, and C. Ponticelli. 1981. Renal disease in essential mixed cryoglobulinaemia: long-term follow-up of 44 patients. Q. J. Med. 50:1–30.
10. Tracy, R. P., R. A. Kyle, and D. S. Young. 1984. Two-dimensional gel electrophoresis as an aid in the analysis of monoclonal gammopathies. Hum. Pathol. 15:122–129.

Chapter 24

Gene Rearrangements Applied to Diagnostic Immunopathology

JEFFREY COSSMAN, AJAY BAKHSHI, AND STANLEY KORSMEYER

A valuable contribution to the diagnosis and classification of lymphoproliferative disease is the elucidation of specific cellular lineage and the demonstration of monoclonality. A wide variety of lineage-associated cell surface markers, usually identified by monoclonal antibodies, are often sufficient to classify a lymphoid neoplasm as being B or T cell in type (see chapter 120). In practice, monoclonality has been demonstrable within B-cell neoplasms where a secreted immunoglobulin has a restricted electrophoretic mobility, as in myeloma, or where cell-associated immunoglobulin has a single light-chain type, as in most non-Hodgkin's lymphomas and some lymphocytic leukemias. A lymphoid population that is shown to be monoclonal, and therefore derived from a single progenitor cell, is usually considered neoplastic in the appropriate clinical setting.

The process of making surface and secreted immunoglobulin is preceded by a DNA rearrangement which combines the separated gene segments responsible for the final immunoglobulin molecules. Such rearrangements are mandatory in B cells and only rarely occur in non-B-cell lineages. Gene recombination provides the organism with a mechanism to create antibodies with a vast range of antigen specificities from a limited amount of genetic information. Because the pattern of immunoglobulin gene rearrangement of a B cell is faithfully reproduced in its progeny, cells of a clonal B-cell neoplasm will all show the same gene configuration. Immunoglobulin gene rearrangements serve as clonal markers at the DNA level and do not require the final expression of the antibody product for their detection. Recently, candidate genes for both the α and β chains of the heterodimeric T-cell receptor have been cloned. These genes are organizationally similar and bear evolutionary homology to the immunoglobulin gene locus. This locus must undergo a DNA rearrangement in any T cell bearing an antigen receptor and thus serves as a T-cell-associated clonal marker at the DNA level. Finally, a host of chromosomal translocations which are uniquely or at least commonly associated with leukemias and lymphomas have been described. These recombinations involve certain genetic loci (for example, c-*myc* in Burkitt's lymphoma and c-*abl* in chronic myelogenous leukemia) and result in changes in the location of restriction enzyme sites encompassing these loci. As sites of chromosomal translocation become better defined, it should be possible to identify DNA rearrangements in many additional malignancies. In this chapter we describe how rearrangements are detected in the immunoglobulin genes. The methods described here, however, are applicable to the T-cell receptor genes and the genetic loci involved in interchromosomal translocations.

Immunoglobulin gene assembly

To understand the basis for immunoglobulin gene analysis, we will review here the molecular genetic process by which heavy-chain and then light-chain gene subsegments are assembled during early B-cell development. Initially, the genes encoding immunoglobulins lie along the chromosomes as widely separated segments. The process of forming a functional immunoglobulin gene is accomplished by a rearrangement which combines, at the DNA level, the separated gene segments responsible for the final immunoglobulin molecule. An example is the human κ-light-chain gene, shown in Fig. 1, in which one of many available variable (V_k) regions is juxtaposed with one of five joining (J_k) segments. This V_k/J_k rearrangement codes for the entire variable portion of the κ-light-chain protein. This rearranged allele is then transcribed into RNA, where the intervening sequence between V_k/J_k and C_k is removed by RNA splicing. This processed RNA is then translated into the κ-light-chain protein. The heavy-chain variable-region peptide is similarly constructed but contains additional information corresponding to the third hypervariable region (or complementarity determining region), which is contributed in part by an additional diversity gene subsegment. In addition to these movable genetic elements, this system utilizes flexibility at the sites of recombination and somatic mutation within the variable region to vastly expand the antibody repertoire from a limited amount of germ line material (reviewed in references 4 and 7).

The process of V/J (or V/D/J) joining at the DNA level generates a marker unique to an individual cell which can be detected by Southern blot analysis. These DNA rearrangements produce a change in the location of restriction endonuclease sites surrounding the gene, as is schematically depicted for the κ gene in Fig. 1. A restriction endonuclease is an enzyme which reproducibly cuts DNA only at sites where a specific set of nucleic acid bases recognized by that enzyme are aligned (for example, GGATCC for *Bam*HI) (Fig. 2). A DNA rearrangement such as V/J joining alters the location of such restriction sites and thus alters the size of the *Bam*HI fragment containing the κ gene. To demonstrate such alterations, high-molecular-weight DNA is prepared from the nuclei of the lymphoid cells, digested to completion with the appropriate restriction enzyme, size fractionated by agarose gel electrophoresis, and transferred to nitrocellulose paper. The nitrocellulose blots are then hybridized with radiolabeled DNA probes of the human immunoglobulin genes capable of detecting germ line and rearranged alleles. After these blots are washed at the appropriate stringency, the sizes of the restriction enzyme fragments bearing the immunoglobulin gene are visual-

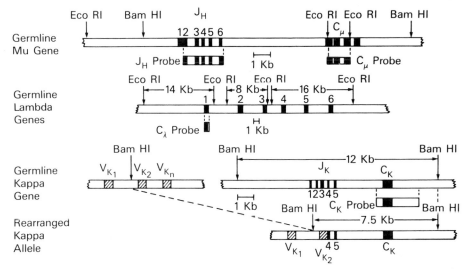

FIG. 1. Restriction map of the germ line heavy, κ, and λ genes plus a rearranged κ allele. The location of restriction enzyme sites used for the detection of immunoglobulin gene rearrangements are indicated. The corresponding cloned gene fragments (probes) are shown below each restriction map. As shown, rearrangement of a κ gene joins together one of many Vκ genes, with one of five $J_κ$ genes ($V_{κ2}$ joins $J_{κ4}$ in this case). The consequence of this recombination is an alteration of the BamHI restriction fragment site 5' (left) of the $J_κ$ region. This results in a BamHI restriction fragment length different from germline, in this case 7.5 kb as compared to a germ line 12-kb $C_κ$-BamHI fragment. If comigration of rearranged and germ line fragments is suspected, additional restriction enzymes can be used. For example, the J_H probe can detect heavy-chain gene rearrangements when either EcoRI or BamHI is used. Heavy-chain gene rearrangements are also detectable with a $C_μ$ probe that hybridizes with genomic DNA digested with BamHI. Digestion with EcoRI divides the λ locus into four restriction fragments that hybridize with the $C_λ$ probe. In most individuals, fragments of 5, 8, 14, and 16 kb are seen but restriction fragment length polymorphisms occur (see the text).

ized by autoradiography (Fig. 2). By running DNA from test lymphoid cells in parallel with a control source of DNA known to have germ line immunoglobulin genes (placenta or fibroblast DNA) it can be determined whether rearrangements have occurred.

CLINICAL USES AND INTERPRETATION

Demonstration of monoclonality

The presence of a rearranged immunoglobulin gene band on the Southern blot indicates that a monoclonal cell population is present. To have such a uniformly migrating DNA band (restriction fragment), the restriction enzyme sites flanking the hybridizing genomic (cellular) DNA must be identical from cell to cell. A homogeneous restriction fragment size would be expected only from a genetically uniform cell population. By contrast, a polyclonal B-cell population, such as from a normal lymph node or peripheral blood, would contain a mixture of B cells with heterogeneous immunoglobulin gene rearrangements and restriction fragment sizes. If no single clone predominates, no rearranged band would be detected among normal B cells since none would occur at a sufficient frequency for detection.

A word of caution concerning monoclonality: the Southern blot technique is sensitive and a rearranged band can be seen even when the clonal population represents only 1 to 5% of the total cells. Thus, it is conceivable that a band could be detected in a nonmalignant cell population. Such bands might, for example, represent regulated clones responding to antigenic challenge. Indeed, a monoclonal subpopulation of B cells was found in a lymph node from a patient with the Wiskott-Aldrich syndrome who had no evidence of lymphoma despite careful follow-up (1). Researchers should proceed with caution when interpreting a rearranged band in certain clinical settings such as an immunosuppressed host or a possible Epstein-Barr virus infection. Note: it is important to remember that the determination of clonality as detected by an immunoglobulin gene rearrangement is not, by itself, diagnostic of malignancy.

Determination of cellular lineage

It is sometimes difficult to determine the lineage of a malignant tumor. This could be because of the admixture of large numbers of nonneoplastic cells or it could be due to purely technical reasons. It may also be because the malignant cells, although committed to a particular lineage, are not yet differentiated enough to express surface markers solely restricted to a given lineage. The elucidation of specific lineage, however, has been of crucial importance in advancing our understanding of the biology, pathogenesis, and indeed the therapy of these malignancies.

Analysis of immunoglobulin gene configuration can be used to demonstrate the B-cell origin of neoplastic cells. Hematopoietic and nonhematopoietic cells which pursue other than a B-cell pathway of development usually retain their immunoglobulin genes in the germ line form. However, exceptions to this rule do occur for heavy-chain genes, which can occasionally be rearranged in T cells or myeloid cells. Light-chain genes have uniformly been retained in their germ line form within T, myeloid, monocytic, and

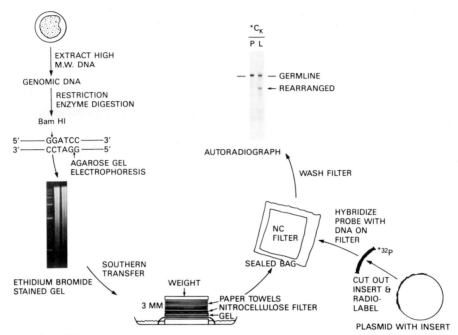

FIG. 2. Genomic (Southern) blot analysis of gene rearrangement. The Southern blot technique is used to determine whether a monoclonal population of cells with a rearranged immunoglobulin gene is present. High-molecular-weight DNA is extracted from the cells and then digested with an appropriate restriction enzyme such as *Bam*HI, which recognizes a 6-base-pair sequence. This digests the DNA into fragments of many sizes. These fragments are size separated by electrophoresis on an agarose gel, and the distribution of the various fragments is visualized by ethidium bromide and UV illumination. Molecular weight markers (λ phage DNA digested with *Hin*dIII) are run in an adjacent lane (left). The Southern transfer consists of placing a wet nitrocellulose filter directly over the gel, which allows DNA in the gel to transfer onto the nitrocellulose paper. To detect the location of specific gene sequences, for example, human immunoglobulin C_κ, the filter is placed in a bag along with a radiolabeled probe (cloned C_κ DNA). The probe hybridizes to complementary single-stranded sequences embedded in the filter, and, after washing, the location of the hybridized probe is observed by autoradiography. By running a known germ line control, such as placenta (P), in parallel with the lymphocytes (L), it can be determined whether a rearranged allele is present. In the example shown, rearrangement of one κ-light-chain gene has occurred and produced a *Bam*HI restriction enzyme fragment that includes C_κ sequences smaller than the restriction enzyme fragment obtained from germ line DNA. It can be concluded from this Southern blot analysis that a monoclonal B-cell population was present.

promyelocytic cells. Thus, the detection of simultaneously rearranged heavy- plus light-chain genes within a lymphoid neoplasm serves as a strong marker for B-cell lineage commitment. For example, it was possible to show that the so-called non-T-non-B acute lymphoblastic leukemias were really a developmental series of precursors of B cells committed to B-cell differentiation at the immunoglobulin level. Similarly, lymphoid blast crisis episodes of chronic myelogenous leukemia represent stages in the development of B-cell precursors. In addition, the leukemic cells of hairy cell leukemia demonstrate the appropriately rearranged and expressed immunoglobulin genes of a mature B-cell stage of development.

It is sometimes difficult to determine the lineage of a cell of hematopoietic derivation by routine immunological and cytochemical methods. When immunophenotypic analysis is unclear, as in some non-Hodgkin's lymphomas, molecular and genetic analysis can reveal the monoclonal B-cell nature of these neoplasms (1–5). Other types of tumors considered to be undifferentiated morphologically and lacking phenotypic characteristics of carcinoma, lymphoma, sarcoma, etc., are appropriate candidates for immunoglobulin gene rearrangement analysis. If rearrangements are found in this situation it can be concluded that the neoplasm is a B-cell-type lymphoma (1).

It must be remembered, however, that heavy-chain gene rearrangements may occur in some T cells. Thus, without other evidence, one cannot be absolutely certain that a neoplasm is B-cell type when only a heavy-chain gene is rearranged and all four light-chain alleles are germ line. Additional analysis of B- or T-cell-restricted surface antigens, in addition to seeking rearrangements of the T-cell antigen receptor, may help resolve these difficulties.

Follow-up of lymphoid malignancies

An additional application of this analysis would be the serial examination of clonal B-cell populations. This sensitive and specific marker could be used to determine both clonal evolution and early recurrence after therapy of a B-cell clone when the immunoglobulin rearrangement serves as a tumor-specific marker. Thus, the examination of two separate lymphoid blast crisis episodes from a patient with chronic myelogenous leukemia revealed that the clonally affected pluripotent stem cell precursors in chronic myelogenous leukemia are capable of sequential differentiation steps of heavy- and then light-chain gene rearrangements (2). Serial examination of bone marrow specimens from patients with B-cell neoplasms in remission may allow the early detection of recurrences before routine histologic or tumor-associated markers are capable of detecting disease.

Technical cautions

Choice of DNA probes. (See Fig. 1.) The J_H probe has the greatest overall utility when looking for heavy-chain gene rearrangements. At times the constant-region genes (C_μ, C_γ, etc.) may be deleted by heavy-chain class switch and a constant-region probe (such as C_μ) may not show a band. Some of the J_H regions will still be present after V/D/J recombination and a heavy-chain class switch and will hybridize with the J_H probe. The C_κ and C_λ probes indicated in Fig. 1 are sufficient to detect rearrangements of their corresponding genes.

Comigration: false-negative. A rearrangement may at times yield a restriction fragment approximately equal in size to the germ line form of the gene, and the two fragments then comigrate in the gel. This gives a false impression for a lack of rearrangement, and additional enzymes must be used to exclude this possibility. Usually one other enzyme is sufficient (see Fig. 1).

Polymorphisms: false-positive. Genetic polymorphisms occur in the C_λ gene. DNA from most individuals show EcoRI bands of 5, 8, 14, and 16 kilobase pairs (kb) on a Southern blot. However, other patterns occur and should not be considered rearrangements until they are shown not to be polymorphic. These restriction fragment length polymorphisms alter the 8-kb EcoRI fragment to produce bands of 13, 18, or 23 kb. If these size fragments appear, a non-B-cell source of DNA (T cells, fibroblasts, etc.) must be obtained from the individual to reveal the true germ line pattern of λ genes.

TEST PROCEDURES

Extraction of high-molecular-weight DNA

Materials. The buffer consists of 0.25 M sucrose, 50 mM Tris (pH 7.5), 25 mM KCl, and 5 mM $MgCl_2$ (Triton X-100 to be added to sucrose buffer as required). Phenol is prepared as follows. Redistilled phenol (Fluka Chemical Corp.), stored frozen at −20°C, is melted at 68°C. 8-Hydroxyquinolone is then added to a final concentration of 0.1%. The solution is extracted several times with an equal volume of buffer (1 M Tris [pH 8.0] followed by 0.1 M Tris [pH 8] and 0.2% β-mercaptoethanol until the pH of the aqueous phase is >7.6). This solution is stored at 4°C under equilibrium buffer for up to 1 month.

Method

1. Draw 20 ml of blood with EDTA (heparin may interfere with subsequent restriction enzyme digestion) in a 50-ml Falcon tube. Centrifuge out plasma at 1,000 × g for 12 min.

2. Wash cells once in phosphate-buffered saline and once in sucrose buffer (chilled).

3. Dilute cells to 10 ml per tube with chilled sucrose buffer. Mix.

4. Add 30 ml of 0.25% Triton-sucrose buffer. Vortex gently.

5. Incubate mixture 5 to 6 min on ice.

6. Centrifuge at 800 × g for 12 min in a chilled (2 to 4°C) centrifuge. Discard supernatant.

7. Resuspend pellet in 25 ml of 0.25% Triton-sucrose buffer. Vortex gently. Incubate on ice for 8 min.

8. Centrifuge at 800 × g for 10 min in a chilled centrifuge.

9. Wash pellet twice with 20 to 30 ml of sucrose buffer (without Triton X-100), centrifuging at 800 × g for 5 to 10 min.

10. Gently resuspend pellet in 5 ml of sucrose buffer. Then add 0.25 ml of 0.4 M EDTA (tetra sodium; pH 7.5), 0.7 ml of 10% sodium dodecyl sulfate (SDS) while vortexing, and 2 mg of proteinase K per tube (2-mg/ml stock), and incubate for 3 h at 37°C. This solution should be liquid. If it is too viscous, add additional increments of buffer EDTA, SDS, and proteinase K.

11. Adjust solution to 0.5 M NaCl with 5 M NaCl.

12. Extract two times (until protein is removed) with PCI (100 ml of phenol, 100 ml of chloroform, 1 ml of isoamyl alcohol) as follows: add an equal volume, shake vigorously, centrifuge at 3,000 × g for 10 min, and take top aqueous phase.

13. Extract two to three times with chloroform or until interface is clear (no more protein extracted). Take top aqueous phase.

14. Add 2.5 volumes of cold 95% ethanol in 50-ml Falcon tubes, and store at −20°C (for up to 2 days).

15. Centrifuge at 4,000 × g for 15 min in a chilled centrifuge (4°C). Pour off ethanol and air dry samples (make sure DNA pellet does not fall or slip out).

16. Resuspend in 10 mM Tris–0.5 mM EDTA. Refrigerate for 1 to 2 days to allow adequate time for the DNA to resuspend. Read the optical density at 260 nm, and adjust the DNA concentration to 0.5 µg/µl.

This method works very well for whole blood and cell lines. Other methods for extracting high-molecular-weight DNA should be used for frozen or fresh chunks of tissue.

Restriction enzyme digestion of DNA and agarose gel electrophoresis

To detect single-copy sequences, 10 µg of total mammalian DNA must be applied to a single gel slot. The DNA is digested with the appropriate enzyme using an initial concentration of 5 U of DNA per µg for 1 to 2 h at 37°C in the buffer suggested by the manufacturer (Boehringer Mannheim Biochemicals; New England BioLabs, Inc.; Bethesda Research Laboratories, Inc. [BRL]). At the end of this period it is useful to check for completeness of digestion by running 0.5 µg of the DNA on a minigel (BRL).

The restricted DNA is then size separated on an agarose gel (SeaKem agarose). The agarose is dissolved in electrophoresis buffer by bringing it to a boil in a microwave oven. The agarose is cooled to 50°C before pouring gel (pouring the gel when it is too hot can easily warp the electrophoresis apparatus). The gel may be poured on a glass plate (20 by 20 cm) with a lucite comb or with the apparatus and combs provided by the manufacturer (BRL; International Biotechnologies, Inc.). The gel is then covered with Tris-acetate buffer (50× Tris acetate buffer; 242 g of Tris, 57.1 ml of glacial acetic acid, and 37.2 g of disodium EDTA [pH 7.2]).

Load 10 to 20 µg of DNA per sample well with 1/10 volume of tracking dye (50% glycerol, 0.25% bromophenol blue). Voltage gradients are usually between 0.5 and 5 V/cm. High resolution of high-molecular-weight DNA is achieved at low voltage gradients. Higher voltage gradients are used on small DNA fragments (<2 kb) to increase mobility, thus reducing the amount of diffusion. Most frequently for immunoglobulin genes we use 1 V/cm for 24 to 36 h with Tris-acetate buffer. The mobility of DNA is almost inversely proportional to the log of the molecular length. To determine the sizes of the bands observed after autoradiography, size markers are run alongside the restricted genomic DNA (for example, lambda phage is digested with HindIII).

The electrophoresed DNA and markers can be visualized by staining the gel with 0.5 μg of ethidium bromide per ml and photographing the fluorescence after exposing the gel to UV light at 260 nm. (Note: ethidium bromide is a mutagen; therefore, gloves should be worn while handling it.) It is useful to place a ruler alongside the gel so that the distance that any given band of DNA has migrated can be read directly from the photographic image.

Transfer of DNA from agarose gels to nitrocellulose paper

1. After the gel is photographed, denature the DNA by soaking the gel in several volumes of 1.5 M NaCl and 0.5 M NaOH for 1 h at room temperature with constant shaking.

2. Neutralize the gel by soaking it in several volumes of a solution of 1 M Tris hydrochloride (pH 8.0) and 1.5 M NaCl for 1 h with shaking. (The transfer may be accomplished by neutralizing the gel after denaturation with 1 M ammonium acetate and 0.02 M NaOH and transferring in this same buffer instead of 10× SSC ["10×" means 10 times the concentration of 1× SSC; 1× SSC is 0.15 M NaCl plus 0.015 M sodium citrate].)

3. Drape a piece of Whatman 3MM filter paper wetted with 10× SSC around a piece of plexiglas or a stack of glass plates as shown (Fig. 1). Fill the dish with 10× SSC (20× SSC: dissolve 175.3 g of NaCl and 88.2 g of sodium citrate in 800 ml of water; adjust pH to 7.0 with a few drops of 10 N NaOH; adjust volume to 1 liter). Smooth out all air bubbles with a glass rod (10-ml glass pipette).

4. Invert gel, place on damp 3MM paper, and remove all air bubbles between 3MM paper and gel.

5. Cut a piece of nitrocellulose paper (Schleicher & Schuell BA 85 or Millipore HAHY) to the gel dimensions and float on a solution of 2× SSC until it wets completely from below. Then immerse the filter in 2× SSC for 2 to 3 min. If unevenly wet at the end of this period, use a new piece of nitrocellulose since the transfer will be unreliable. Wear gloves while handling nitrocellulose because it is sensitive to oil.

6. Place the wet nitrocellulose on top of the gel, once again carefully removing all air bubbles. Wet two pieces of Whatman 3MM paper and place them over the nitrocellulose filter.

7. Stack paper towels (5 to 10 cm) on the 3MM paper, put a glass plate on top of the stack, and weigh it down with a 500-g weight. Prevent short circuiting of the flow (with glass rods or Saran Wrap) of liquid from the reservoir through the gel and nitrocellulose paper.

8. Allow transfer for about 12 to 24 h. Small fragments of DNA (<1 kb) transfer within 1 to 2 h, whereas fragments greater than 15 kb take 15 h or more.

9. Remove paper towels and Whatman papers. Mark the positions of the gel slots on the nitrocellulose paper. Carefully lift off the nitrocellulose and soak in 6× SSC for 5 min. Dry at room temperature on a sheet of 3MM paper.

10. Place dried filter between two sheets of 3MM paper. Bake for 2 h at 80°C under vacuum. Store filter at room temperature under vacuum.

Radiolabeling DNA probes

The genomic fragments to be radiolabeled may first be separated from the pBR host into which they are cloned. The $C_κ$ fragment, for example (Fig. 1), is prepared from the plasmid by restriction with EcoRI, separation of the 2.5-kb EcoRI $C_κ$ region from the 4.2-kb pBR host by agarose-polyacrylamide gel electrophoresis, and then elution of the 2.5-kb fragment from the gel (by electroelution, electrophoresis onto DEAE paper, etc.). This fragment is then extracted with phenol-chloroform two times, ethanol precipitated, and finally resuspended at 0.1 μg/μl in Tris-EDTA. The fragment can then be radiolabeled by nick translation or random priming. The latter method is easier and more efficient.

1. Combine 50 to 200 ng of DNA with water to a final volume of 6.75 μl in an Eppendorf tube. Boil at 100°C for 2 min. Plunge tube into an ice bath and, when cool, centrifuge in an Eppendorf tube briefly to pellet the droplet.

2. To the denatured (single-stranded) probe add 1 μl of 10-mg/ml bovine serum albumin, 1.25 μl of 0.1-U/ml hexamer (P-L Biochemicals, Inc.), 5 μl of [^{32}P]CTP, 10 μl of 2.5× reaction buffer (0.5 M HEPES [N-2-hydroxyethylpiperazine-N'-2-ethanesulfonic acid; pH 6.6], 12.5 M MgCl$_2$, 0.025 M β-mercaptoethanol, 0.125 M Tris hydrochloride [pH 8.0], and a 50-μl solution of dGTP, dATP, dTTP), and 1 μl of Klenow fragment (BRL; Boehringer-Mannheim) of DNA polymerase.

3. Incubate at room temperature for at least 2 h (can be allowed to stand overnight).

4. Heat inactivate Klenow fragment at 68°C for 1 min. Add 150 μl of 10 mM EDTA–0.1% SDS.

5. Extract once with phenol-chloroform.

6. Separate labeled probe from free nucleotides by either column chromotography or spin columns.

Hybridization of Southern blots and autoradiography

The hybridization and washing conditions depend on the extent of homology between the probe and the sequences to be detected. The conditions described below are for detecting single-copy genes in genomic DNA using a completely homologous cloned genomic probe. An alternate method is described in reference 6.

1. For a 40-ml final volume, dissolve 4 g of dextran sulfate in 14.28 ml of water and add 16 ml of deionized formamide (Fluka), 8 ml of 20× SSC, 0.14 ml of 2 M Tris (pH 7.6), 0.4 ml of 2-mg/ml salmon sperm DNA, and 0.32 ml of 100× Denhardt solution (10 g of Ficoll,

10 g of polyvinyl pyrrolidone, 10 g of bovine serum albumin fraction V, and water to 500 ml; filter through a Nalgene filter and store at −20°C in 25-ml portions).

2. Soak the filters in the mixture described above, and then prehybridize at 40°C for 3 to 4 h in a heat-sealable plastic bag.

3. Denature probe (0.1 to 1.0 ml) by first adding 0.5 ml of 2-mg/ml salmon sperm DNA carrier and then 50 μl of 10 N NaOH. After vortexing the mixture for a few seconds, add 140 μl of 2 M Tris (pH 7.6) and 0.5 ml of 1 N HCl to neutralize. Add 20 ml of hybridization mix to denatured probe (use 50 μl/cm^2 of filter).

4. After prehybridization, cut open plastic bag, remove prehybridization fluid, and add the hybridization solution (at 40°C) to the bag. Squeeze as much air as possible from the bag. Seal the cut edge with a heat sealer.

5. Incubate the bag at 40°C for 12 to 16 h.

6. Remove the bag from the water bath, cut along three sides, and put the filters in 2× SSC–0.1% SDS at room temperature. Leave for 20 min, with occasional gentle agitation. Transfer to a fresh dish with the fresh 2× SSC–0.1% SDS. Repeat this process twice.

7. Finally, wash the filters twice for 30 min each in 0.1× SSC–0.1% SDS at 50°C with occasional gentle agitation.

8. Dry the filter at room temperature on Whatman 3MM filter paper. Tape the filters onto Whatman 3MM paper, and mark the gel slot origin with radioactive ink. Wrap the sample in Saran Wrap and apply it to X-ray film (with or without an intensifying screen) to obtain an autoradiographic image.

LITERATURE CITED

1. **Arnold, A., J. Cossman, A. Bakhshi, E. S. Jaffe, T. Waldmann, and S. J. Korsmeyer.** 1983. Immunoglobulin gene rearrangements as unique clonal markers in human lymphoid neoplasms. N. Engl. J. Med. **309:**1593–1599.

2. **Bakhshi, A., J. Minowada, A. Arnold, J. Cossman, J. P. Jensen, J. Whang-Peng, T. A. Waldmann, and S. J. Korsmeyer.** 1983. Lymphoid blast crises of chronic myelogenous leukemia represent stages in the development of B cell precursors. N. Engl. J. Med. **309:**826–831.

3. **Korsmeyer, S. J., A. Arnold, A. Bakhshi, J. V. Ravetch, U. Siebenlist, P. A. Hieter, S. O. Sharrow, T. W. LeBien, J. H. Kersey, D. G. Poplack, P. Leder, and T. A. Waldmann.** 1983. Immunoglobulin gene rearrangement and cell surface antigen expression in acute lymphoblastic leukemias of T cell and B cell precursor origins. J. Clin. Invest. **71:**301–313.

4. **Korsmeyer, S. J., A. Bakhshi, A. Arnold, K. A. Siminovitch, and T. A. Waldmann.** 1984. Genetic rearrangements of human immunoglobulin genes, p. 75–95. In M. I. Greene and A. Nisinoff (ed.), The biology of idiotypes. Plenum Publishing Corp., New York.

5. **Korsmeyer, S. J., W. C. Greene, J. Cossman, S. M. Hsu, J. P. Jensen, L. M. Neckers, S. L. Marshall, A. Bakhshi, J. M. Depper, W. J. Leonard, E. S. Jaffe, and T. A. Waldmann.** 1983. Rearrangement and expression of immunoglobulin genes and expression of TAC antigen in hairy cell leukemia. Proc. Natl. Acad. Sci. U.S.A. **80:**4522–4526.

6. **Maniatis, T., E. F. Fritsch, and J. Sambrook (ed.).** 1982. Molecular cloning: a laboratory manual. Cold Spring Harbor Laboratory, Cold Spring Harbor, N.Y.

7. **Tonegawa, S.** 1983. Somatic generation of antibody diversity. Nature (London) **302:**575–581.

Chapter 25

Section D. Complement and Immune Complexes

Introduction

PETER H. SCHUR

It has been traditional to present the subjects of complement and immune complexes together. This reflects the historical definition of complement as the heat-labile factor in normal serum that interacts with immune complexes. This interaction was first recognized as the killing of either (antibody-) sensitized bacteria or erythrocytes. The last 50 years have seen the isolation and characterization of the 18 proteins that make up the serum complement system. The role of complement in immune complex disorders has been determined. However, scientists do not sit still. They have demonstrated that there are many types of immune complexes, each with different biological properties, and that only some of them interact with ("fix") complement. Although serum complement is often consumed by immune complexes, other mechanisms may account for low serum levels, such as poor synthesis, activation by complex polysaccharides and bacteria, or genetic reasons. While we now talk of the 18 serum complement components, genetic studies have demonstrated further heterogeneity of these proteins. These allotypes may be associated with particular diseases, which may tell us more about their function. Some complementologists have also become molecular biologists and have isolated DNA se-quences (clones) that control specific complement component structure. Analysis of complement DNA has demonstrated greater heterogeneity within this system than have studies in which specific components were analyzed as proteins.

Although earlier studies examined the complement binding sites of immunoglobulins, more attention has recently focused on cellular receptors of complement. This "complement" system is complex. It is involved in immune complex clearance, phagocytosis, cytotoxicity, chemotaxis, leukocyte respiration, and secretion. There are receptors for complement components on erythrocytes, polymorphs, monocytes, lymphocytes, mast cells, and even glomerular podocytes. At least three receptors are recognized: CR1, CR2, and CR3. Another cellular protein, delay-accelerating factor (DAF), is also involved in modulating complement cellular interactions and is species specific.

Thus the complement system keeps growing. In this section we have addressed a number of the well-characterized components of the system and its cousin, immune complexes, and how the laboratory-oriented physician and scientist can measure complement and immune complexes and determine what they mean in biological phenomena and in disease.

Chapter 26

Complement†

SHAUN RUDDY

"Complement" originally meant a heat-labile factor in normal serum required to complete the killing of bacteria coated with antibody. The complement system now includes 18 plasma proteins which mediate a variety of inflammatory effects in addition to bacteriolysis. All of the complement proteins have now been purified to homogeneity (Table 1), and their functions are known. Recognition of activating agents by either of two proteolytic pathways (Fig. 1) leads to a final common sequence which assembles the membrane attack complex (Fig. 2). The classic activation pathway—so called because it was discovered first—is triggered primarily by immune complexes formed from the union of immunoglobulin G or M antibodies with their antigens. The alternative pathway—phylogenetically the more primitive—is activated principally by repeating polysaccharides and similar polymeric structures. Activation by either pathway generates enzymes with identical specificity: both pathways cleave the third complement component, C3, releasing the 8,000-molecular-weight activation peptide C3a from the remainder of the molecule, C3b. Both pathways also lead to cleavage of C5 and assembly of the membrane attack complex from the terminal sequence (C5b-C9). Proteins of the classic pathway and the terminal sequence are called components and are symbolized by the letter C followed by a number, e.g., C1, C4, C2, C3, C5, C6, C7, C8, and C9. Proteins of the alternative pathway are termed factors and are symbolized by letters, e.g., B, D, and P. Enzymatically active forms are indicated by a bar over the letter or number, e.g., C1s, D̄. Cleavage fragments are noted with suffixed lowercase letters, e.g., C3a and C3b. Control proteins are symbolized by contractions of their trivial names, e.g., C1 inhibitor, C4 binding protein (C4BP), C3b inactivator (I), and β1H globulin (H).

Classic activation pathway

In the classic activation pathway, the first component, C1, exists in serum as a calcium-dependent complex of three glycoprotein molecules, C1q, C1r, and C1s; these molecules are present in equimolar concentrations. The C1q molecule bears six recognition units for sites on the Fc portions of immunoglobulins. The binding of two or more recognition units on C1q induces a rearrangement in C1r, converting it to an active protease which cleaves both itself and C1s. The natural substrates of the active C1s protease are C4 and C2. Both are cleaved, releasing activation peptides, with the major fragments being incorporated into a magnesium-dependent enzyme complex, C42, the classic pathway C3 convertase. Normal serum contains an α-2 neuraminoglycoprotein which complexes with both C1s and C1r, irreversibly block-

†This paper is publication no. 224 from the Charles W. Thomas Fund.

ing the activities of these proteases, thereby preventing the activation of C1s or the cleavage of C4 and C2. Control of the assembly of C42 is effected by two plasma proteins: C4BP and C3b-C4b. C4b generated by the action of C1s on C4 is further cleaved by I in the presence of C4BP into two inactive fragments, C4c and C4d.

Alternative activation pathway

Polysaccharides such as those found in the coats of yeasts, pneumococci, or many gram-negative bacteria induce cleavage of C3 and assembly of the membrane attack complex by a mechanism which is independent of the classic pathway. In a reaction which is strikingly similar to that of the classic pathway, four factors participate in the formation of the alternative pathway convertase. Factor D, C3, and factor B are the homologous proteins for C1s, C4, and C2, respectively. An extra protein, properdin, serves to stabilize the magnesium-dependent complex enzyme C3 convertase, C3bBb, which is identical to C42 in its capacity to cleave C3 and C5 and to initiate the terminal sequence. Just as cleavage of C4 to C4b reveals a site for interaction with C2, cleavage of C3 to C3b permits its participation in a complex with factor B. Cleavage of C3b-bound B by D yields C3bBb. Unlike C1, factor D already exists in plasma in its active form. Control of proteolysis is limited by the availability of substrate: D acts only on B which has complexed with C3b and not on free or unbound B. A positive feedback or amplification loop is built into the alternative pathway. C3b, the product of the cleavage reaction catalyzed by C3bBb, is itself capable of complexing with additional B, rendering it susceptible to cleavage by D, thereby producing additional C3bBb. Uncontrolled cycling of this loop is prevented by the following reactions: (i) H dissociates the C3bBb complex, rendering it inactive, and (ii) I further degrades C3b in the presence of H, yielding C3c and C3dg. Agents which trigger the alternative pathway do so by protecting the newly formed C3bBb from dissociation and degradation by these two control proteins. These agents increase the formation of the alternative pathway convertase by transforming an inefficient fluid-phase reaction into fruitful solid-state assembly of the enzyme complex. In the fluid phase, a small amount of C3 is continuously being hydrolyzed at its internal thiolester bond, permitting B to complex with it and become susceptible to cleavage by D. This reaction generates small amounts of C3 convertase and produces small amounts of C3b. Surfaces which activate the alternative pathway provide a haven on which the small amount of C3b produced by the fluid-phase reactions can be deposited and protected from the action of H and I, thereby shifting the slow fluid-phase reaction to an amplified solid-state cleavage.

TABLE 1. Proteins of the complement system

Complement system and components	Mol wt	Serum concn (μg/ml)	Cleavage fragments
Classic activation pathway			
C1q	385,000	70	
C1r	190,000	34	
C1s	174,000	31	
C4	209,000	430	C4a, C4b, C4c, C4d
C2	117,000	30	C2a, C2b
Alternative activation pathway			
Properdin	220,000	25	
$\overline{D}$	23,500	2	
B	100,000	240	Bb, Ba
C3	180,000	1,300	C3a, C3b, C3c, C3d, C3g
Terminal sequence			
C5	206,000	75	C5a, C5b
C6	128,000	60	
C7	121,000	55	
C8	153,000	80	
C9	79,000	160	
Control proteins			
C$\overline{1}$INH[a]	105,000	150	
I	88,000	35	
H	150,000	360	
C4BP	590,000	400	

[a] C1INH, C1 inhibitor.

Terminal sequence

The terminal sequence is illustrated in Fig. 2. C3b provides a binding site for native C5, making it susceptible to cleavage by either the classic or alternative pathway convertases. The products of this reaction are the 11,000-molecular-weight activation peptide, C5a, and the remainder of the molecule, C5b. Activated C5b has a specific metastable binding site for C6 and combines with it to form C5b6, which reacts with C7. Binding of the nascent complex of C5b67 to cell membranes is the first step in assembling the membrane attack complex. Reaction with C8 initiates membrane damage, but formation of a stable transmembrane channel requires the addition of multiple molecules of C9, possibly in polymeric form, to the complex. The C5b-C9 complex is inserted through the lipid bilayer of the cell membrane, with hydrophobic residues on the exterior in contact with the lipid bilayer, and leads to osmotic lysis of the cell.

Synthesis and metabolism of complement proteins

Although in vitro culture studies have detected synthesis of C4, C2, C3, B, D, and properdin by peritoneal macrophages, in vivo studies have tended to identify the liver as the primary, if not sole, source of synthesis. Patients with severe hepatic failure have marked depressions of the levels of C4 and C3 in serum, and impaired synthesis of C3 has been measured directly in metabolic turnover studies.

Measurements of the fractional catabolic rates of C4, C3, C5, and B indicate that complement proteins are among the most rapidly metabolized of all plasma proteins. The mean fractional catabolic rates in nor-

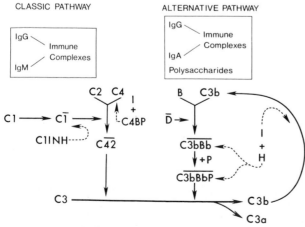

FIG. 1. Pathways for complement activation.

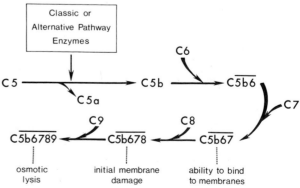

FIG. 2. Assembly of the membrane attack complex.

mal individuals are in the range of 50% of the plasma pool over 24 h. Synthetic rates are significantly correlated with levels in serum, indicating that in normal individuals, the rate of synthesis is the major determinant of concentration in plasma. Levels in plasma reflect the balance between catabolism and synthesis. Increased synthetic rates induced by an inflammatory condition may produce elevated levels of complement proteins. When the disease progresses to a state in which increased utilization of complement proteins is occurring, levels may then fall into the normal range. For this reason, serial determinations of levels in an individual patient are often much more informative than measurements at isolated times.

Complement genetics

With the exception of properdin, which is X linked, the synthesis of complement proteins is encoded by genes inherited in an autosomal codominant fashion. Congenital deficiency is the consequence of inheritance of a null gene, which codes for nonsynthesis of the protein and is allelic with the normal structural gene. Inheritance of C4 is complicated by the existence of two adjacent loci, C4A and C4B, which are separated by about 10 kilobases of DNA. At both of these loci, null (Q0) alleles are common, and levels in serum roughly correspond to the number of expressed C4 genes. Individuals homozygous for null alleles at both loci (C4AQ0,BQ0/C4AQ0,BQ0) are rare, but those with one, two, or three null alleles and levels in serum equal to three-fourths, one-half, or one-fourth of the normal mean occur more frequently. The C4 genes are located on the sixth chromosome, in the region of the major histocompatibility complex, between the HLA-D/DR and HLA-B loci. The genes are about 30 kilobases downstream from the genes for C2 and factor B, the homologous proteins of the classic and alternative pathways, which are separated from each other by less than 2 kilobases.

The relatively high frequency of null alleles coding for nonsynthesis of complement protein causes aberrations in the distribution of concentrations in plasma in the normal population. Undoubtedly this situation occurs in the case of C4. It is difficult to distinguish individuals who inherit a null allele at one of the two C4 loci, and who therefore have approximately 75% of the normal mean, from individuals who have four fully functional genes. Even those who are heterozygous null at both loci and would be expected to have a level in plasma which was 50% of normal are often difficult to identify. The predicted result is a much broader range of normal in the population. Partly because of these null alleles, the normal range for most complement proteins is quite broad, usually ±50% of the normal mean.

METHODS OF MEASUREMENT

Functional assays have been devised to measure groups of components, e.g., those of the classic and alternative activation pathways and the terminal sequence, or individual components, e.g., C1, C4, C2, and C3. Immunochemical assays for individual complement proteins or fragments of these proteins are also available and are more commonly used (8).

Total hemolytic complement assay

The total hemolytic complement assay (also called the CH_{50} assay) is the traditional method for the determination of complement in serum or other body fluids. It measures the ability of the test sample to lyse 50% of a standard suspension of sheep erythrocytes (E) coated with optimal amounts of rabbit antibody in a reaction that includes the entire classic activation pathway as well as the terminal sequence. These antibody-coated erythrocytes (EA) are incubated with various dilutions of the test specimen for a time sufficient to complete the reaction, the mixtures are centrifuged, and the percent hemolysis is determined from spectrophotometric measurements of hemoglobin released into the supernatant by the lysed cells. When percent lysis is plotted against input amount of serum, a typical sigmoid curve, resembling a cumulative normal distribution, results. Values in the range from 10 to 90% are linearly transformed either by plotting on probit graph paper or by using the Von Krogh transformation. The volume of serum containing 1 CH_{50} unit, i.e., a volume corresponding to 50% hemolysis, is determined graphically, and from this value the number of CH_{50} units per milliliter of test specimen is calculated. The actual number of CH_{50} units obtained per milliliter is a function of the number of EA in the test system, the relative concentrations of the reactants, the ionic strength of the buffer system, and many other variables. Either of two systems is commonly employed in clinical laboratories: the method of Kent and Fife (4), which measures the lysis of 0.6 ml of a 1% suspension of EA in a total volume of 1.5 ml, or the method of Mayer (7), which measures the lysis of 1.0 ml of a 5% suspension of EA in a total volume of 7.5 ml. Although the exact limits of a normal population must be determined by assays in the laboratory in which the test is being performed, normal CH_{50} values for the Kent and Fife method are usually in the range of 125 to 300 U/ml, and values for the Mayer method are 25 to 50 U/ml.

Because the alternative pathway induces the lysis of unsensitized rabbit erythrocytes, the activity of this pathway in conjunction with the terminal sequence may be assessed by substituting rabbit erythrocytes for E and omitting the antibody. Selectivity for the alternative pathway is improved by the addition of a chelating agent such as ethylene glycol tetraacetic acid with excess magnesium, which eliminates the calcium-dependent function of C1, but permits the assembly of the magnesium-dependent C3bBb.

Effective molecule titrations of individual components

Molecule titrations of individual components also involve the lysis of E, but these titrations are designed with purified components and stable intermediate complexes of the immune hemolytic system. The test sample supplies the missing component in a hemolytic system in which all other components are present in excess either on the cell or in the fluid phase. The result is a stoichiometric titration in which the average numbers of hemolytic sites formed per cell are calculated by application of the Poisson distribution. The number of effective molecules of the component being measured is calculated from the dilution required to generate an average of one site per cell and the number of cells in the reaction mixture.

Radial immunodiffusion

Antibodies specific for each of the complement proteins are available, and, with the exception of factor D, concentrations of these proteins in plasma are high enough to permit their detection by the simple technique of single radial immunodiffusion. An appropriate dilution of a monospecific antibody is incorporated into a buffered agar gel, holes are punched in the gel, and test material is placed in the holes. As the antigenic complement protein diffuses into the gel containing the antibody directed against it, a ring of immune precipitation forms. The size of the ring increases as diffusion continues, until the source of antigenic complement protein contained in the well is exhausted, and equilibrium is reached. At this point, the area of the precipitin ring is proportional to the concentration of complement protein originally placed in the well. Known concentrations of complement proteins are placed in some of the wells in the gel, and a standard curve relating ring area to concentration is constructed. The concentration in the test specimen is obtained by interpolating its ring area on the standard curve.

Nephelometric immunoassays

When a specific antibody interacts with antigen, complex formation occurs, and the intensity of light scatter increases. Although changes in dilute solutions may not be visible to the naked eye, they can be measured with an appropriate nephelometric apparatus. A number of systems for the analysis of such reactions have been marketed during the past 10 years. Some incorporate a laser light source for a high degree of collimation and detection at a narrow angle of scatter, with measurements made at equilibrium, when the formation of complexes has proceeded to completion; at this point the intensity of light scatter is proportional to the antigen concentration. Other systems measure the rate of change of light scatter during the complex formation; i.e., the maximum rate of change occurs at the kinetic equivalence point and is a linear function of antigen concentration. All of the systems include a high degree of automation, with sample handling and data analysis under microprocessor control.

Detection of activation or cleavage products

The limited proteolytic reactions of the complement system give rise to a number of activation peptides or degradation fragments. For example, the anaphylatoxins C4a, C3a, and C5a are N-terminal peptides liberated from C4, C3, and C5. In the alternative pathway, the fragment Ba is released from factor B when it is elevated by factor D. Degradation of C4b by factor I in the presence of C4BP produces C4c and C4d. Similarly, degradation of C3b by factor I in the presence of H or cell surface C3b receptors yields C3c and C3dg. Detection of such reaction products, whose concentrations in plasma or interstitial fluids are normally close

to zero, may provide more sensitive indices of complement activation during disease than a fall in the concentration of a particular component in plasma. Since detection of the fragments often employs an antibody which reacts with determinants on the native molecule, the intact complement protein must first be removed from the sample by differential precipitation with either polyethylene glycol or dilute acid. The remaining fragments are then detected by immunoprecipitation or radioimmunoassay, depending on the concentrations at which they must be identified.

Among these assays, sensitive and reproducible methods for the detection of nanogram quantities of the anaphylatoxin peptides (C3a, C4a, and C5a) have been developed. The plasma of patients undergoing extracorporeal circulation transiently contains elevated levels of C5a which are temporally associated with the leukopenia and depressed pO_2 observed during the initiation of this procedure (3). Synovial fluid from patients with rheumatoid arthritis or gout have markedly increased levels of C3a, whereas the level of C5a is within normal limits. Measurements of C3a may provide a more sensitive index of in vivo complement activation than those of C5a because the latter peptide is avidly bound to receptors on leukocytes and is thereby rapidly cleared from the circulation.

Although C3b and its derivative C3c are rapidly catabolized, C3d (or possibly C3dg) appears to have a much longer half-life in plasma. A number of methods for the detection of circulating C3d depend on precipitation of the larger and less soluble native C3, C3b, iC3b, and C3c with polyethylene glycol, followed by various methods to measure the residual soluble C3d. Elevated levels of C3d have been found in plasma from patients with systemic lupus erythematosus or rheumatoid arthritis and with parasitosis, as well as in synovial fluid from patients with rheumatoid arthritis. Levels of C3d have been used to monitor clinical activity in systemic lupus erythematosus, although in rheumatoid arthritis they are not any better than measurements of C-reactive protein in plasma.

Comparison of methods

Measurement of the total hemolytic complement activity is a useful procedure for detecting homozygous deficiency of a component or factor, but does not exclude all abnormalities of individual components, either congenital or acquired. Large variations in the levels of certain proteins may not be reflected as an abnormal CH_{50} value. In addition to this lack of sensitivity, the CH_{50} value, when it is subnormal, provides no information on the mechanism of the depression. In patients with impaired host defenses suspected due to complement deficiency, the CH_{50} assay is a useful screening test.

Immunoassays measure the complement protein as antigen, without regard to whether or not it is active. Excepting certain kindreds with hereditary angioedema, in which the synthesis of nonfunctional but antigenically intact C1 inhibitor is inherited, the difference between the results of functional and immunochemical determinations in plasma is not clinically important. Functionally inactive products of the component sequence are cleared very rapidly from the plasma, so that precipitation of a component in an in vivo reaction is usually reflected by depressed levels in serum as measured by either functional or antigenic assays. In the case of closed body spaces such as the synovial, pleural, pericardial, and subarachnoid spaces, clearance of spent complement protein proceeds at a much slower rate, so that considerable divergence between the results of functional and immunoassays may be observed.

Immunoassays are reasonably priced, and in most cases they provide information equivalent to functional assays. The technique of radial immunodiffusion is simple and reliable. Kits for the measurement of C3, C4, and factor B are available from a number of reagent suppliers, and it is not difficult to prepare immunodiffusion plates by the procedure described below, given a source of monospecific antibody. Nephelometric procedures are much more rapid and less laborious than radial immunodiffusion. For laboratories at medical centers involved in the analysis of large numbers of specimens, the high initial expense of the equipment and the relatively high continuing expense of the reagents are offset by decreases in labor costs. The precision of nephelometry is approximately the same as that of radial immunodiffusion, with coefficients of variation in the range of 5 to 10% (2).

CLINICAL INDICATIONS

Complement measurements should be performed whenever utilization due to a complement-activating disease is suspected or whenever hyposynthesis due to inherited deficiency is a possibility. Clinically, the former usually presents as a rheumatic disease, and the latter presents as recurrent infection due to impaired host defenses. Immunoassays for individual components, e.g., C4 and C3, are most useful in monitoring patients with immunologic diseases, whereas functional assays which screen for the activities of several components are more likely to detect inherited deficiencies. The precise clinical indications for complement measurements are not agreed upon.

INTERPRETATION

Sample collection and storage

Most instances of contradictory or uninterpretable results obtained from complement assays are traceable to improper handling or storage of specimens. Because complement proteins are heat labile, any sample which will be subjected to a functional assay must be collected and preserved with care that exceeds that available in routine clinical pathology laboratories. The results of immunoassays may also be altered by excessive exposure to heat; the antigens associated with C1q and C5 are especially heat labile. C3 and C4 are cleaved into smaller, but still antigenic, fragments which diffuse more rapidly and yield artifactually high values in radial immunodiffusion, although the increase does not usually exceed 10%. Values obtained by nephelometry, which is not influenced by diffusion, remain unchanged if the antiserum used is directed principally against the most common antigens of these proteins and not against those selectively represented in the native or intact

molecule. Improper sample collection often produces spurious elevations in assays for activation or cleavage products.

Blood obtained by clean venipuncture should be allowed to clot for about 1 h at room temperature, centrifuged at 4°C, and frozen in aliquots at −70°C in an electric freezer. It is important that clotting occur at room temperature, because at 0°C, cold activation of the complement system may occur, with resultant loss of activity. Although storage at −20°C may preserve hemolytic activity overnight, comparative studies have demonstrated diminutions in activity after 30 days at −20°C, even in lyophilized samples, with continued deterioration over the ensuing 2 months. Repeated freezing and thawing of a specimen are also deleterious to the activity. If circumstances are such that the proper handling or storage of a specimen cannot be ensured, the inclusion of one or more normal control specimens in the processing and storage procedure may provide an index to the adequacy of handling. If the quality of the specimen processing is in doubt, the examination of the mobility in immunoelectrophoresis of serum C3 is a useful screening test. If part or all of the C3 is converted to the electrophoretically fast form, C3c, handling was probably improper, since the finding of circulating C3c in the plasma in vivo is an extremely rare event.

Standardization

The Complement Standardization Subcommittee and the Biometrics Subcommittee of the International Union of Immunological Societies have conducted a multinational study of four processed, freeze-dried serum pools (10). Several immunologic methods were used to determine the analytic suitability of each candidate preparation. The analysis was restricted to antigenic activity and total hemolytic complement, the number of collaborators who provided data for effective molecule titrations being too small. The mean coefficients of variation between duplicate assays performed in the same laboratory were approximately 5% for immunoassays and 10% for functional assays. When the differences in relative potency of the four preparations were examined, most of the variance was due to differences among collaborators, with some laboratories consistently reporting higher potencies for all measurements. Overall, the coefficient of variation was approximately 10%. One preparation was selected and recommended for acceptance by the World Health Organization Expert Committee on Biological Standardization, to be defined as containing 100 IU/ml. The primary standard has been made available to major reagent suppliers and to local laboratories for the preparation of secondary standards. Such a standard for immunoassay of C3 and C4 is available from the Biological Products Program, Center for Infectious Diseases, Centers for Disease Control, Atlanta, Ga.

This agreement on international standardization has not had wide effects on clinical practice in the United States, as judged by comparative surveys. While comparisons of ratios between values of two standards obtained by the same laboratory indicated an acceptable degree of precision, the accuracy, as judged by absolute values (milligrams per deciliter) obtained for the same standard in different laboratories, showed a much higher degree of variation. The absolute values reported were highly dependent on the technique used, suggesting an inadequate standardization of reagents. A survey conducted in 1984 by the College of American Pathologists demonstrated that even for the same technique, absolute values reported were highly dependent on the reagent supplier. For example, 46 laboratories using the same kit for radial immunodiffusion reported a concentration of 19.5 ± 4.9 mg/dl (mean ± standard deviation) for a C3 test sample, whereas 30 other laboratories using a kit from another supplier reported a value of 31.0 ± 2.5 mg/dl.

Normal range

In view of the very large differences in normal population means reported by various suppliers of reagents, even for the most commonly measured of the components, and the likelihood of genetically determined true differences among populations, the normal range for each component should be determined by the systematic examination of a normal population in the laboratory performing the measurement.

Complement proteins are acute-phase reactants, and levels tend to increase with intercurrent illnesses, so that a brief medical history is required to determine the normality of the individuals selected as controls. A tendency for levels to be elevated in females who are either pregnant or using oral contraceptives has been noted, and such persons should be excluded from any normal control series. In neonates, levels of most components are less than those in adults, but this aberrancy disappears within a few weeks. Levels tend to rise slightly in aged individuals, but the differences are not sufficiently large to be clinically significant.

The ranges of normal complement protein concentrations are quite broad, ordinarily approximately ±50% of the normal population mean. In part, this reflects the inclusion of individuals with one or more null alleles for the protein being measured, since it is often impossible to identify such individuals without family studies. Values are usually not symmetrically distributed about the mean but are skewed toward higher levels. Logarithmic transformation of the data is often required to obtain a normal distribution and permit statistically correct calculation of the 95% confidence limits for the population.

The broad range of normal, the relatively poor standardization from laboratory to laboratory, and the relatively high coefficient of variation of replicates from the same laboratory all make the interpretation of an isolated value from an individual very difficult. At the very least, such interpretation should be made with reference to a normal control population collected and analyzed by the laboratory that performed the test. Measurements of levels in serum in a few normal individuals over several years indicate that the level of any component for a particular individual tends to be set within much narrower limits than the broad range of normals. Trends in levels, even within the normal range, observed in serial measurements for a single individual over time are, therefore, often more meaningful than comparison of an isolated determination with levels in a normal group.

Increases in concentrations in plasma

The most frequent abnormality in complement determinations is an elevated level. This elevation is due to increased synthesis and occurs as part of the acute-phase response. It is accompanied by characteristic changes in the levels of other plasma proteins, most notably increases in C-reactive protein, serum amyloid A protein, alpha-1 acid glycoprotein, and haptoglobin and decreases in transferrin and albumin levels. Elevations in levels of total hemolytic activity, C3, and C4 in plasma occur regularly in the active phase of virtually all rheumatic diseases including rheumatoid arthritis, systemic lupus erythematosus, dermatopolymyositis, scleroderma, rheumatic fever, ankylosing spondylitis, and temporal arteritis. In these diseases elevated levels are frequent, so that a level at the lower limit of normal may be inappropriate and indicate in vivo complement activation. Other conditions in which elevated levels have been observed include acute viral hepatitis, myocardial infarction, cancer, diabetes, pregnancy, sarcoidosis, amyloidosis, thyroiditis, inflammatory bowel disease, typhoid fever, and pneumococcal pneumonia. The magnitude of the increase in complement protein rarely exceeds twofold, compared with increases as high as 100- to 1,000-fold with C-reactive protein.

Decreased concentrations due to hypercatabolism

Any disease associated with circulating immune complexes is likely to lead to acquired hypocomplementemia, including systemic lupus erythematosus, rheumatoid arthritis, subacute bacterial endocarditis, hepatitis B surface antigenemia, pneumococcal infection, gram-negative sepsis, viremias such as measles, or recurrent parasitemias such as malaria. Essential mixed cryoglobulinemia, a disease characterized by arthritis or arthralgias, cutaneous vasculitis, and nephritis, is invariably accompanied by profound hypocomplementemia due to classic pathway activation by the immune complexes which occur in this disease. In contrast to most immune complex diseases, which have evidences of classic pathway activation such as a low C4 level, type II membranoproliferative glomerulonephritis is associated with normal levels of C4 and low levels of C3, factor B, and properdin, indicating direct activation of the alternative pathway. The responsible mechanism involves circulating C3 nephritic factor, an autoantibody directed against the alternative pathway C3-cleaving enzyme, which combines with this enzyme and stabilizes it, favoring positive feedback into the amplification loop.

Systemic lupus erythematosus. Total hemolytic complement levels are depressed at some time in most patients with systemic lupus erythematosus, whereas levels are generally normal in patients with discoid lupus. As a rule, complement depressions are associated with increased severity of disease, especially renal disease. Component analyses have demonstrated low levels of C1, C4, C2, and C3. Serial observations often reveal decreased levels preceding clinical exacerbations; reductions in C4 occur before reductions of C3, other components, and total hemolytic complement activity (9). As attacks subside, levels return toward normal in the reverse order, with C4 tending to remain depressed longer, even when the patient appears to be doing well clinically. The clinical usefulness of monitoring complement levels in patients with systemic lupus is controversial. Opinions range from those recommending complement measurements enthusiastically to those who find no value in these tests. Authors of studies with more detailed clinical characterizations of patients and longer follow-ups tend to conclude that complement determinations are useful adjuncts in the management of patients with known systemic lupus erythematosus and that they are useful tools in the diagnosis of this disease (6, 11). The hemolytic activity of C4 in cerebrospinal fluid is labile, and measurements are not helpful in the diagnosis of central nervous system lupus unless base-line levels, made while the patient has no central nervous system involvement, are available. Levels of complement in synovial fluid are usually profoundly depressed in patients with systemic lupus erythematosus.

Rheumatoid arthritis. Levels of total hemolytic complement activity, C3, and C4 in serum are usually normal or elevated in patients with rheumatoid arthritis. Depressed levels are associated with extra-articular manifestations of the disease, particularly vasculitis. Such patients usually also have a high titer of rheumatoid factor in their serum, circulating immune complexes which are detectable by C1q-binding assays, and often small amounts of antinuclear antibody. Levels of complement in synovial fluid are low in patients with rheumatoid arthritis when the levels are measured by activity determinations, and depression of the level of total hemolytic complement activity, C4, or C2 is most frequently found in patients with positive tests for rheumatoid factor. Levels of complement component protein measured in synovial fluid by radial immunodiffusion are usually normal, due to the presence of antigenically intact but functionally inactive complement fragments which have not been cleared from the joint space. Cleavage fragments of C3 in synovial fluid include C3c and C3d, high proportions of C3d in relation to total C3, electrophoretically converted forms of C3, and increased C3a by radioimmunoassay. The clinical significance of complement measurements in synovial fluid is marginal. The only functional assay widely available is the assay for total hemolytic complement activity, and it is by no means uniformly subnormal in cases of rheumatoid arthritis, nor is the finding of a depressed level unique to rheumatoid arthritis. In one study, the sensitivity of the CH_{50} assay for the diagnosis of seropositive rheumatoid arthritis was determined to be 70%, and the specificity was only 66%. The finding of a depressed level of total hemolytic complement activity in synovial fluid is not correlated with disease duration.

Depressed levels due to hyposynthesis

Acquired deficiency. Severe liver disease, with impaired hepatic synthesis of plasma proteins, is occasionally associated with depressed complement levels. Protein-calorie malnutrition has the same effect.

C1 inhibitor deficiency: hereditary angioedema. Depressed levels of total hemolytic complement activity, C4, and C2 may be manifestations of an underlying deficiency of C1 inhibitor. Afflicted individuals experience lifelong and recurrent swelling of the subepithelial tissues of the skin and the upper respiratory and gastrointestinal tracts. Family history may not be positive. Clinical attacks of edema are accompanied by the appearance of free active C1 in the plasma and by falls in the levels of C4 (which are subnormal even during asymptomatic intervals) to undetectable. Diagnosis is most simply and reliably made by the C4 level; a normal value virtually excludes the diagnosis. Some kindreds synthesize an abnormal C1 inhibitor protein that is reactive in immunoassays but devoid of the ability to inhibit the C1 enzyme, so that direct immunoassays for C1 inhibitor may not detect all cases. Diagnosis is clinically important so that precautions can be taken to prevent death from laryngeal edema and because the disease is treatable by the administration of nonmasculinizing androgenic steroid hormones.

Congenital deficiencies and impaired host defense. The role of C3 in host defenses against pyogenic microorganisms is evident from the severe recurrent infections that afflict individuals who are homozygously deficient for this component. Complete deficiency of factor I or factor H also leads to uncontrolled cycling of the alternative pathway amplification loop and secondary hypercatabolism and depletion of C3. Such individuals also have recurrent pyogenic infections. Recurrent neisserial infections, either meningococcal or gonococcal, occur in individuals homozygously deficient for any of the constituents of the membrane attack complex (C5, C6, C7, C8, or C9), indicating the importance of bacteriolysis in host defense against these agents.

Congenital deficiency and rheumatic disease. Homozygous deficiencies of the early-reacting components, i.e., C1, C4, or C2, are clearly associated with an increased frequency of rheumatic diseases such as systemic lupus erythematosus (1). Ordinarily this disease is milder, has less renal and more extensive and disfiguring skin involvement, and has a weakly positive or negative antinuclear antibody test, though exceptions, including patients with florid lupus glomerulonephritis, have been reported. A complete list of the complement deficiencies reported with associated rheumatic diseases is included in Table 2. Some of the associations may reflect the fact that patients with rheumatic disease tend to have their complement levels measured more frequently than do normal individuals. In the case of systemic lupus erythematosus, however, a case control study demonstrated that C2 deficiency was significantly more prevalent among patients than among a group of control blood donors. Since patients with C1 and C4 deficiency, as well as those with acquired classic pathway defects due to C1 inhibitor deficiency, have been reported to have systemic lupus erythematosus, it seems likely that impaired processing of immune complexes may be involved.

REAGENTS

Functional assays

Day-to-day variations in assay sensitivity are minimized by constancy of supply of reagents. For example, most laboratories engaged in complement re-

TABLE 2. Complement deficiencies associated with rheumatic diseases

Deficient protein	Disease
C1q	Glomerulonephritis; poikiloderma congenita
C1r	Glomerulonephritis; lupuslike syndrome
C1s	Lupuslike syndrome
C1INH[a]	Discoid lupus; systemic lupus; lupuslike syndrome
C4	Systemic lupus; Sjogren's syndrome
C2	Systemic lupus; discoid lupus; polymyositis; Henoch-Schonlein purpura; Hodgkin's disease; vasculitis; glomerulonephritis; common variable hypogammaglobulinemia
C3	Vasculitis; lupuslike syndrome; glomerulonephritis
C5	Systemic lupus; neisserial infections
C6	Neisserial infections
C7	Systemic lupus; rheumatoid arthritis; Raynaud's phenomenon and sclerodactyly; vasculitis; neisserial infection
C8	Systemic lupus; neisserial infections
C9	Neisserial infection

[a] C1INH, C1 inhibitor.

search maintain their own sheep for a supply of E and use samples from a single standardized pool of rabbit antibody to E for years at a time. Alternatively, arrangements with a single commercial supplier to provide sheep blood on a regular basis and the purchase of sizeable quantities of a single lot of rabbit antibody avoid the problem of changing reagents frequently. Even such apparently trivial matters as a change in the source of gelatin used as a carrier protein in diluent buffers or in the way in which glassware is cleaned and rinsed may cause aberrant results.

A large number of commercial sources of E and of rabbit antibody to E are listed in *Linscott's Directory of Immunological and Biological Reagents* (5). More specialized materials, including functionally pure complement components, i.e., with very low contamination with other components, are available from Cordis Laboratories, Miami, Fla. Cordis also supplies E coated with complement components for use in effective molecule titrations of individual human component activities and appropriate reagents for developing the reactions. Alternatively, Cordis performs titrations on individual test specimens in their laboratory.

Immunoassays

Radial immunodiffusion kits for the most commonly performed component measurements are widely available from commercial suppliers, although considerable savings in cost can be achieved by purchasing the antiserum and preparing the immunodiffusion plates by the technique outlined below. Nephelometric systems for use by clinical pathology laboratories are marketed by several competing companies. Sources of antibodies specific for human complement proteins are listed in *Linscott's Directory* (5). Inventories of antisera against a wide variety of complement proteins are maintained by Atlantic Antibodies,

Scarborough, Maine, Calbiochem-Behring, San Diego, Calif., California Immunodiagnostics, San Marcos, Calif., Miles Laboratories, Napierville, Ill., and Serotec Ltd., Bicester, England. Kits for radioimmunoassay of $C4a_{desArg}$, $C3a_{desArg}$, and $C5a_{desArg}$ are sold by Upjohn Diagnostics Division of The Upjohn Co., Kalamazoo, Mich.

TEST PROCEDURES

Total Hemolytic Complement Assay

The following method is that of Kent and Fife as modified by Peter Schur.

Reagents

5% Gelatin. Dissolve 5 g of gelatin (Difco Laboratories, Detroit, Mich.) in 100 ml of distilled water at 56°C. Add NaN_3 to a final concentration of 0.1%. Dispense the solution in 10-ml portions, stopper with cotton, autoclave, and store at 4°C. Prior to use, heat for 5 min at 37°C.

TBS. (i) 10× Stock solution. To make triethanolamine-buffered saline (TBS), dissolve 75 g of NaCl in 700 ml of distilled water; add 177 ml of 1.0 N HCl, 28 ml of triethanolamine, 1.2 ml of 4.16 M $MgCl_2$, and 1.2 ml of 1.25 M $CaCl_2$; bring the solution to 1,000 ml; and store it at 4°C.

(ii) "TBS without." Dilute 10× stock solution 1/10 with H_2O, adjust it to pH 7.3 to 7.4, and store it at 4°C.

(iii) "TBS with." Dilute stock solution 1/10 with H_2O, adding 10 ml of 5% gelatin before bringing the solution to a 1,000-ml volume. Maintain the solution at 4°C, discarding it after 24 h.

EA

1. Wash sheep cells in 10 volumes of "TBS without" three times, carefully aspirating buffy coat at the interface each time.
2. Measure the packed cell volume, and suspend E in 40 volumes of "TBS with."
3. Lyse the E suspension by diluting it 1/20 in distilled H_2O, read the optical density at 541 nm (OD_{541}), and adjust the suspension by further addition of buffer such that the OD of the lysate is 0.495 to 0.505. This is a 2% E suspension. It can be used without further washing for 24 h. E will keep for a week or more, but they require further washing and spectrophotometric restandardization.
4. Slowly, with swirling, add an equal volume of the appropriate dilution of rabbit anti-E antibody to the E suspension. Mix the solution by pouring it back and forth between two flasks six times, and allow it to sit at room temperature for 10 min. This EA suspension can be used for up to 24 h, provided it is kept cold.

Assay

1. Remove test sera and normal human serum standard from a −70°C freezer, and defrost them at 4°C for about 2 h.
2. Prepare a 1/50 dilution of serum in "TBS with" (1/25 dilution for serum with known low activity).

3. Maintaining all reagents at ice bath temperature, prepare a series of tubes for each test serum containing 0.0, 0.2, 0.3, 0.4, 0.5, 0.7, and 0.9 ml of the 1/50 serum dilution and sufficient "TBS with" to bring the final volume in each tube to 0.9 ml. For each set of assays, prepare three tubes with 0.9 ml of H_2O in place of serum dilutions (100% lysis).

4. Resuspend the EA, and add 0.6 ml of suspension to each tube.

5. Thoroughly mix the contents of the tubes, and incubate them in a 37°C water bath for 30 min. Shake the racks every 10 min to maintain the EA in suspension.

6. Remove the EA to an ice bath, and add 0.5 ml of "TBS with" to all tubes.

7. Centrifuge the tubes for 5 min at 2,500 rpm.

8. Read the OD_{541} of the supernatant.

Calculations

1. Correct the observed OD of each tube for spontaneous lysis of the EA by subtracting from it the OD of the tube containing only the EA in "TBS with," i.e., 0.0 ml of serum dilution.

2. The proportion of cells lysed (y) is calculated as follows: y = corrected OD of tube/corrected OD with 100% lysis.

3. Calculate $y/(1 - y)$.

4. Plot $y/(1 - y)$ against the volume of serum dilution for each tube on log-log graph paper. The points for tubes with $0.8 < y > 0.2$ should fall on a straight line.

5. Determine the volume in milliliters at which $y/(1 - y)$ equals 1.0. This volume corresponds to 50% hemolysis.

6. CH_{50} = dilution factor used (e.g., 50 or 25)/volume in milliliters at 1.0 intercept.

7. A standard serum with a known CH_{50} value should be titrated in parallel with the test specimen, and the value should be observed for the latter adjusted for any variation in sensitivity indicated by the titration of the standard serum.

Immunodiffusion Assay for Third Component (C3)

Reagents

Stock Veronal (5×). Dissolve 42.5 g of NaCl, 1.875 g of sodium barbital, and 2.875 g of barbituric acid in 1,000 ml of distilled water. At 4°C, the pH should be 7.4 to 7.6.

Immunodiffusion buffer. Dilute 5× Veronal 1/5 in water. Add 0.086 M EDTA (pH 7.5) to a final concentration of 0.003 M.

3% Agar. Heat 50 ml of immunodiffusion buffer in boiling water on a hot plate with a magnetic stirrer. When the water is boiling, slowly add 1.5 g of agar. Continue heating the water until the solution is clear and the agar is dissolved. Agar may be stored at 4°C and reheated in boiling water as needed.

Antiserum to C3. Antiserum to C3 is available commercially.

Preparation of immunodiffusion plates

1. Melt 3% agar in boiling water, and cool it to 56°C.

2. Place the appropriate dilution of antiserum in 1.5 ml of immunodiffusion buffer in a test tube at 56°C. The dilution will depend on the strength of the antiserum and must be determined by trial and error.

3. Add 1.5 ml of the molten 3% agar to the test tube.

4. Agitate the tube briefly at 56°C, and add 3 ml of mixture to a petri dish (50 by 15 mm) on a level surface. Allow the mixture to cool until it is solidified, and store it in a moist chamber at 4°C. Shelf life is several weeks.

Procedure

1. In solidified agar gel, punch 1.5-mm-diameter holes at least 12 mm equidistant from each other.

2. Aspirate agar gel from the punched holes with a fine-tip transfer pipette attached to a vacuum line.

3. Fill the holes in the gel with test serum and standard C3 source diluted 1/1, 1/2, 1/4, and 1/8. The holes are filled when the surface of the sample is level with the surface of the agar gel. Set up each plate in duplicate.

4. Place the plate in a humid atmosphere at room temperature for 48 to 72 h.

5. Invert the plates, and measure the ring diameter in two directions at right angles to each other with a measuring magnifier. (Faint rings can be sharpened by brief exposure of the plates to 1% tannic acid when the rings become visible.)

6. Multiply ring height by width. Plot this value against the concentration of C3 standard to construct a standard curve.

7. Interpolate ring sizes of the test sample on the standard curve.

This work was supported by research grants AI 13049 and AM 18976 from the National Institutes of Health and by an Arthritis Clinical Research Center grant from the Arthritis Foundation.

It is a pleasure to thank O. M. Lee for her expert editorial assistance.

LITERATURE CITED

1. **Agnello, V.** 1978. Complement deficiency states. Medicine **57**:1–23.

2. **Alexander, R. L., Jr.** 1980. Comparison of radial immunodiffusion and laser nephelometry for quantitating some serum proteins. Clin. Chem. **26**:314–317.

3. **Chenoweth, D. E., S. W. Cooper, T. E. Hugli, R. W. Stewart, E. H. Blackstone, and J. W. Kirklin.** 1981. Complement activation during cardiopulmonary bypass: evidence for generation of C3a and C5a anaphylatoxins. N. Engl. J. Med. **304**:497–503.

4. **Kent, J. F., and E. H. Fife.** 1963. Precise standardization of reagents for complement fixation. Am. J. Trop. Med. **12**:103–116.

5. **Linscott, W. D.** 1984. Linscott's directory of immunological and biological reagents, 3rd ed. W. D. Linscott, Mill Valley, Calif.

6. **Lloyd, W., and P. H. Schur.** 1981. Immune complexes, complement and anti-DNA in exacerbations of systemic lupus erythematosus (SLE). Medicine **60**:208–217.

7. **Mayer, M. M.** 1961. Complement and complement fixation, p. 133–240. *In* E. A. Kabat and M. M. Mayer (ed.), Experimental immunochemistry. Charles C Thomas, Publisher, Springfield, Ill.

8. **Ruddy, S.** 1985. Complement, p. 137–162. *In* A. S. Cohen

(ed.), Laboratory diagnostic procedures in the rheumatic diseases, 3rd ed. Grune & Stratton, Orlando, Fla.

9. **Schur, P. H.** 1983. Complement studies of sera and other biologic fluids. Hum. Pathol. **14:**338–342.

10. **van Es, L., S. J. Smith, P. H. Schur, G. Hauptman, W. Leskovar, P. Spath, G. Fust, P. Lachmann, U. Rother, R. A. Thompson, and T. B. L. Kirkwood.** 1981. International collaborative study of four candidate reference preparations for the antigenic and hemolytic measurement of human serum complement components. J. Biol. Stand. **9:**91–104.

11. **Weinstein, A., B. Bordwell, B. Stone, C. Tibbetts, and N. F. Rothfield.** 1983. Antibodies to native DNA and serum complement (C3) levels. Application to diagnosis and classification of systemic lupus erythematosus. Am. J. Med. **74:**206–216.

Chapter 27

Methods for Allotyping Complement Proteins

DEBORAH MARCUS AND CHESTER A. ALPER

Overview

Extensive genetic polymorphism has been found in many complement components during the past two decades. The complement system is divided into two well-defined pathways, the classical and alternative, and has several inhibitors. The classical pathway contains nine components, with the first component consisting of three subcomponents, i.e., C1q, C1r, C1s, and, in sequence of activation, C4 and C2. The proteins of the alternative pathway are B, D, C3, and P (properdin). Activation of either the classical or alternative pathway results in the assembly of C3 and C5 convertases which then lead to the formation of the membrane attack complex containing C5, C6, C7, C8, and C9. Inhibitors of the complement system include I (C3b-C4b inactivator), its cofactors H and C4BP (C4 binding protein), and CT inhibitor. In addition, cell surfaces bear CR1 (C3b-C4b receptor), which also serves as a cofactor of I-mediated inactivation of C3b, and decay-accelerating factor or DAF.

Inherited structural variants of complement components are studied by techniques which detect differences in net surface charge resulting from amino acid substitutions. Two methods commonly used to separate proteins are high-voltage agarose gel electrophoresis, as described by Laurell and Niléhn (5), to detect variations in electrophoretic mobilities, and isoelectric focusing in thin-layer polyacrylamide gel (3), a sensitive system capable of detecting slight differences in isoelectric points.

Proteins can be visualized by one of the following methods. Functional overlay gels can be used in which antibody-sensitized sheep erythrocytes (EA) are combined with animal or human complement-deficient serum (either natural or artificially produced) (4). With C2, dilute normal human serum can replace C2-deficient serum as a reagent because C2 is the limiting factor in the classical pathway. Specific proteins can also be studied by immunofixation electrophoresis, which uses the insolubility of antigen-antibody complexes to visualize the particular protein of interest (2). This technique is described in greater detail in chapter 21.

Human plasma contains C3 at a relatively high concentration, and because of this, C3 can be detected directly after prolonged agarose gel electrophoresis by a simple total-protein stain. Most of the typings can be carried out on whole serum or EDTA plasma without prior purification, with the exception of analyses of C4BP and H, which require immunoprecipitates to isolate the proteins. Only small volumes of sample (5 to 15 μl per test) are required for most assays.

Sample collection and storage

Special care should be taken during the collection and storage of samples for complement testing be-cause of the instability of these proteins at room temperature or at 4 or $-20°C$. Serum samples are obtained from whole blood which has been allowed to clot at room temperature for 30 min and then placed at 4°C for 1 h or until ready to process. When plasma is required, EDTA (1.5 mg/ml of blood) should be used as an anticoagulant. The EDTA chelates Mg^{2+} and Ca^{2+} and inhibits the activation and conversion of complement components. Samples should be placed immediately on wet ice or at 4°C and should be processed within 24 h of collection. Multiple samples should be made for each donor to minimize repeated freezing and thawing that could alter the proteins. Complement proteins appear to be stable for an indefinite time when stored at $-80°C$.

Linkage of the complement components

It has been well documented that the four loci coding for the three proteins B, C2, and C4 are located in the major histocompatibility complex (MHC), between HLA-B and -DR and very close to HLA-DR, on the short arm of chromosome 6. No crossing-over events at meiosis have been observed within the complement gene region. The genes which code for these complement proteins are inherited as a unit, and their haplotypes, given in arbitrary order of BF, C2, C4A, and C4B alleles, have been given the name complotypes. As a unit, some complotypes demonstrate significant linkage disequilibrium with HLA-B and HLA-DR. Such haplotypes, which show limited HLA-A and other MHC allele variation, have been named extended haplotypes.

Other complement gene linkages include C6-C7, C3BRM (encoding the C3b-C4b receptor)-FH (for factor H)-C4BP (for C4 binding protein) on chromosome 1, C3-Lu-Le-H-Apo E-APO CI-Apo CII-Dm-Pep D on chromosome 19, and C8I and the locus for C1q B chain on chromosome 1.

Finally, complotyping is often informative in bone marrow transplant family studies. When analyzed as a unit, complotypes comprise a large number of combinations of alleles and are second only to HLA-B in number of known polymorphisms. Complotyping is helpful when HLA-DR typing and interpretation of MLC reactions are difficult. Complement typings require small blood sample volumes compared with those for HLA testing and, because of the fact that complement antisera react with all variants, are useful in studies of different ethnic groups for whom HLA reagents are at present still incomplete.

CLINICAL INDICATIONS

There are at least three situations in which the allotyping of complement proteins is clinically useful: as MHC markers for certain diseases, in the confirmation of inherited deficiency states of complement proteins, and as an adjunct to HLA typing in the identification of family donors for organ or tissue transplantation. Those MHC-encoded complement genes with increased relative risks for a variety of diseases are, in general, relatively infrequent alleles on extended haplotypes. For example, *BF*F1* on [HLA-B18 DR3 F1C30] increased in type 1 diabetes and membranous glomerulonephritis, *C4B*3* on [HLA-B15 (62) DR4 SC33] increased in rheumatoid arthritis and type 1 diabetes, and *C4B*31* on [HLA-Bw47 DR7 FC0,31] increased in salt-losing 21-hydroxylase deficiency congenital adrenal hyperplasia. Allotyping in family members of complement proteins thought to be hereditarily deficient in patients is useful (in conjunction with assays of concentrations in serum) in showing null complement alleles. In Caucasians the allele responsible for C2 deficiency, *C2*Q0*, has a carrier frequency of around 1% and is usually part of an extended haplotype [HLA-B18 DR2 S042] (1). Deficiencies of classical pathway components, particularly C4 or C2, are often associated with systemic lupus erythematosus, whereas patients with deficiencies of C3, I, or H are particularly susceptible to infection by pyogenic bacteria. Patients with hereditary deficiency of C5, C6, C7, C8, C9, or P are particularly prone to meningococcal or gonococcal systemic infection (6). Differences in immunofixation patterns of C̄1 inhibitor have been shown in some forms of hereditary angioneurotic edema in which patients' sera contain normal or elevated levels of a nonfunctional molecule with altered electrophoretic mobility.

The nomenclature used in this chapter conforms to that of the International Society of Human Genetics (7). The alleles are written as an italicized locus name, an asterisk, and one or more italicized letters or numbers or both, e.g., *C6*A*. Null alleles are designated Q0 for quantity zero.

The methods for studying structural variation in complement components are grouped into three sections. In the first group, isoelectric focusing is used to separate proteins, and functional hemolytic overlays are the detection system. In the second group, proteins separated under specific conditions during electrophoresis are analyzed by patterns developed by immunofixation. Complement components in the third group are partially purified by immunoprecipitation, isofocused in polyacrylamide gels, and stained with a protein-staining dye. Inheritance of all complement variants is autosomal codominant except for dysfunctional C̄1 inhibitor, which is inherited as a dominant trait.

STUDY OF COMPLEMENT POLYMORPHISMS BY ISOELECTRIC FOCUSING AND FUNCTIONAL DETECTION SYSTEMS

For more information, see reference 4.

Stock solutions

Acrylamide stock solution for 5% gels with 0.2 M taurine (1 liter). Dissolve 66.6 g of acrylamide (Bio-Rad Laboratories, Richmond, Calif.), 1.6 g of bisacrylamide (Bio-Rad), and 33.3 g of taurine (Sigma Chemical Co., St. Louis, Mo.) in 1 liter of distilled water. Filter the solution, and store it for a maximum of 2 weeks at 4°C.

Note. Acrylamide is highly neurotoxic. Special care should be taken to avoid inhalation and absorption through the skin.

Acrylamide solution stock (2×) for 5% gels with urea and 0.2 M taurine (1 liter). Dissolve 133.2 g of acrylamide (Bio-Rad), 3.2 g of bisacrylamide (Bio-Rad), and 66.6 g of taurine (Sigma) in 1 liter of distilled water. Filter the solution, and keep it for a maximum of 2 weeks at 4°C.

Note. Acrylamide is highly neurotoxic. Special care should be taken to avoid inhalation and absorption through the skin.

Riboflavin (1 mg% [mg/100 ml]; 200 ml). Dissolve 2 mg of riboflavin (Bio-Rad) in 200 ml of distilled water.

Note. This reagent is light sensitive, and storage should be in a dark bottle at 4°C.

$MgCl_2$ stock (1.5 M) and $CaCl_2$ stock (1.5 M). *Note.* $MgCl_2$ and $CaCl_2$ are hygroscopic and should be prepared by making an appropriate dilution of an approximately 2 M solution for which the density of 1 ml has been determined and the true molarity has been interpreted from the table "Concentrative Properties of Aqueous Solutions" in the *Handbook of Chemistry and Physics* (8).

0.2 M EDTA (pH 7.4; 1 liter). Dissolve 74.4 g of disodium EDTA in 600 ml of distilled water. Titrate with 10 N NaOH to pH 7.4. Bring to 1 liter with water.

VBS-EDTA (pH 7.4; 1 liter). For Veronal-buffered saline (VBS)-EDTA, dissolve 1.02 g of sodium barbital and 8.3 g of NaCl in approximately 500 ml of distilled water. Add 3.46 mg of 1 N HCl and 50 ml of 0.2 M EDTA (pH 7.4). Bring to 1 liter with distilled water.

5× VBS + Mg^{2+} + Ca^{2+} (pH 7.4; 1 liter). Dissolve 41.5 g of NaCl and 5.1 g of sodium barbital in approximately 500 ml of distilled water. Add 17.3 ml of 1 N HCl, 1.6 ml of 1.5 M $MgCl_2$ stock, and 0.49 ml of 1.5 M $CaCl_2$ stock. Bring to a volume of 1 liter with distilled water.

GVBS + Mg^{2+} + Ca^{2+} (500 ml). Dissolve 0.5 g of gelatin (Fisher Scientific, Springfield, N.J.) in 400 ml of boiling water. Bring to room temperature, and add 100 ml of 5× VBS + Mg^{2+} + Ca^{2+} to make gelatin-VBS (GVBS).

H_3PO_4 (5%; 100 ml). Add 5.8 ml of 85.5% phosphoric acid (Fisher) to distilled water, and bring to a final volume of 100 ml.

Ethanolamine (5%; 100 ml). Add 5 ml of monoethanolamine to distilled water, and bring to a final volume of 100 ml.

0.01 M phosphate–0.02 M EDTA (pH 5.6; 1 liter). Add 1.38 g of monobasic sodium phosphate to 100 ml of distilled water. Titrate with 10 N NaOH until the pH reaches 5.6. Dissolve 7.44 g of disodium EDTA in acetate buffer. Readjust the pH to 5.6. Bring to a final volume of 1 liter in distilled water.

General Methods

Preparation of EA (approximately 300 ml)

1. Fill two centrifuge tubes with a total of 30 ml of sheep erythrocytes (E), aged 2 weeks.
2. Wash the E four times with VBS-EDTA at 3,000 rpm (IEC centrifuge PR2) for 10 min.
3. Wash the E three times with GVBS + Mg^{2+} + Ca^+ at 3,000 rpm for 10 min.

4. Resuspend the E with GVBS + Mg^{2+} + Ca^{2+} to a volume 10 times that of the packed cells.

5. Lyse 0.1 ml of the cell suspension with 2.4 ml of distilled water.

6. Read the total hemolysis at 541 nm with distilled water as the blank.

7. Correct the cell concentration until the absorbance reads 0.420 by using the following formula: optical density (OD) of $V_1/(0.420 \times V_1) = V_2$, where V_1 is the present volume of E, and V_2 is the final volume. The final cell concentration is 10^9 cells per ml.

8. Dilute the rabbit anti-sheep hemolysin to a predetermined titer with GVBS + Mg^{2+} + Ca^{2+}.

9. Add an equal volume of antibody solution dropwise with gentle mixing to the final volume of cell suspension.

10. Store at 4°C for a maximum of 2 weeks.

Titration of anti-sheep cell hemolysin

1. Prepare a twofold serial dilution of anti-sheep hemolysin (Colorado Serum Co., Denver, Colo.), i.e., 1:100, 1:200, 1:400, 1:800, 1:1,600 . . . 1:12,800, in VBS-EDTA.

2. Add 0.1 ml of E to 0.1 ml of hemolysin dilution. Mix gently on a vortex mixer.

3. Wash the E four times with VBS-EDTA.

4. Wash the E three times with GVBS + Mg^{2+} + Ca^{2+}.

5. Add 0.2 ml of guinea pig complement. Use either a 1:35 dilution of fresh guinea pig serum in GVBS + Mg^{2+} + Ca^{2+} or a 1:20 dilution of commercially available lyophilized serum (these dilutions are suggestions and should be determined by experimentation). For positive and negative controls, substitute a guinea pig serum dilution with 0.2 ml of distilled water and 0.2 ml of GVBS + Mg^{2+} + Ca^{2+}, respectively.

6. Bring the final volume of the cell suspension to 1.5 ml with GVBS + Mg^{2+} + Ca^{2+}.

7. Mix gently, and incubate for 60 min at 37°C.

8. Centrifuge, and measure the OD of the supernatant at 541 nm.

9. Correct the OD by subtracting the negative control.

10. Calculate percent lysis by the formula (OD corrected/OD of positive control) × 100%.

11. Determine the highest dilution with maximum lysis, and use a solution twice as concentrated to sensitize the E.

Preparation of 5% thin-layer polyacrylamide gels with 0.2 M taurine

1. Prepare a mold with a 1-mm spacer placed between two clean glass plates that have been rinsed, first with ethanol and then distilled water, and dried.

2. To prepare one gel, add to a sidearm flask 10 ml of acrylamide stock; 0.5 ml of carrier ampholytes (40%, wt/vol; LKB Instruments, Inc., Rockville, Md.) at the desired pH range; 0.1 ml of ampholytes (40%, wt/vol; LKB) at pH 3.5 to 10; and, added last because of its light sensitivity, 2.7 ml of 1 mg% riboflavin.

3. Degas the solution for 2 min, and pour it into the mold without trapping in the gel any air in the form of bubbles, which will inhibit polymerization.

4. Place the mold under fluorescent light until it is polymerized.

5. Store the mold at 4°C for up to 2 weeks.

Preparation of 5% thin-layer polyacrylamide gels with 0.2 M taurine and 3.1 M urea

1. This step is as described for the previous method.

2. To prepare one gel, add to a sidearm flask 5.8 ml of 2× acrylamide stock and 2.9 g of urea. Dissolve with mixing and low heat. Add 0.5 ml of ampholytes (40%, wt/vol; Bio-Rad) at pH 6 to 8, 0.1 ml of ampholytes (40%, wt/vol; LKB) at pH 3.5 to 10, and 1.35 ml of 1 mg% riboflavin. Adjust the volume to 13.3 ml with distilled water.

3.–4. Perform steps 3 and 4 as described for the previous method.

Preparation of hemolytic overlay

1. Remove the gel from the isoelectric focusing apparatus.

2. Prepare the mold with the isoelectric focusing gel, 2-mm spacer, and clean glass plate (final thickness of overlay, 1 mm).

3. Place 5 ml of EA suspension in the centrifuge tube.

4. Wash the suspension two times with VBS + Mg^{2+} + Ca^{2+}.

5. Add 14.5 ml of 0.6 g% (g/100 ml) agarose in GVBS + Mg^{2+} + Ca^{2+} at 60°C.

6. Add an appropriate volume of complement-deficient serum.

7. Mix gently on a vortex mixer, and pour.

8. Incubate at 37°C until the pattern is fully developed.

Preparation of zymosan-treated serum

1. Add 1 g of zymosan (Sigma) to 200 ml of 0.85 g% NaCl and boil it for 0.5 h.

2. Centrifuge the solution, and decant the supernatant.

3. Add 1 liter of 0.85 g% NaCl to bring the final concentration to 0.1 g% zymosan.

4. Measure the zymosan suspension so that the total volume is two times that of the serum to be treated. Centrifuge the suspension, and decant the supernatant.

5. Add the serum to the zymosan precipitate, and incubate it with mixing for 1 h at 37°C.

6. Centrifuge the suspension to separate the serum from the zymosan, and collect the supernatant.

C2 typing

Patterns are observed after C2-induced hemolysis in overlay gels on isoelectric focusing gels. The most frequent pattern consists of two major and several minor bands (Fig. 1). This pattern has been given the designation C (for common). Several rare variants are seen as displacements of the major bands and develop more slowly and with lesser intensity. Depending on their relative position with respect to the common variant, these bands are named B (for basic) or A (for acidic).

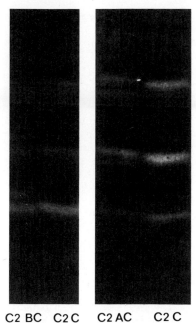

C2 BC   C2 C   C2 AC   C2 C

FIG. 1. C2 patterns produced by isoelectric focusing in polyacrylamide gel overlay containing EA and dilute normal human serum.

Inherited complete deficiency occurs in about 1 in 10,000 normal Caucasians. C2 is encoded by a single locus, and variants are inherited as autosomal codominant traits. Close linkage has been observed between the locus for C2 and the loci for BF, C4A, and C4B, and these loci are located near HLA-DR on the short arm of chromosome 6.

Procedure

1. Prepare a 5% thin-layer polyacrylamide gel (20 by 10 by 0.1 cm) containing 0.2 M taurine and ampholytes with the desired pH range of 5 to 8.

2. Apply 15 µl of serum or EDTA plasma to 5- by 15-mm pieces of Whatman no. 1 filter paper. Place the serum- or plasma-soaked paper across the 10-cm end of the gel, approximately 2 cm from the anode.

3. Apply 5% H_3PO_4 to the anode and 5% ethanolamine to the cathode.

4. Place the gel on the apparatus at 4°C, and focus for approximately 16 h at 450 V.

5. After the proteins on the gel have completely focused, prepare the hemolytic overlay by adding 0.5 ml of C2-deficient serum. Normal human serum at 1/100 (vol/vol) dilution may be substituted for C2-deficient serum, because C2 is normally the limiting factor in the classical pathway.

C5 typing

Many ethnic groups have been examined (Table 1), including Americans, English, Portuguese, and West Africans, with no evidence of polymorphism in the fifth component of complement. A polymorphism for C5 has, on the other hand, been described for Melanesian and related peoples. Serum samples are placed on an isoelectric focusing gel containing 1 M urea, and patterns are visualized by a C5-induced hemolytic overlay. Two alleles, *C5*1* and *C5*2*, are observed.

Eight bands of lysis are present, with an additional cathodal band in the heterozygote. Inheritance of the variant is as an autosomal codominant trait.

Procedure. (i) Preparation of isoelectric focusing gel

1. Prepare a 5% polyacrylamide gel (20 by 10 by 0.1 cm) containing 0.2 M taurine, 1 M urea, and carrier ampholytes with the desired pH range of 5 to 8.

2. Apply 10 µl of serum sample to 5- by 15-mm Whatman no. 1 filter paper. Place the serum-soaked paper across the 10-cm end of the gel, approximately 2 cm from the anode.

3. Apply 5% H_3PO_4 to the anode and 5% ethanolamine to the cathode.

4. Place the gel on the apparatus at 4°C, and focus for approximately 16 h at 45 V.

5. After focusing is complete, wash the gel for 0.5 h in 1 liter of phosphate-buffered saline (PBS) to remove urea.

6. Drain the gel, and apply the overlay.

(ii) Preparation of C5 detection gel

1. Wash 5 ml of EA two times with VBS + Mg^{2+} + Ca^{2+}.

TABLE 1. Frequencies of complement component alleles in the major races

Component	Allele	Frequency in:			
		Caucasians	Blacks	Orientals	Melanesians
BF	S	0.8055	0.437	0.890	
	F	0.1755	0.512	0.110	
	F1	0.0095	0.051		
	S1	0.0095			
C2	C	0.95			
	B	0.04			
	A	0.01			
C3	S	0.77	0.93		
	F	0.22	0.06		
C4A	1	0.002			
	2	0.056			
	3	0.636			
	4	0.078			
	5	0.002			
	6	0.034			
	Q0	0.176			
C4B	1	0.737			
	2	0.110			
	3	0.026			
	Q0	0.115			
C5	1	1.00			0.93
	2	0.00			0.07
C6	A	0.61	0.56	0.59	
	B	0.37	0.38	0.35	
	R	0.015	0.06	0.05	
C7	1	0.98[a]			
	2	<0.01[a]			
	3	<0.01[a]			
C81	A	0.649	0.700	0.655	
	B	0.348	0.246	0.345	
	A1	0.003	0.054		
C82	A	0.952			
	B	0.044			
	A1	0.004			
C4BP	1	0.98			
	2	0.02			
H	1	0.691			
	2	0.302			
	3	0.006			

[a] Estimates given by the authors.

2. Add 9 ml of VBS + Mg^{2+} + Ca^{2+} to the packed cells.

3. Add 1 ml of zymosan-treated serum, and mix the solution for 75 s at 37°C.

4. Add 0.2 ml of Antrypol (suramin sodium; Mobay Chemical Corp., FBA Pharmaceuticals, New York, N.Y.) at a concentration of 50 mg/ml, and mix it for 1.5 min at 37°C.

5. Centrifuge the EA, and wash them with VBS + Mg^{2+} + Ca^{2+}.

6. Add 14.5 ml of 1.0% agarose in GVBS + Mg^{2+} + Ca^{2+} and 0.5 ml of C5-deficient mouse serum at 60°C to the packed cells.

7. Mix gently on a vortex mixer, and pour over the isoelectric focusing gel.

C6 typing

A common polymorphism can be found in C6 patterns produced by overlaying isoelectric focusing gels with a C6-sensitive hemolytic overlay. Two common and several rare alleles have been described with isoelectric points between 6.0 and 6.5. The common variants are named according to their relative positions, with the more cathodal named B (basic) and the more anodal named A (acidic).

The homozygous patterns consist of a major central band surrounded by two minor bands (Fig. 2). The heterozygous pattern is the sum of the two homozygous patterns, with two major bands of equal intensity surrounded by two of lesser intensity. Several other minor bands are also observed throughout the pattern.

(i) Procedure

1. Prepare a 5% thin-layer polyacrylamide gel (20 by 10 by 0.1 cm) containing 0.2 M taurine and carrier ampholytes producing a gradient between pH 5 and 8.

2. Apply 15 μl of serum or EDTA plasma to 5- by 15-mm pieces of Whatman no. 1 filter paper. Place the serum- or plasma-soaked paper across the 10-cm end of the gel, approximately 2 cm from the anode.

3. Apply 5% H_3PO_4 to the anode and 5% ethanolamine to the cathode.

4. Place the gel on the apparatus at 4°C, and focus for approximately 16 h at 450 V.

5. After the gel has completely focused, prepare the hemolytic overlay, adding 0.5 ml of C6-deficient rabbit serum.

(ii) Alternative method.

A second method for detecting C6 is worth mentioning because it allows analysis of C6 without the necessity of obtaining homozygous C6-deficient serum. Briefly, C6 is detected after thin-layer polyacrylamide isoelectric focusing and electrophoretic transfer to nitrocellulose by using anti-human C6 and then a peroxidase-conjugated antibody to animal immunoglobulin. The results obtained by this method were identical to those previously reported under the conditions of a hemolytic assay.

C7 typing

A genetic polymorphism exists in the seventh component of complement, particularly in Orientals. Three alleles have been described, i.e., *C7*1*, which is the most common, *C7*2*, and *C7*3*. Bands are visualized after isoelectric focusing in thin-layer polyacryl-

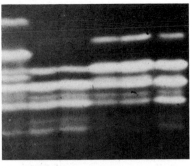

FIG. 2. C6 patterns produced by isoelectric focusing in polyacrylamide gel with development in an agarose gel overlay containing EA and C6-deficient rabbit serum. The patterns are for the following types of C6 in lanes 1 through 6, respectively: A plus rare basic variant, A, A, B, B, and AB.

amide gels and a detection overlay with C7-induced lysis.

Procedure. (i) Preparation of isoelectric focusing gel

1. Prepare a 5% polyacrylamide gel (20 by 10 by 0.1 cm) containing 0.2 M taurine and carrier ampholytes with a gradient between pH 5 and 7.

2. Apply 5 μl of serum samples to 5- by 5-mm Whatman no. 1 filter paper. Place the serum-soaked paper across the 10-cm end of the gel, approximately 2 cm from the anode.

3. Apply 5% H_3PO_4 to the anode and 5% ethanolamine to the cathode.

4. Place the gel on the apparatus, and focus for approximately 16 h at 450 V, with resistors, at 4°C.

(ii) Preparation of C7 detection gel

1. Prepare $C\overline{56}$ euglobulin by treating serum from parturient women with zymosan (as described above). Incubate the serum with zymosan overnight at room temperature.

2. Dialyze the serum against 0.01 M phosphate–0.02 M EDTA buffer (pH 5.6).

3. Collect the euoglobulin (precipitate), which contains $C\overline{56}$, C8, and C9.

4. Prepare a detection gel containing 1 g% agarose (Indubiose A37) in PBS–0.01 M EDTA, 0.5% guinea pig erythrocytes (preparation described above in section on E except that the cells are not sensitized with antibody), and a suitable concentration of $C\overline{56}$ euglobulin. Pour at 60°C.

5. Incubate the gel at 37°C until patterns develop fully.

C8

C8 is a 151,000-dalton molecule consisting of three subunits, alpha, gamma, and beta. The alpha chain is covalently bound to the gamma chain by disulfide linkage, and these two chains are in weak association, by a noncovalent bond, with the beta chain. Two loci have been described as encoding for C8. The designations given to the two loci are *C81*, coding for the alpha-gamma chains, and *C82*, coding for the beta chain. No close linkage has been found between these two loci.

Deficiency states have been described for both C81 and C82. In C81 deficiency, no C8 alpha-gamma chains are detected, yet C8 beta chains are present. In C82 deficiency, C8 alpha-gamma chains are detected in the absence of C8 beta chains.

It should be noted that prolonged storage of EDTA plasma (not serum) produces an anodal shift in the pattern of either the C81 or C82 typings.

C81 typing

The polymorphism of C81 can be studied by C8 alpha-gamma chain-induced lysis after isoelectric focusing using gels containing 3.1 M urea. Patterns are produced with pIs between 6.2 and 6.5. Two common and one rare allele have been described with the designations A (acidic), B (basic), and A1 (more acidic). The homozygous pattern consists of a major band with three flanking bands of unequal intensity (Fig. 3). The heterozygous pattern is the sum of the two homozygous patterns, with two central bands of equal intensity surrounded by three bands of differing intensity.

Procedure

1. Prepare a 5% polyacrylamide gel (20 by 10 by 0.1 cm) containing 0.2 M taurine, 3.1 M urea, and carrier ampholytes producing a gradient between pH 6 and 8.

2. Dilute the serum or EDTA plasma samples 1:4 with PBS. Apply 5 μl of sample dilution to 5- by 5-mm Whatman no. 1 filter paper. Place the sample-soaked papers across the 10-cm end of the gel, approximately 2 cm from the anode.

3. Apply 5% H_3PO_4 to the anode and 5% ethanolamine to the cathode.

4. Place the gel on the apparatus at 4°C, and focus for approximately 16 h at 450 V with resistors.

5. After the gel has completely focused, remove the urea by soaking the gel in VBS + Mg^{2+} + Ca^{2+} for 1 h.

6. Prepare the hemolytic overlay with 0.5 ml of C8 alpha-gamma-chain-deficient human serum.

C82 typing

C82 typing is done by a technique similar to the one described above for C81. Bands of hemolysis are analyzed after isoelectric focusing with gels containing 3.1 M urea. The most common pattern has been given the name B (for basic) and consists of a major band surrounded by two less-intense bands. A rare pattern showing the heterozygous state AB consists of the B pattern plus an additional, more anodal band (Fig. 4). The very rare homozygous A (for acidic) pattern is similar to the B pattern but is in a more anodal position. C82 is encoded by a single locus and is inherited as an autosomal codominant trait unlinked to *C81*.

Procedure

1. Step 1 is the same as that described above for C81.

2. Apply 15 μl of serum or EDTA plasma to 5- by 15-mm pieces of Whatman no. 1 filter paper, approximately 2 cm from anode.

3.–4. Steps 3 and 4 are the same as steps 3 and 4 described above for C81.

5. Prepare the hemolytic overlay by adding 0.5 ml of C8 beta-deficient human serum.

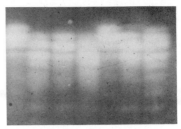

FIG. 3. C81 (α-γ) patterns produced by isoelectric focusing in polyacrylamide gel in the presence of 3.1 M urea and development in an agarose gel overlay containing EA and C8 α-γ-deficient human serum. Patterns are for the following types of C81 in lanes 1 through 7, respectively: B, AA1, A, AA1, B, A, and AB.

An alternative procedure is immunoblotting with anti-C8 for C81 and C82.

STUDY OF COMPLEMENT POLYMORPHISMS BY ELECTROPHORESIS

Stock solutions

VB + 2 mM Ca^{2+} (pH 8.6; 1 liter). For Veronal buffer (VB) with Ca^{2+}, dissolve 8.8 g of sodium barbital (Fisher), 1.4 g of barbituric acid (Fisher), and 0.6 g of calcium lactate (Fisher) in distilled water by heating, and bring to a final volume of 1 liter.

VB + 5 mM EDTA (pH 8.3; 1 liter). Dissolve 8.9 g of sodium barbital (Fisher), 1.4 g of barbituric acid (Fisher), and 1.9 g of disodium EDTA (Fisher) in distilled water by heating, and bring to a final volume of 1 liter.

Tris glycine barbital (pH 8.8; 1 liter). Dissolve 22.6 g of Tris (Sigma), 28.1 g of glycine (Fisher), 6.6 g of sodium barbital, and 1.0 g of barbituric acid in distilled water by mixing, and bring to a final volume of 1 liter.

10× 0.1 M phosphate–5 mM EDTA (pH 6.8; 1 liter). Dissolve 65.6 g of $NaH_2PO_4 \cdot H_2O$ (Fisher), 137.5 g of $Na_2HPO_4 \cdot 7H_2O$ (Fisher), and 18.8 g of disodium EDTA in distilled water by mixing, and bring to a final volume of 1 liter.

VBS + Mg^{2+} + Ca^{2+} (pH 7.4) and 0.2 M EDTA (pH 7.4). Stock solutions of VBS + Mg^{2+} + Ca^{2+} (pH 7.4) and 0.2 M EDTA (pH 7.4) are described above under Study of Complement Polymorphisms by Isoelectric Focusing and Functional Detection Systems.

Stain solution (2 liters). Dissolve 5 g of Coomassie brilliant blue (Schwarz/Mann, Cambridge, Mass.) by mixing it in a solution containing 900 ml of methanol, 900 ml of distilled water, and 200 ml of acetic acid.

Destain solution (2 liters). Mix 900 ml of methanol, 900 ml of distilled water, and 200 ml of acetic acid.

General Methods

Sample application for agarose gel electrophoresis with mask

1. Apply the samples by using a mask which is made of a piece of Mylar (FMC Corp., Marine Colloids

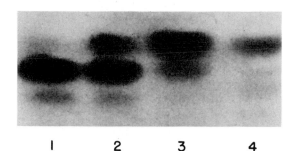

FIG. 4. C82 (β) patterns produced by isoelectric focusing in polyacrylamide gel in the presence of 3.1 M urea and development in an agarose gel overlay containing EA and C8 β-deficient human serum. Patterns are for the following types of C82 in lanes 1 through 4, respectively: A, AB, B, and B (known to be genotypically *C81*B/C81*Q0*).

Div., Rockland, Maine) with slits (1 cm by 0.5 mm) cut horizontally.

2. The gel underneath the mask is partially dried with Whatman no. 1 filter paper.

3. The mask is placed so that the sample application is approximately 2 cm from the edge of the gel.

4. A piece of Kimwipe is gently wiped across the slots to blot up excess liquid.

5. A small volume of sample is placed to cover each slot.

6. Allow the sample to diffuse into the gel for the amount of time predetermined for each method.

7. The excess sample is blotted from the top of the mask with Whatman no. 1 filter paper, and the mask is removed.

Immunofixation electrophoresis

1. Prepare a 0.1-cm-thick gel in appropriate gel buffer.

2. Apply the samples with a mask.

3. Place the gel on the electrophoresis apparatus, and run the apparatus under given conditions.

4. After electrophoresis is complete, remove the gel from the apparatus, and smear approximately 1 ml of antibody, or dilution of antibody, across the surface of the gel.

5. Incubate the gel for 1 h in a moist chamber at room temperature.

6. Press the gel, and wash it in PBS overnight.

7. Rinse the gel with tap water, and stain it with a protein-staining dye.

Staining procedure

1. Dry the gel completely with forced hot air.

2. Place the gel in staining solution for 20 min.

3. Place the gel in destain solution until blue bands appear on a clear background. Change the destain solution if necessary.

4. Dry the gel with forced hot air.

C3 typing

The genetic polymorphism of C3 was the first described for the complement components. C3 variants differ in charge at pH 8.6 and can be resolved and

separated from other plasma proteins after prolonged agarose gel electrophoresis in the presence of 2 mM Ca^{2+}. The concentration of C3 is higher than that of most other complement components and can be visualized, after electrophoresis, by total protein fixation in methanol-water-acetic acid and then staining, without the use of antibody. C3 produces a simple pattern comprising a single band for the homozygote and two bands for the heterozygote, with each of the latter bands having half the intensity of the homozygote band (Fig. 5).

Two common and several rare alleles have been described. The nomenclature is based on their relative mobilities. The most common allele in the three major races is S (for slow). In Caucasians, F (for fast) is also commonly observed as well as the rare alleles S0.6 (for slower), F1 (for faster), and F0.8 (for a variant with a mobility which lies 80% of the distance between F and F1).

Complete deficiency of the third component is rare. C3 is encoded by a single locus.

Procedure

1. Prepare a gel (20 by 10 by 0.1 cm) containing 0.8 g% agarose ME (Marine Colloids) in VB + 2 mM Ca^{2+} (pH 8.6).

2. Apply serum or EDTA plasma samples with a mask on the 20-cm end of the gel for 10 min.

3. Place the gel on the electrophoresis apparatus with the sample application near the cathode. Use five pieces of Whatman no. 1 filter paper for each wick.

4. Set the power supply at 350 V and 75 mA. Continue electrophoresis until a hemoglobin A marker has migrated 6 cm towards the anode.

5. After electrophoresis is complete, remove the gel from the apparatus, and place it in a fixing solution containing methanol-water-acetic acid (45:45:10, vol/vol/vol; see above, under Destain solution, for exact amounts) for 20 min.

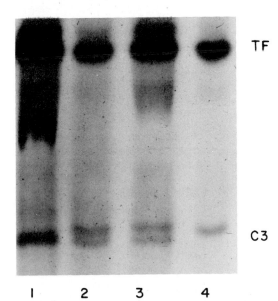

FIG. 5. C3 patterns produced by agarose gel electrophoresis at pH 8.6 in calcium-containing buffer and with protein staining. Patterns are for the following types of C3 in lanes 1 through 4, respectively: S, FS, FS, and F. The anode was at the top.

6. Press the plate to remove excess buffer salts.

7. Dry the gel, and stain it by the staining procedure.

Immunofixation electrophoresis may be used as an alternative method. Samples are diluted 1:3 with PBS, applied, and run under the same electrophoretic conditions as described above for C3 typing. After electrophoresis is complete, the gel is removed from the apparatus, smeared with approximately 1 ml of goat anti-human C3 (Atlantic Antibodies, Scarborough, Maine), and incubated for 1 h in a moist chamber at room temperature. The gel is then pressed, washed, and stained as described above for immunofixation electrophoresis.

BF typing

Properdin factor B was earlier known as GBG (glycine-rich beta-glycoprotein) and C3PA (C3 proactivator). It is highly polymorphic and can be detected after prolonged agarose gel electrophoresis and immunofixation. The homozygous pattern consists of three visible bands. The center band is the most intense and is surrounded by two minor bands. The heterozygous pattern is the sum of two homozygous patterns and consists of two major bands of approximately equal intensity surrounded by two minor bands (Fig. 6).

The variants are named after their mobility in relation to the anode, i.e., F (for fast), S (for slow), F1 (for faster), and S1 (for slower). BF is encoded by a single locus, and variants are inherited as autosomal codominant traits.

Procedure

1. Prepare a gel (20 by 10 by 0.1 cm) containing 0.8 g% agarose ME (Marine Colloids) in VB + 2 mM Ca^{2+} (pH 8.6).

2. Apply serum or EDTA plasma samples with a mask on the 20-cm end of the gel for 10 min.

3. Place the gel on the electrophoresis apparatus with the sample application near the cathode. Use five pieces of Whatman no. 1 filter paper for each wick.

4. Set the power supply at 350 V and 75 mA. Continue electrophoresis until a hemoglobin A marker has migrated 6 cm towards the anode.

5. After electrophoresis is complete, remove the gel from the apparatus, and smear it with approximately

1 ml of goat anti-human properdin factor B (Atlantic Antibodies).

6. Incubate the gel for 1 h in a moist chamber at room temperature.

7. Press, wash, and stain the gel as described above in the procedure for immunofixation electrophoresis.

C4 typing

The genetic polymorphism of the fourth component of complement has proved to be an informative tool in studying the short arm of chromosome 6. C4 is the most polymorphic of all the complement components, with many common alleles at each of its two closely linked loci, *C4A* (for acidic) and *C4B* (for basic).

Six common variants have been described for the *C4A* locus and three common variants at the *C4B* locus (Fig. 7 and 8). Many rare variants at both loci have been observed. Rodgers "blood group" activity has been associated with the *C4A* locus, and Chido activity has been associated with *C4B*. Null alleles for one or the other C4 locus (but not both) are common on individual chromosomes. These null alleles are designated *C4A*Q0* and *C4B*Q0* and result in common half-null C4 haplotypes (*C4A*3 C4B*Q0* and *C4A*Q0 C4B*1*, for example). The doubly null haplotype *C4A*Q0 C4B*Q0* is rare, and homozygotes (even rarer) are totally C4 deficient.

C4 has a relatively complex polymorphism and requires the use of three different techniques. Each individual technique and its purpose will be described.

Detection of C4 variants by immunofixation electrophoresis. C4 patterns can be visualized after prolonged agarose gel electrophoresis by using a discontinuous buffer system and immunofixation. It is necessary to pretreat the samples with neuraminidase to remove sialic acid before electrophoresis. The patterns produced show three bands for each variant, and depending on the mobility, some overlap may occur between variants.

Procedure

1. Dilute neuraminidase type VI (Sigma) with 0.1 M phosphate–5 mM EDTA (pH 6.8) to a final concentration of 40 U/ml (i.e., 10 U in 250 μl).

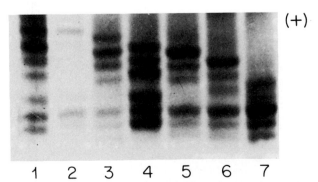

FIG. 7. C4 patterns produced by agarose gel electrophoresis at pH 8.8 of neuraminidase-treated plasma and immunofixation with anti-C4. Patterns are for the following types of C4: lane 1, A6, 4, B2, 1; lane 2, A6, B1; lane 3, A5, 3, B1, Q0; lane 4, A4, B2; lane 5, A3, 3, B1, Q0; lane 6, A2, B1; lane 7, A1, Q0, B1, 1. The anode was at the top.

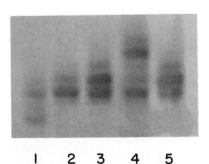

FIG. 6. BF patterns produced by agarose gel electrophoresis at pH 8.6 followed by immunofixation with anti-B and protein staining. Patterns are for the following types of BF in lanes 1 through 5, respectively: SS1, S, FS, F1S, and FS. The anode was at the top.

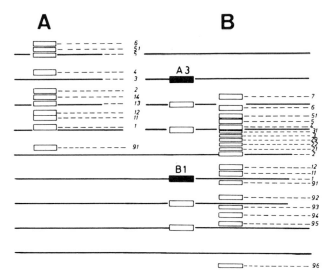

FIG. 8. Diagram showing C4 variants. Each variant is shown by its most anodal band. The anode would be at the top.

2. For each sample, add 4 µl of neuraminidase solution to 10 µl of EDTA plasma.

3. Dialyze against 0.1 M phosphate–5 mM EDTA (pH 6.8) overnight at 4°C.

4. Prepare 0.1 g% agarose (ICN Pharmaceuticals Inc., Irvine, Calif.) solution containing 35 ml of Tris glycine barbital buffer (pH 8.8), 0.5 ml of 0.2 M EDTA (pH 7.4), and 60 ml of distilled water.

5. Pour the gel (20 by 15 by 0.1 cm) with hot agarose solution.

6. Apply the total sample volume with a mask across the 20-cm end of the gel for 20 min.

7. Place the gel on the electrophoresis apparatus (Bio-Rad) with the sample application at the cathode. Use five pieces of Whatman no. 1 filter paper for each wick.

8. Set the power supply at 600 V maximum and 75 mA at constant current. Continue electrophoresis until a hemoglobin S marker has migrated 10 cm towards the anode.

9. After electrophoresis is complete, remove the gel from the apparatus, and smear it with approximately 1 ml of goat anti-human C4 (Atlantic Antibodies) diluted 2 parts antibody to 1 part VBS-EDTA.

10. Incubate the gel for 1 h in a moist chamber at room temperature.

11. Press, wash, and stain the gel as described above for immunofixation electrophoresis.

Detection of C4A versus C4B variants by a functional hemolytic assay. Some rare variants may have mobilities intermediate between or overlapping those of the common variants produced by either the *C4A* or *C4B* locus. To further define these variants it may be necessary to perform an additional test which selects for C4B hemolytic activity. C4B variants have 5 to 10 times the hemolytic activity of C4A variants, as a rule. Activated C4B preferentially acylates –OH groups, and activated C4A acylates –NH$_2$ groups.

EA and artificially produced C4-deficient guinea pig serum are incorporated into a gel and layered onto a C4 agarose gel after completion of electrophoresis.

Bands of hemolysis are selectively produced from C4B variants only (Fig. 9). Other variants seen by immunofixation, and producing little or no functional activity under these conditions, are usually products of *C4A*.

Two additional tests can be used to determine whether the C4 gene product is from the *C4A* or *C4B* locus. In appropriate individuals (those with a null allele on the other chromosome for the locus in question), Rodgers *(C4A)* or Chido *(C4B)* serological reactivity may be tested for. The individual serum is incubated with either human anti-Rodgers or human anti-Chido to test for inhibition of agglutination with appropriate positive erythrocytes.

Analysis of molecular weight differences in the alpha chain of C4 can be an alternative method to distinguish C4A from C4B variants. Immunoprecipitates are produced from neuraminidase-treated plasma and run under denaturing conditions on a 10% polyacrylamide gel (acrylamide/bisacrylamide, 1:0.006). The alpha chain of any C4A variant produces a single band with a molecular weight of 96,000. All C4B variants produce a single band with an apparently lower-molecular-weight alpha chain of 94,000.

Procedure

1.–8. Steps 1 through 8 are as described above for the detection of C4 variants by immunofixation electrophoresis. Prepare the hemolytic overlay 1 h before completion of electrophoresis.

9. Prepare hydrazine solution by adding 7.5 µl of hydrazine (K & K Laboratories, Inc., Plainview, N.Y.) to 5 ml of distilled water.

10. Add 0.1 ml of hydrazine solution to 0.5 ml of guinea pig serum (GIBCO Laboratories, Grand Island, N.Y.), and incubate the mixture for 60 min at 37°C (guinea pig serum is previously divided into aliquots and stored at −80°C) to produce C4-deficient guinea pig serum.

11. Wash 7.5 ml of EA two times with VBS + Mg^{2+} + Ca^{2+}.

12. After electrophoresis is complete, remove the gel from the apparatus, and prepare the mold with gel, 1.5-mm spacer, and clean glass plate.

13. Add 20 ml of 0.6 g% agarose ME (Marine Colloids) in GVBS + Mg^{2+} + Ca^{2+} and treated guinea pig serum to packed cells at 60°C.

14. Mix the solution gently on a vortex mixer, and pour.

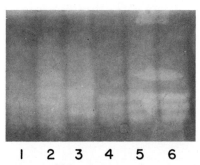

FIG. 9. Patterns of hemolysis in gel produced after agarose gel electrophoresis. Only C4B patterns are seen. Patterns are for the following C4B types in lanes 1 through 6, respectively: 1; 3, 1; 3, 2; 1; 1; and 1.

15. Incubate the gel at 37°C until patterns are developed.

Detection of null alleles in heterozygotes

C4 null genes in the homozygous state are easily identified by the absence of bands in either the C4A or C4B region after immunofixation electrophoresis. The detection of half-null C4 haplotypes in heterozygotes, however, requires the quantification of all gene products and analyses of their ratios, by either visual inspection, crossed immunoelectrophoresis, or densitometric scanning of the immunofixation pattern.

For crossed immunoelectrophoresis, samples treated with neuraminidase are subjected to electrophoresis just long enough to separate the C4A region from the C4B region. The gel is then removed from between the lanes, with only the gel of the sample lanes remaining on the plate. A second gel containing anti-human C4 (Atlantic Antibodies) is poured around the sample lanes. The plate is turned 90° and run in the second direction.

After the staining, peaks are visible and can be quantitated by placing the gel on 1-mm graph paper and counting the squares under the peaks. The following five different patterns can be observed (Fig. 10): A = B, B only, A only, A > B, and B > A. Patterns in Fig. 10, lanes 2 and 3, indicate samples that are from subjects homozygous deficient at one of the C4 loci. The sample producing an A peak only is from a homozygote for C4B*Q0. The sample producing a B peak only is from a homozygote for C4A*Q0. The individual producing the pattern in which B < A has

one haplotype in which C4A and C4B are expressed and another haplotype in which only C4A is expressed and C4B is null. One C4A is null of four possible C4 genes in the pattern B > A.

A = B is an ambiguous pattern which cannot distinguish between the phenotypes containing no null genes and those containing one null gene at each locus on opposite chromosomes. This distinction can usually be resolved by family studies.

An alternative method for the detection of null alleles is to analyze the C4 alpha chain after sodium dodecyl sulfate-polyacrylamide gel electrophoresis on immunoprecipitates as described above. Null alleles can be identified by comparing the relative ratios of the alpha-chain bands.

In Caucasians, 1 or 2% of C4 haplotypes show duplications of C4A or C4B. The presence of these duplications renders the preceding considerations more complicated.

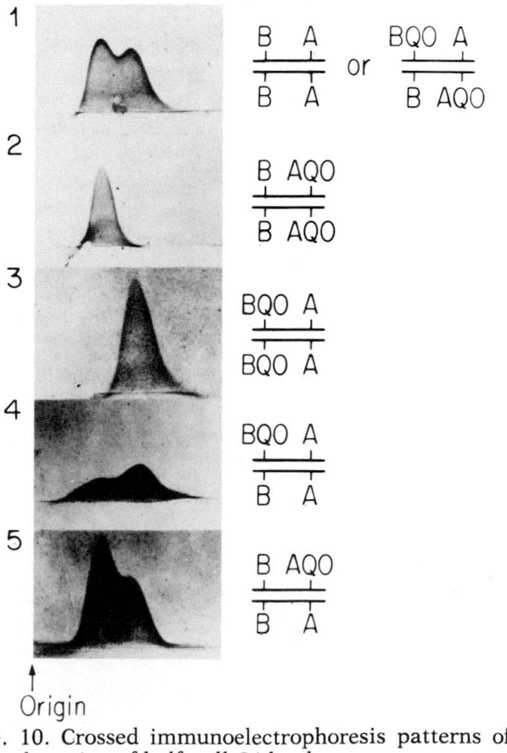

Procedure

1.–3. Steps 1 through 3 are as described above for the detection of C4 variants by immunofixation electrophoresis.

4. Prepare a gel (20 by 10 by 0.1 cm) containing 0.8 g% agarose LE (Marine Colloids) in VB + 5 mM EDTA (pH 8.3).

5. After dialysis is complete, apply the total sample volume with a mask for 20 min.

6. Place the gel on the apparatus, with the sample application across the 20-cm end of the gel near the cathode. Use five pieces of Whatman no. 1 filter paper for each wick.

7. Set the power supply at 300 V and 75 mA, and continue electrophoresis until hemoglobin A marker has migrated 6 cm.

8. After electrophoresis is complete, remove the gel from the apparatus. Cut and remove the gel between lanes, leaving the gel of the sample lanes on the plate.

9. Prepare the mold with the remains of the first gel, 1-mm frame, and clean glass plate.

10. Pour the second gel, embedding lanes from the first gel in 0.8 g% agarose ME (Marine Colloids) containing VB + 5 mM EDTA (pH 8.3) and 0.24% (vol/vol) goat anti-human C4 (Atlantic Antibodies) at 60°C. Allow the gel to cool. Note. The concentration of anti-C4 may be adjusted for proper peak height and antigen/antibody ratio.

11. Turn the gel 90°, and place it on the electrophoresis apparatus.

12. Set the power supply at 200 V and approximately 10 mA. Run the apparatus overnight.

13. Press, stain, and destain the gel (omit the wash).

C1̄ inhibitor

C1̄ inhibitor has not been shown to be polymorphic in normal individuals. Decreased activity of the inhibitor has been found in patients with hereditary angioneurotic edema. Two types of C1̄ inhibitor deficiencies have been described. In one type, the levels of C1̄ inhibitor are decreased (85% of random patients), and in the other type, normal or increased levels of a dysfunctional C1̄ inhibitor molecule usually differ in electrophoretic mobility from normal (Fig. 11). Inheritance of susceptibility to angioneurotic edema is an autosomal dominant trait.

FIG. 10. Crossed immunoelectrophoresis patterns of C4 for the detection of half-null C4 haplotypes.

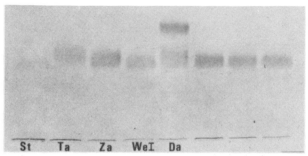

FIG. 11. C$\overline{1}$ inhibitor patterns after agarose gel electrophoresis of whole serum at pH 8.6 and immunofixation with anti-C$\overline{1}$ inhibitor. Patterns are as follows: St, low-antigen hereditary-angioedema patient; Ta, Za, WeI, and Da, dysfunctional-protein hereditary-angioedema patients. Note that patient Da has four times the normal level of C$\overline{1}$ inhibitor. The extra-rapid-mobility band is a complex of the latter protein with albumin. The three right-hand patterns are normal sera treated with C$\overline{1}$s in excess, with antigen-antibody complexes, and with nothing and are indistinguishable.

Procedure

1. Prepare a gel (20 by 10 by 0.1 cm) containing 0.8 g% agarose ME (Marine Colloids) in VB + 2 mM Ca^{2+} (pH 8.6).

2. Apply whole serum across the 20-cm end of the gel with a mask for 10 min.

3. Place the gel on the electrophoresis apparatus, with the sample application near the cathode.

4. Set the power supply at 300 V and approximately 75 mA. Continue electrophoresis until the bromphenol blue-albumin marker has migrated 10 cm.

5. After electrophoresis is complete, remove the gel from the apparatus, and cover the gel with approximately 1 ml of goat anti-human C$\overline{1}$ inhibitor (Atlantic Antibodies).

6. Incubate the gel for 1 h in a moist chamber at room temperature.

7. Press, wash, and stain the gel as described above for immunofixation electrophoresis.

COMPLEMENT POLYMORPHISMS OF IMMUNOPRECIPITATED PROTEINS AFTER ISOELECTRIC FOCUSING UNDER DENATURING CONDITIONS

Stock solutions

0.1 M acetate buffer (pH 4) containing 1 M NaCl and 0.1% NP-40 (100 ml). Dissolve 245 mg of sodium acetate · 3H$_2$O (or 148 mg of sodium acetate anhydrous) and 5.8 g of NaCl (Fisher) in 90 ml of distilled water. Add 470 µl of acetic acid and 0.2 ml of Nonidet P-40 (NP-40). Bring to a final volume of 100 ml with distilled water.

0.1 M Tris hydrochloride (pH 8) containing 1 M NaCl and 0.1% NP-40 (100 ml). Add 1.2 g of Tris (Sigma) to 50 ml of distilled water. Titrate with 1 N HCl until pH 8.0 is reached. Add 5.8 g of NaCl and 0.1 ml of NP-40 (Sigma). Bring to a final volume of 100 ml.

Sample buffer containing 8 M urea, 1% NP-40, 10% beta-mercaptoethanol, and 4% ampholytes (pH 3.5 to 10, pH 4 to 6, and pH 6 to 8; 1:4:4) (10 ml). Dissolve 4.8 g of urea (Schwarz/Mann) in 5 ml of distilled water. Add 0.1 ml of NP-40, 1 ml of beta-mercaptoethanol (Sigma), 0.11 ml of ampholytes (LKB) at pH 3.5 to 10, 0.44 ml of ampholytes (LKB) at pH 4 to 6, and 0.44 ml of ampholytes (LKB) at pH 6 to 8. Bring to a final volume of 10 ml.

Acrylamide stock for 4.5% gels (100 ml). Dissolve 29.4 g of acrylamide (Bio-Rad) and 0.6 g of bisacrylamide (Bio-Rad) in distilled water, and bring to a final volume of 100 ml.

4 M urea containing 0.5% NP-40 and 0.2% ampholine (100 ml). Dissolve 24 g of urea in 50 ml of distilled water. Add 0.5 ml of NP-40, 60 µl of ampholytes (LKB) at pH 3.5 to 10, 225 µl of ampholytes (LKB) at pH 4 to 6, and 225 µl of ampholytes (LKB) at pH 6 to 8. Bring to a final volume of 100 ml.

0.02 M NaOH (100 ml). Add 80 mg of NaOH pellets gradually, with mixing, to 100 ml of distilled water.

5% H$_3$PO$_4$. See above under Study of Complement Polymorphisms by Isoelectric Focusing and Functional Detection for a description of 5% H$_3$PO$_4$.

Ammonium persulfate stock (1 ml). Add 200 mg of ammonium persulfate (Bio-Rad) to 1 ml of distilled water. (*Note.* Make a fresh solution each day.)

Fixing solution (300 ml). Mix 80 ml of methanol, 20 ml of acetic acid, and 200 ml of distilled water.

Staining solution (1 liter). Add 1.5 g of Coomassie brilliant blue R (Sigma) to 1 liter of a mixture of 380 ml of methanol, 76 ml of acetic acid, and 543 ml of distilled water.

C4BP typing

Genetic polymorphisms can be observed in C4 binding protein after neuraminidase treatment, immunoprecipitation, and isoelectric focusing under complete denaturing conditions.

Two alleles have been identified, i.e., *C4BP*1*, with a pI of 6.65, and *C4BP*2*, with a pI of 6.60 (Fig. 12). Inheritance of variants is autosomal codominant.

Multiple bands representing heavy and light chains from polyclonal immunoglobulins are visualized across a wide area of the basic end of the gel and are ignored.

Procedure. (i) Preparation of immunoprecipitates

1. Treat serum or EDTA plasma with neuraminidase (as described above for C4 typing).

2. Mix 100 µl of neuraminidase-treated plasma with 100 µl of anti-human C4 binding protein. (*Note.* Antiserum was made by the authors; no vendor is given.)

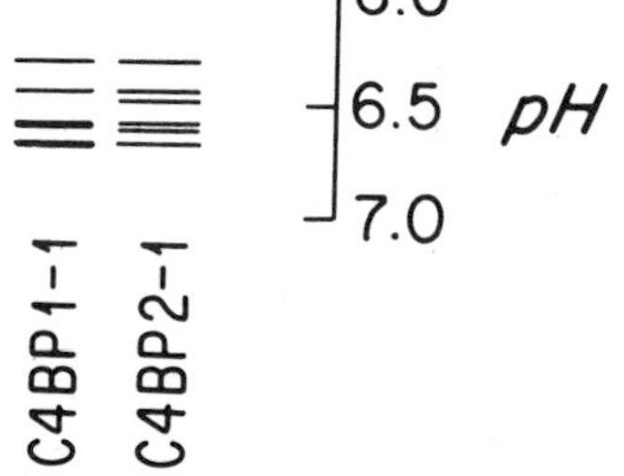

FIG. 12. Diagram of variants of C4 binding protein detected by isoelectric focusing of dissociated specific precipitates.

3. Incubate the plasma for 10 min at room temperature.

4. Add 1 ml of 0.1 M acetate buffer at pH 4 containing 1 M NaCl and 0.1% NP-40. Mix the solution on a vortex mixer, and centrifuge it for 5 min at 10,000 rpm.

5. Aspirate the supernatant, and wash the precipitate in 0.1 M Tris hydrochloride (pH 8) containing 1 M NaCl and 0.1% NP-40. Centrifuge for 5 min at 10,000 rpm.

6. Aspirate and dissolve the precipitates in 100 ml of sample buffer, and boil the tubes for 2 min.

(ii) Preparation of isoelectric focusing gel

1. Prepare a mold (20 by 20 by 0.15 cm), and seal it with agarose.

2. Prepare a gel containing 4.5% acrylamide, 1.7% NP-40, 8 M urea, 2% ampholytes (pH 3.5 to 10, pH 4 to 6, and pH 6 to 8; 1:4:4), and 0.02% ammonium persulfate. Add 11.25 ml of acrylamide stock for 4.5% gels, 1.28 ml of NP-40 (Sigma), 36.0 g of urea, 0.42 ml of ampholytes at pH 3.5 to 10, 1.67 ml of ampholytes at pH 4 to 6, and 1.67 ml of ampholytes at pH 6 to 8. Bring to a final volume of 75 ml. Degas for 15 min, and add 75 μl of ammonium persulfate stock.

3. Pour immediately, and form wells at the upper end with a comb.

4. After polymerization, remove the combs and bottom spacer, and wash the wells with distilled water.

5. Place the gel on a vertical gel electrophoresis apparatus.

6. Equilibrate the wells with sample buffer for 5 to 10 min.

7. Add samples (maximum, 100 μl) to the wells, and overlay the samples with 4 M urea containing 0.5% NP-40 and 0.2% ampholytes.

8. Place 0.02 M NaOH in the cathode reservoir and 0.1 M H_3PO_4 in the anode reservoir. H_3PO_4 solution should be degassed just before use.

9. Set the power supply at 400 V and 10 mA constant current. Run the power for 15 h at room temperature.

10. After isoelectric focusing is complete, place the gel in fixing solution, and incubate it for 60 min.

11. Place the gel in staining solution until bands appear.

H typing

H was previously known as human factor H and beta 1H. Patterns are developed after neuraminidase treatment, immunoprecipitation, and isoelectric focusing under denaturing conditions. Multiple bands representing heavy and light chains from polyclonal

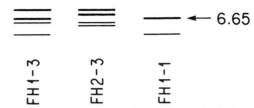

FIG. 13. Diagram of variants of factor H detected by isoelectric focusing of dissociated specific precipitates.

immunoglobulins are visualized over a wide area of the basic end of the gel and are ignored.

Two common variants, FH1 and FH2, and one rare variant, FH3, have been observed (Fig. 13). H is encoded by a single locus, and variants show autosomal codominant inheritance.

Procedure. The procedure is as described above for C4BP except that anti-human beta 1H (Calbiochem-Behring, La Jolla, Calif.; Miles Laboratories, Inc., Elkhart, Ind.) is substituted for anti-human C4BP.

LITERATURE CITED

1. **Alper, C. A., Z. L. Awdeh, D. D. Raum, E. Fleischnick, and E. J. Yunis.** 1984. Complement genes of the human major histocompatibility complex: implications for linkage disequilibrium and disease associations, p. 50–91. *In* G. S. Panayi and C. S. David (ed.), Immunogenetics. Butterworths, London.

2. **Alper, C. A., and A. M. Johnson.** 1969. Immunofixation electrophoresis: a technique for the study of protein polymorphism. Vox Sang. **17:**445–452.

3. **Awdeh, Z. L., A. R. Williamson, and B. A. Askonas.** 1968. Isoelectric focusing in polyacrylamide gel and its application to immunoglobulins. Nature (London) **219:**66–67.

4. **Hobart, M. J., P. J. Lachmann, and C. A. Alper.** 1975. Polymorphism of human C6, p. 575–580. *In* H. Peeters (ed.), Protides of the biological fluids. Pergamon Press, Inc., Elmsford, N.Y.

5. **Laurell, C.-B., and J.-E. Niléhn.** 1966. A new type of inherited serum albumin anomaly. J. Clin. Invest. **45:**1935–1945.

6. **Raum, D., V. H. Donaldson, F. S. Rosen, and C. A. Alper.** 1980. Genetics of complement. Curr. Top. Hematol. **3:**111–174.

7. **Shows, T. B., C. A. Alper, D. Bootsma, M. Dorf, T. Douglas, T. Huisman, S. Kit, H. P. Klinger, C. Kozak, P. A. Lalley, D. Lindsley, P. J. McAlpine, J. K. McDougall, P. Meera Khan, M. Meisler, N. E. Morton, J. M. Opitz, C. W. Partridge, R. Payne, T. H. Roderick, P. Rubinstein, F. H. Ruddle, M. Shaw, J. W. Spranger, and K. Weiss.** 1979. International system for human gene nomenclature 1979. Cytogenet. Cell Genet. **25:**96–116.

8. **Weast, R. C.** 1982. Handbook of chemistry and physics, 63rd ed. CRC Press, Inc., Boca Raton, Fla.

Chapter 28

Assays for Detection of Complement-Fixing Immune Complexes: Raji Cell, Conglutinin, and Anti-C3 Assays†

ARGYRIOS N. THEOFILOPOULOS AND M. TERESA AGUADO

Both exogenous and endogenous antigens can trigger pathogenic immune responses which result in immune complex (IC) disease. Because circulating ICs play such an important part in many diseases, including autoimmunity, neoplasms, infectious diseases due to bacteria, viruses, and parasites, and other unclassified disorders, the demonstration of ICs in tissues and biological fluids has achieved rising prominence (9, 10). Two main approaches have been used to demonstrate the occurrence of ICs in human and animal diseases: analysis of tissue specimens and analysis of various biological fluids.

Immunological methods for detecting soluble ICs directly in body fluids are divided into two main groups: antigen-specific tests (i.e., detection of a specific antigen complexed with antibody) and, by far the larger and more useful group, antigen-nonspecific tests. The provocative antigen of a pathogenic immune response is rarely known, but if it is, ICs composed of the known antigen and corresponding antibody are easily detected in the circulation. If one suspects a specific viral disease, the host's serum can be tested for ICs containing the viral antigens by immunoprecipitation with an antiserum to host immunoglobulin or antiserum to host complement, a reaction which markedly decreases the titers of virus or viral products in the supernatant. However, when the viral antigen is present in such large quantities that only a small proportion binds to antibody, titers of circulating antigen may not decrease appreciably during immunoprecipitation. In this case, precipitation should be preceded by sucrose density gradient fractionation or gel filtration to separate the large quantities of free antigen from the small quantities of antibody-bound antigen. The fractions obtained should be analyzed by methods such as radioimmunoassays to define the distribution of the known antigenic substance. Fractions containing antigenic material heavier than free, non-immunoglobulin-bound antigen should then be separated, and the antigen should be tested for its association with host immunoglobulin or complement. This association becomes evident if the antigen is removed by immunoprecipitation with anti-immunoglobulin or anti-C3 or by absorption to Sepharose-immobilized anti-immunoglobulin, anti-C3, or staphylococcal protein A. We have followed these steps in demonstrating circulating gp70 (retroviral envelope antigen)–anti-gp70 complexes under conditions of large antigen excess in mice with autoimmune syndromes (3).

Because of the enormous diversity of antigens involved in circulating ICs, it is doubtful that antigen-specific assays will ever find widespread use in clinical immunological studies. Therefore, there has been a growing interest in and use of antigen-nonspecific techniques (Table 1). Current antigen-nonspecific techniques and their application to diseases have been discussed in detail elsewhere (9, 10). Our laboratory has developed the following three assays for the detection of complement-fixing ICs: the Raji cell assay (11), the conglutinin assay (2), and the anti-C3 assay (7; M. T. Aguado, J. D. Lambris, G. C. Tsokos, R. Burger, D. Bitter-Suermann, J. D. Tamerius, F. J. Dixon, and A. N. Theofilopoulos, submitted for publication).

RAJI CELL ASSAY

Nature of Raji cells

Raji cells, a cultured human lymphoblastoid cell line, are derived from a Burkitt's lymphoma. The Raji cell assay is based on the observation that ICs containing complement attach to the large numbers of receptor sites on the Raji cell surface for epitopes expressed on C3d and iC3b (CR2 receptors) and C1q. Because Raji cells are devoid of membrane-bound immunoglobulin, the technique quantitates cell-bound ICs by measuring uptake of radioactive antibody to immunoglobulin G (IgG) in the complexes. Although the Raji cells contain IgG Fc receptors, these receptors are of low avidity and do not interfere with the test.

Cell culture conditions

Raji cells are cultured in Eagle minimal essential medium supplemented as described by Theofilopoulos et al. (11). Cell cultures are placed in sterile Erlenmeyer flasks (the cell culture volume should not exceed one-fifth of the total flask volume) at a density of 2×10^5 cells per ml. The flasks are tightly stoppered, incubated at 37°C on a gyratory shaker (New Brunswick Scientific Co., Inc., Edison, N.J.), and passaged twice weekly. Although no alterations of Raji cell membrane receptors have been observed in our laboratory, it is advisable to check the identity of the cells periodically by studying the profile of their surface receptors. As mentioned above, Raji cells are devoid of membrane-bound IgG, have IgG Fc receptors of very low affinity, and have CR2 and C1q receptors.

Assay method

Antiserum to human IgG is prepared in rabbits, and the IgG fraction is isolated by ammonium sulfate

†Publication no. 3824-IMM from the Department of Immunology, Scripps Clinic and Research Foundation, La Jolla, CA 92037.

TABLE 1. Antigen-nonspecific methods for detecting circulating immune complexes

Physical techniques
    Analytical ultracentrifugation
    Sucrose density gradient centrifugation
    Gel filtration
    Ultrafiltration
    Electrophoresis and electrofocusing
    Polyethylene glycol precipitation
    Cryoprecipitation
    Nephelometric assays

Methods based on IC biologic characteristics
    Complement techniques
        Microcomplement consumption test
        Assays based on the interactions of ICs with purified
        C1q: C1q precipitation in gels, C1q deviation test,
        C1q-polyethylene glycol assays, C1q solid-phase
        assays
        Conglutinin assays
        Anti-C3 solid-phase assays
    Antiglobulin techniques
        Rheumatoid factor tests
        Other antiglobulin tests
    Cellular techniques
        Platelet aggregation test
        Inhibition of antibody-dependent cellular cytotoxicity
        Intracytoplasmic staining of polymorphonuclear
        leukocytes
        Release of enzymes from eosinophils and mast cells
        Macrophage inhibition assay
        Rosette inhibition tests
        Raji cell assay
    Binding to staphylococcal protein A

precipitation followed by fractionation on an anion-exchange chromatography column (DEAE-cellulose 52; Whatman Chemical Separation Ltd., Maidstone, England). Antiserum from reputable commercial sources may also be used. The IgG fraction of the antiserum is brought to 5 mg/ml, and 1 ml is labeled with ^{125}I, using 100 µg of chloramine-T and 3,000 µCi of ^{125}I. After iodination and dialysis, the antiserum is diluted to 1 mg/ml with phosphate-buffered saline (PBS) to give a specific activity of about 3×10^5 cpm/µg. Raji cells are harvested after 72 h of culture, and portions of 2×10^6 cells in 200 µl of medium are placed in 1.5-ml plastic Eppendorf conical tubes (Brinkmann Instruments, Inc., Westbury, N.Y.; catalog no. 22-36-411-1). One milliliter of Spinner medium (Eagle minimal medium without Ca^{2+} and Mg^{2+}) is added to each tube, and the cells are centrifuged at $800 \times g$ for 8 min. Supernatant fluids are aspirated, and the cell pellets are resuspended in 50 µl of Spinner medium. Serum to be tested is diluted fourfold in 0.15 M NaCl (physiological saline), and 25 µl is added to the Raji cells. After a 45-min incubation period at 37°C with gentle shaking by hand every 5 to 10 min, the cells are washed three times with Spinner medium. After the final wash, the cells are allowed to react for 30 min at 4°C, with gentle shaking every 5 to 10 min, with ^{125}I-labeled rabbit anti-human IgG diluted with Spinner medium containing 10 g of human serum albumin (HSA) per liter. The optimal amount of radiolabeled anti-IgG to be used in the assay is determined as described previously (11). After incubation, the cells are washed three times, supernatant fluids are completely aspirated, and cell pellet radio-

activity is determined in a gamma counter. All assays are done in duplicate. The amount of uptake, expressed as absolute counts, percentage of the input, or micrograms of antibody, is referred to a standard curve of radioactive antibody uptake by cells incubated with normal human serum (complement source) containing various amounts of aggregated human IgG (AHG). The quantity of ICs in serum is equated to an amount of AHG after correction for the dilution factor and is expressed as micrograms of AHG equivalent per milliliter of serum. The soluble AHG is formed from a solution of 6.5 mg of Cohn fraction II or isolated human IgG per ml of physiological saline, heated at 63°C for 30 min, and centrifuged (1,500 × g, 15 min) to remove insoluble large aggregates. This preparation is then diluted with buffer to obtain a final concentration of approximately 1.6 mg/ml. Portions (0.5 ml) of this preparation are stored at −70°C and can be used for as long as 1 month.

Standard curve

Fifty-microliter portions of AHG (80 µg of protein) are serially diluted (11 twofold dilutions) in saline. Subsequently, 50 µl of a twofold dilution of normal human serum (source of complement), freshly obtained or stored at −70°C, is added to each dilution of AHG, mixed carefully, and incubated at 37°C for 30 min. Thereafter, 25 µl of each mixture is added to 2×10^6 cells in duplicate (fourfold final dilutions of serum containing from 20 µg to about 20 ng of AHG); the mixture is incubated, washed, and reacted with radiolabeled antibody. Radioactivity is then counted as with the test sera. A base line of radioactive antibody uptake (background) by cells incubated with 25 µl of a fourfold dilution of normal human serum, used as source of complement in the reference curve, is also established.

Standard preparations of IgG aggregates and of tetanus toxoid–human anti-tetanus toxoid ICs have recently been developed under the auspices of the International Union of Immunologists and are available through the Swiss Red Cross Blood Transfusion Service (6).

Interpretations and comments

Serum to be tested in the Raji cell assay should be used fresh or stored at −70°C and not frozen and thawed more than three or four times. The sensitivity of the assay is about 6 µg of AHG per ml of serum. In each group of sera to be tested, normal control sera handled under identical conditions should be included, and the mean ± two standard deviations of the concentrations of ICs in the normal population should be established. Our studies have shown that only 3% of normal subjects have IC concentrations exceeding 12 µg of AHG equivalent per ml of serum. Of patients with autoimmune, infectious, and malignant diseases, 42 to 97% were found to be positive for ICs (Table 2). High concentrations of Raji cell-bound IgG, presumably in the form of complexes, were observed in patients with autoimmune diseases (systemic lupus erythematosus, rheumatoid vasculitis), with a mean of 100 to 300 µg of AHG equivalent per ml, and intermediate concentrations were found in patients

TABLE 2. Raji cell radioimmunoassay for ICs in human sera

Diagnosis[a]	No. of cases	% Positive	µg of AHG equivalent/ml (mean ± SD)
SLE	121	82	264 ± 296
RA-vasculitis	26	50	189 ± 252
Periarteritis nodosa	6	90	102 ± 139
Infective endocarditis	28	97	90 ± 109
Serum hepatitis	34	53	53 ± 77
MS	67	49	44 ± 35
SSPE	6	50	58 ± 32
DHF	24	62	62 ± 15
Malignancies	610	42	89 ± 103
Hospitalized patients	60	8	39 ± 12
Normal patients	120	3	21 ± 8

[a] Abbreviations: SLE, systemic lupus erythematosus; RA, rheumatoid arthritis; MS, multiple sclerosis; SSPE, subacute sclerosing panencephalitis; DHF, dengue hemorrhagic fever.

with bacterial (infective endocarditis) and viral (hepatitis, subacute sclerosing panencephalitis, dengue hemorrhagic fever) diseases, as well as in those with malignancies, with a mean of 50 to 100 µg of AHG equivalent per ml. In follow-up studies of patients with systemic lupus erythematosus, serum hepatitis, infective endocarditis, and malignancies, good correlation was found between IC concentrations and disease activity, as evidenced by clinical and serological criteria. The results of these studies have been reviewed (9, 10).

The Raji cell technique is easy to perform, is reproducible, and requires only small amounts of serum. Moreover, antigens related to the diseases under study can be demonstrated on the Raji cell surface-bound immune complexes by immunofluorescence and radiolabeled-antibody techniques. The major disadvantages of the Raji cell technique are (i) false-positive results due to the presence of noncomplexed IgG-type antilymphocyte antibodies and (ii) interaction of autoantibodies in serum with cytoplasmic or nuclear antigens liberated from dead cells. We believe that warm reactive IgG antilymphocyte antibodies, if present in the serum, are in low amounts and low affinity and react poorly with Raji cells under our experimental conditions. This conclusion is based on the following observations: (i) very little or no IgG from systemic lupus erythematosus sera binds at 37°C to Raji cells with blocked Fc and complement receptors; (ii) $F(ab')_2$ fragments from systemic lupus erythematosus serum IgG bind very poorly to Raji cells as observed by immunofluorescence, and then only when the fragments are used in a concentration similar to that in undiluted serum; (iii) there is no correlation between IC concentrations as assessed by the Raji cell assay and cytotoxic titers in sera of patients with systemic lupus erythematosus; and (iv) results obtained with the Raji cell assay for various human sera correlate with those obtained by noncellular techniques such as the conglutinin and Clq methods.

The second theoretical disadvantage can be overcome by using the immunofluorescence Raji cell test described previously. In this test, Raji cells in suspension are incubated with the pathological sera, washed, and then reacted with fluorescein-conjugated antibody to human IgG. When 50 serum samples from patients with systemic lupus erythematosus and other disorders were tested by both the Raji cell radioimmunoassay and the Raji cell immunofluorescence assay, all but one of the samples were positive in both tests, and the intensity of surface immunofluorescence paralleled the quantity of ICs determined by the Raji cell radioimmunoassay. Of course, this technique does not exclude the possibility of IC formation in vitro as a result of cell damage during the collection of the serum or during the test itself.

Critical steps of the Raji assay are as follows: (i) before attempting to detect ICs in sera, one must determine the optimal amount of radiolabeled antibody to be used in the assay, and (ii) to obtain reproducible results, one should use the same number of cells per test, the same preparation of AHG in the standard curve, and the same preparation of anti-immunoglobulin antibody. Modifications of the Raji cell assay, which use glutaraldehyde-fixed cells and enzyme-conjugated (rather than radiolabeled) anti-immunoglobulin as the final reagent, have also been devised.

CONGLUTININ ASSAY

Conglutinin is an unusual protein (molecular weight, 750,000) that occurs naturally in the sera of certain ruminants, including cattle. It has a high affinity for IC-fixed C3. Information regarding its molecular structure and binding specificity confirms that bovine conglutinin is not an immunoglobulin and therefore is distinct from immunoconglutinins, which are found in essentially all species. Conglutinin has the important property of producing strong agglutination of sheep erythrocytes coated with antibody and complement. The binding of conglutinin to ICs is complement and Ca^{2+} dependent and appears to be specific for a fragment (iC3b) of the third complement component (C3). The interaction of conglutinin with complement-fixing ICs can be inhibited or, more importantly, reversed by chelators of divalent cations, such as EDTA, and by sugars with acetamido groups, e.g., N-acetyl-D-glucosamine. Based on the affinity of conglutinin for IC-fixed C3, a solid-phase radioimmunoassay was developed to detect complement-fixing ICs in serum (2). The technique currently used in our laboratory is given below.

Isolation of conglutinin

Conglutinin may be purified from bovine serum. It is essential that many cows be screened with the conglutinination reaction, using antibody and complement fixed to horse erythrocytes, to find one cow with a relatively high titer. Individual titers can vary from about 1/8 to 1/2,096; the cows we use have titers of 1/256 to 1/512. Sera are heated at 56°C for 60 min before use.

As a first step, we autoclave 0.45 kg of bakers' yeast in 2 volumes of PBS for 30 min at 120°C. The particles are washed with PBS until the supernatant fluid is clear and then are suspended in 500 ml of 0.2 M Tris (pH 8.6). The suspension is reduced with 0.2 M 2-mercaptoethanol for 3 h at 37°C and then alkylated with a 10% molar excess of iodoacetamide in an equal volume of 0.2 M Tris (pH 7.2). After four additional washes with PBS, the yeast is autoclaved again as described above. The mixture is then washed twice with PBS–0.1 M EDTA and 12 more times with PBS. The preparation can be stored for months at 4°C in 0.2 M Tris (pH 7.2) with added NaN_3 (1 g/liter). Before use, this mixture must be washed in PBS containing 0.2 mM $CaCl_2$.

Approximately 3 liters of heat-inactivated (56°C, 30 min) bovine serum is mixed with 0.11 kg (dry weight) of processed yeast for 1 h at room temperature. The yeast-conglutinin complex is then washed extensively (about 12 times) with PBS–0.2 mM $CaCl_2$ until successive washes have a more or less constant absorbance at 280 nm. The conglutinin is then eluted four times with 200 ml of PBS–0.01 M EDTA–25 mM N-acetyl-D-glucosamine. The combined eluates are centrifuged (20,000 rpm, 10 min, in a Beckman Ti 75 rotor) to remove yeast fragments, and then the conglutinin is precipitated as a euglobulin by dialysis for 2 days against three 6-liter changes of 10 mM phosphate (pH 5.5).

The precipitated euglobulin, collected by centrifugation, is redissolved in 10 ml of 0.15 M NaCl, and a small amount of crystalline NaCl is added to speed the dissolution. Undissolved material is removed by centrifugation at 20,000 rpm for 30 min. The soluble material is recentrifuged at 75,000 rpm for 1 h. The supernatant containing the conglutinin is further purified by anion-exchange chromatography, using DEAE-cellulose 52 (Whatman) and an initial buffer (pH 8.0) of 33 mM phosphate, 33 mM NaCl, and 6.7 mM EDTA. The conglutinin is eluted from this column with a linear gradient made with the initial buffer and a final buffer (pH 8.0) of 50 mM phosphate, 200 mM NaCl, and 10 mM EDTA. Conglutinin-containing fractions are identified by the conglutination reaction and precipitated as a euglobulin as described above. The final yield is about 10 to 25% of the initial activity, and the preparation has no contaminants, or only one, as determined by double immunodiffusion against anti-whole bovine serum. Based on nitrogen determination, a pure conglutinin preparation has an absorbance at 280 nm of 0.83 (1 g/liter of solution in PBS). The final conglutinin, after passage through membrane filters (Millipore Corp., Bedford, Mass.), may be stored in PBS (with NaN_3 preservative) at 4°C for more than 1 year.

The purification of bovine conglutinin has been improved based on the relative resistance of this protein to pepsin digestion (5). Conglutinin is purified as described above by absorption on yeast, and then the preparation is treated with 2% (wt/wt) pepsin at 4°C for 18 h and filtered on agarose A-5m (Bio-Rad Laboratories, Richmond, Calif.). Briefly, the yeast eluate is dialyzed overnight against 0.5 M NaCl at 4°C and then dialyzed for 2 additional hours against 0.001 N HCl–0.5 M NaCl (pH 3.0) at 4°C. To this eluate, a fresh solution of 0.5 mg of pepsin A (Worthington Diagnostics, Freehold, N.J.) per ml of 0.01 N HCl is added to reach a final concentration of 2% (wt/wt, enzyme/substrate ratio) pepsin A, and the mixture is stirred for 18 h at 4°C. The reaction is stopped by raising the pH to 7.2 and stirring the solution for 15 min at room temperature. The hydrolysate is concentrated by vacuum dialysis against PBS–0.01 M EDTA (pH 7.2) until the optical density at 280 nm is higher than 2.0. The concentrate is then centrifuged at 12,000 rpm for 15 min and applied to an agarose A-5m column (5 by 90 cm). The high-molecular-weight fractions contain the conglutinin; these fractions are pooled and concentrated by vacuum dialysis against PBS (pH 7.2) until a concentration of 0.5 mg/ml is achieved. This modification of the conglutinin purification gives fewer protein aggregates (by avoiding the euglobulin precipitation) and increases the yield up to approximately 60%.

Assay method

We perform the conglutinin assay in flexible plastic microtiter plates (Dynatech Laboratories, Inc., Alexandria, Va.; catalog no. 1-220-25) as follows. Plates are washed with distilled water and dried. Each well is loaded with 100 μl of conglutinin in borate-buffered saline (BBS). The concentration of conglutinin used is about 1 μg/ml, but this must be determined carefully for each preparation (see below). Plates are incubated for 5 h at room temperature and washed twice with BBS. A 200-μl portion of BBS containing 0.2 mM $CaCl_2$ and 5 g of bovine serum albumin (BSA) per liter (BBS-Ca-BSA) is added to each well, and incubation is continued for another hour. The plate is then chilled to 4°C, the BBS-Ca-BSA is aspirated, and the serum samples (see below) are loaded into the wells. After incubation overnight at 4°C, the plate is washed five times with BBS-Ca, and 100 μl (2 μg) of ^{125}I-labeled goat anti-human IgG is added in BBS-Ca-BSA (in this case, 20 g of BSA per liter). The antibody used is affinity purified (gamma-chain specific) and lactoperoxidase radioiodinated to a specific activity of about 3 × 10^5 cpm/μg. The plate is incubated for 3 h at 4°C and washed five times with BBS-Ca, and then individual wells are cut for counting.

To prepare the serum samples for testing, 20 μl of each sample is diluted with 400 μl of BBS–Ca–2% BSA, and duplicate 100-μl portions are added to the assay plate. A standard curve, similar to that in the Raji assay, is prepared by making serial twofold dilutions of AHG (40 μg to 2 ng) in 50-μl volumes, each incubated with 25 μl of normal human serum for 15 min at 37°C. Each standard is then diluted with 500 μl of BBS–Ca–2% BSA, and duplicate 100-μl portions are added to the plate. Results are expressed, as in the Raji assay, as micrograms of AHG equivalent per milliliter of serum, by reference to the standard curve.

Before a given batch of conglutinin is used, it is essential to determine the optimal concentration to add to the wells of the plate. This is done by running preliminary assays with a standard curve prepared as described above and a control curve prepared in a parallel fashion with heat-inactivated (56°C, 30 min) normal human serum. Several dilutions of conglutinin are tested, for example, 200-, 300-, 400-, and 500-fold dilutions. If too little conglutinin is used, the assay sensitivity declines greatly. However, too much conglutinin causes the assay to detect AHG in the absence of active complement. Although the optimal range is usually quite narrow, it remains stable from day to day.

TABLE 3. Conglutinin and Raji cell assays for ICs in human sera

Diagnosis[a]	No. of cases	Conglutinin assay		Raji cell assay	
		% Positive (>35 µg/ml)	µg of AHG equivalent/ml (mean ± SD)	% Positive (>20 µg/ml)	µg of AHG equivalent/ml (mean ± SD)
Infective endocarditis	119	52	104 ± 80	68	90 ± 109
MS	52	58	65 ± 37	54	45 ± 35
SLE	124	21	109 ± 81	62	264 ± 296
Vasculitis	26	38	245 ± 474	50	189 ± 252
Glomerulonephritis	21	10	55 ± 8	19	28 ± 4
Malignancies	138	7	109 ± 104	64	69 ± 83
Normal	111	4	59 ± 17	4	21 ± 8

[a] Abbreviations: MS, multiple sclerosis; SLE, systemic lupus erythematosus.

Interpretations and comments

The values obtained by the conglutinin assay in a panel of sera correlated well with the results obtained by the Raji cell assay in the same panel of sera (Table 3). The advantages of the conglutinin assay are that only soluble, stable reagents are used and many sera may be assayed concurrently.

Further clinical experience is needed to determine the ultimate value of the assay, but we have had the most impressive results to date with sera from patients with infective endocarditis and vasculitis. Theoretically, the conglutinin assay should only detect large ICs that have fixed C3. The presence of lipopolysaccharide, DNA, aggregated IgG, or antibodies directed towards cellular components should not interfere with the results. On the other hand, the narrow specificity of the conglutinin assay may be a disadvantage in some situations. Complexes that do not have surface iC3b may not be detected, since, upon the rapidly occurring conversion of IC-fixed C3b to C3dg by the C3b-converting factors (factor I, factor H, and C3b receptors), interaction with conglutinin is minimal. Therefore, ICs that have been in the circulation for long periods might escape detection by this method.

ANTI-C3 ASSAY

As mentioned above, although the Raji cell and conglutinin assays are useful indicators of IC-like materials, these reagents may give false results. Therefore, we developed another assay in which most of the C3-fixing ICs are specifically detected. In this assay, an anti-C3 antibody is fixed to a solid matrix, serum samples and standards are allowed to interact, and the amount of immunoglobulin bound to the solid-phase matrix through the C3–anti-C3 reaction is measured by a second reaction with radiolabeled or enzyme-conjugated anti-immunoglobulin. The assay, which initially utilized a polyclonal anti-C3 antibody (7), has recently been improved by using monoclonal antibodies (mAbs) recognizing neoantigenic determinants on C3c or C3d (Aguado et al., submitted). By using this modification, C3-fixing ICs in biologic fluids can be characterized with regard to the C3 fragment they express. The test is simple and reproducible, and the sensitivity is about the same as that of the Raji and conglutinin assays (6 to 12 µg of AHG per ml of serum).

Characterization of anti-C3 mAbs

Several anti-C3 mAbs have recently been developed in various laboratories (1, 4, 8), and these mAbs have been further characterized in our laboratory with regard to their C3 fragment specificity by using the following two techniques. (i) U-shaped microtiter wells (Dynatech Laboratories) are coated with 50 µl of C3 fragments (C3b, iC3b, C3c, C3d), free sites are blocked with 150 µl of 1% HSA–BBS, and serial dilutions (50 µl) of the murine mAbs are allowed to react for 30 min at room temperature. Plates are washed three times, and 50 µl of peroxidase-conjugated goat anti-mouse IgG is added. After 30 min of incubation at 37°C and color development, plates are read at 412 nm in a Dynatech MR600. (ii) Microtiter wells are coated with mAbs, nonreacting sites are blocked with 1% HSA–BBS (pH 7.5), and serial dilutions of radiolabeled C3 fragments are added. After 2 h of incubation at 37°C, plates are washed five times, and wells are cut and counted. The C3 fragment specificities of the mAbs identified by these procedures are given in Table 4.

To determine if an anti-C3 mAb is able to recognize neoantigens in the C3 molecule (i.e., to discriminate

TABLE 4. C3 fragment specificity of anti-C3 mAbs

mAb	Reference or source	C3 fragment specificity	Location of reactive epitope
mAb-4	4	C3b, iC3b, C3c	C3c
mAb-105	1	iC3b, C3c	C3c
mAb-BRL	Bethesda Research Laboratories, Inc., Gaithersburg, Md.	C3b, iC3b, C3c	C3c
mAb-3	4	C3b, iC3b, C3d	C3d
mAb-130	8	iC3b, C3d	C3d
mAb-Ortho	Ortho Diagnostics, Inc., Raritan, N.J.	C3b, iC3b, C3d	C3d

Use the OD of the normal human serum pool as 0 µg of AHGG per ml. Using linear regression analysis, draw a line through the respective points. Use this curve to determine microgram equivalents of AHGG per milliliter for the patient samples.

mRF inhibition assay

The mRF inhibition assay is a competitive inhibition radioimmunoassay in which the amount of mRF reactive substance in the sample is quantitated by inhibition of binding of radiolabeled mRF to an IgG-Sepharose substrate. The C1q inhibition assay is based on the same principles (5).

1. Test samples are run in duplicate. Serum samples are diluted 1:10 in binding buffer (75 mM Tris, 10 mM EDTA, 1% BSA [pH 7.4]). Nonspecific binding is determined by running a control sample containing only binding buffer and ^{125}I-mRF. The level of 100% binding is determined by tubes containing ^{125}I-mRF and IgG-Sepharose. A standard curve for AHGG (6 to 200 µg/ml) is included.

2. To the test samples (0.1 ml) add 0.1 ml of ^{125}I-mRF (2 µg/ml; specific activity, 0.1 µCl/mg), and vortex them.

3. Add 0.25 ml of a 1.23% suspension of IgG-Sepharose.

4. Add 0.55 ml of binding buffer, seal the tubes, and incubate them overnight (16 to 18 h) with rotation.

5. Centrifuge the tubes at 500 rpm (2 min), and aspirate the supernatant. Wash the pellet three times with buffer (0.4 M NaCl, 0.1 M EDTA [pH 7.4]). Recap the tubes, and count in a gamma counter.

6. Percent inhibition is calculated as follows: percent inhibition = (cpm 100% bound − cpm nonspecific binding) − (cpm test sample − cpm nonspecific binding) × 100. Results by comparison with the standard curve can be expressed in equivalent AHGG concentrations.

Nephelometric detection of immune complexes with mRF

The nephelometric mRF assay measures the increased light scatter from an incident laser beam to detect immune complexes bound to mRF. This method has the advantage of being rapid and simple; however, the necessary equipment is expensive (8).

1. Serum samples are diluted 1:25 with PBS (pH 7.3), and isolated mRF (5 µl) in PBS (14 mg/ml) is added to achieve a final volume of 0.5 ml. The samples are incubated at room temperature for 1 h. The resulting precipitate is quantitated by laser nephelometry.

2. All samples are assayed in duplicate. The standard curve is prepared with known amounts of AHGG diluted in normal human serum; the threshold of detection is 6 µg/ml.

LITERATURE CITED

1. **Agnello, V.** 1983. Assessment of the new immune complex assay technology. *In* K. J. Isselbacher and R. D. Adams (ed.), Harrison's principles of internal medicine: update 4. McGraw-Hill Book Co., New York.
2. **Avrameas, S., T. Ternynck, and J. Guesdon.** 1978. Coupling of enzymes to antibodies and antigens. Scand. J. Immunol. 8(Suppl. 7):7–23.
3. **Bahr, E., and D. Drahovsky.** 1984. Rapid three step purification procedure for isolation of the C1q component of human complement and its use in solid phase binding assay. J. Immunol. Methods 69:43–50.
4. **Bentwich, Z., N. Bianco, L. Jager, V. Houba, P. Lambert, W. Knapp, N. Rose, M. Seligmann, R. Thompson, G. Torrigiani, and A. de Weck.** 1981. Use and abuse of laboratory tests in clinical immunology: critical considerations of eight widely used diagnostic procedures. Clin. Exp. Immunol. 46:662–674.
5. **Gabriel, A., and V. Agnello.** 1977. Detection of immune complexes: the use of radioimmunoassays with C1q and monoclonal rheumatoid factor. J. Clin. Invest. 59:990–1001.
6. **Nydegger, U., and S. Svehag.** 1984. Improved standardization in the quantitative estimation of soluble immune complexes making use of an international reference preparation. Results of a collaborative multicentre study. Clin. Exp. Immunol. 58:502–509.
7. **Pohl, D., J. Gibbon, C. Tsai, and S. Roodman.** 1980. Isolation and purification of human C1q from plasma. J. Immunol. Methods 36:13–27.
8. **Whitsed, H., W. McCarthy, and P. Hersey.** 1979. Nephelometric detection of circulating immune complexes using monoclonal rheumatoid factor. J. Immunol. Methods 29:311–321.
9. **Williams, R.** 1980. Immune complexes in clinical and experimental medicine, p. 167–194. Harvard University Press, Cambridge, Mass.
10. **Zubler, R., G. Lange, P. Lambert, and P. Miescher.** 1976. Detection of immune complexes in unheated sera by a modified ^{125}I C1q binding test. J. Immunol. 116:232.

Chapter 30

Section E. Lymphocyte Enumeration

Introduction

NOEL L. WARNER AND JOHN L. FAHEY

One of the greatest recent advances in diagnostic immunology has been the use of fluorescence-activated flow cytometry instrumentation, which combines many new developments in laser, optic, fluid, and electronic technology with the development of monoclonal antibodies against immune cells. While the gains from this new innovation have not yet been fully realized, the impact is already a major one.

Flow cytometry with monoclonal antibodies has allowed identification and quantification of subsets of the major lymphocyte populations and even further subdivisions that differ in biologic function, maturation stage, and activation. Additional characterization is possible. This technology provides an analytic capacity and a reproducibility that were not previously available.

Fluorescence-activated flow cytometry is becoming established in the routine evaluation of the immune system in any disease where immune disorders may play a role. These include immune deficiency diseases of all types and particularly acquired immunodeficiency syndrome, autoimmune diseases, and situations such as transplantation immunology where immunosuppression is required. It is also important in the assessment of neoplastic diseases of the lymphoid system and, very likely, will become routine in other neoplastic diseases to assess reactive changes in the immune system or side effects of chemotherapeutic agents. The present status of the use of flow cytometry in these disorders is outlined in this section.

A striking advance has been a general association of surface markers (phenotypic features) with functional properties. This delineation is far from complete, and assumptions that functional changes do parallel numerical changes in broad phenotypic groups are sometimes inappropriate since the functional cells constitute only a small fraction of each phenotype group. It is likely that future developments will enable a more precise association between functional feature and phenotypic detail. Currently, however, numerical (and maturation) changes can reflect significant alterations in the immune system.

In this section the role of the fluorescence microscope in detecting T and B cells as well as characterizing complement receptors on immune cells is presented by Winchester and Ross. In the following chapter, Jackson and Warner outline the principles and techniques of cell preparation, staining with monoclonal antibody, and fluorescence-activated flow cytometry. The various uses of flow cytometry are covered in the succeeding chapters: characterizing T-cell changes in disease, covered by Giorgi; characterizing B-cell changes, discussed by Ault; and detection of antibodies to platelets, discussed by Corash and Rheinschmidt.

One of the consequences of rapid developments in a field is a plethora of names and terms. In an effort to establish a standardized nomenclature for the lymphoid population, an international committee has recommended a terminology based on clusters of differentiation (CD). This is outlined in Table 1 of the chapter by Jackson and Warner.

These chapters present the state of the art. Interested scientists and technologists, however, will need to consult reviews and other relevant literature in the coming years to keep abreast of developments in this rapidly moving field.

Chapter 31

Methods for Enumerating Cell Populations by Surface Markers with Conventional Microscopy

ROBERT J. WINCHESTER AND GORDON D. ROSS

Immunologic phenotypes

The application of immunologic techniques to the detection of molecules differentially expressed on particular cell lineages has revolutionized the characterization of cells. Cellular lineage, stage of maturation, and degree of activation or modulation in respect to various stimuli can now be determined. For example, despite the seeming morphological uniformity of lymphocytes, the methods described in this chapter make possible the division of these cells into a number of subpopulations reflecting their state of maturation and functional differentiation on the basis of differing membrane surface structures that serve as population markers. Moreover, in each of the hematopoietic lineages, leukemic cells representing particular stages of differentiation can be characterized according to phenotype. In some instances these data have already been correlated with therapy and outcome.

In blood the typical B lymphocyte has readily detectable clonotypic membrane immunoglobulin (mIg) that is similar in extramembrane structure to serum immunoglobulin. T lymphocytes lack these molecules. Conversely, the typical blood T lymphocyte is primarily characterized by the molecules that are receptors for nominal antigen. These receptors are general homologs to the immunoglobulin molecules but are relatively difficult to detect by conventional reagents. In addition, there are a variety of different molecules on B and T cells and their subsets that are recognized by monoclonal antibodies. T-cell subsets are discussed further in chapters 32 and 33.

Among the other nucleated cells in blood, monocytes and granulocytes are principally distinguished from lymphocytes by their phagocytic function, physical separability by adhesion or density, and characteristic appearance, as well as by a variety of surface structures recognized by either monoclonal antibodies or receptor-ligand interactions.

Differentiation

The meaning of a differentiation-specific molecule or antigen is illustrated in Fig. 1. If it is taken that there are approximately 40,000 genes encoding distinct products, of which roughly 10,000 are engaged in "housekeeping" functions essential for the life of the cell, 30,000 genes remain which code for products that function in specialized ways. The determination that a cell will be committed to a certain pathway of differentiation necessitates the expression of a number of different molecules that subserve the specific functions of the cell. Since there are well over 300 readily distinguishable cell types by conventional histology, a rough estimate indicates that approximately 100 different kinds of distinctive molecules

may be present in or on cells in a particular lineage. Of these, the characterization of only a small number by monoclonal antibodies will probably suffice to make diagnostic distinctions of practical significance.

This chapter covers the methods for detecting these structures and enumerating the cells that bear them based on the use of microscopy. The choice of monoclonal antibodies and the distribution of the antigens detected by them is covered in chapter 32 on the use of flow cytometry. The methods described here are (i) immunofluorescence to demonstrate the binding of monoclonal antibodies and (ii) rosette techniques.

Monoclonal antibodies

The reliance on polyclonal antibody preparations and related techniques described in the previous editions of this manual has been largely replaced by the use of monoclonal antibodies, which offer immense superiority for almost every application. The use of F(ab')$_2$ reagents in the second stage of immunofluorescence has been recommended as a uniform approach in the two-stage technique utilizing unlabeled monoclonal antibodies in the first stage. Similarly, microstaining procedures using 96-well trays have been emphasized because large panels of monoclonal reagents are commonly needed in cell phenotype analysis.

Technique and interpretation

There are two kinds of problems that recur in the methods used in this chapter and in the interpretation of their results. The first is how to measure unambiguously the presence of a particular marker without technical interference, and the second is the proper inference concerning lymphocyte type that is to be made from the finding of a given marker.

The choice of methods used to determine surface markers has been greatly simplified by the introduction of monoclonal antibody technology. However, a number of pitfalls must still be avoided. The basic methods described in detail here represent the most simplified methods that retain the necessary specificity for determining the population markers and avoid the major technical problems. Each of the determinations is relatively specialized and varies in its difficulty and demand for special equipment; however, most of them can be performed with commercially available starting reagents and equipment.

CLINICAL INDICATIONS

Lymphocyte assessment

Several clinical areas requiring lymphocyte assessment are discussed below.

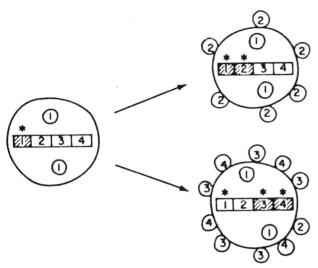

FIG. 1. Selective gene activation during differentiation.

First, the determination of malignant proliferation may require, in addition to an evaluation of peripheral blood, an analysis of bone marrow aspirates or lymphocytes obtained from lymph node or other biopsies.

B lymphocytes give rise to a spectrum of lymphoproliferative malignancies that vary in character from acute lymphocytic leukemia, chronic lymphocytic leukemia, and Waldenström's macroglobulinemia through a variety of lymphomas to multiple myeloma. Monoclonality, usually evidenced by exclusive staining for κ or λ chains, is the hallmark of these malignancies. In the case of pre-B cells, the heavy chains and subsequently the light chains are evident only upon intracellular staining. The cells of each of these neoplasms can be thought of as analogous to a step in the differentiation of the B lymphocytes from primitive cell to mature plasma cell. A smaller number of acute and chronic leukemias and lymphomas arise from T cells at different stages of differentiation and within the several alternative T-lymphocyte lineages. These are usually best recognized because they represent a predominance of a single subpopulation or differentiation stage, such as the T4 leu3 helper population.

It is generally accepted that there exists a normal stage of differentiation analogous to the phenotype of the leukemic cell. In this view, the leukemic cell is frozen at a stage of maturation. There are a considerable number of antibodies that recognize specific stages of cells in differentiation. Nevertheless, one should be prepared to find exceptions to the rule that certain antigens are found only in specific stages of the leukemic process. Also, repetition of testing during the course of therapy can contribute to a more precise determination of therapeutic response.

A second area of clinical application is suspected deficiency of the immune system. Attention is usually directed to the immune deficiencies because of recurrent or unusual infections, unexplained fever, weight loss and lymphadenopathy, or the presence of certain risk factors that predispose a patient to immune deficiency. A variety of acquired (such as acquired immune deficiency syndrome [AIDS]) and inherited differentiation failures and functional defects are included in this group. However, the most common immune deficiencies are those that accompany normal aging processes and to which only limited attention has been directed. The assessment of both lymphocyte markers and the accessory cells of the immune system such as monocytes, coupled with the appropriate test of lymphocyte function, should permit an accurate definition of the nature of the more gross cellular defects and a prediction of the most probable complications facing the patient. These tests will ultimately form the basis of an approach to correct or compensate for the deficiency.

A third principal area requiring lymphocyte assessment includes a wide variety of acute and chronic diseases associated with evidence of some alteration in the immune system. Here, the use of a variety of antibodies directed to activation antigens permit analysis of the state of compartments of the immune system. In some diseases, such as infectious mononucleosis, the objective of the study is to characterize the cellular response to a known organism. In other infections, such as leprosy or parasitic diseases, the objective is to define the elements of an ineffective immune response.

Autoimmune and other diseases of unknown etiology, such as rheumatoid arthritis, systemic lupus erythematosus, and sarcoidosis, are studied primarily to uncover features of the abnormal immune response that might in turn lead to a better understanding of the nature of these diseases. A number of abnormalities have been found that have yet to be fully interpreted, including appreciation of the quantity and reactivity of autoreactive antilymphocyte antibodies.

Studies of synovial and other fluids such as pleural effusions occurring during rheumatoid arthritis have revealed considerable changes in the composition of the lymphocyte populations compared with peripheral blood. It is interesting that the ability to determine T-cell activation antigens such as interleukin-2 (TAC) receptors or Ia antigens has given insight into the degree to which the immune system is "activated" in a disease.

Mononuclear and polymorphonuclear phagocyte assessment

The study of surface markers that characterize cells of the monocyte or granulocyte lineage indicates that their principal application is in three areas. The first of these areas is the analysis of the surface phenotype of myeloid leukemias in order to define the lineage and stage of differentiation of the leukemia and ultimately to devise categories for therapy and prognosis.

Second, these reagents permit analysis of the nature of reacting or infiltrating cells in a variety of situations, ranging from joint tissues to pulmonary alveolar macrophages. It is interesting that certain products of stimulated lymphocytes or monocytes have the property of altering or modulating the phenotype and function of the resident cells where the immune response occurs. For example, interferon-γ is capable of inducing a variety of cells to express Ia antigens. The presence of Ia-positive endothelial or fibroblastoid cells would presumably greatly influence the resultant immune response in terms of cell trafficking and perhaps antigen presentation.

The third area of application is the identification of patients who have increased susceptibility to bacterial infections and a genetic deficiency of the phosphorylated neutrophil-monocyte membrane antigen family known as CR_3/LFA-1/p150,95 (7). Several patients with this newly recognized type of genetic deficiency have now been described, and new cases may be diagnosed easily by using the appropriate monoclonal antibodies.

Lastly, the state of circulating granulocytes and monocytes in terms of their functional properties is beginning to be studied by measuring the cell phenotype, as illustrated by the alterations in CR_3 expression induced by the complement component fragment C5a.

TEST PROCEDURES AND REAGENTS

The common features of each category of assay will be presented first, followed by sections covering particular techniques and the preparation of the specific reagents. These will be preceded by a general section discussing the preparation of cells for analysis and other special considerations.

Cell preparation

Density separations. The Ficoll-Hypaque method described in chapter 38 is used to separate mononuclear cells from polymorphonuclear cells. This method is used with blood, other fluids, or dissociated tissue cells. The large majority of cell types from dissociated tissue are isolated along with the mononuclear cell fraction. In general, particular care should be directed to obtaining yields of 70% or greater to ensure representative results. Attention to the force and duration of centrifugation and the way in which supernatants are poured or aspirated off is important. A total cell count with differential of the material before density centrifugation should be used on all samples to permit calculation of the actual cell count. Viability should approach 100%. The procedure need not be carried out under sterile conditions, although the reagents must be kept free from bacterial or fungal contamination. If desired, neutrophils may be obtained from the erythrocyte pellet fraction of the Ficoll-Hypaque gradient. After all supernatant fluid is aspirated, the erythrocytes are selectively lysed by adding an ammonium chloride solution, and the remaining neutrophils are washed into the desired staining medium.

Blood samples from other than normal individuals might require modification of the cell preparation procedure. For example, in rheumatoid arthritis or other similar inflammatory states, platelets and monocytes are increased and tend to form clumps. Also, erythrocytes will more frequently be found to contaminate the mononuclear cell layer. The biologic basis of this phenomenon is not completely understood, but includes entrapment and cell-cell interaction, as well as changes in erythrocyte density. Therefore, it may be necessary to deplete the erythrocytes first by sedimenting the cells in 5% dextran (75,000 molecular weight or by simply allow the high erythrocyte sedimentation rate usually found in these samples to accomplish the preparation of leukocyte-rich

plasma by permitting the sample tube to sediment undisturbed for 30 min.

Lysis of erythrocytes contaminating these cell pellets usually makes subsequent analysis simpler and so should be almost routine. However, it must be cautioned that some cell surface systems and certain leukemia cell types are sensitive to lysis.

Lysis of erythrocytes. With blood samples of 30 to 100 ml, the erythrocyte pellet is lysed at room temperature with 50 ml of ammonium chloride solution in a plastic conical tube. For 1 liter of lysing solution, dissolve 8.3 g of NH_4Cl, 37 mg of disodium EDTA, and 1 g of $KHCO_3$ in 1 liter of water, and adjust the pH to 7.3 just before each use.

Tissue preparation. Tissues are dissociated by a variety of methods that range from teasing to enzyme digestion. For soft tissues, such as lymph nodes, the following procedure should be used.

1. Place about 1 g or less of the tissue in a petri dish, and add a medium containing glucose until the dish is about one-quarter full. Either phosphate-buffered saline (PBS) containing glucose (5 mg/ml) (PBS-G) or HEPES (N-2-hydroxyethylpiperazine-N'-2-ethanesulfonic acid)-buffered medium such as RPMI 1640 is suitable. However, media buffered only by the bicarbonate system will lose CO_2 and become alkaline, injuring the cells. The medium is made 0.1 mg/ml in DNase II to depolymerize DNA released by cell destruction, and heparin (25 to 50 U/ml) is added.

2. Tease the tissue using two disposable tuberculin syringes as handles fitted with a 26-gauge or larger needle. With a minimum of practice the tissue can be nearly completely dissociated in 1 to 10 min.

3. The cell suspension is transferred to a plastic culture tube (15 by 100 mm), and any clumps of cells are allowed to settle for 1 to 2 min.

4. The suspension is filtered through a Nytex-50 membrane (50 μm, mesh size). This can be accomplished in two ways. In one method, a disk of Nytex membrane is cut to fit in a Millipore Swinnex filter holder. This can be autoclaved if sterilization is required. The cell suspension is taken up in a Luer-Lok syringe and with minimal pressure is gently passed through the membrane. In the second method, squares of the Nytex membrane are securely fastened to the top of 50-ml plastic tubes using disposable plastic electrical cable dressing clamps. The cells are gently pipetted on top of the membrane with a Pasteur pipette, taking care not to direct the stream from the pipette tip directly toward the membrane. In both procedures the 50-μm (mesh size) membrane filtration system is washed with two 10- to 20-ml portions of PBS-G or the equivalent to give an adequate cell yield.

5. The resulting cells are washed twice by centrifugation using PBS-G or equivalent buffer.

6. Note that if the tissue cannot be readily teased apart because it is fibrous, digestion with collagenase (Worthington Diagnostics, Freehold, N.J.) and hyaluronidase (Worthington) is performed by adding the enzymes to RPMI 1640 at a concentration of 1 mg/ml. DNase is added at a concentration of 0.01 mg/ml. This solution may be sterilized by filtration through a Millipore filter (0.22 μm, pore size). The tissue is first minced using scissors. This can be accomplished by placing 1 g of tissue in a test tube (12

by 75 mm) with 1 ml of enzyme solution and mincing the tissue into cubes of approximately 1 mm with fine scissors having a blade length of about 1.5 cm. The minced tissue is transferred to a small (50-ml) Spinner culture flask or trypsinizing flask (Bellco Glass, Inc., Vineland, N.J.) using 10 ml of enzyme mixture at room temperature. The flask is incubated at 37°C on a magnetic stirrer. The progress of the digestion is closely monitored by examination of the flask and by preparing a slide if necessary. The optimal time must be determined for each tissue and varies from a few minutes to an hour or more. The digest is then passed through the Nytex membrane as described above.

Monocyte labeling

The lymphocyte preparations obtained from Ficoll-Hypaque are primarily depleted of erythrocytes and mature polymorphonuclear leukocytes. Thus, monocytes compose approximately one-third of the cells isolated from the blood of a normal individual by this method. The monocytes, if not properly identified as such, can simulate positively reacting cells in several of the assays and might lead to serious errors of interpretation (see below).

One way of solving this problem is to label the monocytes by latex bead ingestion. This is particularly useful for accurate determinations of lymphocyte structures when one is gaining experience with the morphological distinction of monocytes and lymphocytes in the phase microscope. The labeling procedure also has the advantage of permitting cold-reactive antilymphocyte antibodies found in various diseases with autoimmune features to be eluted as described below.

1. Suspend the mononuclear cell preparation to approximately 10^7 cells per ml in Hanks balanced salt solution (HBSS) supplemented with 20% heat-inactivated fetal calf serum.

2. Add 1 drop (25 μl) of a freshly centrifuged 1% suspension of latex particles per 4×10^6 to 5×10^6 cells.

3. Incubate the mixture at 37°C for 45 min with occasional mixing to keep the cells in suspension.

4. Wash the cells three times with 40 to 50 ml of HBSS or PBS, using low-speed centrifugation at 200 $\times$ g for 10 min so that free, uningested latex particles do not pellet and are discarded in the wash supernatants. This condition simulates the differential centrifugation used to remove platelets from the cell pellets.

5. Monitor a drop of the cell suspension to determine whether there are fewer than one free latex particle per 5 to 10 cells; if not, an additional wash is necessary.

6. If monocytes are abundant, clumps of monocytes can form that trap other cells and thus interfere with analysis; such clumps can usually be disrupted by vigorous blending in a Vortex mixer.

7. Some points on the discrimination between lymphocytes and monocytes are included in the section on fluorescence analysis (see below).

Latex reagent

Latex (polystyrene) particles 1.1 μm in diameter are available from several suppliers (Dow Diagnostics, Midland, Mich.; Sigma Chemical Co., St. Louis, Mo.;

Difco Laboratories, Detroit, Mich.) as a 10% suspension. They are washed three times in PBS by centrifugation at 15,000 $\times$ g for 10 min and are stored as a 1% suspension in PBS at 4°C. Just before use, they are resuspended vigorously with a Vortex mixer and centrifuged at 50 $\times$ g for 2 min, and the samples of the reagent are removed from the supernatant without disturbing the small pellet of clumped latex particles. Latex particle clumps may cause cell aggregation and cell loss during washing and are not easily separated from cells by subsequent washing procedures.

Preparation of PBS (pH 7.4)

To prepare 20 liters of PBS, combine the following: 160 g of NaCl, 4 g of KCl, 23 g of anhydrous Na_2HPO_4 (dibasic salt), and 4 g of KH_2PO_4 (monobasic salt). Solubilize the salts in distilled H_2O and bring up to volume with additional H_2O. Bottle the preparation after filtering it through a 0.45-μm (pore size) filter and then autoclave. Glucose (5 mg/ml) may be added as needed according to the application (PBS-G).

Antilymphocyte antibodies

Antilymphocyte antibodies and other substances found in certain pathological states can cause serious interference with the assays. They confer polyclonal immunoglobulin staining on cells (12) and may block access of certain antigens to staining by monoclonal antibodies. If their presence is suspected, such as in patients with systemic lupus erythematosus, Sjögren's syndrome, or AIDS, this effect can usually be minimized by carrying out the latex incubation procedure or an equivalent incubation at 37°C in the absence of autologous serum and washing with buffers warmed to 37°C. In certain uncommon circumstances, overnight incubation in a medium such as RPMI 1640 supplemented with 10% fetal calf or normal human serum may be necessary to allow shedding of absorbed antibody (12).

FLUORESCENCE MICROSCOPY ANALYSIS

The staining procedure differs according to whether the primary antibody is tagged with a fluorochrome (direct immunofluorescence) or whether a developing antibody that is tagged with a fluorochrome is needed to detect the binding of the first-stage antibody (indirect immunofluorescence). Since the indirect procedure essentially involves a repetition of the direct staining reaction, both types of reactions can be performed in an integrated procedure after the critical washing steps. This integrated procedure is commonly done using panels of monoclonal antibodies that include directly labeled and unlabeled reagents. The cells bearing Fc receptors can also be enumerated by the same procedure using incubation with soluble aggregates of human immunoglobulin G (IgG) in the first stage and development with a fluorochrome-labeled anti-human IgG reagent (3, 11). The staining reaction is performed either in tubes or in a 96-well microtray.

When a sample is to be divided for parallel analysis by flow cytometry and microscopy, the tube method is usually used unless the flow cytometer is equipped with a microsampling device, in which case the microtray method is preferable. The procedure for staining is given first, followed by sections on the reagents.

Staining procedure, tube method

The tube method is used when there are relatively few samples (<10) or in the uncommon situation where the extensive washing steps are important to remove all traces of an antibody.

1. Mononuclear cell preparations, previously incubated with latex if appropriate and washed as described above, are given a final wash with 1% bovine serum albumin (BSA) in PBS containing 0.02% sodium azide (PBS-BSA) and are resuspended at a concentration of 10^7 cells per ml in PBS-BSA. The staining is usually done at room temperature, although, as noted below, for special purposes 4°C is sometimes used (see sections below on microtray staining and antilymphocyte antibodies).

2. A 25-μl amount of cell suspension is placed in a plastic tube (12 by 75 mm).

3. Aggregated human IgG (10 μl) at 0.5 mg/ml is added to minimize Fc receptor uptake of any murine antibodies. This is especially important with those of the IgG2b class. This step would obviously be avoided if the presence of cell surface IgG was being evaluated.

4. Then 10 μl of the appropriate monoclonal antibody reagent is added. The cells are mixed with the added reagent. This can be done by quickly and forcibly rubbing the tip of the test tube over the bottom of a plastic-coated wire test tube rack.

5. After a 30-min incubation, 2 ml of PBS-BSA is added and the cells are centrifuged for 1 min in a desk top serofuge or equivalent instrument.

6. After centrifugation, the wash is poured out with a continuous motion, the tube top is blotted while inverted, and the pellet is resuspended in residual fluid as described above before the next portion of wash solution is added.

7. The cells are washed three times. After each centrifugation, any residual foam is aspirated away before the supernatant is poured off. At this point the staining reaction is complete if a directly conjugated antibody was used, and the cells can be fixed and slides made as described below for step 10. If the first-stage reagent was unlabeled, the labeled second-stage antibody is added to develop the reaction.

8. Suspend the pelleted cells and add 10 μl of aggregated human IgG at 0.5 mg/ml to minimize Fc receptor uptake of any complexes that may form.

9. Typically, 10 μl of an appropriate dilution of, for example, fluorescein isothiocyanate-labeled antimouse immunoglobulin reagent in the form of F(ab')$_2$ fragments is added. The remainder of the incubation and washing procedure is performed again exactly as described for the first-stage reagent and involves repeating steps 5, 6, and 7.

10. At this point the cells may be fixed by suspending the pellet in the residual fluid and adding 75 μl of a solution of 1% paraformaldehyde in PBS.

11. Incubate for 5 min.

12. The fixative is washed away by adding 2 ml of PBS without BSA and centrifuging as described in step 5.

13. The wash is not poured off until immediately before making the slide; then the top of the tube is briefly pressed against a towel to dry it. The pellet is resuspended with several forcible strokes across the test tube rack.

14. Then 5 μl of a 50% solution of glycerol in PBS is added.

15. A Pasteur pipette is quickly put in the tube, and a column of 0.5 to 1.0 cm of cell suspension is removed by capillary action and expressed on the slide by thumb pressure. Eppendorf pipettes can also be used to aspirate 20 μl of cell suspension. The purpose of these final maneuvers is to achieve a cell density of 15 to 25 per oil immersion field.

16. After 15 to 20 s, a 12-mm-diameter number 1 thickness circular cover glass is placed on the drop and pressed firmly down with the eraser of a pencil. The edges are sealed with a high-quality, quick-drying clear nail polish if the sample is to be kept for a day or more. Otherwise the glycerol suffices to keep the fluid in the cell's environment.

17. The slides are examined according to the instructions at the end of the microtray procedure section (see below).

Reagents

It is important to filter all reagents to remove bits of debris, primarily glass or plastic residues, that would otherwise interfere with pressing the cover slip to expel residual liquid. If the debris is not removed, focusing is rendered difficult, the sample dries out more readily, and the cells flow from one part of the slide to another. PBS is prepared as described above. It is rendered 2% (M/vol) with BSA and 0.02% (M/vol) with sodium azide and filtered (0.45 μm, pore size) for PBS-BSA.

Microtray procedure

This method is ideally suited for studying reaction with a panel of monoclonal antibodies. If flow cytometry is used in parallel with fluorescence microscopy, the instrument can be equipped with a microsampling device.

1. Nonsterile conical-bottom microtest plates (Becton Dickinson Labware, Oxnard, Calif.) are stored free of dust particles. The well margins may be labeled with a black indelible marking pen, making certain that the dye cannot interfere with the fluorescence reaction.

2. A sample (100 to 150 μl) of a cell suspension containing 0.5×10^5 to 1.5×10^5 cells in PBS-BSA is added to each of the wells. The plate is covered with a clean plastic lid and centrifuged at 1,200 rpm in a Beckman J6 centrifuge for 1 min. The centrifuge must be equipped with plate carriers. Acceleration and rotor radius should be taken into account when adapting this method to other machines.

3. The plate is carefully removed from the plate carrier and inverted over the sink, and the supernatant is thrown out. This maneuver is not particularly forceful and is best described as a gradually accelerating motion with an abrupt precise stop. Monitor the number of cells by an inverted microscope or other means while perfecting this discarding technique.

Briefly blot the still inverted plate on a paper towel, and return it to an upright position.

4. Tap the plate to suspend the cells, but avoid inadvertent transfer between wells. Here it is necessary to determine whether the remainder of the reaction should be performed on ice using chilled buffers. Lymphocyte staining can usually be done at room temperature, but monocyte and granulocyte staining is better when performed at 4°C. The cold temperature, however, favors Fc receptor interactions.

5. Add 25 μl of the appropriate dilution of a monoclonal antibody in PBS-BSA. Known positive and negative controls should also be done. Include murine myeloma proteins of each isotype without known antibody activity as negative controls, as well as a PBS control in indirect fluorescence.

6. When large numbers of the same plate are used, it is convenient to invert steps 4 and 5. The antibodies are plated out in 25-μl volumes in PBS-BSA containing 0.4% sodium azide; the plates are then covered with tape and flash frozen for storage at −70°C. Then 25 μl of a cell suspension is added to each thawed plate. The plates are centrifuged for 30 s at 1,000 rpm to concentrate the cells in the antibody.

7. The wells are covered with tape, and the cells are mixed with the antibodies by gentle tapping.

8. The plates are incubated 20 to 30 min at room temperature and then washed by the addition of 200 μl of PBS-BSA-N$_3$ followed by centrifugation at 1,200 rpm for 1 min. The supernatant is discarded as described above. A minimum of four washes is used; the number is increased if more cells are used in the staining procedure. A multiwell Titer Tek pipette assists in these washes.

9. A portion (10 μl) of the appropriate dilution of the second-stage antibody is added. For example, the working dilution of a commercial antibody F(ab')$_2$ preparation (e.g., from Cappel Laboratories, West Chester, Pa.) is usually in the range of 1:25 to 1:50.

10. The procedure described above for steps 5, 7, and 8 is repeated. After the last wash the supernatant is discarded. The cells may be fixed by incubating them for 5 min with 10 μl of 1% paraformaldehyde in PBS as described above followed by centrifugation and removal of the supernatant. Ten microliters of 50% glycerol in PBS that has been membrane filtered (0.22 μm, pore size) is added to each well.

11. Approximately 20 μl of the sample is transferred to a clean microscope slide and allowed to stand for 1 to 2 min. Up to 5 droplets may be placed at different positions on the slide to facilitate examination of a panel of reagents. A 12-mm-diameter round number 1 cover slip is placed on the droplet. After 2 to 5 min the cover slip is gently pressed flat with a pencil eraser, and any extra fluid is blotted with a Kimwipe.

12. When parallel flow cytometry is performed it is preferable to dilute the sample with an additional 10 μl of PBS-glycerol.

Microscopy. The slides are examined with a high-resolution oil immersion objective. A 63× objective with a 1.3 NA is commonly used. Phase optics alternating with the incident fluorescent illumination of a Ploem-type device are used to identify the cell type and to perform the fluorescence analysis. It is absolutely critical to optimally align the fluorescence microscope. In our experience the most common cause of

erroneous readings occurs from the lack of recognition that fluorescence illumination is inadequate (8). A total of 100 to 500 cells are counted, depending on the percentage of positive cells encountered and the desired accuracy. Cells with homogeneous cytoplasmic staining due to early cell death are not counted. They are readily recognized by the absence of the circumferential ring of fluorescence and greater fluorescence intensity in the cell center. Practice in the discrimination of dead cells should be acquired. This is most readily done by oscillating the fine-focus knob to move the focal plane through the cell, which emphasizes the difference between surface and internal staining.

The intensity of fluorescence is scored by using the following convention: ±, vague faint fluorescence which may or may not be positive but seems different from the control and has a rim distribution; tr, a trace of reliable and definite surface staining but at the weakest level consistent with certitude; 1+ to 4+, grades of increasingly strong fluorescence. A score of 4+ is probably equivalent to 200,000 to 500,000 molecules expressed per cell surface and is taken to be the fluorescence given by an anti-Ia reagent on a typical lymphoblastoid B-cell line (10). If there is a wide range of staining this would be indicated by, for example, scores of 2+ to 4+. If there is a minor 4+ bright-staining population with the majority of cells at only 1+ this would be indicated by 1+(4+). Some practice, most readily acquired by performing plateau estimates (see below), is required to perform these estimates.

Discrimination of lymphocytes from monocytes is essential and requires some practice. The majority (usually 90 to 95%) of monocytes will have ingested latex particles, and these are seen to be clearly within the cytoplasm. However, up to 5% of cells shown to be monocytes by specialized criteria fail to ingest latex. These monocytes may be recognized by an irregular ruffled profile of the cell membrane, granular cytoplasm, and an indistinct nuclear membrane. Alternatively, occasionally one or two latex particles can be found adhering to the surface membrane of a typical lymphocyte. These are not excluded from the lymphocyte population.

Intracytoplasmic staining

1. This method is designed for a Shandon Cytospin cytocentrifuge, although similar models give equivalent results. Place holder filter and slide in position. Take care to align the hole in the filter paper with the opening in the holder. The frosted side of the slide is positioned to the center. Be certain the slide is clean or the cells and antiserum will not adhere and spread.

2. Add 1 to 2 drops of BSA-PBS to each well.

3. Add 10,000 to 50,000 cells to each well in 20 to 100 μl (usually 1 to 2 drops) of medium plus 10% fetal calf serum or PBS-BSA.

4. Cytocentrifuge at 350 rpm for 5 min. Remove the holder and slide as a unit carefully, without smearing the cell area.

5. Separate slide and blotter.

6. Mark the location of the cells on the back of the slides with a Diamond pencil.

7. Place slides into a Copland jar without allowing them to become overly dry.

8. Add a solution of absolute ethanol (95 ml)–glacial acetic acid (5 ml) that has been kept at −20°C.

9. Incubate slides at −20°C in the freezer for 20 min.

10. Pour off the fixative and save it. Replenish the fixative periodically, e.g., weekly if used daily.

11. Wash slides three times with PBS. This can be done by placing the jar on a magnetic stirrer and using a small stirring bar at the bottom of the jar. Allow 30 min for each final change and 1 to 3 min for the first two washes.

12. Dry the outside area of the slides carefully with a Kimwipe, excluding the area containing the cells, which should be kept moist.

13. Put 1 drop of PBS-BSA containing the appropriate dilution of the antibody on top of the staining area. Make sure the liquid does not spread too far to the side. If this reagent is directly conjugated, proceed to step 16.

14. If a second-stage antibody is required, wash the slides three times in PBS as described in step 11, allowing 1 to 3 min for each wash.

15. Proceed as with steps 12 and 13, adding appropriate amounts of the second-stage antiserum (usually on the order of a 1:50 dilution or higher) and spreading it by tilting.

16. Incubate slides in a moist chamber for 15 to 20 min.

17. Wash slides four times in PBS as described in step 11, including one 15-min wash with stirring.

18. Dry slides carefully, excluding the cell area.

19. Add 1 drop of 100% glycerol, and put a number 1 cover slip (22 by 22 mm) on the drop.

20. Absorb excess glycerol with a Kimwipe.

Reagents for determining Fcγ receptors

See references 3 and 11.

Two different fluorescence techniques are described, the first involving soluble immune complexes of IgG antibody and antigen and the second involving soluble aggregates of IgG formed by heat denaturation. The principle involved in the first method is the formation of fresh immune complexes with an IgG antibody that is conjugated to a fluorochrome. These immune complexes bind to the Fcγ receptor, and cells are identified by their positive fluorescence. Nearly any antigen-antibody system could in principle be used. However, it is important to note that some immune complex systems exhibit preferential binding to Fcγ receptors on T-cell subpopulations, B-cells, or other cell types.

Soluble aggregates formed by limited heat denaturation of IgG tend to have a broader range of specificity for Fcγ receptors, presumably because of their heterogeneity in size and subclass. In addition, they are simpler to use. However, the aggregates of certain preparations tend to precipitate out of solution and so must be prepared at frequent intervals with interim restandardization of the optimal aggregate concentration. Whichever method is used, it should be determined whether the assay may be preferentially detecting either B-cell or non-B-cell Fcγ receptors. This can be ascertained by observation of the proportion of fluorescein-stained cells that double stain for either a B-cell marker or a T-cell marker.

The following is an example of one particular immune complex system. The antigen is rabbit IgG obtained as Cohn fraction II (FII) and is made up in PBS-BSA at 10 mg/ml. The antibody is whole sheep anti-rabbit IgG conjugated to either fluorescein or tetramethyl rhodamine. The antibody should be batch absorbed with human IgG insolubilized on Sepharose beads to prevent cross-reacting antibodies from directly reacting with human immunoglobulin. The optimal ratio of antigen will vary according to the strength of the antiserum and is found empirically. Dilutions of the antigen are made at 0.01, 0.05, 0.10, and 0.20 mg/ml in PBS-BSA. To each separate tube containing cells, 25 μg of the antibody conjugate is added, followed by 25 μg of the antigen solution. The procedure of incubation, washing, slide preparation, and examination described above is then carried out. The optimal amount of antigen is selected by determining the concentration which gives the highest percentage of stained cells. This standardization curve should show a distinct maximum zone, with higher and lower concentrations of antigen giving lower values. Preference is given to a concentration that produces a fine granular pattern of staining. In some instances, additional concentrations of antigen must be explored if there is doubt that the maximum has been reached. Since the high dilutions of antigen, less than perhaps 0.01 mg/ml, are not stable, they should be prepared freshly each day from an intermediate dilution. A known standard cell preparation should be run periodically to verify the system. Although normal peripheral blood cells can be used, the use of a lymphocyte preparation from a patient with chronic lymphatic leukemia or a B-cell line such as Daudi will greatly simplify the standardization and control of the procedure.

As an alternative method, heat-aggregated human IgG may be used as a reagent to detect Fcγ receptors instead of immune complexes. Commercially available FII (primarily IgG) is heat aggregated; the aggregates are then incubated with Fcγ receptor-bearing cells, and the bound complexes are detected by the addition of an anti-human IgG conjugated to a fluorochrome. IgG at 10 mg/ml is dissolved in and dialyzed against two changes of 0.15 M NaCl. The solution is carefully heated to 63°C for 10 min. The resulting aggregates are partially purified by slowly adding sodium sulfate to a final molarity of 0.62. The precipitated aggregates are harvested by centrifugation and dissolved by dialysis against PBS containing 0.02% sodium azide. The final concentration is then adjusted to 0.5 mg/ml, rendered 2% in BSA, and stored at 4°C. Alternatively, commercially prepared aggregated IgG used for nephelometric determination of rheumatoid factor (e.g., from Hyland Laboratories, Costa Mesa, Calif.) has proven to be of equivalent efficacy. Detection of lymphocytes binding aggregated IgG is performed by incubating the lymphocytes with 25-μl volumes of doubling dilutions of the aggregated IgG preparation for 30 min. The cells are washed three times with ice-cold PBS-BSA and then treated with 25 μl of fluorescent whole anti-IgG reagent in a manner similar to that used for the detection of mIg. The simplest method of staining for Fc receptors involves preparing an extra tube or well of cells and adding the same aggregated IgG used to block Fc receptor binding of the antibody systems. Pilot experiments should be performed to determine whether the amount of aggregates is on a saturating plateau.

Reagents for determining mIg on B cells

The primary factors influencing the choice of methods are listed below.

1. IgD and IgM compose the dominant mIg classes on peripheral blood B cells and chronic lymphocytic leukemia cells. IgA and IgG account for a minority of less than 1/10 of these mIg-positive cells (9). IgM and IgD occur together on the majority of mIg-positive cells. Cells from other sites, e.g., tonsil, lymphomas, or leukemias, differ in maturity and consequently in the immunoglobulin class that is expressed on the surface or intracytoplasmically.

2. The presence of the Fc receptor for IgG introduces strong constraints on the methods since any immune complexes formed with minute residual amounts of serum immunoglobulin will confer positive staining due to formation and uptake of immune complexes (8, 9). In addition, aggregates present in the antiserum preparation will be nonspecifically taken up and similarly produce false-positive staining. The use of a panel of monoclonal antibodies separately specific for κ, λ, μ, δ, α, and γ, is used for general determination of isotype preponderance. The total number of immunoglobulin-bearing cells is measured by using a pool of these reagents.

VALIDATION OF AN IMMUNOFLUORESCENCE SYSTEM

The use of monoclonal antibodies has greatly simplified the assessments involved in determining the adequacy of immunofluorescent staining. Nevertheless, standardization of each reagent must be performed to determine both specificity and sensitivity of the system. In the procedures described above, the antibody solution volume of 10 μl was recommended but the concentration was not specified.

The critical test used to determine the quantity of antibody is termed the plateau test and involves serial dilution of the staining reagent and assessment of the percentage and type of cells stained. Analysis of the plot of percentage of stained cells versus increasing concentration of antibody obtained by such an experiment reveals four regions as follows.

(i) The amount of reagent bound on the cell surface is insufficient to be detected.

(ii) There is an ascending slope where increasing members of cells are detected. The fact that the number of molecules of antigen varies from cell to cell implies that until a saturating quantity of antibody is used, those cells with a lesser amount of antigen could be scored as negative because their fluorescence is below the threshold recognized as being positive. Complex competition, multivalence considerations, and antibody affinity influence the distribution of fluorescence on a per cell basis.

(iii) When saturation is achieved, a plateau is reached where the percentage and intensity of stained cells is constant and independent of antibody concentration. All immunofluorescence should be performed within this working range.

(iv) As the concentration of antibody is increased, further "nonspecific" effects may become evident in which additional cells are stained because of a variety of physicochemical or immunologic phenomena. The latter include Fc receptor interactions through formation of immune complexes that secondarily bind to cells expressing Fcγ receptors. This is especially apparent in indirect immunofluorescence assays.

The performance of this test varies according to the reagent system employed.

Directly labeled single antibody. For example, testing a directly conjugated pan-T-cell monoclonal antibody, e.g., leu1, is straightforward. Use mononuclear cells in which monocytes are labeled by latex ingestion, note the recommended working quantity of reagent to be added per unit of cells in the product literature, and add 1/10, 1/5, 1, and 5 times this volume. Stain the cells and then count the percentage of positive cells, recording the intensity of staining and whether the monocytes are stained. However, if an antibody to antigen present on a minor subpopulation of cells in normal blood is titrated by this procedure, it should be remembered that the plateau concentration will be higher in a pathological sample where nearly all of the cells express the antigen. Flow cytometric analysis performed in parallel with linear amplification is helpful.

Indirect immunofluorescence. This system is inherently more intricate because the two independent variables of primary monoclonal antibody and fluorochrome-tagged developing antibody necessitate a two-dimensional checkerboard of dilutions to optimize staining. Moreover, there is the potential that residual excess of the first-stage reagent can interfere with the second-stage reagent by binding to it in the aqueous phase. This results in a decrease in available antimurine developing antibody and possibly in the formation of immune complexes that bind to Fc receptors resulting in nonspecific staining. The formation of such complexes is recognized by, for example, inappropriate monocyte or B-cell staining when a T-cell-specific primary reagent is used.

Usually a hybridoma supernatant contains enough antibodies (20 to 40 μg/ml) so that a 10-μl portion has sufficient antibodies to stain 10^6 cells. When ascites are used it is imperative to dilute the samples to 1:10,000 or more. This should be a working dilution with which to start. At higher concentrations of ascites there are frequent examples of preparations that contain additional polyclonal antilymphocyte antibodies. These stain all of the cells and yield confusing results.

Fc receptor problems. These are most readily recognized by using cell preparations that contain monocytes or granulocytes, cells with high-affinity Fcγ receptors. Any staining of a monocyte by, for example, an anti-immunoglobulin reagent is clear evidence of an immune complex Fc receptor problem.

Two-color immunofluorescence. In instances of increasing frequency it is of interest to determine whether two molecules are coexpressed on the same cell. This is a trivial problem if both reagents are independently labeled with different fluorochromes. The standardization is simply that described above for a directly labeled reagent performed independently with the added control of using both reagents together. If only one is directly conjugated to a fluorochrome such as rhodamine, the binding of the monoclonal antibody must be detected using indirect immunofluorescence. Here the sequence of staining should be as follows: (i) addition of unlabeled first monoclonal antibody, (ii) development of antimurine reagent tagged with fluorochrome, (iii) quenching of available unreacted combining sites on the developing antibody by adding the unlabeled monoclonal antibody again, and (iv) addition of the directly labeled second monoclonal antibody. Washing steps are interposed between each reagent addition. In control experiments, it is necessary to assess that the percentage of cells stained by each reagent independent of the other yields the same result when the entire staining sequence is performed. It is obvious that inadequate quenching will result in binding of the second monoclonal antibody to the cells which bound the first monoclonal reagent.

ANTI-MOUSE F(ab')$_2$-FRAGMENT DEVELOPING REAGENTS

An important advance in increasing the immunofluorescence specificity was the recognition that whole antibodies could bind to cells containing Fc receptors through their Fc regions and that this introduced serious problems (12). F(ab')$_2$ reagents were advanced to solve this problem (9). The Fc regions of the developing anti-mouse immunoglobulin antibodies used in these procedures are removed by pepsin digestion, and the resulting fragments are conjugated with fluorochrome. This minimizes the potential uptake of any immune complexes formed during staining from residual monoclonal antibody and removes the requirement for ultracentrifugation before each staining. One has the option of purchasing or preparing the F(ab')$_2$ reagents since they are widely available from commercial sources. However, in either instance their quality should not be assumed without verifying both specificity and sensitivity as described above. The method of F(ab')$_2$ fragment preparation and conjugation, while containing a number of steps, is basically a series of simple chromatographic preparations that are readily standardized and do not require fraction collectors, pumps, or monitors.

Preparation of F(ab')$_2$ reagents

1. A 30- to 50-ml amount of a very strong rabbit antiserum raised against a pool of murine antibodies of differing isotypes is mixed with an equal volume of a saturated solution of ammonium sulfate.
2. After standing for 1 h at 4°C the precipitate is harvested by centrifugation at 10,000 rpm for 15 min in a Sorvall SS34 rotor.
3. This precipitate is dissolved in 10 to 15 ml of 0.05 M NaCl$_2$–0.01 M phosphate buffer (pH 7.5) and dialyzed against two changes of 500 ml of this buffer.
4. It is then passed over a DEAE-cellulose column equilibrated with the same buffer.
5. Only the fall-through material is collected. This rabbit IgG fraction is concentrated to about 10 mg/ml for digestion with pepsin to yield the F(ab')$_2$ fragments.
6. The total protein content is measured, and the solution is rendered approximately 0.1 M in sodium acetate buffer (pH 4.1) by adding 3 M stock solution.

7. The solution is dialyzed against 0.1 M sodium acetate buffer (pH 4.1) for 1 to 2 h at room temperature.
8. Then 2 mg of pepsin per 100 mg of IgG is added, and the mixture is incubated at 37°C for 18 h.
9. The mixture is neutralized by adding Trizma base (1.0 M) and dialyzed against 0.01 M sodium phosphate buffer (pH 7.5) using several changes of buffer.

Note: The optimal ratio of pepsin to IgG may vary with some pepsin preparations and with antibody preparations that have undergone long-term storage, so that in some instances this standard 2% ratio may result in overcleavage and loss of antibody activity. For this reason, it is advisable to make a pilot study in which small amounts of the specific antibody preparations are treated with various amounts of pepsin; then, after neutralization, the antibody is examined for both cleavage and immunoprecipitation activity in an Ouchterlony plate and compared to the untreated antibody. Occasionally it has been observed that as little as 0.1% pepsin produces complete cleavage of IgG to F(ab')$_2$ in only 6 h at 37°C and that the standard conditions with 2% pepsin significantly reduce antibody activity. The activity of pepsin is also very much dependent upon the acidity of the reaction mixture. If the pH is lowered to 3.2 instead of 4.1, then complete pepsin cleavage may occur in as little as 1 h, and, conversely, if a pH of 4.5 is used instead of 4.1, then as much as 4 to 6% pepsin may be required for the 18-h treatment. Accuracy of pH readings is therefore essential for consistent results with the same preparation of pepsin.

The species of the IgG also influences susceptibility to pepsin digestion, and, in comparison to rabbit IgG, it is more difficult to obtain satisfactory results with goat IgG because F(ab')$_2$ fragments are formed in higher yield. This tendency is diminished if the goat immunoglobulin fraction is digested using 0.2 M acetate buffer (pH 4.3).

10. After treatment with pepsin, the sample is dialyzed against the buffer used in step 3 and then passed over a DEAE-cellulose column equilibrated with the same buffer, and the fall-through peak is retained. If gel filtration techniques with fraction collectors are available, it is preferable to omit the last DEAE-cellulose chromatography step and to apply the neutralized digest to a G-150 Sephadex (or S-200 Sephacryl) column equilibrated with 0.05 M phosphate buffer (pH 7.3) and 0.5 M NaCl. By using a 1.5-m column length and slow flow column, this gel filtration step will eliminate any undigested 150,000-molecular-weight material, as well as any Fab fragments, along with the other smaller fragments removed on DEAE-cellulose chromatography. The F(ab')$_2$ fragments will elute in a large peak following the void volume and any undigested IgG.
11. At this point or at any other point in the procedure, the sample volume can be reduced by adding ammonium sulfate to half saturation and dialyzing the precipitate against the appropriate buffer, in this case 0.15 M NaCl.
12. The reconcentrated preparation of F(ab')$_2$ fragments should then be tested for contaminating uncleaved IgG by immunodiffusion analysis versus an Fc fragment-specific antiserum. With preparations of

rabbit F(ab')$_2$, small amounts of contaminating IgG can be removed by passage through a column of protein A-agarose.

Conjugation with fluorochrome

1. The optical density of each sample is measured at 280 nm and divided by 1.35 to obtain the protein concentration in milligrams per milliliter.

2. A known volume of the rabbit F(ab')$_2$ preparation containing about 100 mg is adjusted to a concentration between 5 and 10 mg/ml.

3. A 0.1-ml amount of 1.0 M sodium bicarbonate-sodium carbonate (pH 9.5) buffer is added per ml of protein solution, and the mixture is put in a small beaker with a small magnetic stirring bar gently turning.

4. A 1.0-mg/ml suspension of tetramethyl rhodamine isothiocyanate or fluorescein isothiocyanate in 0.15 M saline is prepared by adding 5 to 10 mg of fluorochrome, followed by saline, to a plastic test tube and finely suspending the reagent by ultrasound. In a Branson ultrasound machine the microtip unit is used to deliver 60 to 70 W/cm^2 for three 30-s intervals (9).

5. A volume of the fluorochrome suspension sufficient to give 0.035 mg of rhodamine fluorochrome or 0.012 mg of fluorescein fluorochrome per 1.0 mg of protein is added dropwise. After being covered with Parafilm, the mixture is stirred in a 4°C room overnight.

6. Unconjugated fluorochrome is removed by passing the mixture over a column (3 by 25 cm) of G-50 Sephadex equilibrated with 0.01 M phosphate buffer (pH 7.5) at a rate of no greater than 1 ml/min.

7. The first colored peak obtained is then applied to a column (1 by 15 cm) of DEAE-cellulose equilibrated with 0.01 M phosphate buffer (pH 7.5).

8. The fall through is reserved but usually contains hypoconjugated F(ab')$_2$ fragments and gives weak staining.

9. The major peak of conjugated antibodies is obtained by elution with 0.01 M phosphate buffer (pH 7.5) which has been rendered 0.125 M in NaCl.

10. The yield should be greater than 50% and with some sera can be above 90% (1).

11. Conjugate still remaining on the column is usually hyperconjugated and can nonspecifically adhere to cells by charge-charge interactions; a 0.15 M NaCl elution can be attempted if significant material remains on the column, but the possibility of nonspecific staining should be carefully evaluated.

12. The conjugate is made 2% in BSA and dialyzed against PBS containing azide.

DE-52 (Whatman, Inc., Clifton, N.J.) and DEAE-Sephacel (Pharmacia Fine Chemicals, Piscataway, N.J.) are convenient forms of DEAE-cellulose that require only washing with the phosphate buffer before use. Stock solutions of 1.0 M sodium chloride and 0.5 M sodium phosphate buffer are both maintained, and dilute solutions are prepared on the day of use by accurate dilutions to prepare the buffers for this isolation and conjugation.

The conjugation step requires additional comment (1, 5, 12). Tetramethyl rhodamine isothiocyanate is chosen as a superior fluorochrome for the demonstration of surface immunoglobulin for a variety of technical reasons; however, the conjugation is sometimes more difficult to perform satisfactorily than with fluorescein. Lot-to-lot variations result in appreciably different solubility properties, shelf life, and ultimate conjugation efficiency of tetramethyl rhodamine isothiocyanate. Also, the fluorochrome is hygroscopic, and water uptake not only diminishes solubilization but may cause hydrolysis of the isothiocyanate linkage.

It is recommended that new lots of fluorochrome be tested on dialyzed human or rabbit FII IgG in trial conjugation procedures and that it be determined whether they give a suitable yield of properly conjugated IgG in order to avoid wasting antibody preparations. The technical service divisions of the manufacturer can be of assistance in solving problems that arise. We have had satisfactory results with fluorochromes obtained from BBL Microbiology Systems, Cockeysville, Md.

Absorption with human immunoglobulin

It is critical to absorb the second-stage reagent, e.g., goat anti-mouse immunoglobulin, with human IgG and IgM to prevent cross-reactions with human immunoglobulin on the surface of B cells. The human immunoglobulin should be insolubilized on CNBr-activated Sepharose beads to prevent the formation of soluble complexes during absorption. Similarly, if antibodies from species other than mice are to be used, all combinations of potentially undesirable cross-reactions should be eliminated by absorption. It should be emphasized that complete specificity of fluorescent reagents, established by other standard immunologic criteria such as immunodiffusion or intracellular staining, does not ensure that a reagent is suitable for lymphocyte surface staining.

ASSAYS INVOLVING ROSETTE FORMATION

E-rosette assay (spontaneous sheep erythrocyte rosettes)

Delicate rosettes formed between T lymphocytes and sheep erythrocytes are formed during incubation at 4°C. There are a number of methodological variations in use. The procedure outlined below gives a high level of E-rosette-forming cells. This classic rosette assay has for many years been the primary method used to identify T cells. Currently this assay is used to prepare purified T or T-depleted (E$^-$) cells which are then used for assays where the marker to be investigated is found on both B cells and certain T cells (for example, Ia antigens). Alternatively, the expression of the sheep E receptor can be monitored by immunofluorescence with monoclonal antibodies specific for the sheep E receptor such as OKT11 (Ortho Diagnostics, Raritan, N.J.), Leu 5 (Becton-Dickinson, Paramus, N.J.), or T11 (Coulter Electronics, Inc., Hialeah, Fla.).

1. In a plastic, capped test tube (12 by 75 mm) place 0.1 ml of 0.5% sheep erythrocyte suspension and 10^6 mononuclear cells in 0.1 ml of HBSS.

2. Add 1 drop of sheep erythrocyte-absorbed heat-inactivated human serum.

3. Centrifuge slowly (50 × g) for 5 min, and place the tubes in a refrigerator (4°C) overnight or for at

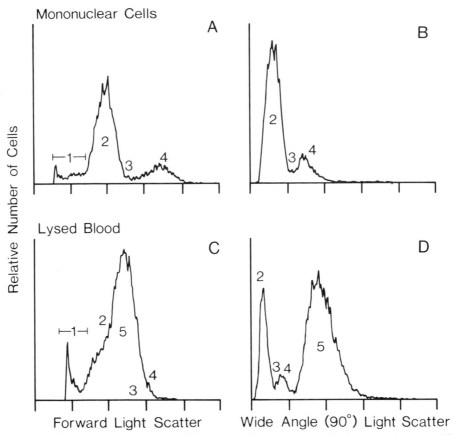

FIG. 1. Single-parameter frequency histograms of human leukocytes. (A and B) PBMC (prepared by Ficoll-Hypaque separation); (C and D) lysed blood cells; (A and C) low-angle forward scatter; (B and D) side or wide-angle (90°) light scatter. Component designations: (1) erythrocytes, dead cells, and debris; (2) lymphocytes; (3) LGLs; (4) monocytes; (5) PMNs. Dead cells are not discriminated from live cells by side scatter or volume. Dead cells display less forward scatter than their live counterparts.

a. It is important that anti-mouse immunoglobulin is absorbed with insolubilized human serum prior to use, as the cross-reaction between mouse immunoglobulin and human immunoglobulin results in background staining of monocytes and B cells with surface immunoglobulin.

b. For mouse IgM monoclonal antibodies, it is important to have either anti-mu or sufficient anti-L chain present to detect all positively labeled cells.

c. In the biotin systems, avidin conjugated with phycoerythrin, fluorescein, or Texas red is added as the second step. Do not use biotin-containing media (e.g., RPMI 1640) with avidin second steps.

Two-color indirect staining. Two-color indirect staining is used for biotin-labeled antibodies, with either fluorescein or phycoerythrin conjugates.

1. Add the directly labeled monoclonal antibody and biotin-labeled monoclonal antibody simultaneously to 10^6 mononuclear cells.

2. Incubate the cells for 20 min at 4°C, and wash them as described above.

3. Add approximately 1 μg of avidin conjugate, and incubate the cells for 20 min. Wash the cells as

described above, and suspend them for flow cytometry analysis.

Excess biotinylated antibodies and avidin nonspecifically stain monocytes and frequently lymphocytes. Therefore, careful attention should be paid to the amounts of biotinylated antibody and avidin used. It is also advantageous to include biotinylated nonreactive immunoglobulin as a control.

Setting up for either direct or indirect two-color staining in the laboratory should include preliminary experiments including single as well as dual labeling. Inclusion of fluorescinated, phycoerythrin, and biotinylated isotype controls is important, since cell preparations vary a great deal in their "stickiness" (e.g., mitogen- or antigen-activated cells [blasts] bind more nonspecifically than resting lymphocytes). These controls are also important for setting of markers for determination of the percentages of labeled cells, for assessment of antigen density, and for comparisons of certain machine settings on the flow cytometer.

Fluorescence analysis of monocytes with Fc receptors makes isotype controls mandatory. It is not uncommon to see an IgG2a mouse monoclonal control show fluorescence five to seven times that of background autofluorescence.

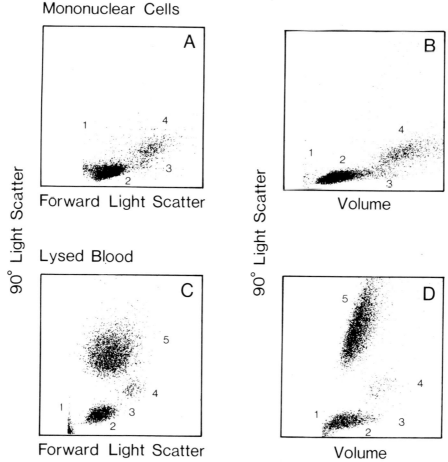

FIG. 2. Simultaneous two-parameter dot displays of human leukocytes. Component designations: (1) erythrocytes, dead cells, and debris; (2) lymphocytes; (3) LGLs; (4) monocytes; (5) PMNs. Dead cells are not discriminated from live cells by side scatter or volume. Dead cells display less forward scatter than their live counterparts. The volume parameter is measured by changes in electrical resistance as is done on some flow cytometers. Each dot plot includes 10,000 events. Thus panels A and B have 6,000 to 9,000 lymphocytes, and panels C and D have 2,000 to 4,000 lymphocytes.

Some combinations of monoclonal antibodies which may compete or interfere sterically with each other on the surface of the cell may require careful attention to marker settings, since fluorescence intensity in the mixed reagents may be lower than that for the single-color direct staining of the same cells.

Paraformaldehyde fixation of stained leukocytes

Fixation of the stained cells with paraformaldehyde preserves cellular integrity and fluorescence for up to 5 days. There is some loss of fluorescence which may be unacceptable with some reagents and for cytometers with lower sensitivity.

1. At the conclusion of immunofluorescence staining, if protein (bovine serum albumin or calf serum) was present in the last step, wash the cells with protein-free medium.
2. Aspirate the supernatant fluid, leaving approximately 50 μl above the cell pellet.
3. Resuspend the cells in the pellet.
4. Add 50 μl of cold 1% paraformaldehyde in PBS (see below, Reagents).

5. Mix the solution immediately. Failure to mix at once and vigorously will result in cell clumping and loss of viability.
6. Store the solution at 2 to 8°C in the dark. The osmolarity of this solution is higher than that of PBS, and the addition of PBS or other media before fixation is complete will distort and damage the cells.
7. When the cells are ready to be analyzed, add 0.5 to 1.0 ml of 0.5% paraformaldehyde for analysis. Alternatively, wash solution may be used for suspension if the cells have been fixed for at least 4 h.

Flow Cytometry Analysis of Stained Peripheral Blood

Characterization and identification of the leukocytes by light scatter or cell volume or both

When a focused beam of laser or lamp arc light intercepts a cell passing from or through a flow chamber, the light is absorbed and scattered at both low (forward) and wide (approximately 90°) angles (side scatter), both of which can be measured (5). Since the cells are suspended in an isotonic electrolyte solution, cell volume may also be determined by changes in electrical resistance.

Human leukocytes have characteristic and identifiable scatter and volume properties which, with the aid of electronic sensors, can be used to classify the leukocytes into lymphocytes, monocytes, and granulocytes. Erythrocytes, platelets, dead cells, and debris are usually also separable by these criteria. The data may be displayed as frequency histograms or as simultaneous two-parameter dot displays. Some examples are shown in Fig. 1 and 2.

With PBMC, a single scatter parameter can be used to electronically isolate and analyze cells. This process is usually referred to as "gating." Thus it is possible to analyze lymphocytes separately from monocytes with various degrees of overlap (Fig. 1A and B). Large lymphocytes are intermediate in scatter. However, for the analysis of lysed whole blood (Fig. 1C and D), no one parameter is sufficient, since the many PMNs present are intermediate in low-angle scatter and volume between lymphocytes and monocytes and overlap to various degrees with monocytes in 90° scatter. The simultaneous two-parameter data (Fig. 2) show that this type of analysis is far more sensitive and accurate in the discrimination of these leukocyte subpopulations than is single-parameter analysis. Either forward light scatter or volume can be combined with 90° scatter, and each event can be shown on a two-dimensional dot plot. PMNs, erythrocytes, and debris can be readily separated from lymphocytes and monocytes. This type of separation is required if large lymphocytes (which include the natural killer [NK] cells and some activated cells) are to be analyzed in the lymphocyte gates without accompanying monocytes. The setting of gates to analyze the desired populations varies from one instrument to another. Indeed, the x and y axes may also be reversed, but the principles remain the same.

All the facts mentioned above assume that the instrument has been aligned and fine tuned to maximum scatter and fluorescence sensitivity and that some stable calibration indicator, e.g., glutaraldehyde-fixed chicken erythrocytes or fluorescent particles (3, 5), has been run to ensure reproducibility. This alignment and fine tuning should be done before and after each run. Variable gain and photomultiplier tube settings on the instrument should not be used indiscriminately and randomly to correct improper alignment (3, 5).

Figure 3 illustrates a method of checking that the gates set with scatter and volume parameters include all positively labeled cells. This technique utilizes cells stained with antibodies directed toward various leukocyte subsets. The cells are analyzed with simultaneous fluorescence and scatter or volume parameters so that the labeled cells in question are separated from negative cells. After the scatter gates for one parameter are selected, the data for that parameter and the appropriate fluorescence are displayed as simultaneous dot plots, and the gate settings are checked. B cells and helper-inducer (CD4) lymphocytes, which are (or appear to be) smaller than most lymphocytes, are shown in Fig. 3A. Conversely, the result of setting gates to ensure that NK cells (which are larger) are not excluded is also shown (Fig. 3B) with anti-CD16 (Leu 11c). It is also possible to use an antibody (anti-T200 [HLe-1]) which stains all leukocytes to separate (or correct for) any debris or eryth-

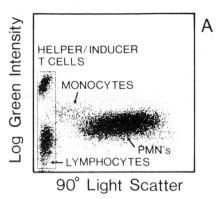

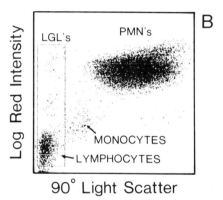

FIG. 3. Gating of lysed blood cells. (A) Stained with fluorescein-conjugated anti-CD4 (Leu 3a). The gates (or box) are set on 90° scatter to include all of the positively and negatively stained lymphocytes. Helper-inducer T cells are positively stained, as are monocytes. The few monocytes which have overlapped will be gated out by forward light scatter. Green fluorescence of PMNs is due to autofluorescence, which is greater than that of the unstained lymphocytes. (B) Stained with phycoerythrin–anti-CD16 (Leu 11c). The large lymphocytes are included in the lymphocyte box set on 90° scatter. Note two populations of low- and high-density positive cells. PMNs have high reactivity because anti-Leu 11 reacts with these cells as well.

rocytes which may not have been clearly resolved from small lymphocytes. (See chapter 34 for an example.) For PBMC, either of the scatter parameters or volume may be selected for this checking process, but wide-angle scatter is needed if lysed blood is being analyzed. After the gates are set with simultaneous two-parameter data, if monocytes continue to overlap into settings which include large granular lymphocytes (LGLs), a correction can be made by an increase in the scatter gain to increase the apparent resolution or by the use of monocyte-specific antibodies.

Selection of marker settings and determination of positively stained cells for single-color histograms

In the above section on staining, the use of controls was strongly urged. Some preparations have cells whose Fc receptors bind the controls and appear as a distinct population of stained lymphocytes despite careful gating. Isotype controls will detect these cells, and the fluorescence-scatter gating described above

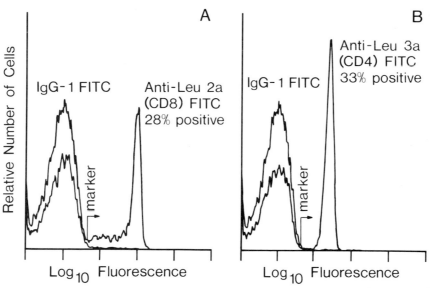

FIG. 4. Frequency histograms of stained PBMC. Markers are set to determine percentage of positive cells. (A) Lymphocytes stained with anti-CD8 (Leu 2a) FITC and control IgG1 FITC. Percentage of lymphocytes above control marker is 0.9. Percentage of positive lymphocytes is 28. (B) Lymphocytes stained with anti-CD4 (Leu 3a) FITC and control IgG1 FITC. Percentage of lymphocytes above the control marker is 0.4. Percentage of positive lymphocytes is 33.

may indicate by size if they are B cells or LGLs. If so, the values obtained should be corrected; e.g., if they are B cells, percentages are subtracted from T-cell percentages, but not from B-cell determinations, always using the appropriate number for the isotype. The problems that occur with immune complexes and the Fc receptor binding are discussed in chapter 31.

When no apparent Fc binding is seen, control marker settings should be placed where 1% or less of the cells are registered as positive. If controls are not available, unstained cells (or second-step reagent for indirect fluorescence) must be used, and it must be kept in mind that a 5% or greater error may occur. With a well-calibrated instrument, it will be found that marker settings do not vary more than 5 of 256 channels on a 5-decade log scale.

Figure 4A illustrates an example of a marker setting when there is no clear-cut distinction between positive and negative cells (anti-CD8), and Fig. 4B (anti-CD4) illustrates a more easily discriminated histogram.

Fluorescence compensation and marker settings for two-color analysis

Two-color analysis has added immensely to the knowledge of lymphocyte subsets. It may also complicate the lives of many individuals whose enthusiasm outstrips their caution.

Many cells which were classified as doubly marked turned out to be nonspecifically labeled, and improper filter combinations lost others which were truly doubles. It is important to know the spectral characteristics of the labeled reagents and the filters used to eliminate or pass both fluorescence signals for the instrument employed.

It cannot be overemphasized that isotype controls are even more important in two-color than in single-color analysis. If initial modifications to instrument

settings are usually performed on unstained cells, to place the gated negative population in the bottom left corner of the fluorescence display, interactions between differing isotypes (IgG2 and IgG1 or IgG2 plus IgG2) and differing amounts of each isotype can shift the unstained cells in either direction, e.g., towards red or green or both. This shift can lead to improper marker settings and incorrect percentages. Therefore, fine tuning requires a mix of controls in approximately the best combination. We routinely mix the maximum amount of each color of isotype control that is being used in an experiment. Selection of color and reagents can dramatically reduce the number of controls; e.g., if an attempt is made to put all IgG1 and IgM antibodies in green, where there is a minimum of expected background, then only one green control will be required.

When filters for phycoerythrin are used to optimally detect red fluorescence, they allow a significant amount of fluorescein signal to pass into the red detector. This result is due to fluorescence emission from fluorescein that extends into higher wavelengths (580 nm). Since the use of barrier or pass filters that exclude these fluorescein isothiocyanate (FITC) emissions will concomitantly reduce the sensitivity of the red detection (maximum for phycoerythrin, 575 nm), electronic or computer compensation is preferred.

There is usually minimal red intrusion into the green channels. Electronic compensation of lymphocyte-gated or mononuclear cells labeled with phycoerythrin (red)-labeled anti-CD11 (C_3bi receptor) and fluorescein (green)-labeled anti-CD8 (suppressor-cytotoxic T cells) is shown in Fig. 5. Uncompensated data show that almost all (31.46 to 32.38%) of the suppressor, cytotoxic cell population is in the upper right or doubly labeled quadrant (Fig. 5A). When the data are properly compensated, two doubly labeled populations are seen, i.e., a set of low-density (less label) cells and a set of high-density CD8 and low-

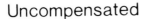

Uncompensated

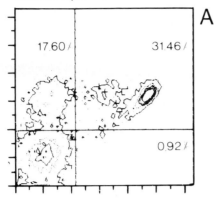

A

Compensated

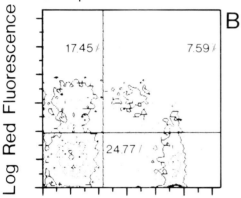

B

Log Red Fluorescence

Overcompensated

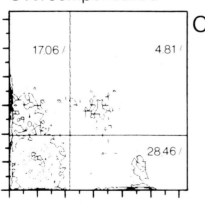

C

Log Green Fluorescence

FIG. 5. Two-color immunofluorescence analysis of mono-nuclear cells stained with anti-CD11 (C₃bi receptor-Leu 15) (*y* axis) and anti-CD8 (Leu 2a) (*x* axis) and gated on lymphocytes plus LGLs. The four quadrant settings were based on appropriate isotype controls (IgG1 and IgG2).

density CD11. These latter cells are lost if the instrument is overcompensated. To set compensations, either single- or two-color-labeled cells may be used. If single-color reagent control tubes are available, samples with medium to bright intensities are suggested, whereas for experiments without these controls, a tube labeled with a pair of reagents that have minimal overlap (e.g., CD4-CD8 or helper-suppressor) should be employed.

For marker settings if isotype controls are available, the single-color rules apply, e.g., no more than 1% positive cells in each of the three positive quadrants, with less than 2% total. A tendency to see 1% or more in the doubles area generally suggests some monocyte contamination or nonspecific binding.

Figure 5B shows properly compensated, two-color analysis with two significant populations of doubly labeled cells. Anti-CR3 (complement receptor-C₃bi) labeled with phycoerythrin is plotted on the *y* axis, while anti-CD8 (Leu 2a) labeled with fluorescein is plotted on the *x* axis. In addition to the negative cells and CR3$^+$-only cells (NK subset), there are two CR3$^+$CD8$^+$ subsets, i.e., one of low-density CD8 cells (NK subset) and one of high-density CD8 cells (in vitro T-cell suppressor activity). The remainder of the suppressor-cytotoxic subset is found in the green-only quadrant. It is quite obvious that overcompensation could lose the bright CD8$^+$CR3$^+$ subsubset (Fig. 5C).

REAGENTS

Wash solutions

Dulbecco PBS. Dulbecco PBS (0.01 M) is used for washing and staining. A 10× stock solution with azide should be stored at 2 to 8°C.

Dissolve in 1 liter of glass-distilled H₂O the following:

2.0 g of KH₂PO₄
2.0 g of KCl
21.6 g of Na₂HPO₄ · 7H₂O
80 g of NaCl
5 g of NaN₃

A 10× PBS solution without azide can be obtained commercially (GIBCO Laboratories).

To prepare a 1× solution, dilute the 10× solution 100 ml to 1 liter. Filter through a 0.22-μm filter. Check the pH (it should be 7.2 to 7.5), as pH changes during staining and analysis will alter fluorescence.

PBS-bovine serum albumin. Dissolve 2 g of bovine serum albumin (radioimmunoassay grade) in 100 ml of 1× PBS. Filter the solution.

PBS-newborn calf serum. Add 2 ml of newborn calf serum (GIBCO, etc.) to 100 ml of 1× PBS. Filter the solution.

Hanks balanced salt solution. Hanks balanced salt solution is available from GIBCO.

Ammonium chloride lysing buffer

A 10× stock solution of ammonium chloride lysing buffer should be stored at 2 to 8°C.

8.29 g of NH₄Cl
1.09 g of KHCO₃
37.0 mg of disodium EDTA

QS to 100 ml with glass-distilled H₂O.

For a 1× solution, dilute 10 ml of the 10× solution to 100 ml with 1× PBS. Filter the solution. The pH should be 7.3 to 7.4. Store the solution at room temperature. Use within 1 week. Check the pH and adjust it if necessary.

Paraformaldehyde fixative

A 2% stock solution of paraformaldehyde fixative should be stored at 2 to 8°C. Dissolve 2.0 g of *p*-formaldehyde (Eastman Kodak Co.) in 100 ml of 1× PBS at no more than 60°C. Excess temperature converts *p*-formaldehyde to formaldehyde and may increase the background fluorescence of cells.

For a 1× stock solution, dilute 1 part 10× solution with an equal volume of 1× PBS. Store the solution at 2 to 8°C. Use within 1 week. Do not use unbuffered saline.

Density gradient separation medium

For density gradient separation medium, use Ficoll-Hypaque (Pharmacia Fine Chemicals), Histopaque (Sigma Chemical Co.), or Leuco-paque (Litton Bionetics).

LEUCO-Prep

LEUCO-Prep is available from Becton Dickinson and Co.

SUMMARY

Immunofluorescence staining of peripheral blood CSA and analysis by flow cytometry places two responsibilities on a laboratory. The first is to prepare, stain, and present for analysis a clean preparation of cells which truly represents those found in the original blood sample. The second is to have a properly maintained, stable, optimally aligned and calibrated instrument. It is necessary for all those concerned to be aware of these dual responsibilities and the limitations of the instrument being employed.

LITERATURE CITED

1. **Ault, K. A., J. H. Antin, D. Ginsburg, S. H. Orkin, J. M. Rappaport, M. L. Keohan, T. Martin, and B. R. Smith.** 1985. Phenotype of recovery lymphoid cell population after marrow transplantation. J. Exp. Med. **161**:1483–1502.
2. **Bayer, E., and M. Wilcheck.** 1978. The avidin-biotin complex as a tool in molecular biology. Trends Biochem. Sci. **3**:N257.
3. **Parks, D. R., L. L. Lanier, and L. A. Herzenberg.** 1985. Flow cytometry and fluorescence activated cell sorting (FACS), p. 107–117. *In* D. M. Weir (ed.), Handbook of experimental immunology. C. V. Mosby Co., St. Louis.
4. **Reinherz, E. L., B. F. Haynes, L. M. Nadler, and I. D. Bernstein (ed.).** 1985. Leucocyte typing, vol. 2. Springer-Verlag, New York.
5. **Steinkamp, J. A.** 1984. Flow cytometry. Rev. Sci. Instrum. **55**:1375–1400.

Chapter 33

Lymphocyte Subset Measurements: Significance in Clinical Medicine

JANIS V. GIORGI

The number and functional capacity of circulating peripheral blood leukocytes reflects the overall state of immune competence of an individual. In a variety of clinical situations, tests for granulocyte, lymphocyte, and monocyte number and function have become routine in the diagnosis of disease and in monitoring immunosuppressive and immunorestorative treatments. In recent years, flow cytometric tests for lymphocyte subsets have begun to take their place as useful diagnostic and prognostic indicators in several clinical situations, including bone marrow and organ transplantation, diagnosis of leukemias and lymphomas, and evaluation of immune deficiency disorders. Flow cytometric measurements allow the enumeration of different types of lymphocytes which are known to have distinctive functional activities.

The techniques available to enumerate lymphocytes of various types have improved as a result of the development of monoclonal antibodies against cell surface differentiation antigens. These reagents are especially valuable when used in conjunction with flow cytometry to define lymphocyte cell surface phenotypes. T lymphocytes, B lymphocytes, and natural killer (NK) cells, as well as subsets of these populations, can be discriminated. The close correlation of lymphocyte phenotype with function results in part from the fact that some of the molecules in the cell membrane of lymphocytes play a role in the specific functions that these cells perform. Such functions include recognition of antigen or other cells in the immune system, regulation of the immune response, cytotoxicity, and a variety of other cellular interactions. Many of the monoclonal antibodies against lymphocytes react with molecules which play a role in one or more of these functions of lymphocytes. Other monoclonal antibodies which are valuable in characterizing lymphocyte subpopulations react with receptors for soluble molecules which regulate the immune system. Overall, the cell surface phenotype of lymphocytes may reflect their lineage, differentiation state, and immunological potential.

Flow cytometry and monoclonal antibodies have provided unique and useful information in several clinical areas, which are discussed later in this chapter. The full clinical potential of lymphocyte enumeration by flow cytometry has not yet been realized, however. As more reagents that delineate additional specific cell populations become available, improvements in the diagnostic and prognostic value of flow cytometry will be forthcoming.

PRACTICAL CONSIDERATIONS

Advantages of flow cytometry in clinical medicine

Flow cytometry in conjunction with monoclonal antibody staining has a number of advantages over alternative methods of lymphocyte enumeration. The technique is quick, precise, reproducible, and quantitative. Furthermore, it can be subjected to stringent quality control and standardization. Another advantage is that a very small blood volume, sometimes as little as 0.05 ml, is required for each test. After the initial purchase of equipment, the test is relatively inexpensive. In addition, flow cytometric methods are less labor intensive than many alternative cellular immunology assays.

Other samples besides peripheral blood can be analyzed, including the cells in bone marrow, ascitic or pleural fluid, cerebrospinal fluid, or urine. The principles of staining and analyzing these samples are similar to those for whole blood, although each requires specialized handling.

Setting up a flow cytometry facility

The choice of which flow cytometer to purchase depends upon what types of flow cytometric analyses the laboratory intends to perform. Each machine currently on the market has certain advantages. For example, the FACS Analyzer (Becton Dickinson Immunocytometry Systems, Mountain View, Calif.) is very simple to install and maintain and permits dual-color fluorescence analysis for a low price. The Ortho Spectrum III (Ortho Diagnostics Systems, Inc., Raritan, N.J.), when fully operational, requires relatively little operator adjustment of the machine from day to day and allows rapid throughput of whole blood samples. The EPIC C (EPICS Div., Coulter Corp., Hialeah, Fla.) and the FACStar (Becton Dickinson) are extremely versatile and permit both fluorescence analysis and cell sorting. Other flow cytometers with additional options are also on the market. In shopping for the best choice for a particular laboratory, consider the type of data storage provided, the type of data analysis and printout available, the cost of annual service contracts (including coverage for laser replacement), and the ease of daily standardization and use. Most flow cytometers require installation of dedicated electrical lines and specialized plumbing. Some people also suggest that a way to dim the room lights is useful to facilitate viewing the cathode ray tube video display.

The technical aspects of working in a flow cytometry laboratory fall into two separate areas. One is the preparation of cells for analysis, including separation of mononuclear cells, adjustment of cell concentrations, and staining with monoclonal antibodies. The second is the operation of the flow cytometer. Individuals who perform flow cytometry work can utilize training and skills in both areas. Courses in biology and hematology are valuable, and familiarity with immune changes characteristic of disease facilitates interpretation of the results from unusual samples. In addition, some mechanical aptitude is needed to maintain the flow cytometry equipment.

Training in sample preparation and analysis is provided as part of the purchase price of the flow cytometers by the companies which make them. Additional training in how to set up a flow cytometry laboratory to perform clinical testing is available from several different sources. One of the best is a course offered by specialists in the clinical applications of flow cytometry. Announcements of these courses can be found in *The Journal of Immunology*.

An excellent reference on the principals of flow cytometry with particular emphasis on analysis of cell surface fluorescence is an article by Parks and Herzenberg (26). Another outstanding reference which discusses a variety of topics relevant to applications of flow cytometry is a book by Shapiro (28). In addition, the journal *Cytometry* is a source for information on current methods, results, and applications in this rapidly developing field.

Monoclonal antibodies for routine clinical enumeration of lymphocyte subpopulations

The nomenclature adopted by the International Leukocyte Differentiation Antigen Workshop (8) is used in this chapter to designate the antigens with which various monoclonal antibodies react. A comprehensive list of this nomenclature, including the names of several vendors who sell monoclonal antibodies, can be found in Table 1 of chapter 32.

Routine lymphocyte subset evaluation in the clinical flow cytometry laboratory usually includes enumeration of the two major functional T-cell subsets, using reagents against CD4 and CD8, and enumeration of total T cells. Total T-cell enumeration may be done using a pan-T-cell reagent (CD3 or CD6) or a reagent against the sheep erythrocyte receptor (CD2). Enumeration of T cells by sheep erythrocyte rosetting is a standard procedure in clinical laboratories (19), so the use of monoclonal antibodies against CD2 to quantitate T cells was a natural evolution of this procedure. The use of OKT11 (Ortho) in combination with the Ortho Spectrum III is cleared by the Food and Drug Administration as an alternative for T-cell enumeration by sheep erythrocyte rosetting. However, some NK cells also express the CD2 antigen (14). CD3, a molecule which is part of the receptor for antigen on T cells, is an antigen which is exclusive to mature T cells (27). Fitc-Leu4 (Becton Dickinson), which reacts with the CD3 antigen, is cleared by the FDA for in vitro diagnostic use to enumerate T cells by fluorescence microscopy or flow cytometry. Antibodies against CD5 are no longer used as pan-T-cell markers because they are sometimes expressed on B cells (3). One minor point is that some people do not have the part of the CD4 molecule which reacts with OKT4 (Ortho) (16). Since the CD4 cells from these people are functional and do react with most other monoclonal antibodies against CD4, including OKT4A, one of these other reagents should be chosen for the routine quantitation of CD4 levels.

In addition to enumeration of total-T, CD4, and CD8 cells, enumeration of B cells or NK cells may be of interest. For example, if the patient has an immuno-globulin abnormality, evidence for the presence of B cells can be sought by using monoclonal antibodies against CD19 or CD20. Enumeration of NK cells may be of interest during immunosuppressive treatment or after bone marrow transplantation. Since NK cells bear the Fc receptor, one of several monoclonal reagents, including one against the CD16 antigen (e.g., Leu11 [Becton Dickinson]), can be used. Other subsets may be evaluated by dual-color fluorescence. The functional features of certain subpopulations of lymphocytes which are defined by dual-color fluorescence can be found in Table 3 of chapter 32.

Saturating concentrations of monoclonal antibodies should always be used. If the flow cytometer is calibrated each day and the same lot of a reagent is used over a period of time, changes in the intensity of staining with each monoclonal antibody can be employed as an indicator of the relative amount of each antigen that is expressed on lymphocytes in different individuals. In general, a higher intensity of staining indicates that more of the antigen is present on the cell surface. The intensity of staining can yield valuable information since cells which stain with high or low intensity with certain monoclonal reagents may belong to different functional subpopulations. For example, dimly stained CD8 cells are a subset of NK cells (21), whereas brightly stained CD8 cells are classic "cytotoxic/suppressor" cells. Alternatively, cells which stain with high or low intensity with a particular monoclonal antibody may represent different stages of maturation or activation. Thus, thymocytes have more CD2 than do peripheral T cells, and after activation, even more CD2 antigen is expressed.

Lymphocyte subset values: percentages, absolute values, and the CD4/CD8 ratio

As described in detail by Jackson and Warner in chapter 32, right angle and forward angle scatter are usually used to identify the lymphocyte population when a cell sample is analyzed on a flow cytometer. An electronic gate is set around the lymphocytes, and the fluorescence emission from these cells (usually between 500 to 10,000 cells per sample when a single fluorochrome is being used) is stored. Fluorescence is usually displayed as a histogram of fluorescence intensity versus frequency, and the percentage of positively stained cells is determined by setting a cursor or marker on the histogram, using an appropriate control sample to select the placement of the cursor. The "absolute" number of each lymphocyte subset can be calculated by multiplying the percentage value obtained from the flow cytometer by the number of lymphocytes in a given volume of blood. For example, the value may be expressed as number of cells per cubic millimeter. In general, the absolute value for each lymphocyte subset is more informative than the percentage, since absolute values indicate which subset is elevated or decreased. The number of lymphocytes can be derived from a leukocyte count and leukocyte differential. Since the value reported as the number of lymphocytes can radically affect the absolute value which is calculated, good quality control should be exercised in obtaining the leukocyte count and differential evaluation.

TABLE 1. Reference values for T-lymphocyte subsets[a]

Percentile	CD3 (total T)		CD4 (T-helper/inducer)		CD8 (T-suppressor/cytotoxic)		CD4/CD8 ratio
	% of lymphocytes	No./mm³	% of lymphocytes	No./mm³	% of lymphocytes	No./mm³	
Median	72	1,258	45	756	25	450	1.73
5	59	558	31	350	17	147	0.84
10	61	714	37	441	18	205	1.19
90	80	1,800	53	1,243	33	709	2.61
95	81	1,948	55	1,334	38	812	3.05

[a] From the UCLA Medical Immunology Laboratory, UCLA School of Medicine, Los Angeles, Calif.

The ratio of CD4 to CD8 cells is sometimes used to concisely express the status of the immune system. The validity of this expression is controversial. The major objection is that the CD4 and CD8 subsets are now known to be made up of several diverse and distinct cell populations: the CD4 population, which is traditionally called the helper/inducer population, also contains cells with suppressor activity; the CD8 population, which is traditionally called the suppressor/cytotoxic population, contains cells with helper activity. Thus, the functional distinction between the CD4 and the CD8 populations is not as clear as originally thought. In addition, the ratio does not indicate which subset is elevated or depressed. Nevertheless, the CD4/CD8 ratio has diagnostic or prognostic significance (or both) in many clinical situations when it is considered together with the absolute values of the lymphocyte subsets, the individual's clinical status, and other laboratory values.

Establishing a reference range for lymphocyte subset values

National or international standards for normal levels of the various lymphocyte subsets have not been established, so each laboratory must generate its own reference range. The reference range for the UCLA Medical Immunology Laboratory for the major T-cell subpopulations is shown in Table 1.

A reference range can be created by quantitating the number of different types of lymphocytes (based on cell surface antigen expression) in blood specimens collected from a large group of healthy men and women. If individuals are tested more than once, only the first set of values is used to calculate the reference range. Ordinarily, blood samples from people between 18 and 50 years of age are used to generate the reference range, since full immunocompetence is considered to exist during this time. Individuals who have had a recent illness should be excluded from the group used to generate the reference range since their cell subset values may be altered by their recent illness.

Absolute values and percentages for lymphocyte subset levels do not usually approximate a bell-shaped curve or normal distribution. Consequently, the reference range for each subset is established by arranging the values from the reference population in order of magnitude and then defining the "control" or reference range as those values that fall between the 5th and 95th percentiles. Values below the 5th or above the 95th percentile are reported as falling outside the reference range. The median is usually utilized as a measure of central tendency for lymphocyte subset levels.

The representation of the various lymphocyte subsets in healthy populations is broad. The biologic variables that are correlated with the representation in the peripheral blood of lymphocyte subpopulations include age, race, gender, and environmental influences, including season, drugs, and smoking (2). The absolute numbers of the major T-cell subsets in healthy children are significantly higher than adult values, predominantly due to the relative lymphocytosis during the first few years of life (4). In addition, a higher percentage of CD4 cells has been reported in infants than in adults (31). Finally, in elderly people, a slight decrease in the percentage of CD8 cells has been reported (25).

In addition to these variables, there is circadian fluctuation in the level of circulating lymphocytes, particularly the CD4 cells, throughout the day (24). This alteration correlates with a fluctuating corticosteroid level. Thus, the percentage and number of circulating CD4 cells drop between 8:00 a.m. and noon, about 4 h after the circulating corticosteroid level peaks. The CD4 level then gradually increases in the afternoon and remains high throughout the night, even if sleep deprivation occurs. The average fluctuation in absolute CD4 levels throughout the day is 15 to 20% but can be as high as 50%.

Despite such variability in measurements in healthy individuals, the effects of disease and immunological intervention such as organ transplant, immunological disease, immunosuppression, and lymphoid malignancy can be so profound and specific that alterations in lymphocyte subsets in affected individuals often fall well outside the reference range.

Control populations for specific clinical evaluations

To interpret the significance of lymphocyte subset levels in specific clinical situations, individuals should be compared with groups who are closely matched in age, stage of disease, treatment, and other relevant variables. The distribution of values in the matched population may differ significantly from the values in the laboratory's healthy reference population. Obviously, conclusions about changes in subset values resulting from disease or intervention will be influenced by what control group is used for comparisons.

Longitudinal studies are particularly valuable to evaluate changes in an individual's immune system

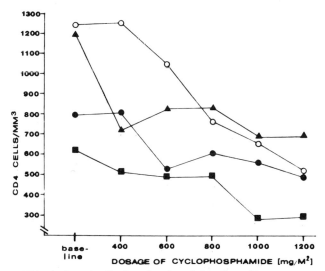

FIG. 1. Longitudinal evaluation of the effect of immunosuppressive therapy on the CD4 levels in four multiple sclerosis patients given escalating doses of cyclophosphamide once a month over 5 to 7 months. Each symbol represents one patient, the base line represents the mean of three measurements for each person, and the points during therapy represent the mean of two to four measurements taken in the month following administration of the indicated dose of cyclophosphamide. These data were provided by D. J. Moody.

over time. Since each individual has a unique cell subset profile, changes in the immune system induced by therapy or disease progression can be evaluated by comparing that person's values with his or her own values obtained before therapeutic intervention or before disease progression. Three base-line measurements should be obtained for each individual (20). This increases the chance of documenting significant changes that have occurred. An example of the results of a longitudinal study in which individuals' own base lines were used to evaluate changes induced by therapy is shown in Fig. 1.

Handling of a sample in the clinical flow cytometry laboratory

Blood for lymphocyte phenotyping can be collected into anticoagulant contained in a Vacutainer (Becton Dickinson). Ordinarily, a 3-, 7-, or 15-ml blood sample is obtained, depending on the expected lymphocyte yield, the number of antibodies that will be tested, and convenience. Heparin, citrate, or EDTA can be used. If EDTA is used, a leukocyte count and differential can be performed on the same specimen. The blood should be kept at room temperature, not refrigerated, and processed as soon as feasible. The tube can be left sitting upright or lying on its side until processing begins, but the cells should be completely resuspended by inverting the tube several times before removing a sample to stain. Most cell subsets can be quantitated accurately if measurements are made within 24 h after the blood is drawn, but significant changes occur by 48 h. In clinical laboratories, an accession number is usually assigned to facilitate record keeping.

Either whole blood, buffy coat, or Ficoll-Hypaque-purified mononuclear cells can be stained. With a few

exceptions, the different cell preparations all give similar results when stained with the same monoclonal antibodies. The exceptions include situations in which the monoclonal antibodies also bind to other cells in the peripheral blood; for example, staining on lymphocytes is weak with Leu11 (CD16), Leu15 (CD11), and Leu8 (all from Becton Dickinson) and TQ1 (Coulter Corp.) when the amount of reagent that is recommended by the company to stain Ficoll-Hypaque-purified mononuclear cells is used to stain whole blood. This is because these reagents are bound by other cells, particularly granulocytes which express the relevant antigens. Adding more Leu8, TQ1, or Leu15 will allow lymphocyte antigen sites to be saturated with these monoclonal antibodies, but the density of the Fc receptor (the antigen with which Leu11 reacts) is so much higher on granulocytes than it is on NK cells that quantitation of Leu11-staining lymphocytes requires that a mononuclear cell preparation be used.

Care should be taken that selective loss of lymphocytes does not occur when the samples are prepared for analysis. Additional steps to appropriately prepare samples may need to be performed in special circumstances. Depending on a patient's disease or treatment, the cells may need to be incubated or washed to remove inhibitory factors which could prevent the monoclonal antibodies from binding, or the cells may need to be concentrated more than usual in cases of severe leukopenia.

After the cells are stained, they are then further processed to prepare them for analysis on the flow cytometer. It is critical that all the erythrocytes be lysed or removed during this process. Erythrocytes and lymphocytes have similar right and forward scatter, and any erythrocytes which remain may decrease the apparent percentage of lymphocytes during the analysis. Lysis of erythrocytes is usually accomplished by adding NH_4Cl. If the cells are fixed in paraformaldehyde, this is done after staining, washing, and removing all residual erythrocytes.

Analysis on the flow cytometer to evaluate the percentage of cells stained with the monoclonal antibody should be done according to the protocols for lymphocyte enumeration provided by the manufacturer of each machine. "Gating" must be done so that the relevant cells are included in the analysis and irrelevant cells are excluded. For lymphocyte enumeration, both small lymphocytes and large granular lymphocytes must be included, while monocytes and erythrocytes are excluded. An antileukocyte or antimonocyte antibody can be used to evaluate whether gating is appropriate for specific situations. Results should be evaluated to determine whether the value obtained for each lymphocyte subset is reasonable. For example, the CD3 value should be approximately the sum of the CD4 and CD8 values, and the cumulative percentages of NK cells, B cells, and T cells should not exceed 100%. Any values which are suspect should be repeated. Reflex panels needed to further characterize lymphocyte populations should be done within 24 h.

Laboratory precautions for working with human blood

Precautions for working with human blood have recently been reiterated by the Centers for Disease

Control (6). All human blood specimens should be viewed as potentially infectious and treated with equal caution. Exposure by mouth, aerosols, or skin contact, especially to open cuts or abrasions, should be avoided. Gloves should be worn for handling specimens but should be removed so as not to contaminate items outside the work area. A 1:10 dilution of 5.25% sodium hypochlorite (household bleach) in water should be used to decontaminate work areas. Centrifuges should be cleaned weekly or more often if needed to remove blood spills.

Tubes should be capped when centrifuged; further protection is provided by placing covers over the centrifuge carriers. Specimen processing, i.e., pipetting blood into tubes, aspirating supernatants, etc., should be done in a biological safety hood, preferably with vertical laminar flow designed to protect the operator. When the rubber plug is removed from the Vacutainer tubes, an alcohol-coated wipe or piece of gauze should be used to cover the plug to prevent spraying of blood droplets; a tissue should be used under the plug when it is set down on the floor of the hood.

All reusable glass items should be soaked in a 1:10 dilution of bleach for several hours to decontaminate them before they are washed. Supernatant media from cell washings should be removed by vacuum suction into a sidearm flask filled with 10 ml of undiluted bleach for every 100 ml which the flask holds. These fluids can be poured down the sink after they are autoclaved. All blood, paper products, and disposable glass and plastic ware should be autoclaved before general disposal.

Laboratory accidents are dangerous potential sources of contamination, especially if broken glass is involved. Spilled blood should be flooded with a 1:10 dilution of bleach, covered with an absorbent material, and left for 10 min. This material should be cleaned up with paper towels or other disposable absorbent material, using the 1:10 dilution of bleach. The towels and other materials should be autoclaved and discarded. Centrifuge spills should be treated similarly. If the centrifuge is on when the accident occurs, turn off the instrument and allow it to stop completely before opening it. Disinfectants which have been found to be effective against LAV/HTLV-III include 0.2% sodium hypochlorite, 1% glutaraldehyde, and 25% ethanol (30).

When the flow cytometer is used to evaluate lymphocytes, modifications to reduce aerosol exposure are in order. These modifications include the use of a closed flow cell rather than stream-in-air for analysis. In addition, Plexiglas shields should be designed to direct any aerosols which do form away from the operator.

SPECIFIC CLINICAL SITUATIONS

Laboratory indications for lymphocyte subset evaluation by flow cytometry include (i) increased or (ii) decreased lymphocytes as determined by leukocyte and differential count, (iii) immunoglobulin abnormalities, and (iv) positive serology with the presence of antibodies to HTLV-III/LAV. Clinical indications include (i) suspicion of leukemia, (ii) persistent lymphadenopathy, (iii) viral, fungal, or protozoal in-

fections that accompany immune deficiency, (iv) repeated infection, (v) suspicion of acquired immune deficiency syndrome (AIDS) or an AIDS-related disorder, (vi) bone marrow transplantation and subsequent immune regeneration, (vii) immune reconstitution for immune deficiency disorders, and (viii) immunosuppressive drug regimens for organ transplantation or autoimmune diseases.

In many of these situations, the number and types of T cells are of interest. T cells, in addition to serving as effector cells for a variety of cell-mediated interactions, are also responsible for regulation of the homeostatic balance of the immune system. To operate effectively, the different T-cell subsets must be within specific minimum and maximum levels. Changes in these levels may reflect either the response of a healthy immune system to immunological challenge or an alteration which is consistent with a disorder of the immune system.

Several applications of lymphocyte subset enumeration and evaluation are outlined below, with examples of results that might be expected and how these results would be interpreted. In addition, Table 2 lists lymphocyte subset changes which occur in some clinical situations that are frequently encountered.

Primary immunodeficiency disorders

In cases of suspected primary immunodeficiency, the clinician is attempting to define the cellular basis for an individual's inability to handle an infection. Tests on granulocyte, monocyte, lymphocyte, and complement levels and function are indicated. If the lymphocytes are found to be reduced in number or if the types of infections suggest a lymphocyte defect, lymphocyte subset enumeration should be performed to determine which of the subsets are reduced.

There is considerable variety in the type of lymphocyte defects that may be found in patients with primary immunodeficiencies. Often these patients have recurrent infections with specific pathogens. In some patients there are deficiencies in the numbers of T cells, CD4 cells, CD8 cells, B cells, or NK cells that can be detected by using monoclonal antibodies in conjunction with flow cytometry evaluation. However, in other cases of clinically diagnosed primary immunodeficiency, no abnormalities in lymphocyte subset numbers are apparent, although in vitro functional activity may be defective. It is likely that further characterization of lymphocyte subsets by using some of the more recently developed reagents, including those which further subdivide the CD4 and CD8 populations of lymphocytes, will indicate that certain subsets are absent in these immunodeficiencies or that the lymphocytes lack functionally essential cell surface molecules. It is likely that specific abnormalities are present in each case of immunodeficiency. If the discrete cellular defect can be identified, the information will aid in the further classification of immunodeficiency disorders, allow the evaluation of therapeutic intervention, and add to our understanding of how the immune system develops and functions.

The cellular defects that underlie specific primary immunodeficiencies may be difficult to distinguish from the effects of infectious agents on the immune

TABLE 2. Characteristic lymphocyte subset alterations in peripheral blood[a]

Clinical disorder or treatment	Change frequently observed
Autoimmunity	
Multiple sclerosis	Both CD8 decrease and no change have been reported
Systemic lupus erythematosus	CD4 and CD8 decreases have been reported
Drugs[b]	
ATG	Immediate depletion of T lymphocytes of all subclasses
Azathioprine	Decrease in NK cells
Corticosteroids	Preferential decrease in CD4 lymphocytes
Cyclophosphamide	Depression of CD4 and B cells with chronic administration
OKT3, T12	Immediate clearance of T cells from the circulation
Infection	
AIDS	Chronic CD4 decrease
CMV mononucleosis	Transient CD4 decrease, CD8 increase that lasts months to years
EBV mononucleosis	CD8 increase that returns to normal during convalescence
Measles	Transient CD4 decrease that returns to normal during convalescence
Malaria (*P. falciparum*)	Transient CD4 decrease that rebounds during recovery
Severe bacterial infections	Relative increase in CD4 cells
Tuberculosis, progressive	Chronic relative CD4 decrease
Other	
Sarcoidosis (with high-intensity alveolitis)	CD4 cells decreased in the peripheral blood and increased in the lung (18)

[a] This table lists profound changes which are often observed in the majority of people in these situations. There is considerable heterogeneity, however. The effect of drugs given to treat disease is often a confounding variable.

[b] Effects may vary with dosage and route of administration.

system, since certain infections can themselves cause marked changes in lymphocyte subsets. The changes may last for months after the clinical infection has subsided. Because immunodeficiency is often diagnosed as a result of the presence of persistent infection, it is not always possible to determine whether changes in lymphocyte subsets in immunodeficiency reflect the underlying immune defect or the response of the immune system to infection.

The cellular defects in clinically diagnosed severe combined immune deficiency syndrome have been studied extensively by flow cytometry analysis with monoclonal antibodies. These studies show that many affected children lack circulating mature T cells that express CD3; others have some or normal levels, but these cells fail to function normally in tests of cellular immunity, including mixed leukocyte culture and proliferation to T-cell mitogens. There is often reduced expression of CD2, CD4, and CD8 antigens on T cells, although immature T cells which express CD1 or stain with OKT10 (Ortho) are present (10). B cell and NK cells and activity may be present or not. Bone marrow transplantation has been used successfully to treat children with severe combined immune deficiency syndrome. The recovery of the lymphcoyte subsets in these children can be followed flow cytometrically (Fig. 2).

AIDS and HTLV-III/LAV infection

AIDS usually occurs in individuals who belong to one of several high-risk groups. However, AIDS may be suspected in an individual who develops severe cellular immune deficiency without another known cause. The etiologic agent of AIDS is a T-lymphotropic virus known as HTLV-III/LAV. This virus can cause profound immune deficiency accompanied by the loss of CD4 lymphocytes. Clinical tests for AIDS and AIDS-

related complex are described in detail elsewhere in this volume. The information here is focused to assist in the interpretation of the T-cell subset changes as they relate to the diagnosis of AIDS or individuals in high risk-groups, and in evaluating disease progression or the results of immunorestorative therapy.

Individuals who are at high risk for AIDS, including homosexually active males and hemophiliacs, often have characteristic immunological changes unrelated to HTLV-III/LAV infection which set them apart, immunologically, from a reference population (13). The most frequent change is an elevation in the CD8-bearing T lymphocytes, which results in a low CD4/CD8 ratio in many of these individuals. Some of these individuals are seropositive for HTLV-III/LAV, but many are seronegative. Thus, the cause of an increased CD8 level may be the HTLV-III/LAV infection or may be normal host immune responsiveness to other elements. Repeated serious infections in homosexually active males and intravenous drug abusers, as well as reactivation of cytomegalovirus (CMV), may be responsible for the elevated CD8 cells in some of these high-risk individuals.

In individuals with clinical signs suggestive of AIDS and in individuals who are seropositive for HTLV-III/LAV antibody, T-subset analysis is an important indicator of the extent of destruction of the immune system by the virus. A severe decrease in CD4 cells to below the 5th percentile of the reference range and a low CD4/CD8 ratio (also to below the 5th percentile) serve as markers of disease in AIDS-related complex or in frank AIDS accompanied by opportunistic infection or Kaposi's sarcoma. In addition, the CD8 number is frequently increased during the early stages of the development of AIDS. Dual-color immunofluorescence studies indicate that specific subsets within the major T-cell classes are altered in AIDS. An example of the differences between the subsets of lymphocytes

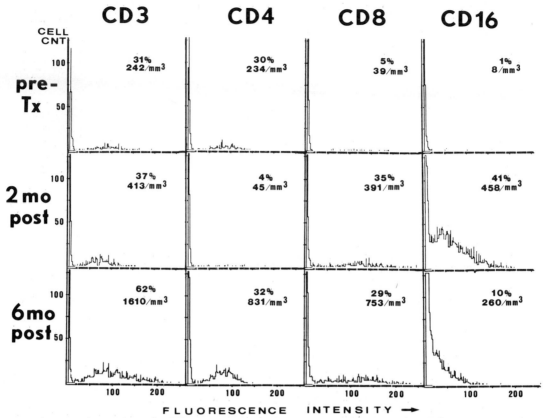

FIG. 2. Lymphocyte subset values of a child diagnosed as having severe combined immune deficiency syndrome and treated with bone marrow transplantation at 8 months of age. CD3 (Leu4), CD4 (Leu3), CD8 (Leu2), and CD16 (Leu11) values were measured before transplant and at 2 and 6 months after transplant. The histograms were generated on an Ortho Spectrum III; in the upper right-hand corner of each histogram is the percentage and absolute number (cells per mm³) of each lymphocyte subset. Evidence of restored T-cell function was found 6 months after transplant.

present in a control subject and those present in a patient with AIDS is shown in Fig. 3.

AIDS is known to occur in infants and children. The T-cell subset abnormalities in children usually resemble those in adults; i.e., the absolute number of CD4 cells is quite low, despite a normal or near-normal total T-cell number. Most of the T cells are CD8 cells, and frequently many of these cells bind OKT10 antibody. There usually are known risk factors which suggest that AIDS may be a possibility in a child with this immune deficiency. These risk factors include intravenous drug use by the mother or father and transfusions received by the child due to premature birth or other causes.

T-cell subset measurements have prognostic value in patients who are infected with HTLV-III/LAV. Patients who have lower values of CD4 cells and lower CD4/CD8 ratios when they first seek medical care have a poorer prognosis than patients who have higher values for these parameters. Patients who have high proportions of T lymphocytes which express OKT10, mostly on CD8 cells, have a poorer prognosis than patients with lower OKT10 percentages. Progressive deterioration of the immune system, as well as the immunorestorative effects of immunomodulating drugs, can be assessed quantitatively by monitoring patients with AIDS over a period of months or years. Values in a particular patient can be compared over time to evaluate changes in specific T-cell subsets. A decrease in CD4 cells over time is associated with progressive deterioration of the immune system. On the other hand, an increase in CD4 cells would be expected if immunorestorative therapy was working successfully.

Infections

There is considerable variability in the type of T-cell subset alterations which result from infections. In most cases, the relevance of these changes to the infectious process itself and to the host's recovery from infection have not been completely defined.

The alterations have been defined best for herpes-type viruses. Infection with these viruses are known to have profound effects on the immune system. CMV and Epstein-Barr virus (EBV) infections induced a marked rise in the number of circulating CD8 cells. In CMV infection there is also a transient decrease in the number of circulating CD4 cells. With both CMV and EBV, the absolute increase in CD8 cells may be as much as 10-fold. In EBV mononucleosis, the elevated CD8 levels fall to normal during convalescence (11), whereas elevations after CMV infection may last months to years (5). Functionally these cells have suppressive activity in vitro, but they may have a role in vivo in recovery from the infection.

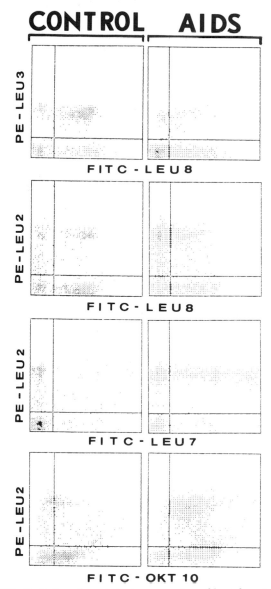

FIG. 3. Cell surface antigen expression of lymphocytes in the peripheral blood of a healthy control and an AIDS patient. The cells were stained with phycoerythrin (PE)-labeled Leu3 (CD4) or Leu2 (CD8) and fluorescein (Fitc)-labeled Leu8 or Leu7 or OKT10 plus fluorescein-labeled goat anti-mouse immunoglobulin. The histograms were generated on an EPICS C. Green fluorescence is shown on the horizontal axis, and red fluorescence is shown on the vertical axis; there are 1,000 cells in each histogram. Note that the AIDS patient has a deficiency of both Leu3$^+$ Leu8$^-$ and Leu3$^+$ Leu8$^+$ cells, a relative increase in Leu2$^+$ Leu8$^-$ cells, and marked increases in both Leu2$^+$ Leu7$^+$ and Leu2$^+$ OKT10$^+$ cells. Most controls look similar to the pattern on the left, whereas there is considerable heterogeneity in the subsets in different AIDS patients.

Immune challenge with tetanus vaccination (12), measles infection (1), and *Plasmodium falciparum* malaria (32) have all been reported to cause a transient decrease in the absolute number of CD4 cells. Advanced active pulmonary tuberculosis is accompanied by a persistent decrease in the relative number of CD4 cells, although no decrease was found in newly diag-

nosed cases (29). In contrast, some bacterial infections, particularly endocarditis caused by *Staphylococcus aureus* or *Klebsiella pneumonia* (15), may result in relative increases in CD4 cells, with CD4/CD8 ratios as high as 20. In contrast, superficial infections with these organisms cause less marked alterations in T-cell subsets.

Although the changes in T-cell subsets which accompany infection are not usually diagnostic, the effects of infection on the immune system need to be considered in interpreting T-cell subset results.

Renal transplantation

T-cell subset measurements are used in renal transplantation to monitor the effects of immunosuppressive therapy on the immune system and to assist in the evaluation of whether graft failure due to immune rejection is occurring. A monoclonal antibody against one of the pan-T-cell markers is usually used, and the CD4 and CD8 values are obtained. A leukocyte count and differential should be done so the absolute values can be calculated. The dosage of immunosuppressive drugs needed to depress an individual transplant patient's T cells can be adjusted on the basis of how each person responds to his or her immunosuppressive regimen. Lymphocyte enumeration is usually done every few days immediately after transplantation and then less frequently. Quantitation of lymphocyte numbers is particularly important when the mechanism of action of the drug depends on reducing the number of T lymphocytes. With most drugs, the absolute level of T cells should be kept below some safe level to decrease the likelihood of a rejection episode. For example, with anti-thymocyte globulin the levels should be kept around 150 CD3 cells per mm^3 immediately after transplantation, to prevent graft rejection (9). This level will vary somewhat, especially if the drug inhibits the function of the cells rather than reducing their number. After the graft has been in place for some time, the number of circulating mature T cells can be higher without risk of rejection, presumably because specific suppressive mechanisms develop.

One specific application of the monitoring of drug effects on the immune system of renal transplant patients involves evaluating in vivo treatment with monoclonal antibodies to reverse acute graft rejection. Monoclonal antibodies against T-cell antigens, including CD3 and CD6, have been used successfully to reverse acute allograft rejection. Enumeration of T cells is performed to determine whether depletion of the T cells has been accomplished and when T cells return to the circulation. Extensive studies on patients treated with these drugs have provided valuable insight into the mechanism of action of these monoclonal antibodies in vivo.

T-cell subsets can also be evaluated in transplant patients to determine whether graft failure may be due to one of two major forms of acute cell-mediated allograft rejection. This can be done if frequent sequential measurements of CD4 and CD8 are available. If a rise in creatinine occurs and no other cause can be identified, then graft rejection is probable. If the patient has a relatively high peripheral blood CD4/CD8 ratio (greater than 1.0) and there is interstitial damage to the kidney as determined by biopsy, then it is likely that the rejection episode is a case of typical acute rejection that will respond to antirejection therapy with pulse steroids or ATG. However, if the patient has a low CD4/CD8 ratio (usually less than 0.5) and biopsy reveals primarily glomerular and vascular damage, then a type of rejection is probably under way which does not respond to conventional rejection treatments. This type of rejection is associated with a high rate of infectious complications, and appropriate treatment includes reducing the dosage of conventional immunosuppressive drugs (7). In this clinical situation, the CD4/CD8 ratio guides the therapy administered.

Monitoring the effects of drugs on the immune system

An application of flow cytometry which began with renal transplantation, but which now has broader application, is the use of T-cell subset analysis to monitor the effects of immunosuppressive and immunomodulating drugs on the composition of the immune system. An example of such monitoring is the analysis of T-lymphocyte levels to adjust the dosage of ATG which is needed to suppress T cells to a certain level. In autoimmune diseases, reduction of B cells is frequently the goal, and the dosage of a drug may be adjusted accordingly. Such determinations can be used to adjust the dosage of drugs which affect minor subpopulations of T lymphocytes defined by two-color immunofluorescence. Current studies indicate that immunosuppressive and immunomodulating drugs usually have differential effects on subsets within the major T-cell subpopulations. This information will broaden the application of T-cell subset enumeration in monitoring the effects of drugs in individual patients.

Leukemia and lymphoma phenotyping

In recent years, extensive studies on the cell surface phenotype of leukemias and lymphomas of various histologic types have been performed in order to try to correlate the immunological stage of these tumors to tissue morphology, prognostic outcome, and successful therapeutic intervention. A few general principles have been derived from these studies, but the issues are complex and many remain unresolved.

From a practical standpoint, two applications of flow cytometry are now standard for the diagnosis of these types of malignancies. One application is the use of flow cytometry in conjunction with monoclonal antibodies to identify the immunological origin of tumors, in particular, to distinguish B-cell, T-cell, and myeloid malignancies. This application makes use of reagents which identify a variety of lineage-associated antigens, including the common acute lymphocytic leukemia antigen (CALLA; CD10) (17). A second standard application, which is still in the developmental stages, is to use appropriate reagents to distinguish monoclonal proliferations of malignant cells from reactive immunological processes.

Most lymphoid malignancies are of B-cell origin. B-cell malignancies were originally identified by expression of surface immunoglobulin. Although this allows B-cell tumors of intermediate maturation state to be detected and characterized, early and late stages are missed using this property alone, since pre-B cells and plasma cells do not express surface immunoglobulins. Consequently, the battery of monoclonal antibodies to cell surface antigens of B cells which is now available offers an alternative and complementary scheme to identify B-cell tumors.

The most useful monoclonal antibodies for phenotyping B-cell neoplasms are those directed against CALLA. This antigen is a 100,000-molecular-weight molecule which is found on pre-B cells and early B cells during normal differentiation and, in addition, on about 80 to 90% of acute lymphocytic leukemias. It assists in distinguishing these malignancies from myeloid malignancies.

Used together, CALLA and a reagent against more mature B cells, e.g., monoclonal antibodies against CD19, CD20, or CD24, will identify most B-cells malignancies. A number of other monoclonal antibodies which in combination identify cells in discrete stages of differentiation are also of interest in classifying the maturation state of B-cell leukemias, but the diagnostic value of such fine characterization has not yet been realized.

Those lymphoid malignancies which are T cells are usually more aggressive, have poorer prognoses, and require different treatment. There is tremendous heterogeneity in the antigenic markers which T-cell malignancies may express. However, most express the pan-T-cell antigen CD7 which has been identified by reactivity with the monoclonal antibodies known as Leu9 (Becton Dickinson) or 3A1 (8, 22). In addition, most express some other T-cell antigens as well. Such antigens relate to the maturational phase of the tumor and thus may eventually serve as guides to different treatment regimens. Immature T-cell malignancies usually also express immature T-cell antigens such as CD1 or OKT10 and may simultaneously express CD4 and CD8 antigens. In addition, many express other pan-T-cell antigens (CD2 or CD5). Reactivity with CD2 identifies those tumors which historically would have been identified as T cells due to their property of rosetting sheep erythrocytes. Mature T-cell malignancies usually express the various pan-T antigens (CD2, CD3, CD5, CD7) but lack immature markers. They may express the CD4 or CD8 antigen but, like mature normal T cells, do not simultaneously express both.

Sometimes the analysis of suspensions of cells stained with monoclonal antibodies can be used to distinguish between monoclonal and polyclonal proliferations and between malignancies and reactive processes. One special clinical situation in which this is elegantly demonstrated is in identification of monoclonal proliferations of B cells which are surface immunoglobulin positive. This method is described in detail in chapter 34. Other situations in which the distinction between polyclonal proliferation and malignancy must be made are usually more difficult, but support for monoclonal proliferation can sometimes be obtained by using flow cytometric techniques.

The practical application of flow cytometric analysis to leukemia and lymphoma phenotyping is technically complex because of the wide variation of specimen types and usually unavoidable contamination of the tumor sample with normal cells. One common type of contamination is residual erythrocytes which may remain in the lymphocyte interphase during Ficoll-Hypaque purification of the mononuclear cells. When samples are analyzed on a flow cytometer, erythrocytes fall in the same light scatter region as lymphocytes. Consequently, the complete elimination of erythrocytes is necessary in order to properly evaluate the expression of lymphocyte markers, since percentages will be lowered by such contamination. Brief treatment of the tumor cell pellet with distilled water, followed by the addition of an equal volume of double-strength medium, usually lyses the erythrocytes without damaging the tumor cells.

An additional source of contamination which is more difficult to deal with is the presence of normal cells in the tumor preparation. Thus, bone marrow specimens frequently contain peripheral blood, and lymphoma tissue suspensions may contain the cells from surrounding normal tissue or reactive immune cells which have infiltrated the tumor. An estimate of the degree of contamination of bone marrow specimens with peripheral blood is useful in interpreting the results of flow cytometry analysis. Such an estimate can be made for most specimens by using the monoclonal antibodies which react with mature T-cell subsets, taking into consideration the fact that CD8 and CD4 cells are mutually exclusive and add up to approximately the number of CD3 cells in mature blood. If the values for reactivity with monoclonal antibodies against the CD3, CD4, and CD8 antigens were, respectively, 25, 15, and 10%, the contamination of the bone marrow specimen with peripheral blood would be around 30%, and the highest value that one could expect with a reagent against a B-cell antigen or CALLA would be 70%. A few lymphoid tumors will be of mature T-cell origin and express CD3 as well as either CD4 or CD8 antigen, but most will have characteristics which allow their profile to be clearly distinguished from that produced by peripheral blood. In the case of lymphomas, it is particularly useful to combine flow cytometric studies with immunohistologic and morphologic examination of tissue sections. Some of these techniques are described by Jaffe and Cossman in chapter 120.

Bone marrow transplantation

Bone marrow transplant is given to reconstitute the immune system in cases of immune deficiency or after bone marrow ablation performed to treat leukemia. Many of the same principles which apply to renal transplantation and to leukemia and lymphoma phenotyping are also relevant to bone marrow transplantation, although the clinical questions are somewhat different. The applications of flow cytometry in the field of bone marrow transplantation include evaluation of the donor marrow before transplant and serial studies of the blood and marrow of the patient after transplant.

Flow cytometry is used before transplant to evaluate the presence of cells in donor bone marrow which might cause a graft-versus-host reaction in the recipient (23). Usually, allogeneic bone marrow is treated to remove mature T cells in order to prevent the graft-versus-host reaction. T-cell depletion is often accomplished by either lectin-affinity purification or a method that utilizes a monoclonal antibody which

reacts with a specific T-cell subset. An example of the latter type of depletion might call for incubating the bone marrow with antibody against CD2 and then reacting it with magnetic beads coated with goat anti-mouse immunoglobulin. After the depletion procedure, the composition of the remaining bone marrow can be determined by staining it with fluorescein isothiocyanate-labeled monoclonal antibodies and evaluating the reaction flow cytometrically. Cells which were coated with the CD2 monoclonal antibody but not removed during the depletion procedure can be detected by using fluorochrome-labeled goat anti-mouse immunoglobulin serum.

After transplant, the major application of lymphocyte enumeration is to determine whether the immune system of the transplant recipient is reconstituting. The recovery of minor subpopulations of lymphocytes can be followed by obtaining serial peripheral blood samples from the patient. The first lymphocytes to return are NK cells which express the CD8 antigen. These cells also express the CD16 antigen (with which Leu11 reacts) and do not express the CD3 antigen. Subsequently, mature T cells return that express CD3 as well as CD4 or high-density CD8. These cells are functionally active and herald the reconstitution of the individual's immune system.

The applications of flow cytometry in the field of bone marrow transplantation are continuing to evolve. Methods are needed for determining whether there is a recurrence of malignancy and whether the graft-versus-host reaction will occur.

Conclusion

The use of T-cell subset enumeration is expanding. Clearly, the use of multicolor analysis to define the subsets of lymphocytes more precisely will be of increasing value as the functional capacity of these subsets becomes better defined. Ideally, specific reagent combinations which can be used to diagnose and evaluate particular disease states and stages should be developed so that more precise descriptions of each disorder can be accomplished.

LITERATURE CITED

1. **Alpert, G., L. Leibovitz, and Y. L. Danon.** 1984. Analysis of T-lymphocyte subsets in measles. J. Infect. Dis. **149:**1018.
2. **Burton, R. C., P. Ferguson, M. Gray, J. Hall, M. Hayes, and Y. C. Smart.** 1983. Effects of age, gender, and cigarette smoking on human immunoregulatory T-cell subsets: establishment of normal ranges and comparison with patients with colorectal cancer and multiple sclerosis. Diagn. Immunol. **1:**216–223.
3. **Caligaris-Cappio, F., M. Gobbi, M. Bofill, and G. Janossy.** 1982. Infrequent normal B lymphocytes express features of B-chronic lymphocytic leukemia. J. Exp. Med. **155:**623–628.
4. **Campbell, A. C., C. Waller, J. Wood, A. Aynsley-Green, and V. Yu.** 1974. Lymphocyte subpopulations in the blood of newborn infants. Clin. Exp. Immunol. **18:**469–482.
5. **Carney, W. P., R. H. Rubin, R. A. Hoffman, W. P. Hansen, K. Healey, and M. S. Hirsh.** 1981. Analysis of T-lymphocyte subsets in cytomegalovirus mononucleosis. J. Immunol. **126:**2114–2116.
6. **Centers for Disease Control.** 1982. Acquired immune deficiency syndrome (AIDS): precautions for clinical and

laboratory staff. Morbid. Mortal. Weekly Rep. **31**:577–580.

7. **Colvin, R. B.** 1984. Flow cytometric analysis of T cells: diagnostic applications in transplantation. Ann. N.Y. Acad. Sci. **428**:5–13.

8. **Committee on Human Leukocyte Differentiation Antigens, IUIS-WHO Nomenclature Subcommittee.** 1984. Differentiation human leukocyte antigens: a proposed nomenclature. Immunol. Today **5**:158–159.

9. **Cosimi, A. B., R. B. Colvin, R. C. Burton, R. H. Rubin, G. Goldstein, P. C. Kung, W. P. Hansen, F. L. Delmonico, and P. S. Russell.** 1981. Use of monoclonal antibodies to T-cell subsets for immunologic monitoring and treatment in recipients of renal allografts. N. Engl. J. Med. **305**:308–314.

10. **Davies, E. G., R. J. Lavinsky, M. Butler, R. M. Thomas, and D. C. Linch.** 1983. Lymphocyte subpopulations in primary immunodeficiency disorders. Arch. Dis. Child. **58**:346–351.

11. **De Waele, M., C. Thielemans, and B. K. G. Van Camp.** 1981. Characterization of immunoregulatory T cells in EBV-induced infectious mononucleosis by monoclonal antibodies. N. Engl. J. Med. **304**:460–462.

12. **Eibl, M. M., J. W. Mannhalter, and G. Zlabinger.** 1984. Abnormal T-lymphocyte subpopulations in healthy subjects after tetanus booster immunization. N. Engl. J. Med. **310**:198–199.

13. **Fahey, J. L., H. Prince, M. Weaver, J. Groopman, B. Visscher, K. Schwartz, and R. Detels.** 1984. Quantitative changes in T-helper or T-suppressor/cytotoxic lymphocyte subsets that distinguish acquired immune deficiency syndrome from other immune subset disorders. Am. J. Med. **76**:95–100.

14. **Fast, L. D., J. A. Hansen, and W. Newman.** 1981. Evidence for T cell nature and heterogeneity within natural killer and antibody-dependent cellular cytotoxicity (ADCC) effectors: a comparison with cytolytic T lymphocytes (CTL). J. Immunol. **127**:448–452.

15. **Fishman, J. A., K. M. Martell, and R. H. Rubin.** 1983. Infection and T-lymphocyte subpopulations: changes associated with bacteremia and the acquired immunodeficiency syndrome. Diagn. Immunol. **1**:261–265.

16. **Fuller, T. C., J. E. Trevithick, A. A. Fuller, R. B. Colvin, A. B. Cosimi, and P. C. Kung.** 1984. Antigenic polymorphism of the T4 differentiation antigen expressed on human T helper/inducer lymphocytes. Hum. Immunol. **9**:89–102.

17. **Greaves, M. F.** 1981. Monoclonal antibodies as probes for leukemic heterogeneity and haematopoetic differentiation, p. 19–32. *In* W. Knapp (ed.), Leukemia markers. Academic Press, Inc., New York.

18. **Hunninghake, G. W., and R. G. Crystal.** 1981. Pulmonary sarcoidosis: a disorder mediated by excess helper T-lymphocyte activity at sites of disease activity. N. Engl. J. Med. **305**:429–434.

19. **Jondal, M., G. Holm, and H. Wigzell.** 1972. Surface markers on human B and T lymphocytes. I. A large population of lymphocytes forming nonimmune rosettes with sheep red blood cells. J. Exp. Med. **136**:207–215.

20. **Korn, E. L., F. Dorey, C. A. Spina, and J. L. Fahey.** 1984. The use of three baseline values in intervention studies: application to evaluation of immune modulation therapies. Immunobiology **167**:431–436.

21. **Lanier, L. L., A. M. Le, J. H. Phillips, N. L. Warner, and G. F. Babcock.** 1983. Subpopulations of human natural killer cells defined by expression of the Leu-7 (HNK-1) and Leu-11 (NK-15) antigens. J. Immunol. **131**:1789–1796.

22. **Link, M., R. Warnke, J. Finlay, M. Amylon, R. Miller, J. Dilley, and R. Levy.** 1983. A single monoclonal antibody identifies T-cell lineage of childhood lymphoid malignancies. Blood **62**:722–728.

23. **Martin, P. J., J. A. Hansen, and E. D. Thomas.** 1984. Use of flow microfluorometry in bone marrow transplantation. Ann. N.Y. Acad. Sci. **428**:14–25.

24. **Miyawaki, T., K. Taga, T. Nagaoki, H. Seki, Y. Suzuki, and N. Taniguchi.** 1984. Circadian changes of T lymphocyte subsets in human peripheral blood. Clin. Exp. Immunol. **55**:618–622.

25. **Nagel, J. E., F. J. Chrest, and W. H. Adler.** 1981. Enumeration of T lymphocyte subsets by monoclonal antibodies in young and aged humans. J. Immunol. **127**:1286–1288.

26. **Parks, D. R., and L. A. Herzenberg.** 1984. Fluorescence-activated cell sorting: theory, experimental optimization, and applications in lymphoid cell biology. Methods Enzymol. **108**:197–241.

27. **Reinherz, E. L., S. C. Meuer, K. A. Fitzgerald, R. E. Hussey, H. Levine, and S. F. Schlossman.** 1982. Antigen recognition by human T lymphocytes is linked to surface expression of the T3 molecular complex. Cell **30**:735–743.

28. **Shapiro, H. M.** 1985. Practical flow cytometry. Alan R. Liss, Inc., New York.

29. **Shiratsuchi, H., and I. Tsuyuguchi.** 1984. Analysis of T cell subsets by monoclonal antibodies in patients with tuberculosis after in vitro stimulation with purified protein derivative of tuberculin. Clin. Exp. Immunol. **57**:271–278.

30. **Spire, B., F. Barré-Sinoussi, L. Montagnier, and J. C. Chermann.** 1984. Inactivation of lymphadenopathy associated virus by chemical disinfectants. Lancet **ii**:899–901.

31. **Thomas, R. M., and D. C. Linch.** 1983. Identification of lymphocyte subsets in the newborn using a variety of monoclonal antibodies. Arch. Dis. Child. **58**:34–38.

32. **Whittle, H. C., J. Brown, K. Marsh, B. M. Greenwood, P. Seidelin, H. Tighe, and L. Wedderburn.** 1984. T-cell control of Epstein-Barr virus infected B cells is lost during *P. falciparum* malaria. Nature (London) **312**:449–450.

Chapter 34

Flow Cytometric Evaluation of Normal and Neoplastic B Cells

KENNETH A. AULT

The use of flow cytometry to evaluate normal and neoplastic B lymphocytes has assumed increasing importance in both immunological research and clinical diagnosis. B cells offer some unique opportunities for flow cytometric evaluation as well as some unique problems. In this discussion we will review the current status, some future possibilities, and also some pitfalls of B-cell evaluation.

Markers for B cells

Far and away the most distinctive and useful marker for B cells is their surface immunoglobulin (sIg). This sIg is present on all mature B cells and is the receptor for specific antigen. The earliest definable B-cell precursors contain cytoplasmic immunoglobulin M (IgM) but do not express it on their surface. To date, this "pre-B" stage has been studied only with fluorescence microscopy to evaluate the cytoplasmic staining. The difficulty in using flow cytometry at this stage is in obtaining specific labeling of the cytoplasmic immunoglobulin and at the same time excluding the presence of sIg. It seems likely that dual labeling in flow systems will soon overcome this difficulty and permit direct measurement of pre-B cells.

All later stages of B cells express sIg in various amounts. The majority of B cells express sIgM and sIgD. Smaller numbers express one of the other heavy-chain types such as IgG and IgA. It is clear that some B-cell subsets differ in the relative amounts of sIgM and sIgD that they express. However, the distinction of B-cell subsets on the basis of heavy-chain class is difficult, usually requiring dual labeling of sIgM and sIgD on the same cells. In addition, there appears to be a relatively smooth transition between B-cell subsets so that they cannot be clearly resolved on this basis. In addition, neoplastic B cells can seldom be distinguished from normal B cells on this basis, since most neoplastic B cells also express various amounts of sIgM and sIgD. Only when a population of neoplastic B cells happens to express predominantly sIgG or sIgA can their presence be suspected. As differentiating B cells approach the plasma cell stage, they gradually lose most of their sIg and once again must be identified on the basis of large amounts of cytoplasmic immunoglobulin.

In contrast to the variable heavy-chain class of the sIg, each B cell and all of its progeny express only one light-chain class and only one immunoglobulin variable region antigen-binding site. Antigenic specificities located at or near the antigen-binding site are known as "idiotypes." Since the antigen-binding site is unique to each antibody, these idiotypic markers are also very specific for a particular clone of B cells. Thus both light-chain class and imunoglobulin idiotype can be considered "clonal" markers for B

cells. Of the two, idiotype is much more specific, but at present much more difficult to identify. Normal human B cells are nearly equally divided between those expressing kappa and lambda light chains. Since a neoplastic clone of B cells may express only one light chain, the presence of these clones can often be detected by an imbalance of light-chain expression in a population of B cells. This imbalance forms the basis for a clinically useful method of distinguishing monoclonal B-cell proliferations as described below. Recently it has become more practical to make anti-idiotypic antibodies that are truly clonal markers for B cells. As this technique becomes more widespread, it may dramatically improve our ability to detect clonal proliferations. However, this work has already resulted in the unexpected and disturbing finding that a significant proportion, perhaps 10 to 20%, of B-cell neoplasms may consist of two or more clones (7). If this phenomenon is widespread, it could significantly complicate the job of defining neoplastic B cells.

Despite the obvious value of sIg in studying B cells, there are several pitfalls that must be avoided. The most serious is the problem of "cytophilic" immunoglobulin on lymphocytes of all kinds. Normal B cells, all natural killer cells, activated T cells, and all phagocytic cells have Fc receptors which bind, with various avidities, soluble immunoglobulin (see chapter 31). Thus, it is imperative to demonstrate that the sIg which is being measured is synthesized by the cell in question. Usually such cytophilic immunoglobulin is mostly IgG, but IgM can also bind in this way. In most cases a brief (1-h) incubation of the cells at 37°C in the absence of human immunoglobulin is sufficient to remove most cytophilic immunoglobulin (10). In other cases the definitive technique is to remove all of the sIg by using proteolytic enzymes such as pronase and then show the regeneration of sIg by the B cells during an overnight incubation. This precaution is most important when a patient is known to have a serum "M component" consisting of monoclonal immunoglobulin. Binding of the M component to lymphocytes of all kinds will create the illusion of a large population of monoclonal B cells.

Several technical issues associated with the detection of sIg on B cells should be noted. The first is the phenomenon of capping and shedding of sIg. When sIg is cross-linked by the binding of an anti-immunoglobulin antibody, it rapidly undergoes a transition from a fairly uniform distribution on the membrane to a clumped distribution known as patching. Patching takes place even in the cold and in the absence of metabolic activity. It is a reflection of the intrinsic mobility of the sIg molecules in the lipid membrane. If the cells are allowed any metabolic activity at all, a second phenomenon takes place in which all of the sIg is brought to one pole of the cell. This movement is called capping, and it takes place within 5 min at 37°C or within 10 to 20 min at room temperature. At the same time that capping is taking place, a significant amount of label is being lost from the cell surface by the shedding of sIg–anti-immunoglobulin complexes. In addition, some of the complexes are internalized by the cell and degraded (6). The result is a rapid loss of labeling which can make detection of sIg very difficult if the cells are not maintained strictly in the cold throughout the labeling and washing process. This capping and shedding phenomenon is much less prominent with other surface structures and, interestingly, is frequently very abnormal in malignant B cells (3).

The second issue concerns the problem of Fc receptor binding of immunoglobulin to B cells and other cells. Many cells of the immune system, notably B cells, activated T cells, natural killer cells, monocytes, and macrophages, have surface structures capable of binding immunoglobulin. This capability raises two problems. First, an anti-immunoglobulin antibody being used to detect sIg on B cells may very well label passively bound immunoglobulin on many other kinds of cells. Second, an anti-immunoglobulin may bind to these other cells nonspecifically because it will bind to the Fc receptor. For these reasons, studies of B-cell sIg must always include measures to remove the passively bound immunoglobulin, and the antibodies should be pepsin digested to remove their Fc region so that they will not bind nonspecifically. The latter procedure is particularly important when rabbit antibodies are used and seems to be less of a problem when goat antibodies or mouse monoclonal antibodies are used.

A growing number of monoclonal antibodies are now being produced which recognize structures found on B cells. Although these structures do not constitute clonal markers, they may be especially useful in defining the maturation stage of a B-cell population and may be used to suggest clonality if a disproportionate number of B cells express one set of such markers. Very recently, monoclonal antibodies have been found that may recognize structures of considerable functional importance, such as receptors for growth factors. These markers may be useful in defining B-cell populations that are capable of unregulated growth. Such an approach may be a new way of defining neoplastic B cells other than by their clonality.

CLINICAL INDICATIONS

There are several clinical situations in which the evaluation of B cells is indicated. The most clear-cut situations are the immunodeficiency states and the lymphocytic neoplasms.

Immunodeficiency includes a heterogeneous group of disorders, some congenital and some acquired. Frequently, there is hypogammaglobulinemia or agammaglobulinemia. These diseases are summarized elsewhere (5). In any instance in which there is a disorder of immunoglobulin production, there is an indication for enumerating B cells and, if they are present, determining their subtypes. In many cases normal B-cell numbers will be found despite severe defects in antibody production. The proper functioning of the immune system requires coordinated inter-

action of T cells, B cells, and macrophages as well as a properly structured environment in the lymphoid tissue. Defects in any of these compartments or in their interactions may result in immunodeficiency.

A more subtle indication arises in patients who have recurrent infections with pyogenic organisms but do not have a quantitative immunoglobulin disorder. It is possible in these cases that there is a defect in B-cell function which impairs the ability to produce some specific antibodies but does not interfere with immunoglobulin production in general. Unfortunately, it is very difficult to demonstrate such specific B-cell defects by present methods.

In the case of the neoplastic B-cell disorders, the situation is much clearer. At least 80% of all non-Hodgkin's lymphoid neoplasms are of B-cell origin. Thus, in any case in which lymphoma is suspected, a careful evaluation of B-cell markers is in order. In most cases this evaluation will mean examination of biopsied tumor tissue by the standard techniques of immunopathology. However, in an increasing number of cases, examination of lymphoid cells in suspension, i.e., in blood or in pleural, ascitic, or cerebrospinal fluid, becomes an important part either of establishing the diagnosis of lymphoma or of its staging. In addition, flow cytometric evaluation of cell suspensions made from tissue specimens can be an important adjunct to conventional morphological evaluation.

A particularly interesting case in which evaluation of B cells is in order is the patient with unexplained lymphocytosis. Frequently, morphological examination of the lymphocytes will lead to the suspicion that the lymphocytosis is due to a reactive process (atypical lymphocytes) or a lymphoproliferative disorder (such as chronic lymphocytic leukemia, hairy cell leukemia, or Sezary syndrome). However, the distinctions between reactive and neoplastic changes are not always clear and are always subjective. Flow cytometric evaluation of B-cell markers is frequently very helpful.

In general the evaluation of lymphoid cells in a clinical sample will proceed along these lines. First, are the lymphocytes of B- or T-cell type? In rare instances they may not fall into either category and will instead be of the type known variously as "null" cells or natural killer cells. If they are of B-cell type a distinction must then be made between a clonal, oligoclonal, or polyclonal proliferation. The last is most likely not a malignant process, but may be caused by chronic antigenic stimulation, autoimmune disease, etc. The presence of a single clone of B cells in excess is generally taken as indication of malignancy, although this concept may be changing, as mentioned above. Fortunately we have at our disposal good methods for determining clonality in the B-cell series.

When this line of reasoning is extended, the laboratory work-up will generally consist of using markers for T and B cells, each marker having as broad a specificity as possible. A generally accepted marker for T cells is the sheep erythrocyte rosette receptor, which can be evaluated either by a rosetting assay or by using one of the monoclonal antibodies that are specific for the receptor. A similar widely accepted marker for B cells does not yet exist, but a few monoclonal antibodies have sufficiently broad specificity to make them useful in this regard. The most frequently used monoclonal antibodies are Leu12 (Becton-Dickinson and Co., Paramus, N.J.) for CD10 and B1 (Coulter Electronics, Inc., Hialeah, Fla.) for CD20. The presence of sIg is the most reliable marker, if it is reasonably certain that cytophilic immunoglobulin has been eliminated.

Once it has been determined that there is a B-cell proliferation, the question of clonality can be approached by evaluating the sIg heavy- and light-chain isotypes. For reasons discussed above, the light chains are usually more useful. It is likely that the techniques for examining immunoglobulin genes may supplant the use of surface markers in this determination in the near future (2).

Finally, in some cases it may be of use to determine the presence of a specific subset of B lymphocytes. An excellent example of this is the B-cell subset that expresses the 67-kilodalton protein (CD5) recognized by the monoclonal antibody Leu1, T1, or OKT1 (p67). This subset of B cells is rare in normal people but is the usual type of B cell found in chronic lymphocytic leukemia and in the immunodeficiency state after bone marrow transplantation.

The presence of the "T-cell" antigen on a subset of B cells brings up a very important point about the use of monoclonal antibodies to identify cell types, especially abnormal cell types. There are a number of examples of the unexpected presence or absence of marker antigens on abnormal cells. B cells can express the p67 antigen previously thought to be restricted to T cells. Conversely, a number of B-cell neoplasms (approximately 10%) lack markers such as B1 which are otherwise excellent pan-B-cell reagents. Thus, in general, it is necessary to know a great deal about the markers chosen for laboratory testing, to keep up with current literature on the subject of markers, and, most importantly, to use more than one marker to classify a cell.

In many laboratories it is now possible to assess two markers simultaneously in each cell by using two-color immunofluorescence and flow cytometry. This method greatly reduces the chance of misclassifying a cell type with a single marker. It is likely that most of the marker studies of the future will make use of this technique which, with the proper instrumentation, is no more difficult than single-marker studies.

For the purposes of this chapter, two techniques will be described. The first technique is the use of two-color immunofluorescence to subclassify B cells. This discussion will also serve to illustrate the technique used for any evaluation of monoclonal antibody markers. The second method is the clonal excess or kappa-lambda method for evaluation of light-chain labeling of B cells. In each case, the method currently in use in our laboratory will be described. There are many possible variations on these methods, some of which will be mentioned briefly.

DUAL-LABELING IMMUNOFLUORESCENCE

A detailed discussion of this technique can be found in chapter 32 or reference 8. Lymphocytes are prepared by standard Ficoll-Hypaque gradient separation with any of a number of commercial preparations. It is very desirable to remove monocytes. This is best done by preincubating the cells with carbonyl iron (e.g., Lymphocyte Separator Reagent; Technicon Instruments Corp., Tarrytown, N.Y.). A mixture of 4 parts heparinized blood to 1 part iron solution incubated on a rotating platform for 1 h at 37°C works well to allow phagocytosis of the iron by monocytes and polymorphonuclear leukocytes. When the blood is subsequently separated by Ficoll-Hypaque, the monocytes will sink to the bottom. Alternatively, the separated mononuclear cells can be incubated overnight in cell culture medium in plastic flasks. The monocytes will adhere to the plastic, and the lymphocytes can be removed by gently washing with warm medium.

In an alternative technique, whole blood is used instead of Ficoll-Hypaque cells. This technique requires that the erythrocytes be lysed by one of the very effective lysing reagents which are now commercially available. This method also requires that the flow cytometer be used to eliminate monocytes and polymorphonuclear leukocytes from the analysis. This method works well with normal samples but may cause various degrees of difficulty when used with abnormal samples. It does, however, have the advantage that there is no risk of losing abnormal cells during the Ficoll-Hypaque step.

The lymphocytes are then counted, and between 5×10^5 and 1×10^6 cells are placed into each of three tubes. One tube will be a negative control, one will be a postive control which will also allow adjustment of the flow cytometer, and the third will contain the doubly labeled cells. There can obviously be more than one such tube if different combinations of antibodies are to be used.

Each tube is then labeled. When dual labeling is being done, the two antibodies can be added simultaneously. The amounts to be added are determined either by the instructions of the manufacturer or by previous titrations carried out in the laboratory. The latter method is always preferable when a new antibody preparation is to be used. A typical example would be 5 μl of each antibody added to the cells in a total volume of about 100 μl. In general, the labeling should be done at ice temperature. The presence of sodium azide in the antibody mixture makes the possibility of metabolism of the antibody or shedding of the bound antibody less likely, but strict observance of cold conditions is preferable, especially for the labeling of B cells.

The cells are incubated with the antibodies for 20 min, with occasional agitation. They are then washed twice with ice-cold saline and suspended in about 0.5 ml of saline. They can then be fixed by the addition of 0.5 ml of 2% paraformaldehyde in saline. The fixed cells can be left in the paraformaldehyde solution and will remain stable for at least 1 week. Such fixed samples should be stored in the cold and dark.

At this time by far the best choices of fluorochromes for double labeling are fluorescein and phycoerythrin. A very large variety of monoclonal antibodies is available conjugated to fluorescein, and a growing number are available conjugated to phycoerythrin. This combination has the great advantage that both fluorochromes can be excited by a single wavelength of light (488 nm). Other combinations, such as fluorescein and Texas red, require two light sources and, although

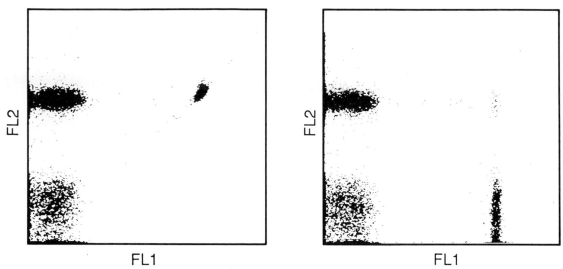

FIG. 1. Fluorescein- and phycoerythrin-conjugated beads (Calibrite, Becton Dickinson) analyzed on a flow cytometer. This dot plot display shows each bead as a dot whose position corresponds to the amount of green (fluorescein) fluorescence on the horizontal axis, and orange (phycoerythrin) fluorescence on the vertical axis. The beads can be used to illustrate the principles of electronic compensation for two-color fluorescence. Left, Analysis of the beads after the flow cytometer is fully adjusted for optimal sensitivity but without electronic compensation. Unlabeled beads fall in the lower left corner. The phycoerythrin-conjugated beads fall along the vertical axis, showing that they have orange fluorescence but minimal green fluorescence. The fluorescein-conjugated beads, however, fall in the upper right, showing that they have both substantial green and orange fluorescence. This is due to the leakage of the fluorescein emission through the filters used in the orange channel. Right, Electronic compensation has been adjusted to eliminate the orange component of the fluorescein emission. Now the three bead populations lie in the appropriate positions, and a small number of truly double-fluorescent (green and orange) beads can be seen in the upper right. These are actually pairs of beads, one green and one orange, bound to each other.

quite workable, are not likely to find their way into clinical use because of the greater complexity of instrumentation. The emission of fluorescein is measured at 535 nm and that of phycoerythrin at 580 nm. Either a laser or mercury arc-based flow cytometer can be used with equal results. All of the instrument manufacturers now have filter combinations suitable for these fluorochromes. Regardless of the filters chosen, there will very likely be a certain amount of "spillage" of the signal from fluorescein into the phycoerythrin channel because the emission spectrum of fluorescein has a long "tail" that extends beyond 580 nm. For this reason a control is needed to set the internal compensation of the flow cytometer as described below.

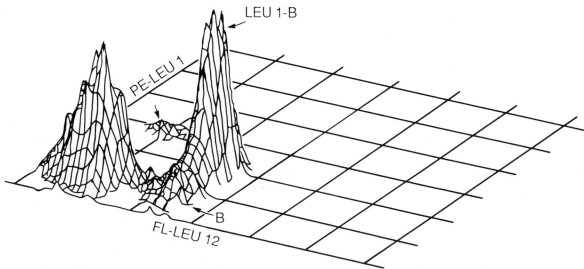

FIG. 2. Flow cytometric data presented in the form of a three-dimensional graph in which the fluorescein and phycoerythrin fluorescence is shown in the horizontal plane and the number of cells is plotted vertically. Data are from a bone marrow transplant recipient and show a large number of cells labeling for both Leu12, a B-cell-specific monoclonal antibody, and Leu1. The populations of normal T and B cells are clearly shown. The unlabeled cell populations are largely natural killer lymphocytes and erythroid cells.

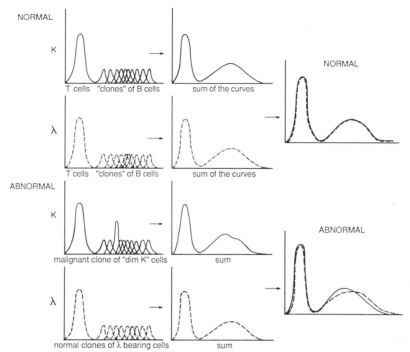

FIG. 3. A theoretical explanation for the method of detecting monoclonal B lymphocytes described in the text. The total curve for labeling of kappa or lambda B cells is assumed to be made up of a series of "clones" of B cells, each clone expressing a different level of sIg (and thus light chain). In the normal situation, the resulting distribution of each light chain is the same. When an abnormal clone is present, there will be a change in shape of one of the two curves. Thus the presence of the abnormal clone is detected by comparing the two light-chain distribution curves for any difference in their shapes. This method is independent of the absolute number of B cells of each light-chain class.

It should be pointed out that only direct immunofluorescence is preferred for dual labeling. Although it may be possible in certain cases to devise protocols with indirect labeling (i.e., fluoresceinated second antibodies or biotin-avidin systems), these protocols introduce complexity and the need for several more controls to detect the possibility of unwanted cross-labeling.

The negative control in this type of assay is best chosen as a fluorochrome-conjugated monoclonal mouse immunoglobulin of the same isotype as the monoclonal in use. Such control reagents are now commercially available. The positive control should consist of an antibody that will be strongly positive on a large number of cells in the sample. Antibodies that recognize T-cell subsets (such as Leu2 and Leu3 or T4 and T8) serve well. We use a combination of fluorescein-HLE and phycoerythrin-LeuM3, both from Becton-Dickinson. This combination has the advantage that all of the lymphocytes will be strongly labeled with HLE, whereas any residual erythrocytes will not be labeled, and any residual monocytes will be labeled with the LeuM3. The positive control is used for two purposes: (i) to set "gates" on the flow cytometer which include all of the lymphocytes but eliminate monocytes and erythrocytes; and (ii) to set the compensation of the cytometer to eliminate any spillage from the fluorescein into the phycoerythrin channel. This step is easily accomplished by adjusting the compensation until the large population of HLE-labeled cells lie against the appropriate axis (Fig. 1). If any erythrocytes or monocytes lie within the chosen gates, they can be enumerated with this control.

Finally, the test samples are run, the dual-parameter data are collected, and the number of cells falling into each subset is analyzed. The exact methods will depend on the instrument in use.

Work done in our laboratory has indicated that in any given population analyzed by this method, the estimate of the proportion of cells can be obtained with a coefficient of variation of ±10% in routine studies of 20,000 cells, even for populations amounting to 5% of the total. The lower limit of detection of rare subpopulations of cells is usually around 1%, limited by the presence of background labeling in the negative control.

Figure 2 shows examples of double labeling with fluorescein-Leu12, which is a pan-B-cell antibody, and phycoerythrin-Leu1, which recognizes the p67 protein mentioned above. This study was done in a marrow transplant patient and clearly shows the presence of two distinct populations of B cells, one being Leu1 negative and the other having amounts of Leu1 less than that found on T cells. The significance of these cells in transplant patients remains to be determined, but their presence may explain the prolonged immunosuppression seen in these patients (1a). Similar cells are found in the majority of cases of chronic lymphocytic leukemia.

KAPPA-LAMBDA METHOD OF DETECTING CLONAL B CELLS

Details of the kappa-lambda method of detecting clonal B cells can be found in references 1 and 9. It is

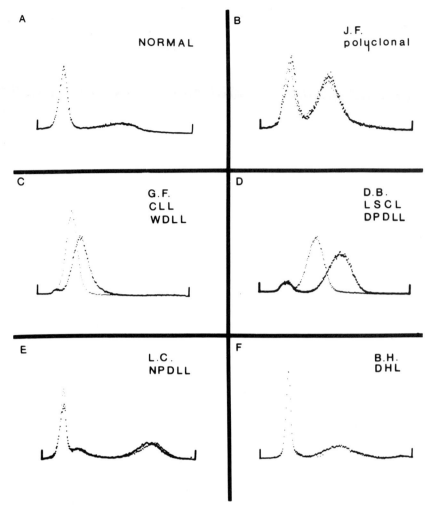

FIG. 4. Examples of normal and abnormal kappa-lambda analyses. (A) Normal, with the two curves identical. (B) Results from a patient with a large number of B cells, but with no difference between the two curves, suggesting the presence of a polyclonal B-cell proliferation. (C and D) Results from patients with chronic lymphocytic leukemia (CLL) or lymphosarcoma cell leukemia (LSCL) in which the presence of a large population of cells labeling with one light chain is clearly evident. (E and F) Results from patients with nodular, poorly differentiated lymphocytic lymphoma (NPDLL) or diffuse histiocytic lymphoma (DHL), with small differences in the two curves revealing the presence of an abnormal clone. This type of finding is very common in lymphoma patients even in the absence of any morphologically identifiable abnormal circulating cells.

a sensitive technique for detecting small numbers of clonal B cells in a population of normal B cells. It depends on the fact that the presence of a clone of B cells will alter the distribution of fluorescence intensity of either the kappa or the lambda labeling but not both. In other words, if a clone of B cells expresses lambda light chains, it will be labeled by antibodies to lambda but not to kappa. The test is set up so that the labeling of normal B cells by anti-kappa and anti-lambda results in identical fluorescence intensity distributions. This is not to say that there are necessarily equal numbers of kappa- and lambda-bearing B cells, but that the distribution of fluorescence intensity is the same for both (Fig. 3).

In practice, the cells are prepared as described above with the important addition of at least a 1-h incubation at 37°C in medium containing fetal calf serum but no human serum. This step substantially reduces the contribution of cytophilic immunoglobulin. The cells are placed in three tubes. One tube will serve as the control, and one tube each will be labeled with anti-kappa and anti-lambda. An indirect labeling protocol is necessary for this method to obtain identical labeling with both antibodies.

This method does not lend itself to the use of monoclonal antibodies since it is very important that the labeling with each antibody be identical. We use rabbit anti-human kappa and lambda from Accurate Scientific Co., Westbury, N.Y. These antibodies should be directed against intact light chains, not free light chains, and they should be digested with pepsin to obtain F(ab')$_2$ fragments. Details for performing this digestion can be obtained from manuals of immunological methods (4). The second antibody is a fluoresceinated goat anti-rabbit immunoglobulin obtainable from a number of sources. The exact amount of antibody to be used must be determined by titration on normal-blood B cells. Saturating doses of both the first and second antibodies must be used. In general we have found that about 50 μl of a solution containing 0.5 mg of antibody protein per ml is about right for labeling 10^6 cells.

The control tube receives no first antibody. The other two tubes receive either anti-kappa or anti-lambda. The tubes are incubated on ice for 20 min and then washed three times. This method is much more demanding than most monoclonal antibody labeling methods. Careful attention to the amount of antibody, the temperature, and the washing is essential. The cells must be kept very cold during the washing. Even a brief exposure to room temperature will markedly reduce the labeling due to capping and shedding of the antibodies. After being washed, all three tubes receive the second antibody, followed by another incubation and two washes. The cells can then be fixed as described above.

The flow cytometric evaluation of this sample must also be done carefully. First, the kappa sample is run, and data from at least 50,000 cells are collected in histogram form. Next, the lambda sample is run similarly. It is absolutely critical that there be no change in the cytometer between the two samples. If there is any visible difference between the two histograms, the kappa tube should be rerun to determine if the difference is reproducible. Finally, the control tube is run to determine the level of unstained cells.

The evaluation of these data requires a computer program which performs a statistical test for the difference in the shape of the two histograms. The B-cell regions of the two histograms are first normalized, and then the two curves are compared. There are several mathematical approaches to this comparison. The one we have used is based on the Kolmogorov-Smirnov test for goodness of fit between the two curves. A complete description of this method is beyond the scope of this chapter but can be found in reference 11. The output of the computer program is a number which is proportional to the degree of difference between the two curves. The normal amount of variation must be determined by running a group of normal samples. Variations above this level can be taken as evidence for the presence of a clone of B cells. This variation has been called clonal excess.

Experiments in which clonal (malignant) B cells are added to normal blood have indicated that this method is capable of routinely detecting a 10% population of clonal B cells among normal B cells. In some cases the method is sensitive to as few as 1% or even 0.1% clonal cells. In general the method is more sensitive for clonal cells that label brightly with one of the antibodies.

Figure 4 shows examples of the results of this method for a variety of lymphoproliferative diseases. In our hands this method is superior to any other for detecting the presence of clonal B cells in blood, body fluids, and cell suspensions from tissues. It does not work well on bone marrow, due to high levels of nonspecific labeling and autofluorescence in myeloid cells. It must be emphasized that the presence of clonal B cells in a sample does not imply that they are malignant B cells. Thus this approach must not be used to diagnose lymphoma unless there is other evidence for a malignant process. It is useful, however, for confirming the presence of malignant cells, staging, and monitoring the patient during and after treatment. A more complete discussion of the clinical implications of this method can be found in reference 7a.

In summary, the evaluation of B-cell subsets such as Leu1-B cells is still in its infancy, but there is little doubt that the ability to identify subsets of B cells will be as important as our ability to identify subsets of T cells. In addition, the ease with which one can identify and study the B-cell antigen receptor and its role as a tumor-specific marker will lead to both diagnostic and therapeutic advances for the B-cell lymphomas.

LITERATURE CITED

1. **Ault, K. A.** 1979. Detection of small numbers of monoclonal B lymphocytes in the blood of patients with lymphoma. N. Engl. J. Med. **300**:1401–1405.
1a. **Ault, K. A., J. H. Antin, D. Ginsburg, S. H. Orkin, J. M. Rappeport, M. L. Keohan, P. Martin, and B. R. Smith.** 1985. The phenotype of recovering lymphoid cell populations following marrow transplantation. J. Exp. Med. **161**:1483–1502.
2. **Cleary, M. L., G. S. Wood, R. Warnke, J. Chao, and J. Sklar.** 1984. Immunoglobulin gene rearrangements as a diagnostic criterion of B cell lymphomas. Proc. Natl. Acad. Sci. USA **81**:593–597.
3. **Cohen, H. J.** 1975. Human lymphocyte surface immunoglobulin capping: normal characteristics and anomalous behavior of chronic lymphocytic leukemic lymphocytes. J. Clin. Invest. **35**:84–93.
4. **Mishell, B. B., and S. M. Shiigi (ed.).** 1980. Selected methods in cellular immunology. W. W. Freeman and Co., San Francisco.
5. **Rosen, F. S., M. D. Cooper, and R. J. P. Wedgwood.** 1984. The primary immunodeficiencies. N. Engl. J. Med. **311**:235–242.
6. **Schreiner, G. F., and E. R. Unanue.** 1976. Membrane and cytoplasmic changes in B lymphocytes induced by ligand-surface immunoglobulin interaction. Adv. Immunol. **24**:37.
7. **Sklar, J., M. L. Cleary, K. Thielemans, J. Gralow, R. Warnke, and R. Levy.** 1984. Biclonal B cell lymphoma. N. Engl. J. Med. **311**:20–27.
7a. **Smith, B. R., M. Towle, E. Luther, N. J. Robert, and K. A. Ault.** 1984. Circulating monoclonal B lymphocytes in non-Hodgkin's lymphoma. N. Engl. J. Med. **311**: 1476–1481.
8. **Warner, N. L., J. Y. Kimura, and D. J. Recktenwald.** 1983. Multiparameter flow cytometry analysis of normal and neoplastic human lymphocytes with Leu monoclonal antibodies. *In* F. Dammaco, G. Doria, and A. Pinchera (ed.), Monoclonal antibodies. Elsevier Biomedical Press, New York.
9. **Weinberg, D. S., G. S. Pinkus, and K. A. Ault.** 1984. Cytofluorometric detection of B cell clonal excess: a new approach to the diagnosis of B cell lymphoma. Blood **63**:1080–1087.
10. **Winchester, R. J., S. M. Fu, T. Hoffman, and H. G. Kunkel.** 1975. IgG on lymphocyte surfaces: technical problems and the significance of a third cell population. J. Immunol. **114**:1210.
11. **Young, I. T.** 1977. Proof without prejudice: use of the Kolmogorov-Smirnov test for the analysis of histograms from flow systems and other sources. J. Histochem. Cytochem. **25**:935–941.

Chapter 35

Detection of Platelet Antibodies with a Fluorescence-Activated Flow Cytometric Technique

LAURENCE CORASH AND MARGARET RHEINSCHMIDT

Thrombocytopenia may occur as the sole manifestation of a disease or secondary to another disorder. The management of either primary or secondary thrombocytopenia depends on the correct identification of the causal pathophysiologic processes. Over the past decade a number of research laboratories have provided data that strongly support the hypothesis that primary isolated thrombocytopenia in adults, idiopathic thrombocytopenia purpura, is immune mediated and in many cases may be more correctly termed autoimmune thrombocytopenia purpura (3). The development of assays to directly measure platelet-associated immunoglobulin (PAIg) corroborated earlier studies that suggested that this disorder is due to the deposition of immunoglobulin on the platelet surface, leading to abnormal clearance of sensitized platelets. The ability to directly measure PAIg, in contrast to the earlier tests for the presence of serum antiplatelet factors, increased the sensitivity for identification of patients with suspected platelet immune destruction. However, the increase in sensitivity also raised new questions about the specificity of PAIg (4). It is now well recognized that increased PAIg can be seen in thrombocytopenia associated with a wide variety of disorders, including systemic lupus erythematosus (4), lymphoma (4), carcinoma (7), Hodgkin's disease (1), acquired immunodeficiency syndrome (AIDS) (6), and Hashimoto's thyroiditis (2). It is unknown in most cases whether the PAIg observed in either autoimmune thrombocytopenia purpura or these secondary disorders is specifically directed against a platelet antigen or is nonspecifically deposited on the platelet surface as part of an immune complex. Several recent reports of studies using immunoblot techniques have identified PAIg directed against integral platelet proteins glycoprotein Ib (9) and the glycoprotein IIb/IIIa complex (10). Other studies using sensitive techniques for the detection of cell-associated immunoglobulin have also provided evidence that the elevated PAIg is specific for immune-mediated platelet destruction in patients with classical immune thrombocytopenia and that it is not found in patients with nonimmune thrombocytopenia (5). The pathophysiology of immune-mediated platelet destruction is probably not the same in all disorders; for example, the AIDS-related thrombocytopenia may be due to immune complex disease (8).

A number of different techniques to measure PAIg have been described. Each of these techniques requires the isolation of platelets from whole blood, which may be difficult in patients with severe thrombocytopenia. The ideal assay technique should be sensitive enough to allow the use of small numbers of platelets, be simple to perform in a routine laboratory, permit storage of samples so that assays can be performed in a batch mode, and yet yield data with sensitivity and specificity equivalent to those of the best technique available. The assay described in this chapter appears to meet many of these criteria in that it requires small numbers of cells, avoids the use of radioisotopes, can be performed in a batch mode with sample storage, and utilizes instrumentation with which a multiplicity of different tests can be performed. It also exhibits adequate sensitivity and specificity for the detection of PAIg.

CLINICAL INDICATIONS

Measurement of PAIg is useful for both diagnostic and therapeutic purposes. It is indicated for patients who present with isolated thrombocytopenia without an antecedent history of a hematologic disorder and in whom a physical examination does not indicate the presence of any other systemic disorders. In the appropriate setting, patients with the classical clinical presentation of autoimmune thrombocytopenia purpura may not require a bone marrow examination if the PAIg test is positive. Measurement of PAIg is indicated for thrombocytopenia during pregnancy, since maternal autoimmune thrombocytopenia may lead to neonatal thrombocytopenia if the antibody is immunoglobulin G (3). Measurement of PAIg is indicated for patients with systemic lupus erythematosus who develop thrombocytopenia or qualitative platelet function defects during the course of their disease. Both of these situations may require specific diagnoses to determine alternative therapeutic approaches. The onset of thrombocytopenia which cannot be explained by decreased platelet production in patients with malignant lymphoproliferative disorders (1, 4) or carcinoma (7) is an indication for measurement of PAIg because it may indicate that a different therapeutic strategy is needed. Patients with other autoimmune disorders, such as Hashimoto's thyroiditis, may benefit from the measurement of PAIg, especially when symptoms of platelet dysfunction arise (2). Patients who present with qualitative platelet dysfunction but a normal platelet count may require measurement of PAIg to document the etiology of their hemostatic disorder. Patients with thrombocytopenia during the course of AIDS and the AIDS-related disorders should have PAIg determined to document the presence of immune platelet destruction.

PAIg can also be measured by using an indirect test with the patient's serum and a normal donor target platelet. This technique may be useful to detect the presence of drug-dependent platelet antibodies in order to decide which pharmacologic agents are safe in patients with suspected drug-induced thrombocytopenia. The indirect assay for PAIg is also useful to detect maternal antibodies directed against fetal paternal platelet antigens in neonatal alloimmunization. A similar approach may also be used to select platelet donors for patients who are refractory to random donor platelet support.

TEST PROCEDURE

Rationale

Cell-associated immunoglobulin is detected on the surface of intact, washed, fixed platelets isolated from the patient's blood. Normal platelets contain 100 to 200 molecules of immunoglobulin G per platelet; this number increases severalfold in patients with immune-mediated platelet destruction (5). Cell surface immunoglobulin is detected by using a biotinated goat anti-human immunoglobulin antibody F(ab')$_2$ fragment directed against three heavy-chain classes (G, M, and A). The F(ab')$_2$ fragment is used to prevent nonspecific sticking of the anti-human immunoglobulin Fc portion and the platelet Fc receptor. The detection system consists of avidin labeled with fluorescein isothiocyanate, and fluorescence is measured with a fluorescence-activated flow cytometer (FACS Analyzer; Becton Dickinson Inc., Mountain View, Calif.). A paired negative control with biotinated goat anti-rabbit immunoglobulin F(ab')$_2$ fragments may be analyzed for each sample; however, based on our experience that this control was consistently negative, it was eliminated from the test routine. Appropriate positive and negative control samples are analyzed with each assay run and must meet specific criteria. The criteria for a positive result are based on a large normal control population study, and the specificity and sensitivity for the assay were determined by a prospective study of patients with clinically documented diagnoses of either immune or nonimmune thrombocytopenia.

This assay may also be used to detect serum antiplatelet antibodies by an indirect test. Washed, fixed, normal donor target platelets are preincubated with the patient test serum, washed free of unbound serum, and analyzed by the same procedure as in the direct assay. Parallel control sera with and without known antiplatelet antibodies are analyzed simultaneously to serve as positive and negative controls.

Specimen collection and platelet isolation

Whole blood is collected into acid-citrate-dextrose (ACD) anticoagulant vacuum tubes (no. 4606, Vacutainer ACD; Becton Dickinson Vacutainer Systems, Rutherford, N.J.). The specimen is stable at room temperature for 24 h. If the patient's platelet count is greater than 50,000/μl, one tube (8.5 ml) is adequate. If the platelet count is less than 50,000/μl, then 17.0 ml of whole blood is drawn to ensure adequate cell numbers. A normal control blood sample is drawn and processed in parallel to the patient sample.

Five milliliters of ACD-blood is transferred to a polypropylene plastic tube (Falcon no. 2059; Becton Dickinson Labware, Oxnard, Calif.), to which 2 ml of buffered saline-glucose containing 13 mM sodium citrate and 10 mM EDTA is added. The contents of the tube are mixed by gentle inversion and centrifuged at 600 × g for 3 min at 20°C. After centrifugation, the supernatant, consisting of diluted platelet-rich plasma (PRP), is removed with a plastic pipette without disturbing the erythrocyte interface and the buffy coat, which is rich in lymphocytes. The diluted PRP is conserved in a second Falcon no. 2059 tube. The volume of the residual erythrocyte pellet is restored to 7.0 ml, and the contents of the tube are mixed and centrifuged again under the same conditions. The second supernatant is removed as described above and pooled with the first supernatant. The procedure is repeated once more, and all of the supernatant fractions are pooled. If two full ACD collection tubes are processed, this procedure requires four platelet wash tubes. The procedure results in greater than 95% platelet recovery with virtually no leukocyte contamination and minimal erythrocyte contamination.

The pooled PRP is centrifuged at 2,000 × g for 10 min at 20°C to produce a platelet pellet. The platelet-poor supernatant is discarded, and the pellet is suspended in 1.0 ml of 1% ammonium oxalate. A 1-ml Eppendorf pipette is used to gently suspend the platelet pellet, and then 4.0 ml of additional ammonium oxalate is added to the suspended platelet. If multiple tubes were required to pellet the dilute PRP, then the individual pellets are combined at this point. The platelets are incubated for 5 min at room temperature to lyse erythrocytes and then pelleted at 2,000 × g for 10 min. The platelets are suspended in 1.0 ml of 1% paraformaldehyde solution (PFA), dispersed by gentle pipetting with an Eppendorf tip, brought to a final volume of 3 ml with 1% PFA, and incubated at room temperature for 5 min. The platelets are pelleted at 2,000 × g for 10 min, the supernatant is discarded, and the pellet is dispersed in 1 ml of Tyrodes buffer containing 10 mM EDTA and 0.5% bovine serum albumin (Tyrodes-EDTA-BSA) and brought to a final volume of 5 ml with the same buffer. The platelets are then pelleted and resuspended in Tyrodes-EDTA-BSA two more times under the same conditions as before. After the final centrifugation, the platelets are resuspended in 1 ml of Tyrodes-EDTA-BSA and stored at 4°C until analyzed. PFA-fixed, washed platelets are stable at 4°C for 30 days.

Preparation of platelets for analysis in the direct test

The platelet concentration of both the control and the patient samples is adjusted to 200,000 cells per μl with Tyrodes-EDTA-BSA. Twenty-five microliters of platelet suspension is placed into each of two 1-ml polystyrene centrifuge tubes, and 50 μl of biotinated goat anti-human immunoglobulin diluted 1:20 in Tyrodes-EDTA-BSA is added. The dilution of this reagent may vary with different immunoglobulin lots. Each new lot is assayed in comparison to the previous lot, and the dilution is adjusted based on the positive control to provide a consistent result. After their contents are mixed, the tubes are incubated on ice for 30 min, 1.0 ml of Tyrodes-EDTA-BSA is added to each tube, and the tubes are centrifuged at 2,000 × g for 5 min. The supernatant fraction is discarded, and the cells are washed twice more with Tyrodes-EDTA-BSA. After the second wash, 50 μl of avidin-fluorescein diluted 1:20 in Tyrodes-EDTA-BSA is added to the resuspended platelet pellet and incubated on ice for

30 min. This step is followed by three washes under the same conditions as for the first label step. At the end of the final wash, the platelets are suspended in 1.0 ml of Isoton II (Coulter Electronics, Inc., Hialeah, Fla.) and transferred to a plastic tube. Platelet suspensions are stored on ice until analyzed. Samples must be analyzed on the same day that they are labeled with fluorescein, but previously washed fixed platelet suspensions are usable for 30 days.

Preparation of control platelets for analysis

The negative control sample consists of a platelet suspension prepared from a normal donor and processed in parallel to the patient sample. The positive control sample is composed of normal platelets which have been sensitized by incubation with serum containing multiple HLA antibodies from patients who have received long-term platelet support. The same procedure as for the indirect test may be used (see below). Positive control platelets are prepared in a batch mode and can be used for up to 5 months with stable results. This permits comparison of daily positive controls over a 1-month period to evaluate assay sensitivity.

Operating conditions for the Becton Dickinson FACS Research Analyzer

The PAIg assay is performed with the 50-μm orifice. Instrument settings are as follows: for volume, current 0.5, log mode, and threshold minimum; for fluorescence, photomultiplier tube 600, log mode, and threshold off. The alignment is adjusted with glutaraldehyde-fixed chicken erythrocytes to obtain maximum sensitivity. The variable gain of the FL-1 channel is adjusted with 2.0-μm-diameter beads (Duke Scientific Corp., Palo Alto, Calif.) so that the fluorescence mean of the beads lies within channels 43 to 47 and the fluorescence mean of the chicken erythrocytes lies above channel 200. Volume gates are set at channels 20 and 255. This excludes debris below the normal platelet size distribution. A flow rate of 300 to 500 events per s is maintained, and 10,000 events are analyzed in the single-parameter mode. FL-1 markers are set at channels 0 and 255. The FL-1 mean is recorded, and a sample with a mean channel which lies 2 standard deviations beyond the normal control mean ($n = 100$) is considered positive. One positive control and at least one negative control are run in duplicate with each assay run. The fluorescence mean of the negative control must lie between channels 58 and 71, and the fluorescence mean of the positive control must lie between channels 110 and 126. This may vary with different lots of reagents but has been constant in our laboratory for the past year. The volume distribution curve for each patient sample must be symmetrical and free of debris, with a well-defined left side. If the controls or the volume distribution curve is not acceptable, then the test must be repeated.

Preparation of platelet samples for the indirect test

Platelets are isolated and prepared as for the direct test from a normal subject with blood type O. The platelet count is adjusted to 200,000/μl with Tyrodes-EDTA-BSA. The target platelets (0.025 ml) are resuspended in 0.1 ml of test serum and incubated at room temperature for 30 min. After incubation, 1.0 ml of Tyrodes-EDTA-BSA is added and the sample is centrifuged at 2,000 × g for 5 min. The supernatant is discarded, and the platelets are washed in Tyrodes-EDTA-BSA one additional time. A negative control is run by using the serum sample from a pool of 20 blood type AB, untransfused male donors previously screened to rule out cytotoxic antibodies (Medical Specialty Laboratories, Boston, Mass.). The assay is performed as for the direct test.

Preparation of samples for the indirect test to detect drug-dependent antibodies

Target platelets are isolated as described above, fixed, and stored at 4°C until needed. The suspected drug must be obtained in soluble form and is diluted to 2 mM in normal saline. Patient and control sera are serially diluted with either normal saline or normal saline containing 2 mM drug so that the final concentration of the drug is 1 mM. Target platelets are incubated with the patient and control sera containing either normal saline or normal saline plus drug and are analyzed as for the indirect test. A positive result is defined by the same criteria as for the direct assay.

REAGENTS

Buffered saline with glucose and citrate

Combine 6.832 g of NaCl, 4.0 g of sodium citrate, 2.0 g of glucose, 1.22 g of disodium phosphate, 0.218 g of potassium phosphate, and 3.36 g of disodium EDTA. Bring to 1 liter with deionized water, adjust the pH to 7.4 with 1 N NaOH, and store in the cold.

1% Ammonium oxalate

Dissolve 1 g of ammonium oxalate in 100 ml of deionized water.

Tyrodes EDTA-BSA

Combine 8.0 g of NaCl, 0.2 g of KCl, 0.065 g of sodium phosphate, 0.184 g of magnesium chloride, 0.1 g of sodium bicarbonate, 1.0 g of glucose, and 3.36 g of disodium EDTA. Bring to 1 liter with deionized water, add 5 g of bovine serum albumin, adjust the pH to 7.1 with 1 N NaOH, and store in the cold.

4% PFA

Add 4 g of PFA to 100 ml of Tyrodes buffer, heat to 70°C, and add 1 N NaOH dropwise to dissolve the PFA. Filter the solution and store in the cold.

1% PFA

Add 1 part 4% PFA to 3 parts Tyrodes buffer. Adjust the pH to between 7.2 and 7.4 with 1 N HCl immediately before use. Store cold. The solution is good for 1 week.

TABLE 1. Sensitivity and specificity of the FACS assay for detection of PAIg[a]

Clinically documented diagnosis	No. PAIg positive	No. PAIg negative
Immune thrombocytopenia	92	6
Nonimmune thrombocytopenia	4	69

[a] Sensitivity, 93.8%; specificity, 94.5%; prevalence, 57.3%; positive predictive value, 95.8%; negative predictive value, 92.0%. Samples were submitted from patients with a positive history of thrombocytopenia or qualitative platelet dysfunction. Clinical diagnosis is based on bone marrow aspirate, clinical course, and response to therapy.

Immunologic reagents.

Goat anti-human immunoglobulin conjugated to biotin [F(ab')$_2$ fragment]. Store at −80°C in 0.05-ml aliquots; do not refreeze the aliquots.
Avidin-fluorescein conjugate. Store at 2 to 8°C.

INTERPRETATION

The diagnostic efficacy of the technique described here has been evaluated by a prospective study of 171 patients who presented with either a laboratory finding of thrombocytopenia or a clinical suspicion of a qualitative platelet defect based on a prolonged template bleeding time. The clinical diagnosis was established for each patient independent of the determination of PAIg. The clinical diagnosis of immune-related thrombocytopenia was based on a bone marrow examination and the subsequent clinical course in response to therapy. The diagnosis of qualitative platelet dysfunction was based on an abnormal template bleeding time and platelet aggregation studies. The results of this study are summarized in Table 1. This study indicates that both the sensitivity and the specificity of this test are acceptable. A parallel study to evaluate the indirect test has not yet been performed. It must be kept in mind that this test does not provide specific information as to the nature of the immunoglobulin deposited on the platelet surface. PAIg may represent antibody directed against specific platelet antigens (9, 10) or immune complexes nonspecifically absorbed to the platelet surface or an Fc receptor site

(8). However, while the results of this technique are nonspecific, the technique does make it possible to analyze eluates (R. B. Stricker, D. I. Abrams, L. Corash, and M. A. Shuman, Blood 64:241a, 1984) obtained from positive platelet preparations by the indirect test procedure in order to further define the specificity of the cell-associated immunoglobulin. Fab fragments can also be prepared from these platelet immunoglobulin eluates and then tested in the indirect assay to discriminate between Fab- and Fc-dependent binding. Thus, this technique offers the potential to serve as a sensitive screening test and as a tool to subsequently define antibody specificity.

LITERATURE CITED

1. **Hassidim, K., R. McMillan, M. S. Conjalka, and J. Morrison.** 1979. Immune thrombocytopenia purpura in Hodgkin's disease. Am. J. Hematol. **6:**149–153.
2. **Hymes, K., M. Blum, H. Lackner, and S. Karpatkin.** 1981. Easy bruising, thrombocytopenia, and elevated platelet immunoglobulin G in Graves's disease and Hashimoto's thyroiditis. Ann. Intern. Med. **94:**27–30.
3. **Karpatkin, S.** 1980. Autoimmune thrombocytopenia purpura. Blood **56:**329–343.
4. **Kelton, J. G., P. J. Powers, and C. J. Carter.** 1982. A prospective study of the usefulness of the measurement of platelet associated IgG for the diagnosis of idiopathic thrombocytopenic purpura. Blood **60:**1050–1053.
5. **LoBuglio, A. F., W. S. Court, L. Vinocur, G. Maglott, and G. M. Shaw.** 1983. Immune thrombocytopenia purpura. Use of a 125-I-labeled antihuman IgG monoclonal antibody to quantify platelet-bound IgG. N. Engl. J. Med. **309:**459–463.
6. **Morris, L., A. Distenfeld, E. Amorosi, and S. Karpatkin.** 1982. Autoimmune thrombocytopenic purpura in homosexual men. Ann. Intern. Med. **96:**714–717.
7. **Schwartz, K. A., S. J. Slichter, and L. A. Harker.** 1982. Immune mediated platelet destruction and thrombocytopenia in patients with solid tumors. Br. J. Haematol. **51:**17–24.
8. **Walsh, C. M., M. A. Nardi, and S. Karpatkin.** 1984. On the mechanism of thrombocytopenic purpura in sexually active homosexual men. N. Engl. J. Med. **311:**635–639.
9. **Woods, V. L., Y. Kurata, R. R. Montgomery, P. Tani, D. Mason, E. H. Oh, and R. McMillan.** 1984. Autoantibodies against platelet glycoprotein Ib in patients with chronic immune thrombocytopenia purpura. Blood **64:**156–160.
10. **Woods, V. L., E. H. Oh, D. Mason, and R. McMillan.** 1984. Autoantibodies against the platelet glycoprotein IIb/IIIa complex in patients with chronic ITP. Blood **63:**368–375.

Chapter 36

Section F. Cellular Components

Introduction

ROSS E. ROCKLIN

This section deals with various techniques currently available for evaluating the cellular components of the immune response in humans. The cell types which contribute to the cellular hypersensitivity reaction include lymphocytes, macrophages, and granulocytes. The techniques described in this section are used to assess in vivo and vitro cellular function in patients who may have certain types of recurrent infections (fungal, mycobacterial, and pyogenic), depressed cellular immunity (acquired immunodeficiency syndrome, sarcoidosis, and cancer), or autoimmune disease (glomerulonephritis and thyroiditis).

At present, the best in vivo screening procedure that the clinician can employ to evaluate cellular hypersensitivity is still the 24- to 48-h skin test (chapter 37). The development of one or more positive cutaneous responses to environmental antigens such as purified protein derivative of tuberculin, monilia, streptokinase-streptodornase, or mumps, or the new sensitization to a contact allergen such as dinitrochlorobenzene, usually indicates intact cellular immunity. A positive delayed skin test response results from lymphocyte-macrophage interaction as well as certain components of the inflammatory response. In vitro testing in such patients will not usually provide more information. However, polymorphonuclear leukocyte function is not evaluated by delayed hypersensitivity skin testing, and therefore such tests would not detect defects in this system. Failure to respond to a battery of environmental antigens or to be sensitized to a new antigen is referred to as cutaneous anergy and is associated with depressed cellular immunity and lowered resistance to infection. Since cutaneous anergy may result from abnormalities in the lymphocyte, the macrophage, or both, the in vitro tests are valuable in defining the level of the defect. The following chapters in this section describe techniques for the qualitative and quantitative evaluation of lymphocyte, macrophage, and polymorphonuclear leukocyte functions. Basophil and eosinophil functions are covered in section J.

The tests which quantify lymphocyte function detect the ability of lymphocytes to proliferate, produce mediators, mount cytotoxic responses, and regulate immune responses. The enumeration of lymphocyte subpopulations (T cells and B cells) is covered in section E. Lymphocyte proliferative responses can be evaluated by using nonspecific mitogenic stimulants such as phytohemagglutinin, concanavalin A, or pokeweed mitogen, and by specific stimuli such as soluble antigens (chapter 38). The nonspecific activation of lymphocytes measures both T-cell and B-cell function, although the kinetics of these responses differ. In contrast, specific antigenic challenge appears to measure only T-cell function. By using autologous as well as homologous serum in the cultures, one can also determine whether the patient's serum contains factors which may interfere with the proliferative response.

The elaboration of soluble mediators by lymphocytes and monocytes indicates that these cells are capable of producing factors which alter the function of a variety of cells involved in cellular immune reactions. Some examples include migration inhibitory factor (chapter 39), leukocyte inhibitory factor (chapter 39), chemotactic factor (chapter 40), interferon (chapter 41), T-cell growth factor or interleukin-2 (chapter 42), and interleukin-1 (chapter 46). The production of these mediators, as well as their unique biological assay systems, is described in the indicated chapters. Although the elaboration of these factors can be shown to correlate with in vivo delayed hypersensitivity in humans, they do not necessarily measure the function of a particular cell type (T or B cells).

The ability of lymphocytes to act as cytotoxic "killer" cells, in response to either allogeneic target or malignant cells, is covered in chapters 43 and 44. Measurement of these responses has clinical relevance in transplant and cancer patients. T-cell regulation of immunoglobulin synthesis or antibody production, as well as lymphocyte proliferation, has been found to have clinical application (chapter 45). Excessive or diminished regulation of these immune responses can result in disorders in humoral or cell-mediated immunity, or both.

Whenever possible, the clinician should measure more than one in vitro test of lymphocyte function, since each assay may detect a distinct subpopulation of cells. Furthermore, the present evidence indicates that lymphocytes are compartmentalized; that is, cells in the blood may be functionally different from those in the lymph nodes or spleen. Therefore, sampling of blood lymphocytes alone may not yield representative results. An evaluation should include quantitation of the numbers of T and B cells, determination of proliferative responses to mitogens and specific antigens, measurement of at least one lymphocyte mediator, and determination of a cytotoxic response. If any of these functions are found to be abnormal, then assessment of suppressor cell activity would be indicated. It should be pointed out that the precise role of suppressor cells in disease is presently an area of active investigation, and some of the data are still preliminary.

Assessment of macrophage and polymorphonuclear leukocyte function is performed by measuring the ability of these cells to ingest particles, kill microorganisms, and respond to certain stimuli by increased directed movement (chemotaxis); by identifying certain surface receptors; and by determining the response of these cells to lymphocyte mediators. These procedures are covered in chapters 47, 40, and 46, respectively.

Because of their complexity, not all of these in vitro assays are carried out in most clinical laboratories; they are restricted at present to research centers which specialize in basic and applied investigation. Moreover, because of the nature of these assays (that is, they are biological phenomena and subject to considerable variation), the results should be interpreted with caution. Therefore, in an individual patient a negative result should be repeated to confirm abnormal cellular function. For this reason, these tests are more useful when applied to the study of groups or populations of patients with certain diseases rather than to individual patients. Although they are not usually diagnostic, these tests are of value clinically for the purposes of identifying certain pathogenetic factors and monitoring the results of therapy and the clinical course of patients with depressed cellular function.

Chapter 37

Delayed Hypersensitivity Skin Testing

C. EDWARD BUCKLEY III

Skin tests are among the most useful tools of the clinical immunologist. Tests of delayed cutaneous hypersensitivity, along with the number of circulating peripheral blood lymphocytes and the immunoglobulin concentrations in serum, are the indicated initial studies used to evaluate patients with immune disorders. Delayed skin tests provide a generally accepted cost-effective way to evaluate cellular immunity in patients (6). Patients with quantitatively normal delayed cutaneous hypersensitivity do not need costly in vitro studies of cellular immunity. Despite their clinical utility and the importance of containing health care costs, very few well-characterized delayed skin test antigens are available. Indeed, delayed skin test antigens and other clinically useful immunogens can be viewed as orphan drugs. The clinical immunologist is obliged to appropriate antigens prepared for other purposes to implement delayed skin testing. No critically evaluated, generally acceptable standard method for testing exists. This chapter reviews our current understanding of delayed hypersensitivity skin testing and presents a critical discussion of the methods and circumstances under which useful, safe clinical tests can be accomplished. Easily accomplished standard methods for performing skin tests, measuring reactions, and recording observations are described. Several methods for interpreting and reporting results are presented and discussed.

BASIC CONCEPTS

Many different natural and man-made substances can provoke inflammation of living tissues. Systemic exposure to these substances can cause disease and death. Despite this potential for injury, skin tests can often be performed successfully with minimum risk by using small quantities of the substance. A skin test consists of the purposeful local application of a substance which can provoke a cutaneous inflammatory reaction. The local reaction provides a visible representation of the subject's general ability to react to the substance. Skin tests are usually initiated with sequentially increased quantities (doses) of the potentially harmful substance. This process can elicit two kinds of cutaneous reactions. Skin tests with compounds, including the natural products of bacteria, can elicit a threshold dose which causes a local destructive reaction in all subjects tested. This type of inflammation is called a toxic reaction. Skin tests with reactive doses of phytohemagglutinin, croton oil, and sodium lauryl sulfate provide examples of toxic reactions. Skin tests with other compounds identify a threshold dose which provokes an inflammatory reaction in a restricted number of subjects. The nontoxic nature of the reaction is deduced from the failure of many subjects to react to the compound. Those subjects who react are considered hypersensitive or allergic to the compound.

This simple distinction between hypersensitivity and toxic reactions is extremely important. The detection of a hypersensitivity reaction permits four important deductions about the compound. These deductions provide the basis for the experimental and clinical use of hypersensitivity reactions. First, the substance used to induce the reaction is immunogenic. Second, the substance used to elicit the skin test reaction is antigenic. Third, those subjects with hypersensitivity reactions have been previously exposed and sensitized to the antigen. Fourth, the resulting hypersensitivity reaction is specific for the antigen. A fifth ambiguous deduction is also possible; individuals who do not react to the antigen either (i) have not been previously exposed or (ii) lack the immune mechanisms needed to become sensitized or react to the antigen. Clinical concern is focused on this last possibility. These patients often have impaired immune function.

Almost a century lapsed between Jenner's 1798 description of the delayed papular erythematous skin lesion of persons revaccinated for smallpox as a "reaction of immunity" and Koch's 1890 description of local induration and swelling after the subcutaneous injection of tuberculin (15). Our current understanding of cutaneous hypersensitivity reactions developed during the following century and shares an intimate, romantic relationship with our understanding of allergy and host resistance to the tubercle bacillus. Clinical awareness of the diagnostic utility of the direct tuberculin skin test stems from Epstein's studies of tuberculous children in 1891. Studies over the next three decades led to the development of the percutaneous skin test by Von Pirquet and Schick in 1903 and the direct intradermal (intracutaneous) test by Mantoux in 1910. The Mantoux skin test (10) remains the standard method for clinical and epidemiologic studies of tuberculosis and mycotic diseases and the clinical assessment of delayed cutaneous hypersensitivity.

These early studies failed to distinguish between the meaning of the early and late components of the cutaneous hypersensitivity reactions. This distinction followed the classic passive transfer studies of Zinsser and Mueller (17), who showed that cutaneous allergy to tuberculin and related bacterial antigens could be separated into two types of hypersensitivity reactions. Each hypersensitivity reaction is named for the time of occurrence after antigen challenge. Immediate hypersensitivity reactions occur within 24 h after antigen challenge. Delayed hypersensitivity reactions occur 48 h or more after antigen challenge. Immediate hypersensitivity reactions are initiated by antibodies and reflect the function of humoral immune mechanisms. Delayed hypersensitivity reactions are initiated by lymphocytes and reflect the function of cellular immunity. The tuberculin reaction is the classic prototype of delayed cutaneous hypersensitivity.

Much evidence indicates that several different humoral and cellular mechanisms contribute to the expression of hypersensitivity reactions. The classic time-dependent separation of antibody- and cell-initiated hypersensitivity reactions suggested by Zinsser may not be completely valid. Studies by Dienes and Mallory and by Jones and Mote (7) revealed evidence of a different kind of cellular hypersensitivity reaction. Although this reaction shows histopathologic features characteristic of the tuberculin-type delayed cutaneous hypersensitivity reaction, it differs in its early onset, the histologic presence of a basophil component, and scant numbers of infiltrating polymorphonuclear leukocytes (4, 5). The cutaneous mononuclear- and basophil-enriched cell infiltrate begins to form 2 to 4 h after antigen challenge and reaches maximum intensity in 24 to 72 h. The intensity of the basophil infiltrate varies among species and is least in humans. Unlike the tuberculin reaction, the Jones-Mote or cutaneous basophilic hypersensitivity reaction tends to subside after the onset of immediate hypersensitivity and the production of circulating immunoglobulin G (IgG) antibodies. Reactions to chemical contact allergens, the prototype of cutaneous basophilic delayed hypersensitivity, do not generate circulating antibodies. This hypersensitivity reaction can also be produced by the repeated injection of protein antigens in the absence of mycobacterial adjuvants, poison ivy, drugs, viruses, allografts, and insect bites. Like the tuberculin reaction, cutaneous basophilic hypersensitivity is T-cell dependent and can be passively transferred with cells. Interestingly, tuberculin skin tests in guinea pigs which have been adoptively sensitized with lymphocytes from animals with active tuberculin hypersensitivity produce a cutaneous basophilic reaction to tuberculin instead of the classic tuberculin reaction. In contrast to tuberculin hypersensitivity, Jones-Mote hypersensitivity is relatively susceptible to desensitization and the pharmacologic effect of corticosteroids. Cutaneous basophil-type reactions can be passively transferred with cell-fixed antibodies, such as IgE, in guinea pigs (1), mice (12), and humans (14).

CLINICAL CONCEPTS

The antigens used to produce delayed hypersensitivity can also cause immediate hypersensitivity. An awareness of the different attributes of immediate and delayed cutaneous hypersensitivity reactions is technically important. Considerable overlap exists in the time of occurrence of the manifestations of cutaneous hypersensitivity reactions. Attributes of the cutaneous reaction and the time of observation are used to discriminate between the immediate and delayed components of cutaneous hypersensitivity. Adverse immediate hypersensitivity reactions can also occur. In monitoring the safety of antigens, the arbitrary selection of skin test reactions ≥40 mm in diameter at any time of observation provides a plausible conservative criterion for an adverse reaction (16). An awareness of the characteristics of immediate as well as delayed cutaneous hypersensitivity is needed to evaluate the antigens used for delayed hypersensitivity skin tests.

Cutaneous antigen reactions

Although infrequent, large reaginic hypersensitivity reactions can occur 15 to 30 min after skin tests with microbiologic antigens. Reaginic hypersensitivity is caused by vasodilation and increased vascular permeability at the site of antigen challenge and typically results in a large, flat, erythematous flare reaction and a pale, central, elevated edematous wheal. Rare instances of anaphylaxis have occurred after challenge with antigens used to elicit delayed hypersensitivity. Reaginic reactions are frequently followed by a late cutaneous reaction, manifested by circumscribed erythema and edema 4 to 12 h after antigen challenge. This reaction differs from the flare and wheal in that the erythema usually lies within the area of edema. The late cutaneous reaction, a cutaneous basophilic reaction caused by cytophilic IgE antibodies, can persist, but usually subsides by 24 h after testing. Although unusual, severe Arthus hypersensitivity reactions, manifested by local warmth, erythema, edema, petechiae, and even necrosis and ulceration, can occur 24 h after antigen challenge. This reaction is caused by circulating IgG and IgM complement-fixing antibodies. The occurrence of a severe Arthus reaction at 24 h can obscure the subsequent cool, firm, palpable cutaneous induration characteristic of delayed hypersensitivity. In addition to the delayed induration, local vesicles, bullae, and ulceration can occur 48 to 96 h after antigen challenge. The cutaneous changes associated with severe delayed reactions can persist for as long as 2 weeks.

Histopathology

Local delayed hypersensitivity reactions to contact allergens and microbiologic antigens share similarities and exhibit distinct differences (5). The route of antigen challenge contributes to differences in the distribution of histopathologic changes and in the time of maximum reactivity. The histopathologic distribution of tissue changes and the 4- to 6-day time of maximum reactivity after epicutaneous challenge with contact allergens and tine tests differ from the more focal tissue changes and the 2- to 3-day time of maximum reactivity induced by the standard Mantoux intradermal antigen injection (9). The retarded development of epicutaneous tests hazards the interpretation of tine-induced reactions at 24 and 48 h as delayed hypersensitivity reactions. Species differences in the number and tinctoral properties of cells in tissue infiltrate are other sources of variability. Skin test reactions occur more quickly and the basophil infiltrate is more intense in guinea pigs than in humans. Despite this species difference, the 24-h skin test in sensitized guinea pigs is used to standardize skin test antigens for human use. Even within a single species, such as humans, variation exists in the cellular composition of the delayed cutaneous hypersensitivity reaction (4). The following brief description of findings represents a synopsis of observations in humans.

The initial changes produced by antigen challenge are microscopic evidence of local edema and dilation of the small arterioles, capillaries, venules, and lymphatics (5). Changes observed as early as 2 to 4 h include hypertrophy of the cells of involved vessels, endothelial cell and pericyte hyperplasia, and thickening of the vascular basement membrane. Individual endothelial cell necrosis can occur. A perivenular infiltrate of small and large lymphocytes develops by 4 to 6 h. Basophilic leukocytes, the only granulocytes seen in contact allergen reactions, are initially detected in the lumen of involved vessels and by 3 to 4 h are present in the evolving perivascular cuffs. An earlier, less intense basophil infiltrate also occurs as a part of the tuberculin reaction. The early perivascular changes are followed and accompanied by a less intense, diffuse, intervascular infiltrate composed of lymphocytes, variable numbers of monocytes, and basophils. In the tuberculin skin tests, the perivascular changes reach a maximum in 2 to 3 days and can assume a nodular pseudogranulomatous appearance. In contrast, the basophil infiltrate observed with strong reactions to contact allergens in intervascular tissues reaches maximum intensity in 4 to 6 days. The tuberculin reaction is usually accompanied by a prominent polymorphonuclear granulocytic infiltrate and differs in this way from the cutaneous basophilic reaction. The basophil infiltrate is usually sparse with weak reactions and may not be detectable even after challenge with contact allergens. With contact allergens, the tissue changes primarily involve the vessels in the superficial vascular plexus at the junction of the papillary and reticular dermis. With tuberculin, the changes extend into the deep dermis and can involve the subcutis with relative sparing of the epidermis.

The tuberculin skin test has been studied with hybridoma antisera to specific cell phenotypes (11). Approximately 75 to 90% of the mononuclear cells in the perivascular aggregates bear phenotypic markers of T lymphocytes or monocytes. The ratio of cells with the T-helper cell phenotype to cells with the T-suppressor cell phenotype is increased and exceeds the ratio of cells with similar phenotypes in the peripheral blood 6 h after antigen challenge. By 12 to 24 h, the dermal interstitium becomes infiltrated with T lymphocytes and monocytes. Cells bearing the T-helper cell phenotype are more numerous. In the epidermis, lymphocytes bearing the helper and suppressor phenotypes occur in approximately equal portions. Studies of lymphocyte receptor phenotypes consistent with cell activation, such as transferin and interleukin 2, suggest that cell activation does not occur until approximately 48 h after antigen challenge.

Nonresponders and anergy

Everyone is normally exposed and sensitized to many antigens. Modern prophylactic immunization practices result in the purposeful exposure to antigens from microorganisms responsible for diphtheria, tetanus, pneumococcal pneumonia, mumps, influenza, and other virus infections. In addition, natural exposure results in sensitization to antigens prepared from streptococci, staphylococci, and certain common fungi, and to other ubiquitous antigens. Skin tests elicit delayed cutaneous hypersensitivity to these antigens in most healthy subjects. An adequately exposed healthy subject who does not exhibit a delayed cutaneous reaction to an antigen is called a nonresponder to the antigen.

Deductions about the nonresponder status of a subject are most easily made when the individual has been exposed to an antigen dose that produces sensitization in most normal subjects. This deduction is completely valid only after prospective immunization with a potent antigen. Deductions about the responder status of a subject can also be made when several nonresponders to the same ubiquitous antigens are detected among closely related members of the same family. For example, a plausible genetic contribution to shared nonresponsiveness to poison ivy can often be identified among healthy exposed family members. Finally, deductions about the nonresponder status of a subject can be made from the failure to react to a large number of antigens which elicit delayed reactions in most normal individuals.

Additional important deductions can often be made about the nonresponder status of patients. The nonresponder status of a patient is most evident when the specific impairment of the delayed skin test reaction is directed toward a microorganism responsible for active infection. This type of impairment of delayed cutaneous hypersensitivity is called anergy. Classically, anergy is defined as unresponsiveness to a specific antigen. The occurrence of a negative tuberculin skin test in a patient with active tuberculosis is an example of "tuberculin anergy." Patients are also clinically categorized as anergic when they exhibit an improbable degree of impairment of delayed cutaneous hypersensitivity to a large number of test antigens. Delayed cutaneous anergy can occur in patients who have known prior exposure, intact immediate hypersensitivity, and circulating antibodies to or circulating immune complexes containing the antigen. The occurrence of delayed cutaneous anergy and circulating antibodies to the same antigen is called an immune deviation.

SKIN TEST STRATEGIES AND ANTIGENS

The detection of delayed cutaneous hypersensitivity is dependent upon prior sensitization. Appropriate antigens are an important component of any skin test strategy. Table 1 provides a representative list of antigens, categorized by intended purpose and potential source. The ability of these antigens to elicit delayed cutaneous hypersensitivity reactions in patients and in healthy subjects is well documented. Despite these reports, the use of these antigens for delayed hypersensitivity skin tests has not been formally approved by regulatory agencies. This means that the interpretation of the results of skin tests with these antigens must be based on generally available information. The only antigens formally approved for delayed hypersensitivity skin tests are provided as a tine test panel (Multitest; Merieux Institute, USA, Miami, Fla.). Because of the differences in the time of development and tissue distribution of epicutaneous reactions (9), reactions reported at 24 or 48 h with this device (8) may not be comparable to the delayed reactions elicited by the standard Mantoux intradermal skin test. Tables 2 and 3 summarize quantitative information about Mantoux tests with recall antigens. The clinical use of these antigens for delayed skin tests represents a generally accepted extension of laboratory science.

Two general strategies are used to solve the problem of prior exposure and sensitization: (i) prospective

TABLE 1. Antigens used to assay delayed cutaneous hypersensitivity[a]

Antigen and use	Product name	Concn supplied	Skin test dilution	Suggested source[b]
Diagnostic delayed skin tests				
Coccidioidin	Spherulin	1:100[c]	Neat	2
	Coccidioidin	1:100[c]	Neat	8
Histoplasmin	Histocyl	1:100	Neat	2
	Histoplasmin	1:100	Neat	11
Mumps virus	Mumps skin test antigen	20 CFU/ml	Neat	4
Tuberculin		50 TU/ml[c]	Neat	5, 11
Immunization				
Diphtheria toxoid		30 Lf/ml	Neat	11, 12, 14
Tetanus toxoid		10 Lf/ml	Neat	10, 12, 13, 14
Staphylococcal	Staphage Lysate		1:5	3
Allergenic skin tests				
C. albicans	Monilia	1:10 (wt/vol)	1:500	9
	C. albicans	1:10 (wt/vol)	1:1,000	1, 6, 9
Trichophyton sp.	Dermatophyton	1:10 (wt/vol)	1:30	9
	Trichophyton	1:10 (wt/vol)	1:1,000	1, 6, 9
Compounds adapted for delayed hypersensitivity testing				
Streptococcal	Varidase[d]	Lyophilized	100 U of SK/ml[e]	10
	SK	Lyophilized	375 U of SK/ml[e]	7

[a] TU, Tuberculin units; Lf, flocculation units, SK, streptokinase.

[b] Antigen sources: (1) Allermed, San Diego, Calif.; (2) Berkeley Biologicals, Berkeley, Calif.; (3) Delmont Laboratories, Inc., Swarthmore, Pa.; (4) Eli Lilly & Co., Indianapolis, Ind.; (5) Squibb-Connought, Princeton, N.J.; (6) Greer Laboratories, Lenoir, N.C.; (7) Hoechst-Roussel Pharmaceuticals, Somerville, N.J.; (8) Iatric Corp., Phoenix, Ariz.; (9) Hollister-Stier Laboratories, Spokane, Wash.; (10) Lederle Laboratories, Pearl River, N.Y.; (11) Parke Davis & Co., Morris Plains, N.J.; (12) Sclavo, Wayne, N.J.; (13) E. R. Squibb & Sons, Inc., Princeton, N.J.; (14) Wyeth Laboratories, Philadelphia, Pa. Information obtained from J. R. Boyd, ed., *Facts and Comparisons, 1984*, J. B. Lippincott, St. Louis, 1984, and G. K. McEvoy, ed., *The American Hospital Formulary Service*, American Society of Hospital Pharmacists, Bethesda, Md., 1984.

[c] Bioequivalent.

[d] No longer available.

[e] Prepared by weighing.

immunization before the skin tests, and (ii) skin tests with ubiquitous antigens. Advantages of the first strategy include the certainty of prior antigen exposure and the ability to test both the afferent and efferent portions of the immune response. Experimental use has been made of contact allergens, keyhole limpet hemocyanin, tetanus and diphtheria toxoids, and other antigens used for prophylactic immunization. The major disadvantage of prospective immunization is the prolonged time needed to induce sensitization and determine the ability of the patient to react. The second approach, tests with a panel of ubiquitous antigens, is used in the routine clinical evaluation of patients. Advantages of this strategy include the relatively short 3-day interval needed to complete the tests and the ability to simultaneously assess prior sensitization to pathogens. Disadvantages include the need for accurate information about prior exposure and sensitization in a reference population, the inability to test the afferent part of the immune response, and the occurrence of adverse reactions to antigen doses capable of eliciting a high prevalence of delayed cutaneous reactions.

Contact allergen skin tests

Contact allergens, such a dinitrochlorobenzene, are the most frequently used antigens in clinical tests involving prospective sensitization and challenge (3). There are several reasons for this choice. Contact allergen tests provide an uncomplicated assessment of cellular immunity. The tests can be easily accomplished with reagents and equipment generally available in most clinics. The procedure is relatively free of adverse effects when precautions are taken to avoid exposure of personnel to the contact allergen and when excessive sensitizing doses are avoided in patients with intact immunity. When the test is positive, the outcome can be easily interpreted. Problems arise only in the presence of a negative test, which can occur in approximately 1 of 10 normal subjects sensitized with the 500-μg dose of dinitrochlorobenzene.

Recall antigen skin tests

The most frequently used strategy relies on skin tests with naturally occurring antigens. These ubiquitous antigens are also called recall antigens, because they elicit evidence of prior antigen exposure and sensitization. Recall antigen skin tests can be used in two ways: (i) sequential testing, based on measurements of reactions to serial tests with sequential increases in the dose of the same test antigen, and (ii) antigen panel testing, based on the assessment of reactions to specific antigens which have a known

TABLE 2. Summary of reports of delayed cutaneous recall antigen reactivity

Type of subject and reference no.[a]	C. albicans		Mumps		Varidase		Trichophyton		Tuberculin (PPD)		Tetanus toxoid		Coccidioidin	
	Positive	No. tested	Positive	No. tested	Positive	No. tested	Positive	No. tested	Positive	No. tested	Positive	No. tested	Positive	No. tested
Normal subjects														
1	50	151					32	151	74	168				
2	117	208	182	208	158	208	126	208	108	208				
3	39	100	78	100	55	100	28	100	16	100			19	100
4	60	68	35	68	50	68	19	68	12	68				
5	24	38	29	38	33	38								
6	8	12	11	12	7	12	10	12	3	12				
7	70	81			50	81	40	81			31	81		
8	8	47	22	47			35	47	14	47			11	47
Total	376	705	357	473	353	507	290	667	227	603	31	81	30	147
(% positive)	(53.3)		(75.5)		(69.6)		(43.5)		(37.6)		(38.3)		(20.4)	
Patients														
9	73	79	71	79			54	79	56	79				
10	58	85	50	85					17	85	24	75		
11	474	752	304	752			466	752	248	752			90	752
4	56	73	27	73	35	73	9	73	13	73				
Total	661	989	425	916	35	73	529	904	334	989	24	75	904	752
(% positive)	(66.8)		(46.4)		(47.9)		(58.5)		(33.8)		(32.0)		(12.0)	

[a] Adapted from data presented by: (1) J. E. Sokal and N. Primikiros, Cancer **14**:597, 1961; (2) D. Lamb et al., J. Immunol. **89**:555, 1962; (3) L. E. Spitler, *in Manual of Clinical Immunology*, 1st ed., American Society for Microbiology, 1976, p. 60; (4) P. G. Simpson et al., S. Med. J. **69**:424, 1976; (5) T. F. Hogan et al., Cancer Immunol. Immunother. **10**:27, 1980; (6) E. C. Keystone et al., Clin. Exp. Immunol. **40**:202, 1980; (7) E. H. Gordon et at., J. Allergy Clin. Immunol. **72**:487, 1983; (8) H. Lichtenstein et al., J. Am Gerontol. Soc. **30**:447, 1982; (9) W. W. Schier et al., Am. J. Med. **20**:94, 1956; (10) D. L. Palmer and W. P. Reed, J. Infect. Dis., **130**:132, 1974; (11) J. C. Delafuente et al., J. Am. Med. Assoc. **249**:3209, 1983.

probability of reacting in a reference population. The main differences between these two test methods are the time and expense involved in demonstrating delayed cutaneous reactivity with sequential testing and the frequency with which a prior test with the same or other antigens can alter the patient's subsequent ability to react. The production of "booster reactions" after tests with tuberculin and histoplasmin is well documented. Impaired reactivity or desensitization to subsequent challenge with the same antigen can also occur. Both effects hazard the interpretation of sequential testing.

Sequential testing. Sequential testing is most applicable to patients who can be followed and subjected to repeat tests. The main advantage of the method is the limited discomfort produced by the injection of a single antigen. Sequential tests with one antigen, such as *Candida albicans*, are frequently used in infants and children who are normally less reactive and are likely to have easily detectable defects in cellular immune function. The same method can also be used in ambulatory clinics and in nursing home populations, where rapid detection of cellular immunity is not needed. The identification of a definite delayed (48- to 72-h) cutaneous hypersensitivity reaction is sufficient to demonstrate intact cellular immunity. The antigen concentration at which the test antigen becomes positive is important. High skin test antigen concentrations can produce a toxic inflammatory reaction. For example, skin tests with high doses of tuberculin can produce a toxic cutaneous reaction in unsensitized

neonates. This test strategy requires prior knowledge that the maximum antigen dose actually detects delayed hypersensitivity in appropriate controls.

Antigen panel testing. Antigen panel testing makes use of several antigens to determine the chance that the patient has impaired delayed cutaneous hypersensitivity. This approach is applicable to the rapid evaluation of hospitalized adult patients with subtle alterations in cellular immunity. The major disadvantages of this method are the discomfort of multiple skin tests and the need to determine reactivity to the antigen panel in a reference population. Geographic and demographic differences exist in the prevalence of sensitization to recall antigens. Antigen panels should maximize the chance of detecting positive reactions in patients drawn from the population tested.

Antigen selection

Published reports of recall antigen testing have been limited to a relatively small number of antigens. Table 2 reveals a modest degree of variability among the outcomes of reported studies. Several factors contribute to this variation. The number of subjects tested in many studies was small. Differences also exist in the methods used, the criteria selected for a positive test, the time (24 to 48 h) of observations, and the potency or concentration of similar antigens. Despite these limitations, Table 2 reveals a similar range of reactivity among healthy subjects and patients. This outcome is not surprising. The number of reac-

TABLE 3. Cutaneous hypersensitivity reactions to selected antigens[a]

Antigen and dose (manufacturer)	No. of subjects	Diam (mm)	% Patients responding at:				
			0.25 h	6 h	24 h	48 h	72 h
Mumps, 0.1 ml, neat (Eli Lilly & Co.)	4,431	≥2	98.7	83.0	78.9	59.6	47.1
		≥5	94.2	65.2	64.2	36.6	24.0
		≥10	42.1	27.6	37.1	15.3	7.6
C. albicans, 0.1 ml, 1:1,000 (Hollister-Stier Laboratories)	8,878	≥2	99.2	61.1	60.5	50.1	42.3
		≥5	93.8	33.8	46.3	37.3	28.9
		≥10	36.6	13.5	29.1	16.6	10.1
Varidase, 0.1 ml, 100 U of SK (Lederle Laboratories)	7,009	≥2	99.1	60.6	60.5	48.9	40.7
		≥5	91.9	29.3	44.4	37.5	29.2
		≥10	21.3	8.3	27.9	21.7	15.0
PPD, human, 0.1 ml, 50 TU (Squibb-Connought)	8,878	≥2	98.9	65.1	53.4	38.1	31.7
		≥5	90.6	31.0	37.6	27.2	23.4
		≥10	14.3	9.6	20.8	15.3	12.7
Trichophyton, 0.1 ml, 1:1,000 (Greer Laboratories)	6,512	≥2	99.0	63.4	46.8	33.7	29.6
		≥5	92.7	35.6	31.5	23.8	20.5
		≥10	35.4	16.8	19.8	12.0	9.3
Histoplasmin, 0.1 ml, 1:1,000 (Duke Medical Center)	8,847	≥2	99.1	58.1	31.6	14.2	11.5
		≥5	91.4	24.6	15.2	9.3	8.3
		≥10	15.8	5.2	6.9	4.8	4.0
Coccidioidin, 0.1 ml, 1:100 (Cutter Laboratories)	8,876	≥2	98.9	59.0	32.9	8.6	5.0
		≥5	90.1	26.4	15.0	3.6	2.5
		≥10	15.4	3.4	3.8	1.3	0.8
Blastomycin, 0.1 ml, 1:1,000 (Duke Medical Center)	8,873	≥2	98.8	54.2	25.3	6.5	3.9
		≥5	88.6	20.4	8.6	2.3	1.5
		≥10	15.7	2.9	2.0	0.6	0.3

[a] Note the marked variation in the number of reactors related to the time of observation and the size of reaction categorized as positive. These sources of variation are equivalent to the range of variability among reports by different investigators presented in Table 2. The antigens used in these tests are described in reference 16. SK, Streptokinase; TU, tuberculin units.

tors and the average size of positive reactions to skin test antigens are relatively insensitive to minor changes in antigen concentration or potency. Simultaneous skin tests with 10-fold-different concentrations of the same antigen in sensitive subjects elicits no more than a 30 to 50% increase in the size of the average reaction to the higher concentration. This increase in average reaction size is accompanied by an increased number of reactors. As with many other biologic phenomena, the sizes of skin test reactions appear log-normally distributed with respect to antigen concentration. The experience summarized in Table 2 identifies several generally available antigens and the reactor rates expected in recall antigen testing.

Table 3 lists the distribution of the sizes of positive reactions to eight antigens used in patients sampled from the southeastern United States. The observations in Table 3 are the outcome of clinical studies in more than 8,000 patients during the interval from 1970 to 1979 (16). Each patient was tested with a minimum of three generally available antigens adapted as recall antigens, with tuberculin, and with antigens derived from the three major pathogenic fungi. The number of patients and the percentage with reactions ≥2, ≥5, and ≥10 mm in diameter at each time of observation are presented. Note the similarity between the range of percentages of patients with

≥5-mm reactions at 24 and 48 h and the percentage of reactors summarized in Table 2. The information presented in Table 3 indicates that a part of the reaction variation in Table 2 could be related to the use of different times of observation. The choice of a categorical reaction size provides another potential source of variation. Both arbitrary decisions have a profound effect on the number of positive reactors and are more important than minor differences in antigen potency.

The observations summarized in Table 3 do not represent healthy subjects. Large numbers of comparable observations in healthy subjects are not generally available to the hospital-based immunologist. Despite this problem, the observations in Table 3 can be used to define the expected distribution of skin test response in reactor patients. Several observations suggest that the distribution of reaction sizes among patients is comparable to the range of reaction sizes in healthy subjects. Periodic studies of much smaller numbers of healthy subjects with the same antigens revealed that the average sizes of the reactions observed among skin test-positive patients at 6, 24, and 72 h are slightly but significantly larger than those detected in healthy subjects (2). The average sizes of the reactions detected at 0.25 and 48 h in healthy subjects and patients are not significantly different. Despite the significant differences, 97% of all observed

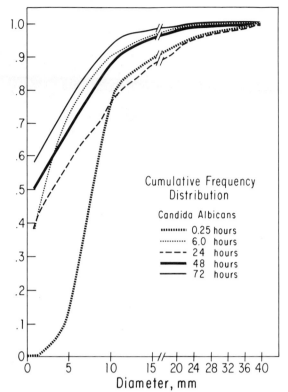

FIG. 1. Summary of the outcome of all immediate and delayed cutaneous reactions detected at 0.25, 6, 24, 48, and 72 h in 8,878 patients tested with 0.1 ml of a 1:1,000 (wt/vol) concentration of an allergenic glycerinated extract of a culture filtrate of *C. albicans*. The lines represent the cumulative frequency distribution of all measured reactions at each time of observation. Even though a substantial majority of reactions ranged in size from 2 to 16 mm, and 50% reactivity ≥2 mm in diameter was elicited at 48 h, an appreciable prevalence of adverse (≥40-mm) immediate and delayed reactions was detected (see text and Table 4). An increase in the antigen dose would shift the curve toward the right and increase the number of reactors (≥2-mm diameter) and the number of adverse reactors (≥40-mm diameter). This figure illustrates the way adverse immediate and delayed reactors limit the useful dose of recall antigens. The selection of an optimal safe recall antigen dose is important in clinical testing.

reactions in healthy subjects at all times of observation fell within the 1st to 99th percentile ranking of reactions detected in skin test-positive patients. A similar low prevalence of nonresponders has been reported in tests with antigen panels in healthy subjects (6).

Antigen dose

Once an appropriate antigen has been selected, attention must be focused on the choice of an optimal dose for clinical testing. Figure 1 provides a quantitative illustration of the pitfalls and limitations encountered in selecting an optimal recall antigen dose. The antigen was a single lot of a glycerinated allergenic extract of a culture filtrate of *C. albicans*. The skin tests were done on patients during the interval from 1970 to 1979 with 0.1-ml intradermal injections of a

1:1,000 (wt/vol) extract. A quantitative assessment of the possibility of adverse immediate and delayed hypersensitivity reactions is an important part of the selection of an optimal recall antigen dose. Prior experience with this antigen in more than 100 subjects revealed that the dose selected elicited a remarkable number of delayed cutaneous hypersensitivity reactions and fewer than 3% adverse reactions (≥40 mm) at all times of observation.

Figure 1 presents a quantitative assessment of the same antigen dose as the cumulative frequency distribution of reactions observed 0.25, 6, 24, 48, and 72 h after antigen challenge in 8,878 patients. By inspection, more than 85% of all detected reactions were ≤16 mm in diameter. Between 40 and 60% of the patients tested had no detectable reaction (<2 mm) at 6, 24, 48, and 72 h. Only the size of the reaginic immediate hypersensitivity wheal (at 0.25 h) exhibited a sigmoid dose-response relationship, involving almost 90% of the patients tested and reactions ranging from 2 to 16 mm in diameter. A second distribution of larger reaginic reactions was detected in approximately 10% of the patients tested. Approximately 2% of the patients tested had reactions of ≥40 mm, and these were most prevalent at 0.25 and 24 h after antigen challenge. An inflection also exists in the distribution curve of delayed 48- to 72-h reactions of >10 mm in diameter. A small number of large delayed reactions occurs in this second distribution of reactors. The observations presented in Fig. 1 illustrate how adverse hypersensitivity reactions limit the utility of this recall antigen dose. With an ideal diagnostic skin test antigen dose, this second distribution of adverse immediate and delayed reactions would be very small or would not occur. Antigens available for recall antigen testing, such as the antigen illustrated in Fig. 1, approach but do not attain this ideal distribution of reaction sizes.

Very little attention has been directed toward the occurrence of adverse reactions to recall antigens. Table 4 summarizes the percentages of skin test reactions ≥40 mm in diameter observed during tests with the antigen shown in Fig. 1 and the remaining antigens presented in Table 3. Among the recall antigens, the total number of observed adverse reactions at all times was lowest with the mumps skin test antigen.

TABLE 4. Adverse cutaneous hypersensitivity reactions to selected antigens

Antigen	% Patients with adverse reactions at[a]:					Total adverse reactions
	0.25 h	6 h	24 h	48 h	72 h	
Mumps	0.27	0.11	0.11	0.13	0.00	0.62
C. albicans	0.99	0.12	1.12	0.24	0.02	2.49
Varidase	0.06	0.03	0.77	1.03	0.46	2.35
PPD, human	0.06	0.02	0.28	0.23	0.09	0.68
Trichophyton	0.89	0.73	1.23	0.20	0.05	3.10
Histoplasmin	0.09	0.02	0.06	0.09	0.05	0.31
Coccidioidin	0.02	0.00	0.02	0.01	0.01	0.06
Blastomycin	0.03	0.00	0.01	0.02	0.00	0.06

[a] All reactions ≥40 mm in diameter at each time of observation were categorized as adverse reactions. Total adverse reactions are summed over all times of observations. Adverse reactions limit the maximum effective dose of available recall antigens used for delayed hypersensitivity skin tests.

The prevalence of adverse reactions to the mumps antigen compares favorably with tuberculin (PPD). Adverse reactions to the pathogenic fungi occurred in 0.06 to 0.31% of the observations. Tests with fungal and bacterial antigens adapted as recall antigens produced detectable adverse reactions at 2.35 to 3.10% of the times of observation. Less than 30% of the observed adverse reactions occurred at 48 and 72 h. Most of the morbidity induced by the test procedure occurred before the optimal time for evaluation of the standard Mantoux skin test.

The shape of cumulative distribution curves, such as those presented in Fig. 1, also provides a basis for estimating the effect of an increase in the antigen dose. It is possible to increase the number of delayed cutaneous reactors to recall antigens by increasing the antigen dose. An increase in the *C. albicans* antigen dose would shift the cumulative distribution curves shown in Fig. 1 to the right. By inspection and interpolation of the distribution of reactions detected 48 h after antigen challenge, it is possible to estimate that an antigen dose capable of yielding reactions ≥ 2 mm in diameter in 80% of the patients tested would also increase the number of adverse reactions to approximately 10% of the patients tested. This high prevalence of adverse reactions is clinically unacceptable. In some studies, a high prevalence of adverse reactions has occurred when excessive doses of *C. albicans* were used. The choice of an optimal antigen dose for clinical testing involves a careful evaluation of the prevalence of adverse immediate and delayed hypersensitivity reactions as well as an assessment of the number of delayed reactors in a reference population.

Pathogen skin tests

Skin tests with antigens from pathogenic microorganisms can be done at the same time as recall antigen skin tests. Skin test reactions ≥ 2 mm in diameter to tuberculin and the pathogenic fungi also provide evidence of intact cellular immunity; reciprocally, a positive recall antigen reaction increases the utility of a negative pathogen skin test. This use of pathogen reactions differs from the ≥ 5-mm delayed (48-h) reaction to histoplasmin, coccidioidin, and blastomycin needed to identify sensitization. A low level of cross-reacting skin test reactivity to *Mycobacterium intercellulare* and other atypical mycobacteria is prevalent in the United States. A tuberculin (PPD) skin test reaction ≥ 10 in diameter at 48 or 72 h is needed to identify sensitization to *Mycobacterium homonis*, the human tubercle bacillus. The selection of a ≥ 10-mm reaction diameter for the interpretation of a positive tuberculin skin test is based on epidemiologic studies done more than 40 years ago on tuberculin sensitivity in patients and in healthy young military recruits. The detection of a positive (≥ 10-mm diameter) tuberculin skin test is advocated as a basis for initiating antituberculous therapy in healthy subjects.

The use of the tuberculin skin test is also advocated as a screening procedure for tuberculosis among hospitalized patients. The diagnostic reliability of the tuberculin skin test in patients with active tuberculosis was established more than 50 years ago. This experience was based on studies in predominantly young adult patients who had sufficient innate resistance to survive their infection long enough to establish a microbiologic diagnosis and gain admission to a sanatorium. Currently hospitalized patients differ from this patient sample. Aged patients and those with recent onset of infection, compromised immunity, or impaired innate resistance were not adequately represented in this past clinical experience. Many recent reports indicate that a single negative tuberculin skin test may be misleading in sick patients. Active tuberculosis, per se, can impair the ability to express delayed cutaneous hypersensitivity. In sick patients, the interpretation of a "positive" tuberculin reaction of any size and the possible need for antituberculous therapy can best be made on the basis of clinical judgment about the specific illness (13) and corroboration by a microbiologic diagnosis. The central problem in the use of diagnostic skin tests in sick patients is the clinical uncertainty about the particular patient's ability to exhibit a delayed cutaneous hypersensitivity reaction. A single negative pathogen skin test does not exclude sensitization. A negative pathogen skin test is meaningful only if the patient shows evidence of intact delayed cutaneous hypersensitivity. The positive controls provided by simultaneous skin tests with recall antigens help circumvent this problem.

CLINICAL INDICATIONS FOR SKIN TESTING

Immune disorders

The clinical diseases in which skin tests are used to detect impaired delayed cutaneous hypersensitivity are almost encyclopedic. Striking degrees of impaired cellular immunity and delayed hypersensitivity occur in the rare primary immunity deficiency disorders. Less severe degrees of impaired delayed hypersensitivity occur in the more common immune disorders, such as atopy, unexplained inflammation associated with evidence of autoimmunity, and reticuloendothelial neoplasms. Mechanical impairment of lymphocyte circulation and impaired delayed cutaneous hypersensitivity occur in Milroy's disease and intestinal lymphangiectasis. Variable degrees of impaired delayed cutaneous hypersensitivity also occur in patients with cancer, where the magnitude of the impairment appears to be related to survival (2).

Infectious diseases

Impaired delayed cutaneous hypersensitivity also occurs in infectious diseases. The most striking impairment occurs in the chronic dimorphic or bipolar forms of infection caused by intracellular microorganisms. The term bipolar means that the infection can exhibit extreme divergence in its clinical form and outcome. Infections of this type include Whipple's disease, chronic coccidioidomycosis, lepromatous leprosy, cryptococcosis, aspergillosis, and, less often, tuberculosis. Patients with the unusual chronic form of the infection exhibit a remarkable difference between their humoral and cellular responses to antigens from the infecting organism. The occurrence of intact or augmented humoral immunity and delayed cutaneous anergy to the same antigen in these patients is called an immune deviation. A similar difference between humoral and cellular immunity to specific antigens can also occur in noninfectious diseases, such as sarcoidosis, certain rheumatic disorders, and Hodgkin's disease. Tests of delayed cutaneous hypersensitivity and the detection of an immune deviation provide information about the guarded prognosis of these patients.

Nonspecific impairment

A relatively nonspecific form of impairment of delayed hypersensitivity occurs during the course of viral infections and after viral immunization. Nonspecific effects such as the inflammation resulting from conditions which produce leukocytosis (gram-negative sepsis, pancreatitis) and uremia can impair delayed hypersensitivity. Psychobiologic effects, which operate through the neural-immunologic axis, including hypnosis, grief reactions, circadian changes, and the effect of prolonged immobilization, can also alter delayed hypersensitivity. Finally, iatrogenic impairment of immunity produced by treatment with corticosteroids, cytotoxic agents, antimitotic drugs, and radiation therapy results in a nonspecific decrease in both humoral and cellular immunity.

Aging and nutrition

The degree of physiologic impairment associated with inadequate nutrition and advanced age can impair delayed hypersensitivity (2). Disease-associated impairment can be superimposed on innate and nutritional causes of impaired delayed cutaneous hypersensitivity. All three causes of impairment can increase the patient's susceptibility to infection. Tests of delayed cutaneous hypersensitivity have been used to prospectively evaluate the patient's immune status, the risk of infection after surgery, survival potential, and the adequacy of nutrition. Although it is not always possible to clearly know which of these several causes of impaired resistance are primarily responsible for decreased delayed cutaneous hypersensitivity, skin tests can be used to provide a global assessment of the magnitude of impairment. Retrospective judgments about the probable cause of impairment can be made on the basis of the response to intervention.

General indications

The clinical indications for the use of delayed cutaneous hypersensitivity skin tests in patients include (i) evaluation of the possibilities of anergy or immune deviation and (ii) quantitation of delayed hypersensitivity to validate a negative pathogen reaction, follow a disease process, or assess the outcome of therapy. The demonstration of delayed cutaneous anergy lacks specificity for a particular disease process. The diagnostic utility of tests of delayed cutaneous hypersensitivity lies not in the identification of a particular disease, but in the ability to exclude a spectrum of diseases that are associated with anergy. The actual diagnosis must be made on the basis of other attributes of the illness in the particular patient. At a pragmatic level, the demonstration of a single positive delayed skin test with a pathogenic or recall antigen

provides direct evidence of intact cell-mediated immunity. Despite this interpretation, the demonstration of a single positive test cannot be used to exclude an illness which is associated with delayed cutaneous anergy. The degree of impairment in many diseases is not absolute. For example, recall antigen reactions can be detected in patients with sarcoidosis. A quantitative appraisal is needed. At best, the demonstration of a lack of normal reactivity identifies a condition which may be consistent with a spectrum of diseases. In contrast, the demonstration of a quantitatively normal level of delayed cutaneous hypersensitivity can be used to avoid more costly in vitro tests of cell-mediated immunity.

INTERPRETATION OF SKIN TESTS

Quantitative assessments of cutaneous hypersensitivity provide a measure of the maximum level of immune function. The direct skin test is a miniature localized stress test. The initial local concentration of antigen produced by a skin test is extraordinarily high in relation to the local tissue concentration of antibodies and immune cells. At a constant antigen dose, the size of the local reaction is limited by the patient's ability to recruit the immune mechanisms responsible for the observed reaction. Large reactions occur in exquisitely sensitive patients and are clinically important when directed toward specific pathogens or antigens responsible for allergic diseases. Small or absent reactions suggest impaired immune function. The detection of decreased hypersensitivity does not identify the cause of the impairment. As with other stress tests, such as exercise tests of cardiovascular and respiratory functions, several mechanisms can contribute to the observed impairment. The demonstration of altered hypersensitivity provides an objective basis for pursuing other studies in the patient. A quantitatively normal level of delayed cutaneous hypersensitivity suggests that alterations in the mechanisms responsible for cellular immunity are small and of little pathophysiologic significance.

Interpretive problems

Irrespective of the method used to evaluate test results, the interpretation of test results will depend upon (i) the degree of independence among reactions to the test antigens and (ii) information about the nonresponder frequency in an appropriate reference population. An awareness of how these prior observations limit the interpretation of test results is important. The independence of observations to panels of antigens is a difficult problem. Cross-reactivity exists among the antigenic products of microorganisms, such as recall antigens. The extent of this lack of independence of observations can be evaluated as associations (correlation coefficients) between measured reactions to antigens (16). Among seven of the eight antigens presented in Table 3, many small significant positive correlations exist among immediate (0.25-, 6-, and 24-h) hypersensitivity reactions. Small significant correlations are much weaker and less frequent among delayed (48- and 72-h) hypersensitivity reactions. The pattern of correlations indicates that the 24-h skin test reaction is more related to the

0.25- and 6-h than to the 48- and 72-h skin test reactions. Subtraction of each subject's averaged ability to react to all seven antigens from each observed reaction yields small significant negative correlations predominantly between the 48- and 72-h reactions. The positive correlations among immediate hypersensitivity reactions to the recall antigens represent either broadly shared cross-reactivity or each subject's general innate ability to exhibit an immediate reaction. Cross-reactivity is least among recall antigens with the 48- to 72-h Mantoux-type skin test reaction. The 48-h Mantoux-type skin test reaction provides the best specific measure of delayed cutaneous hypersensitivity.

The number of nonresponders detected with test antigens presents a second interpretive problem. For example, experimental studies suggest that sensitization with an optimal 500-μg dose of the contact allergen dinitrochlorobenzene and subsequent challenge with a 50-μg test dose may fail to elicit a positive reaction in 10% of healthy subjects. This chance of not knowing that the patient is anergic may be unacceptably high. The problem of interpreting a negative skin test is not restricted to contact allergens. Recall antigens also have a finite probability of not reacting in an appropriate reference population. In the interpretation of test results, it is necessary to know that the number of skin test antigens is sufficient to yield an improbable chance occurrence of a healthy nonresponder. For example, the mumps skin test antigen is frequently used as a potentially positive control in conjunction with the tuberculin skin test. The tuberculin skin test can be interpreted as a true negative when the mumps skin test is positive. Patients who fail to react to both antigens are often called anergic. Table 5 presents an estimate of the reliability of this assessment based on the information presented in Tables 2 and 3. The chance (p) of measurable skin test reactions to tuberculin and the mumps skin test antigen is known. The probability of nonreaction to each antigen (q) is equal to $1 - p$ and can be calculated. The probability of nonreaction to both antigens can be estimated from the product of the probabilities of nonreaction to each antigen. Table 5 indicates that healthy subjects and patients will fail to react to the combined mumps control and tuberculin 15 and 25% of the time, respectively. Several important conclusions about the interpretation of skin tests can be drawn from this illustration. First,

neither skin tests with a single contact allergen nor tests with one recall antigen and tuberculin provide a reliable assessment of anergy. Second, the product of the probability of nonreaction to recall antigens can be used to estimate the number of test antigens needed for the reliable identification of anergic patients. The magnitude of this problem can be evaluated by a similar appraisal of the probability of a nonresponder to successive additions of the test antigens listed in Table 3. Using reactions ≥2 mm in diameter as a positive test at 48 h, four recall antigens and tuberculin are needed to reduce the chance of a nonresponder to less than 1 in 20. In contrast, the chance of a nonresponder with a reaction ≥5 mm in diameter as a positive test at 48 h is less than 1 in 10 with all eight antigens. The categorical use of the smallest measurable reaction and multiple antigens provides the best discrimination of anergic patients.

Interpretive methods

The results of delayed skin tests can be formulated for interpretation in three ways. First, the number of tests with reactions equal to or greater than an arbitrarily selected reaction diameter can be counted and compared with observations in the reference population. This simple method has been extensively used in experimental studies involving groups of patients. Even though a single ≥5-mm reaction diameter can be more reliably identified than a ≥2-mm reaction diameter, the gain in discrimination provided by the smaller diameter may be more important than uncertainty about detecting small reactions. The occasional identification of a 2-mm reaction diameter is relatively unimportant when tests are done with multiple antigens or compared among a group of patients. In contrast, the use of a ≥5-mm reaction diameter as a positive test is clearly justified when a single antigen is used in an individual patient. Despite these precautions, counts of the number of positive tests elicited by antigen doses which are reasonably free of adverse reactions may not reliably identify patients with subtle degrees of impaired delayed cutaneous hypersensitivity. Because of this problem, formulations focused on the size of skin test reactions are more helpful.

A second method of formulation and interpretation can be based on the sum of the measured reaction diameters to all antigens. The summed reaction size is obtained by addition and ranked in relation to a similar formulation of observations in the reference population. This pragmatic, nonparametric approach to the problem of identifying different degrees of impaired delayed cutaneous hypersensitivity is useful. Depending on the size of the reference population, observations in an individual patient can be interpreted in relation to the appropriate quartile, decile, or other descriptor of the reference population. This type of assessment provides the physician with an estimate of the chance that observations similar to those made in the patient might be found in the reference population. This method of evaluation has the advantage of not requiring extensive computation beyond a critical appraisal of the reference population.

Finally, the average and the standard deviation of the logarithms of the diameter of positive reactions

TABLE 5. Estimated chance of nonreaction to two skin test antigens

Subjects and antigens	Reactors (p)	Nonreactors (q)	Nonreactors to both antigens
Healthy persons[a]			
PPD	0.376	0.624	0.152
Mumps	0.755	0.245	
Patients[b]			
PPD	0.381	0.619	0.250
Mumps	0.596	0.404	

[a] Estimates based on the number of reactors with reaction diameter ≥ 5 mm at 24 or 48 h, as presented in Table 2.

[b] Estimates based on the number of reactors with reaction diameter ≥ 2 mm at 48 h, as presented in Table 3.

procedure is done properly, the skin will dimple on slight pressure or movement of the tip of the needle.

2. Inject the 0.1-ml antigen volume into the skin. The patient will feel a transient burning discomfort when this is done if the location of the site of antigen injection is truly intracutaneous. The injection should produce a 5- to 10-mm wheal. The failure to obtain a wheal indicates that the antigen has been placed subcutaneously. Although a subcutaneous injection is less than ideal, if the antigen is located close to the dermis the resulting reaction will not be very different. The injection need not be repeated.

3. Repeat the procedure for each antigen until the test panel is completed. Inform the patient when the last skin test is done.

4. Remain with the patient for a minimum of 15 min after each test procedure to detect evidence of a severe local or systemic immediate reaction. The records of the test and appropriate demographic and epidemiologic information can often be obtained during this interval. Inform the patient of the time at which the reactions to each test will be inspected and measured.

5. Also inform the patient that it is not necessary to endure a severe local reaction for the test to be meaningful. If severe discomfort occurs, the patient should be advised either to inform the ward staff or his or her own physician or to call a phone number provided by the testing laboratory.

Time of test observations. The time of observation will depend on the information to be obtained from the tests. The skin test reactions present 48 h after antigen challenge provide the best assessment of specific sensitization, delayed hypersensitivity, and cell-mediated immunity. Hour 48 is the standard time to observe, measure, and record delayed skin test reactions.

Earlier observations (at 0.25 to 24 h) of immediate hypersensitivity skin test reactions can be measured when evaluating novel skin test antigens or setting up a safe, reliable antigen panel, and these observations can be used to identify adverse reactions ($\geq$40 mm in diameter). The 24-h skin test reaction should not be categorized as a delayed skin test reaction. Reactions detected at 72 h can be observed, but they should be recorded separately from the 48-h reactions.

Reaction measurements. Crossed, bisecting, perpendicular (orthogonal) diameters of each skin test reaction should be measured to the nearest millimeter. A millimeter rule or appropriate caliper should be used. Usually, the largest diameter is measured first and is used to select the bisecting perpendicular diameter. Both diameters are recorded.

(i) Hour 0.25 reactions. The diameters of the flare and wheal reactions detected 15 to 20 min after testing can be used to identify anaphylactic hypersensitivity to the test antigen. This observation is especially important in the identification of those test antigens capable of provoking adverse allergic reactions.

(ii) Hour 6 reactions. The crossed diameters of the erythema and edema produced by the test antigens are measured and recorded. The 6-h reaction probably provides the least ambiguous assessment of a late cutaneous reaction to the test antigen.

(iii) Hour 24 reactions. The crossed diameters of the erythema and edema are measured and recorded. Adverse reactions and other complex changes can occur at 24 h. Rarely, severe reactions lead to vesiculation, central petechiae, and early suppurative changes consistent with an Arthus-like immediate hypersensitivity. Although this type of severe local reaction is unusual, unusually large 24-h reactions can either mimic or obscure later reactions, and their occurrence should be noted.

(iv) Hour 48 reactions. The crossed diameters of the area of induration should be measured and recorded. Induration is defined as palpable thickening of the skin and is independent of residual visible erythema and swelling. A ballpoint pen can be used to trace inward from both sides of the reaction toward the central part of the test site until local skin resistance is identified. The distance between the points at which resistance is identified can be used as a measurement of the diameter of induration. Trained observers can usually obtain equally reliable measurements of induration by direct palpation of the reaction size.

(v) Hour 72 reactions. The crossed diameters of the area of induration should be measured and recorded. The 72-h reaction often provides the best opportunity to detect and estimate delayed cutaneous hypersensitivity when the test antigen has elicited a large 24-h reaction.

ADVERSE TEST REACTIONS

Occasionally, skin tests can cause a nervous reaction or fainting. This unusual response is not dangerous and can be treated with appropriate medications, reassurance, and a brief rest.

Rarely, skin tests cause allergic symptoms in exquisitely sensitive patients. A remote risk of anaphylaxis exists. Anaphylaxis is a mixture of intense itching and hives, congestion of the breathing passages, and asthma. Anaphylaxis is extremely rare with the antigen doses used for skin testing. The severe allergic reactions would also likely occur after a chance exposure to the same antigen. When elicited in the hospital or clinic environment, the systemic reaction can be stopped by prompt treatment. The immediate availability of treatment with 0.1 to 0.3 ml of 1:1,000 adrenaline and parenteral antihistamines makes the circumstances in which skin tests are done the safest way to find out if a patient has exquisite reaginic hypersensitivity to an antigen.

Positive skin test reactions are manifested by an area of local tenderness, redness, and swelling which reaches a maximum in 3 days and usually subsides completely within a week. Exquisitely sensitive patients can develop severe local reactions at the test site. In addition to a large area of edema and tender, painful erythema, the test site can exhibit blister formation and even tissue necrosis. The local tissue destruction can produce scar formation and changes in pigmentation similar to that of a smallpox vaccination scar. Local lymphadenopathy and systemic symptoms such as fever can occur. Severe local skin test reactions can be controlled by the topical application of corticosteroid creams or the local injection of corticosteroid into the site. The administration of parenteral systemic corticosteroids is also effective but is rarely necessary to control a local reaction.

LITERATURE CITED

1. **Askenase, P. W.** 1973. Cutaneous basophilic hypersensitivity in contact-sensitized guinea pigs. I. Transfer with immune serum. J. Exp. Med. **138:**1144–1155.
2. **Buckley, C. E., III, and D. H. White.** 1979. Aging and immunocompetence skin testing, p. 444–449. *In* H. Orimo, K. Shimada, M. Iriki, and D. Maeda (ed.), Recent advances in gerontology. Proceedings of the 11th International Congress of Gerontology. Excerpta Medica, Amsterdam.
3. **Catalona, W. J., P. T. Taylor, and P. B. Chrieten.** 1972. Quantitative dinitrochlorobenzene contact sensitization in a normal population. Clin. Exp. Immunol. **12:**325–333.
4. **Dvorak, H. F.** 1976. Cutaneous basophil hypersensitivity. J. Allergy Clin. Immunol. **58:**229–240.
5. **Dvorak, H. F., M. C. Mihm, Jr., A. M. Dvorak, R. A. Johnson, E. J. Manseau, E. Morgan, and R. Colvin.** 1974. Morphology of delayed type hypersensitivity reactions in man. I. Quantitative description of the inflammatory response. Lab. Invest. **31:**111–130.
6. **Gordon, E. H., A. Krouse, J. L. Kinney, E. R. Steihm, and W. B. Klaustermeyer.** 1983. Delayed cutaneous hypersensitivity in normals: choice of antigens and comparison to in vitro assays of cell-mediated immunity. J. Allergy Clin. Immunol. **72:**487–494.
7. **Jones, T. D., and J. R. Mote.** 1934. The phases of foreign protein sensitization in human beings. N. Engl. J. Med. **210:**120–123.
8. **Kniker, W. T., C. T. Anderson, and M. Roumiantzeff.** 1979. The multi-test system: a standardized approach to evaluation of delayed hypersensitivity and cell-mediated immunity. Ann. Allergy **43:**73–79.
9. **Konttinen, Y. T., V. Bergroth, K. Visa-Tolvanen, S. Reitamo, and L. Forstrom.** 1983. Cellular infiltrate in situ and response kinetics of human intradermal and epicutaneous tuberculin reactions. Clin. Immunol. Immunopathol. **28:**441–449.
10. **Mantoux, C.** 1908. Intradermo-reaction de la tuberculine. C. R. Acad. Sci. (Paris) **147:**355–357.
11. **Platt, J. L., B. W. Grant, A. A. Eddy, and A. F. Michael.** 1983. Immune cell populations in cutaneous delayed-type hypersensitivity. J. Exp. Med. **158:**1227–1242.
12. **Ray, M. C., M. D. Tharp, T. J. Sullivan, and R. E. Tigelaar.** 1983. Contact-hypersensitivity reactions to dinitrofluorobenzene mediated by monoclonal IgE anti-DNP antibodies. J. Immunol. **131:**1096–1102.
13. **Snider, D. E.** 1982. The tuberculin skin test. Am. Rev. Respir. Dis. **12:**108–118.
14. **Solley, G., G. Gleich, R. Jordan, and A. Schroeter.** 1976. The late phase of the immediate wheal and flare skin reaction. Its dependency upon IgE antibodies. J. Clin. Invest. **58:**408–420.
15. **Turk, J. L.** 1975. Delayed hypersensitivity. North-Holland Publishing Co., Amsterdam.
16. **Woodruff, W. W., III, C. E. Buckley III, H. A. Gallis, J. R. Cohn, and R. W. Wheat.** 1984. Reactivity to spherule-derived coccidioidin in the southeastern United States. Infect. Immun. **43:**860–869.
17. **Zinsser, H., and J. H. Mueller.** 1925. On the nature of bacterial allergies. J. Exp. Med. **41:**159–177.

Chapter 38

Lymphocyte Proliferation

ANNETTE E. MALUISH AND DOUGLAS M. STRONG

Lymphocyte proliferation or transformation is the process whereby new DNA synthesis and cell division takes place in lymphocytes after a stimulus of some type, resulting in a series of changes. The lymphocytes increase in size, the cytoplasm becomes more extensive, the nucleoli are visible in the nucleus, and the lymphocytes resemble blast cells. The term "blast transformation" is also sometimes applied to this process. Lymphocytes from immunized animals and humans proliferate in response to antigens to which they are sensitized. This in vitro response correlates with the existence of delayed-type hypersensitivity in the host. Lymphocyte proliferation also occurs in response to different histocompatibility antigens when leukocytes from two donors are mixed in a mixed leukocyte culture. Mitogens, including pokeweed mitogen, phytohemagglutinin (PHA), and concanavalin A, will induce proliferation in normal cells in culture.

The first report of mitogen-induced lymphocyte proliferation was a report by Nowell in 1960 (6) in which the proliferation of lymphocytes in response to PHA was described. Since then, lymphocyte proliferation in response to mitogens, antigens, and allogeneic mixed leukocytes has been widely used in the study of lymphocyte biology.

Evaluation of lymphocyte proliferation can be quantitated by determination either of the percentage of lymphoblasts or of increased DNA synthesis. This evaluation may be achieved by the addition of a radiolabeled precursor of DNA (usually tritiated thymidine) to the culture medium and the subsequent detection of the amount of radioactivity incorporated into the cells. The methodology of these assays is the same regardless of the species or source of the lymphocytes or the form of stimulus used to induced proliferation. The assay involves the in vitro culture of a lymphocyte population in the presence or absence of a selected stimulus for various periods of time. The changes induced in the stimulated groups are compared with changes in the unstimulated cell populations. Radiolabeled amino acids are used most commonly for these comparisons, as they offer a means of quantitating the changes in a simple, reproducible manner. The use of automated harvesting procedures results in greater reproducibility and ease of performance of the assay.

In this chapter we will describe the lymphocyte proliferation assay for human peripheral blood lymphocytes, although the principles apply also to studies of lymphocytes from other sources. The assay system described here is a miniaturized assay performed in 20-μl volumes rather than in the 200-μl volumes of the more commonly used assay (4). The miniassay was first described by Farrant et al. (2) and offers the particular advantage of requiring very few cells to quantitate proliferative responses. The general principles of performance, standardization of results, and data interpretation described herein for the miniassay apply also to the more commonly used assay which is performed in the standard manner. However, the optimal conditions for other cell types and other assay systems need to be established. The methods for determining these optimal conditions will be discussed in detail in a later section of this chapter.

CLINICAL INDICATIONS

The lymphocyte transformation test has a broad range of applications, including assessment and monitoring of congenital immunological defects; assessment of either immunosuppressive or immunoenhancing therapies; determination of histocompatibility matching in transplantation; identification of serum or plasma factors which may suppress or enhance reactivity; diagnostic testing for detection of previous exposure to a variety of antigens, allergens, or pathogens; and determination of a variety of lymphokines. For additional information on applications and pitfalls, several reviews are available (3, 5, 7, 8).

Lymphocyte transformation in patients with congenital immunological defects ranges from complete lack of function, as in severe combined immunodeficiency disease and DiGeorge syndrome, to a partial deficit, as in ataxia telangiectasia, Wiskott-Aldrich syndrome, and chronic mucocutaneous candidiasis, to normal reactivity, as in X-linked hypogammaglobulinemia. A wide variety of acquired conditions has been shown to have impaired lymphocyte transformation. These conditions include a variety of bacterial and viral infections as well as chemotherapy and autoimmune diseases such as Sjögren's syndrome and systemic lupus erythematosus. A variety of other clinical conditions have also been shown to affect lymphocyte transformation, including surgery and anesthesia, stress, aging, malnutrition, a variety of malignancies, uremia, and major burns, to mention a few.

Lymphocyte transformation has also been used to monitor sequential samples from patients undergoing a variety of immunoenhancing or immunosuppressive therapies in the treatment of disease states. This approach is especially sensitive when patients show nearly complete deficits before initiation of therapy, such as in immunodeficient subjects requiring bone marrow transplantation. Patients undergoing immunoenhancing therapy with lymphokines such as recombinant interferon or the interleukins for cancer can be monitored for increased reactivity after therapy.

An equally important application of this assay has been its use as a diagnostic tool for detecting immunological memory for a variety of antigens or pathogens. Soluble antigens such as tetanus toxoid, purified protein derivative, streptokinase-streptodornase, etc., have been commonly used to assess immunological recall of antigens to which most individuals have been exposed. In addition, standard immunization to these antigens, followed by assay at an appropriate time after inoculation, can be used to assess the ability of an individual to respond to an appropriate challenge. In some instances, it has been shown that in vitro proliferation in response to a variety of pathogens is the only way to detect prior immunity, due to the lack of serum antibodies. Antigens from infectious agents used in stimulation of lymphocyte preparations can be prepared as the soluble form, whole organisms, or infected cell lines (such as of cytomegalovirus- or rubella-infected cells). Furthermore, antigens responsible for allergies have also been shown to stimulate specific lymphoproliferative responses in vitro. This system has been used to test a variety of potential antigens responsible for autoimmune disorders as well as other clinical conditions in which the antigen responsible for the disorder was unknown.

Another important application has been in the field of transplantation. The mixed lymphocyte reaction has been shown to be the corollary to the homograft reaction in transplantation. A series of antigens coded for within the major histocompatibility complex has been shown to be responsible for the stimulation. As a result, the mixed lymphocyte reaction has been used for matching in both whole-organ and bone marrow transplantation. Definition of the HLA-D complex has progressed to the use of genotypically homozygous lymphocyte donors as stimulating cells for the assignment of HLA-D specificities. Cells primed in vitro to homozygous cells will proliferate in an accelerated way when challenged by similar antigens on untyped cells. In addition, sera from transplant recipients or multiparous women have been used to block this reactivity, leading to the definition of the so-called HLA-D-related (HLA-DR) serological specificities. These so-called class II antigens have been found on B cells and monocytes and are responsible for the stimulation of T-helper cells in this reaction. The class I antigens (HLA-A, HLA-B, and HLA-C) are recognized by the T-cytotoxic-suppressor cells in this reaction. Although various subsets of T cells initiate the reactivity, the generation of a variety of lymphokines eventuates in up to 35% of the cells in the mixture responding during the reaction. There are continued attempts to define the genetic basis for susceptibility to a variety of diseases which can be predicted on the basis of HLA-D or HLA-DR specificity. The use of monoclonal antibodies and gene probes has helped to delineate the polymorphism of the major histocompatibility complex.

The detection in serum of antibodies to HLA-DR-stimulating determinants is representative of an approach that has been used to define a variety of specific and nonspecific serum factors which suppress the lymphoproliferative response. Since there has been such a variety of inhibitory factors defined, this approach does not generate very significant information unless clearly defined proteins are used in attempts to suppress the reaction.

The functional capacity of a variety of subpopulations of lymphocytes can also be used to more exactly define particular functional defects. Lymphoproliferation has also been used to assay soluble mediators of immunity, such as the interleukins. For example, cultured T cells that are dependent on interleukin-2 can be used as target cells for assaying interleukin-2 in supernatants of stimulated cells. T-suppressor cells also can be assayed by their ability to suppress a known lymphoproliferative level.

A greater understanding of the diversity of lymphocyte and monocyte subpopulations that exist in the immune response has been accelerated by the advent of hybridoma technology and the definition of specific monoclonal antibodies against such subsets. It has been shown that approximately 15 to 20% of the T-helper cell population, as defined by the T4 cell surface marker, is entirely responsible for the proliferation to specific antigens, the mixed lymphocyte reaction, and the ability to induce B cells to produce immunoglobulin. These reactions also require monocytes, and thus lymphoproliferation includes a variety of cell types. Anti-idiotype antibodies to specific T-cell receptors also induce proliferation in T-cell subpopulations.

Although this assay has been used in a variety of applications, both clinically and experimentally, the day-to-day variability and the inherent problems of the assay require that careful standardization and quality control be included to ensure meaningful interpretation of results. As in most biological reactions, a clear-cut dose-response curve is present for the responding cell population, as well as for the dose of stimulating mitogens, antigens, cells, etc. The adaptation of this assay in a miniature form has allowed a greater number of these variables to be determined, thus bringing more meaningful information to the clinician.

INTERPRETATION OF DATA

Assays of lymphocyte proliferation in response to mitogens and alloantigens offer a potentially sensitive indicator of altered lymphocyte function due to disease or therapy. However, there are wide differences of opinion among investigators as to the criteria to be used to express data, define depressed responses, and assess biological (as opposed to technical) fluctuations. Many criteria have been adopted arbitrarily, and differences in methods of data calculation and expression may well account for some conflicting reports. The most commonly used measures of proliferation (reviewed by Dean et al. in reference 1) are net counts per minute (Δcpm) for tritiated thymidine incorporation, stimulation index (SI), and relative proliferation index (RPI).

Studies on individuals rather than on populations pose problems in comparing data from experiment to experiment. For longitudinal responses of individual patients, although the use of cryopreserved cells can alleviate the problems of assay-to-assay variability, the method of data calculation is very important. Each of these methods with its associated advantages and disadvantages will be addressed.

Some laboratories express the proliferative response as Δcpm, calculated as cpm in stimulated cultures minus cpm in control cultures. The major drawback with this method of calculation is that there may be wide variation between lots of mitogens, even from day to day. It is impossible to be completely accurate in dilutions of mitogens over a period of time, and variations in mitogen concentration can contribute substantially to differences in cpm. Other assay-associated factors will also affect the cpm on a daily basis. These problems do not allow accurate analysis of longitudinal trends and can lead to problems even in population-based studies unless elaborate plans ensure the correct randomization of samples for each assay. This is not practical in studying fresh patient samples.

SI is calculated as experimental, stimulated cpm/control, unstimulated cpm. This calculation is heavily influenced by changes in the unstimulated cpm, and this method is less than satisfactory for a number of reasons. The variation in SI among normal donors is large and does not correlate well with Δcpm or RPI, due to considerable variations in baseline unstimulated values, which strongly affect the SI but not the other calculations. An elevated baseline value will depress the SI, and Dean et al. (1) report that such elevated values occur more frequently or are more variable in cancer patients. The baseline incorporation of tritiated thymidine may be altered by factors other than the intrinsic ability of the cells to respond to a stimulus, such as culture conditions or in vivo stimulation by autologous non-T cells or antigens. The determination of a cutoff point for diagnosis of a depressed response is problematical for these reasons.

The use of the RPI overcomes many of the difficulties described for these methods. The RPI is defined as the ratio of Δcpm (cpm in experimental cultures containing stimulus minus control, unstimulated cpm) of a test individual (e.g., a cancer patient) to the mean Δcpm of lymphocytes from a panel of normal donors tested simultaneously in the assay.

$$RPI = \frac{\Delta cpm \text{ of test individual}}{\text{mean } \Delta cpm \text{ of normal individuals} \atop (>3) \text{ tested simultaneously}}$$

Thus, the RPI value can be considered as a proportion of the mean response of normal individuals. Because the RPI is a proportion of the normal response, it is clear that the choice of "normals" is very important when a "depressed" response is defined. In studies in our laboratories, we use a panel of 3 normal donors chosen to have reactivity in the midrange of at least 10 donors tested. Cells are obtained from these donors by leukapheresis, and large numbers of aliquots (>200) are cryopreserved from each donor. These same three normals are used in every assay for the determination of the RPI. When other normal donors are tested, the RPI of these donors ranges from 0.65 to 1.8, with 90% of the values falling between 0.75 and 1.65. A response is considered depressed if it falls below 0.75.

The RPI has been shown to give a smaller coefficient of variation among normal donors and in serial testing of normals than the other methods of calculation and is a sensitive measure of altered responses. The use of a panel of cryopreserved normals provides a stable and consistent base from which a relative response can be confidently calculated.

REAGENTS

Stimulants

All stimulants must be kept in sterile vials, and dilutions must be made with sterile media.

PHA (Sigma Chemical Co., St. Louis, Mo.) is dissolved in phosphate-buffered saline and kept frozen at −20°C at a concentration of 100 μg/ml. PHA is kept frozen in small aliquots, and a fresh aliquot is thawed for use each time it is needed.

Concanavalin A (Sigma) is handled the same way as PHA, but is kept frozen at a concentration of 500 μg/ml.

Pokeweed mitogen (GIBCO Laboratories, Grand Island, N.Y.) is diluted with medium and frozen at −20°C in small aliquots before being used.

Tetanus toxoid, 5 flocculation activity units per ml (Merrell Laboratories, Cincinnati, Ohio)

Streptokinase-streptodornase, 125 U/ml (Lederle Laboratories, Pearl River, N.Y.)

Purified protein derivative, 5 μg/ml (Parke, Davis & Co., Detroit, Mich.)

Candida albicans, 1:100 dilution of glycerine-saline extract (Hollister-Stier, Spokane, Wash.)

Mixed leukocyte culture (MLC). The stimulators for the MLC consist of a pool of leukocytes from six normal donors. The leukocytes are mononuclear cells obtained by Ficoll-Hypaque separation of peripheral blood. To measure the proliferation of the test lymphocytes in response to this stimulus, it is necessary to prevent proliferation of these stimulating cells. If this is not done, these cells will proliferate in response to the test lymphocytes, incorporate the radionucleotide marker, and make the test results impossible to interpret. To prevent such proliferation, the cells can be treated with mitomycin C or irradiation. The ability of cells to induce proliferation is dependent on a mismatch of the major histocompatibility antigens, and thus some cells will stimulate more effectively than others. The stimulators are prepared by pooling the cells from six normal donors. To ensure maximum stimulation, 8 to 10 normal donors are tested individually for the ability to stimulate proliferation in three other normal donors, and the six which give the best stimulation are used for the pool. This pool of cells is cryopreserved in aliquots of 10^6 cells with a controlled-rate freezer, and the cells are irradiated in the frozen state with 7,500 rads. Sufficient cells for 1 month are irradiated at one time.

For blood collection and cell preparation

Disposable syringes and needles for venipuncture
Preservative-free heparin
Ficoll-Hypaque

Medium

The bottles of medium should be prepared (one with serum, one without serum).

RPMI 1640 without L-glutamine (Biofluids no. 102)..500 ml
L-Glutamine (100×), 200 mM (GIBCO no. 320-5030)..................................5 ml/500 ml
HEPES (N-2-hydroxyethylpiperazine-N'-2-ethanesulfonic acid) buffer, 1 M (GIBCO no. 380-5630)
....5 ml/500 ml
Sodium pyruvate (100×), 100 mM (GIBCO no. 320-1360)..........................5 ml/500 ml
Nonessential amino acids (GIBCO no. 320-1140)
....5 ml/500 ml

(Sodium pyruvate and nonessential amino acids should be made up first with plain RPMI 1640 at a 1:100 dilution [0.1 ml into 9.9 ml of medium]. Nonessential amino acids should be added last to prevent discoloration of the medium.)

2-Mercaptoethanol......................5 ml/500 ml

(2-Mercaptoethanol is made up from a stock solution which is kept refrigerated, 35 μl is added to 10 ml of medium, and then 0.5 ml of this mixture is added to the bottle of medium.)

Garamycin, 50 mg/ml (M. A. Bioproducts, Walkersville, Md., no. 22-740 A)............0.5 ml/500 ml

Human AB serum, 10% protein source (GIBCO formula no. 79-0279)..................55 ml/500 ml

Assay reagents

[3H]thymidine (Schwartz-Mann); specific activity, 6 Ci/mmol, 1 mCi/ml

Beckman scintillation fluid (ready soluble)

Water for use with harvesting system

Equipment and other materials

Coulter Counter (Coulter Electronics, Inc., Hialeah, Fla.).

Accuvettes

Isoton II

Isoterge II

Zap-O-Globin II, azide free

Hamilton syringes, 10 and 1 μl (Hamilton Co., Reno, Nev.)

Monoject needles, 25 gauge, 5/8 in. (ca. 1.6 cm) (for use with Hamilton syringes)

Sterile 100-μl Hamilton disposable pipette tips

Pipet-Aid automatic pipettor

Sterile disposable pipettes (1, 5, and 10 ml)

Clay Adams pipettes and sterile tips, for 10, 20, 25, and 30 μl

Nunc vials (1 ml). These are convenient for [3H]thymidine dilution.

1-ml syringe with needle

96-well flat-bottom plates with lids (Linbro; Flow Laboratories, McLean, Va.) for making dilutions

Terasaki microtest cell culture plates, 60 wells (Falcon no. 3034)

Square Integrid petri dish, 100 by 15 mm (Falcon no. 1012)

Sterile gauze pads

Beckman TJ-6 centrifuge

Water bath at 37°C

5% CO_2 wet incubator at 37°C

Packard Tri-Carb 460C liquid scintillation counter

Biovials for counting

Brandel Micro-Harvesting System (no. MC-60)

TECHNICAL PROCEDURES

The techniques required in the procedures for determining cellular proliferation demand careful and precise attention to detail. Although laminar-flow hoods do decrease the incidence of bacterial contamination, this equipment does not diminish the need for good sterile technique. In fact, the maintenance of sterile conditions is mandatory for these assays, since the lymphoid cells are cultured over a 3- to 5-day period. Any bacterial contamination will cause a distortion in the results, either by interfering with the response of the lymphoid cells to the various mitogens or by causing excess label to be incorporated into the bacterial DNA.

The advantages of using a miniaturized system are numerous. However, this type of assay system requires precision work and careful practice before optimal results can be consistently achieved. To obtain reliable results, technicians must pay strict attention to plating details and use finely calibrated Hamilton syringes, to dispense both the 10- and 1-μl volumes accurately. In addition, minimal distractions during the setting up of the assay are crucial to ensure the maximum precision and attention necessary for the success of the assay.

Cell preparation

Peripheral blood. Human peripheral blood is obtained by venipuncture. Blood can be defibrinated or heparinized with 20 to 50 U of preservative-free sodium heparin per ml. Lymphocytes can be separated from the heparinized blood by several methods. The simplest of these is the use of sedimentation ($1 \times g$). Blood is either placed in tubes or left in the syringes and placed in an incubator at 37°C for 30 min to 1 h. If a syringe is used, it should be placed with the needle up to allow easier removal of the leukocyte-rich plasma. The tubes or syringe should be placed at a slight angle to increase the surface area, which results in fast sedimentation. For those blood samples that take an excess of time to sediment, sedimentation can be accelerated by the addition of sterile dextran (6% [vol/vol] in sterile normal saline). The leukocyte-rich plasma is expressed when the erythrocytes have sedimented. It is important not to leave the blood to sediment for longer than 1 h, as many of the lymphocytes will sediment onto the erythrocyte layer and the yield from the plasma will be reduced. Cells are recovered from the plasma and washed free of plasma components by centrifugation in the appropriate medium. Leukocyte counts are performed by standard hematological techniques, either manually or with a Coulter Counter.

The more commonly used procedure is for separation of the mononuclear cells by density gradient centrifugation of whole blood. This procedure is performed by carefully layering whole blood diluted 1:2 with sterile saline over Ficoll-Hypaque. Optimal results are obtained by layering no more than three times the volume of diluted blood onto a given volume of Ficoll-Hypaque. This procedure can be performed in tubes of narrow diameter (15-ml conical tubes) or wider diameter (50-ml conical tubes), depending on the volume of blood to be separated. The diluted blood is added to the gradient by gently pipetting with the tubes held at an angle or by pouring the blood onto the Ficoll-Hypaque. This latter method requires a lot of practice and is not recommended for beginners. To obtain good separations, it is critical that a clear separation be kept between the dense Ficoll-Hypaque and the blood layer before centrifugation. The tubes are centrifuged for 30 min at room temperature at 400 $\times$ g. Care should be exercised when the tubes are removed from the centrifuge so that the layers are not disturbed. For this reason it is advantageous not to use the brake on the centrifuge, so that the deceleration at the end of the centrifugation is not too rapid. The mononuclear cells will appear as a white band between the plasma and the Ficoll-Hypaque. The erythrocytes and polymorphonuclear cells will have sedimented through the Ficoll-Hypaque to the bottom of the tubes.

Both methods provide lymphocytes capable of reacting in the lymphoproliferation assay, but there are several advantages of the Ficoll-Hypaque separation method. Sedimentation at $1 \times g$ results in a significant contamination with erythrocytes and neutrophils, which may be as great as 50% of the total cells. This contamination may lead to reduced proliferative responses, which may be incorrectly interpreted as depressed function, rather than to the less than optimal conditions associated with the contaminating cells. For sequential studies, it is often desirable to cryopreserve cells, and this procedure is more reliable if the erythrocytes and neutrophils are removed before cryopreservation. Separation by Ficoll-Hypaque results in a mononuclear cell preparation free of contaminating erythrocytes and neutrophils. If it is not possible to perform cell separations with Ficoll-Hypaque, the neutrophils can be removed by passage of the cell suspension over sterile glass beads or nylon wool. However, these surfaces retain adherent phagocytic cells and will also retain monocytes. If all monocytes are removed, the resultant population will not respond unless some monocytes are added back to the cultures. On the other hand, there have been reports of monocytes being inhibitory for lymphoproliferative responses in some cancer patients, and this technique offers the capability of investigating findings of depressed reactivity in some instances. Techniques for the removal of adherent cells can be used to investigate questions related to the effects of various populations on the proliferative response, but for routine use, Ficoll-Hypaque preparations are the most convenient.

Cryopreserved cells. For many reasons, the use of cryopreserved cells is advantageous in lymphoproliferative assays. It is not always convenient to set up the assay as soon as blood samples are drawn, nor is it always possible to have blood drawn on the convenient days! Cryopreservation of the cells allows assays to be set up at convenient times and also plays an important role in quality control of assays. For sequential studies of lymphocyte function on individual patients, cryopreservation of cells at each time point, followed by simultaneous assay of all samples at the completion of the study, reduces the concern for potential assay-to-assay variability. The methodology for cryopreservation is described in detail by Strong et al. (9). Mononuclear cells separated from whole blood by Ficoll-Hypaque density centrifugation are washed and suspended at room temperature in RPMI 1640 plus 20% heat-inactivated fetal calf serum. An equal volume of freezing medium (complete RPMI 1640 plus 15% dimethylsulfoxide [DMSO]) is added dropwise. This gives a final freezing suspension of complete RPMI 1640 plus 10% fetal calf serum plus 7.5% DMSO. This mixture is pipetted into ampoules which are then transferred to a controlled-rate freezer. It is important that cells remain in the freezing mixture for a minimum time before being frozen. Once frozen, the ampoules must be transferred for storage to the vapor phase of liquid nitrogen. When required, the cells are thawed by the following procedure.

Immediately after removing the cells from the freezer, thaw them rapidly with shaking in a 37°C water bath. Just before the last ice crystal has melted, remove the vial from the water bath. With a 1-ml disposable pipette, transfer the contents of the vial to a 15-ml round-bottom tube (Corning 25760). The cell suspension should be gently added down the side of the tube. Place the tube at room temperature, and immediately start the dilution procedure to remove the DMSO. Using RPMI with human AB serum, begin by gently adding 1 drop of complete medium down the side of the round-bottom tube. Repeat the addition, doubling the volume each time (i.e., 2, 4, 8, 16, 32 drops, etc.) until a DMSO concentration of 4% is achieved. Gently mix the cells and medium after each addition. Fill the round-bottom tube to a 15-ml volume with medium. Centrifuge the cell suspension for 10 min at speeds which generate no more than $200 \times g$. Pour off (or aspirate off) the medium. Gently resuspend the cells in remaining medium. Resuspend in complete RPMI with human serum concentration, and count the cells. Do not mix or pipette the cells vigorously, since cells that have been frozen are initially more sensitive to mechanical stress than fresh cells are.

CULTURE CONDITIONS

Before setting up the assay, the medium should be warmed to 37°C, and all plates, tubes, and accuvettes for the Coulter Counter should be labeled.

Cell suspension (from fresh blood or cryopreserved cells) should be adjusted to 2×10^6 cells per ml in medium containing 10% serum. Serum is necessary in the medium for optimal proliferation of the cells, and pooled human AB serum is the most reliable source. Not all lots of human AB serum support optimal growth of cells, and in fact, some lots are inhibitory.

Several lots should be tested to find one lot supportive of optimal growth. It is advisable to request samples, test them, and reserve one complete lot for use in this assay. Heterologous serum, such as calf or horse serum, should be avoided, as it is often somewhat stimulatory even in the absence of other stimuli.

It is possible to detect proliferation under serum-free conditions in response to potent mitogens, but antigen-induced proliferation is not detected. Serum concentrations in excess of 40% have been reported to prevent detection of a proliferative response, due to nonspecific immunosuppressive factors. The use of pretested human AB serum at a concentration of 10% is satisfactory for most situations.

The length of time of the cultures for each type of stimulus is determined, and the optimal time is used. This time should be determined periodically and needs to be examined when any aspect of the technique is altered. Seemingly minor changes such as a new brand of plates, different batch of serum, or new incubator may make a significant difference in the assay. It is important to remember that this assay is very sensitive to environmental changes; incubator doors should not be opened often, as the fluctuations in CO_2 levels that result can be harmful to the cells.

ASSAY PROCEDURES

Cultures are set up at three concentrations of responder cells, since in some cases depressed responses may be observed only at suboptimal concentrations. Dilutions are performed in the 96-well plates. The three final dilutions should be 2×10^6, 1×10^6, and 0.5×10^6 cells per ml. These result in 2×10^4, 1×10^4, and 0.5×10^4 cells per well in the Terasaki plates.

The volumes used are very small, and it is necessary to work efficiently to prevent drying out of the wells.

The mitogen or medium controls are plated first in a predetermined pattern on the plate in 10-μl volumes with Hamilton syringes and sterile tips. As the volumes are small, it is necessary to work quickly and to replace the lid on the plate while refilling the syringe. The mitogens, antigens, or stimulator cells for the MLC are plated at the concentration determined to be optimal in the system. (See below for determination of optimal stimulus concentration.) The responding cells at the three different concentrations are plated next, with 10-μl volumes. Once both cells and stimuli are plated, the plates are gently inverted. The 20-μl hanging drop is retained by surface tension. Each plate is placed in a square petri dish, with a gauze pad moistened with sterile water in the bottom. This system is used to ensure adequate humidity for the plates.

The petri dishes are then transferred to a 37°C water-jacketed incubator gassed with 5% CO_2 to maintain a pH of 7.2 to 7.3. At 18 h before the time of harvesting the assay, the plates are removed from the incubator, gently returned to the normal position, and pulsed with 1 μl of [³H]thymidine. They are then inverted again and returned to the incubator for the remainder of the culture time. The actual time for pulsing should be determined for each laboratory and depends to some extent on the specific activity of the [³H]thymidine used. A detailed description of this determination is given by Farrant et al. (2). These authors describe a 2-h pulse time with [³H]thymidine of 2 Ci/mmol specific activity. In our hands, 16 to 18 h is the optimum with [³H]thymidine of a specific activity of 6 Ci/mmol.

Harvesting of the assay requires the use of a harvester designed specifically for use with Terasaki plates. Essentially, the harvester contains wells over which filter disks are cut, with a dry Terasaki plate as a cutter. The culture plate (still in the inverted position) is presented to the harvester, and suction is applied below the filter disks. The culture plate is discarded, and the disks with the transferred cellular material are washed under suction with distilled water. The disks are transferred to counting vials and dried in an oven or at room temperature. Once the disks are dried, scintillation fluid is added, and the disks are counted for tritium in a liquid scintillation counter.

Determination of optimal conditions

Optimal DNA synthesis in response to mitogens is usually detected in 2 to 4 days, whereas 5 to 7 days are necessary to detect optimal responses to antigens and mixed allogeneic leukocytes. Under suboptimal conditions (either low cell numbers or low concentrations of mitogen), the response to mitogens also peaks after 4 days, which suggests a relationship between the number of responding cells and the rate of DNA synthesis. Although there are times when it is important to gather information obtained under suboptimal conditions, it is essential that these conditions be established in parallel with determination of optimal conditions. Suboptimal proliferation can result from inadequate numbers of cells, incorrect (either too short or too long) incubation times, incorrect concentrations of mitogens or antigens, or inhibitory medium or sera. Each of these factors must be addressed individually, and the optimal conditions must be identified for each variant. Up to certain limits, increasing numbers of cells will result in a linear increase in proliferation. However, too many cells will actually appear as depressed proliferation, as nutrients are used up rapidly and cells are then unable to continue to proliferate. A similar pattern is observed when cultures are allowed to incubate for longer than optimal periods of time. As shown in Fig. 1, increased proliferation is observed in 3-day cultures with PHA with cell numbers from 0.5×10^4 to 2×10^4 cells per well, but when 4×10^4 cells per well are plated, the proliferative response is markedly reduced. Similarly, if the cultures are incubated with PHA for 5 days, then proliferation of cells plated at 2×10^4 cells per well is significantly lower than 1×10^4 cells per well and is also significantly lower than the parallel cultures harvested at 3 days. Mitogen concentration is also an important consideration, and the optimum must be established for each laboratory.

Figure 2 shows a PHA curve. This curve is determined by using a range of concentrations of PHA in a 3-day assay and should be determined with each new lot of mitogen. It is advisable to determine the curve on 3 to 5 normal donors before making the final determination of the concentration to be used. As can be seen from the curve, there is a range of concentrations which produces good proliferation, and it is

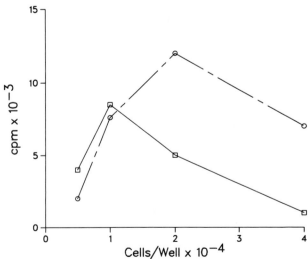

FIG. 1. Lymphocyte proliferation of peripheral blood mononuclear cells expressed as cpm in cultures incubated with PHA for 3 days (○) or 5 days (□).

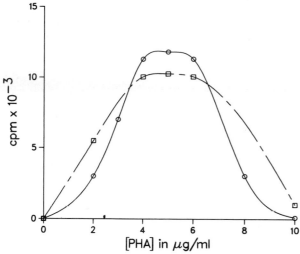

FIG. 2. Lymphocyte proliferation of peripheral blood mononuclear cells expressed as cpm in cultures incubated for 3 days with various concentrations of PHA. Donor 1, ○; donor 2, □.

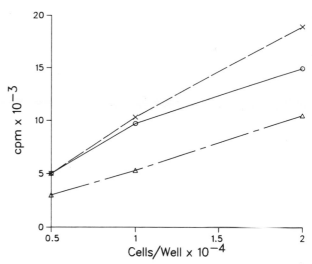

FIG. 4. Lymphocyte proliferation of peripheral blood mononuclear cells expressed as cpm in cultures containing 0.5×10^6, 1×10^6, or 2×10^6 cells per well and PHA at a concentration of 5 μg/ml. Cultures were set up in medium containing 10% human AB serum obtained from three sources. Source 1, △; source 2, ○; source 3, ×.

important to define the concentration which will give good proliferation on all normal donors.

There are other difficult-to-define factors which influence lymphocyte proliferation. Two major sources of problems are serum and medium. It is clear that all sources of medium are not identical. RPMI 1640 from three manufacturers are compared in Fig. 3. We are unable to determine the reasons for the different effects, but it is clear that media from various sources vary, and this fact is confirmed by repeat testing of these products. Different batches of sera are also clearly different (Fig. 4) and need to be evaluated. The effects observed may be due to the presence of nonspecific immunosuppressive factors such as an α-macroglobulin or the competitive binding of stimulants by other serum constituents.

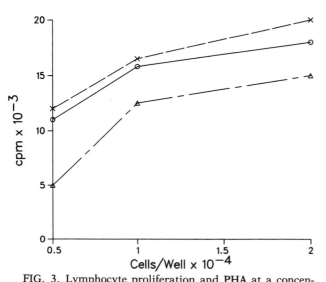

FIG. 3. Lymphocyte proliferation and PHA at a concentration of 5 μg/ml. Cultures were set up in RPMI 1640 medium from three sources. Source 1, △; source 2, ○; source 3, ×.

The determination of optimal conditions represents a considerable investment of time, but unless this determination is made, subsequent data cannot be considered valid.

Controls and quality assurance

Lymphoproliferative assays are subject to change as the result of sometimes minor changes in the assay. A rigorous system of controls for quality assurance is absolutely essential.

Routine checks on all equipment should be performed monthly. Incubators should be checked for accuracy of temperature and CO_2 level. It is not sufficient to rely on the dials on the incubator; they need to be confirmed with thermometers and CO_2 calibration devices. Background counts of empty vials must be checked on beta counters, and if these counts show a sudden increase, the cause should be found and eliminated. Hamilton syringes also need to be calibrated, as small changes in the syringes may result in large changes in the final assay.

In the assay itself, the cells with medium alone (no mitogen or MLC) serve as the control for the level of stimulation. The unstimulated control gives certain information about the cell population and is used to calculate the degree of stimulation. Quality control of the reagents and assay conditions is achieved by the inclusion of a set of standard cells. A large number of cells are obtained by leukapheresis, and many aliquots are cryopreserved. We recommend the use of three standards to be included every time the assay is set up. As the aliquots are all cryopreserved at one time, the freeze procedure is constant, and with practice, the thawing procedure also will be constant. Any variations observed from day to day will therefore be the result of differences in the assay.

Over a period of time, data from all three standards are collected, and any variability from the pattern seen for any of the standards may point to a problem with an assay. If, for example, two of the three standards behaved normally, then the problem may have been in the thawing of the one standard. If, however, two or three standards were aberrant, then the situation needs to be investigated. This is why we recommend three standards, but two or even one are better than none! If both the unstimulated control and stimulated values are high, these values could be due to contamination. Although plates may be purchased as sterile, they can be subsequently contaminated. In contaminated medium, the unstimulated control may be up to 10 times its normal value. If only the stimulated wells have unusually high counts, check the [³H]thymidine. Low counts are not often seen, but they may reflect either medium prepared without the addition of all the essential nutrients or contamination by mycoplasma. A result that shows no counts above background is usually because the plates were not pulsed.

We routinely include one row of unstimulated standards on each plate to check plate-to-plate variation. Such variation is rarely seen, but the row is an additional control which is sometimes useful if unexpected results are seen.

Different incorporation rates are frequently found when more than one technician sets up similar assays. Repeat testing of the standards over time is, however, remarkably consistent for each technician. Although the mean cpm may be different for different technicians, the RPI is very constant, and this is one of the reasons that expression of the data in this form is desirable.

Standardization of the procedure is best accomplished by the use of cryopreserved materials. Even with the most rigorous quality control, there is still some interassay variability, and for sequential studies in patients, this variability can be minimized by the use of cryopreserved cells and simultaneous testing.

Sequential studies to monitor therapy should include at least three baseline (pretherapy) samples. These samples allow the determination of a more accurate baseline value (taken as the mean of the pretherapy determination) from which to assess any subsequent changes. With both adequate quality control of the assay and the establishment of limits of day-to-day fluctuations in activity, alterations in activity can be observed which may be confidently interpreted as being the result of treatment.

This project has been funded at least in part with federal funds from the Department of Health and Human Services under contract number NO1-CO--23910 with Program Resources, Inc.

LITERATURE CITED

1. **Dean, J. H., R. Connor, R. B. Herberman, J. Silva, J. L. McCoy, and R. K. Oldham.** 1977. The relative proliferation index as a more sensitive parameter for evaluating lymphoproliferative responses of cancer patients to mitogens and alloantigens. Int. J. Cancer **20:**359–370.

2. **Farrant, J., J. C. Clark, H. Lee, S. C. Knight, and J. O'Brien.** 1980. Conditions for measuring DNA synthesis in PHA stimulated human lymphocytes in 20μl hanging drops with various cell concentrations and periods of culture. J. Immunol. Methods **33:**301–312.

3. **Greaves, M. F., J. J. T. Owen, and M. C. Raff.** 1973. T and B lymphocytes, origins, properties and roles in immune responses. American Elsevier Publishing Company, Inc., New York.

4. **Hartzman, R. J., M. Segall, M. L. Bach, and F. H. Bach.** 1971. Histocompatibility matching. VI. Miniaturizations of the mixed leucocyte culture test: a preliminary report. Transplantation **11:**268–273.

5. **Ling, N. R., and J. E. Kay.** 1975. Lymphocyte stimulation. North Holland Publishing Co., Oxford.

6. **Nowell, P. L.** 1960. Phytohemagglutinin: an indicator of mitosis in cultures of normal human leucocytes. Cancer Res. **20:**462–466.

7. **Oppenheim, J. J., S. Dougherty, S. C. Chen, and J. Baker.** 1975. Utilization of lymphocyte transformation to assess clinical disorders, p. 87–109. In G. N. Vyas (ed.), Laboratory diagnosis of immunological disorders. Green and Stretton, New York.

8. **Oppenheim, J. J., and D. L. Rosenstreich.** 1976. Lymphocyte transformation: utilization of automatic harvesters, p. 573–577. In B. R. Bloom and J. R. David (ed.), In vitro methods in cell-mediated and tumor immunity, Academic Press, Inc., New York.

9. **Strong, D. M., J. R. Ortaldo, F. Pandolfi, A. Maluish, and R. B. Herberman.** 1982. Cryopreservation of human mononuclear cells for quality control in clinical immunology. I. Correlations in recovery of K- and NK-cell functions, surface markers, and morphology. J. Clin. Immunol. **2:**216–221.

nonadherence index =

$$\frac{\text{mean counts in presence} \quad - \quad \text{mean control}}{\text{mean control counts}} \times 100$$

It has been shown that with peripheral blood leukocytes from more than 95% of control subjects, the difference in nonadherence to two unrelated tumor extracts is less than 30%. Therefore, a nonadherence index of more than 30 is considered significant.

MATERIALS

Migration inhibition assays

Materials for preparing lymphokines
Sterile plastic syringes, 50 ml (Becton-Dickinson and Co., Paramus, N.J.)
Butterfly needle, 19 by ⅞ in., 12-in. tubing (Abbot Hospitals, Inc., North Chicago, Ill.)
Needle, 18 gauge (American Pharmaseal Laboratories, Glendale, Calif.)
Heparin (1,000 U/ml), grade I (Sigma Chemical Co., St. Louis, Mo.)
Dextran 70, 6% (wt/vol) in saline (Pharmacia Diagnostics, Piscataway, N.J.)
Conical centrifuge tubes, 50 ml (no. 2070; Becton Dickinson Labware, Oxnard, Calif.)
Lymphocyte separation medium (Bionetics Laboratory Products, Kensington, Md.)
Tissue culture medium, RPMI 1640 (other tissue culture media may be suitable)
Penicillin, 10,000 U/ml, and streptomycin, 10,000 μg/ml (Irvine Scientific, Santa Ana, Calif.)
HEPES buffer (GIBCO Laboratories, Grand Island, N.Y.)
L-Glutamine (Irvine Scientific)
Nalgene filter (Nalge Corp., Rochester, N.Y.)
ConA (Miles Biochemicals, Elkhart, Ind.)
PHA (Burroughs Wellcome Co., Greenville, N.C.)
Purified protein derivative of tuberculin (Parke-Davis Pharmaceutical, Detroit, Mich.)
Plastic tissue culture flasks, 175 ml (Becton Dickinson Labware)

Materials for purification of monocytes
Percoll (Pharmacia Fine Chemicals, Piscataway, N.J.)
Fetal calf serum (Flow Laboratories, Inc., McLean, Va.)
Polycarbonate centrifuge tubes, 50 ml (Ivan Sorvall, Inc., Norwalk, Conn.)
Hanks balanced salt solution

Materials for indirect macroagarose assay
Agarose (Litex Corp., Glostrup, Denmark)
Medium 199, 10× (Irvine Scientific)
Plastic petri dishes, 49 by 9 mm (Millipore Corp., Bedford, Mass.)
Gel punch, 2.5 mm (Bio-Rad Laboratories, Richmond, Calif.)
Drummond microdispenser, 10 μl (Drummond Scientific Co., Broomall, Pa.)

Materials for indirect agarose microdroplet assay
Seaplaque agarose (FMC Corp., Marine Colloids Div., Rockland, Maine)
Hamilton Luer lock syringe, 50 μl (Fisher Scientific Co., Pittsburgh, Pa.)

Hamilton repeating 1-μl dispenser (Fisher)
Clay Adams Intramedic Luer stub adapter, 20 gauge (James W. Daly, Inc., Lynnfield, Mass.)
Linbro microtiter tissue culture plate, 96 flat-bottom wells (Flow Laboratories)
Plaque viewer with 50× lens (Bellco Glass, Inc., Vineland, N.J.)

LAI assays

Materials for preparing tumor extracts (antigens)
Small scissors and forceps
Stainless steel spatulas
Stainless steel mesh, 10 by 10 cm (80 mesh)
Plastic petri dishes, 60-mm diameter
Motor-driven glass homogenizer (plunger type; Arthur H. Thomas Co., Philadelphia, Pa.)
Phosphate-buffered saline, 0.15 M, pH 7.2 to 7.4
Material for preparing human blood leukocytes
Ammonium chloride solution, 0.15 M
Materials for hemocytometer LAI test
Hemocytometers (Arthur H. Thomas Co.)
Cover slips, no. 1 (24-mm square)
Petri dishes, 150-mm diameter
Beakers, 150 to 200 ml
Microscope (10× eyepieces, 10× and 40× objectives)
Materials for test tube LAI test
Kimax Glass Test Tubes, 20 ml (16 by 150 mm, Arthur H. Thomas Co.)

COMMENTS

Migration inhibition assays

In assessing LIF or MIF production by sensitive lymphocytes, false-positive results may occur since there may be nonlymphokine factors which directly inhibit random migration. These factors include antigen-antibody complexes and antigen by itself. This may be more of a problem when interpreting the results of a direct migration inhibition assay. There is a small (10%) incidence of false-negative results in which the indicator cells do not respond to LIF or MIF because of individual variation. In such cases the assay should be repeated with another set of indicator cells to confirm deficient lymphocyte function. Nevertheless, population studies are recommended for the investigation of a disease rather than dependence on individual results. A positive result for LIF or MIF activity in response to antigen stimulation may indicate lymphocyte sensitization but may also result from nonspecific mitogenic activity of the specific antigen. Furthermore, lymphocyte sensitization does not necessarily imply a cause-and-effect relationship between antigen sensitivity and the pathogenesis of the disease.

LAI assays

LAI assays have phases that are evaluated subjectively, so it is essential that samples be coded during the technical performance and calculations. Statistical analysis of data has variously involved either calculations of degrees of significance between the control and test adherences or use of a nonadherence index with significance defined as an index greater than 95% of that of the control population.

No information exists on the components of the tumor extract responsible for LAI. It appears to be stable for up to 6 months at −50°C and maybe even longer lyophilized or in the presence of protease inhibitors. BFs appear to have a shorter storage life, and it is recommended that serum be assayed soon after its collection.

LITERATURE CITED

1. **Bendtzen, K.** 1976. Some physiochemical properties of human leukocyte migration inhibitory factor (LIF). Acta Pathol. Microbiol. Scand. Sect. C **84**:471–476.
2. **Bloom, B. R., and B. Bennett.** 1966. Mechanism of a reaction in vitro associated with delayed-type hypersensitivity. Science **153**:80–82.
3. **Clausen, J. E.** 1971. Tuberculin-induced migration inhibition of human peripheral leukocytes in agarose medium. Acta Allergol. **26**:56–80.
4. **David, J. R.** 1966. Delayed hypersensitivity in vitro. Its mediation by cell-free substances formed by lymphoid cell-antigen interaction. Proc. Natl. Acad. Sci. U.S.A. **56**:72–77.
5. **Gmelig-Meyling, F., and T. A. Waldmann.** 1980. Separation of human blood monocytes and lymphocytes on a continuous percoll gradient. J. Immunol. Methods **33**:1–9.
6. **Halliday, W. J., A. E. Maluish, and W. H. Isbister.** 1974. Detection of anti-tumor cell mediated immunity and serum-blocking factors in cancer patients by the leukocyte adherence inhibition test. Br. J. Cancer **29**:31–35.
7. **Halliday, W. J., and S. Miller.** 1972. Leukocyte adherence inhibition: a simple test for cell-mediated tumor immunity and serum blocking factors. Int. J. Cancer **9**:477–783.
8. **Harrington, J. T., and P. Stastny.** 1973. Macrophage migration from an agarose droplet: development of a micro-method for assay of delayed hypersensitivity. J. Immunol. **110**:752–759.
9. **Holt, P. G., P. J. Fimmel, L. M. Finlay-Jones, and R. L. Flower.** 1979. Evaluation of the microplate leukocyte adherence inhibition test and its reproducibility, sensitivity, and relationship to other tests of cellular immunity. Cancer Res. **39**:564–569.
10. **Holt, P. G., L. M. Roberts, P. J. Fimmel, and D. Keast.** 1976. The LAI microtest: a rapid and sensitive procedure for the demonstration of cell mediated immunity in vitro. J. Immunol. Methods **8**:277–288.
11. **Maluish, A. E., and W. J. Halliday.** 1975. Quantitation of anti-tumor cell-mediated immunity by a lymphokine-dependent reaction using small volumes of blood. Cell. Immunol. **17**:131–140.
12. **Marti, J. H., N. Grosser, and D. M. P. Thomson.** 1976. Tube leukocyte adherence inhibition assay for the detection of antitumor immunity. II. Monocyte reacts with tumor antigen via cytophilic anti-tumor antibody. Int. J. Cancer **18**:48–57.
13. **McCoy, J. L., J. H. Dean, and R. B. Herberman.** 1977. Human cell-mediated immunity to tuberculin as assayed by the agarose micro-droplet leukocyte migration inhibition technique: comparison with the capillary tube assay. J. Immunol. Methods **15**:355–371.
14. **Rocklin, R. E.** 1974. Products of activated lymphocytes: leukocyte inhibitory factor (LIF) distinct from migration inhibitory factor (MIF). J. Immunol. **112**:1461–1466.
15. **Rocklin, R. E.** 1975. Partial characterization of leukocyte inhibitory factor by concanavalin A-stimulated human lymphocytes (LIF). J. Immunol. **114**:1161–1165.
16. **Rocklin, R. E., O. L. Meyers, and J. R. David.** 1970. In vitro assay for cellular hypersensitivity in man. J. Immunol. **104**:95–102.
16a. **Rocklin, R. E., and A. M. Urbano.** 1978. Human leukocyte inhibitory factor (LIF): use of benzoyl L-arginine ethyl ester to detect LIF activity. J. Immunol. **120**:1409–1414.
17. **Thompson, D. M. P.** 1979. Demonstration of the tube leukocyte adherence inhibition assay with coded samples of blood. Cancer Res. **39**:627–629.
18. **Tsang, P. H., J. F. Holland, and J. G. Bekesi.** 1982. Central role of T lymphocytes in specific recognition of tumor antigens in Cr^{51} leukocyte adherence inhibition. Cell. Immunol. **73**:365–375.
19. **Weiser, W. Y, D. K. Greineder, H. G. Remold, and J. R. David.** 1981. Studies on human migration inhibitory factor: characterization of three molecular species. J. Immunol. **126**:1958–1962.
20. **Wright, S. D., and S. C. Silverstein.** 1982. Tumor-promoting phorbol esters stimulated C3b and C3b′ receptor-mediated phagocytosis in cultured human monocytes. J. Exp. Med. **156**:1149–1164.

Chapter 40

Leukocyte Chemotaxis

EUFRONIO G. MADERAZO AND PETER A. WARD

One important characteristic of phagocytic leukocytes is their capacity to move in response to chemotactic stimuli. This response is an essential part of host defense against infection (9). Leukocyte locomotion is either random or chemotactic. Random locomotion is multidirectional (i.e., the tendency of the cell to move in one direction is equal to the tendency to go in any other direction), whereas chemotaxis is unidirectional movement in response to a concentration gradient of a chemical attractant. Random locomotion is either unstimulated or stimulated. Stimulated random movement (also called chemokinetic) occurs when a chemoattractant interacts with a leukocyte but in the absence of a concentration gradient (e.g., the cells are uniformly bathed in a solution containing the chemoattractant). Under these conditions, the cell engages in considerably more movement than do "resting" cells, but the movement is nonoriented, so the result is no net movement (i.e., the movement tends to be circular). To differentiate these responses in leukocytes from responses of other cells, the terms leukotaxis and leukokinesis may be used. The most important known source of chemotactic factors in vivo is the complement system, from which is derived the C5a chemotactic fragment and factor Ba (a fragment of factor B resulting from action by factor D). Other plasma-derived mediators with chemotactic activity include the Hageman factor-dependent chemotactic factors, kallekrein and plasminogen activator, and by-products of arachidonic acid metabolism via both the lipoxygenase pathway (12-hydroxy-Δ5,8,10,15-eicosatetraenoic acid) and the cyclo-oxygenase pathway (prostaglandins and thromboxanes). Cell-derived chemotactic factors include lymphocyte, monocyte, and polymorphonuclear leukocyte products (9). Certain tissue, bacterial, and viral products contain C3- and C5-cleaving enzymes which can indirectly result in the liberation of complement-derived chemotactic factors (9). In addition, bacteria and viruses may betray their presence to body defenses by liberating preformed low-molecular-weight chemotactic metabolites. Limited studies that indicate bacterial chemotactic factors to be small peptides have led to the discovery of the chemotactic activity of N-formylmethionyl peptides. These peptides are now available commercially for use in the laboratory. Studies of leukocyte locomotion have uncovered the presence of regulators of the chemotactic system. These regulators include the chemotactic factor inactivator (9), the cell-directed inhibitor (9), and the leukokinesis-enhancing factor (8), all of which are normal constituents of human serum, where they are present in trace amounts.

The chemotactic factor inactivator interacts directly with chemotactic factors to bring about their inactivation. Elevations of serum chemotactic factor inactivator have been observed in patients with Hodgkin's disease, cirrhosis, sarcoidosis, lepromatous leprosy, hairy cell leukemia, and systemic lupus erythematosus. The cell-directed inhibitor acts directly on both polymorphonuclear cells and monocytes to inhibit locomotion and, to some extent, phagocytosis. Elevations of cell-directed inhibitor activity in serum have been associated with abnormal leukocyte locomotion and have been observed in patients with cirrhosis, in those with cancer, in those who sustained major trauma, in many hospitalized seriously ill patients, and in some patients with recalcitrant periodontitis. Although cell-directed inhibitor activity has been associated with immunoglobulins A and G, this activity does not usually parallel immunoglobulin levels in serum. The leukokinesis-enhancing factor is responsible for the chemokinetic effect of normal serum and directly stimulates the locomotory responses of granulocytes and, to a lesser extent, monocytes. This factor appears to antagonize the effects of cell-directed inhibitor on leukocyte function. A deficiency of leukokinesis-enhancing factor in serum has been associated with less serious recurrent or chronic infections in several patients (8).

GENERAL INDICATIONS FOR LEUKOTACTIC TESTING

In vitro leukocyte migration assays are performed to determine the extent to which leukocytes can respond to chemotactic, as well as to chemokinetic, stimuli. Disorders of locomotion are often found in patients with histories of chronic, recurrent bacterial infections. Locomotory disorders may be due to internal abnormalities in leukocytes, to defects in the plasma substrate system (e.g., deficiency of complement), or to abnormal levels of regulators. Cellular defects may be either acquired or familial; examples are diabetes mellitus and the Chediak-Higashi syndrome, respectively. Leukocyte migration testing is most frequently done on the blood neutrophils, since these are abundant and readily obtainable. Blood monocytes, which are isolated in adequate amounts only with more difficulty, can also be studied. In addition, it is possible to test serum for the generation of leukotactic factors or for the presence of inhibitors. Advantages of these techniques include the in vitro nature of the assay and the ready availability of test material by venipuncture. The major disadvantage is the requirement for experienced laboratory personnel and the somewhat time-consuming nature of the assay. Chemotaxis of basophils or eosinophils does not yet have sufficient clinical relevance for routine testing in clinical laboratories.

TEST PROCEDURES

Two different quantitative techniques for in vitro assessment of leukocyte migration are available: the micropore filter method (7) and the "under agarose" technique (2). In the micropore filter method, the cells placed on a filter are allowed to migrate into the channels of the filter. The number of migrating cells or the distance of migration into the filter (or both) is then analyzed. In the agarose method, cells placed in a central well are allowed to migrate under the agarose toward peripheral wells containing either a blank (medium alone) or a chemoattractant. As in the micropore filter assay, the number of responding cells or the distance of migration (or both) can be used to assess the response. The agarose method has gained acceptance because of its simplicity and its amenability to special staining procedures, which permits identification of specific types of cells (e.g., eosinophils and basophils) in preparations containing a mixture of leukocytes. We have continued to utilize the micropore filter method almost exclusively in clinical studies because with recent modification the filter method requires a shorter incubation period (1.5 h versus 2 to 3 h for the agarose method). Moreover, a number of investigators with extensive experience using both methods have expressed disappointment over the lack of sensitivity of the agarose method (the agarose method is approximately 50 to 100 times less sensitive than the micropore filter method) (4, 6). In addition, there is considerable day-to-day and technician-to-technician variability with the agarose method. Migration through micropores may also more closely resemble leukocytic migration in tissues (particularly through the capillary wall). Thus, one explanation offered for the relative insensitivity of the agarose technique in detecting abnormal chemotaxis inChediak-Higashi leukocytes is the greater influence of cell deformability on migration through pores of filters than on that under agarose. Finally, the micropore filter assay can be modified to use whole blood in situations in which only small volumes of blood can be obtained, such as in the pediatric population (5). Consequently, despite the apparent usefulness of the agarose method for certain experimental studies, clinical experience with it is still limited, and more extensive studies comparing its sensitivity and usefulness for detecting abnormalities in patients will be needed. Therefore, we continue not to recommend it for regular use in the clinical setting. The "under agarose" method will not be discussed in this chapter. Those interested in details are referred to the work of Chenoweth et al. (2).

Quantitation of chemotactic response can also be accomplished by measurement of lysosomal enzymes released during interaction of neutrophils and chemotactic attractant (3, 6). This is possible because chemotactic and lysosomal enzyme release curves are closely parallel. Another method, which uses time-lapse video of neutrophils migrating in response to chemotactic factor in a Zigmond chamber (10) and then assessment of directionality and speed of migration by multiple vectorial analyses has been found to be too variable to be quantitative (E. G. Maderazo and C. L. Woronick, unpublished data).

Leukocytes

The neutrophil is the most commonly tested cell for locomotory responses. Leukocytes are obtained by gravity sedimentation of erythrocytes in anticoagulated blood (50 U of preservative-free heparin per ml) in an inverted syringe into which the blood has been drawn. Hetastarch-induced sedimentation of erythrocytes can also be used for nonsedimenting blood samples (usually from normal male volunteers) by using 1 part of 6% hetastarch in saline (McGaw Laboratories, Irving, Calif.) to 5 parts of whole blood; sedimentation is carried out in a 50-ml plastic centrifuge tube since leukocytes adhere to glass surfaces. The yields of neutrophils will vary with the leukocyte count of the donor and with conditions of sedimentation, but 5 to 10 ml of blood usually provides adequate numbers of neutrophils. Once the leukocyte-rich suspension is obtained, the cells are gently pelleted by centrifugation ($500 \times g$) for 10 min and then are suspended in medium 199 at a concentration of 5×10^6 neutrophils per ml. The protocol given in Table 1 describes a typical assay and normal values.

For monocyte chemotaxis, special fractionation of blood with a Ficoll-Hypaque gradient is required (1).

Chemotactic factors

In testing for chemotactic responsiveness, several chemotactic preparations can be used. The first is the culture supernatant obtained by overnight growth of Escherichia coli in medium 199. Bacteria are removed by centrifugation, and the pH is adjusted to neutrality with 1 M NaOH. Bacterial chemotactic factor can be

TABLE 1. Protocol for neutrophil locomotion work-up[a]

Upper chamber (cells + serum)	Lower chamber (factor)	Normal values (LI_{20})[b]	Functions to be tested
N + none	None	31.1 ± 5.2	Unstimulated response
P + none	None		
P + none	ZSn		Chemotaxis, complement-derived chemotactic factor, and chemotactic factor inactivator
N + none	ZSn	45.5 ± 9.2	
N + none	ZSp		
N + none	ZSnS	58.1 ± 10.2	
N + N	None	53.0 ± 5.9	Chemokinesis, elevated cell-directed inhibitor or lowered leukokinesis-enhancing factor activity
N + P	None		
P + N	None		

[a] Abbreviations: N, normal cells or serum; P, patient's cells or serum; ZSn, zymosan-activated normal serum; ZSp, zymosan-activated patient's serum; ZSnS, stabilized zymosan-activated normal serum (see text).
[b] See Table 2 for LI_{20}. $n = 22$ normal volunteers.

frozen in small portions for storage. Each batch is tested for potency, and the least amount producing maximum activity is used (usually involving a 1:10 dilution). The second preparation of chemotactic factor, activated serum containing the C5 chemotactic fragment, is generated in fresh normal human serum by addition of zymosan (5 mg of zymosan per ml of serum) with incubation of the mixture for 20 to 30 min at 37°C. Activated serum can be stabilized by addition of 1 M of ε-aminocaproic acid and by heat inactivation at 56°C for 1 h to inhibit inactivation of the C5 chemotactic fragment by chemotactic factor inactivator and other serum enzymes. The activated serum can be stored at −80°C in small portions for future use. A 3% solution in medium 199 is used in the lower chamber. The third preparation of chemotactic factor consists of 10^{-6} M N-formylmethionylleucylphenylalanine, a synthetic chemotactic peptide which is now available commercially. This preparation is stored in small batches at a concentration of 10^{-2} M dissolved in stock (14 M) dimethyl sulfoxide.

The advantage of bacterial chemotactic factor is its easy availability, but activity of $E. coli$ varies considerably between strains, and many strains do not produce potent chemotactic factors. Moreover, we have observed deterioration of chemotactic activity in bacterial supernatant even after short storage at −80°C. Activated serum is easily available, but activity in individual sera is variable. A great advantage of using activated serum is that with a few experiments one can check several functions: (i) chemotactic responsiveness of the patient's cells versus control cells, (ii) ability to generate chemotactic activity in the patient's serum versus control serum, and (iii) chemotactic factor inactivator activity in the patient's serum versus control serum (Table 1). The advantages of the synthetic chemotactic peptide N-formylmethionylleucylphenylalanine are its convenience and the fact that it is standardized.

Chemotactic chambers

Several types of chambers are available; one utilized frequently is the clear acrylic chamber (Fig. 1). When assembled with a 13-mm-diameter micropore filter in place, this chamber consists of an upper chamber and a lower chamber, which are separated by the filter. The upper chamber contains cells suspended in a maximum volume of 0.7 ml, whereas the volume of the lower chamber is 1.5 ml. There are several advantages of this type of chamber over the stainless-steel chemotactic chambers: (i) the small upper chamber volume requires fewer cells, a particular advantage in studies with humans and especially with infants; (ii) the chamber has fewer parts; (iii) 13-mm-diameter filter paper is more convenient and less expensive, and a pair (duplicates) can be mounted on a single glass slide and covered with a single cover slip (22 by 40 mm); and (iv) expensive tuberculin syringes and needles for injection of contents into the lower compartment are not required.

Preparation of chemotactic chambers

The chamber is prepared by placement of a filter that is 13 mm in diameter with 5-μm porosity. The

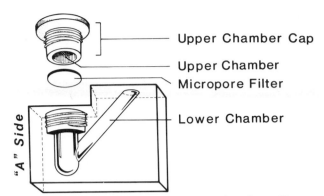

FIG. 1. Clear acrylic chemotactic chamber that utilizes a 13-mm-diameter micropore filter (Ahlco Corp., Meriden, Conn.).

upper chamber cap is placed and tightened slightly over the filter. With the "A side" of the chamber positioned downwards (to avoid trapping air under the filter on filling), the lower compartment is half filled with the appropriate reactants. Cell suspension (0.1 ml containing 5×10^{-5} neutrophils) is added to the upper compartment, which is then filled completely with medium 199. The lower chamber is then completely filled with the previously added reactant. The sequence as outlined is important when chemotactic factor is used in the lower chamber, since complete filling of the lower chamber before the upper chamber will lead to leakage of chemotactic factor through the filter into the upper chamber.

Incubation

The prepared chambers are incubated in air at 37°C. The optimal incubation is one that will allow the fastest-migrating cells to reach beyond halfway through but not completely through the thickness of the filter. Incubation periods that allow only shallow penetration into the filter will not detect defects except for the most obvious ones. In our laboratories, chambers not containing serum or plasma in the upper compartment are incubated for 90 min, and those containing serum or plasma are incubated for 60 min. These precautions to prevent cells from completely migrating through the filter are needed to avoid the variability produced by cell loss due to detachment of cells from the distal surface of the filter.

Protocol

The usual complete protocol for assessment of neutrophil migration is shown in Table 1.

Staining

After incubation, the filters are removed, placed in staining cassettes (Fig. 2) without being allowed to dry, and quickly fixed in absolute isopropyl alcohol for at least 30 s. (Filters dry quickly, and if they are allowed to do so, cell outlines will be lost. This can be avoided by dipping the filter into the alcohol before placement in the cassette.) The filters are then stained

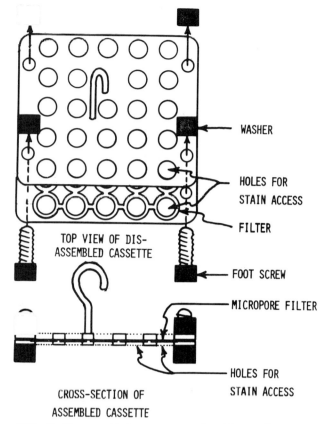

FIG. 2. Brass staining cassette for 13-mm-diameter micropore filters (Ahlco Corp., Meriden, Conn.).

ities, at least in our experience, are not limited to defective mass migration. The third method ("cell distance" or "microsectioning" technique) is the method of choice in our laboratory. In this method the cells are counted at every 10-μm interval from the proximal-surface cell monolayer to the distal surface. The number of cells counted at each level is multiplied by the distance of that level from the proximal surface. The products obtained are added, and the sum is divided by the total number of cells counted. The number obtained, which is the average distance migrated per cell, is called the locomotion index or, if chemotactic factor was used in the lower compartment, the leukotactic index (LI). A sample calculation of LI and two variations is illustrated in Table 2. Three or more fields are evaluated, and the mean LI for each duplicate or triplicate filter is calculated. When using an automatic particle counter, we start our counts at 20 μm to minimize machine error resulting from multiple counts of particles on the proximal surface (mostly lymphocytes and monocytes) whose shadows could still be seen from the 10-μm level. The resulting index is called LI_{20}. Normal controls are evaluated simultaneously with each experiment, and a cumulative normal value (Table 1), which may vary according to the filters being used, is maintained in our laboratory. Only indices lower than 2 standard deviations of the normal mean are considered abnormal. Thus, with the present batch of filters, inhibitions of greater than 33% for unstimulated, 40% for chemotaxis, and 20% for chemokinesis are abnormal. Although inconvenient, it is preferable to repeat the tests before calling the results abnormal.

Assessment of monocyte chemotaxis

Monocytes respond chemotactically most effectively to the C5 fragment and to a product of antigen-stimulated lymphoid cells (9). In clinical medicine two different aspects of monocyte chemotaxis are

in hematoxylin for 2 min, rinsed in water again, dehydrated successively in several vessels containing absolute isopropyl alcohol for 30 s each, and finally cleared in xylene for 5 to 10 min. The stained filters are then mounted on slides with Permount and covered with a thin cover slip.

Assessment of cell migration

Many methods of assessing the results of cell migration have been described. In general, they fall into three types (7). The first method involves counts of the number of cells that have arrived at a preselected distance, such as the distal surface. This method is sensitive in detecting differences in nonstimulated and chemotactic responses. However, it is susceptible to bias and suffers from a larger coefficient of variation. The second method ("leading-front" technique) measures the distance migrated by the faster-migrating cells. This method is less susceptible to the problems of the first method, but it cannot detect abnormalities of mass migration, and the assumption that the faster-moving population represents the total cell population (on which the validity of this procedure as a method for assessing leukocyte migration is based) may not be true, since subpopulations of cells with varied migration characteristics have been noted. Although these objections appear serious, the leading-front technique is still useful because of its simplicity, the speed with which it can be accomplished, and the fact that most human leukocyte migration abnormal-

TABLE 2. Sample calculation of LI[a]

Distance from origin (μm) (A)	No. of cells (B)	A × B
0 (monolayer)	15	0
10	37	370
20	13	260
30	12	360
40	10	400
50	9	450
60	8	480
70	7	490
80	6	480
90	4	360
100	0	0
Total count from 0 μm (for LI_0)	121	3,650
Total count from 20 μm (for LI_{20})	69	3,280

[a] LI = $\Sigma(A \times B)/\Sigma(B)$. LI_0 = 3,650 ÷ 121 = 30.2 μm (improves detection of mass migration effect of chemotactic factors; use purified neutrophils instead of mixed leukocytes if automatic particle counter is to be used). LI_{20} = 3,280 ÷ 69 = 47.5 μm (preferable if mixed leukocyte suspension is used instead of purified neutrophils and counting is done with an automatic particle counter).

usually studied: the monocytes themselves and the chemotactic factors produced from lymphoid cells, particularly in patients with suspected underlying immunological dysfunction (deficiency states). If monocyte function is to be studied, the cells must be fractionated from blood by the Ficoll-Hypaque method. In monocyte studies several modifications are necessary, such as (i) use of cellulose micropore filters of 8-μm porosity, (ii) use of the C5 chemotactic fragment or the lymphocyte-derived monocyte chemotactic factor as the attractant, and (iii) incubation of the chamber for 3 h. For screening studies of monocyte function, only unstimulated and chemotactic responses are usually necessary.

REAGENTS

Chemotaxis chambers and staining cassettes

Clear acrylic chemotactic chambers (Fig. 1) and staining cassettes (Fig. 2) are obtained from Ahlco Corp., Meriden, Conn.

Micropore filters

The cellulose nitrate filters used are 13 mm in diameter and of 5-μm porosity (catalog no. SM 113 24.013; Sartorious Filters, Inc., Hayward, Calif.). Since values change with filters from other lots and since some lots of filters are not suitable for leukocyte migration studies, we pretest various lots and select the most suitable (i.e., least variability and values closer to cumulative normal mean) for purchase. Polycarbonate filters are only 10 μm thick and therefore are not suitable for the microsectioning technique.

Culture medium

Medium 199 is made by reconstituting 10 ml of the concentrated medium (TC medium 199, 10×), which can be obtained from any tissue culture supplier, with 10 ml of 1.4% sodium bicarbonate, 1.75 ml of 1 M MOPS [3-(N-morpholino)propanesulfonic acid] adjusted to pH 7.3, and enough deionized water to make 100 ml. Other buffers can be used, but of the buffers tested, MOPS showed the least change in pH during incubation at 37°C. With Tris hydrochloride, for example, the medium (initially pH 7.3) became excessively alkaline (pH 7.8) during incubation for 1 h.

Chemotactic factors

Chemotactic factors are discussed above. Zymosan, which is used to activate serum, and the chemotactic peptide formylmethionylleucylphenylalanine are available from Sigma Chemical Co., St. Louis, Mo., and other biochemical companies.

Hematoxylin

Hematoxylin stain can be obtained from Fisher Scientific Co., Medford, Mass. We use the "Gill formulation" because it stains only the cell nucleus and not the cytoplasm; thus, better contrast between the cells

(nuclei) and background is obtained—a definite advantage, particularly if an automated particle counter is utilized for counting.

Automatic particle counters

Several systems are now available in the market, and three of these systems have been evaluated in our laboratories: Alpha-500 Image Analysis System, Bausch & Lomb, Rochester, N.Y.; Optomax Image Analyser, Micromeasurements, Burlington, Mass.; and the Artek Counter model 980, Artek Systems Corp., Farmingdale, N.Y. All systems performed satisfactorily. Other systems with built-in calculators or computers are extremely expensive and beyond the means of most small laboratories. Also available with the Bausch & Lomb Image Analysis System are an Automatic Focus Hardware (catalog no. 37–20–47), Automatic Stage Control (catalog no. 37–20–70), and an interface for Hewlett-Packard 9825A tabletop computer (catalog no. 37–20–35 or Hewlett-Packard 9832A 16 BIT I/O). Once focused on the monolayer cells, the system can be programmed to perform the counting and calculation of the LI automatically for each field. With the proper programs and if the system is interfaced (Hewlett-Packard 98034A HP-1B interface) with a printer (Hewlett-Packard 2631A printer) and a plotter (Hewlett-Packard 9872A plotter), results can be recorded in table form or plotted instantaneously.

LITERATURE CITED

1. **Boyum, A.** 1968. Isolation of mononuclear cells and granulocytes from human blood. Scand. J. Clin. Lab Invest. **21**(Suppl. 97):77–89.
2. **Chenoweth, D. E., J. G. Towe, and T. E. Hugli.** 1979. A modified method for chemotaxis under agarose. J. Immunol. Methods **25**:337–353.
3. **Fantone, J., R. M. Senior, D. L. Kreutzer, M. Jones, and P. A. Ward.** 1979. Biochemical quantitation of the chemotactic factor inactivator activity in human serum. J. Lab. Clin. Med. **93**:17–24.
4. **Gallin, J. I., and P. G. Quie (ed.).** 1978. Leukocyte chemotaxis: methods, physiology, and clinical implications, p. 40–41. Raven Press, New York.
5. **Krause, P. J., R. M. Pock, C. L. Woronick, and E. G. Maderazo.** 1983. Simplified micropore filter assay of neutrophil migration using whole blood. J. Infect. Dis. **148**:881–885.
6. **Kreutzer, D. L., J. T. O'Flaherty, F. W. Orr, H. J. Showell, E. L. Becker, and P. A. Ward.** 1979. Quantitative comparison of various biological responses of leukocytes to different chemotactic factors. Immunopharmacology **1**:39–47.
7. **Maderazo, E. G., and C. L. Woronick.** 1978. Micropore filter assay of human granulocyte locomotion: problems and solutions. Clin. Immunol. Immunopathol. **11**:196–211.
8. **Maderazo, E. G., C. L. Woronick, and P. A. Ward.** 1979. Leukokinesis-enhancing factor in human serum: partial characterization and relationship to disorders of leukocyte migration. **12**:382–395.
9. **Ward, P. A.** 1974. Leukotaxis and leukotactic disorders. Am. J. Pathol. **77**:520–538.
10. **Zigmond, S. H.** 1977. Ability of polymorphonuclear leukocytes to orient in gradients of chemotactic factors. J. Cell Biol. **75**:606–616.

Chapter 41

Biological and Immunological Assays of Human Interferons

SIDNEY E. GROSSBERG, JERRY L. TAYLOR, RUTH E. SIEBENLIST, AND PATRICIA JAMESON

The interferons (IFNs) constitute a class of natural cell products that stimulate antiviral resistance in cell cultures and animals (1; S. E. Grossberg in L. M. Pfeffer, ed., *Mechanisms of Interferon Actions*, in press). The definition of IFNs as proteins that can make cultured cells resistant to virus infection rests on a biological assay (4). The three major types of human IFNs (Hu IFNs), designated alpha, beta, and gamma, differ in their amino acid sequences and their physical, pharmacological, and biological properties, as well as in their antigenic structure. This last characteristic not only makes it possible to distinguish them by neutralization with their specific antibodies but also has made feasible the development of immunoassays employing monoclonal as well as polyclonal antibodies in competitive binding or sandwich-type assays (4).

Some of the salient distinguishing biological, genetic, and physicochemical properties of the Hu IFN-α, Hu IFN-β, and Hu IFN-γ types are listed in Table 1. Only the Hu IFN-α type has a large number of distinguishable subtypes, the nomenclature for some of which is given in Table 1, footnote *a*.

The mechanisms for the production and the action of IFNs are distinct and unrelated. These soluble, hormonelike proteins are produced in response to virus infections or to stimulation of immunocompetent as well as other somatic cells by a great variety of quite different nonviral materials. Some typical inducers as well as some cell types which are involved in producing IFNs of different types are also listed in Table 1. The genetic loci for production of Hu IFN-α and Hu IFN-β are located primarily on human chromosome 9, and those for Hu IFN-γ are located on chromosome 12. The complex cellular reactions which ensue when cells are treated with Hu IFN-α or -β occur after binding to a plasma membrane receptor coded for by a locus on human chromosome 21; indeed, cells (fibroblasts or monocytes) taken from patients with trisomy 21 (Down's syndrome) show heightened responses to Hu IFN treatment (1, 3, 4, 6; Grossberg, in press).

In addition to their antiviral effects, IFNs have exceedingly diverse biological activities. These effects depend in part upon the particular specialized cell under study and the cellular product or function being measured. The alterations in cell phenotype include inhibition of growth, differentiation (e.g, bone marrow stem cells), delayed hypersensitivity, allograft rejection, and lectin-stimulated lymphocyte proliferation, as well as enhancement of IFN production (so-called priming effect), human leukocyte surface antigen (HLA) expression (e.g., β_2-microglobulin), phagocytosis, cytotoxic lymphocyte action (e.g., natural killer cell activity), and immunoglobulin E (IgE)-mediated histamine release. In Tables 2 and 3 are summarized the inhibitory and stimulatory actions of Hu IFN-α and Hu IFN-β on cells of the immune system (6; Grossberg, in press).

The lymphokine Hu IFN-γ appears to have more potent cellular effects than Hu IFN-α or Hu IFN-β, the activities of which can be enhanced by simultaneous treatment with Hu IFN-γ. The more notable stimulatory activities of Hu IFN-γ include macrophage activation (which appears to copurify with macrophage-activating factor), production of interleukins 1 and 2, and an increase in receptors for interleukin 2. Hu IFN-γ has a marked inhibitory effect on cell growth, and this antiproliferative activity is enhanced by simultaneous treatment with Hu IFN-α or Hu IFN-β (6; Grossberg, in press).

CLINICAL INDICATIONS

The situations in which the measurement of IFNs may be undertaken include the evaluation of immune function in immune-related diseases (3), e.g., immune deficiency syndromes, including acquired immune deficiency syndrome (AIDS), and the so-called collagen diseases, such as rheumatoid arthritis and lupus erythematosus. In the last instance, antibodies to IFN have been described in a patient with lupus nephritis that were present not only in the circulation but also in the renal tubules (1).

In clinical trials of Hu IFN efficacy with either the natural products or those derived by recombinant DNA technology, it is essential to monitor IFN levels. IFN has been shown to have a therapeutic benefit in viral infections such as herpes, varicella, and hepatitis B, as well as varicella-zoster in immunosuppressed patients. Among the tumors on which Hu IFN has been shown to have a beneficial effect are osteosarcoma, multiple myeloma, Kaposi sarcoma, and certain lymphomas, as well as viral papillomas in the larynx and on the skin. Antibodies to IFN occur in some patients receiving exogenous IFN (Grossberg, in press).

The different types of IFN can be identified by neutralization tests with specific antibody in the biological assays described below and, for Hu IFN-α, by demonstration of resistance or lability of biological activity to acid (pH 2).

INTERPRETATION

There is a great variety of IFN bioassays, which vary with respect to cell-virus combinations and the methods for determination of virus growth (viral antigen, enzyme, nucleic acid, infectivity) or effects (destruction of cells). These methods and the definition of terms used in describing the features of IFN assays are reviewed in reference 4. The practical and theoretical

TABLE 1. Distinguishing characteristics of Hu IFNs by type

Characteristic	Hu IFN-α	Hu IFN-β	Hu IFN-γ
Former designation	Leukocyte (Type I)	Fibroblast (Type I)	Immune (Type II)
Genes			
Number	13[a]	1 or 2	1
Chromosomal location	Chromosome 9[b]	Chromosome 9	Chromosome 12
Number of amino acids	166	166	146
Glycosylation	No	Yes	Yes
Acid stability	Yes[c]	Yes	No
Synergistically active	γ	γ	α and β
Receptors in common	β	α	Not α or β
Most common producer cells[d]	B, M, Null	Fibroblasts	T
Inducers[e]	Viruses, double-stranded RNA, allogeneic cells, B-cell mitogens	Viruses, double-stranded RNA, allogeneic cells, B-cell mitogens	T-cell mitogens, antigens, tumor cells

[a] The corresponding designations for DNA-derived Hu IFN-α subtypes named in the literature in two different ways are: $\alpha_1 = \alpha D$; $\alpha_2 = \alpha A$; $\alpha_5 = \alpha G$; $\alpha_6 = \alpha K$; $\alpha_7 = \alpha J$; $\alpha_8 = \alpha B$.

[b] Loci scattered throughout chromosome 9.

[c] Acid-labile IFN-α can occur in serum of patients with diseases of the immune system (e.g., AIDS and lupus erythematosus).

[d] B, Bone marrow-derived lymphocytes; T, thymocyte-derived lymphocytes; M, monocytes-macrophages; Null, non-B, non-T lymphocytes.

[e] Some inducers may stimulate the production of more than one IFN type from a given cell population.

considerations in the selection of a given type of IFN assay for a particular purpose are also described therein. It is essential that the IFN assay be relatively precise and reproducible, such that a titer can be reliably reported in International Units (IU) per milliliter of original material. Since IFN assays vary considerably in their sensitivity to IFNs, the assay chosen must be calibrated by the proper use of World Health Organization International Reference Standards for the specific IFN type that might be found in the clinical sample (8). These reference preparations, as well as corresponding polyclonal antibodies, can be obtained from the National Institute of Allergy and Infectious Diseases, National Institutes of Health, Bethesda, Md. It should be noted that the reference preparation of one type cannot be substituted for another. The manner of assay calibration is described below.

Several immunoassays have been described (reviewed in reference 4). They require either pure IFN or antibody to pure IFN without contaminating antibodies to other antigens. The calibration of antigen content in relation to units of biological activity remains a problem to be resolved; such measurements have not yet been made for International Reference Preparations of IFN. Data from our laboratory (unpublished) and from Chang et al. (2) suggest that the immunoassay described below for Hu IFN-γ measures biologically active IFN. It is obvious that biologically inactive IFN molecules can still be antigenic and react in some radioimmune or enzyme-linked immunosorbent assays. Immunoassays for IFNs appear to be superior to bioassays in terms of rapidity and reproducibility, but they can be only as specific as the purity of the labeled IFN or immunoglobulins employed.

TABLE 2. IFN immunomodulation: stimulatory effects of IFN on immune system functions[a]

Macrophages
  Phagocytosis
  Spreading
  Cytotoxicity against tumor cells
  Cytotoxicity against virus-infected cells
  Macrophage-activating factor (IFN-γ)
T lymphocytes
  Cytotoxicity
  Suppression
B lymphocytes
  Antibody production (IFN given after antigen)
NK cells
  Cytotoxicity (in vitro and in vivo)
K cells
  Cytotoxicity (antibody dependent)
Basophils
  IgE-mediated histamine release
Antigen expression
  Histocompatibility antigens
  Fcγ receptors
  Tumor-associated antigens (e.g., carcinoembryonic)

[a] Reprinted from Grossberg (in press) with permission.

TABLE 3. IFN immunomodulation: inhibitory effects of IFN on immune system functions[a]

Delayed-type hypersensitivity responses (to chemicals, viruses, or cellular [erythrocyte] antigens)
  Afferent pathway
  Efferent pathway
  Graft-versus-host reaction (allograft survival promoted)
Monocyte-to-macrophage differentiation
T lymphocytes
  Proliferation (due to mitogens, antigens, allogenic lymphocytes)
  Production of leukocyte migration inhibition factor
B lymphocytes
  Proliferation
  IgG, IgM, and IgE antibody production (IFN given with or before antigen) (primary or secondary response)
Granulocytes
  Migration inhibition (by mitogen or antigen)
Antigen expression
  Fcμ receptors
NK cell target cell sensitivity
Hematopoietic (bone marrow) cell proliferation

[a] Reprinted from Grossberg (in press) with permission.

TEST PROCEDURES: VIRUSES AND CELLS

Three IFN assays are described that are suitably sensitive and provide objectively measured endpoints. The first two microtiter assays measure the biological (antiviral) activity of Hu IFN-α, Hu IFN-β, and Hu IFN-γ and the third, a radioimmunoassay, measures the presence of Hu IFN-γ antigen. The two biological assays utilize encephalomyocarditis (EMC) virus, a rodent virus, and A549 cells, a human lung carcinoma cell line shown to be sensitive to all three Hu IFN types (4, 5).

Growth of A549 cells

A549 cells are grown in Dulbecco modified Eagle minimal essential medium containing 4.5 g of glucose per liter (DMEM-glu) and 10% heat-inactivated newborn calf serum (NCS). The cells are subcultured weekly at a 1:7 split ratio, with 0.01% trypsin to disperse cells.

Preparation of EMC virus stock

Mouse L cells are grown in Eagle minimal essential medium in a Hanks balanced salt solution (HBSS) base (MEMH) containing 10% fetal bovine serum (FBS) previously heated at 56°C for 30 min. Confluent monolayers of L cells in 800-cm^2 roller bottles, each containing about 8×10^7 cells, are infected with 5×10^9 PFU of EMC virus (titrated in L cells) in 5 ml of MEMH with 2% FBS per bottle. After a 1-h adsorption of EMC virus, MEMH containing 10% FBS is added, and cultures are incubated at 36°C for approximately 18 h. To harvest the virus, cultures are frozen, thawed, and centrifuged at $350 \times g$ for 10 min. The supernatant fluid is dispensed in 1-ml quantities into glass screw-capped vials and stored at −80°C.

Plaque titration of EMC virus

A549 cell suspensions with 5×10^5 cells per ml in DMEM-glu with 10% NCS are dispensed, 1 ml per well, onto 12-well plastic plates. The following day, serial 10-fold dilutions of virus are made in GLB (0.5% gelatin and 0.25% lactalbumin hydrolysate in HBSS). Medium is removed from monolayers, cells are washed with GLB, and 0.1 ml of each virus dilution is added to wells in triplicate. After a 1-h incubation at 36°C for virus adsorption, cultures are overlaid with 1 ml of MEMH containing 4× concentrations of vitamins and 2× concentrations of amino acids, 0.8% Bacto-Agar (Difco Laboratories, Detroit, Mich.), 5% NCS, 10 mM BES [N,N-bis(2-hydroxyethyl-2-aminoethanesulfonic acid], 15 mM HEPES (N-2-hydroxyethylpiperazine-N'-2-ethanesulfonic acid), 10 mM TES [N-tris(hydroxymethyl)methyl-2-aminoethanesulfonic acid], 0.14% tryptose phosphate broth, and 400 μg of DEAE-dextran per ml. After 24 h, a second agar overlay of 1 ml, lacking DEAE-dextran but containing 0.0067% neutral red, is added to each well. Cultures are incubated for 24 h more, and clear plaques in the red background monolayer are counted to calculate the virus titer (PFU per milliliter) of the original virus stock.

Plaque titration of EMC virus in L cells is performed as in A549 cells, except that L cells are planted in MEMH, and FBS is used in all media.

TEST PROCEDURES: BIOASSAYS

Hemagglutinin yield reduction assay

For more information see reference 5.

Day 1. A549 cell suspensions, with 2.5×10^5 cells per ml, are dispensed into flat-bottomed 96-well plates, with 0.2 ml per well.

Day 2. IFN samples are diluted in serial two- or threefold steps in DMEM-glu with 2% NCS (maintenance medium) in 96-well plates. Medium is removed from wells, and 100 μl of an IFN dilution is added to each well. Each plate includes a row of wells containing no IFN and a row of wells containing a dilution series of a laboratory IFN standard preparation for each type of IFN being assayed. The laboratory standards must have been previously calibrated against the appropriate International Reference IFN Standards.

Day 3. EMC virus is diluted in maintenance medium to approximately 2×10^7 PFU/ml (as measured in A549 cells). This concentration of virus gives an approximate multiplicity of infection of 7 PFU per cell; the sensitivity of the assay can be increased somewhat by decreasing the multiplicity of infection to about 1. Medium is removed from wells, and the cells are washed twice with HBSS. Each well is infected with 30 μl of EMC diluted in maintenance medium, and the plates are incubated for 1 h at 36°C for virus adsorption. Cells are washed three times with HBSS, and 125 μl of maintenance medium is added to each well. During virus adsorption and incubation, pH must be maintained in the range of 7.3 to 7.8 for maximum virus replication.

Day 4. After 16 to 24 h, cultures are frozen and thawed, and EMC virus yield is measured by titration of viral hemagglutinin (HA). The HA diluent (borate-potassium chloride-bovine serum albumin) is composed of 3.09 g of boric acid and 8.95 g of KCl per liter of water, adjusted to pH 7.2 with NaOH. At the time of use for dilution of virus-infected cell culture materials, bovine serum albumin is added to 0.02%. Human type O erythrocytes are diluted with saline (0.85% NaCl) and centrifuged at $350 \times g$ for 10 min. The erythrocyte pellet is suspended in fresh saline, and the washing procedure is continued until the supernatant fluid is clear (approximately three washes). The pellet is suspended in saline to achieve a 10% (vol/vol) suspension. This erythrocyte suspension is then diluted 1:12 in HA diluent for addition to virus dilutions in the HA test.

HA procedure. Virus from each row of the infected A549 cell plate is diluted by 12 steps in serial twofold dilutions (0.05 ml of virus in 0.05 ml of diluent) in a round-bottomed 96-well plate, by using a Titertek or other multiple dilution device, and 0.05 ml is discarded from the last row. To each well of the diluted virus, 0.05 ml of erythrocytes is added. Plates are held at room temperature for approximately 1 to 2 h. The last dilution at which HA is detected is recorded. The dilution well number is equal to the $\log_2$ of the HA titer (reciprocal of the virus dilution).

Cytopathic effect dye uptake assay

In the cytopathic effect (CPE) dye uptake assay, cells can be dispensed into the IFN dilutions.

Chapter 43

Lymphocyte-Mediated Cytotoxicity

C. B. CARPENTER

The best-described cell-mediated component of the effector immune response is produced by subsets of cytotoxic T lymphocytes (CTL). These cells injure target cells bearing specific antigens to which clones of CTL are directed. When cell preparations processed directly from blood or lymphoid tissue contain cytotoxic activity, the term lymphocyte-mediated cytotoxicity has been used to describe the CTL phenomenon, while the in vitro priming of cells before testing has often been called a cell-mediated lympholysis assay, especially when the allogeneic mixed lymphocyte response is used to generate CTL against alloantigens. There is fundamentally no difference in the assay for lymphocyte-mediated cytotoxicity or cell-mediated lympholysis effector cells. They require intimate contact with target cells, and injury is usually measured by release of cytoplasmic ^{51}Cr from the target cells.

CYTOTOXIC T LYMPHOCYTES

T lymphocytes bear surface molecules related to the functional programs of various subsets (1). In general, human CTL obtained after in vivo immunization or in vitro culture with antigen are included within the T8$^+$ (leu 2$^+$) subset. T8 also marks suppressor T cells, and some CTL have been found which are of the T4$^+$ (leu 3$^+$) subset; hence, the phenotypes defined by mouse anti-human monoclonal antibodies do not uniquely define CTL. There is, however, some symmetry with regard to the interaction of CTL with histocompatibility antigens. Alloimmunized CTL, clonally reactive with class I histocompatibility antigens, are generally T8$^+$, whereas class II directed CTL are generally T4$^+$. In addition to CTL-target cell attachment via the T-cell receptor for antigen, the T8- or T4-bearing molecules appear to provide an additional binding site, increasing both the strength and specificity of interaction (4). A few individual clones derived from lymphocyte cultures have been found which show dissociation of this phenotype-target symmetry, but the general rules apply when dealing with populations of immunized cells.

Certain restrictions on CTL-target cell interactions have been demonstrated when the antigen is not an HLA molecule. For example, a virus-infected cell can be lysed by CTL having specificity to viral antigen, but only if at least one class I antigen of the target cell is shared with the CTL (6). Such genetic restriction indicates that the antigen receptor on the CTL must also recognize an element of self. In this concept, a virus-altered self structure is what is recognized by the CTL recognition site(s). The allogeneic response appears to perceive allodeterminants of another individual as if they were altered self. Further study of the T-cell receptor complex will be needed to resolve the relationship of alloimmunity to immunity against microorganisms and other antigens.

Mechanisms of lysis

The cytolytic reaction itself is a complex series of events, the first of which is specific binding of target cells by CTL (3). For this initial step, magnesium but not calcium ions are essential. The binding of CTL to target cells is an energy (glucose)-dependent process, as cytolysis can be arrested by substitution of 2-deoxy-D-glucose. In addition, binding is inhibited by cytochalasin B and colchicine, chemicals known to interfere with the lymphocyte contractile microfilaments. Electron microscopic studies of CTL-target cell binding have revealed that a portion of the plasma membranes averaging 150 nm in span is involved in the interdigitation of the CTL and target cell membranes.

The physical state of the cell surface membrane is important for CTL-target cell binding. Local anesthetics such as procaine and lidocaine reversibly inhibit binding, as does alteration of cholesterol synthesis, suggesting that nonspecific intercellular membrane interactions are necessary for the binding process.

Operationally, binding of CTL to target cells is followed by a second phase whereby the target cell membrane is damaged. CTL can lyse target cells from as early as 10 min to more than 3 h after CTL-target cell binding. Furthermore, the lytic process is unidirectional; i.e., target cell killing has no effect on the viability of the effector cell. It is known that cytolysis occurs as a linear function of time, and the number of target cells destroyed is directly proportional both to the number of effector lymphocytes in the assay system and to the number of target cells. Analyses of target cell destruction have shown that cytolysis results from collision between a single lymphocyte and a single target cell. Moreover T-cell-mediated destruction is a cyclic phenomenon in which the lymphocyte has the capacity to detach itself from the initial target cell and proceed to injure additional target cells.

Whatever the lytic mechanism, the effector cell seems to require for its lytic activity ongoing protein synthesis, as inhibitors of RNA-protein metabolism suppress cytolysis, although clearly there is no necessity for continuous synthesis of DNA or cell replication. Alterations in the level of intracellular cyclic nucleotides have been shown to modulate events. Agents which augment intracellular cyclic AMP (i.e., prostaglandins) uniformly suppress lysis, whereas elevation of cyclic GMP by cholinergic agonists leads to an increase in the cytolytic process. Insulin also has an augmenting effect, due perhaps to the raising of cyclic GMP levels.

If secretion of a cytolytic compound is involved in target cell injury, it has been clearly shown that this product is not lymphotoxin. No evidence of lymphotoxin release has ever been found in the supernatant of CTL cultures or after sonic fragmentation of sensitized effector cells.

Somewhat less is known about the actual lesion produced in the target cell. Lysis of an entire target cell population does not appear to be instantaneous, inasmuch as released cellular constituents continue to accumulate in the culture medium for a considerable time after the onset of target cell interaction. Therefore, the lytic process can be treated as a series of individual lethal events. Although release of intracellular components from the target cell can be totally arrested by lowering the surrounding temperature, damaged target cells will disintegrate once the temperature is increased. This fact illustrates the irreversibility of target cell damage once a critical stage has been reached. Several hypotheses have been proposed to explain the lytic event. During CTL-target cell interaction, local changes in the target cell membrane may cause leakage of intracellular K^+ and influx of Na^+ ions and water, resulting in osmotic swelling and lysis. Alternatively, the firm adhesion of CTL to target cells may produce tangential shear forces on the membrane, leading to rupture. A third proposal involves activation of a membrane-bound phospholipase, causing removal of one fatty acid from phosphatidylcholine and resulting in the formation of lysophosphatidylcholine, a strong detergent and a potent cytolytic agent.

A correlation between lytic capacity and the number of cells in a CTL-containing population capable of binding to target cells has been demonstrated by utilizing the CTL-target cell conjugation technique and the ^{51}Cr release assay (2). In the conjugation technique, mixtures of CTL and target cells are cocentrifuged at room temperature and then vigorously suspended, and the number of CTL target clusters is determined microscopically. By utilizing this technique, the increase in cytolytic activity that follows alloimmunization has been shown to be due to increases in the concentration of CTL rather than to variation in the activity of individual CTL.

Cold target inhibition

The specificity of CTL activity may be examined by the methodology of cold target cell inhibition. In this procedure a population of immune T cells is incubated with ^{51}Cr-labeled target cells bearing the immunizing surface antigens. Next, these immunized T cells are mixed with equal volumes of ^{51}Cr-labeled target cells and unlabeled target cells. The amount of isotope released into the extracellular medium will be reduced by about one-half compared with a mixture in which all of the target cells are tagged. However, when the labeled target cells are mixed with other unlabeled cells bearing antigens to which the cells have not been immunized, there is no reduction in lysis as expressed by extracellular ^{51}Cr.

ASSAY FOR DIRECT LYMPHOCYTE-MEDIATED CYTOTOXICITY

Preparation of effector and target cells

Draw 10 ml of heparinized blood from the recipient for effector cells. Draw 10 ml of heparinized blood from the donor for target cells. Divide the blood into three sterile 10-ml test tubes, dilute with 2 parts sterile Hanks balanced salt solution to 1 part blood, and mix by inversion. Add 2 ml of Ficoll-Hypaque at room temperature by underlayering with a pipette. Centrifuge at $400 \times g$ for 15 min. Remove the interfaces, dilute with wash medium (RPMI 1640 medium with penicillin, streptomycin, and HEPES [N-2-hydroxyethylpiperazine-N'-2-ethanesulfonic acid] buffer, pH 7.3) at room temperature (three interfaces plus 2 ml of wash medium per tube), and centrifuge at $250 \times g$ for 10 min. Suspend each pellet in 10 ml of wash medium, and centrifuge at $200 \times g$ for 10 min.

Phytohemagglutinin blasts. Although freshly prepared peripheral blood lymphocytes can be used as CTL targets, sensitivity is improved if activated blasts are employed, principally because they are more susceptible to lysis. The background spontaneous release of ^{51}Cr may also be higher with blast cells, however. Phytohemagglutinin (PHA) blasts must be prepared in advance. They can be used between 3 and 6 days after initiation of the PHA culture.

1. To target cells at $10^6/ml$, add PHA to a concentration of 0.5 µg/ml.
2. Culture at 37°C in a humidified atmosphere of 5% CO_2–95% air.
3. On the day of assay, wash the cells at $200 \times g$ for 10 min, and proceed with ^{51}Cr labeling.

Note. PHA blasts are very fragile and should not be vigorously vortexed. Cryopreservation of PHA blasts is even more hazardous. It is wise to save some nonstimulated target cells in case PHA blasts prove to be of poor viability on the day of assay.

Other target cells. Cell lines, especially virally transformed, are usually used for the study of CTL against viruses. Each cell line may have peculiarities of culture and handling.

Labeling target cells

Resuspend 1×10^6 to 3×10^6 target cells in 0.2 to 0.4 ml of RPMI 1640 medium. Add 500 µCi of buffered ^{51}Cr solution. Add 3 drops of fetal calf serum or normal human serum to keep the pH neutral. Incubate and rock the suspensions at 37°C for 1 h. After incubation, add 8 ml of medium and centrifuge for 10 min at 1,500 rpm. Change the tubes and wash twice more. Adjust to 10^5 cells per ml in 10% normal human serum-RPMI 1640 medium.

Test procedure

1. Prepare a 10% normal human serum-RPMI 1640 solution (10% NHS-RPMI).
2. Set the test up with quadruplicate wells in a round-bottom microtiter plate, as follows.

Maximum release:
   150 µl of distilled water
   50 µl of target cells in 10% NHS-RPMI
Spontaneous release:
   150 µl of 10% NHS-RPMI solution
   50 µl of target cells in 10% NHS-RPMI
Experimental wells:
   100 µl of recipient cells in 10% NHS-RPMI
   50 µl of 10% NHS-RPMI solution
   50 µl of target cells in 10% NHS-RPMI

The number of target cells (5,000) may be reduced if labeling efficiency is high. Some workers are able to use as few as 1,000 cells.

Maximal release may also be assessed by lysis of target cells with detergent, such as by adding 150 μl of a 1:100 dilution of Triton-X or undiluted Isoterge.

Dilution of recipient cells is essential to generate a dose-response curve of lysis. Volumes are kept constant, and cells are diluted to represent final attacking/target cell ratios of 100:1, 50:1, 25:1, and lower in some cases. For 5,000 target cells in a final volume of 200 μl, these stock concentrations are 5×10^6, 2.5×10^6, and 1.25×10^6.

3. Centrifuge the plate at $100 \times g$ for 5 min.

4. Incubate the plate at 37°C for 4 h.

5. To harvest the plate, centrifuge it at $400 \times g$ at 4°C for 10 min. Remove 100 μl from each well, and place this volume in 2 ml of scintillation fluid for the counting of ^{51}Cr in a scintillation counter.

6. Calculate the percent specific lysis on the basis of the counts per minute in the wells as follows:

$$\% \text{ Specific lysis} = \frac{E - S}{M - S} \times 100$$

where E is the experimental counts per minute, S is the spontaneous counts per minute, and M is the maximum counts per minute.

Data can be expressed as the maximal percentage of specific ^{51}Cr release at 100:1 or by calculation of lytic units. A lytic unit is the number of effector cells which produce 50% lysis $\times 10^3$ and is derived from the dose-response curve. It is not truly an absolute number, as it can vary with the number of target cells used and conditions of the assay; however, when conditions are standardized, the lytic unit is a useful method for comparisons. When the percentage of specific lysis is plotted against the log of attacking/target cell ratio, a straight line is obtained from which the 50% lysis point is extrapolated.

Interpretation

Specific lysis of ≥5% may be considered a positive result. The use of Student's t test to yield a >95% confidence limit between the experimental and spontaneous release values is also recommended. Typical results are shown in Table 1.

Serum preparation

Draw 10 ml of blood from the recipient into a nonheparinized test tube to clot. Allow the blood to clot, remove the clot from the test tube, and centrifuge the clot at $400 \times g$ for 10 min. Remove the serum with a pipette, and place it in a test tube in a 56°C water bath for 45 min to inactivate it. Recipient serum can be used at this point.

Prepare normal human serum by pooling the serum from at least three normal males and passing it through a 0.45-μm Nalgene filter. Divide the serum into sterile 3-ml portions, and freeze it for later use.

ASSAY FOR CELL-MEDIATED LYMPHOLYSIS FROM AN IN VITRO MIXED LYMPHOCYTE CULTURE

The cellular products of an in vitro immune response, such as the allogeneic mixed lymphocyte response, can be assayed for the presence of CTL by methods similar to those described above. Cells are taken from culture, washed, and incubated with appropriate ^{51}Cr-labeled target cells for the standard 4-h incubation (5). Such an assay shows the capability of a patient to generate CTL, either against a specific donor in the case of a transplant or against a pool of randomly chosen individuals. This pool is used as a control for intact inducer and effector phases of the cellular immune response; for example, it can be used as a control on the CTL response to a virus to show whether or not the patient is nonspecifically suppressed. Frozen aliquots of pooled peripheral blood lymphocytes from three to six normal individuals can be prepared in advance for such a purpose.

1. Generation of effector cells in MLR. Cultures are set up in bulk in 3-ml sterile plastic tubes containing 1 ml of 1.5×10^6 gamma-irradiated (3,000 rads) stimulator cells and 1 ml of 1.5×10^6 responder cells, all in NHS-RPMI 1640, HEPES buffer, penicillin, streptomycin, and L-glutamine.

2. Harvest the cells at 6 days, wash them, and use them as effector cells as in the direct lymphocyte-mediated cytotoxicity assay.

3. If PHA-treated target cells are to be used, these cultures are started 3 days before the planned cell-mediated lympholysis assay.

Notes and troubleshooting

1. The longer the cells are chromated, the better the labeling. If total counts per aliquot of target cells are low, try longer incubation times on a rocking platform at 37°C.

2. If target cells are not used immediately after ^{51}Cr labeling, hold them at 4°C in McCoy medium. (RPMI 1640 can be toxic to cells at 4°C.)

3. Either a gamma counter or a beta liquid scintillation counter can be used, although efficiency is generally better with a liquid system. Use a solvent system capable of accepting the necessary aqueous volume (e.g., Liquiscint).

4. High spontaneous release (SR) indicates low viability of target cells or inadequate washing of targets after washing. The SR should be 5 to 25% of the maximal release (MR). If the SR is >60% of the MR, then the assay must be considered a technical failure.

5. Low MR can be due to an inadequate incubation time or a mistake made in adding the lysing reagent. Also, ^{51}Cr preparations must be used when fairly fresh, their specific activity should be greater than 300 mCi/mg, and their concentrations should be at >1 mCi/ml.

TABLE 1. Typical values in lymphocyte-mediated cytotoxicity assay

Attacking/ target cell ratio	Assay values (cpm) in:			% Specific ^{51}Cr release
	Experimental release	Spontaneous release	Maximum release	
100:1	835	234	3,015	29
50:1	625	234	3,015	14
25:1	373	234	3,015	5

REAGENTS AND SUPPLIES

RPMI 1640 medium

0.005 M HEPES (*N*-2-hydroxyethylpiperazine-*N'*-2-ethanesulfonic acid; Calbiochem-Behring, San Diego, Calif.)

Penicillin (5,000 U) and streptomycin (5,000 μg/ml) stock. Add to 1% final dilution in RPMI 1640.

L-Glutamine, 200 mM (29.2 mg/ml) stock. Add to 1% final dilution.

Hanks balanced salt solution, sterile

Ficoll-Hypaque solution (Pharmacia Diagnostics, Piscataway, N.J.)

Normal human serum. Pooled human male blood group AB preferred. Fetal calf serum, screened for nontoxicity to human lymphocytes in culture, is an alternative. Sera are heat inactivated at 56°C for 1 h before use.

Sterile plastic culture tubes, for cell washing and preparation. Nunc polystyrene 10 ml (100 by 15 mm) and 3 ml (70 by 11 mm) (Vanguard International, Neptune, N.J.)

Sodium chromate ^{51}Cr, (>300 mCi/mg) (New England Nuclear Corp., Boston, Mass.)

Microtiter plates, 96 well, round bottom, sterile (Costar, Cambridge, Mass.)

Phytohemagglutinin P (Burroughs-Wellcome Corp., Research Triangle Park, N.C.)

Isoterge (Coulter Electronics, Inc., Hialeah, Fla.)

Liquiscint (National Diagnostics, Somerville, N.J.)

LITERATURE CITED

1. **Lanier, L. L., E. G. Engleman, P. Gatenby, G. F. Babcock, N. L. Warner, and L. A. Herzenberg.** 1983. Correlation of functional properties of human lymphoid cell subsets and surface marker phenotypes using multiparameter analysis and flow cytometry. Immunol. Rev. **74:**143–160.

2. **Martz, E.** 1975. Early steps in specific tumor cell lysis by sensitized mouse T lymphocytes. I. Resolution and characterization. J. Immunol. **115:**261–267.

3. **Martz, E.** 1977. Mechanism of specific tumor-cell lysis by alloimmune T lymphocytes: resolution and characterization of discrete steps in the cellular interaction. Contemp. Top. Immunobiol. **7:**301–361.

4. **Reinherz, E. L., S. C. Meuer, and S. F. Schlossman.** 1983. The delineation of antigen receptors on human T lymphocytes. Immunol. Today **4:**5–7.

5. **Schendel, D. J., R. Wank, and B. Dupont.** 1979. Standardization of the human in vitro cell-mediated lympholysis technique. Tissue Antigens **13:**112–120.

6. **Shaw, S., G. M. Shearer, and W. E. Biddison.** 1980. Human cytotoxic T-cell responses to type A and type B influenza viruses can be restricted by different HLA antigens. J. Exp. Med. **151:**235–245.

Chapter 44

Natural Killer Cell Activity and Antibody-Dependent Cell-Mediated Cytotoxicity

RONALD B. HERBERMAN

One of the major mechanisms by which the immune response deals with foreign or abnormal cells is to damage or destroy them. Such immunologic cytotoxicity may lead to complete loss of viability of the target cells (cytolysis) or an inhibition of the ability of the cells to continuc growing (cytostasis). Immunologic cytotoxicity can be manifested against a wide variety of target cells. These include malignant cells, normal cells from individuals unrelated to the responding host, and normal cells of the host that are infected with viruses or other microorganisms. In addition, the immune system can cause direct cytotoxic effects on some microorganisms, including bacteria, parasites, and fungi. Immunologic cytotoxicity is a principal mechanism by which the immune response copes with and often eliminates foreign materials or abnormal cells. Cytotoxic reactions are frequently observed as a major component of an immune response that develops after exposure to foreign cells or microorganisms. In addition, there is increasing recent evidence that cytotoxic reactions represent a major mechanism for natural immunity and resistance to such materials. In most instances, cytotoxicity by immune components requires the recognition of particular structures on the target cells; in addition, the targets need to be susceptible to attack by the immune components. Some cells are quite resistant to immunologic cytotoxicity, and this appears to represent a major mechanism by which they can escape control by the immune system.

There are a variety of mechanisms for immunologic cytotoxicity. The two main categories are antibody- and cell-mediated cytotoxicity. Within cell-mediated cytotoxicity, a multiplicity of effector cell types and mechanisms can be involved. The characteristics and functions of cytotoxic T lymphocytes (CTL) are described elsewhere in this manual. This chapter will emphasize information related to natural killer (NK) cells and antibody-dependent cell-mediated cytotoxicity (ADCC), discuss the similarities and differences between these effectors, and compare their characteristics with those of CTL.

NATURAL KILLER CELLS

NK cells were discovered about 12 years ago during studies of cell-mediated cytotoxicity. Although investigators expected to find specific cytotoxic activity of tumor-bearing individuals against autologous tumor cells or against allogeneic tumors of similar or the same histologic type, appreciable cytotoxic activity was also observed with lymphocytes from normal individuals. With the wide array of recent studies related to natural cell-mediated cytotoxicity, there has been considerable diversity in the terminology related to the effector cells, and consequently some confusion in the literature. However, at a recent workshop devoted to the study of NK cells, a consensus definition for these effector cells was developed (4). NK cells were defined as effector cells with spontaneous cytotoxicity against various target cells; these effector cells lack the properties of classical macrophages, granulocytes, or CTL; and the observed cytotoxicity does not show restriction related to the major histocompatibility complex. This definition is sufficiently broad to include not only "classical" NK cells but also other natural effector cells such as natural cytotoxic cells. The workshop participants agreed that the observations relating to the development of cytotoxic cells in culture (e.g., lectin-activated killers, anomalous killers) remain difficult to interpret and that, for the moment, it is best to categorize separately cultured or activated cells with cytotoxic reactivity that cannot be classified as CTL.

Until recently, the cells responsible for NK activity could be defined only in a negative way, i.e., by distinguishing them from typical T cells, B cells, or macrophages. However, it is now possible to isolate highly enriched populations and show that the NK activity is closely associated with a subpopulation of lymphocytes, morphologically identified as large granular lymphocytes (LGL), that comprise about 5% of peripheral blood lymphocytes and 1 to 3% of total mononuclear cells. LGL, which contain azurophilic cytoplasmic granules, can be isolated by discontinuous density gradient centrifugation on Percoll. LGL are nonphagocytic, nonadherent cells that lack surface immunoglobulin or receptors for the third component of complement but contain cell-surface receptors for the Fc portion of immunoglobulin G (IgG) (3, 4). This latter quality allows them to bind antibody-coated target cells and mediate ADCC, a function previously attributed to the K (killer) cell. Hence, the same cells (i.e., NK and K cells) seem able to mediate both forms of cytotoxicity, with NK activity due to NK receptors discrete from the Fc receptors that interact with target cell-bound antibody.

Approximately one-half of human NK cells and LGL express detectable receptors for sheep erythrocytes, as measured by rosette formation at 4°C. However, some monoclonal antibodies to the sheep erythrocyte receptor react with a considerably higher proportion of LGL. Analogously, a proportion of mouse NK cells express Thy 1 antigens, and most rat NK cells express OX-8 and some other T-cell-associated markers. Thus, although NK cells are clearly not thymus dependent (since high levels of activity have been detected in athymic nude mice or in neonatally thymectomized mice), they share many characteristics associated with CTL and other T cells.

Although LGL appear to account for most NK activity in humans, other primates, and rodents, not all

LGL possess measurable NK activity. One possible explanation for the lack of detectable cytotoxic activity in some LGL is that the array of target cells tested has not been sufficient to reflect the entire repertoire and that some LGL may recognize and lyse only a limited variety of target cells. Despite this potential limitation, tests of human LGL against several NK-susceptible target cell lines in a single-cell cytotoxicity assay result in the estimate that in most normal individuals, after activation of the cells with interferon, 75 to 85% of the LGL are capable of killing at least one NK-susceptible target cell line. The nature of the other 15 or 20% of the LGL, with no detectable cytolytic activity, is unclear. They may represent a distinct subset of cells that inherently lack this functional capability, or they may simply be at a noncytolytic stage of differentiation or activation.

In regard to the converse issue, of whether all NK cells are LGL, the available data are not conclusive. However, as discussed above, LGL account for a high proportion of detectable NK activity, and in the conventional assays for cytotoxic activity, cell populations depleted of LGL show little if any NK activity.

Some cell surface antigens, particularly those detected by monoclonal antibodies, have been found on virtually all NK cells. They therefore help to characterize the phenotype of these effector cells. For example, most human NK cells react with the following antibodies: (i) several monoclonal antibodies (B73.1, 3G8, Leu 11) reactive with Fc receptors for IgG on LGL (3G8 and Leu 11 also are strongly expressed on granulocytes); (ii) rabbit antisera to the glycolipid asialo GM$_1$, which also react with monocytes and granulocytes; (iii) OKT10, which also reacts with most thymocytes and activated lymphocytes; and (iv) OKM1, which also reacts with monocytes and macrophages, granulocytes, and platelets. Removal of cells bearing any of these markers, either by treatment with antibody plus complement or by negative-selection immunoaffinity procedures, results in a depletion of most or all detectable NK activity.

NK cells can also be characterized by a lack of expression of certain cell surface markers. For example, human NK cells have no detectable surface reactivity with monoclonal antibodies to pan-T-cell antigens such as Leu 1 or OKT3 or to T-helper antigens as defined by OKT4 or Leu 3. Human NK cells also do not express surface antigens detected by a number of monocyte-specific reagents such as MO2 and Leu M1.

In contrast to a pattern of features common to most or all CTL, NK cells and also LGL in general are rather heterogeneous with respect to other monoclonal antibody-defined markers. Human NK cells react to a variable extent with monoclonal antibodies directed against the sheep erythrocyte receptors (Lyt 3, OKT11, Leu 5), with only about half of the NK cells in some experiments giving positive results. Only a portion of human NK cells have been shown to react with a variety of other monoclonals, including 3A1 (on most CTL and other T cells and 50 to 60% of LGL), HNK1 (on 40 to 60% of NK cells), and OKT8 (on the suppressor-cytotoxic T lymphocytes and 10 to 30% of LGL). About 25% of the LGL react with monoclonal antibodies against Ia framework (HLA-DR) determinants.

Although most NK cells and LGL are nonadherent to plastic or nylon wool, a subset of these cells show some adherence. For instance, when human myelomonocytic cells are isolated by means of their adherence to plastic, the small percentage of contaminating cells is disproportionately composed of LGL. Although this subpopulation of cells shares the adherence property with myelomonocytic cells, it retains the morphology and cell surface characteristics of LGL. The phenotype of human adherent NK cells has been shown to be OKT3$^-$ OKT10$^+$ OKT11$^+$ OKM1$^+$ Leu M1$^-$ B73.1$^+$. Such cells thus contrast with typical adherent monocytes, which only react with OKM1 and Leu M1.

In summary, NK cells have a characteristic phenotype. For example, most human NK cells and LGL can be described as OKT3$^-$ OKT4$^-$ OKT10$^+$ B73.1$^+$ OKM1$^+$ Leu M1$^-$. Thus, these cells have a readily definable and general phenotype which sets them apart from all other lymphoid cell types. The heterogeneity in cell surface phenotypes extends to only a few markers, e.g., with human NK cells: OKT8, HNK1, Ia, and OKT11.

There is increasing evidence that NK cells play a major role in natural resistance against tumors, particularly against the metastatic spread of tumor cells (3). They have also been shown to be involved in natural resistance against infections by certain viruses (especially herpesviruses), fungi (Cryptococcus), and parasites (especially trypanosomes). In addition, and as a probable corollary of the ability of NK cells to react against the subpopulation of normal bone marrow cells, including the colony-forming units, NK cells appear to play an important role in rejection of grafts of foreign bone marrow cells, and they may also be involved in regulation of normal hematopoiesis in the autologous individual. Similarly, in view of the demonstrated ability of LGL to secrete appreciable levels of a variety of cytokines, it seems likely that the cell population may have important immunoregulatory functions in addition to its direct cytotoxic activities.

ANTIBODY-DEPENDENT CELL-MEDIATED CYTOTOXICITY

Immunologic cytotoxicity also can be mediated by a collaboration between immune or natural antibodies and certain immunologic effector cells. Known as ADCC, this collaboration appears to be a potent mechanism for elimination of some microorganisms and may also be involved in the destruction of tumors and other foreign cells. ADCC usually consists of binding of immunoglobulins of the G class to target cells, followed by the binding of certain types of effector cells to the target cells by means of cell surface receptors for the Fc portion of IgG. After such binding, lysis of the targets may result. Several distinct cell types with Fc receptors have been shown to be capable of mediating ADCC. These include macrophages, granulocytes, and a lymphocyte subpopulation initially termed the K cell and recently shown to be mediated by LGL. LGL appear to be responsible for most ADCC activity against tumor target cells and other nucleated human target cells.

Assays for ADCC could have two useful clinical applications. The first would be to assess the functional activities of the particular subpopulations of effector cells. This might be a helpful addition to the usual array of assays used to assess cellular immune competence in patients with various diseases. Although little information on this application is available, the results thus far have been of some interest. A population of cancer patients was found to have significantly depressed K-cell activity, but depression did not correlate with stage of disease. However, in some other cancer patients and in some patients with various other diseases, levels of ADCC against tumor target cells have been reported to be in the normal range, even in patients with depressed NK activity. Thus, although LGL appear to be responsible for both forms of cytotoxicity, the levels of NK and ADCC reactivity are not necessarily concordant.

The other main clinical application for ADCC has been the study of specific antibody reactivity against alloantigens, viruses, or tumor cells. Studies of sera from potential graft recipients for antibodies active in ADCC may be a useful addition to the more usual cross-matching procedures. Such antibodies have been detected in the sera of some patients undergoing hyperacute graft rejection. The sensitivity for detection of alloantibodies in the sera of those patients and in multiparous women has been greater than that seen in complement-dependent cytotoxicity assays. In addition, much of the cell-mediated cytotoxic reactivity of immune individuals against virus-infected target cells has been attributed to ADCC.

An in vivo role for ADCC in resistance against tumors or microbial infections has not been clearly established. However, it is quite possible that NK cells and other effectors with the capability of exerting ADCC mediate their in vivo effects by this mechanism as well as by their direct cytotoxic reactivity. The recent demonstration of in vivo antitumor effects by some IgG monoclonal antibodies has lent support to the possible importance of ADCC. The monoclonal antibody-induced resistance did not appear to be dependent on complement, and therefore collaboration with LGL or macrophages for ADCC seems likely.

REGULATION OF CYTOTOXIC ACTIVITY OF EFFECTOR CELLS

Interferon (IFN) has been shown to augment potently the activity of NK cells. In vivo administration to mice or rats of a variety of IFN inducers, or of IFN itself, led to rapid boosting of NK activity. Similarly, incubation in vitro of human or rodent lymphoid cells or of purified LGL with IFN induced considerable augmentation of NK activity. Almost all of the proteins with antiviral activity that have been studied, including various species of IFN-α, IFN-β, and IFN-γ, have had the ability to increase NK activity significantly. The one exception found to date has been IFN-α J, which, although apparently able to bind to LGL, induced no boosting of NK activity after treatment of human NK cells for several hours, and induced low levels of boosting after overnight incubation (7). In addition, there have been considerable quantitative differences in the efficacy of boosting by the various species of IFN. Some species have been shown to be high-level boosters, with greater than 50% increase in NK activity by less than 50 U of IFN,

whereas other IFN species have been found to have low-level boosting activity, with an increase in NK activity by 50% only seen with 500 U or more of IFN.

Detailed studies on the mechanisms by which IFN augments NK activity have recently been considerably facilitated by the ability to identify morphologically and purify human NK cells. With some target cells, but not with others, one action of IFN is to convert pre-NK cells into cells able to recognize and bind to the targets. In addition, IFN pretreatment has caused an accelerated rate of lysis of bound target cells. IFN has also been shown to increase interactions with target cells by increasing the degree of recycling, i.e., facilitating the interaction with, and lysis of, multiple target cells during the cytotoxicity assay. Yet another aspect of the effect of IFN on the interactions between NK cells and targets, recently demonstrated, is the ability of IFN to protect certain target cells from lysis by NK cells.

NK cells have also been shown to respond to interleukin 2 (IL-2) and can be maintained in culture. However, cytolytic activity has been observed against NK-susceptible target cells not only in clear-cut situations in which the cell cultures were initiated with highly purified LGL which retain their morphologic and cytotoxic characteristics, but also when the cultures were initiated with unseparated lymphoid populations. Since the relationship of the generated cytotoxic effector cells to NK cells remains somewhat unclear, it seems best to refer to such activities as activated killer cells.

Recently, lymphokine-activated killer cells have been described (1) which share many of the characteristics of the previously described culture-activated NK-like cells. Lymphokine-activated killer cells have been activated after a short period of culture in vitro with highly purified IL-2 and display cytotoxic activity against a variety of autologous, allogeneic, and xenogeneic tumors. These cells lack markers typical of fresh NK cells (i.e., they have been reported to be OKM1$^-$ OKT10$^-$ OKT11$^-$) and appear devoid of cytolytic activity before culture. The exact relationship between NK cells and lymphokine-activated killer cells requires further investigation.

In addition to its ability to promote the proliferation of T cells, LGL, and possibly other cytotoxic effector cells, IL-2 has been found to strongly stimulate both human and mouse NK activity (8). Endogenous production of IL-2 may be responsible, or at least required, for maintenance of spontaneous human NK activity, since preincubation of human LGL with monoclonal antibodies to IL-2 for about 20 h resulted in a complete loss of NK activity, which could be reversed by addition of IL-2. The IL-2 boosting of NK activity appears to result from a direct interaction of the lymphokine with LGL. This boosting was observed with Tac antigen-negative LGL and was not abrogated by monoclonal anti-Tac antibodies. Thus, it appears that the Tac antigen is not involved in this immunoregulatory effect of IL-2 on NK cells, whereas it is required for IL-2-induced proliferation of LGL as well as T cells. These results suggest that LGL may express receptors for IL-2 which are distinct from Tac and which mediate the boosting of cytotoxic reactivity. This Tac-independent interaction of IL-2 with LGL also results in the secretion of IFN-γ.

INTERACTIONS BETWEEN EFFECTOR AND TARGET CELLS WHICH LEAD TO CYTOTOXICITY

As a result of efforts to dissect the mechanisms involved in the interactions between cytotoxic effector cells and target cells, it has been possible to define a sequence of events which appear to be required for the lytic process. These steps were first described for CTL, and subsequently a similar sequence has been shown to be involved in NK activity (4). The main stages can be identified as: (i) recognition of target cells by effector cells; (ii) binding of effectors to targets; (iii) activation of lytic machinery of effector cells; (iv) lytic effects on target cells, often referred to as the "lytic hit"; and (v) effector cell-independent dissolution of the targets.

The recognition event appears to be dependent on two types of structures, the cell surface recognition receptors on the effector cells and the antigens or other structures on the target cells which need to be recognized. There has as yet been little documentation of the nature of the recognition receptors on NK cells. The main issue currently is whether NK cells have structures directly analogous to the T-cell receptor. The available data suggest that NK activity is dependent on a different type of receptor.

There is also little definitive information about the nature of the target structures recognized by NK cells. NK cells react against a wide variety of syngeneic, allogeneic, and xenogeneic tumor cells. Susceptibility to cytotoxic activity is not restricted to malignant cells; fetal cells, virus-infected cells, and subpopulations of normal lymphoid or hematopoietic stem cells (thymus cells, bone marrow cells) are susceptible to lysis by NK cells. In contrast to cytolytic T lymphocytes, NK cells demonstrate no known MHC restriction. In fact, they have strong reactivity against MHC-deficient targets (e.g., K562), and their activity is not inhibited by antibodies against MHC determinants. Differentiation antigens may be a major type of target-cell structure recognized by NK cells. Studies with maturational agents and with a wide variety of target cells indicate that undifferentiated cells are generally more susceptible NK targets. In further support of this possibility, normal lymphoid cells are totally insensitive to NK lysis, whereas a subpopulation of relatively immature hematopoietic thymus and bone marrow cells is susceptible to cytolysis.

A central issue in the study of the specificity of NK cells is whether one common target structure is recognized by all NK cells or whether subsets of NK cells recognize a variety of target-cell structures. The available data indicate that distinct subsets of NK cells appear to possess different patterns of reactivity, rather than nonselective reactivity of each NK cell against the wide array of susceptible targets (6).

After the requisite recognition of target cells by effectors and their binding together to form conjugates, a complex series of events are initiated which lead to the lysis of the target cells. Many of the early biochemical changes in the effector cells and the clear definition of a Ca^{2+}-dependent step have been found to be similar for CTL and NK cells. However, the actual mechanism underlying the lethal hit has been difficult to identify.

A recent major advance in our understanding of the possible mechanism involved in lysis by NK cells has come from studies with cytoplasmic granules isolated from LGL (2). Observations of human LGL-target cell conjugates by electron microscopy indicated the secretion of granules in close proximity to the target cell membrane. To evaluate directly the possible role of such granules in the lytic mechanism, they were isolated from rat LGL leukemias with NK activity. Granules containing β-glucuronidase and other lysosomal enzymes were purified on Percoll gradients and shown to have potent calcium-dependent lytic activity not only against tumor target cells but also against a wide variety of normal cells, particularly sheep erythrocytes. A potent protein cytolysin could be solubilized from the LGL granules. It was possible to isolate such highly cytolytic granules from normal rat and human LGL as well as from the rat leukemic LGL, whereas lysosomal granules isolated from liver, granulocytes, and a variety of other cell types had no detectable cytolytic activity. To determine whether the potent granule cytolysin was responsible for the lytic activity of NK cells, rabbit antibodies were prepared against the purified granules from rat leukemia cells. These antibodies and $F(ab')_2$ fragments prepared from them were able to block the cytolytic activity of purified LGL granules and also of rat NK cells. The antibodies were also found to cross-react with human NK cells and at least partially block their NK and ADCC activities.

The granule-induced lytic activity was found to be associated with the formation of ringlike structures on the surface of the target cells, which were detectable by electron microscopy. The LGL granules and the solubilized cytolysin could also be shown to lyse liposomes, and the affected liposomes had porelike structures inserted into their lipid bilayer. These porelike lesions, which were demonstrated by electron microscopy, were quite similar to those previously observed with target cells lysed by NK cells or by K cells and were shown to be cylindrical structures 15 nm in diameter. The appearance and other features of the lesions were very similar to, but about twice the diameter of, the previously described channels produced by the membrane attack complex of complement. It is also noteworthy that the ringlike structures associated with cytotoxicity by LGL are very similar to those described on target cells affected by CTL.

Taken together, the available evidence would fit well into the following sequence: NK cells and perhaps also CTL, upon recognition of, and binding to, target cells, are triggered to release the granule-associated cytolysin, which can insert into the target cell membrane and lead to the death of the targets.

ASSAY PROCEDURES

Materials

Assay medium. A variety of media can be utilized for suspending the target cells and effector cells. The cell culture medium in which the target cells are normally passaged is suitable for the assay. A quite satisfactory medium is RPMI 1640 medium supplemented with 5% fetal bovine serum, 25 mM HEPES (N-2-hydroxyethylpiperazine-N'-2-ethanesulfonic acid) buffer, penicillin (100 μg/ml), and streptomycin (100 μg/ml).

For enrichment of NK and K cells, density gradients of Percoll (Pharmacia Fine Chemicals, Piscataway, N.J.) have been used. The osmolality of the Percoll must be adjusted to 285 mosmol/kg of water with 10×-concentrated phosphate-buffered saline.

IFN. Crude or partially purified human IFN preparations (either α, β, or γ) have been found to be satisfactory. In addition, comparable results have been obtained with homogeneous human natural or recombinant IFNs.

IL-2. Culture supernatants containing IL-2 or partially purified IL-2 have been satisfactory, but for definitive studies of the effects of IL-2 in the absence of other cytokines, homogeneous natural or recombinant IL-2 is preferable.

Assay for NK and ADCC activities

Effector cells. Human peripheral blood mononuclear leukocytes of normal, adult donors or of patients are separated from heparinized blood by centrifugation on a Ficoll-Hypaque density gradient in a 50-ml graduated conical plastic centrifuge tube (Falcon Plastics, Los Angeles, Calif.). This procedure provides mononuclear cells with a yield of greater than 95% and viability greater than 90%. The cells are washed twice (centrifugation first at $390 \times g$ for 10 min and second at $200 \times g$ for 8 min) with Hanks balanced salt solution (without serum) and suspended to the desired concentration in assay medium. Monocytes can be effectively removed from the mononuclear cell suspension by adherence to nylon wool or Sephadex G-10 (Pharmacia). For separation by adherence to nylon wool, up to 10^9 leukocytes in 10 ml of warm medium (37°C) can be added to a prewarmed column containing 5 g of scrubbed nylon-wool fibers. After incubation at 37°C for 45 min, the column is flushed with 100 ml of assay medium. Alternatively, up to 10^8 leukocytes can be added to a column of 5 ml of packed Sephadex G-10, prewashed with Hanks balanced salt solution. After incubation at room temperature for 15 min, the column is flushed with 50 ml of Hanks balanced salt solution. The nonadherent cells (containing <1% monocytes) are collected (centrifugation at $390 \times g$ for 7 min) and suspended in assay medium.

For detailed characterization or mechanistic studies, it is very helpful to work with enriched populations of effector cells. LGL, separated on discontinuous Percoll density gradients, have been found to account for virtually all of the NK and ADCC activities. Separation of the LGL with high cytotoxic activity and almost devoid of other lymphoid cell types is particularly advantageous for characterization of the effector cells and for examination of the mechanism of augmentation of function.

To obtain highly purified LGL, nonadherent mononuclear cells are separated on Percoll density gradients. A discontinuous gradient of Percoll is prepared by carefully layering a series of fractions with various concentrations of Percoll (from 37 to 60%) into a 15-ml conical test tube (no. 2095, Falcon). These fractions are made by mixing Percoll (osmolality adjusted to 285 mosmol/kg of water; this can usually be obtained by mixing 27.81 ml of Percoll with 2.19 ml of 10×-concentrated phosphate-buffered saline) with RPMI 1640 medium, supplemented with 10% fetal bovine

TABLE 1. Construction of discontinuous Percoll density gradient for purification of LGL

Fraction	Density (refractive index at 25°C)	Usual vol of Percoll (μl) in a 6-ml mixture
1	1.3432	2,500
2	1.3436	2,700
3	1.3440	2,850
4	1.3443	3,000
5	1.3446	3,150
6	1.3450	3,300
7	1.3470	4,000

serum and 5 mM HEPES (adjusted to 280 to 285 mosmol). The proportions of Percoll and medium in each fraction are given in Table 1. It is essential that the density of each fraction, as measured with a refractometer, be correct. If the density of the osmolality-corrected Percoll is 1.125 g/ml and that of the medium is 1.0284 g/ml, then the fractions can be made by mixing the volumes of Percoll indicated in Table 1 with medium to give a total volume of 6,000 μl. The gradient is constructed with 2.5 ml of the first three fractions and 1.5 ml of the last four, added in order of decreasing density.

For separation of peripheral blood lymphocytes, 5×10^7 cells in 1.5 ml of medium are placed on the top of the gradient, which is then centrifuged at $550 \times g$ for 30 min at room temperature. Acceleration and deceleration should be slow. Fractions are then collected from the top with a Pasteur pipette. Most LGL and the associated NK and ADCC activities should be in fractions 2 and 3 (peak in fraction 3), whereas most of the cells recovered should be in fraction 6 or 7 (5 to 15% of input cells in fractions 2 and 3 and 40 to 70% in fractions 6 and 7, with usual overall recovery of 90%).

Augmentation of cytotoxic activity with IFN or IL-2

A total of 2×10^6 to 10×10^6 lymphocytes or LGL in 1 ml of assay medium are incubated at 37°C with IFN or IL-2. Optimal and consistent augmentation of NK activity by IFN-α or -β is achieved with incubation for 60 to 180 min. Routinely, 1,000 U of IFN is used, but lower concentrations can be effective. Dose-responsive effects are usually observed between 100 and 1,000 U. For augmentation of NK activity with IFN-γ or IL-2, or for augmentation of ADCC activity, overnight incubation is usually required for optimal results. After incubation with the augmenting agent, the cells are washed with medium and suspended at the concentrations needed for the cytotoxicity assay. The presence of IFN during the assay is not desirable, since it may decrease the sensitivity of the target cells to lysis.

Assay for NK activity. The untreated or treated effector cells are tested for cytotoxic activity in a 4-h ^{51}Cr release assay. Various target cells are suitable, but K-562, a tumor cell line derived from a patient with chronic myelogenous leukemia in blast crisis, has usually been found to be most sensitive for measurement of NK activity. The target cells (2×10^6 to 4×10^6 in 0.6 ml of assay medium) are labeled with 150 μCi of ^{51}Cr (as sodium chromate; New England Nuclear Corp., Boston, Mass.) for 45 to 60 min. Cells are washed (centrifugation at 285 × g for 8 min), suspended in assay medium, and adjusted to the desired concentrations. Target cells (5×10^3 per reaction) are mixed with effector cells (ranging from 5×10^5 to 5×10^3 cells per reaction), with resultant 100:1 to 1:1 effector-to-target cell ratios (E:T), in Linbro U-bottomed 96-well microtiter plates. Plates with reaction mixtures of 0.1 ml of targets and 0.1 ml of effectors are incubated, with lids on, in a 5% CO_2-air atmosphere for 4 h at 37°C. All reactions are performed at least in triplicate. Autologous controls (unlabeled target cells added, in place of effector cells, to the labeled targets) are employed for base-line release values in all experiments. The supernatants can be conveniently harvested with the Titertek Harvesting System (Flow Laboratories, Rockville, Md.). Radioactivity in the supernatants is counted in a gamma scintillation counter. The percentage of isotope released from the target cells is calculated by the following formula:

$$\text{Percent release} = \frac{\text{cpm released from cells during incubation}}{\text{total cpm incorporated into cells}} \times 100$$

The percent specific cytotoxicity (a) is calculated as $a = b - c$, when b is the percent release in the experimental group and c is the percent release in the autologous control.

Assay for ADCC

Untreated or treated effector cells are tested for ADCC in the same 4-h ^{51}Cr release assay described above for NK activity. The differences between the tests involve the use of other target cells, coated with IgG antibodies. The percent ADCC is calculated by subtracting the percent cytotoxicity against the non-antibody-coated target cells from that obtained with antibody-coated targets.

A variety of target cells can be used for ADCC. However, for optimal interpretation of results, a target cell line that is highly resistant to NK activity should be used. When target cells with some degree of susceptibility to NK activity are used, higher NK levels will be seen in the interaction of IFN- or IL-2-treated effector cells with the non-antibody-coated target cells. Thus, it would be difficult to discriminate the contribution of augmented NK and ADCC activities against antibody-coated target cells. For studies of ADCC in my laboratory, some mouse T-cell lymphomas (YAC-1, RBL-5, RL♂1, EL-4) have been very useful, since they are resistant to human NK activity and are highly sensitive to ADCC when coated with a rabbit anti-mouse T-cell serum.

The source of antibody used to sensitize the target cells may also be an important factor in the demonstration of ADCC. Consistent ADCC activity has been seen with rabbit antibodies, whereas only some human antibodies or mouse monoclonal antibodies give positive results.

Analysis of data

Positive results in the cytotoxicity assay are generally defined as experimental release of radioactivity being significantly higher than the base-line, autologous control (Student's t test, $P < 0.05$). In most studies, it is necessary to make quantitative comparisons between levels of cytotoxic reactivity in various experimental groups. Three main types of comparisons are usually required, as follows.

(i) Within experiments, one frequently needs to compare the spontaneous levels of NK activity by a donor's cells with the levels of reactivity after pretreatment of the cells. Pretreatment of effector cells with IFN or IL-2 usually results in appreciable augmentation of NK activity at all ratios of effector cells to target cells. However, the degree of boosting of activity varies substantially among normal donors, and no augmentation may be observed with effector cells from some patients. Various methods can be used to analyze the degree of augmentation. The percent cytotoxicities of treated and untreated cells, at one effector/target cell ratio, can be compared. Such a comparison lends itself well to determination of the significance of the difference between the two points by Student's t test. Alternatively, lytic units (LU) for each cell population can be calculated. An LU is defined as the number of effector cells needed to give a certain level of cytotoxicity (e.g., 30%). Calculation of the number of LU per 10^7 cells provides an overall quantitative expression of the data for the entire dose-response curve of each group. Then the differences between the treated and untreated cells can be expressed as the percentage of activity in the treated population relative to the untreated, or as the difference in LU between the treated and untreated cells. Comparison of LU between groups provides the best quantitative assessment of the degree of augmentation of reactivity. Comparison of percent cytotoxicity values at one effector/target cell ratio can give misleading results, particularly if one or both of the points are not on the linear portion of the dose-response curve. However, there are also some limitations to the use of the LU method. Valid calculations of LU can only be determined from the linear portion of the cytotoxic dose-response curve. Also, LU from two experimental groups can only be compared if the slopes of the dose-response curves are parallel. Usually treatment of IFN or IL-2 does result in a curve of augmented cytotoxicity that is parallel with that for the untreated effecter cells.

(ii) In many other situations, it is necessary to compare the levels of cytotoxicity of one group of individuals with those of another group, e.g., comparison of reactivity of patients with a given disease or treatment with that of normal donors. Such comparisons can be performed on the basis of the percent cytotoxicity of each donor at the same effector-to-target cell ratio or, preferably, on the basis of the LU of reactivity. The latter type of calculation needs to be modified from that described above to allow satisfactory comparisons of data from different experiments, even when the slopes of dose-response curves vary (9). Since the cytotoxic reactivity data from patient groups are often not distributed normally, statistical comparisons between groups should be done with a nonparametric method, e.g., Kruskall-Wallis or Wilcoxon tests.

(iii) In an increasing number of studies of clinical treatments of patients with various diseases, serial monitoring of cytotoxic reactivity is performed. The objective is to determine whether the treatment can produce a significant alteration from the pretreatment levels of NK activity, ADCC activity, or both. For correct interpretation of results, it is necessary to utilize the proper study design and procedures for data analysis. First, it is necessary to determine, by repeated testing before treatment, an individual's base-line level of reactivity and the degree of test-to-test variation. Then the levels of reactivity during and after treatment can be compared with the pretreatment limits of variability. As an example, this approach has been utilized to analyze the effects of IFN on NK activity in cancer patients (5).

LITERATURE CITED

1. **Grimm, E. A., A. Mazumder, H. Z. Zhang, and S. A. Rosenberg.** 1982. Lymphokine activated killer cell phenomenon. Lysis of natural killer resistant fresh solid tumor cells by interleukin 2-activated autologous human peripheral blood lymphocytes. J. Exp. Med. **155**:823–830.
2. **Henkart, P., M. Henkart, P. Millard, R. Blumenthal, and C. W. Reynolds.** 1985. The role of cytoplasmic granules in NK cell cytotoxicity, p. 305–322. *In* R. B. Herberman and D. M. Callewaert (ed.), Mechanisms of cytotoxicity by NK cells. Academic Press, Inc., Orlando, Fla.
3. **Herberman, R. B. (ed.).** 1982. NK cells and other natural effector cells, p. 1566. Academic Press, Inc., New York.
4. **Herberman, R. B., and D. M. Callewaert (ed.).** 1985. Mechanisms of cytotoxicity by NK cells. Academic Press, Inc., New York.
5. **Maluish, A. E., J. R. Ortaldo, J. C. Conlon, S. A. Sherwin, R. Leavitt, D. M. Strong, P. Weirnik, R. K. Oldham, and R. B. Herberman.** 1983. Depression of natural killer cytotoxicity following in vivo administration of recombinant leukocyte interferon. J. Immunol. **131**:503–507.
6. **Ortaldo, J. R., and R. B. Herberman.** 1984. Heterogeneity of natural killer cells, p. 359–394. *In* W. E. Paul, C. G. Fathman, and H. Metzger (ed.), Annual review of immunology, vol. 2. Annual Reviews Inc., Palo Alto.
7. **Ortaldo, J. R., R. B. Herberman, C. Harvey, P. Osheroff, Y.-C. Pan, B. Kelder, and S. Pestka.** 1984. A species of human α-interferon that lacks the ability to boost human natural killer activity. Proc. Natl. Acad. Sci. U.S.A. **81**:4926–4929.
8. **Ortaldo, J. R., A. T. Mason, J. P. Gerard, L. E. Henderson, W. Farrar, R. R. Hopkins III, R. B. Herberman, and H. Rabin.** 1984. Effects of natural and recombinant IL-2 on regulation of IFN gamma production and natural killer activity: lack of involvement of the Tac antigen for these immunoregulatory effects. J. Immunol. **133**:779–783.
9. **Pross, H. F., M. T. Baines, P. Rubin, P. Shragge, and M. S. Patterson.** 1981. Spontaneous human lymphocyte mediated cytotoxicity against tumor target cell. IX. The quantitation of natural killer cell activity. J. Clin. Immunol. **1**:51–63.

Chapter 45

Assays for Suppressor Cells

JOSEPH B. MARGOLICK AND ANTHONY S. FAUCI

It has become clear over the past few years that a major mechanism of regulation of normal immunologic reactivity is the balance between positive and negative influences in the form of helper and suppressor cells. In animal models, suppressor cells have been the focus of a great deal of interest since they have been demonstrated to play a critical immunoregulatory role in a number of systems including immunologic tolerance, antigenic competition, cell-mediated immune reactions such as delayed hypersensitivity and contact sensitivity to various haptens, antibody responses to T-cell-dependent and -independent antigens, chronic allotypic suppression, and even the control of certain tumors (24). In certain mouse systems, by use of alloantisera against stable cell surface antigens of lymphocyte subpopulations (termed Lyt antigens), a complex feedback-regulated circuit of distinct immunoregulatory T-cell subsets has been identified (2). Abnormalities of certain of these subsets have been shown to be associated with autoimmune phenomena.

In humans, it has now been amply documented that T- and B-cell function is normally modulated by a complex interaction between responder cells, suppressor cells, and suppressor-inducer cells (17, 18, 24). Although we usually consider T cells to be the suppressor cells in most systems, monocytes and even B cells have been demonstrated to be the suppressor cells in certain systems (24). Of particular relevance is the fact that a number of disease states in humans have been shown to be associated with abnormalities of number, function, or both, of suppressor cell systems. To name just a few examples of this everincreasing group, overly active suppressor T cells have been demonstrated in certain patients with common variable hypogammaglobulinemia, isolated immunoglobulin deficiency, and acute infectious mononucleosis (14, 24). The antithesis of this is seen in certain autoimmune diseases, particularly systemic lupus erythematosus, in which quantitative and qualitative deficiencies of suppressor T cells have been described in association with hyperreactivity of B cells (reviewed in reference 5). In addition, adherent suppressor cells, most likely monocytes, have been demonstrated in the polyclonal immunoglobulin deficiency of multiple myeloma (24), in the anergy of Hodgkin's disease (23), and in patients with active sarcoidosis (15).

The present chapter deals predominantly with certain of the commonly used in vitro assays for suppressor cells in humans. Since a large number of human suppressor cell systems have been described over the past few years, this chapter will focus on only a few of the representative assays. These can be used to delineate the normally operable balance between suppressor and helper cells as well as to demonstrate abnormalities in the balance of number, function, or both, of immunoregulatory subpopulations of cells in diseases characterized by aberrancies of immune function.

CLINICAL INDICATIONS

The indications for the use of assays for suppressor cells are generally divided into the clinical settings of (i) hyporesponsiveness of immunologic reactivity demonstrable in vivo or in vitro or (ii) states of immunologic hyperreactivity, usually at the level of the B cell. The former situation is generally seen in patients with manifestations of decreased cell-mediated immunologic reactivity. This is usually first noted in vivo by cutaneous anergy seen in primary immunodeficiency states or in immunologic hyporeactivity secondarily associated with other primary diseases such as Hodgkin's disease (23) and sarcoidosis (15). In addition, and perhaps more impressive from the standpoint of in vitro demonstration, are the states of hypogammaglobulinemia or agammaglobulinemia, either of all immunoglobulin classes or of particular immunoglobulin classes. These can occur in connection with a primary immunodeficiency or in association with another underlying disease.

Immunologic hyperreactivity is most notably represented by the autoimmune diseases such as systemic lupus erythematosus, which are characterized by abnormally accelerated B-cell responses.

TEST PROCEDURES

Procedures directed at the demonstration of abnormally active, naturally occurring suppressor cells most frequently utilize B-cell indicator systems as the assays for the presence of suppressor cells. In these systems, unfractionated mononuclear cells or subpopulations of lymphoid cells are cocultured with allogeneic responder mononuclear cells, and the effect on mitogen-induced function of the allogeneic responder B cells is observed. The mitogen most commonly used is pokeweed mitogen (PWM), and the indicator B-cell function may be the production of intracytoplasmic immunoglobulin (3), supernatant immunoglobulin (24), or hemolytic plaque-forming cells (PFC) (4, 8, 10, 12) or the blastogenesis of B cells (19). In addition, a number of other systems have been successfully employed to detect mitogen-induced and antigen-induced responses by using assays for PFC or supernatant immunoglobulin (6, 21).

Since certain suppressor cells are sensitive to various manipulations such as irradiation (20), cell suspensions or subpopulations of cells which are being assayed for spontaneous suppressor cell activity may be irradiated before coculture with responder cells to determine whether the suppression can be abrogated. In addition, certain suppressor cell populations can be removed from cell suspensions by a number of physical means such as adherence or differential centrifugation of rosetted cells (see below).

In situations in which deficiencies of suppressor cell activity are suspected, induction of suppressor cells by mitogenic stimuli before coculture with responder cells has been extensively utilized (reviewed in references 6, 17, and 24). In this system, responder cells may be assayed for B-cell function by the techniques listed above or for T-cell responses by measuring blastogenic responses to stimulation by various mitogens or by the mixed-lymphocyte reaction (19).

There are a number of other assays for human suppressor cells, such as assaying for cells that either die off in culture (22) or actually evolve after variable periods of time in culture (16).

Finally, there are certain cell surface markers which phenotypically identify cells that have been shown in certain systems to possess suppressor activity. The most important such marker is a surface molecule, termed T8, which is present on human T cells of the suppressor-cytotoxic subset and can be detected by immunofluorescent staining using murine antihuman monoclonal antibodies such as OKT8 (Ortho Diagnostics, Raritan, N.J.) or Leu 2 (Becton-Dickinson, Mountain View, Calif.). However, it should be emphasized that detection of the T8 marker on a cell does not necessarily imply that the cell will express functional suppressor activity.

As mentioned above, given the large number of human suppressor cell systems and assays, it would be impossible to describe each of them in the context of this chapter. We shall thus describe in detail certain representative systems and refer the reader to the references cited above for variations in methodologies seen in other systems.

Assays for spontaneously occurring suppressor cells in unfractionated mononuclear cell suspensions

1. Draw 50 to 100 ml of venous blood from one or more normal individuals and from the patient to be assayed into plastic syringes containing 1 ml of sodium heparin (1,000 U/ml) per 50 ml of whole blood. Dilute the blood 1:1 with phosphate-buffered saline (PBS).

2. Add 30-ml volumes of diluted blood to 50-ml conical plastic tubes and, using a syringe and spinal needle, inject 12 ml of a Hypaque-Ficoll solution under the blood. Alternatively, 30 ml of diluted blood can be layered directly over 12 ml of a Hypaque-Ficoll solution.

3. Centrifuge the tubes at $400 \times g$ for 40 min at room temperature. Aspirate the upper plasma layer and discard it; gently aspirate the mononuclear cell layer at the interface, and pool interface layers from two tubes into a 50-ml plastic conical tube. Resuspend cells by adding RPMI 1640 medium up to 50 ml per tube.

4. Wash the cells at 400 to $500 \times g$ for 10 min at room temperature. Decant the supernatants, combine the cell buttons, suspend the cells in medium, wash them again as above, add medium to 10 ml, and count the cells from each individual.

5. Separately culture (in triplicate) 2×10^6 mononuclear cells from each subject in plastic round-bottom tubes (12 by 75 mm) in 1 ml of RPMI 1640 medium containing 2 mM L-glutamine, 100 U of penicillin per ml, 100 μg of streptomycin sulfate per ml, and 1% gentamicin. Cultures are stimulated either with nothing (control) or with PWM at optimal stim-

ulatory concentrations, usually in final concentrations of 1:100 to 1:2,000 of stock dilution. For determination of PWM-induced PFC, medium is supplemented with 10% pooled human AB or A serum; for PWM-induced intracytoplasmic immunoglobulin, medium is supplemented with human serum as described above or with fetal calf serum; for supernatant immunoglobulin assays, fetal calf serum is used. For the PFC system, the serum is absorbed twice with sheep erythrocytes (SRBC) at 4°C. All cultures are incubated at 37°C in 5% CO_2 in air and 100% humidity for 6 to 7 days for PFC and intracytoplasmic immunoglobulin and for up to 10 to 12 days for supernatant immunoglobulin. Cultures for the determination of PFC are incubated on a rocker platform.

6. At the end of the respective culture periods, cells to be assayed are washed twice in RPMI 1640 medium and are brought to an appropriate concentration in RPMI 1640 medium depending on the assay performed.

The assay for anti-SRBC PFC by the direct hemolysis-in-gel technique (8) has been generally superseded by indirect PFC assays which measure the total number of immunoglobulin-secreting cells, such as the reverse hemolytic PFC assay (4) or the staphylococcal protein A-coated SRBC (SPA-SRBC) assay (12). Here we describe the latter as used in our laboratory.

(i) Preparation of SPA-SRBC. The following conditions have been found to be optimal. SRBC are washed three times with 0.85% NaCl (not PBS). One milliliter of fresh stock $CrCl_3$ (1 mg in 1 ml of 0.85% NaCl) is added to 9.9 ml of 0.85% NaCl, 0.1 ml of stock SPA (5 mg/ml in 0.85% NaCl), and 1 ml of packed, washed SRBC. The mixture is gently shaken at 30°C for 50 min and then centrifuged at $1,000 \times g$ at 4°C. If gross hemolysis is seen, indicating a failure of the SPA to bind to the SRBC, the cells are discarded and the procedure is repeated. The shelf life of SPA-SRBC is 1 to 1.5 weeks.

(ii) Preparation of plaquing plates. Agarose (1,400 mg; Accurate Chemical, Hicksville, N.Y.) is added to 100 ml of distilled water and boiled until dissolved. This solution is added to 100 ml of $2\times$ RPMI prewarmed to 56°C. Volumes of 4 ml of the mixture at 56°C are added to petri dishes (60 by 15 mm; e.g., Falcon no. 3002), and the plates are stored at 4°C until used.

(iii) PFC assay. Lymphocytes are harvested and suspended at a dilution to give approximately 50 to 100 PFC per plate (10^5 to 10^6 per 0.1 ml). The lymphocytes, along with 0.85 ml of agarose-RPMI solution (see above) and 0.06 ml of a 25% solution of SPA-SRBC (see above) in Hanks salt solution, are added to a tube (12 by 75 mm; e.g., Falcon no. 2058) and heated to 47°C in a heating block. The contents of the tube are rapidly vortexed, poured onto an agarose plaquing plate (see above), and swirled. Each plate is then incubated at 37°C for 2 h, after which 1 ml of developing antibody (rabbit anti-human immunoglobulin; Cappel Laboratories, Downington, Pa.; diluted 1:50 to 1:200 in RPMI) or medium (as a control) is added and the plates are incubated for an additional 2 h at 37°C or overnight at 4°C. The developing antibody is removed, and the plate, if refrigerated, is warmed to room temperature. Guinea pig complement (1 ml, absorbed with SRBC) at a dilution of 1:30 to 1:40 in

Veronal-buffered saline is then added for 1 h at 37°C or overnight at 4°C. The complement is then aspirated, and PFC are enumerated with a dissecting microscope; results are expressed as PFC per 10^6 cells plated.

For the intracytoplasmic immunoglobulin assay (3), cells are harvested from the cultures, washed twice in cold PBS, and applied to glass slides by cytocentrifugation. The cytocentrifuge preparations are air dried, fixed in 5% acetic acid–95% ethanol for 15 min at $-10°C$, and washed twice in cold PBS. The slides are then stained with fluorescein-conjugated goat or rabbit $F(ab')_2$ anti-human total immunoglobulins or class-specific immunoglobulin (immunoglobulin G, A, and M) for 40 min at 37°C. The concentration of antiserum should be adjusted for each batch but is generally 0.5 mg/ml. The slides are then washed once with PBS and once with water. A drop of a 1:1 solution of PBS-glycerol is placed on the slide, and a cover slip is applied. The slide is read under oil immersion with a fluorescence microscope. The percentage of cells showing intracytoplasmic fluorescence is noted in a total of 200 counted cells.

For the assay of supernatant immunoglobulin produced by cultured cells, the most frequently used technique is the enzyme-linked immunosorbent assay. This technique is described in detail elsewhere in this volume.

7. Once the B-cell responses of the individual indicator and test suspensions are determined by any of the methodologies listed above, coculture experiments are performed to determine the spontaneously occurring suppressor cell activity of the test cell suspension. Coculture experiments are indicated if the individual tested manifests an abnormally low response.

In coculture experiments the allogeneic indicator and test cell suspensions are cultured together in a 1:1 ratio. Total numbers of cells in culture should remain constant since cell density can clearly affect responses. For example, if individual suspensions are cultured at a density of 10^6 cells per ml, cocultures should contain 0.5×10^6 cells from one individual and 0.5×10^6 cells from the other individual in a total of 1 ml. Results are expressed as the expected response per 10^6 cells of the coculture (calculated by determining the sum of the response per 10^6 cells for each of the subjects when cultured alone) compared with the actual observed response per 10^6 cells of the coculture. Suppression occurs when the ratio of observed to expected responses is significantly less than the mean ratio of observed to expected responses of cocultures between a series of control normal allogeneic cocultures.

Assays for inducible suppressor cells in unfractionated mononuclear cell suspensions

The assays for inducible suppressor cells are directed predominantly at clinical situations in which a deficiency of suppressor cells is likely. In these situations, the cell suspension is usually induced with a mitogen such as concanavalin A (ConA). The "induced" cells are then cocultured with either autologous or allogeneic responder-cell suspensions. The test systems with which the suppressor cells are assayed may reflect a wide variety of in vitro functions. One can use either the PWM-induced B-cell functional assays described above or the T-cell blastogenic responses of the responder suspensions. For example, the induced suppressor cells are assayed for their effects on mitogen-induced blastogenesis or on the allogeneic mixed-lymphocyte reaction (19).

In addition, suppression of PWM-induced B-cell responses by soluble factors derived from ConA-activated T cells has also been reported (10). The clinical importance of these factors, however, is unknown.

For ConA induction of suppressor cells, Hypaque-Ficoll-separated mononuclear cells (see above) at a density of 5×10^6 cells per 2 ml are cultured for 48 h in flat-bottomed plates with 10 μg of ConA per ml or with no ConA. ConA in the solid phase, i.e., bound to Sepharose beads, may also be used to minimize carryover of lectin to subsequent steps. At 48 h, cells are agitated with a sterile rubber policeman and removed from the plates by aspiration. ConA (10 μg/ml) is added to unstimulated cell cultures at the time of harvest to control for the effects of ConA itself carried over with the cells in the subsequent assays. All cells are then washed three times with 0.3 M methyl-α-D-mannopyranoside and once with RPMI 1640 medium to remove any surface-bound ConA. Control cells receive no ConA on culture initiation but are cultured alone for 48 h, pulsed with ConA at harvest, and washed with methyl-α-D-mannopyranoside in the same manner as ConA-generated cells.

Induced suppressor cells and unstimulated (control) cells are then evaluated in coculture experiments, depending on the respective assay. The induced cells may or may not be treated with mitomycin C (40 mg/ml for 1 h at 37°C) or X irradiation (2,000 R) before coculture with the responder cells. In certain systems, the ConA suppressor cells are blocked by mitomycin C or irradiation in their induction or expression, or both (13), whereas in others they may be resistant to mitomycin C and irradiation (19).

If the PWM-induced B-cell functional responder systems are to be evaluated, the control or ConA-generated suppressor cells are cocultured at a 1:1 ratio with responder cells in the presence of PWM for 6 to 7 days, after which time the appropriate assays for B-cell function are performed. Suppressor activity of ConA-generated cells versus control cells is evaluated in the patients being tested, compared with similar activity in a group of normal control subjects.

If the responder system to be evaluated is the mitogen- or mixed-lymphocyte reaction-stimulated lymphocyte blastogenic response, the following protocol is used. Blastogenic responses are assayed in multiwell microtiter plates. In determining effects of suppressor cells on mitogen-stimulated blastogenesis, 0.5×10^5 responder mononuclear cells are cocultured in a well with 0.5×10^5 autologous control cells or ConA-generated cells (irradiated or mitomycin C treated) in 0.2 ml per well in the presence of optimal stimulatory concentrations of phytohemagglutinin or ConA. In determining the effect of suppressor cells on the allogeneic mixed-lymphocyte reaction (19), 0.5×10^5 responder mononuclear cells (or T cells) are cocultured with 0.5×10^5 control or ConA-generated cells which are autologous to the responder cells in the presence of 0.5×10^5 mitomycin C-treated or irradiated allogeneic stimulator cells. Quadruplicate cultures for each point are incubated at 37°C in 5% CO_2 in air at 100% humidity. Four hours before harvesting (3 days and 5 days for mitogen- and allo-antigen-stimulated cultures, respectively), 0.4 μCi of tritiated thymidine (6.7 Ci/mmol) is added to each well. The cells are collected from the wells onto fiberglass filters by use of a semiautomated micro-harvesting device (MASH II). The filters are washed with 10% trichloroacetic acid and 95% alcohol and are placed in 4 ml of Aquasol. The trichloroacetic acid-precipitable radioactivity is counted in a liquid scintillation counter. The arithmetic mean of the counts per minute of quadruplicate cultures is determined, and the degree of stimulation is expressed as the difference in counts per minute per 10^6 lymphocytes between mitogen- or alloantigen-stimulated and unstimulated cultures (Δcpm). Percent suppression is determined by the formula: % suppression = [1 − cpm (S)/cpm (C)] × 100, where cpm (S) is the net counts per minute in cultures to which ConA-activated suppressor cells had been added, and cpm (C) is the net counts per minute in cultures to which control or unactivated cells had been added.

Determination of identity of the suppressor cell population

To determine the identity of the suppressor cell population or subpopulation in either the naturally occurring or induced suppressor cell assays described above, certain fractionation procedures can be performed.

(i) Is the suppressor cell an adherent cell? Before being assayed for suppressor cell capabilities, cell suspensions can be depleted of adherent cells by a number of methods, including passage over Sephadex G-10 columns (7), adherence to glass or plastic surfaces (9), passage through nylon-wool columns (7), or the carbonyl-iron magnet method (9). Since certain glass-adherent suppressor cells may mediate suppression via the production of prostaglandin, the effect of addition of inhibitors of prostaglandins such as indomethacin to cultures can also be evaluated (11).

(ii) Is the suppressor cell a T cell or a non-T cell? Mononuclear cells can be separated into T-cell-enriched and T-cell-depleted fractions by differential centrifugation of erythrocyte-rosetted cells over Hypaque-Ficoll gradients (9).

(iii) Does the suppressor cell belong to a particular T-cell subset? Purified T cells can be subjected to one of the following methods to obtain purified T-cell subsets. For positive selection, the T cells are stained with the appropriate monoclonal antibody and separated using (i) a fluorescence-activated cell sorter or (ii) density gradient centrifugation after rosetting with ox erythrocytes coated with goat anti-mouse immunoglobulin. For negative cell selection, cells to be removed are stained with antibody and either treated with complement or passed over an affinity column containing the appropriate anti-immunoglobulin.

It should be pointed out that in the mitogen-induced suppressor cell systems, such as the one with ConA, the mitogen is capable of inducing heterogeneous subpopulations of cells to suppress within given systems and in different systems (19).

REAGENTS AND SUPPLIES

RPMI 1640 medium; 0.85% sterile saline; PBS (pH 7.4)
Heparin sodium injection USP, 1,000 U/ml
Sterile syringes; sterile needles; trocar (spinal) needles, 13 gauge by 3.25 inches (8.3 cm)
Hypaque-Ficoll solution: 10 parts of 33.9% Hypaque to 24 parts of 9% Ficoll
Penicillin (5,000 U), streptomycin (5,000 μg), and gentamicin (10 mg/ml)
Serum: pooled human A or AB serum; fetal calf serum
Mitogens: PWM (GIBCO Laboratories, Grand Island, N.Y.); ConA, grade IV (Sigma Chemical Co., St. Louis, Mo.); phytohemagglutinin P (Burroughs Wellcome Co., Research Triangle Park, N.C.)
Methyl-α-D-mannopyranoside (A grade, Calbiochem, San Diego, Calif.); mitomycin C (Sigma Chemical Co.)
SPA (Pharmacia Fine Chemicals, Inc., Piscataway, N.J.)
Chromium chloride ($CrCl_3$)
Agarose (Accurate Chemical, Hicksville, N.Y.)
SRBC; ox erythrocytes
Fresh guinea pig serum (complement)
Nonconjugated and fluorescein-conjugated rabbit or goat F(ab')$_2$ anti-human immunoglobulin (Cappel Laboratories, Downington, Pa.)
Acetic acid; ethanol; glycerol
Tritiated thymidine, 6.7 Ci/mmol (New England Nuclear Corp., Boston, Mass.)
Test tubes: conical centrifuge tube with screw cap, 50 ml, polypropylene (Becton Dickinson Labware, Oxnard, Calif.); Falcon no. 2058, 12 by 75 mm, sterile, with caps
Cell culture plates: multiwell, flat-bottomed, with wells 1.5 cm in diameter; microtiter cell culture plates, 96 round-bottomed wells (Linbro Scientific, McLean, Va.)
Pipette tips: 10 drops to 1 ml (Scientific Products, Irvine, Calif.)
Pipettes: 1 ml to 10 ml (Becton Dickinson Labware)
Syringes: 10 ml to 60 ml (Sherwood Medical Industries, St. Louis, Mo.)
Sephadex G-10 (Pharmacia)
Nylon wool (Fenwal Inc., Ashland, Mass.)
Microscope slides; cover slips; plastic petri dishes, 100 by 15 mm (Becton Dickinson Labware)
Microscopes: fluorescence, phase; dissecting microscope
Water bath (Precision Systems, Inc., Sudbury, Mass.); heating block (Lab-Line Instruments, Inc. Melrose Park, Ill.)
Cell harvester, MASH II (Microbiological Associates, Bethesda, Md.)
Scintillation fluid (Aquasol; New England Nuclear Corp.)
Biovials (Beckman Instruments, Inc., Fullerton, Calif.)
Liquid scintillation counter (Beckman Instruments, Inc.)
Incubator: CO_2 (Forma Scientific, Inc., Marietta, Ohio)
Rocker platform (Bellco Glass, Inc., Vineland, N.J.)
Refrigerated centrifuge: CRV 5000 (International Equipment Co., Div. of Damon Corp., Needham Heights, Mass.)
Murine monoclonal antihuman antibodies:
    Anti-T cell: OKT3 (Ortho Diagnostics, Raritan, N.J.); Leu 4 (Becton Dickinson Monoclonal Center, Inc., Mountain View, Calif.)

Anti-helper-inducer T cell: OKT4 (Ortho); Leu 3 (Becton Dickinson Monoclonal Center)

Anti-suppressor-cytotoxic T cell: OKT8 (Ortho); Leu 2 (Becton Dickinson Monoclonal Center)

INTERPRETATION

Assays for suppressor cells measure the presence of populations of cells (usually lymphoid cells) which are capable of inhibiting the functional capabilities of lymphocytes. Abnormalities of suppressor cell function may be associated with hyporesponsiveness of certain immune functions, as in hypogammaglobulinemia, or with hyperresponsiveness of immune function, as in certain autoimmune states such as systemic lupus erythematosus. It should first be pointed out that such abnormalities of suppressor cells may not be the primary cause of the altered immune function, but may be secondary to the underlying immune defect. This is clearly exemplified by the chicken model of "infectious agammaglobulinemia," in which chickens bursectomized and irradiated at the time of hatching subsequently develop suppressor cells capable of suppressing immunoglobulin production when adaptively transferred to sublethally irradiated normal adult chickens (1).

In any event, establishment of the presence of overly active suppressor cell function for the most part lies in the demonstration of hyporesponsiveness of a particular lymphoid cell function such as mitogen-induced immunoglobulin production in an individual's mononuclear cell suspension. One then demonstrates that, by removal of a particular immunoregulatory cell population such as a monocyte or T-cell subset, the test response (antibody production) is normalized. The presence of overly active suppressor cells is then confirmed in experiments in which the hyporesponsive mononuclear cell suspension, or preferably the actual immunoregulatory cell subset (where possible), is cocultured with allogeneic responder cells to demonstrate suppression across allogeneic barriers. It is in this area that substantial caution must be exercised since varying degrees of "allogeneic effect" of such allogeneic cocultures could markedly influence the results. Only when a cell suspension from a given individual consistently suppresses a number of responders in coculture, or when several patients with a given disease consistently suppress in coculture, should one interpret the results as clearly indicating abnormal suppressor cell activity. It should also be pointed out that in human systems we are just beginning to delineate various suppressor cell systems, and most of these are nonspecific. Indeed, there are several types of human suppressor cells, and they may suppress in certain in vitro systems and not in others. It is necessary to assay a number of responder systems for naturally occurring and induced suppressor cells to establish fully the functional status of the immunoregulatory suppressor cell systems in various diseases.

LITERATURE CITED

1. Blaese, R. M., P. L. Weiden, I. Koski, and N. Dooley. 1974. Infectious agammaglobulinemia: transmission of immunodeficiency with grafts of agammaglobulinemic cells. J. Exp. Med. 140:1097–1101.

2. Cantor, H., L. McVay-Boudreau, J. Hugenberger, K. Naidorf, F. W. Shen, and R. K. Gershon. 1978. Immunoregulatory circuits among T-cell sets. II. Physiologic role of feedback inhibition in vivo; absence in NZB mice. J. Exp. Med. 148:1116–1125.

3. Cooper, M. D., A. R. Lawton, and D. E. Bochman. 1971. Agammaglobulinemia with B lymphocytes. Specific defect of plasma cell differentiation. Lancet ii:791–795.

4. Eby, W. C., C. A. Chong, S. Dray, and G. A. Molinaro. 1975. Enumerating immunoglobulin-secreting cells among peripheral human lymphocytes. A hemolytic plaque assay for a B cell function. J. Immunol. 115:1700–1703.

5. Fauci, A. S. 1980. Immunoregulation in autoimmunity. J. Allergy Clin. Immunol. 66:5–17.

6. Fauci, A. S., and R. E. Ballieux (ed.). 1979. Antibody production in man: in vitro synthesis and clinical implications. Academic Press, Inc., New York.

7. Fauci, A. S., J. E. Balow, and K. R. Pratt. 1976. Human bone marrow lymphocytes. Cytotoxic effector cells in the bone marrow of normal individuals. J. Clin. Invest. 57:826–835.

8. Fauci, A. S., and K. R. Pratt. 1976. Activation of human B lymphocytes. I. Direct plaque-forming cell assay for the measurement of polyclonal activation and antigenic stimulation of human B lymphocytes. J. Exp. Med. 144:674–684.

9. Fauci, A. S., K. R. K. Pratt, and G. Whalen. 1976. Activation of human B lymphocytes. II. Cellular interactions in the PFC response of human tonsillar and peripheral blood B lymphocytes to polyclonal activation by pokeweed mitogen. J. Immunol. 117:2100–2104.

10. Fleisher, T. A., W. C. Greene, R. M. Blaese, and T. A. Waldmann. 1981. Soluble suppressor supernatants elaborated by concanavalin A-activated human mononuclear cells. II. Characterization of a soluble suppressor of B cell immunoglobulin production. J. Immunol. 126:1192–1197.

11. Goodwin, J. S., R. P. Messner, A. D. Bankhurst, G. T. Peake, J. H. Saiki, and R. C. Williams. 1977. Prostaglandin-producing suppressor cells in Hodgkin's disease. N. Engl. J. Med. 197:963–968.

12. Gronowicz, E., A. Coutinho, and F. Melchers. 1976. A plaque assay for all cells secreting Ig of a given type or class. Eur. J. Immunol. 7:588–590.

13. Haynes, B. F., and A. S. Fauci. 1977. Activation of human B lymphocytes. III. Concanavalin A-induced generation of suppressor cells of the plaque-forming cell response of normal human B lymphocytes. J. Immunol. 118:2281–2287.

14. Haynes, B. F., R. T. Schooley, C. Payling-Wright, J. Grouse, R. Dolin, and A. S. Fauci. 1979. Emergence of suppressor T cells of immunoglobulin (Ig) production during acute Epstein-Barr virus (EBV)-induced infectious mononucleosis. J. Immunol. 123:2095–2101.

15. Katz, P., and A. S. Fauci. 1978. Inhibition of polyclonal B cell activation by suppressor monocytes in patients with sarcoidosis. Clin. Exp. Immunol. 32:554–562.

16. Lipsky, P. E., W. W. Ginsburg, F. D. Finkelman, and M. Ziff. 1978. Control of human B lymphocyte responsiveness: enhanced suppressor T cell activity after in vitro incubation. J. Immunol. 120:902–910.

17. Möller, G. (ed.). 1983. Functional T cell subsets defined by monoclonal antibodies. Immunol. Rev. 74:1–160.

18. Morimoto, C., E. L. Reinherz, Y. Borel, and S. F. Schlossman. 1983. Direct demonstration of the human suppressor inducer subset by anti-T cell antibodies. J. Immunol. 130:157–161.

19. Sakane, T., and I. Green. 1977. Human suppressor T cells induced by concanavalin A: suppressor T cells belong to distinctive T cell subclasses. J. Immunol. 119:1169–1178.

20. Siegal, F. P., and M. Siegal. 1977. Enhancement by irradiated T cells of human plasma cell production:

dissection of helper and suppressor functions in vitro. J. Immunol. **118**:642–647.

21. **Stevens, R. H., and A. Saxon.** 1978. Immunoregulation in humans. Control of antitetanus toxoid antibody production after booster immunization. J. Clin. Invest. **62**:1154–1160.

22. **Stobo, J. D., S. Paul, R. E. Van Scoy, and P. E. Hermans.** 1976. Suppressor thymus derived lymphocytes in fungal infection. J. Clin. Invest. **57**:319–328.

23. **Twomey, J., A. H. Laughter, S. Farrow, and C. C. Douglass.** 1975. Hodgkin's disease. An immunodepleting and immunosuppressive disorder. J. Clin. Invest. **56**:467–475.

24. **Waldmann, T. A., and S. Broder.** 1977. Suppressor cells in the regulation of the immune response. Prog. Clin. Immunol. **3**:155–199.

Chapter 46

Monocyte and Macrophage Function

LANNY J. ROSENWASSER

Monocytes and macrophages are bone marrow-derived cells that have numerous in vivo and in vitro functions (2, 9). These functions include host defense against microorganisms, interaction with lymphoid components in the generation and effector phase of immune responses, and a scavenger function involved in the removal of necrotic and cellular debris.

The monocyte and macrophage system can be viewed as a continuum with bone marrow precursors leading to progressively more mature cells, beginning with monoblasts and promonocytes within the bone marrow and ending with macrophages within the tissues. Promonocytes undergo division into mature monocytes and enter the blood, where they circulate for a matter of hours. From the blood these cells migrate into tissues and terminally differentiate into mature tissue macrophages. Such mature tissue macrophages may be found throughout the body. They may be found within organs such as the lung as alveolar macrophages, within the liver as Kupffer cells, within the kidney as mesangial cells, and in bone as osteoclasts. In addition, macrophages are also found within the lymph node, spleen, and bone marrow sinusoids, where they interact with lymphoid elements.

During the progressive maturation of these cells, there is an enhanced expression of functional, morphologic, and cell surface characteristics. For example, the phagocytic capacity and the expression of Fc and complement receptors on the surface plasma membrane of macrophages and monocytes appear to increase with the differentiation of the promonocyte through the mature tissue macrophage. The proliferative capacity of these cells, however, concomitantly decreases through this range of maturation. In addition, the differential expression of Ia surface molecules and the ability to produce factors such as interleukin 1 (IL-1) also appears to increase as cells mature from the bone marrow precursor pool of the monocyte/macrophage cell line. Note also that at each stage of differentiation along the monocyte/macrophage lineage one can have a discrete state of activation associated with the particular cell type. For example, peripheral blood monocytes may be present in a resting state or may be activated by exogenous or endogenous activators such as bacterial lipopolysaccharide (LPS) or T-cell products. Similarly, freely migrating macrophages of serosal cavities may be observed in their resident or resting state, or they may be activated by endogenous or exogenous factors. In most instances, studies on the functional capacity of human monocytes and macrophages are derived from in vitro tests of peripheral blood monocytes, and for the purposes of this chapter, all of the ensuing discussion will deal with the isolation and functional testing of peripheral blood monocytes.

This chapter first describes the isolation and culture of peripheral blood monocytes from the venous blood of humans. The techniques used to assess the immunocompetence of monocytes as accessory cells for the activation of T lymphocytes are discussed in detail. This discussion centers on the ability of monocytes to support antigen-induced activation of T cells and to appropriately produce the soluble mediator known as IL-1. In a further exposition of the tests of monocyte function, various assays of monocyte competence in mediating tumor cell-dependent cellular cytotoxicity, microbial killing, production of prostaglandins, and the ability to generate a respiratory burst are addressed.

CLINICAL INDICATIONS

The clinical indications for testing monocyte functions in vitro would be primarily in the evaluation of any patient suspected of having a deficiency of cell-mediated immunity. While other functions of T and B lymphocytes are being covered elsewhere in this manual, the tests of monocyte function described in this chapter should be included in any sophisticated evaluation of patients with cell-mediated immune deficiency and normal number and function of T and B cells.

The tests of accessory function (antigen presentation, IL-1 production) should be the most useful in evaluating immunodeficiency, while the other tests (cytotoxicity, microbial killing, prostaglandin and superoxide generation) would be more useful in the evaluation of patients with unusual infections, such as miliary tuberculosis, and infections with atypical mycobacteria, fungi, protozoans, or other saprophytic microorganisms.

REAGENTS

Ficoll-Hypaque solution or lymphocyte separation medium (Litton Bionetics, Rockville, Md.) gradient material, Percoll gradients (Pharmacia Fine Chemicals, Piscataway, N.J.)

Sterile phosphate-buffered saline (PBS) (GIBCO Laboratories, Grand Island, N.Y.)

Heparin (preservative free), 10 U/ml of venous blood

RPMI 1640 medium (GIBCO)

Hanks balanced salt solution (HBSS) (GIBCO)

Sterile, heat-inactivated fetal calf serum (Sterile Systems, Logan, Utah) or pooled human AB serum (Microbiological Associates, Bethesda, Md.)

Trypticase soy broth and agar (BBL Microbiological Systems, Cockeysville, Md.)

Penicillin, streptomycin, L-glutamine (GIBCO)

Antigens, mitogens

Scopoletin (Sigma Chemical Co., St. Louis, Mo.)

Superoxide dismutase (Sigma)

Prostaglandin radioimmunoassay (Seragen, Boston, Mass.)

MONOCYTE ISOLATION AND CULTURE

Monocytes may be conveniently isolated from peripheral blood mononuclear leukocytes by sequential buoyant density centrifugation over Ficoll-Hypaque, Percoll, or similar gradients and adherence to glass or plastic surfaces. The buoyant density of monocytes is similar to that of other peripheral blood mononuclear leukocytes but is considerably less than that of polymorphonuclear leukocytes and erythrocytes. In separating monocytes from lymphocytes with similar density, advantage is taken of the greater adherent properties of the mononuclear phagocyte.

Heparinized venous blood is diluted with an equal volume of PBS or HBSS, and 15-ml volumes are carefully layered over 3 ml of Ficoll-Hypaque in sterile culture tubes. The diluted blood is added carefully so as to avoid turbulence which would disturb the interface. The tubes are centrifuged at approximately 500 × g at room temperature for 30 min. When the tubes are removed from the centrifuge, a distinct band can be seen between the plasma layer and the Ficoll-Hypaque layer. The top layer containing plasma is pipetted and discarded, and the bottom layer above the Ficoll-Hypaque is harvested with a sterile Pasteur pipette; the top one-third of the Ficoll-Hypaque layer is taken up in addition to the cells. The bands from several tubes are then combined in another tube, and the cells are washed with either HBSS or PBS two or more times by centrifuging at 150 × g for 8 min. This cell pellet should be relatively free of platelets and erythrocytes and should contain about 60 to 80% lymphocytes and 20 to 40% monocytes. The mixture of lymphocytes and monocytes is suspended in RPMI medium with 10% human AB serum or fetal calf serum at a concentration of 1×10^6 or 2×10^6/ml and may be used either for functional assays or for further purification of monocytes. To obtain highly induced monocyte populations, the suspension is added to glass petri dishes and cultured at 37°C for a period of 1 or 2 h. The petri dishes are then washed twice with warm RPMI medium containing serum, followed by a final wash of chilled, serum-free PBS. The nonadherent cells taken from the first wash are pooled, washed, and then used as a source of potentially enriched T and B lymphocytes. The adherent cells are harvested and represent a population of cells that will yield greater than 90% mononuclear phagocytic monocytes by various criteria. After the chilled-PBS wash, the cells can be removed from monolayers with either a rubber policeman or 0.25% trypsin. The cells are then vigorously washed and can be assayed by various functional, morphologic, and enzymatic criteria for their purity as monocytes. Many other methods of obtaining monocytes for culture have been described. The phagocytic properties of monocytes may be used to separate the cells from other peripheral blood mononuclear cells. Such methods include the use of either silica or colloidal iron followed by passage over a magnetic field, countercurrent centrifugation using a cell elutriator, or binding to gelatin- or fibronectin-coated plates. Finally, monoclonal antibodies can be used to positively and negatively select monocytes from the overall peripheral blood mononuclear cell population.

ASSESSMENT OF ANTIGEN PRESENTATION BY MONOCYTES

The ability of macrophages or peripheral blood mononuclear cells such as monocytes to support antigen-specific T-cell proliferation can be measured (1). This is an indirect measurement of the functional capability of class II major histocompatibility complex (MHC) antigens on the surface of macrophages or monocytes. T cells used as indicator cells for antigen-specific proliferation assays are further purified from the nonadherent fraction of the peripheral blood mononuclear cells by passage over a nylon-wool column. These T-cell-enriched populations can be even further purified by a second passage over the nylon-wool adherence column or by passage of the cells over a stepwise Percoll density gradient. These multiply passaged T-cell indicator populations can be further depleted of accessory type functions by treatment with monoclonal antimonocyte reagents or monoclonal anti-class II MHC antigen antibodies.

T-cell proliferation (also see chapter 38) is assessed in microtiter cultures carried out in triplicate in flat- or round-bottomed 96-well microtiter plates in 0.2 ml of complete medium containing pooled, heat-inactivated human AB serum. Various test antigens, such as tetanus toxoid, streptokinase, streptodornase, purified protein derivative of tuberculin, or a combination of these, can be used at varying concentrations. Incubation of antigens, T cells, and monocytes can be carried out over 6 days in a humidified atmosphere of 95% air–5% CO_2 in an incubator kept at 37°C. After 5 days of culture, the plates are pulsed overnight with 1 μCi of tritiated thymidine and harvested at day 6 in a multiple-sample harvester. The ability of the cultured cells to incorporate tritiated thymidine is a good indication of antigen-induced T-cell blastogenesis. The radioactivity is counted in a liquid scintillation spectrometer, and the data can be expressed as either counts per minute (cpm) or Δ cpm, for which the background unstimulated cellular combinations are subtracted. Generally, this is a way of assessing the ability of purified monocytes to support antigen-induced T-cell blastogenesis of cells from sensitized donors. One can also directly test the ability of macrophage-associated antigen to activate T cells by the antigen-pulsing technique, in which monocytes are incubated for 18 h in complete medium in the presence of the antigen at a slightly higher concentration than is used for continuous antigen cultures. At the end of the pulsing period, the cells are vigorously washed with complete medium before use in experiments. This antigen-pulsing technique is a way of directly assessing the ability of monocytes to take up, process, and present antigens to sensitized T cells. A typical experiment, involving T-cell proliferation in response to tetanus toxoid and the role of monocytes, is included in Table 1.

METHOD FOR PRODUCING AND ASSAYING IL-1 ACTIVITY

Cultures of adherent monocytes can be grown in petri dishes with either fresh medium alone or medium containing various concentrations of a stimulus such as endotoxin LPS, or a particular stimulus such

TABLE 1. T-cell proliferation to tetanus toxoid antigen in the presence or absence of monocytes[a]

Antigen concn (μg/ml)	Monocytes	T-cell proliferation (cpm)
None	No	300
10	No	600
20	No	800
50	No	900
None	Yes	1,100
10	Yes	7,000
20	yes	30,000
50	Yes	80,000
50[b]	Yes[b]	50,000

[a] T cells (10^5) were cultured with 2×10^4 monocytes per well. T cells were purified by adherence, nylon-wool column passage, and treatment with anti-HLA-DR and complement.

[b] For an antigen pulse (see the text), 2×10^4 monocytes were cultured with 50 μg of tetanus toxoid per ml for 18 h, washed extensively, and then added to the T-cell culture.

as opsonized heat-killed *Streptomyces albus* bacteria. In addition, T cells that have been activated, or activated T-cell supernatants, can be used in the induction phase of monocyte-derived IL-1. However, the use of T-cell supernatants of activated T cells as IL-1 inducers can be misleading, since they may contain IL-2, another mediator derived from T cells which can also be measured as positive in the thymocyte assay for IL-1, since the proliferation of all T cells requires IL-2. After the monocytes have been cultured as monolayers in petri dishes for 24 to 48 h, the supernatants are collected, centrifuged, filtered (Millipore membrane filter), and then tested in the various forms of IL-1 assay.

The standard IL-1 assay involves the enhancement of murine thymocyte mitogenic responses to phytohemagglutinin (7). The thymus glands of mice are aseptically removed and teased apart between the frosted ends of two sterile glass slides in HBSS. The routine IL-1 assay involves young (6 weeks old) C3H/HeJ mice, since they are endotoxin resistant, although other strains of young mice (including C57BL/6, BALB/c, and CBA) can be used. Cells are vigorously washed and suspended in RPMI 1640 medium supplemented with 100 μg of penicillin per ml, 100 μg of streptomycin per ml, 0.3 mg of fresh L-glutamine per ml, 5×10^{-5} M 2-mercaptoethanol, 10 mM HEPES (*N*-2-hydroxyethylpiperazine-*N'*-2-ethanesulfonic acid) buffer, and 5% fetal calf serum. Thymocyte density is adjusted, and 5×10^6 thymocytes are placed in each well of a flat-bottom microtiter plate. Phytohemagglutinin at 1 μg/ml and an accessory addition to culture such as an appropriate dilution of an IL-1-containing medium are added to obtain a final volume of 200 μl of cells in medium per well. These cultures are incubated for 54 h at 37°C, and the plates are then pulsed with 1 μCi of [³H]thymidine for another 18 h of culture. The plates are harvested in a semiautomated harvester, and [³H]thymidine incorporation is measured by liquid scintillation spectrometry.

Recently, a cloned antigen-specific murine T-cell line that is IL-1 responsive has been identified and adapted for use as a routine IL-1 assay in vitro (4).

However, since these cells are not universally available, the details of this assay will not be outlined.

It is important to note that IL-2 can give a positive reaction in the thymocyte assay and that an independent test of a supernatant's capability to activate IL-2-dependent, IL-1-independent T-cell lines or clones may be necessary to rule out IL-2 contamination of the IL-1-containing supernatant. However, if predominantly monocytes are used as the source of cells producing the supernatant, IL-2 contamination is negligible. A typical IL-1 assay and its results are summarized in Table 2.

MICROBIAL KILLING

The microbicidal capacity of monocytes is generally measured by a method in which the monocytes are allowed to ingest and subsequently kill a measured number of microorganisms (8). Once inside the monocyte, the microorganism is exposed to the microbicidal components of the cell. After an appropriate time, the monocytes are lysed and the intracellular organisms are released and assayed by a colony counting method to determine the number of viable organisms remaining within the cell. Microbial killing is enhanced when resting monocytes undergo activation. The procedure for the microbial killing assay involves preparation of a suspension of adherent monocytes as described above. Bacterial suspensions are prepared using either *Staphylococcus aureus* or *Streptomyces albus* and are cultured for 16 to 24 h at 37°C in Trypticase soy broth. Other organisms, including *Escherichia coli*, *Listeria* sp., *Salmonella* sp., and *Candida albicans*, can also be used with minor modifications of this technique. The bacterial culture is centrifuged, washed twice in PBS, and adjusted to a concentration of approximately 10^8 bacteria per ml by measuring turbidity. The bacterial suspension is eventually diluted with HBSS to obtain a final working concentration of 10^7 bacteria per ml. Autologous or normal pooled AB serum can be used as a source of opsonin for the bacteria. In plastic culture tubes (12 by 75 mm), 0.1 ml of medium, 0.2 ml of bacterial suspension at 10^7 bacteria per ml, and 0.5 ml of monocyte suspension (10^6 monocytes per ml) are mixed. This mixture, along with proper controls, is then incubated for ca. 1 to 2 h at 37°C. Before culturing, a sample of the suspension is taken out for

TABLE 2. IL-1 activity produced by adherent human monocytes stimulated by a phagocytic stimulus

Addition to thymocytes[a]	Δcpm[b]
Medium	2,800
Standard IL-1[c]	12,500
Adherent monocytes[d]	2,500
Stimulated adherent monocytes[e]	16,000

[a] In each experiment, 5×10^5 murine thymocytes were cultured with 1 μg of phytohemagglutinin for 72 h and pulsed with 1 μCi of [³H]thymidine for the final 24 h of culture.

[b] Phytohemagglutinin-induced cpm − control cpm.

[c] A 1/100 dilution of 1 rabbit pyrogen dose per well.

[d] Adherent monocytes were cultured for 24 h.

[e] Heat-killed, opsonized *Streptomyces albus* bacteria were added to the adherent monocyte cultures.

bacterial counts. After the 2-h incubation, the cells are resuspended, and colony counts are performed once more to determine the total amount of bacteria remaining. The tubes are then centrifuged, and colony counts are performed on the supernatant. To perform bacterial counts, 0.1 ml of the solution is mixed with 9.9 ml of water in a Vortex mixer to lyse the monocytes and disperse the bacteria. Serial 10-fold dilutions are then made and cultured on pour plates of Trypticase soy agar. The culture plates are incubated at 37°C for 48 h, and the number of CFU is counted to quantitate the remaining viable bacteria.

The percentage of bacteria killed by the monocytes is then calculated as follows.

(CFU at zero time) − (CFU in 15-min supernatant) = number of viable bacteria in pellet in contact with monocytes (A)

(1-h total CFU) − (CFU in 1-h supernatant) = number of viable cell-associated bacteria at 1 h (B)

$$[(A - B)/A] \times 100 = \% \text{ bacteria killed}$$

PROSTAGLANDIN GENERATION

Monocytes can be stimulated in vitro to generate prostaglandins (3). Fresh human blood mononuclear cells are obtained from Ficoll-Hypaque gradients, washed twice, and suspended in HBSS at 5×10^6 cells per ml with 5% heat-inactivated (56°C, 30 min) human AB serum. Samples (2 ml) of suspension are plated into 16-mm-diameter plastic wells (Costar plates; Linbro, Hamden, Conn.). The plates are placed on a slowly rocking platform at 37°C for 1 h to facilitate monocyte adherence. After incubation, the wells are washed twice with 37°C HBSS to remove nonadherent cells, and microscopic examination should reveal monolayers of spreading cells. When a stimulus of opsonized Streptomyces albus is added, more than 90% of cells reveal ingested bacteria. Wells are washed, and 1 ml of replacement HBSS with supplementing sera is added to the adherent monocytes. The plates are incubated for 1 h in a stationary incubator at 37°C. Supernatants from duplicate wells are aspirated, pooled, immediately centrifuged at $2,000 \times g$, and frozen at −70°C until assayed.

The monocyte supernatants are thawed, diluted, and assayed for prostaglandin E with a radioimmunoassay (Clinical Assays, Cambridge, Mass., and Seragen Assays, Boston, Mass.). No extractions are necessary because the protein content of supernatants is less than 1 mg/ml. Supernatants are adjusted to pH 12.5 with NaOH, boiled for 20 min, neutralized, and assayed in triplicate. Prostaglandin E concentrations are calculated from a standard curve (also in triplicate) constructed for each day of the assay, and results are calculated per milliliter of the original supernatant.

A typical monocyte culture of 10^6 adherent monocytes in a sterile culture well with 1 ml of medium will produce between 25 and 300 pg of prostaglandin E per ml after stimulation. The basal synthesis of prostaglandin E by stimulated monocytes should be between 10 and 20 pg/ml.

GENERATION OF TUMOR CELL-DEPENDENT CELLULAR CYTOTOXICITY

To measure tumor cell-dependent cellular cytotoxicity, purified monocytes, as described earlier, are incubated in a 96-well microtiter plate (5). A total of 2×10^5 monocytes are added to each well in 0.2 ml of medium supplemented with 5% pooled human AB serum. The adherent monocytes in the wells of the microtiter plate are then cultured with and without exponentially growing tumor target cells. An example of a potential tumor target that can be killed by monocytes is the A375 human melanoma cell line. Briefly, exponentially growing target cells are labeled for 24 h with ^{125}I-labeled iododeoxyuridine at a concentration of 0.3 μCi/ml. The tumor cells are then washed twice to remove free isotope, harvested by treatment with 0.25% trypsin EDTA, washed again, and pelleted. The cells are then suspended in complete medium and added to the monocyte monolayer to yield a target-to-effector cell ratio of 1:20. The radiolabeled target cells are then plated alone as a control group. After 24 h the cultures are washed to remove the nonadherent cells. The washing procedure does not affect the plating efficiency. The cells are then refed and cultured for an additional 48 h. Those target cells killed by the monocytes are removed. After 48 h the viable cells remaining in each well are lysed with 0.1 M sodium hydroxide, and the radioactivity of the lysate is measured in a gamma counter. The cytotoxic activity of the monocytes is calculated as follows:

% of stimulated cytotoxicity

$$= 100 - \frac{\text{(cpm in target cells cultured with stimulated monocytes)}}{\text{(cpm in target cells cultured with control monocytes)}} \times 100$$

% of monocyte cytotoxicity

$$= 100 - \frac{\text{(cpm in target cells cultured with monocytes)}}{\text{(cpm in target cells alone)}} \times 100$$

PRODUCTION OF OXYGEN METABOLITES

To assay the production of oxygen metabolites, monocytes are prepared as described previously and then allowed to adhere to 13-mm-diameter cover slips. The cover slips are washed thoroughly by swirling in four successive beakers of PBS at room temperature (6) and then drained on absorbent paper and placed in 16-mm Costar wells containing 1.5 ml of Krebs-Ringer phosphate buffer with glucose, 35 nM scopoletin, 1 U of horseradish peroxidase, and 150 ng of phorbolmyristic acetate as a stimulator of the monocytes. Opsonized zymosan can also be used as a stimulus; 40 mg of zymosan is suspended in 5 ml of PBS with 10% pooled human AB serum. Heat-killed, opsonized Streptomyces albus or Staphylococcus aureus cells can also be used as potential stimulators of the monocytes. Controls and cell-free cover slips are treated in the same way as the cover slips carrying adhered monocytes. The Costar wells are placed in a 37°C water bath for 60 min, the supernatant fluid from the monocytes with the various stimulants is collected,

TABLE 3. Superoxide and hydrogen peroxide release from monocytes stimulated by phorbolmyristic acetate or opsonized zymosan

Time (h) of culture	Release[a] (nmol/mg of protein per h) after stimulation by:			
	Phorbolmyristic acetate[b]		Opsonized zymosan[c]	
	O_2^-	H_2O_2	O_2^-	H_2O_2
0	400	900	200	600
48	200	1,000	150	300
96	20	20	20	20

[a] Mean of triplicates.
[b] At 100 ng/ml.
[c] At 100 particles per cell (monocyte).

and the fluoresence of the supernatants is measured with a fluorometer. The fluoresence observed by the oxidation of scopoletin is directly related to the generation of hydrogen peroxide by the resting or stimulated monocytes. All H_2O_2 release assays are performed with triplicate cover slips.

The cover slips containing adherent monocytes can be further assayed for the measurement of superoxide release. These cover slips are washed and rinsed as described earlier for the peroxide assay and are then transferred to Costar wells containing 0.75 ml of Krebs-Ringer PBS with glucose plus 100 μM ferricytochrome c, with or without 40 mg of superoxide dismutase. After 10 min at 37°C, stimulants such as phorbolmyristic acetate, opsonized zymosan, or opsonized heat-killed *Streptomyces albus* or *Staphylococcus aureus* cells are added. The particles are sedimented by centrifugation. After 60 min of culture at 37°C, the trays are cooled to 4°C and the zymosan and phorbolmyristic acetate are removed by centrifugation. Superoxide release is determined from the optical density at 550 nm of samples without superoxide dismutase minus the optical density at 550 nm of matched samples containing the enzyme. All of these samples are assayed in triplicate. A typical experiment is summarized in Table 3.

LITERATURE CITED

1. **Chu, E. C., L. J. Rosenwasser, C. A. Dinarello, M. Lareau, and R. S. Geha.** 1984. Role of interleukin-1 in antigen specific T cell proliferation. J. Immunol. **132:**1311–1316.
2. **Cline, M. J., R. I. Lehrer, M. C. Territo, and D. W. Golde.** 1978. Monocytes and macrophages: functions and diseases. Ann. Intern. Med. **88:**78–88.
3. **Dinarello, C. A., S. O. Marnoy, and L. J. Rosenwasser.** 1983. Role of arachidonate metabolism in the immunoregulatory function of human LP/LAF/IL-1. J. Immunol. **130:**890–895.
4. **Kaye, J., S. Porcelli, J. Tite, B. Jones, and C. A. Janeway.** 1983. Stimulatory antibodies specific for helper T cell clones. J. Exp. Med. **158:**836–856.
5. **Kleinerman, E. S., A. J. Schroit, W. E. Fogler, and I. J. Fidler.** 1983. Tumoricidal activity of human monocytes activated in vitro by free and liposome encapsulated human lymphokines. J. Clin. Invest. **72:**304–315.
6. **Nakagawara, A., C. F. Nathan, and Z. A. Cohn.** 1981. Hydrogen peroxide metabolism in human monocytes during differentiation in vitro. J. Clin. Invest. **68:**1243–1252.
7. **Rosenwasser, L. J., and C. A. Dinarello.** 1981. Antibody of leukocytic pyrogen to enhance phytohemagglutinin induced murine thymocyte proliferation. Cell. Immunol. **63:**134–142.
8. **Territo, M. C., and M. J. Cline.** 1977. Monocyte function in man. J. Immunol. **118:**187–192.
9. **Unanue, E. R.** 1980. Cooperation between mononuclear phagocytes and lymphocytes in immunity. N. Engl. J. Med. **303:**977–985.

Chapter 47

Phagocytosis

FREDERICK S. SOUTHWICK AND THOMAS P. STOSSEL

Phagocytes important in immunology are polymorphonuclear leukocytes (neutrophils) and the mononuclear phagocytes (monocytes and macrophages). Phagocyte hypofunction is a cause of recurrent pyogenic infection. To combat pyogenic infection, neutrophils and monocytes respond to chemotactic factors by moving toward the source of inflammation, where they have to ingest microorganisms and kill them. Macrophages in filter organisms must ingest and kill microorganisms that flow to them. Many microbes resist ingestion because they are not recognized by phagocytes. Serum interacts with most of these microorganisms and deposits opsonins, principally immunoglobulins or complement proteins or both, on them which render them palatable to the cells. During ingestion, granules in the cytoplasm fuse with the membrane of the vacuole forming around the microbe and discharge their contents into the vacuole. Some of this material ends up in the medium surrounding the phagocyte. Since the granules disappear during this process, it is called degranulation. The granule contents include hydrolytic enzymes, bactericidal proteins, and, in the neutrophil, myeloperoxidase. Myeloperoxidase, in combination with hydrogen peroxide and other oxygen metabolites such as superoxide anions, is extremely active in killing ingested microorganisms (8).

Since susceptibility to infection is determined as much by the exposure to the pathogen as by the status of the host, the clinical presentation of patients with phagocyte abnormalities may vary enormously, and the laboratory analysis is an essential feature in diagnosis. The approach to chemotactic functions is covered in chapter 40 of this manual. This chapter will focus on assessment of ingestion, degranulation, oxygen metabolism, and bactericidal activity of neutrophils. The tests are also applicable to mononuclear phagocytes acquired by techniques described elsewhere in this manual.

Many of the tests commonly used for evaluating neutrophil function have been devised or successfully applied in the setting of clear-cut, usually genetic disorders in which certain neutrophil functions were grossly impaired. Some of these tests are not necessarily applicable to more subtle types of neutrophil dysfunction. The degranulation and oxygen metabolism rates are determined by the magnitude of membrane stimulation, usually the ingestion rate. Therefore, it is important that the measurements of degranulation or oxygen metabolism be correlated with equally precise determinations of the ingestion rate. All tests of phagocyte functions presented here are bioassays which are subject to a large amount of variability. The laboratory performing the tests must be prepared to do adequate numbers of control determinations for comparison with samples from patients and must be conservative in interpreting the results.

EVALUATION OF INGESTION

The ingestion process may be analyzed quantitatively (10, 14). It is preferable to measure the accumulation of particles within cells rather than the disappearance of particles from the extracellular medium. In the former case, uningested particles are usually removed, and therefore it is possible to use saturating quantities of particles. Initial rates of ingestion can then be determined by use of short incubation periods since the base line is zero. When the disappearance of extracellular particles is measured, long incubation periods are required if large particle concentrations are used, since it is difficult to measure small changes in large quantities. This approach is acceptable if the differences in ingestion among various experimental conditions are great. Subtle alterations may go undetected. Certain kinetic data must be obtained for a given test system. These data should include proportionality of ingestion rate to cell concentration, proportionality of ingestion rate to particle concentration at low particle-to-cell ratios, and independence of ingestion rate from particle concentration at high particle-to-cell ratios. This last point is especially important because the ability to demonstrate independence from particle concentration implies that nonspecific adherence of particles to cells is not being confused with true engulfment. Also relevant to this issue is the ability to demonstrate complete inhibition of ingestion by incubating cells and particles together at 0°C or with high concentration of metabolic inhibitors.

When the rate of ingestion of particles requiring opsonization is under investigation, a complex interaction comes into consideration. The opsonic activity of serum is first exerted upon the particle, altering it in such a way that its entry into the cell is facilitated. If all reagents, i.e., cells, opsonin source, and test particles, are incubated simultaneously, the measured rate of ingestion will be a combination of two rates, opsonization and ingestion. Different variables introduced into such a system may influence one process and not the other. Therefore, it is best to design experiments in such a way, e.g., by preincubating the particles with the opsonin source, that the rates may be separated.

EVALUATION OF DEGRANULATION

Degranulation may be assessed by measuring the rate of appearance of granule-associated enzymes in phagocytic vacuoles, in the extracellular medium, or in both. The rate of enzyme appearance in phagocytic vacuoles may be determined in a semiquantitative manner by histochemical techniques, with light or electron microscopy used to visualize the results. Quantitative assessment of intravacuolar degranulation is possible by means of techniques in which phagocytic vacuoles are isolated in pure form and the quantity of granule-associated enzyme in them is compared with the amount of ingested material also in the phagosomes (15). Extracellular degranulation is quantified by measuring granule-associated enzymes appearing in the extracellular medium (16). Although it has not been proven that the extracellular secretion of granule contents is absolutely correlated with intravacuolar degranulation, this approach is the simplest.

EVALUATION OF PHAGOCYTE OXYGEN METABOLISM

It is currently believed that recognition of certain objects and substances by phagocytes activates plasma membrane-associated oxidase enzymes that convert oxygen to one- and two-electron reduction products, i.e., superoxide anions and hydrogen peroxide (2), respectively. The antimicrobial activity of hydrogen peroxide is potentiated by myeloperoxidase. In chronic granulomatous disease, phagocytes fail to produce hydrogen peroxide and other oxygen metabolites (8). The phagocytes have a bactericidal defect, and the patients suffer from recurrent pyogenic infections. In addition to its significance for phagocytic functions related to inactivation of ingested microbes, activation of oxygen metabolism is a useful indirect marker for the ingestion process per se. Quantitative methods for direct measurement of hydrogen peroxide (12) and superoxide anions (4) released into the medium are currently available, as are assays for related processes, including hexose monophosphate shunt activity, Nitro Blue Tetrazolium (NBT; Sigma Chemical Co., St. Louis, Mo.) reduction (3), and iodination (the coupling of radioactive iodide to protein, a reaction catalyzed by hydrogen peroxide and myeloperoxidase) (7).

SPECIFIC TESTS

The tests described here can all be done with a spectrophotometer, obviating the need for use of radioactive materials.

Assay for the rate of ingestion by blood phagocytes (neutrophils, bands, and monocytes) and simultaneous assay of the rate of ingestion and of NBT reduction

Principle. Phagocytic cells isolated from human blood are fed *Escherichia coli* lipopolysaccharide-coated oil droplets containing oil red O. The phagocytes ingest these particles only if the particles are first treated with fresh human serum, which opsonizes them by depositing the C3 component of complement on the particle surfaces in a form that makes them palatable. The rate of ingestion of the opsonized particles by the cells is constant for 5 min. After cells and particles have been incubated for 5 min, the uningested oil particles, because of their low density, are efficiently separated from the cells containing ingested particles by centrifugation; the cells sediment and the unengulfed particles float. Oil red O is extracted from the washed cell pellets with dioxane and is spectrophotometrically measured. This system

measures true ingestion rates as discussed above in the introduction (13).

During ingestion, superoxide anions are formed. When NBT, a yellow redox compound, is present in the extracellular medium, it is swept into the phagocytic vacuole with the ingested particle, and there it is reduced by the superoxide anions. The reduction product of NBT, a purple insoluble formazan, can be extracted with the dioxane solution used to extract the oil red O. The optical density (OD) of the formazan is determined at a different wavelength from that used for oil red O.

Preparation of phagocytes. Blood is collected in acid-citrate-glucose anticoagulant at 2 ml/8 ml of blood. The large amount of anticoagulant prevents platelet clumping which fosters leukocyte agglutination. One duplicate assay can easily be performed with 8 ml of blood, although, if available, 16 ml is preferable. Then 6% dextran 75 in isotonic saline (McGraw Laboratories, Glendale, Calif.) is taken into the syringe (0.5 volume per volume of blood), the syringe is stood on its hub, and the erythrocytes are allowed to settle at room temperature (45 to 60 min usually is required). After settling, the supernatant plasma is expressed through a bent venipuncture needle into 50-ml plastic conical centrifuge tubes (15 ml per tube). A sample is taken for differential count (the morphology is well preserved at this point). Ice-cold 0.8% ammonium chloride (35 ml) is added and the tubes are inverted once and immediately centrifuged (80 × g for 10 min). The ammonium chloride solution lyses remaining erythrocytes. The lysis is relatively inefficient, but it is gentle and has less-damaging effects on the leukocytes than hypotonic lysis. The cell buttons are suspended in ice-cold isotonic saline, pooled, and washed once with isotonic saline (centrifuged at 800 × g for 10 min). If a delay in performing the assay is anticipated, the cells can be kept for several hours in cold saline or plasma; this is better than buffered media with divalent cations, which allow for clumping. The final cell buttons are suspended in any buffered isotonic medium with divalent cations (Krebs-Ringer phosphate, Hanks balanced salt solution, etc.) such that the leukocyte count is about 20,000 to 60,000/mm^3. With experience, the count can be approximated by judging the turbidity of the suspension. A sample is taken for cell count at this time.

Preparation of diisodecylphthalate oil plus oil red O. Approximately 2 g of oil red O (Allied Chemical Corp., Morristown, N.J.) is added to 50 ml of diisodecylphthalate (Coleman, Matheson and Bell, East Rutherford, N.J.) in a large porcelain mortar and is ground with a pestle. The saturated suspension is centrifuged in plastic tubes (top speed in a Sorvall or International clinical centrifuge) to remove dye (which can be reutilized). The dye-containing diisodecylphthalate is stable and can be stored indefinitely at room temperature. Since the amount of dye in the oil varies, a factor is computed which converts OD to milligrams of diisodecylphthalate oil to permit normalization and comparison of results. A 10-μl amount of oil red O-diisodecylphthalate oil is added to 10 ml of dioxane, and the OD at 525 nm is determined. The conversion factor is given by the formula 0.94/OD, where 0.94 is the density of the diisodecylphthalate oil (grams per milliliter) and OD is the actual reading.

Preparation of particles. To prepare the droplets, dissolve 40 mg of *E. coli* lipopolysaccharide O26:B6 (Boivin preparation; catalog no. 3920-25, Difco Laboratories, Detroit, Mich.) in 3 ml of balanced salt solution in a 10- to 15-ml glass or thick-walled plastic test tube, and disperse the lipopolysaccharide by brief sonication (any model of Sonifier will do). Layer 1 ml of the diisodecylphthalate oil-oil red O over the aqueous lipopolysaccharide suspension, and sonicate the mixture. The Sonifier probe should be just below the oil-water interface; the length of sonic treatment is about 90 s, just until the tube becomes hot to touch. The output can be low; the sonic treatment details are unimportant except that it is better to err on the side of treating too long. The final preparation should look like a strawberry milkshake. The particle suspension can be used immediately (after cooling) or can be frozen. Brief sonication after thawing is advisable.

Opsonization. The particles are opsonized, usually just before the ingestion step, by adding an equal volume of fresh human serum and incubating the mixture at 37°C for 25 to 35 min. Maximal C3 deposition has occurred by that time; if the particles are allowed to sit longer in serum, proteolytic activity slowly removes the opsonically active C3. Therefore, the opsonized particles must be kept cold, frozen, or washed (see below) until use. Opsonized particles can be frozen and thawed and are still palatable to the phagocytes.

Ingestion. To assay ingestion, add 0.2 volume of opsonized particle suspension (prewarmed to 37°C) to 0.8 volume of cell suspension (also prewarmed). The reaction can be started by adding either particles to cells or cells to particles. The reaction can be run in siliconized glass 15-ml conical centrifuge tubes in a system with a total volume of 1 ml (in which case 0.2 ml of particles is added to 0.8 ml of cell suspension). After 5 min, during which the tubes are occasionally tapped to keep the ingredients in suspension, add 6 ml of ice-cold isotonic saline containing 1 mM *N*-ethylmaleimide (126 ml/liter), which poisons the cells and stops ingestion. Centrifuge the tubes at $250 \times g$ (1,000 rpm for 10 min in a centrifuge with a 19-cm radius). Dislodge the rim of uningested particles at the top by shaking the tube vertically; discard the supernatant fluid, but do not drain the pellets completely. The small amount of residual supernatant fluid is used to suspend the cell pellet by tapping the bottom of the tube. Add more *N*-ethylmaleimide–saline, and repeat the washing. After the second wash, discard the supernatant fluid, invert the tubes to drain the pellets, and wipe the sides of the tubes with tissue. To disrupt the cell pellets and make the oil red O soluble, add 1 ml or more of dioxane with tapping of the tubes or blending in a Vortex mixer. Centrifuge the extracts at $500 \times g$ for 15 min to remove debris, and read the OD of the extracts in a colorimeter or spectrophotometer at a wavelength of 525 nm against a dioxane blank.

Combined assay of NBT reduction and ingestion. NBT is "dissolved" in balanced salt solution at a concentration of 2 mg/ml. In fact, the solubility of this material is variable, and only about 0.6 mg ends up dissolved in 1 ml. The solution-suspension therefore must be carefully filtered, either through an appara-

TABLE 1. Combined assay of NBT reduction and ingestion

Reagent	Amt (ml) in:	
	Tube 1	Tube 2
Opsonized particles	0.2	0.2
Cell suspension	0.4	0.4
Balanced salt solution	0.4	0
NBT in balanced salt solution	0	0.4

tus with 0.8-μm pores (Millipore Corp., Bedford, Mass.) or through Whatman no. 1 filter paper. If sterile equipment is used, the former technique has the advantage that the filtrate can be considered sterile and stored in lots for longer periods of time than an unsterile solution, since the balanced salt solution promotes microbial growth. It is important that microbial contamination be minimized, since bacteria will enhance NBT reduction by the cells.

Incubations are set up as shown in Table 1. The reaction is started by adding the cells to the other premixed, prewarmed reagents. Tube 1 gives the ingestion rate, and tube 2 gives the NBT reduction rate. The rest of the assay is done as described above except that the NBT-formazan must be extracted with dioxane by heating the tube in a boiling-water bath for 15 to 30 min. The OD of NBT-formazan is read at 580 nm and converted to micrograms of formazan by multiplying the OD by 14.14.

Calculation of results

$$\text{Ingestion rate} = \frac{OD_{525} \times \text{conversion factor}}{\begin{array}{c}\text{time of} \\ \text{incubation}\end{array} \times \begin{array}{c}\text{phagocytic cells in} \\ \text{total system} \times 10^7\end{array}}$$

where the phagocytic cells in the total system include polymorphonuclear leukocytes, bands, and monocytes, and the initial ingestion rate is expressed in milligrams of diisodecylphthalate per 10^7 phagocytes per minute.

To determine NBT reduction, the OD of tube 1 at 580 nm must be subtracted from that of tube 2, since oil red O absorbs somewhat at 580 nm. Thus

Initial NBT reduction rate =

$$\frac{(OD_{580} \text{ of tube } 2 - OD_{580} \text{ of tube } 1) \times 14.14}{\text{time of incubation} \times \text{phagocytic cells} \times 10^7}$$

where the initial NBT reduction rate is expressed in micrograms of formazan per 10^7 phagocytes per minute.

Comments. Depending on the question being asked, one may wish to compare different sera against a set of control cells, to compare the same serum against different cells, or to test a patient's serum and cells together as a screening procedure.

If serum opsonic activity is to be tested in detail, the number of samples can be increased by obtaining 30 to 50 ml of blood from a consenting individual with neutrophilia secondary to acute infection. Since the ingestion rate per cell may be increased in infected

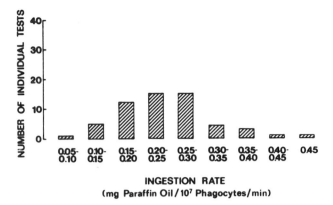

FIG. 1. Frequency distribution of initial ingestion rates by normal blood phagocytes of lipopolysaccharide-coated paraffin oil droplets opsonized with serum from the phagocyte donors.

patients, several control sera (or pooled control serum) should be tested against the test sera, and then the results are compared for that day's determination. External comparisons can be made in that setting by keeping lots of frozen ($-70°C$) control or pooled control sera and including a sample in each run. Obviously, if serum opsonic activity is in question, immunochemical determinations of serum proteins of known opsonic importance (immunoglobulins, early complement components, anticapsular antibodies) should be done.

As discussed above, there is marked variation in test results because of the many factors that contribute to the final value. Figure 1 shows a frequency distribution for ingestion rates of 57 control determinations. In our laboratory we do not consider an initial ingestion rate abnormal if it is greater than 0.05 mg of diisodecylphthalate oil ingested per 10^7 phagocytes per min. The sensitivity of the ingestion assay can be increased, permitting the use of very small quantities of cells, by incorporating radioactive oil (e.g., [^{14}C]octadecane, Amersham Corp., Arlington Heights, Ill.) into the diisodecylphthalate. The dioxane extract is then added to any scintillation counting cocktail and measured for radioactivity (5). As with other micromethods, the effects of errors are magnified compared with procedures using larger quantities.

If one wants to know which cells in a mixture have participated in ingestion, one can make smears of the cell and particle suspension and stain them with Wright stain (a drop of albumin or serum on the slide with the cell suspension improves the morphology). The methanol in the stain dissolves extracellular oil droplets and renders intracellular droplets easily identifiable as lucent vacuoles (1).

Patients with chronic granulomatous disease have ratios of NBT reduction/ingestion that are less than 1.5. In some families the inheritance of this disease is X-linked, and mothers of patients have a population of cells which do not reduce NBT in accordance with the Lyon hypothesis. These "carriers" have reduction/ingestion ratios that range from 1.5 to 3, which does overlap with the lower limit of normal (2.5). The ratios vary enormously and are high in acute inflammatory states. We do not attempt to interpret the

meaning of high reduction/ingestion ratios in our laboratory. Absent NBT reduction has also been found for neutrophils of rare patients lacking neutrophil glucose 6-phosphate dehydrogenase activity (9). These patients behave clinically in a similar way to patients with chronic granulomatous disease.

NBT slide test using phorbol myristate acetate

See reference 11.

Preparation of glass cover slips. Phorbol myristate acetate (Midland Consolidated Corp., Midland, N.Y.) is dissolved in dimethyl sulfoxide at a concentration of 2 mg/ml and kept frozen at $-70°C$ between experiments. This solution is diluted with Krebs-Ringer phosphate to a final concentration of 1 μg/ml, and 0.1 ml is allowed to air dry on cover slips previously boiled in distilled water.

Incubation. Several drops of whole blood obtained by finger-stick or venipuncture are placed on uncoated and phorbol myristate acetate-coated cover slips. The cover slips are then placed in a moist chamber (a petri dish containing saline-soaked gauze works well for this purpose) and incubated at 37°C for 45 min. Clots are gently removed by washing with Krebs-Ringer phosphate solution. The cover slips are then placed on a drop of NBT-serum solution (NBT at 1 mg/ml in 10% serum and Krebs-Ringer phosphate) on a glass slide and reincubated for 20 min at 37°C. The cover slips are then washed, fixed in methanol, counterstained with safranin, and air dried.

Analysis of results. Four hundred polymorphonuclear leukocytes are randomly examined and scored as positive (large dark-blue cells [precipitated formazan]) or negative (small red cells). Generally a normal control is run in parallel with the patient sample.

Comments. This test uses only small quantities of blood, is simple to perform, requires no sophisticated equipment, and generates highly reproducible results. Unlike the OD method described above, which measures NBT reduction by a total population of cells, the NBT slide test allows reliable evaluation of the metabolic function of individual cells. Such data are particularly important for detecting chronic granulomatous disease carriers. Because 99% of polymorphonuclear leukocytes from normal subjects are NBT positive after phorbol myristate acetate stimulation, even chronic granulomatous disease carriers who have a small percentage of defective (NBT-negative) cells can be differentiated from normal individuals by this method (11). Such small differences are undetectable by methods which sample total populations.

Assay of degranulation by measurement of extracellular release of β-glucuronidase activity

Preparation of phagocytes and particles. Peripheral blood phagocytes are prepared as described above. Particles are also prepared and opsonized as described above except that fluorochemical liquid, FC 80 (3M, St. Paul, Minn.), is substituted for the diisodecylphthalate containing oil red O. This heavy liquid results in an emulsion of heavy particles which sediment easily during centrifugation. The effect of these particles on degranulation can be compared with the ingestion rate of paraffin oil particles assayed as described above.

Incubation. About 10^7 leukocytes are incubated in small plastic test tubes (Becton Dickinson Labware, Oxnard, Calif.) in 0.8 ml of balanced salt solution for 5 min in a shaking water bath at 37°C. Opsonized lipopolysaccharide-coated fluorochemical liquid particles, prewarmed at the same time, are added (0.2 ml) to the cell suspensions (zero time). At 15 and 30 min, the tubes are cooled on ice and then centrifuged in a refrigerated centrifuge at 250 × g for 10 min. The supernatant fluid contains the extracellular medium to be assayed for enzyme activity. A 0.5-ml amount of this fluid is aspirated and kept on ice until assayed later the same day or is frozen at −20°C until assayed at a later date. The enzyme is stable in the frozen state for months. Controls to be included in each run are 0.2 ml of balanced salt solution added at zero time in place of opsonized particles and 0.2 ml of particles which have not been opsonized. Each incubation condition should be run at least in duplicate.

Assay of enzyme activity. A substrate mixture is prepared by dissolving 31.5 mg of p-nitrophenyl-β-glucuronide (Sigma) and 100 μl of Triton X-100 (Packard Instrument Co., Downers Grove, Ill.) in 100 ml of 0.05 M sodium acetate-acetic acid buffer, pH 5. The substrate mixture can be kept frozen at −20°C and thawed before each use. Enzyme assay incubations consist of 0.9 ml of substrate mix to which 0.1 ml of sample is added. The mixtures are incubated for 18 h (overnight) at 37°C. The reaction is terminated by addition of 2 ml of 0.1 N NaOH. The OD of the solution is determined spectrophotometrically at 410 nm.

Calculation of results. For the system described, $(OD_{410} \times 20)/1.84 \times 18$ gives the number of nanomoles generated per hour by 10^7 leukocytes at each time of sampling.

As mentioned previously, the results of degranulation assays are best expressed as a function of the initial ingestion rate assayed as described above. The results then can be expressed as degranulation (nanomoles of p-nitrophenyl-β-glucuronide released at a given time per milligram of diisodecylphthalate oil ingested per minute).

Evaluation of neutrophil bactericidal activity

The basis of bactericidal tests is the rapid killing of the test organisms once placed in the cytoplasm of the phagocyte or the removal of the bacteria from the extracellular medium. The method of Maaløe (9) with various modifications (6) has been extensively employed.

The bactericidal assay measures the endpoint of several processes, including opsonization, ingestion, and the metabolic alterations prerequisite for bacterial killing. The limitations of this approach include those mentioned above having to do with separation of ingestion from nonspecific adherence. Because of the diverse number of processes involved, the interpretation of the final killing "rate" is somewhat difficult. Moreover, the test requires prolonged incubation times since the disappearance of viability is determined under nonsaturating conditions. For this reason, agglutination of phagocytes and of bacteria on phagocytes or membranes can occur. A clump of

bacteria will produce a single colony, thus leading to an underestimation of the number of viable organisms actually present. The test is most useful when the anticipated experimental conditions will yield a result that is much different from that of the controls. A description of the technique is included because of its widespread use. It is a tricky, laborious test which should be performed only by those familiar with bacteriological methodology and the pitfalls of interpreting the test.

Reagents

Bacteria grown overnight in Trypticase soy broth (BBL Microbiology Systems, Cockeysville, Md.) (or in other media, depending on the organism), centrifuged, washed, and adjusted in salt solution to an appropriate concentration by turbidimetry at 650 nm
Bovine albumin, 100 mg/liter in distilled water
Nutrient agar

Organisms may be harvested at any phase of the growth cycle. If taken at the early lag phase, populations usually remain stable in phagocytic systems for a period of 1 to 2 h. In contrast, lag-phase organisms will begin multiplying within 1 h and, unless the period of phagocytosis is short, will alter the initial multiplicity of bacteria per phagocyte. It is usually simpler to harvest from liquid media since the bacteria can be collected by centrifugation, are not in large clumps, and may be easily washed. Solutions used to wash and suspend viable organisms are similar to those employed for phagocytes. Certain bacteria are rapidly killed in saline or balanced salt solution. This bactericidal action can be reversed by the addition of as little as 0.01% bovine albumin.

The quantitation of viable populations may be performed by a number of methods. The most rigorous is colony counting after preparing pour plates or streaking a measured sample on the surface of quadrant plates. If the same cultural conditions are employed from day to day, it is easier to assay the OD of the washed suspension at 650 nm and construct a standard curve of OD versus viable units. When late-lag-phase organisms are employed, there may be many nonviable bacteria which influence the nephelometric method but go undetected by plate counts. Under these conditions it is best to do a total particle count with a Petroff-Hausser counting chamber.

Procedure

Phagocytes suspended in balanced salt solution are dispensed to sterile siliconized tubes (15 by 150 mm). Serum and bacteria are then added to appropriate concentrations, the tubes are sealed, and their contents are mixed. Each tube has a total volume of 2.0 ml and contains 20×10^6 to 30×10^6 phagocytes per ml, 1×10^6 to 30×10^6 bacteria per ml, and concentrations of serum ranging from 1 to 50%, depending on the nature of the experiment. It is usually best to employ not more than three bacteria per phagocyte and to use lag-phase organisms which do not multiply readily. The tubes are then incubated at 37°C, either in a reciprocating water bath or end over end in a warm room. At various times from 0 to 3 h or longer, samples are removed for measurement of the total viable bacterial population, the extracellular population, and the cell-associated organisms.

The total count is obtained by diluting 0.01 to 0.2 ml of the suspension in the dilute albumin solution and homogenizing it to disrupt the leukocytes. Homogenization can be performed with a high-speed Teflon pestle in a tight-fitting tube. Serial 10-fold dilutions are then prepared and plated either on the surface of nutrient agar or by pour plate techniques. This procedure liberates most organisms and is an index of both intracellular and extracellular viable bacteria.

Simultaneously, a 1.0-ml sample is taken for evaluation of extracellular and cell-associated microorganisms. This sample is diluted 1:5 with cold salt solution and centrifuged for 3 to 4 min at $45 \times g$. This deposits the leukocytes, leaving a clear supernatant fluid, a sample of which is plated for the extracellular population. The pellet is then suspended in buffer, homogenized, and plated to obtain cell-associated bacteria. The number of viable organisms per milliliter in the original suspension is then calculated, and each of the three bacterial counts per sample is plotted semilogarithmically.

Appropriate controls must be conducted to rule out (i) an extracellular bactericidal effect of the medium (this control can be conducted by incubating bacteria and leukocytes in a stationary system in which contact is minimal) and (ii) major trapping of particles with leukocytes during low-speed centrifugation, which becomes apparent if the difference between total and cell-associated counts at time zero is less than 1 log unit. Under these conditions the "rate" of phagocytosis can be followed for long periods of time, and the influence of components of the medium as well as cell-oriented factors can be evaluated in detail.

This work was supported by the Edwin S. Webster Foundation.

LITERATURE CITED

1. **Altman, A., and T. P. Stossel.** 1974. Functional immaturity of bone marrow granulocytes. Br. J. Haematol. **27**:241–246.
2. **Babior, B. M.** 1978. Oxygen-dependent microbial killing by phagocytes. N. Engl. J. Med. **298**:659–668, 721–725.
3. **Baehner, R. L., L. A. Boxer, and J. Davis.** 1976. The biochemical basis of nitroblue tetrazolium reduction in normal human and chronic granulomatous disease polymorphonuclear leukocytes. Blood **48**:309–313.
4. **Cohen, H. J., and M. E. Chovaniec.** 1978. Superoxide generation by digitonin-stimulated guinea pig granulocytes. A basis for a continuous assay for monitoring superoxide production and for the study of the activation of the generating system. J. Clin. Invest **61**:1081–1087.
5. **Forsgren, A., D. Schmeling, and O. Zettervall.** 1977. Quantitative phagocytosis by human polymorphonuclear leukocytes. Use of radio-labelled emulsions to measure the rate of phagocytosis. Immunology **32**:491–497.
6. **Hirsch, J. G., and A. B. Church.** 1960. Studies of phagocytosis of group A streptococci by polymorphonuclear leukocytes in vitro. J. Exp. Med. **111**:309–322.
7. **Klebanoff, S. J., and R. A. Clark.** 1977. Iodination by human polymorphonuclear leukocytes: a re-evaluation. J. Lab Clin. Med. **89**:675–686.
8. **Klebanoff, S. J., and R. A. Clark.** 1978. The neutrophil: functional and clinical disorders. North Holland Publishing Co., Amsterdam.
9. **Maaløe, O.** 1946. On the relation between alexin and opsonin. Ejnar Munksgaard, Copenhagen.
10. **Mitchell, R. H., S. J. Pancake, J. Noseworthy, and M. L. Karnovsky.** 1969. Measurement of rates of phagocytosis. The use of cellular monolayers. J. Cell Biol. **40**:216–224.
11. **Repine, J. E., B. Rasmussen, and J. G. White.** 1979. An improved nitroblue tetrazolium test using phorbol myristate acetate-coated coverslips. Am. J. Clin. Pathol. **71**:582–585.
12. **Root, R. K., and J. A. Metcalf.** 1977. H_2O_2 release from human granulocytes during phagocytosis. Relationship to superoxide anion formation and cellular catabolism of H_2O_2 studies with normal and cytochalasin B-treated cells. J. Clin. Invest. **60**:1266–1279.
13. **Stossel, T. P.** 1973. Evaluation of opsonic and leukocyte function with a spectrophotometric test in patients with infection and with phagocytic disorders. Blood **42**:121–130.
14. **Stossel, T. P.** 1977. Endocytosis, p. 105–141. *In* P. Cuatrecasas and M. Greaves (ed.), Receptors and recognition, vol. 4. Chapman and Hall, Ltd., London.
15. **Stossel, T. P., R. K. Root, and M. Vaughan.** 1972. Phagocytosis in chronic granulomatous disease and the Chediak-Higashi syndrome. N. Engl. J. Med. **286**:120–123.
16. **Zurier, R. B., S. Hoffstein, and G. Weissmann.** 1973. Cytochalasin B: effect on lysosomal enzyme release from human leukocytes. Proc. Natl. Acad. Sci. U.S.A. **70**:844–848.

Chapter 48

Section G. Host Responses to Bacterial, Mycotic, and Parasitic Diseases

Introduction

STEVEN D. DOUGLAS

It is a great honor to dedicate this section of the manual to the late Erwin Neter (26 May 1909–2 November 1983), Section Editor for the first and second editions. In addition to his many editorial duties, Dr. Neter held many important offices and positions in the American Society for Microbiology and contributed more than 300 original publications which spanned the fields of immunology and microbiology. He made pioneering observations which are highlighted by the first description of enteropathogenic *Escherichia coli*, the discovery of enterobacterial common antigen (EAC), and discoveries related to disease etiologies, chemotherapy, and endotoxins.

A number of new chapters have been added to this section since the previous edition. Major advances in monoclonal antibody production, enzyme-linked immunosorbent assays, and radioimmunoassays have led to the development of improved diagnostic methods.

Chapter 49

Immune Response to *Staphylococcus aureus*

L. JOSEPH WHEAT, RICHARD B. KOHLER, AND ARTHUR WHITE

The detection of antibodies against staphylococcal antigens has been useful in making a diagnosis by serology for patients in whom cultures are either negative or difficult to obtain, such as patients with osteomyelitis, or when cultures are difficult to interpret, such as in sputum cultures from patients with pneumonia or cultures of draining sinuses. In addition, detection of antibodies against staphylococci may aid in differentiation between uncomplicated staphylococcal bacteremias and those that are complicated by metastatic foci or endocarditis. Although patients with serious staphylococcal infections may develop antibodies against a variety of staphylococcal antigens, including ribitol teichoic or lipoteichoic acids, α-hemolysin, or peptidoglycan, most studies have detected antibodies against cell wall teichoic acids of *Staphylococcus aureus* which are alpha- or beta-acetylglucosaminyl ribitol teichoic acids.

Sera from all adults contain antibodies against ribitol teichoic acid of *S. aureus*. Diagnostic tests must distinguish the lower level of antibodies against this acid present in normal subjects from higher levels in patients with serious staphylococcal diseases. Some studies have indicated that teichoic acid antibodies can be detected in a high proportion of normal individuals by the methods commonly employed and therefore have implied that the test has a very high (unacceptable) false-positive rate. If a sensitive method which detects a low level of antibodies in normal individuals is used, quantitation of the antibody content is essential to differentiate between normal low levels of antibody content and high levels in infected subjects.

Both radioimmunoassay (12, 13) and enzyme-linked immunosorbent assay (2, 12, 13) have been utilized for detection of staphylococcal teichoic antibodies, but to date there are no commercial kits available for these methods. Therefore, we shall restrict this discussion to counterimmunoelectrophoresis and agar gel diffusion tests for detection of teichoic acid antibodies. We will also compare the results of commercial kits with those of assays requiring preparation of antigens in individual laboratories.

MATERIALS AND METHODS

Teichoic acid antibody assay (Indiana University)

See reference 10.

The Lafferty strain of *S. aureus* is used. Organisms incubated for 24 to 48 h on Trypticase soy agar (BBL Microbiology Systems, Cockeysville, Md.) are washed in a sterile 0.9% saline solution, suspended at a 20% (vol/vol) concentration, and disrupted for 5 h with a cell disrupter (Bronwill BIO-SONIK sonicator; Blackstone Corp., Jamestown, N.Y.). This ultrasonic extract is used undiluted and has a teichoic acid titer of 1:1,024 against our positive control, commercially available

human pooled immunoglobulin (GAMMA-GEE; Merck Sharpe & Dohme, West Point, Pa.). The teichoic acid content of this ultrasonic extract was estimated to be 529 mg/liter, as determined by radial immunodiffusion by reference to purified ribitol teichoic acid.

Petri dishes (15 by 100 mm) containing 0.9% Noble agar with 7-mm wells spaced 8 mm apart are used for our immunodiffusion method. After addition of 200 μl of the undiluted staphylococcal extract to the central well and serial dilutions of the test serum samples or commercially available human gamma globulin to the peripheral wells, the plates are incubated for 24 h at 37°C. Serum samples that form lines of identity with the human gamma globulin precipitin band nearest the serum well are regarded as positive for teichoic acid antibodies.

ENDO-STAPH Assay

See reference 10.

The teichoic acid antibody assay materials and procedure are described in the package insert and are supplied by Meridian Diagnostics, Inc., Cincinnati, Ohio. The antigen is a partially purified teichoic acid prepared by phenylhydrazine extraction of the Lafferty strain of *S. aureus*. The test antigen used in the assay is standardized to contain 30 mg of teichoic acid per liter, as determined by radial immunodiffusion by reference to the purified ribitol teichoic acid. The positive-control serum sample is prepared by immunizing rabbits with this partially purified ribitol teichoic acid. In immunodiffusion, the control serum sample forms a single precipitin line of identity with test antigen and the purified teichoic acid. A 40-μl portion of the purified antigen is placed in the central well, 40 μl of the rabbit anti-ribitol teichoic acid (positive control) is placed in each of two of the surrounding wells, and 40 μl of the twofold serial dilutions of sera is placed in each of the remaining four wells. The plates are incubated at room temperature for 24 h in Parafilm-sealed petri dishes containing a moist cotton square. The teichoic acid antibody titer is taken as the highest serum dilution forming a precipitin line of identity with the positive-control serum sample.

Counterimmunoelectrophoresis

See reference 9.

A variety of methods utilizing counterimmunoelectrophoresis for detection of *S. aureus* antibodies have been published (12, 13). In published series, the frequency of detectable antibodies by counterimmunoelectrophoresis in sera from uninfected subjects varied from 0 to 100%. This variability is probably due to differences in the antigen preparations and the methods used. Commercial kits for counterimmunoelectrophoresis are available from Diagnostica Inc., Miami,

Fla. Supplied in the kits are antigens and antibody for a positive control, counterimmunoelectrophoresis 10-test plates, and barbital acetate buffer (pH 8.6). Teichoic acids of a sonic extract of the Lafferty strain of *S. aureus* for prepared by published methods (11). The plates for counterimmunoelectrophoresis are 80 by 40 mm with wells 3 mm in diameter and a center-to-center interwell distance of 11 mm. Each serum sample is tested undiluted and at dilutions of 1:2 and 1:4, along with a 1:4 dilution of the positive-control serum and a negative-control serum. After addition of the antigen to the cathodal well and of the test samples to the anodal well, a constant current of 30 mA is applied for 30 min. After electrophoresis the plates are incubated for 5°C for 1 h and then examined for precipitin lines.

RESULTS

In Table 1 are shown data obtained by using a commercial assay (ENDO-STAPH) in patients with staphylococcal infections and in control subjects (10). Complicated bacteremia is defined as bacteremia with metastatic infections confirmed by cultures of bone, kidney, lung, or soft tissue. Uncomplicated bacteremias are those in which a primary site of infection, usually at an access site, is promptly treated and both endocarditis and metastatic infections are excluded. With the ENDO-STAPH assay, more than half of sera from patients with staphylococcal endocarditis and complicated staphylococcal bacteremias had detectable teichoic acid antibodies, but so did a high proportion of sera obtained from control subjects and from subjects without staphylococcal infections (Table 1). Titers of ≥1:4 were present in 16 of 23 sera from patients with staphylococcal endocarditis and in 12 of 20 sera from patients with complicated bacteremias, but only 3 of 17 patients with uncomplicated staphylococcal bacteremia had such titers. None of 21 sera from patients with endocarditis due to other gram-positive organisms had titers of 1:4 or higher. With a titer of ≥1:8 considered positive, sera from 8 of 23 patients with staphylococcal endocarditis and from 8 of 20 patients with complicated staphylococcal bacteremias had

positive titers, but none of 70 sera from control subjects had such titers.

When tested by using an agar gel diffusion test developed at Indiana University Medical Center, none of the control subjects had detectable antibodies (Table 2). Antibodies were detected in 12 of 23 subjects with staphylococcal endocarditis and in 11 of 20 subjects with complicated bacteremia but in only 2 of 17 patients with uncomplicated bacteremia. The difference in the sensitivities of these two assays in detection of antibodies is probably related to the teichoic acid content of the antigen. We have demonstrated (11, 13) that preparations with low concentrations of teichoic acid antigens will detect antibodies present in normal individuals. With higher concentrations of antigens, only elevated concentrations of antibodies are detected.

In Table 3 is shown the frequency with which teichoic acid antibodies can be detected by counterimmunoelectrophoresis at dilutions of 1:4 or greater with the commercially available kit from Diagnostica Inc. (9). Teichoic acid antibody titers of ≥1:4 by counterimmunoelectrophoresis were present in all sera from patients with staphylococcal endocarditis and in 1 of 12 sera from patients with endocarditis due to coagulase-negative staphylococci or other organisms. Titers of ≥1:4 were also present in 8 of 19 sera from patients with complicated staphylococcal bacteremia but in only 2 of 11 sera from patients with uncomplicated staphylococcal bacteremia. None of the 29 sera from normal controls had detectable antibody titers of ≥1:4 by counterimmunoelectropho-

TABLE 2. Indiana University assay

Infection	No. positive/ no. of subjects
Endocarditis	12/23
Complicated staphylococcal bacteremia	11/20
Uncomplicated staphylococcal bacteremia	2/17
Nonbacteremic staphylococcal infections	9/20
Other gram-positive endocarditis	0/21
Other gram-positive infections	0/10
Gram-negative infections	0/19
None	0/20

TABLE 1. ENDO-STAPH assay

Infection (no. of subjects)	No. with titer:		
	Positive	>1:4	>1:8
Staphylococcal endocarditis (23)	20	16	8
Complicated staphylococcal bacteremia (20)	17	12	8
Uncomplicated staphylococcal bacteremia (17)	10	3	0
Nonbacteremic staphylococcal infections (20)	17	10	3
Other gram-positive endocarditis (21)	6	0	0
Other gram-positive infections (10)	2	0	0
Gram-negative infections (19)	4	2	0
None (20)	12	2	0

TABLE 3. Frequency of teichoic acid antibody titers of ≥1:4 with a commercially available counterimmunoelectrophoresis kit

Infection	Frequency
S. aureus endocarditis	13/13
Coagulase-negative staphylococcal endocarditis	0/6
Other endocarditis	1/6
S. aureus bacteremia	
Complicated	8/9
Uncomplicated	2/11
Nonbacteremic *S. aureus* infection	3/19
Nonstaphylococcal disease	3/39
None	0/29

resis, but high titers were present in 3 of 39 subjects without evidence of staphylococcal disease.

INTERPRETATION

Detection of high levels of antibodies against staphylococcal teichoic acids in patients with staphylococcal bacteremia indicates that staphylococcal endocarditis or complicated staphylococcal bacteremia is likely (1–13). Serious staphylococcal infections in patients who have negative blood cultures while on therapy may be detected only by antibody studies. Finally, the development of antibodies may be useful in detecting staphylococcal infections such as osteomyelitis or pneumonia in which cultures are difficult to interpret. A negative test does not exclude staphylococcal disease as the cause of osteomyelitis, pneumonia, etc. Several circumstances should be considered in the evaluation of staphylococcal antibodies. Ten to fourteen days may be required for serological responses against these infections, so the test should be repeated in patients with negative tests (10). Some patients may be unable to mount a serologic response. We have observed impaired responses in patients with chronic renal failure requiring renal dialysis (12, 13). Occasionally, patients with uncomplicated bacteremia without either endocarditis or metastatic infections will have high titers of teichoic acid antibodies, perhaps due to delayed drainage of the primary site (11–13). Finally, elevated titers occur in patients infected with certain organisms known to cross-react with ribitol teichoic acid of *S. aureus*, including diptheroids (12, 13) and *Haemophilus influenzae* (12, 13). With these exceptions, patients with a titer of 1:4 in the ENDO-STAPH test or by counterimmunoelectrophoresis using the Diagnostica kit should be considered to have disseminated staphylococcal infections. A positive result in the absence of prolonged local suppuration mandates a search for endocarditis or metastatic infection. In such a patient, we would treat for at least 4 weeks. Negative results suggest uncomplicated bacteremia and support a shorter duration of therapy. Finally, if clinical findings of endocarditis or metastatic infection are present, prolonged therapy is required irrespective of the teichoic acid antibody titer.

LITERATURE CITED

1. **Bayer, A. S.** 1982. Staphylococcal bacteremia and endocarditis. State of art. Arch. Intern. Med. **142:**1169–1176.
2. **Granstrom, M., I. Julander, and R. Mollby.** 1983. Serological diagnosis of deep staphylococcus aureus infections by enzyme-linked immunosorbent assay (ELISA) for staphylococcal hemolysins and teichoic acid. Scand. J. Infect. Dis. **41:**132–139.
3. **Jackson, L. J., M. I. Sottile, F. G. Aguilar-Torres, T. H. Dee, and M. W. Rytel.** 1978. Correlation of antistaphylococcal antibody titers with severity of staphylococcal diseases. Am. J. Med. **64:**629–633.
4. **Kaplan, M. H., and M. J. Tenenbaum.** 1982. *Staphylococcus aureus:* cellular biology and clinical application. Am. J. Med. **72:**248–249.
5. **Le, C. T., and E. B. Lewin.** 1978. Teichoic acid serology in staphylococcal infections of infants and children. J. Pediatr. **93:**572–577.
6. **Nagel, J. G., C. V. Tuazon, T. A. Cardella, and J. N. Sheagren.** 1975. Teichoic acid serologic diagnosis of staphylococcus endocarditis. Ann. Intern. Med. **8:**13–17.
7. **Tenenbaum, M. J., and G. L. Archer.** 1980. Prognostic value of teichoic acid antibodies in *Staphylococcus aureus* bacteremia: a reassessment. South. Med. J. **73:**140–146.
8. **Tuazon, C. U., J. N. Sheagren, M. S. Choa, D. Marcus, and J. A. Curtin.** 1978. *Staphylococcus aureus* bacteremia: relationship between formation of antibodies to teichoic acid and development of metastatic abscesses. J. Infect. Dis. **137:**57–61.
9. **West, T. E., N. M. Burdash, A. M. Boehm, and M. E. West.** 1984. Evaluation of a commercial counterimmunoelectrophoresis kit for detection of *Staphylococcus aureus* teichoic acid antibodies. J. Clin. Microbiol. **17:**567–570.
10. **Wheat, L. J., R. B. Kohler, M. Garten, and A. White.** 1984. Commercially available (ENDO-STAPH) assay for teichoic acid antibodies. Arch. Intern. Med. **144:**261–264.
11. **Wheat, L. J., R. B. Kohler, and A. White.** 1979. Teichoic acid antibody determination by agar-gel diffusion: effect of using dilute antigen preparation. J. Clin. Microbiol. **10:**138–140.
12. **Wheat, L. J., R. B. Kohler, and A. White.** 1984. Staphylococcal teichoic acid antibodies, p. 177–188. *In* J. S. Remington and M. N. Swartz (ed.), Current clinical topics in infectious diseases 5. McGraw-Hill Book Co., New York.
13. **White, A., L. J. Wheat, and R. B. Kohler.** 1983. Diagnostic and therapeutic significance of staphylococcal teichoic acid antibodies. Scand. J. Infect. Dis. **41:**105–116.

Chapter 50

Immune Responses to Streptococcal Infections

PATRICIA FERRIERI

Among the beta-hemolytic streptococci causing infections in humans, the serological groups A, B, C, and G figure most prominently. Group A streptococci continue to be a focus of interest not only because of their causal role in acute streptococcal pharyngitis and other pyogenic infections, but also because of their association with poststreptococcal sequelae, specifically acute rheumatic fever and acute glomerulonephritis. Serological tests to aid in the diagnosis of a group A streptococcal infection have utilized common extracellular antigens released from the organisms such as streptolysin O, DNase B, nicotinamide adenine dinucleotidase (NADase), hyaluronidase, and streptokinase. For a number of years, the most popular choices for incorporation into an antibody assay were streptolysin O and hyaluronidase. The test for antibody to streptolysin O remains a popular choice among clinicians and serological laboratories and is probably the test most easily performed. In the past decade, increasing interest has led to the introduction of the test for antibody to DNase B because of the greater versatility of this test in assessing immune responses to infections of both the throat and skin (5, 7, 17). In addition, there is a tendency for this antibody to remain elevated, thereby permitting assessment of a previous streptococcal infection in such diseases as Sydenham's chorea, where the latency period is prolonged. The antigens for the antistreptolysin O (ASO) and anti-DNase B (ADB) tests are available commercially, and in the case of the latter system, full commercial kits have been developed in recent years.

The antihyaluronidase test (AHT) can also be performed with commercial reagents, and it also has the versatility of the ADB test in that it is capable of detecting an immunological response to infections of both the skin and the pharynx and subsequent complications such as acute glomerulonephritis. In general, reproducibility has not been as optimal as that seen for the ADB and ASO tests.

Antibodies to somatic group A streptococcal antigens such as the group A polysaccharide antigen, which confers the specific group reaction on group A streptococci, also develop after infection of the throat and skin. Antibodies to this antigen can remain elevated for many months, and in the case of patients with rheumatic fever with valvular involvement and complications, the antibody titer may remain elevated for many years, possibly due to some cross-reaction between heart valve antigens and the streptococcal antigen (1, 3, 5, 17). Reagents for this test are not available commercially, and in a few research laboratories, a radioimmune precipitation technique has been employed for detection of antibodies to this important antigen (1). Recently, an enzyme-linked immunosorbent assay (ELISA) has been described (3).

Reagents for the anti-NADase and antistreptokinase tests are not available commercially. In the case of the anti-NADase test, the enzyme that serves as the antigen poses more problems in purification, potency, and stability of activity. In addition, antibodies to NADase are not as consistent and predictable as those directed against DNase B in patients with streptococcal skin infections and the sequela of acute glomerulonephritis. The application of antibodies to the antigen marker streptokinase is more limited, and the test has not been as reproducible or as sensitive as the ASO and ADB tests.

Antibodies against the type-specific molecule, known as the M protein, of the group A streptococci are of special interest to investigators studying specific immune responses to group A streptococci after throat or skin infections. Various tests such as the classical bactericidal test and opsonophagocytic assays can be used, but these tests are not practical for use in routine clinical laboratories. Since anti-M antibodies can be protective against reinfection of the throat with the same M serotype, a test for these antibodies may be useful in designing protective vaccines against group A streptococci (5, 17).

Detection of antibodies specific for infection with other beta-hemolytic streptococci such as groups B, C, and G is not commonly performed. Since the group-specific carbohydrate of these organisms is distinct for each of them, it is possible to measure antibodies to the group C and G polysaccharide antigens by such techniques as radioimmunoassay. Such a test can provide evidence of a rise in titer and specific confirmation of a preceding infection. Since streptolysin O is produced by group C and G streptococci, an ASO determination can be confirmatory also of documented group C or G streptococcal infection. This possibility has been confirmed in uncommon outbreaks of acute pharyngitis due to these organisms. Similarly, some of the DNases other than DNase B can be produced by these serological groups, and a neutralization test specific for these other species of DNase has been developed in our research laboratory; this test requires control antisera specific for all of the DNases.

Because of the prominent role of group B streptococci in newborn septicemia and meningitis, determination of antibodies to type-specific polysaccharide antigens of the organism is of interest. The polysaccharide antigen may play a role in virulence, and antibodies to these antigens may be protective. Determination of such specialized antibodies in the sera of pregnant women may be indicated in special situations. At present, measurement of these antibodies is either by radioactive-antigen binding tests or by an enzyme-linked immunosorbent assay. The reagents are not available commercially, nor have the procedures been standardized sufficiently for application in a clinical diagnostic laboratory.

The major tests to be discussed in more detail are the ASO and ADB tests and the AHT because of the availability of commercial antigens or even a complete kit to perform the test and because of their contribution to the interpretation of clinical diagnostic problems in group A streptococcal infections. A rapid slide-screening method based on particle agglutination in which erythrocytes are coated with a mixture of several streptococcal extracellular antigens, including streptolysin O, DNase, hyaluronidase, and others, is available commercially and will be discussed first (13).

SCREENING TEST

The Streptozyme test can be used as a simple slide agglutination method to obtain preliminary information on whether a patient has had a group A streptococcal infection (4, 13). A positive screening by further serum dilutions can be used to determine a quantitative value. It should be noted that a single serum determination is not as valuable as the study of sequential specimens obtained during the acute stage of the infection and then timed at intervals after the acute stage and into convalescence. Positive results with Streptozyme have been concordant with positive results for other streptococcal antibody tests such as the ASO and ADB in over 90% of instances (11, 13). However, a negative Streptozyme test does not rule out a group A streptococcal infection, and in circumstances in which a clinical indication requires more substantiation to rule out such a diagnosis, specific tests for antibody to the other extracellular antigens should be performed. Similarly, one may have a positive Streptozyme titer with a negative ASO result because the Streptozyme test is measuring a heterogeneous immune response to several streptococcal antigens.

Test procedure

To perform the test, instructions on the package insert included with the commercial reagents should be followed. The complete kit is available from Wampole Laboratories, Cranbury, N.J.

ASO TEST

The ASO test has been studied extensively in various populations in situations in which group A streptococcal infections are endemic and epidemic (5, 7, 17). The basis of the test is the neutralization of the hemolytic activity of the streptolysin O toxin for erythrocytes by specific antibodies in serum. Since this antigen is produced by nearly all strains of group A streptococci, a significant increase in titer of ASO strongly supports a diagnosis of recent group A streptococcal infection. The principal steps in performing the test are the preparation of dilutions of the patient's serum, addition of a fixed amount of the streptolysin O to each dilution, and incubation of the mixture to permit neutralization of antigen by antibody if present, followed by the addition of a fixed volume of erythrocytes with reincubation of the sample. The presence of specific antibodies directed against streptolysin O is exhibited by the inhibition of hemolysis of the erythrocytes. In most assays in use in various reference laboratories, the endpoint of the ASO neutralization test is the highest dilution of serum exhibiting no hemolysis.

The method of performing microtiter neutralization tests for ASO as described by Klein et al. (12) is widely used in the United States and is highly reproducible. In this method a serum dilution scheme is used in which the intervals are logarithmically spaced at 0.15-log intervals. This equal spacing of the intervals has advantages in the reporting and interpretation of significant results. In our laboratory, a dilution scheme based on approximately 0.1-log intervals is used.

In choosing to perform a microtitration assay over the macro tube test for the ASO determinations, the former test has the advantages of using smaller amounts of serum and reagents as well as increased productivity at a lower cost per test. Reproducibility of the ASO test by microtitration assay is 95% or greater in our laboratory and has been reported as high as 98.1% (13).

Clinical indications

ASO titers are not required on a routine basis in the management of patients with acute streptococcal pharyngitis. In a situation where it is difficult to distinguish between persistent carriage of the group A streptococci and active infection, there may be some value in examining the immune responses to one or more streptococcal antigens. In patients with suspected rheumatic fever, additional information beyond the presence of group A streptococci in the throat is required in meeting the criteria for diagnosis. In most instances, by the time of presentation with this nonsuppurative sequela, the throat culture may be negative. An extremely elevated ASO titer or, more importantly, a significant rise in titer would substantiate a recent streptococcal infection. Since the ASO titer may have fallen by the time of presentation with acute rheumatic fever, examining for antibody to another streptococcal antigen such as DNase B would be of value (2). In acute glomerulonephritis after throat infections, the ASO titer can support the clinical diagnosis, but in acute glomerulonephritis after skin infections, it is uncommon to see a rise in the ASO titer (7, 17).

Among the disadvantages of the ASO test are (i) poor immunogenicity of streptolysin O after streptococcal skin infections; (ii) the tendency for the titer of this antibody to rise more rapidly than and to decline before the ADB titer; (iii) false-positive titers that may be associated with liver disease; (iv) false-positive titers caused by bacterial contamination in the serum specimen, due to bacterial products that may neutralize the hemolytic activity of streptolysin O; and (v) false-positive titers that may be caused by oxidation of the streptolysin O antigen, abrogating its hemolytic activity (9).

ASO MICROTITRATION TEST

Materials

Microtitration equipment is as follows:
0.025- and 0.05-ml calibrated dropper pipettes
0.05-ml microdiluter

Disposable U plates
Vibrator mixer (paper jogger model JIA; Syntron, Homer City, Pa.)
Vertical vibrator (Arthur H. Thomas, Philadelphia, Pa.)
Test-reading mirror
Serological pipettes
Long-tip measuring pipettes
Test tubes (13 by 100 mm)
15-ml conical centrifuge tube
Streptolysin O
Washed erythrocyte suspension
Control serum of known titer
Barbital-gelatin buffered diluent
Cold distilled water

Procedure

The specific details for preparation of the reagents and performance of the ASO test, described in the 2nd edition of this manual, can be followed for the microtitration test as well as the antistreptolysin tube test (9). We always inactivate a lower dilution of serum for 30 min at 56°C before performing the test.

The incorporation of a titered reference serum as a control is advisable for each setup. Although it is not absolutely necessary to include a control serum on each plate in the microtitration test, the advantage of doing so permits one to accept the patient's specimen results on a plate even if the control specimen on another plate is not exactly concordant with the expected result. In my laboratory, sera of low, moderate, and high antibody titers have been standardized, and one of these sera is included on each of three plates in a set. We accept the results of the run if two of the three control sera do not deviate at all from the expected value and if the third serum deviates by only 1 dilution increment (see below).

READING ASO TESTS

A fluorescent lamp and a test-reading mirror should be used for reading the microtitration test, and a fluorescent lamp and a white background are preferable for the tube test. The test results should be considered invalid and the tests should be repeated if any of the following situations is found.

(i) The titer of the reference serum differs by more than 1 dilution from the expected value. Reference sera have been maintained by the Centers for Disease Control, Atlanta, Ga., and these sera have been standardized against an international reference serum available through the World Health Organization.

(ii) The hemolysin control does not exhibit complete lysis of the erythrocytes.

(iii) Hemolysis is seen in the erythrocyte control (this control does not contain any hemolysin).

It is undesirable to see hemolysis in the patient specimen hemolysin control tube or well, since hemolysis indicates the presence of a natural hemolysin in the patient's serum. Although a natural hemolysin may be diluted out at higher dilutions of the serum and may not interfere with the determination of an endpoint, its presence should be investigated.

Reporting of ASO titers

The endpoint in each assay is the highest dilution of serum that has no visible hemolysis; this endpoint is the titer that is reported. The titer can be expressed in terms of either Todd units or international units, since the two measurements are essentially the same (9). If streptolysin O reagent produced in the United States is used in the assay, the number of units would be the same as the titer of that patient's serum (9). An example would be an endpoint of 1:480, which equals a titer of either 480 Todd units if the strength of the hemolysin used in the test was adjusted against the Todd standard or 480 IU if the World Health Organization International Standard was used.

Sources of reagents and materials

Sources of reagents and materials are as follows.
Streptolysin O: Difco Laboratories, Detroit, Mich.; Fisher Scientific Co., Pittsburgh, Pa.; GIBCO Laboratories, Grand Island, N.Y.; and others
Barbital and sodium barbital: Fisher Scientific Co., Pittsburgh, Pa.
Microtitration equipment: Dynatech Laboratories, Inc., Alexandria, Va.
Disposable U plates: Linbro Scientific Co., New Haven, Conn., and Dynatech Laboratories, Inc., Alexandria, Va.

Interpretation

After acute group A streptococcal pharyngitis, an antibody response to streptolysin O may occur in 80% or more of patients. In various population groups, the distribution of ASO titers varies depending on the exposure of the individuals to streptococcal disease. Ideally, the limits of normal antibody titers for a population must be established in each laboratory servicing the population. A significant titer is usually defined as a rise in titer of 2 or more dilution increments between the acute- and convalescent-phase specimens obtained, regardless of the height of the antibody titer. In the scheme of Klein et al. this would be a change of 0.3 log or more (9, 12). If one fixed specimen is dealt with, the interpretation of the titer would depend on the upper limit of normal seen in the population from which the patient originated. Obviously, this value can differ depending on the age of the patient as well as the endemicity of streptococcal disease. The value is highest in school-age children and young adults; most toddlers have low antibody titers compared with those of school-age children. The upper limit of normal value is usually defined as the highest titer that is exceeded by only 20% of a population. In many populations, including our own, an ASO titer of 240 or greater in a school-age patient may suggest a recent group A streptococcal infection (11). One must be very conservative, however, in translating the value of a single titer to any specific disease state. None of the antibody tests discussed is considered diagnostic of a process such as acute rheumatic fever or acute glomerulonephritis; the specific antibody titers must be viewed only as serological aids in the diagnosis of a streptococcal infection. It is difficult to place precisely in time when such an infection may have occurred. Since 15% or more of patients with acute rheumatic fever may not have an elevated ASO titer or demonstrate a rise in titer, it is valuable to carry out a second test such as the ADB test or the AHT after an acute group A streptococcal infection (2, 5). A rise in ASO titer may occur as early as 1 week after the infection, usually peaks at approximately 4 weeks, and then begins to decline. Among patients there is considerable variation in the kinetics of decline of the ASO titer, and the specific titers are altered by other intervening group A streptococcal infections.

ANTI-DNase B TEST

Group A streptococci typically produce four DNases, i.e., A, B, C, and D (16). DNase B is found among nearly all strains of group A beta-hemolytic streptococci, a fact which makes DNase B a valuable biological marker for immune response to infection with these organisms. A few strains of group C and G streptococci may also produce this nuclease. The three nucleases of group B streptococci, on the other hand, are antigenically distinct from the nucleases of group A streptococci. Among the four major nucleases of group A streptococci, antigenic distinctions are found, and specific antibodies can be produced in animals to allow a distinction to be made and to verify the purity of an enzyme preparation. The ADB test is also a neutralization test utilizing the enzyme DNase B as the antigen in the test.

Various dilutions of the patient's serum are made, and a fixed amount of the enzyme is added, with incubation, to allow an antigen-antibody reaction to take place. Addition of the substrate DNA is followed by reincubation. If polymerized DNA is coupled to a dye such as methyl green, it is possible to assess whether digestion or depolymerization of the DNA has taken place or has been inhibited by the neutralization of the enzyme by specific antibody. When the DNA-methyl green complex is intact and the DNA has not been depolymerized, then the color is retained; if the DNA has been depolymerized by the action of the DNase B in the absence of antibody, then the green color is absent. Another method to assess the integrity of the DNA substrate in the test is the addition of alcohol after the incubations have been completed; the presence of a clot in a tube is an indication that the DNA is intact and therefore antibody is present.

Among the tests that can be performed to determine antibody against DNase B are the tube test using alcohol precipitation with clot formation, a microtitration method (10, 15) with in-house preparation of purified DNase B as well as the other reagents, and a commercial kit for performance of a tube test. The latter system incorporates a color indicator to assess when the DNA is depolymerized or inhibited by the presence of specific antibody.

The ADB microtitration test has the advantage of requiring smaller amounts of serum and other reagents, requiring less time to perform, and therefore being more cost effective. Requirements for carrying out either a tube test or a microtitration test, if the reagents are to be made in the clinical laboratory, include familiarity with enzyme purification, possession of a control antibody specific for DNase B (and containing no antibodies to other nucleases) to standardize the working enzyme dilution, preparation of the DNA-methyl green complex, and standardization of a human reference serum for inclusion in the test.

An enzyme-linked immunosorbent assay has been developed to measure antibodies to DNase B (6). This assay requires a purified enzyme for the antigen source. At present the assay is not in use as a routine assay.

Clinical indications

Since large amounts of DNase B are produced by strains of streptococci of throat and skin origin, antibody responses to this enzyme are common and may appear after infections at either site (7). Therefore, this antibody test can be valuable in documenting an antecedent group A streptococcal infection in patients with acute rheumatic fever and in patients with acute poststreptococcal glomerulonephritis after infection of either the throat or the skin (2, 5, 17). Because the antibody levels to DNase B rise later than antibodies to streptolysin O and because the ADB titers decline over a period of several months, this test is a valuable tool in substantiating a preceding group A streptococcal infection in patients with Sydenham's chorea, presenting after a relatively long latency period. For all of these reasons, the ADB test can be viewed as the antibody test of choice if only one test is available.

Another advantage of the ADB test versus the ASO test is that falsely elevated titers due to nonspecific inhibitors in the serum are not a problem.

MICROTITRATION TEST

Materials

Microtitration equipment is as follows (as described for the ASO microtitration test):
Vibrator mixer
Serological pipettes
Long-tip measuring pipettes
Test tubes (13 by 100 mm)
15-ml conical centrifuge tube
DNase B
DNA-methyl green
Standardized control serum
Buffered diluent

Procedure

The procedure is as described in the 2nd edition of this manual (9).

Since some patients may have intrinsic DNase activity in their sera, the 1:10 dilution can be inactivated at 63 to 65°C for 30 min. This dilution should be cooled in an ice bath before the other serum dilutions are made.

Reagents

Directions for making the buffer solution can be found in the 2nd edition of this manual (9).

DNase B

To obtain a homogeneous preparation of the DNase B, avoid using the crude supernatants of growth of a good enzyme-producing strain. A simplification of the preparation and purification of the enzyme has been described by Slechta and Gray (16) by ammonium sulfate precipitation of supernatant fluids of growth of the organism followed by batch adsorption to DE-23 microfibrous DEAE-cellulose. With this technique, a homogeneous enzyme is obtained, as assessed by neutralization with specific rabbit antisera as well as by gel electrophoretic analysis. Electrophoretic analysis may suffice to show a single peak of enzyme activity; a second cycle of adsorption with fresh ion-exchange cellulose would decrease considerably any chance of slight contamination of nuclease B with any of the other nucleases.

Determining the working dilution of the enzyme is essential with a reference serum of known antibody titer. Whenever a new preparation of enzyme or DNA-methyl green substrate is used for the first time, this determination should be made. The enzyme prepared as described can be stored at −20°C or may be lyophilized, being stable at least 1 year if it is lyophilized and frozen at −20°C.

If a highly active preparation of enzyme is obtained, a stock solution of a 1:10 dilution can be stored for several months at 4°C. With such a preparation, a 1:100 dilution could be prepared approximately every 5 days and stored at 4°C; it is imperative, however, that the daily working dilution be made up from the 1:100 dilution immediately before use in the test. Contamination of the enzyme must be avoided. With a highly active enzyme preparation, we have been able to freeze at −70°C a working dilution (greater than 1:1,000) for several months without deterioration. For the average preparation of enzyme, it may not be possible to proceed in this way. If a commercial kit is used, the reconstitution and storage of the enzyme must be precisely as described in the product brochure. On a daily basis, any remaining working enzyme preparation should be discarded, regardless of the source of the enzyme. The determination of the appropriate working dilution of the enzyme is by titration of a reference serum to obtain the precise expected value.

DNA-methyl green substrate

The DNA-methyl green substrate can be prepared as described by Klein et al. (10) but with a word of caution; i.e., depending on the source of the DNA and the degree of polymerization and purity, the amount put into solution can vary somewhat. The coupling of the DNA to the methyl green dye can also be influenced by the preparation and nature of the DNA substrate.

The DNA-methyl green substrate may be lyophilized and stored under vacuum at 4°C, or it may be kept after rehydration for several weeks at 4°C.

Sources of reagents and materials

Sources of reagents and materials are as follows.
ADB test kit (tube test): Wampole Laboratories, Cranbury, N.J.
DNA, highly polymerized from calf thymus: Sigma Chemical Co., St. Louis, Mo.; Worthington Diagnostics, Freehold, N.J.; and Calbiochem-Behring, La Jolla, Calif.

Methyl green dye (C.I. 42590): Fisher Scientific Co., Pittsburgh, Pa.
Imidazole (finest grade): Sigma Chemical Co., St. Louis, Mo., and Calbiochem-Behring, La Jolla, Calif.
Microtitration equipment, disposable U plates, and vibrator mixer, as described for the ASO test.

Interpretation

As indicated for normal values of ASO, the ADB titers vary with the age of the patient, area of origin, and endemicity of group A streptococcal infection. Titers of 240 or greater in a school-age patient and 120 or greater in an adult patient are viewed as elevated in many parts of the country. As for other antibody tests, a single serum specimen is not as valuable as obtaining acute- and convalescent-phase serum specimens to look for a significant rise in titer. Independent of the magnitude of a titer, a rise in titer of 2 (0.3 log by the system of Klein et al. [10]) or more dilution increments between specimens should be considered significant. The kinetics of the rise of the ADB titer reveal a delay compared with the titer of ASO, reaching a peak 4 to 8 weeks after infection and remaining elevated for several months. This test is frequently valuable in clinical entities with a long latent period between the acute streptococcal infection and development of a nonsuppurative complication. It should be emphasized that an elevated ADB titer, although indicative of a recent infection, is not diagnostic of acute rheumatic fever or acute glomerulonephritis. Since the ADB titers may remain elevated for a long time, a patient may present with an illness unrelated to a streptococcal infection but possess an elevated ADB titer. Caution must be used in linking an elevated titer to any specific diagnostic process. It must also be emphasized that, in examining multiple specimens obtained from a patient on different dates, all the sera should be examined in the same assay to diminish technical variation that might occur in any laboratory on a day-to-day basis. Since about 20 to 25% of patients with group A streptococcal infections may not show an immunological response for a specific antigen, it would be advantageous to test for more than one antibody. For example, by using three antibody tests, an elevated titer for at least one antibody can be demonstrated in about 95% of all patients with acute rheumatic fever or poststreptococcal nephritis (2).

AHT

The AHT is also based on a neutralization assay in which the extracellular enzyme, hyaluronidase, is used as the antigen for measuring antibody. Specific antibody to this enzyme inhibits the digestion of a potassium hyaluronate substrate. If antibody to hyaluronidase is present in a serum, it neutralizes the enzymatic breakdown of the substrate, permitting a clot to form when 2 N acetic acid is added to the assay mixture. If the hyaluronidase enzyme is not inhibited by antibody present in the serum specimen, the substrate will be digested, and no clot will form. The endpoint or titer of the serum is the reciprocal of the highest dilution of serum containing a definite clot. A reaction giving a threadlike appearance should not be considered a clot. The reagents for performing the mucin clot test are available in a commercial kit or can be purchased separately. The standard tube dilution test can be adapted to a microtiter technique to enhance the accuracy of reading the endpoints (14). By adding a dye such as India ink to the microtiter system, it is easier to read the clots, since they are rather small. In every assay, a standard serum with a known antihyaluronidase titer should also be tested.

Clinical indications

The AHT can be viewed as a second test if the ADB test is not available in a laboratory. Since the AHT can detect antibodies after group A streptococcal infections of the skin (as well as throat), the AHT is superior to the ASO test for substantiating a preceding group A streptococcal infection in patients presenting with skin-related acute glomerulonephritis. Similar to the ADB test, the AHT is not influenced by factors that may cause false-positive titers in the ASO test. However, reproducibility of the AHT is not as good as that of the ASO and ADB antibody tests.

Test procedure

To perform the test, follow the directions in the package brochure included with reagents for the test.

Source of reagents

The hyaluronidase enzyme, the hyaluronate substrate, and the standard serum or the complete AHT kit can be obtained from Difco Laboratories, Detroit, Mich.

Interpretation

Since the test is carried out by performing twofold dilutions of the patient serum, beginning with a dilution of 1:32, a significant rise in titer between acute- and convalescent-phase serum specimens is considered a fourfold (two-tube) or greater rise in titer.

LITERATURE CITED

1. **Appleton, R. S., B. E. Victorica, D. Tamer, and E. M. Ayoub.** 1985. Specificity of persistence of antibody to the streptococcal group A carbohydrate in rheumatic valvular heart disease. J. Lab. Clin. Med. **105:**114–119.
2. **Ayoub, E. M., and L. W. Wannamaker.** 1962. Evaluation of the streptococcal desoxyribonuclease B and diphosphopyridine nucleotidase antibody tests in acute rheumatic fever and acute glomerulonephritis. Pediatrics **29:**527–538.
3. **Barrett, D. J., M. Triggiani, and E. M. Ayoub.** 1983. Assay of antibody to group A streptococcal carbohydrate by enzyme-linked immunosorbent assay. J. Clin. Microbiol. **18:**622–627.
4. **Bisno, A. L., and I. Ofek.** 1974. Serologic diagnosis of streptococcal infection. Am. J. Dis. Child. **127:**676–681.
5. **Ferrieri, P.** 1981. *Streptococcus,* p. 54–60. *In* F. Milgrom, C. J. Abeyounis, and K. Kano (ed.), Principles of immunological diagnosis in medicine. Lea & Febiger, Philadelphia.
6. **Gerber, M. A., E. D. Gray, P. Ferrieri, and E. L. Kaplan.** 1980. Enzyme-linked immunosorbent assay of antibodies in human sera to streptococcal DNase B. J. Lab. Clin. Med. **95:**258–265.
7. **Kaplan, E. L., B. F. Anthony, S. S. Chapman, E. M. Ayoub, and L. W. Wannamaker.** 1970. The influence of the site of infection on the immune response to group A streptococci. J. Clin. Invest. **49:**1405–1414.
8. **Kaplan, E. L., and L. W. Wannamaker.** 1975. Dynamics of the immune response in rabbits immunized with streptococcal extracellular antigens: comparison of the Streptozyme agglutination test with three specific neutralization tests. J. Lab. Clin. Med. **86:**91–99.
9. **Klein, G. C.** 1980. Immune response to streptococcal infection (antistreptolysin O, antideoxyribonuclease B), p. 431–440. *In* N. R. Rose and H. Friedman (ed.), Manual of clinical immunology, 2nd ed. American Society for Microbiology, Washington, D.C.
10. **Klein, G. C., C. N. Baker, B. V. Addison, and M. D. Moody.** 1969. Micro test for streptococcal antideoxyribonuclease B. Appl. Microbiol. **18:**204–206.
11. **Klein, G. C., C. N. Baker, and W. L. Jones.** 1971. "Upper limits of normal" antistreptolysin O and antideoxyribonuclease B titers. Appl. Microbiol. **21:**999–1001.
12. **Klein, G. C., E. C. Hall, C. N. Baker, and B. V. Addison.** 1970. Antistreptolysin O test. Comparison of micro and macro technics. Am. J. Clin. Pathol. **53:**159–162.
13. **Klein, G. C., and W. L. Jones.** 1971. Comparison of the Streptozyme test with the antistreptolysin O, antideoxyribonuclease B, and antihyaluronidase tests. Appl. Microbiol. **21:**257–259.
14. **Murphy, R. A.** 1972. Improved antihyaluronidase test applicable to the microtitration technique. Appl. Microbiol. **23:**1170–1171.
15. **Nelson, J., E. M. Ayoub, and L. W. Wannamaker.** 1968. Streptococcal antidesoxyribonuclease B: microtechnique determination. J. Lab. Clin. Med. **71:**867–873.
16. **Slechta, T. F., and E. D. Gray.** 1975. Isolation of streptococcal nuclease B by batch adsorption. J. Clin. Microbiol. **2:**528–530.
17. **Wannamaker, L. W.** 1981. Immunology of streptococci, p. 47–92. *In* A. J. Nahmias and R. J. O'Reilly (ed.), Immunology of human infection. Plenum Publishing Corp., New York.

Chapter 51

Immune Response to *Streptococcus pneumoniae*

GERALD SCHIFFMAN

The immune response to *Streptococcus pneumoniae* is primarily concerned with antibody directed against the 84 capsular polysaccharides. Antibodies to the capsular polysaccharides confer type-specific immunity to infection. The immune response directed to other antigens present on the pneumococcus, such as C-polysaccharide and various proteins, plays at best only a minor role in protection. Many attempts have been made to find a common antigen which could produce antibody to all or most of the serotypes involved in infection. To date, such attempts have not been successful. The type-specific antibodies have been studied in great detail to determine methods for maximizing the immune response and the persistence of antibody, as well as to determine protective levels. Since the immune response to the pneumococcus can be induced either to the polysaccharide itself (released from a focus of infection into the bloodstream of the patient or by immunization with the currently available vaccine) or to particulate bacteria present during a bacteremic phase of infection, the isotypes involved can be either immunoglobulin M (IgM) or IgG. Radioimmunoassay (RIA) has been widely used for the measurement of immune response to *S. pneumoniae* in humans. This method is based on total binding and includes the sum of all isotypes involved in the immune response. The results of assays performed by RIA have been correlated with quantitative precipitin measurements, passive hemagglutination, and mouse protection tests (12). In addition to the correlation with other methods, RIA is specific, sensitive, and rapid. The other most popular methods include enzyme-linked immunosorbent assay (ELISA) and passive hemagglutination. These assays involve twofold dilution steps and hence do not have the precision of the RIA.

The immune response to *S. pneumoniae* in mice has been shown to be T-cell independent. If the response in humans involves the same mechanisms, then the immune response to pneumococcal antigens would be a measure of the B-cell functions of the immune system. The pneumococcal vaccine as presently available consists of 23 serotypes which cause 90% of pneumococcal infections in the United States and Europe. This vaccine (10) consists of serotypes 1, 2, 3, 4, 5, 6B, 7F, 8, 9N, 9V, 10A, 11A, 12F, 14, 15B, 17F, 18C, 19A, 19F, 20, 22F, 23F, and 33F. If the immune response to the vaccine is measured quantitatively, then the vaccinee receives not only the benefit of increased protection against infection but also an evaluation of B-cell function (11).

CLINICAL INDICATIONS

An assessment of the antibody response to pneumococcal vaccine in high-risk patients, as well as an estimate of a protective level of antibody, has been made (9). High-risk patients include the aged and those with cardiopulmonary disease, traumatic splenectomy, Hodgkins' disease, sickle cell disease, renal transplants, nephrotic syndrome, or cirrhosis. The vaccine has been recommended for these high-risk patients. After immunization, evaluation of the immune response provides information on the B-cell function of the patient. The RIA is the procedure of choice since it is quantitative, measures all isotypes, is specific, and requires less than 1 ml of serum. Other procedures are useful for a qualitative answer to whether antibodies are produced or not. If the determination of isotypes is required, the ELISA is the procedure of choice.

INTERPRETATION

Table 1 lists antibody levels pre- and postimmunization for 12 of the most common serotypes measured. Preimmunization antibody levels increase with age. Infants up to 2 years of age usually have less than 100 ng of antibody nitrogen per ml. Responses to the vaccine are minimal up to about 5 years of age for serotypes 6A, 14, 19F, and 23F. Normal adults have preimmunization levels which vary with serotype. The values in Table 1 were obtained from pooled sera of 20 individuals 20 to 29 years of age. After immunization, the immune response varies with age; children under 2 years of age respond poorly. Levels produced by 20 selected high-responding adults after pneumococcal vaccination are shown in Table 1. Those over 65 constitute a heterogenous group. Some individuals respond poorly but the majority respond well to vaccine (11). Any condition which suppresses the B-cell function of the immune response will decrease antibody production. These conditions include immunodeficiencies, illnesses (e.g., multiple myeloma), drugs (e.g., chemotherapeutic agents), therapy (e.g., radiation), and surgery (e.g., splenectomy). The reductions in antibody production caused by these and other conditions may result in a decreased response to immunization levels. These decreases may be for all serotypes or may be restricted to some of the serotypes. At present it is estimated that 200 to 300 ng of antibody nitrogen per ml is protective. Patients who are being considered for reimmunization should have their antibody levels determined since side reactions to the vaccine have been associated with high levels of circulating antibody (3).

RIA

Preparation of labeled antigens

See reference 12.

Intrinsic labeling. Stock cultures of *S. pneumoniae* of the types required for assay are grown in fresh beef heart infusion medium and subcultured on blood agar to ensure purity. A 1-ml amount of the culture is then

TABLE 1. Antibody concentrations in pre- and postimmunization sera of 20 young, healthy adults

| Sera | ng of antibody N/ml to pneumococcal serotype: | | | | | | | | | | | |
	1	3	4	6A	7F	8	9	12	14	18	19F	23
Preimmunization	285	125	181	40	170	599	38	795	179	450	521	316
Postimmunization	2,563	3,010	3,919	1,975	2,713	2,528	1,250	4,750	2,049	4,179	1,487	2,252

used to inoculate 50 ml of medium containing 2 mCi of [U-^{14}C]glucose (240 mCi/mmol). The culture is allowed to grow at 37°C for 18 h. Indicator (0.5% phenol red in 95% ethanol) is added, and the culture is neutralized with 3 N NaOH added dropwise. Sodium deoxycholate is added to a final concentration of 1.0 mg/ml. The lysed culture is neutralized as needed and dialyzed against a minimum of 10 volumes of deionized water. The dialysate is changed a minimum of three times. The nondialyzable capsular polysaccharide is recovered by lyophilization and purified by alcohol fractionation. Five milliliters of 5% sodium acetate is used to dissolve the lyophilized preparation. After removal of insoluble material by centrifugation, 2.5 ml of absolute ethanol is added with mixing. The precipitate is allowed to form for 18 h at 4°C and is then centrifuged. An additional 2.5 ml of ethanol is added to the supernatant, and the procedure is repeated two additional times. The precipitates are assayed for total number of incorporated counts and precipitability with specific antiserum by the method described below. Additional purification consists of gel filtration on Sepharose 4B, fractionation with ammonium sulfate, and ion-exchange chromatography on diethylaminoethyl cellulose.

External labeling. Purified polysaccharide of the type required for RIA can be labeled by iodination of a phenolic group introduced to tyramine to polysaccharide treated with cyanogen bromide (6). The polysaccharide containing iodinated phenolic groups can be readily separated from unincorporated iodide by dialysis or gel filtration on Sephadex G-100.

Technique

Antibodies to the 23 serotypes present in the currently licensed pneumococcal vaccines can be assayed as follows. Radiolabeled capsular polysaccharide, prepared as described above, is diluted to give a solution containing 20,000 cpm/ml. Twenty-five microliters of serum is mixed with 0.5 ml (10,000 cpm) of the labeled antigens and incubated at 37°C for 15 min. The antigen-antibody complexes are precipitated by addition of 0.5 ml of ammonium sulfate saturated at 37°C. Centrifugation is performed at 27,000 × g at 4°C for 15 min (Farr technique). The resulting pellet is suspended in 50 μl of 10% aqueous Triton X-100 (Rohm & Haas Co., Philadelphia, Pa.), 10 ml of scintillant is added, and the activity is measured in a liquid scintillation counter. Specific dilutions of a serum standardized by quantitative precipitin are treated in the same fashion. A curve is constructed by plotting the counts per minute in excess of that in a blank sample containing no antibody against the amount in nanograms of antibody nitrogen added. Antibody nitrogen per milliliter in the test serum is determined by reference to the standard curve. Each assay in-

cludes control tubes containing samples of the reference antibody as well as tubes containing labeled antigen only. The within-assay coefficient of variation of standard samples measured repeatedly was 2.1 to 4.3% over the range of concentrations assayed (13).

Reagents

Diluent: phosphate-buffered saline (pH 7.4) containing 2.5% fetal calf serum and 0.25% phenol
Ammonium sulfate solution saturated at 37°C
Labeled polysaccharide antigens prepared as described above
Scintillant: 4.4 g of PPO (2,5-diphenyloxazole; National Diagnostics, Sommerville, N.J.) per liter of a mixture of 2 parts toluene and 1 part Triton X-100 (Rohm & Haas)

Studies have been performed which indicate that both 7S and 19S immunoglobulins bind all radioactive pneumococcal antigens tested. In addition, protection of mice against lethal challenge of virulent pneumococci was exhibited by binding proteins, presumably IgM and IgG, in both the 7S and 19S fractions. It remains to be determined whether there exists a class of immunoglobulins, IgA, IgD, or IgE, which may bind radioactive antigen but do not protect. Values determined by RIA are in general agreement with values determined by other methods (12). These other methods include quantitative precipitin, mouse protection tests, indirect hemagglutination, and opsonization.

OTHER METHODS

Indirect hemagglutination

The procedure of Amman and Pelger (1) has been widely used for indirect hemagglutination. Human type O+ erythrocytes are coated with purified pneumococcal polysaccharides after chromic chloride treatment. Amounts of 50 μl of washed packed erythrocytes are pipetted into test tubes (12 by 75 mm). A 100-μl amount of pneumococcal polysaccharide antigens (2 mg/ml in saline) is added while the tube is being gently shaken; then 100 μl of chromic chloride (0.375 M diluted 1:5, 1:10, or 1:20 in saline) is added, and the tubes are shaken for 4 min. The cells are then washed three times and suspended in 0.01 M phosphate-buffered saline (pH 7.2) containing bovine serum albumin and glucose.

The diluent consists of 100 ml of phosphate-buffered saline, 1.6 ml of 30% bovine serum albumin, and 100 ml of glucose.

The coated cells are used in microtiter plates. The serum samples are diluted in the usual manner. After antigen-coated cells and antibody are mixed, the plates are sealed with tape, agitated, and incubated in a horizontal position for 2 h at room temperature. The plates are then centrifuged at 1,000 rpm for 3 min. After centrifugation, the plates are elevated at a 60° angle for 10 min, and the "rundown pattern" is read.

Application. The indirect hemagglutination method expresses antibody titer as fold increases. The fold increase for a given pair of sera depends on the sensitivity of the method. The sensitivity is increased with decreasing coating of the erythrocytes by polysaccharide. The method measures both IgG and IgM antibody, although the amount of agglutination mole for mole has not been determined. Repeated freezing and thawing or prolonged storage of serum at −20°C did not affect the titers. The method appears to be simple, reproducible, and inexpensive, and it can be utilized to determine the antibody response after immunization in large population studies.

ELISA

The ELISA is widely used for the detection of antibody against protein antigens. It has been difficult to apply the technique to bacterial polysaccharide antigens. The procedure, which depends on the adsorption of antigen to plastic tubes and then specific binding of antibody to the adsorbed antigen, allows antibody bearing an enzyme to react with the antigen-antibody complex in proportion to the amount of complex present. The enzyme is then allowed to react with a substrate for a defined period of time, and the product of the enzyme-substrate reaction is measured. The reason this procedure has not been easily applied to the measurement of pneumococcal polysaccharide antigens is that polysaccharide antigens do not readily bind to plastic. The procedure of Berntsson et al. (2) will be described. In this procedure, coating of the plastic with the polysaccharide antigen is achieved by the use of polystyrene tubes purchased from Hegerplastic AB, Stallarholmen, Sweden. Optimal concentrations of the antigen vary between 0.01 and 0.002 mg/ml. An antibody value is defined as the extinction at 400 nm after the enzyme has reacted for 100 min when the serum is diluted 1:1,000. Alkaline phosphatase is conjugated to anti-human IgG and IgM purchased from Nodick Co., Copenhagen, Denmark.

The procedure described by Gray (7) uses horseradish peroxidase conjugated to anti-IgG. The substrate, H_2O_2, is allowed to react with o-phenylenediamine at 24°C for 30 min. Absorbance at 450 nm is determined with a Brinkmann PC1000 fiberoptic spectrophotometer with a 1-cm light path. The procedure was standardized by using sera quantitated by the RIA method described above. The method is simple, rapid, and sensitive, and it utilizes small amounts of polysaccharide antigens.

Discussion. The ELISA technique is ideally suited for immunoglobulin class determination and undoubtedly will be used for this purpose in the near future. The introduction of automatic equipment for coating, washing, and reading large numbers of tubes will be important if the ELISA is to achieve the potential of which it is capable.

CIE

Pneumococcal antigens can be detected in body fluids (saliva, serum, cerebrospinal fluid, urine) from patients with pneumococcal infections by counterimmunoelectrophoresis (CIE), using antisera that contain antibodies against 82 pneumococcal types (omnisera) as well as monospecific antibody (4, 5, 8). CIE performed with rabbit anticapsular antibody is capable of detecting antigen in concentrations as low as 0.1 to 1.0 µg/ml, or 0.2 ng per test, for pneumococcal polysaccharide types 1, 2, 3, 4, 5, 8, 12, and 18 (8).

In the procedure described by Coonrod and Rytel (4), glass slides (8 by 10 cm) are coated with 13 ml of 1% agarose dissolved in Veronal buffer (pH 8.2, ionic strength, 0.05). Slides are stored at 5°C in a moist chamber and used between 24 and 96 h after preparation. Parallel wells 3 mm in diameter are cut 3 mm apart (edge to edge). Wells are filled with 20 µl of solution. The slide is placed in the center of an electrophoresis chamber with the antibody-containing wells on the anodic slide. The slide is attached by paper wicks (Whatman no. 3) to reservoirs containing Veronal buffer as described above. The chamber is attached to a power source, and a constant voltage of 2.5 V/cm is applied across the slide for 1 h. Slides are examined for precipitin bands immediately after electrophoresis and after cooling at 5°C.

Discussion. CIE has been used to correlate circulating capsular polysaccharide with bacteremia in pneumococcal pneumonia. Antigenemia correlated strongly with bacteremia: 12 of 20 bacteremic patients showed antigenemia, whereas 26 patients negative for bacteremia did not show circulating antigen (8). Pneumococcal polysaccharide dissolved in serum or human urine was detected by CIE with the same sensitivity as when the polysaccharide was dissolved in saline (4).

Types 7 and 14 are much more difficult to detect because of lack of charge. The procedure is at best semiquantitative but is rapid and specific.

LITERATURE CITED

1. **Ammann, A. J., and R. J. Pelger.** 1972. Determination of antibody to pneumococcal polysaccharides with chromic chloride-treated human red blood cells and indirect hemagglutination. Appl. Microbiol. **24:**679–683.
2. **Berntsson, E., K. A. Broholm, and B. Kaijser.** 1978. Serological diagnosis of pneumococcal disease with enzyme-linked immunosorbent assay (ELISA). Scand. J. Infect. Dis. 10:177–181.
3. **Borgono, J. M., A. A. McLean, P. P. Vella, A. F. Woodhour, I. Canepa, W. L. Davidson, and M. R. Hilleman.** 1978. Vaccination and revaccination with polyvalent pneumococcal polysaccharide vaccines in adults and infants. Proc. Soc. Exp. Biol. Med. **157:**145–154.
4. **Coonrod, J. D., and M. W. Rytel.** 1973. Detection of type-specific pneumococcal antigens by counterimmunoelectrophoresis. I. Methodology and immunologic properties of pneumococcal antigens. J. Lab. Clin. Med. **81:**770–786.
5. **Dorff, G. J., J. D. Coonrod, and M. W. Rytel.** 1971. Detection by immunoelectrophoresis of antigen in sera of patients with pneumococcal bacteraemia. Lancet **i:**578–579.
6. **Gotschlich, E. C., M. Rey, R. Triau, and K. J. Sparks.** 1972. Quantitative determination of the human immune response to immunization with meningococcal vaccines. J. Clin. Invest. **51:**89–96.
7. **Gray, B. M.** 1979. ELISA methodology for polysaccharide antigens: protein coupling of polysaccharides for adsorption to plastic tubes. J. Immunol. Methods **28:**187–192.

8. **Kenny, G. E., B. B. Wentworth, R. P. Beasley, and H. M. Foy.** 1972. Correlation of circulating capsular polysaccharide with bacteremia in pneumococcal pneumonia. Infect. Immun. **6**:431–437.

9. **Landesman, S. H., and G. Schiffman.** 1981. Assessment of the antibody response to pneumococcal vaccine in high-risk populations. Rev. Infect. Dis. **3**(Suppl):184–196.

10. **Robbins, J. B., R. Austrian, C. -J. Lee, S. C. Rastogi, G. Schiffman, J. Henrichsen, P. H. Makela, C. V. Broome, R. R. Facklam, R. H. Tiesjema, and J. C. Parke, Jr.** 1983. Considerations for formulating the second-generation pneumococcal capsular polysaccharide vaccine with emphasis on the cross-reactive types within groups. J. Infect. Dis. **148**:1136–1159.

11. **Schiffman, G.** 1983. Pneumococcal vaccine: a tool for the evaluation of the B-cell function of the immune system. Proc. Soc. Exp. Biol. Med. **174**:309–315.

12. **Schiffman, G., R. M. Douglas, M. J. Bonner, M. Robbins, and R. Austrian.** 1980. A radioimmunoassay for immunologic phenomena in pneumococcal disease and for the antibody response to pneumococcal vaccines. I. Method for the radioimmunoassay of anticapsular antibodies and comparison with other techniques. J. Immunol. Methods **33**:133–144.

13. **Siber, G. R., S. A. Weitzman, A. C. Aisenberg, H. J. Weinstein, and G. Schiffman.** 1978. Impaired antibody response to pneumococcal vaccine following treatment for Hodgkins disease. N. Engl. J. Med. **299**:442–448.

Chapter 52

Immune Response to *Neisseria meningitidis*

WENDELL D. ZOLLINGER, BRENDA L. BRANDT, AND EDMUND C. TRAMONT

Four major classes of antigens which can be used in serological assays are present on the cell surface of *Neisseria meningitidis:* (i) a polysaccharide capsule, (ii) outer membrane proteins, (iii) lipopolysaccharides, and (iv) pili. The capsular polysaccharides serve as the basis for classifying meningococci into sero groups, of which thirteen are currently recognized: A, B, C, D, 29E, H, I, K, L, W135, X, Y, and Z. These capsular antigens are quite specific in relation to one another, although partial cross-reactions between groups Y and W135 and between groups Z and 29E have been observed. Nearly all systemic meningococcal disease is caused by groups A, B, C, Y, and W135.

Outer membrane protein and lipopolysaccharide antigens carry both type-specific and cross-reactive determinants which are not unique within each meningococcal serogroup but, with some exceptions, may be found on strains of any serogroup. The type-specific determinants of both the protein and lipopolysaccharide antigens have been used as a basis for subtyping (3). The cross-reactive determinants are shared not only by strains of *N. meningitidis* but also to some extent by strains of other *Neisseria* species. Information about the human immune response to meningococcal pili is limited, but meningococcal and gonococcal pili are known to share some common determinants. Although most of these antigens have been used in studies of the human immune response, clinical experience has mainly been limited to the use of capsular polysaccharide antigens and whole bacteria.

Human meningococcal infections may present a variety of clinical forms: the asymptomatic carrier state, bacteremia, fulminant shock (Waterhouse-Friderichsen syndrome), chronic meningococcemia, meningitis, and localized organ infections (pneumonia, pericarditis, ophthalmitis). No clear-cut difference in serological response appears to characterize a syndrome.

Purified polysaccharide vaccines for serogroups A and C have been licensed and have proven effective in preventing systemic disease caused by meningococci of these serogroups. Serogroup Y and W135 capsular polysaccharides have also been licensed as vaccines and are expected to be effective, but efficacy trials have not been done because the incidence of disease has been too low to perform meaningful field trials. The capsular polysaccharide of group B meningococci has poor immunogenicity, and no vaccine is available for this serogroup. Unfortunately, it is currently responsible for about 50% of all meningococcal disease in the United States.

Three serological tests for antibody and one for antigen will be described in detail because of their ease of performance and general utility in determining the immune response and immune status of individuals and in diagnosing meningococcal infection. These assays include the passive hemagglutination (HA) test which is specific for antibodies to the capsu-

lar polysaccharides; the bactericidal assay, which is particularly important because immunity to meningococcal disease has been strongly correlated with the presence of serum bactericidal antibodies; the solid-phase immunoassays, which are presently recommended for the measurement of antibody to noncapsular antigens; and the particle agglutination assays for capsular antigen, which have utility in rapid diagnosis of meningococcal infections and in establishing a diagnosis that has been masked by antibiotic therapy.

PASSIVE HA TEST

The passive HA test is based upon the ability of antibodies to agglutinate erythrocytes coated with capsular polysaccharide antigen. The assay is specific for the polysaccharide that is used to coat the erythrocytes.

A similar assay may be performed by sensitizing latex particles rather than erythrocytes (7). Although the commercially available, standardized latex particles offer some advantages, this assay is less sensitive than the passive HA test. The radioactive antigen binding assay (Farr assay) is a very sensitive and specific assay for the measurement of antibody response to the capsular polysaccharides (1, 4), but it is best suited to the research laboratory because of the relative complexity of the preparation and standardization of the radioactive capsular polysaccharides.

Clinical indications

The passive HA test serves as a simple, specific test for the detection of group-specific antibody response to infection or polysaccharide immunization.

There are two problems in passive HA (polysaccharide) testing of which the physician should be aware. (i) Infants and young children may not respond to the capsular polysaccharide or may produce only low titers of antipolysaccharide antibody after infection or vaccination. As a result, the passive HA may fail to detect a response. More sensitive assays (such as the radioactive antigen binding assay) are more effective for this age group. (ii) Most sera from normal human adults contain HA antibodies to the B polysaccharide which are of relatively low avidity and which increase in titer with age. Group B meningococcal infections, however, may result in little or no increase in group B HA titer, and the expected mean increase in titer is substantially less than that seen after infections with meningococci of other serogroups.

Interpretation

Passive HA antibody response to infection or immunization occurs in well over 90% of adult subjects. Individual responses, however, vary greatly in magnitude (average of 32- to 128-fold except for group B, whose average is 0- to 16-fold). The passive HA test is most sensitive to the immunoglobulin M (IgM) class of antibodies. Peak serum antibody titers occur 1 to 3 weeks after infection or immunization. After natural infection, antibody titers fall rapidly within 2 months (1), but after vaccination with capsular polysaccharide vaccine (serogroup A, C, Y, or W135), antipolysaccharide titers remain near the peak level for many years. The antibody response to group B polysaccharide, if any, is usually transient (4 to 8 weeks) and involves only antibodies to the IgM class. Since these anti-B polysaccharide antibodies are probably not protective, this assay is of little value in situations involving group B infections. The passive HA test does not correlate with immunity and, therefore, cannot be used for determination of immune status.

Reagents

Sensitized erythrocytes are prepared by using human group O Rh-negative cells which are collected in Alsever solution (0.42% sodium chloride, 0.8% trisodium citrate dihydrate, and 2.05% glucose, adjusted to pH 6.1 with 10% citric acid solution). Cells can be kept for up to 3 weeks if stored at 4°C. Sensitization is carried out by diluting the stock solution of polysaccharide in phosphate-buffered saline (PBS) to the optimal concentration and mixing it with an equal volume of erythrocytes which have previously been washed three times by gently suspending the cells in PBS to a concentration of 4% (vol/vol) and centrifuging at $500 \times g$ for 10 min. The mixture is incubated at 37°C for 30 min with occasional stirring and is then washed three times with PBS to remove excess antigen. After the final wash, the cells are suspended to 0.5% (vol/vol) in PBS containing 0.5% bovine serum albumin. Cells are stored as a 0.5% suspension at 4°C and should be used within 24 h after sensitization. The optimal sensitizing concentration of polysaccharide is determined by grid titration. Serial twofold dilutions of antigen in the range of 5 to 150 µg/ml are used to sensitize small samples of cells which are then tested against replicate serial dilutions of a known positive serum. The lowest concentration which produces the maximum titer and clearest agglutination pattern is used.

Polysaccharide antigens are prepared from liquid cultures of meningococci of the appropriate serogroups (8). Meningococci of the desired serogroup are streaked for isolation onto a Barile-Yaguchi-Eveland agar plate (or other suitable medium) and grown overnight at 37°C in a CO_2 incubator or candle jar. The contents of this plate are used to inoculate 250 ml of liquid medium in a 1-liter Erlenmeyer flask. This culture is grown for 16 to 24 h at 35°C on a rotary shaker operating at about 150 rpm. The organisms are killed, and the polysaccharide in the culture is precipitated by the addition of 2.5 ml of a 10% solution of hexadecyltrimethylammonium bromide in water. The precipitate is collected by centrifugation at $5,000 \times g$ for 15 min. The supernatant is discarded, and the pellet is extracted twice with 10 ml of 0.9 M $CaCl_2$. Insoluble material is removed by centrifugation at $25,000 \times g$ for 15 min. Absolute ethanol is added to the supernatant to a final concentration of 25% (vol/vol), and the mixture is placed at 4°C for 2 h. The precipi-

tate, mostly nucleic acid, is removed by centrifugation, and the supernatant is brought to 75% ethanol (vol/vol) by the addition of cold absolute ethanol. The resulting precipitate is collected by centrifugation at $12,000 \times g$ for 10 min and washed twice by suspending in cold absolute ethanol and repelleting at $12,000 \times g$ for 10 min. The washed pellet is dissolved in about 5 ml of distilled water. This partially purified polysaccharide still contains some protein but is suitable in most instances for use in sensitizing erythrocytes. Further purification can be achieved by cold phenol-water extraction (8). Alternatively, polysaccharides of serogroups A, C, Y, and W135 are commercially available as meningococcal vaccines (Connaught Laboratories, Inc., Swiftwater, Pa., or Merck Sharp & Dohme, West Point, Pa.).

PBS contains 66.6 ml of 0.15 M Na_2HPO_4, 33.3 ml of 0.15 M KH_2PO_4, 8.5 g of NaCl, and distilled water to 1 liter. The pH should be 6.9.

Liquid growth medium contains 10 g of Casamino Acids (technical grade; Difco Laboratories, Detroit, Mich.), 120 mg of KCl, 10.3 g of Na_2HPO_4, and 25 ml of a $40\times$ glucose-magnesium sulfate solution (2.4 g of $MgSO_4 \cdot 7H_2O$ and 20 g of glucose per 100 ml) which is autoclaved separately and added after the medium has cooled.

Barile-Yaguchi-Eveland agar is available from BBL Microbiology Systems, Cockeysville, Md.

Test procedure

Serum is heat inactivated at 56°C for 30 min, after which 11 twofold serial dilutions of 0.05 ml are made in PBS by using disposable microtiter U plates and 0.05-ml dilutors (Dynatech Laboratories, Inc., Alexandria, Va.) or a microliter pipette. Sensitized erythrocytes (0.05 ml) are then added to each well, and the reagents are mixed by briefly placing the plate on a rotary shaker or rotating it by hand on a tabletop. The plates are then placed at room temperature, and the erythrocytes are allowed to settle for 1 to 2 h. Patterns of agglutination are read on a 1+ to 4+ scale, with a 3+ or 4+ agglutination considered positive. A positive control serum, a negative control serum, and an antigen control (PBS in place of serum) are included in each test.

SERUM BACTERICIDAL TEST

The serum bactericidal test measures the ability of serum to kill viable bacteria and may be done either with the intrinsic complement present in fresh serum or with an exogenous source of complement with serial dilutions of the test serum. Because viable bacteria are used, safety precautions must be carefully followed, and results must await overnight incubation. Sterile reagents and technique must be used throughout the procedures since the endpoint is the growth of viable bacteria as colonies.

A modification of the test that is performed in 96-well cell culture plates (8) may be more suitable when many sera must be tested.

Clinical indications

The bactericidal assay is the best measure of the immune status of an individual. It is especially helpful in studies of patients with complement deficiencies and patients with recurrent meningitis or other unusual immunodeficiency syndromes. It may also be useful in establishing the immune status of close contacts of a patient with meningococcal disease. The choice between using a single dilution of fresh serum with its intrinsic complement or determining the titer of the serum with the addition of exogenous complement is dependent on whether one desires to simply determine the immune status or to quantitate the amount of bactericidal antibody present.

The test has several shortcomings which make it difficult to duplicate from laboratory to laboratory. It depends in unknown ways on the media and growth conditions used to grow the meningococci, and it is affected by differences in target strains and complement sources. When the question is the immune status of an individual with respect to group B meningococci, it is important to use human complement, since human anti-B polysaccharide antibodies are bactericidal with rabbit complement but not with human complement and have not been shown to be protective. Bactericidal antibodies (measured with human complement) against group B strains are directed against the antigenically variable subcapsular antigens, so immunity to one group B strain does not necessarily indicate immunity to other group B strains.

Interpretation

Whole viable organisms are used for this assay. Therefore, the antibodies detected are those which are directed against one or more of the surface antigens. In particular, since outer membrane protein and lipopolysaccharide antigens differ among strains of the same serogroup, it is usually necessary to use the strain isolated from a given patient in testing that patient's serological response. Rabbit complement is adequate for studies involving polysaccharide vaccination (serogroups A, C, Y, and W135), and almost any strain of the homologous serogroup is satisfactory for use as the test strain. Both IgG and IgM antibodies participate in the meningococcal bactericidal reaction. IgA antibodies in some sera block the bactericidal activities of IgM and IgG. Normal responses range from 4- to 256-fold antibody increase when paired sera are tested. Antibiotics in the serum will result in a false-positive test, but they will also produce a positive result in the serum control (no complement). When rabbit complement is used, the predominant bactericidal antibodies are those directed against the capsule, and titers are generally higher than with human complement. When determining a person's immune status, however, human complement should be used.

Reagents

Mueller-Hinton broth and agar are available from Difco or BBL.

Gey balanced salt solution (GBSS) for ambient atmosphere without phenol red is obtained from GIBCO Laboratories, Life Technologies, Inc., Chagrin Falls, Ohio).

Gelatin, 10%, is prepared in distilled water with the use of gelatin (Difco).

Undiluted normal human serum (fresh or fresh frozen at $-70°C$), which has been determined by prescreening to lack bactericidal antibodies against the test strain, or 4-week-old-rabbit serum (Rockland, Inc., Gilbertsville, Pa.; Pel-Freez Biologicals, Rogers, Ark.; or Dutchland Laboratories, Inc., Denver, Pa.) may be used as complement. Each lot of complement must be tested against the strain(s) of N. meningitidis used as the test antigen to determine whether the complement alone has antibodies which kill the organism. Each lot of complement is filter sterilized (membrane filter, 0.45-μm pore size) and divided into small volumes (3 ml) which are stored at $-70°C$ for subsequent use. The complement is thawed just before being used in the test and must be kept in an ice-water bath so that it does not lose its activity. A human serum, fresh or fresh frozen at $-70°C$ for less than 1 month, may also be used without added exogenous complement to test for the intrinsic capacity of the serum to kill meningococci.

Test procedure

Organisms for the bactericidal test are prepared by growing N. meningitidis for 16 h at 37°C in a 5% CO_2 atmosphere on Mueller-Hinton agar. Growth from this culture is transferred with a loop into a 250-ml screw-capped nephelometer flask containing 25 ml of Mueller-Hinton broth. Enough organisms are added to give an initial optical density at 650 nm (OD_{650}) of about 0.15 (side arm inside diameter, 1.6 cm). The flask is then incubated at 37°C in a shaking water bath until an OD_{650} of 0.60 is reached (1.5 to 2 h). The organisms are removed from the medium by centrifugation at 3,000 $\times$ g for 10 min in a refrigerated centrifuge. The organisms are next washed once with 25 ml of cold GBSS containing 0.1% gelatin. The pelleted organisms are then suspended in 1 ml of GBSS. On the basis of a standard curve relating optical density to CFU, a sample of this suspension is adjusted to an optical density corresponding to about 3 $\times$ 10^8 bacteria per ml, and then an additional 1:7,000 dilution is made with GBSS as diluent. The growth of the organisms should be so regulated that the bacterial suspension is prepared just before it is used and is kept in an ice bath until needed.

The reaction mixture consists of 0.05 ml of serum dilution, 0.1 ml of GBSS, 0.05 ml of organisms, and 0.05 ml of exogenous complement. The test is performed in sterile plugged test tubes (12 by 75 mm). A 0.1-ml amount of serum previously heat inactivated at 56°C for 30 min and diluted 1:2 in GBSS is added to the first tube. With GBSS as diluent, five serial twofold dilutions are made for the acute or prevaccination sera and eight dilutions are made for the postinfection or postimmunization sera.

To 0.05 ml of serum dilution is added a further 0.1 ml of GBSS, and the tubes are placed in an ice-water bath. To each tube is added 0.05 ml of organism suspension and then 0.05 ml of complement. The reactants are mixed and placed in a shaking water bath at 37°C for 1 h. After incubation, the rack of tubes is placed in an ice bath. The number of viable bacteria is determined as CFU by transferring 20-μl samples of each reaction mixture to Mueller-Hinton agar with a microliter pipette. This sampling is performed in triplicate as follows. Three 20-µl drops are placed across the top of the agar plate, and the plate is tipped so that the drops run down the plate, thus spreading the inoculum. The agar dish is then placed on a flat surface, and the inoculum is allowed to dry.

The following controls are included in each assay: (i) 0- and 60-min plate counts on a sample containing 0.05 ml of organisms, 0.05 ml of heat-inactivated complement, and 0.15 ml of GBSS; (ii) a complement control (0.05 ml of organisms, 0.05 ml of active complement, and 0.15 ml of GBSS) to determine whether the complement alone kills the organisms; (iii) a serum control containing 0.05 ml of a 1:2 dilution of serum, 0.05 ml of organisms, and 0.15 ml of GBSS; (iv) a known positive control serum; and (v) a known negative control serum.

If the individual's fresh serum is to be tested without the addition of exogenous complement, duplicate tubes are set up, each containing 0.1 ml of fresh serum, 0.05 ml of organisms, and 0.05 ml of GBSS. Controls in this case are 0- and 60-min plate counts from a tube containing 0.1 ml of heat-inactivated serum, 0.05 ml of organisms, and 0.05 ml of GBSS. Other parameters of the test remain the same.

The Mueller-Hinton agar plates used for the viability counts are incubated for 16 h at 37°C in a 10% CO_2 atmosphere or a candle extension jar. Colony counts are recorded, and the results of triplicate samples are averaged. With the bacterial inoculum described above, approximately 200 colonies are present in each 20-µl sample plated from control tubes. The serum antibody titer is the greatest dilution in which at least a 50% decrease in the mean number of colonies is observed compared with the number in the zero-time organism control.

SOLID-PHASE IMMUNOASSAY

The solid-phase immunoassays are quantitative, sensitive, and very versatile primary binding assays which are based on the binding of antibody to antigen that has been adsorbed onto the surface of a plastic plate or tube (2, 9, 10). Goat anti-human immunoglobulin labeled with ^{125}I in the solid-phase radioimmunoassay or with an appropriate enzyme in the enzyme-linked immunosorbent assay (ELISA) is used to detect the amount of antibody bound. Once the labeled anti-human immunoglobulin is prepared, antibody to a variety of specific antigens can be measured in a single assay. Membrane protein, exotoxins, and lipopolysaccharides have been found to be excellent antigens for this assay, whereas purified polysaccharides have been less satisfactory due to poor binding to the plastic. With appropriate modifications to enhance binding, however, the assays have successfully been used with polysaccharide antigens.

Clinical indications

The solid-phase immunoassay is best suited for the determination of the immune response to noncapsular antigens such as lipopolysaccharides and the serotype proteins of the outer membrane. Some infections with group B meningococci, especially in young children, may not induce a significant response to the capsular polysaccharide. In these cases a solid-phase im-

munoassay may be used with antigen from the infecting strain to measure the extent of the immune response. The immunoglobulin class of the antibody response may also be analyzed by this assay.

Similar information may be obtained by using either the solid-phase radioimmunoassay or the ELISA. The assays differ mainly in the indicator used. They are affected by most of the same parameters and have essentially the same applications (2, 9). The choice of which assay to use will depend mainly on the availability of the reagents and equipment that are needed. Because it is used in our laboratory, the solid-phase radioimmunoassay is described below, with the differences for the ELISA procedure noted parenthetically.

Interpretation

The specificity of the assay is determined by the antigen used. The outer membrane complex contains the serotype protein antigens, lipopolysaccharide, and some capsular polysaccharide. It will, therefore, react with antibodies directed at all of these antigens. If a sufficiently pure antigen is used, such as lipopolysaccharide, pili, or capsular polysaccharide, only antibodies to that antigen will be detected.

The levels of antibodies to meningococcal outer membrane proteins in children less than 2 years of age are low or undetectable, but they increase with age to a mean adult level of 5 to 10 µg/ml. Antibodies to the outer membrane complex increase 2- to 50-fold as a result of systemic infections and 2- to 10-fold as a result of asymptomatic nasopharyngeal carriage.

Reagents

PBS is Dulbecco's formulation and contains, per liter: NaCl, 8 g; KCl, 0.2 g; Na_2HPO_4, 2.16 g; KH_2PO_4, 0.2 g; $CaCl_2$, 0.1 g; and $MgCl_2 \cdot 6H_2O$, 0.1 g, pH 7.4. When used as diluent for antigens, 0.01% phenol red is added.

PBS-T is PBS which contains 0.05% Tween 20.

Filler is made up of 0.5% bovine serum albumin, 0.5% casein, 0.2% sodium azide, and 0.01% phenol red in PBS. It is stored at room temperature.

Carrier-free $Na^{125}I$ at a concentration of 1 mCi/10 µl is available from New England Nuclear Corp., Boston, Mass., or Amersham Corp., Arlington Heights, Ill.

Affinity-purified heavy-chain specific antibodies to human IgG, IgA, or IgM and the corresponding alkaline phosphatase conjugates are available from several vendors (e.g., Kirkegaard and Perry Laboratories, Gaithersburg, Md., and Cooper Biomedical, Malvern, Pa.). Purified human IgG, IgA, and IgM for use as standards are available from Cooper and from Miles Scientific, Naperville, Ill.

Iodinated second antibody is prepared as follows. Affinity-purified antibodies are most easily iodinated by the Iodobead method, with an appropriate hood and other safety measures. Two Iodobeads (Pierce Chemical Co., Rockford, Ill.) are placed in 200 µl of 0.3 M sodium phosphate buffer (pH 7.4), and 0.6 mCi of $Na^{125}I$ is added. After 5 min, 250 µg of antibody, also in 0.3 M sodium phosphate buffer, is added, and the iodination is allowed to proceed at room temperature for 2 to 15 min. At that time the solution is separated from the beads, and the unbound iodide is removed by passing the sample over a disposable column of Sephadex G-25 (1.5 by 5 cm; PD-10 prepacked column; Pharmacia Fine Chemicals, Inc., Piscataway, N.J.) equilibrated with filler. Fractions are collected manually and monitored with a rate meter. The labeled antibody comes off at the void volume and is followed by the unbound label. The total radioactivity in the void volume divided by the amount of protein labeled (assuming complete recovery) gives an approximate specific activity. The labeled antibody is stored at 4°C and is good for up to 2 months. Before it is used, it is diluted in filler to a concentration of about 1 μg of specific antibody per ml.

For meningococcal antigen, outer membrane complex is prepared from organisms grown as described for the passive HA assay. The 16- to 24-h culture is inactivated with phenol at 0.5% for 1 h, after which the organisms are harvested by centrifugation at $20,000 \times g$ for 15 min. The organisms are suspended in about 10 volumes (pellet volume) of TSE buffer (0.05 M Tris hydrochloride, 0.01 M EDTA, 0.15 M NaCl, pH 7.4) and placed in a water bath at 60°C for 30 min. The suspension is then either blended for 3 min in an Omnimixer (Du Pont Instruments-Sorvall, Newton, Conn.) or placed in a syringe and forced several times through a 23-gauge hypodermic needle. Whole cells and debris are removed by centrifugation at $30,000 \times g$ for 20 min. The resulting supernatant is then centrifuged at $100,000 \times g$ for 2 h. The pelleted outer membrane complex is washed by being suspended in distilled water and repelleted as before. The final pellet of outer membrane complex is suspended in distilled water, assayed for protein, diluted to 1 mg of protein per ml, and stored at −20°C.

Test procedure

1. Antigen is diluted in PBS to 50 μg of protein per ml, and with a microliter pipette, a 25-μl portion is placed in the bottom of each well of a flexible polyvinyl microtiter plate (Dynatech). The plate is then placed in a humidified chamber at 37°C for 1 h. (In the ELISA, 100 μl of antigen at 10 μg/ml in carbonate buffer [pH 9.6] is placed in the wells of a flat-bottom polystyrene 96-well microplate.)

2. The antigen is aspirated from the wells, and 100 μl of filler is put in each well and then aspirated out and replaced by another 100 μl of filler. The plate is placed at 37°C for 1 h. (In the ELISA, 150 μl of filler is used.)

3. Sera to be tested are serially diluted with filler in tubes or in a separate microtiter plate. (We use serial 10-fold dilutions followed by intermediate 3-fold dilutions over the range from 1:10 to 1:10⁴.) The precision of the assay is directly related to the precision of the dilutions.

4. The filler is dumped out of the antigen-coated plate, and the plate is washed twice with PBS either by using a plate washer (e.g., Dynawasher II, Dynatech) or by manually filling the wells with a slow-running stream of buffer from a reservoir and then dumping the solution out. After the last wash, the plate is held upside down and tapped on a paper towel several times to remove any residual liquid. (In the ELISA, PBS-T is used for the washes.)

5. With a microliter pipette, 25 μl of each dilution is transferred to the appropriate antigen-coated well. A blank containing 25 μl of diluent is placed at the end of each dilution series. The plate is then placed in a humidity chamber and left at room temperature overnight. (A volume of 100 μl is used in the ELISA.)

6. The serum dilutions are aspirated from the wells, after which the plate is washed four times with PBS as described in step 4. (PBS-T is used in the ELISA.)

7. Affinity-purified, heavy-chain-specific goat anti-human IgG, IgA, and IgM (or a mixture) labeled with ^{125}I to a specific activity of about 1,000 cpm/ng is diluted in filler to 1 μg of antibody protein per ml, and 25 μl is placed in each well. The plate is then placed in a humidity chamber at room temperature for 8 to 16 h. (In the ELISA, 100 μl of alkaline phosphate-labeled secondary antibody, which is diluted in filler to 1 μg of antibody protein per ml, is placed in the wells.)

8. The plate is washed by aspirating the solution into a radioactive-waste container, adding and then aspirating a drop (about 50 μl) of filler, and then washing the wells five times with PBS as described in step 4. After being dried, the bottom half of each well is cut off with scissors into a tube, and the halves are counted in a gamma counter. (In the ELISA the secondary antibody is aspirated and the wells are washed four times with PBS-T as described in step 4. After residual liquid is removed from the wells, 100 μl of diethanolamine buffer containing 1 mg of p-nitrophenylphosphate [phosphatase substrate] per ml is added, and the plate is incubated at room temperature for 30 min. The reaction is stopped by the addition of 50 μl of 3 N NaOH. A_{405} is read after 30 min.)

In addition to the serum-free control at the end of each dilution series, the following additional controls should be included: (i) a positive high-titered serum and (ii) an antigen-free control in which one or more sera (dilution series) are tested against filler as antigen. This procedure controls for nonspecific binding at the higher serum concentrations and is especially important when serum antibody levels are very low. The higher of the serum- and antigen-free controls is subtracted as background.

For each immunoglobulin class of antibody to be measured, a standard curve relating the net counts per minute of ^{125}I per well (or OD$_{405}$) to the amount of specific antibody bound is generated with each assay (9). This curve is produced by using unlabeled, affinity-purified goat anti-human IgG, IgA, or IgM (or a mixture) at 50 μg/ml in place of antigen to coat three rows of wells. Alternatively, the immunoglobulin fraction of a very high-titered serum may be used. Purified human IgG, IgA, or IgM or a serum containing a known concentration of IgG, IgA, and IgM is diluted in filler to 500 ng of the particular immunoglobulin per ml. Duplicate serial twofold dilutions of this solution are then used in place of serum dilutions for the three rows coated with antibody. The remainder of the assay is performed as described above. A plot of the counts per minute bound per well (or OD$_{405}$) versus the concentration of IgG is then constructed. Normally, the curve will be approximately linear in the range between 5 and 100 ng of IgG per ml. The specific antibody concentration of the unknown is found by selecting the serum dilution which resulted in about

10 to 30% of the maximum (plateau level) counts per minute bound (or OD_{405}), converting the counts per minute to nanograms of antibody bound by use of the standard curve, and multiplying by the reciprocal of the serum dilution. The result—nanograms of antibody bound per milliliter of serum—is a quantitative measure of the binding antibody per milliliter of serum.

PARTICLE AGGLUTINATION

The detection of meningococcal antigens in the cerebrospinal fluid (CSF), serum, urine, and other body fluids has proven a useful tool for establishing a specific etiological diagnosis and is also valuable when previous treatment has masked the specific diagnosis. The principle behind these tests is the reaction of a specific, high-titered meningococcal antiserum with antigen in the body fluid in question. The most commonly used methods include agglutination tests with carrier particles to which the specific antiserum is bound, such as staphylococcal protein A (5) or latex particles (6, 7) and counterimmunoelectrophoresis.

Clinical indications

The particle agglutination assays for the presence of meningococcal antigen in CSF are rapid assays which may be valuable adjuncts to direct microscopic examination and culture in the diagnosis of meningococcal meningitis. There are, however, several problems of which the physician should be aware. The staphylococcal coagglutination test will produce a false-positive reaction when sufficient IgG is present and, therefore, would not be suitable for use with serum. Preabsorption of CSF or other body fluids with stabilized staphylococcal cells eliminates this false-positive reaction. In addition, certain strains of *Escherichia coli* and other normal bacterial flora have capsular antigens that cross-react with meningococcal capsules. For example, *E. coli* K-1 and certain strains of *Moraxella nonliquefaciens* have a capsule that cross-reacts with the group B meningococcal capsule. Finally, the sensitivity of these assays is only slightly better than that of a Gram stain.

Interpretation

In a positive reaction, granular agglutinates are formed while suspension is cleared. Strong coagglutinations are graded 4+ and appear within 20 to 30 tilts. Moderately strong reactions are graded 3+ and appear at a somewhat lower rate. Moderate reactions are graded 2+, and weak reactions are graded 1+. The weak reactions develop slowly and are not obvious until after 50 to 60 tilts. The test is read as negative if a 1+ coagglutination fails to develop within 2 min. Controls with uncoated staphylococci are performed in parallel tests and negate a positive test when coagglutinated. When latex particles are used, results are also read on a 0 to 4+ scale, and any 3+ or 4+ positive test is considered significant.

Reagents

Reagent staphylococci are stabilized staphylococci cultured and prepared as follows. Strain Cowan I of *Staphylococcus aureus* NCTC 8530 is grown overnight on a tryptic soy agar plate, and the contents are used to inoculate 100 ml of tryptic soy broth in a 1-liter Erlenmeyer flask. This culture is grown overnight at 37°C on a rotary shaker operating at 150 rpm. The organisms are harvested by centrifugation and washed twice with PBS by uniformly suspending and pelleting them. The bacteria are then suspended in 0.5% formaldehyde in PBS and kept at room temperature for 3 h. The formaldehyde-treated suspension is then washed four times in PBS and adjusted to a concentration of 10% (vol/vol). The suspension of organisms is then put in a 500-ml flask, stirred in an 80°C water bath for 5 min, and quickly cooled. The bacteria are stable for months when stored at 4°C. A comparable product, Pansorbin, is available from Calbiochem-Behring Corp., La Jolla, Calif.

Antibody-coated staphylococci are prepared by adding 1 ml of a 10% suspension of reagent staphylococci to 0.1 ml of rabbit antimeningococcal serum. After being mixed, the staphylococci are washed twice and suspended to 1% (vol/vol) in PBS containing 0.1% sodium azide.

Antibody-coated latex particles are prepared by adding 1 part latex suspension to 3 parts immunoglobulin fraction of rabbit antimeningococcal serum, mixing the two substances, and placing them in a 37°C water bath for 2 h. (Alternatively, monoclonal antibodies to meningococcal capsular polysaccharide may be used to sensitize the latex particles. The result is a more sensitive and specific test.) The particles are then washed twice with 10 volumes of PBS and suspended in PBS containing 0.5% bovine serum albumin. This suspension can be stored for at least 1 year at 4°C.

Antimeningococcal rabbit sera raised against meningococci of groups A, B, C, X, Y, Z, and W135 are available from Burroughs-Wellcome Corp., Research Triangle Park, N.C., and from Difco.

Several kits based on latex agglutination are commercially available for use in the rapid diagnosis of meningococcal disease (e.g., Directigen, from Hynson, Westcott & Dunning, Baltimore, Md.).

Tryptic soy broth and agar are available from Difco or BBL.

Latex particles are available from Difco (Latex 0.81).

PBS contains 0.15 M NaCl and 0.01 M sodium phosphate, pH 7.4.

Test procedure

The CSF (or other fluid) is preabsorbed by mixing equal volumes of unsensitized staphylococci and CSF and centrifuging at $3,000 \times g$ for 10 min. Two drops of the supernatant are placed on a glass slide, two drops of antimeningococcal reagent staphylococci are then added, and the slide is tilted to and fro and observed for coagglutination for 2 min. Controls with uncoated staphylococci are tested in parallel procedures.

If latex particles are used as the carrier particles, no pretreatment of the CSF is required. To 0.04 ml of CSF is added 0.02 ml of sensitized latex particles on a ringed slide. The slide is then shaken manually or on a rotary shaker at 150 rpm for 3 min, and the agglutination is read with the naked eye.

LITERATURE CITED

1. **Brandt, B. L., F. A. Wyle, and M. S. Artenstein.** 1972. A radioactive antigen-binding assay for *Neisseria meningitidis* polysaccharide antibody. J. Immunol. **108:**913–920.
2. **Carlsson, H. E., and A. A. Lindberg.** 1977. Application of ELISA for the diagnosis of bacterial infections, p. 97–110. *In* T. M. S. Chang (ed.), Biomedical applications of immobilized enzymes and proteins, vol. 2. Plenum Publishing Corp., New York.
3. **Frasch, C. E.** 1979. Noncapsular surface antigens of *Neisseria meningitidis*, p. 304–337. *In* L. Weinstein and B. N. Fields (ed.), Seminars in infectious disease, vol. 2. Stratton Intercontinental Medical Book Corp., New York.
4. **Gotschlich, E. C., M. Rey, R. Triau, and K. J. Sparks.** 1972. Quantitative determination of the human immune response to immunization with meningococcal vaccines. J. Clin. Invest. **51:**89–96.
5. **Olcen, P., D. Danielsson, and J. Kjellander.** 1975. The use of protein A-containing staphylococci sensitized with anti-meningococcal antibodies for grouping *Neisseria meningitidis* and demonstration of meningococcal antigen in cerebrospinal fluid. Acta Pathol. Microbiol. Scand. Sect. B **83:**387–396.
6. **Severin, W. P. J.** 1972. Latex agglutination in the diagnosis of meningococcal meningitis. J. Clin. Pathol. **25:**1079–1082.
7. **Tramont, E. C., and M. S. Artenstein.** 1972. Latex agglutination test for measurement of antibodies to meningococcal polysaccharides. Infect. Immun. **5:**346–351.
8. **World Health Organization.** 1976. Requirements for meningococcal polysaccharide vaccine. World Health Organization Technical Report Series, no. 594, p. 50–75. World Health Organization, Albany, N.Y.
9. **Zollinger, W. D., and J. W. Boslego.** 1981. A general approach to standardization of the solid phase radioimmunoassay for quantitation of class-specific antibodies. J. Immunol. Methods **46:**129–140.
10. **Zollinger, W. D., J. M. Dalrymple, and M. S. Artenstein.** 1976. Analysis of parameters affecting the solid phase radioimmunoassay quantitation of antibody to meningococcal antigens. J. Immunol. **117:**1788–1798.

Chapter 53

Neisseria gonorrhoeae: Role of Antibodies in Diagnosis and Identification

STEPHEN A. MORSE AND DOUGLAS S. KELLOGG

The application of serologic techniques for the detection and identification of *Neisseria gonorrhoeae* has involved three general areas, i.e., antibody detection, confirmation of identity, and antigen detection. These areas are listed in the general historical sequence of their development. The use of serologic techniques rests upon the sensitivity and specificity of the antigen-antibody reaction. These two characteristics are dependent upon (i) the biochemical nature, quantity, and availability of the antigen(s); (ii) the immunoglobulin class, source, and polyclonal or monoclonal nature of the antibodies; and (iii) the type of reaction in which the antigens and antibodies are involved. Serologic tests for gonorrhea were once thought to be of use for individuals for whom culture was unlikely to succeed (e.g., where antibiotics had already been given) and in screening programs. These tests have not been developed to the point where they may be used for routine diagnosis. To understand the problems associated with the serologic diagnosis of gonorrhea, it is necessary to review our current knowledge concerning the human immune response to gonococcal infection.

IMMUNE RESPONSE TO INFECTION

Both humoral and cell-mediated immune responses occur during gonococcal infections. However, reinfections occur frequently, and this reoccurrence has led to the notion of an apparent lack of protective immunity acquired through natural infections. The forms of local treatment practiced before the use of antimicrobial agents were relatively ineffective, and the eradication of gonococci and the cure of the disease were more often the result of the patient's own immune response to a prolonged infection. Nevertheless, repeated episodes of acute gonorrhea were well described before the use of antimicrobial agents. With the availability of antimicrobial agents, the short incubation period and the rapid development of symptoms in most males have usually resulted in prompt treatment. In males, the infection is first confined to the anterior urethra, from which the infecting organisms are regularly, but incompletely, removed by urination. This removal of organisms limits the amount of antigen available to stimulate a protective immune response as well as the time the immune response can operate before removal of the stimulating antigens by treatment. In women, gonorrhea is frequently asymptomatic, so the duration and degree of antigenic stimulation are greater. This difference is evident when one compares the differences between men and women in the detection of antigonococcal antibodies (Tables 1 and 2).

Many antigenic types of *N. gonorrhoeae* can be differentiated based on outer membrane components (proteins, lipopolysaccharide). Buchanan et al. (3) observed that patients with one episode of gonococcal pelvic inflammatory disease were less likely to have a recurrent episode of salpingitis caused by a strain of *N. gonorrhoeae* with the same protein I serotype. They also observed that recurrent gonorrhea without salpingitis was frequently caused by strains with the same protein I serotype. Thus, it is currently unclear whether repeated episodes of gonorrhea indicate multiple gonococcal serotypes with little or no antigenic relatedness between them or whether the host is unable to mount a protective immunologic response against gonococci that invade mucosal surfaces. The immune response to cell envelope antigens also varies in individuals and may be an important factor in the antigenic variation of *N. gonorrhoeae*.

Cell-mediated immune response

The cellular response to gonococcal antigens in patients with gonococcal urethritis has been studied in vitro by the lymphocyte transformation test (35). A blastogenic response was occasionally seen with cells from controls, but was almost always present in various degrees in patients with gonococcal urethritis. Antigen-induced lymphocyte transformation was only slightly greater in patients experiencing a first infection than in controls, whereas the difference was often significant between patients with a history of at least two gonococcal infections and controls. The extent of the blastogenic response in women was much greater than in men, a fact which probably reflects the duration of infection before peripheral blood lymphocytes are obtained. The responsiveness of lymphocytes to gonococcal antigens is relatively short-lived and is often lost within 5 weeks after successful therapy. Of particular significance is the fact that lymphocytes from control and infected subjects exhibited occasional blastogenic responses when stimulated with crude antigen preparations from *Neisseria meningitidis*, nonpathogenic *Neisseria* species, and *Branhamella catarrhalis*. Thus, prior exposure to cross-reacting antigens will affect the cellular response to gonococcal antigens.

Humoral immunity

Antibodies with bactericidal and opsonic activities are produced in response to infection with *N. gonorrhoeae*. Both local and systemic antibody responses have been observed. Bactericidal antibodies which cross-react with *N. gonorrhoeae* can also be elicited during meningococcal infection (6). Normal human serum often contains antibodies which cross-react with antigens from *N. gonorrhoeae* and *N. meningitidis*. Antibodies to gonococci have also been demon-

TABLE 1. Serologic tests for the diagnosis of gonorrhea

Category	Reference	Sensitivity (%)[a]		Specificity (%)		Antigen character
		F	M	F	M	
Complement fixation[b]	Danielsson et al. (8)	36	20	95		Pooled cells from each of six strains of *N. gonorrhoeae* heated at 60°C for 30 min
	Young et al. (36)	56	33	98		Heated (60°C for 30 min) cells of *N. gonorrhoeae* 9
	Oranje et al. (20)	21	10	96	93	Sonic extract of *N. gonorrhoeae* 46695
	Toshach et al. (31)	55	67	88 (68)[c]	85	*N. gonorrhoeae* antigen (unspecified)
Passive hemagglutination[d]	Ward and Glynn (33)	84	46	96	98	Alkali-treated phenol-water-extracted lipopolysaccharides from *N. gonorrhoeae* G1, G36, and G2
Indirect fluorescent antibody	Welch and O'Reilly (34)[e]	79	56	97		Suspension of *N. gonorrhoeae* 9 (piliated)
	Kearns et al. (14)[f]		83		83	Suspension of *N. gonorrhoeae* 9 (piliated)
	Toshach et al. (31)[e]	78	50	95 (69)[c]	94	Suspension of *N. gonorrhoeae* 9 (piliated)
	McMillan et al. (18)[f]	72		95		Suspension of *N. gonorrhoeae* 9 (piliated)
Indirect fluorescent antibody (heated)	Gaafar and D'Arcangelis (10)	95	87	97	100	Gonococcal surface antigen (L-antigen)
	Toshach et al (31)	56 (84)[c]	83	88 (55)[c]	89	L-antigen, a heat-labile, trypsin-sensitive antigen made up of protein (MW, 38,500), carbohydrate (10%, wt/vol), and organic phosphorus (2 to 3%, wt/wt) (15)
Counterimmuno-electrophoresis[d]	Schrader and Gaafar (27)	86	76	88	89	Partially purified antigen from a NaCl extract of *N. gonorrhoeae* B370
ELISA[b]	Brodeur et al. (2)[b]	80[g] (98)[h]		94[g] (0)[h]		Lithium acetate-extracted outer membranes from eight selected strains of *N. gonorrhoeae*

[a] F, Female; M, male
[b] Measures both IgG and IgM antibodies.
[c] Numbers in parentheses are results from a high-prevalence population.
[d] Measures primarily IgG antibodies.
[e] Measures IgG, IgM, and IgA antibodies.
[f] Measures IgA antibodies.
[g] Combined results for male and female patients.
[h] Numbers in parentheses are combined results for male and female patients with history of previous gonococcal infection.

strated in the sera of individuals without a history of gonococcal infection. These antibodies react with lipopolysaccharide, outer membrane protein I, and pili (4) and may be opsonic or bactericidal. Thus, an individual's prior exposure to cross-reactive antigens will influence the extent and nature of his or her response to an initial gonococcal infection.

Kearns et al. (14) determined that both 7S immunoglobulin A (IgA) and secretory IgA (sIgA) antibodies were present in the urethral secretions of 29 of 35 men with uncomplicated gonococcal urethritis. The sIgA antigonococcal antibody appeared early and was present in the urethral discharges of 14 of 16 men who had exhibited symptoms for 1 day or less. The rapid appearance of sIgA was similar in those with first or multiple infections. sIgA antigonococcal antibody is also present in cervicovaginal secretions of infected women (17, 35). Antigonococcal sIgA has also been found in women who had no evidence of infection but were contacts of infected men (17). Thus, the local response is most frequently characterized by a rapid development of antigonococcal sIgA. The levels of sIgA return to normal rapidly after successful treatment.

Antigonococcal IgG (17, 18) and IgM (17) have also been detected in cervicovaginal secretions. McMillan et al. (17) found antigonococcal IgM in the cervical secretions of 29 (39%) of 75 infected women; the IgM antibody was usually associated with infections of less

TABLE 2. Comparison of serologic tests for the detection of antibodies to gonococcal pili

Assay method	Reference	Sensitivity (%)[a]		Specificity (%)	
		F	M	F	M
Radioimmunoassay	Buchanan et al. (4)[b]	86	44	82	86
	Oates et al. (19)[b]	86		87	
Indirect hemagglutination	Reimann et al. (23)[b]	70	61	81	79
	Oranje et al. (20)[b]	58	35	63	78
ELISA	Oranje et al. (20)[c]	45	31	65	86
	Young and Low (37)[b]	57		87	

[a] F, Female; M, male.
[b] Measured anti-pili IgG.
[c] Measured anti-pili IgG, IgM, and IgA.

TABLE 3. Serum immunoglobulin response in uncomplicated gonorrhea

Reference	No. of patients	Sex	Group	% of patients positive for:		
				IgG	IgM	IgA
McMillan et al. (16)[a]	125	Male	Infected	100	45	51
	100	Male	Noninfected	8	3	0
	70	Female	Infected	99	46	56
	70	Female	Noninfected	6	3	0
Ison and Glynn (13)[b]	191	Male	Infected	47	20	43
	84	Male	STD[c] (noninfected)	14	19	39
	106	Male	Normal controls (low risk)	8	10	9
	212	Female	Infected	47	31	45
	94	Female	STD (noninfected)	12	21	20
	131	Female	Normal controls (low risk)	8	18	11

[a] Determined by indirect immunofluorescence with *N. gonorrhoeae* 9 as antigen. A titer equal to or greater than 1:16 was considered positive.

[b] Determined by ELISA with a deoxycholate-extracted outer membrane preparation from *N. gonorrhoeae* H1.

[c] STD, Sexually transmitted disease clinic patients.

than 15 days duration. Antigonococcal IgG was found in the cervical secretions of 73 (97%) of 75 infected women; however, it was also found in 23 (33%) of 70 noninfected women. The IgG is probably the result of transudation of natural serum antibody through the inflamed mucous membrane. Antigonococcal IgG activity decreased slowly after successful treatment. The detection of antigonococcal IgA in cervicovaginal secretions by indirect immunofluorescence has been evaluated as a diagnostic test for gonorrhea (Table 1). The low sensitivity of the test, comparable with that of the Gram stain, and its expense and laboriousness prohibit its use as a routine diagnostic procedure. However, the recent development of highly specific reagents may increase the sensitivity of this assay and make its reevaluation worthwhile.

IgG, IgM, and IgA have been found in the sera of individuals infected with *N. gonorrhoeae* (13, 16). The distribution of the immunoglobulin class of antigonococcal antibodies in sera from infected, noninfected high-risk, and noninfected low-risk populations is shown in Table 3. The percentage of infected individuals with IgG-, IgA-, and IgM-specific antigonococcal antibodies appears to be dependent on the sensitivity of the assay as well as the antigen source. Individuals vary with respect to the titer and class of antigonococcal antibody present in their serum. It is important to note that individuals who belong to high-risk groups, such as patients at clinics for sexually transmitted diseases, or who have a history of gonorrhea often have measurable levels of antigonococcal antibodies (IgG, IgM, and IgA). Serologic tests for gonorrhea have been shown to have lower specificity when used to test patients seen in clinics for sexually transmitted diseases (Table 1).

A small, but significant, proportion of normal controls have serum immunoglobulins which cross-react with *N. gonorrhoeae* (Table 3). This cross-reaction would not be a problem in a population with a high prevalence of gonorrhea. However, Dans et al. (9) pointed out that the predictive value of a positive serologic test with 90% sensitivity and 90% specificity in populations with a 2% prevalence of gonorrhea (low risk) would be only 15%.

One solution to this problem would be to decrease the number of false-positives by using specific anti-gens. The majority of studies employing defined gonococcal antigens have used pili. Pili are polymeric proteinaceous filaments extending from the cell surface of *N. gonorrhoeae* that promote infectivity by binding to epithelial cell surfaces. Gonococcal pili are immunogenic (4, 32); humoral and secretory antibodies are produced in response to natural infection or after immunization. The presence of humoral antibodies to gonococcal pili has been used as an indicator of gonococcal infection. Radioimmunoassay (4, 19), indirect hemagglutination (20, 22–24), and enzyme-linked immunosorbent assay (ELISA; 20, 37) have been used to measure these antibodies. A comparison of serologic tests for the detection of antibodies to gonococcal pili is shown in Table 2. The sensitivities of these tests are higher for females (range 45 to 86%) than for males (range 31 to 61%). The specificities of the tests are similar for both groups. A major factor affecting the sensitivity and specificity of the tests is whether the patient has had a previous gonococcal infection (Table 4). Previous infections apparently increase the sensitivity of the test by enhancing the antibody response to common determinants. At the same time, antibodies to gonococcal pili are long-lived (4), so that previous infections decrease the specificity of the tests.

Cross-reacting antibodies are one of the explanations for the relatively low specificity of assays for antibodies to gonococcal pili. Holmes et al. (12) observed that throat carriage of *N. meningitidis* resulted in antibodies which also cross-reacted with gonococcal pili. The N-terminal amino acid sequence of pili from a group B strain of *N. meningitidis* was found to be identical to that of *N. gonorrhoeae* (11). Other

TABLE 4. Effect of previous gonococcal infections on the serologic diagnosis of gonorrhea with pili antigen[a]

Sex	Previous infection	Sensitivity (%)	Specificity (%)
Male	+	74	65
	−	45	89
Female	+	100	71
	−	61	85

[a] Data from Reimann et al. (23).

gram-negative bacteria possess pili whose N-terminal amino acid sequences are remarkably similar to those of *N. gonorrhoeae* and *N. meningitidis*.

IMMUNOLOGIC IDENTIFICATION OF *N. GONORRHOEAE*

A slide agglutination method for the identification of *N. gonorrhoeae* has been developed to circumvent a variety of problems which have occurred with other procedures used for identifying this organism. This method involves stabilizing cells of *Staphylococcus aureus* (Cowan I) with their covering of protein A intact. The Fc portion of IgG from antigonococcal sera is adsorbed onto the protein A with reactive sites of the antibodies exposed. Reaction of gonococci with this reagent results in a coagglutination reaction between gonococci and staphylococci. Growth of presumptively identified *N. gonorrhoeae* is removed from an 18- to 24-h culture plate, and a dense suspension is made in 0.2 ml of distilled water. This suspension is then heated in a boiling-water bath for 5 min. A drop of this heated cell suspension is added to separate drops of the test reagent (rabbit anti-*N. gonorrhoeae* antibodies bound to the protein A on staphylococci) and the control reagent (nonimmunized rabbit gamma globulin bound to the protein A on staphylococci) on a slide. A positive coagglutination reaction appears after 2 to 3 min of rocking the slide.

A significantly stronger reaction with the test reagent compared with the reaction with the control constitutes a positive result. Equivalent reactions are considered noninterpretable. Limitations of this procedure include the growth medium, age of culture, strain differences, and cross-reactions with some strains of *Neisseria lactamica*.

Coagglutination reagents for the confirmatory identification of *N. gonorrhoeae* are commercially available as the Phadebact test (Pharmacia Diagnostics, Piscataway, N.J.) and the Gono-Gen test (New Horizons, Columbia, Md.). The tests are procedurally identical, but use different antibody sources. The Phadebact test utilizes polyclonal antibodies prepared in rabbits to whole gonococcal cells, whereas the Gono-Gen test utilizes monoclonal antibodies to epitopes on gonococcal protein I.

Early studies demonstrated the utility of the Phadebact coagglutination procedure, but detected a number of noninterpretable or pseudocoagglutination reactions. One problem was associated with gonococcal cells grown on serum-containing medium and could be eliminated by using a serum-free medium and by pretreatment of gonococcal cells with trypsin. Increasing the number of gonococcal cells resulted in a more rapid coagglutination reaction. Cells from 24-h cultures exhibit better reactions than cells from 48-h cultures.

Since 1980, the basic procedure has changed only in its quantitative aspects. The heating (100°C) time has been reduced to 3 to 5 min, the gonococcal cell concentration has been increased, and minimal reactivity levels have been adjusted. Evidence has been conflicting on the influence of gonococcal cultivation time, primary versus subcultured cells, and media composition on test results.

Extensive autolysis occurs when gonococcal cultures are incubated for longer than 24 h. DNA and RNA are released during autolysis and bind to the gonococcal cell surface. Treatment of gonococci with DNase and RNase eliminates the pseudoagglutination observed with older cultures. In addition, conditions favoring autolysis and the release of lipopolysaccharide potentiate the coagglutination reaction. The coagglutination test is equivalent to the fluorescent-antibody test as a method of confirmation. However, 2 to 4% of results are false-negative even with boiled suspensions of cells taken from primary cultures on Martin-Lewis medium.

Coagglutination is a rapid, specific confirmatory test for gonococci that is equivalent to current fluorescent-antibody tests and superior to sugar degradation tests. The use of monoclonal antibodies and a broader range of gonococcal antibodies will make it a widely used test.

ANTIGEN DETECTION FOR THE DIAGNOSIS OF GONORRHEA

The diagnosis of gonorrhea has relied on the isolation and identification of the causative agent, *N. gonorrhoeae*. This process is quite sensitive because a single pair of diplococci can grow into an observable colony. Although culture is very effective (ca. 90%), it is time consuming and subject to losses due to inhibitory media components and environmental conditions. To obviate the problems associated with culture, a variety of serologic tests were developed to detect antibody responses to infection. However, problems associated with their sensitivity and specificity have prevented them from attaining widespread acceptance. Antigen-detection methods have recently been developed for gonorrhea diagnosis to circumvent problems associated with culture and serologic tests. Thornley et al. (29, 30) developed a solid-phase radioisotope-labeled antigen assay which was specific for *N. gonorrhoeae* and *N. meningitidis*. Gonococcal antigens were detected in 31 (74%) of 42 urine sediments from males with urethritis and 10 (71%) of 14 urine sediments from females with cervicitis. Nonspecific binding was low in urine sediments from healthy men but was a significant factor in men with nonspecific urethritis. Soybean trypsin inhibitor reduced or eliminated this nonspecific binding. The low sensitivity of this test was probably due to its use for detecting only the particulate antigen in the urines.

Aardoom et al. (1) examined the use of a solid-phase enzyme immunoassay (EIA) to detect gonococcal antigens (Gonozyme; Abbott Laboratories, North Chicago, Ill.). This procedure used coated beads to capture the antigen, rabbit antibodies to *N. gonorrhoeae*, horseradish peroxidase-labeled goat anti-rabbit IgG, and *o*-phenylenediamine as substrate. Endocervical or urethral specimens on cotton swabs are placed in a storage reagent and diluted with buffer before being tested. The specimens and appropriate positive and negative controls are placed in reaction tray wells, and a specifically sorptive bead is added to each well. The reaction tray is incubated at 37°C for 45 min. The liquid is then aspirated from each well, and the beads are washed with distilled water. Rabbit antibody to *N. gonorrhoeae* is added to each well and incubated as

TABLE 5. Comparison of studies employing antigen detection for the diagnosis of gonorrhea

Reference	Sensitivity (%)		Specificity (%)	
	Males	Females	Males	Females
Thornley et al (29)[a]	74	71		
Rudrick et al. (25)[a]	92	87	98	94
Aardoom et al. (1)[b]	100	87	100	90
Schachter et a. (26)[b]	93	87	100	98
Papasian et al. (21)[b]	97	79	96	87
Stamm et al. (28)[b]	94	78	98	98
Danielsson et al. (7)[b]	87	91	94	100
Burns et al. (5)[b]	100	89	97	94
Martin et al. (15)[c]	91	92	90	95
Young et al. (38)[d]		60		88

[a] Urine specimens.
[b] Swab specimens.
[c] Transported specimens.
[d] Cervical and vaginal washings.

indicated. The aspiration and washing steps are repeated, and a goat anti-rabbit IgG–horseradish peroxidase conjugate is added to each well. Incubation, aspiration, and washing are repeated as indicated. All liquid is removed by blotting, and the beads are transferred to assay tubes. Freshly prepared *o*-phenylenediamine solution is added to each tube, and the tube is incubated at room temperature for 30 min. The reaction is stopped with an acid solution, and A_{492} is measured. Specimens giving an absorbance greater than a calculated cutoff value are considered positive for *N. gonorrhoeae*. The cutoff value is derived from adding the difference between the means of the positive and negative controls (at least 0.800) to the factor 0.190. Specimens giving a reading within ±13% of the cutoff value should be retested.

The limitations of this procedure are affected by the site of specimen origin, duration of infection, and cross-reactions with *N. meningitidis* and *N. lactamica*. Compared with culturing, this procedure is quite sensitive in detecting gonococcal antigens in specimens from males with urethritis and somewhat less sensitive with specimens from female contacts (Table 5). Posttreatment specimens and those from prostitutes had an average specificity of 96%. The sensitivity of this procedure with the different patient groups reflected the relative number of colonies isolated from each group, i.e., the most colonies were observed on cultures from males with urethritis, less from cervical specimens, etc. Rudrick et al. (25) used EIA with uncentrifuged first-voided urine specimens in a comparison with urethral swab specimens from males and a small number of cervical specimens (Table 5). Several other investigators have used the same test and obtained approximately the same results (Table 5). Discordant results between Gonozyme and culture varied for the studies, but on average, results were close enough to indicate trends. False-positive reactions were 4% (range, 0.5 to 8.0%) with male specimens and 6% (range, 2.0 to 9.0%) with female specimens. False-negative reactions were 1% (range, 0.5 to 1.5%) with male specimens and 2.5% (range, 0.5 to 6.0%) with female specimens. Studies involving larger numbers of specimens or clinics or both tended to produce higher levels of discordant results.

With cervical specimens, current EIA procedures (principally the Gonozyme test) have an average sensitivity of 85% and an average specificity of 95%. With male urethral specimens, the sensitivity and specificity average 94 and 98%, respectively. The sensitivity of the test with females (85%) is not high enough for use with high-risk groups. With a low-incidence population, this sensitivity would project a positive predictive value of ca. 30%. Where culture is not available or transport time exceeds 48 h, EIA might be a more effective diagnostic technique than culture. Where penicillinase-producing strains of *N. gonorrhoeae* are present, culture would be necessary; however, EIA tests for beta-lactamase are currently under development. There does not seem to be a consistent relationship between the number of gonococci present in a specimen and the reactivity of the EIA procedure. Seemingly, this lack of correlation indicates that another factor is influencing the correlation of culture and EIA sensitivities, besides those factors taken into account during test development. Distribution of cells or antigen in specimens might account for such discrepancies. Since culture is not 100% sensitive, the specificity will never be 100%. Negative culture results have historical weight behind their acceptance; however, a negative culture is not more accurate than a positive EIA test. As with other methodological developments, antigen detection will have to be used and understood as a separate procedure from culture, which has its own utility in gonorrhea diagnosis.

LITERATURE CITED

1. **Aardoom, H. A., D. de Hoop, C. O. A. Iserief, M. F. Michel, and E. Stolz.** 1982. Detection of *Neisseria gonorrhoeae* antigen by a solid-phase enzyme immunoassay. Br. J. Vener. Dis. **52:**359–362.

2. **Brodeur, B. R., F. E. Ashton, and B. B. Diena.** 1982. Enzyme-linked immunosorbent assay with polyvalent gonococcal antigen. J. Med. Microbiol. **15:**1–9.

3. **Buchanan, T. M., D. A. Eschenbach, J. S. Knapp, and K. K. Holmes.** 1980. Gonococcal salpingitis is less likely to recur with *Neisseria gonorrhoeae* of the same principal outer membrane protein (POMP) antigenic type, p. 266. *In* D. Danielsson and S. Normark (ed.), Genetics and immunobiology of pathogenic *Neisseria*. University of Umea Press, Umea, Sweden.

4. **Buchanan, T. M., J. Swanson, K. K. Holmes, S. J. Kraus, and E. C. Gotschlich.** 1973. Quantitative determination of antibody to gonococcal pili. J. Clin. Invest. **52:**2896–2909.

5. **Burns, M., P. H. Rossi, D. W. Cox, T. Edwards, M. Kramer, and S. J. Kraus.** 1983. A preliminary evaluation of the Gonozyme test. Sex. Transm. Dis. **10:**180–183.

6. **Cremieux, A. D., A. Puissant, R. Ancelle, and P. M. V. Martin.** 1984. Bactericidal antibodies against *Neisseria gonorrhoeae* elicited by *Neisseria meningitidis*. Lancet **ii:**930.

7. **Danielsson, D., H. Moi, and L. Forslin.** 1983. Diagnosis of urogenital gonorrhea by detecting gonococcal antigen with a solid phase enzyme immunoassay (Gonozyme). J. Clin. Pathol. **36:**674–677.

8. **Danielsson, D., N. Thryesson, V. Falk, and J. Barr.** 1972. Serologic investigation of the immune response in various types of gonococcal infection. Acta Dermato-Venereol. **52:**467–475.

9. **Dans, P. E., R. Rothenberg, and K. K. Holmes.** 1977. Gonococcal serology: how soon, how useful, and how much? J. Infect. Dis. **135:**330–334.

10. **Gaafar, H. A., and D. C. D'Arcangelis.** 1976. Fluorescent

antibody test for the serological diagnosis of gonorrhea. J. Clin. Microbiol. **3**:438–442.

11. **Hermodson, M. A., K. C. S. Chen, and T. M. Buchanan.** 1978. *Neisseria* pili proteins: amino-terminal amino acid sequences and identification of an unusual amino acid. Biochemistry **17**:442–445.

12. **Holmes, K. K., T. M. Buchanan, J. L. Adam, and D. A. Eschenbach.** 1978. Is serology useful in gonorrhea? A critical analysis of factors influencing serodiagnosis, p. 370–376. *In* G. F. Brooks, E. C. Gotschlich, K. K. Holmes, W. D. Sawyer, and F. E. Young (ed.), Immunobiology of *Neisseria gonorrhoeae*. American Society for Microbiology, Washington, D.C.

13. **Ison, C. A., and A. A. Glynn.** 1979. Classes of antibodies in acute gonorrhoea. Lancet **i**:1165–1168.

14. **Kearns, D. H., R. J. O'Reilly, L. Lee, and B. G. Welch.** 1973. IgA antibodies in the urethral exudate of men with uncomplicated urethritis due to *Neisseria gonorrhoeae*. J. Infect. Dis. **127**:99–101.

15. **Martin, R., B. B. Wentworth, S. Coopes, and E. H. Larson.** 1984. Comparison of Transgrow and Gonozyme for the detection of *Neisseria gonorrhoeae* in mailed specimens. J. Clin. Microbiol. **19**:893–895.

16. **McMillan, A., G. McNeillage, H. Young, and S. S. R. Bain.** 1979. Serum immunoglobulin response in uncomplicated gonorrhoea. Br. J. Vener. Dis. **55**:5–9.

17. **McMillan, A., G. McNeillage, H. Young, and S. S. R. Bain.** 1979. Secretory antibody response of the cervix to infection with *Neisseria gonorrhoeae*. Br. J. Vener. Dis. **55**:265–270.

18. **McMillan, A., G. McNeillage, H. Young, and S. S. R. Bain.** 1980. Detection of antigonococcal IgA in cervical secretions by immunofluorescence: an evaluation as a diagnostic test. Br. J. Vener. Dis. **56**:203–226.

19. **Oates, S. A., W. A. Falkler, Jr., J. M. Joseph, and L. E. Warfel.** 1977. Asymptomatic females: detection of antibody activity to gonococcal pili antigen by radioimmunoassay. J. Clin. Microbiol. **5**:26–30.

20. **Oranje, A. P., K. Reimann, R. V. W. van Eijk, H. J. A. Schouten, A. de Roo, G. J. Tideman, E. Stolz, and M. F. Michel.** 1983. Gonococcal serology. A comparison of three different tests. Br. J. Vener. Dis. **59**:47–52.

21. **Papasian, C. J., W. R. Bartholomew, and D. Amsterdam.** 1984. Validity of an enzyme immunoassay for detection of *Neisseria gonorrhoeae* antigens. J. Clin. Microbiol. **19**:347–350.

22. **Reimann, K., and I. Lind.** 1977. An indirect haemagglutination test for demonstration of gonococcal antibodies using gonococcal pili as antigen. Acta Pathol. Microbiol. Scand. Sect. C **85**:115–122.

23. **Reimann, K., I. Lind, and K. E. Anderson.** 1980. An indirect haemagglutination test for demonstration of gonococcal antibodies using gonococcal pili as antigen. II. Serological investigation of patients attending a dermatovenereological outpatients clinic in Copenhagen. Acta Pathol. Microbiol. Scand. Sect. C **88**:155–162.

24. **Reimann, K., A. P. Oranje, and M. F. Michel.** 1982. Demonstration of antigenic heterogeneity of *Neisseria gonorrhoeae* pili antigens using human sera in the test system. Acta Pathol. Microbiol. Scand. Sect. C **90**:47–52.

25. **Rudrik, J. T., J. M. Waller, and E. M. Britt.** 1984. Efficacy of an enzyme immunoassay with uncentrifuged first-voided urine for detection of gonorrhea in males. J. Clin. Microbiol. **20**:577–578.

26. **Schachter, J., W. M. McCormack, R. F. Smith, R. M. Parks, R. Bailey, and A. C. Ohlin.** 1984. Enzyme immunoassay for diagnosis of gonorrhea. J. Clin. Microbiol. **19**:57–59.

27. **Schrader, J. A., and H. A. Gaafar.** 1978. Detection of antibodies to *Neisseria gonorrhoeae* by counterimmunoelectrophoresis. Health Lab. Sci. **15**:15–21.

28. **Stamm, W. E., B. Cole, C. Fennell, P. Bonin, A. S. Armstrong, J. E. Herrmann, and K. K. Holmes.** 1984. Antigen detection for the diagnosis of gonorrhea. J. Clin. Microbiol. **19**:399–403.

29. **Thornley, M. J., M. G. Andrews, J. O. Briggs, and B. K. Leigh.** 1979. Inhibitors in urine of radioimmunoassay for the detection of gonococcal antigens. J. Med. Microbiol. **12**:177–185.

30. **Thornley, M. J., D. V. Wilson, R. D. de Hormaeche, J. K. Oates, and R. K. A. Coombs.** 1979. Detection of gonococcal antigens in urine by radioimmunoassay. J. Med. Microbiol. **12**:161–175.

31. **Toshach, S., I. Coull, S. Sigurdson, S. Dublenko, J. Grocholski, and L. Linarez.** 1979. Evaluation of five serologic tests for antibody to *Neisseria gonorrhoeae*. Sex. Transm. Dis. **6**:214–217.

32. **Tramont, E. C., J. C. Sadoff, J. W. Boslego, J. Ciak, D. McChesney, C. C. Brinton, S. Wood, and E. Takafuju.** 1981. Gonococcal pilus vaccine. Studies of antigenicity and inhibition of attachment. J. Clin. Invest. **68**:881–888.

33. **Ward, M. E., and A. A. Glynn.** 1972. Human antibody response to lipopolysaccharides from *Neisseria gonorrhoeae*. J. Clin. Pathol. **25**:56–59.

34. **Welch, B. G., and R. J. O'Reilly.** 1973. An indirect fluorescent antibody technique for the study of uncomplicated gonorrhea. I. Methodology. J. Infect. Dis. **127**:69–76.

35. **World Health Organization.** 1978. *Neisseria gonorrhoeae* and gonococcal infections. Report of a WHO scientific group. Technical Report Series no. 616. World Health Organization, Geneva.

36. **Young, H., C. Henrichsen, and A. McMillan.** 1980. The diagnostic value of a gonococcal complement fixation test. Med. Lab. Sci. **37**:165–170.

37. **Young, H., and A. C. Low.** 1980. Serological diagnosis of gonorrhea: detection of antibodies to gonococcal pili by enzyme-linked immunosorbent assay. Med. Lab. Sci. **38**:41–47.

38. **Young, H., S. K. Sarafian, A. B. Harris, and A. McMillan.** 1983. Non-cultural detection of *Neisseria gonorrhoeae* in cervical and vaginal washings. Med. Microbiol. **16**:183–191.

Chapter 54

Serologic Tests for the Diagnosis of Enterobacterial Infections

R. BRADLEY SACK

Human infections by enterobacteria (genus *Enterobacteriaceae*) encompass the entire range of organ systems, from the gastrointestinal tract to the urinary tract, all body cavities, and all soft tissues. These organisms, which are primarily bowel inhabitants, (i) may be only normal, commensal flora of the gastrointestinal tract, such as *Escherichia coli*, *Klebsiella* spp., and *Proteus* spp., (ii) may be primarily pathogens in the gastrointestinal tract, such as *Shigella* spp., nontyphoidal *Salmonella* spp., and enterotoxigenic *E. coli*, or (iii) may produce a clinically distinct systemic illness by invading the blood stream and other organ systems through a portal of entry in the gastrointestinal tract, for example, *Salmonella typhosa* and *Salmonella paratyphi* A and B. All strains may also act as opportunistic infections outside of their usual bowel habitat, particularly in immunocompromised or otherwise debilitated patients, and particularly in hospital settings.

In nearly all of these clinical settings, the isolation of the microorganism and determination of its antimicrobial sensitivities are crucial to optimum antibiotic therapy. The only exception to this general rule is the acute diarrheal illness produced by enterotoxigenic *E. coli* (ETEC), in which fluid replacement, not antibiotic therapy, is of primary importance.

Serologic diagnosis of all of these infections is theoretically possible, since antibodies are produced in response to the infecting organism. However, for practical purposes, serologic diagnosis is useful clinically in only two instances: (i) the detection of chronic carriers of *S. typhosa*, and (ii) the diagnosis of typhoid fever in endemic areas. These will be discussed in some detail. In other disease syndromes, a relatively specific serologic diagnosis can be made retrospectively and therefore may be of epidemiologic usefulness, such as in diarrheal diseases caused by ETEC. In most clinical syndromes caused by enterobacteria, however, serologic diagnosis is not useful because (i) the incubation period is too short to allow for the development of high titers of antibodies during the acute illness, and (ii) the organisms themselves contain multiple antigens which are cross-reactive, and therefore do not allow for specific identification of the infecting organisms, or are of multiple serotypes, thereby making identification difficult; furthermore, early use of antibiotics may interfere with the normal antigenic load presented for immunologic processing and thus may result in a blunting of the antibody response.

Presumably any infection, either gastrointestinal or systemic, by these organisms will give rise to appropriate mucosal secretory antibodies, serum antibodies, or both in the normal host. The difficulty is determining the appropriate specific antigens against which to measure the antibodies.

This chapter will focus on the serologic diagnosis of infections due to *S. typhosa*, with less attention being given to other members of this genus.

INFECTIONS DUE TO *S. TYPHOSA*

Typhoid fever

Antibodies to *S. typhosa* have classically been measured by the agglutination of patients' sera with suspensions of *S. typhosa*, a process described first by Widal in 1896 (21). Since high titers of antibodies could be detected early in the clinical course of the disease, and because cultures of blood were often more difficult to obtain and probably not of optimum sensitivity, the Widal test assumed the stature of a definitive diagnostic marker for typhoid fever. The test was used diagnostically in two ways; either a single high titer of antibodies during the first week of illness, or a greater than fourfold titer rise in sera taken 1 to 2 weeks apart, was considered diagnostic. As experience was gained in the critical evaluation of the test, however, particularly in the past 30 years when the incidence of typhoid fever was declining markedly in the developed world and antibiotics and immunizations were being widely used, the shortcomings of the test, i.e., its lack of both sensitivity and specificity, were pointed out. As a result, in some contemporary textbooks of infectious diseases, the Widal test is mentioned only to make the reader aware of its unreliability (6).

The major problems with the test are as follows.

False negatives. First, the percentage of patients with known typhoid fever, documented bacteriologically, who develop diagnostic titers of antibodies is unacceptably low in developed countries, ranging from 24 to 60% (2, 9). (This is not true in developing countries where typhoid fever is still endemic; this point will be discussed later.) Second, patients treated with antibiotics early in the course of their disease may not develop a significant titer rise. Third, sera may not be collected at the optimal time periods to demonstrate a diagnostic titer or titer rise.

False positives. First, previous immunizations with typhoid vaccine, or previous infections by *Salmonella* spp. sharing common antigens with *S. typhosa*, may result in prolonged elevations of antibody titers. Also, other nontyphoidal febrile illness or unrelated immunologic disorders may produce significant elevations of antibody titers.

The Widal test is furthermore difficult to standardize, and results vary considerably from one laboratory to another. The use of the Widal test in areas of low typhoid endemicity and sophisticated diagnostic laboratories is therefore not recommended.

TABLE 1. Evaluation of the Widal test in areas of high endemicity for typhoid fever[a]

Year (reference)	Country	Titer considered diagnostic	Sera positive by Widal test			
			Normal persons	Patients with typhoid fever (%)	Patients with fever, nontyphoid (%)	Patients with immunologic disorders (%)
1977 (18)	Sri Lanka	≥1:160		50/53 (94)	1/100 (1)	7/61 (11.5)
1983 (15)	Malaysia	≥1:320	0/300	255/275 (93)	9/297 (3)	
1983 (17)	Thailand	≥1:80	0/79	34/39 (87)		

[a] Burroughs Wellcome Co. bacterial suspensions were used for these studies.

In areas of high typhoid endemicity in developing countries, however, the situation is different, and the diagnostic value of the Widal test has been well documented. In Sri Lanka (18), Malaysia (15), and Thailand (17) recent evaluations have been done which strongly suggest that if the base-line titer in the population is known, and the test is carefully done, the test has both a high specificity and high sensitivity (Table 1). This is probably because of the primed nature of the population, in which antigen stimulation by related *Salmonella* antigens is frequent and therefore a prompt and significant antibody response occurs during the relatively long incubation period of 1 to 2 weeks. Both the O and H titers were found to be useful diagnostically, although the O was considered more reliable. It should be noted that some patients with known immunologic disorders, such as rheumatoid arthritis, gave false-positive tests. Because of the difficulty in obtaining adequate bacteriologic cultures, Pang and Puthucheary (15) believe the Widal test is the only practical one for developing countries.

The test of anti-Vi antibodies for diagnosis of typhoid fever has not been of practical usefulness in either nonendemic or endemic areas (1, 11).

Where adequate bacteriologic facilities are available, the preferred method of diagnosis is clearly by culture. Highly sensitive techniques are now available which include (i) cultures of bone marrow (8), (ii) cultures of the upper small bowel by the string capsule method (7), (iii) cultures of blood clots (13), and (iv) the use of oxgall medium in addition to other standard methods and media.

Chronic carriers of *S. typhosa*

Because chronic carriers harbor *S. typhosa* in the gall bladder and intestinal tract for periods of years, it has been thought that a serologic diagnosis of such infections should be possible. Unfortunately, until the last few years, this was not the case. Studies using the standard Widal agglutination test or crude Vi antigen preparations were neither specific nor sensitive enough for diagnostic use, and detection of carriers was possible only by the obtaining of multiple stool cultures.

In 1972 Wong and Feeley (22) isolated a highly purified Vi antigen from *Citrobacter freundii* which is antigenetically identical to that of *S. typhosa*. Several studies in the past few years (4, 11, 14) have demonstrated the high sensitivity and specificity of this preparation in assays to detect carriers (Table 2). In two outbreaks, individual carriers could be pinpointed by antibody titers as causes of epidemics in the United States (5, 19). Furthermore, there is also evidence that the Vi antibody titer decreases after successful treatment of the carrier state (14) by surgery, antibiotics, or both, thus making possible an independent assessment of the effectiveness of the therapy, in addition to stool cultures.

The Vi antigen has been used in a hemagglutination assay (4, 11, 14), enzyme-linked immunosorbent assay (1, 5), counterimmunoelectrophoresis assay (4), and radioimmune assay (RIA) (4). The passive hemagglutination assay and the enzyme-linked immunosorbent assay seem to have comparable degrees of sensitivity and specificity. The latter assay has an additional advantage because of the stability of the reagents.

The tests. (i) Passive hemagglutination (11). Reagents:

(a) Glutaraldehyde-treated sheep erythrocytes, sensitized with purified Vi antigen (10 μg/ml).
(b) Serum absorbed with normal sheep erythrocytes, then diluted twofold beginning at 1:20.

Procedure: Equal volumes of serum dilutions are added to sensitized and nonsensitized erythrocyte suspensions. Incubation is for 2 h at room temperature and then overnight at 4°C.

(ii) ELISA (1). Reagents:

(a) Burro anti-*S. typhosa* TY-2, diluted 1:5,000 in 0.06 M carbonate buffer (pH 9.6) and mixed with purified Vi antigen to a final concentration of 1 μg/ml.
(b) Patient's sera, serial twofold dilutions in phosphate-buffered saline (PBS)-Tween with 1% fetal calf serum, beginning with 1:20 dilution.
(c) Alkaline phosphatase-conjugated goat anti-human immunoglobulin G, diluted 1:200 in PBS-Tween with 1% fetal calf serum.

TABLE 2. Evaluation of Vi antibodies in the diagnosis of chronic typhoid carriers

Year (reference)	Country	Titer considered diagnostic	Sera positive for Vi antibodies		
			Normals (%)	Convalescent typhoid noncarriers (%)	Typhoid carriers (%)
1980 (14)	United States	≥1:10	0/22	0/6	22/31 (71)
1982 (4)	Hong Kong	≥1:160	2/329 (<1)		12/14 (86)
1983 (11)	Chile	≥1:160	2/59 (3)	3/38 (8)	27/36 (75)

(d) Enzyme substrate (Sigma 104 in diethanolamine buffer, pH 9.5).

Procedure: Burro serum (0.1 ml) with and without Vi antigen is added to wells of U-shaped microtiter plates and incubated for 1 h at 37°C and then overnight at 4°C. Plates are washed with PBS-Tween (PBS with 0.05% Tween 20).

Serial dilutions of sera (0.1 ml) are added to the microtiter plates, incubated for 1 h at 37°C, and then washed three times in PBS-Tween. Conjugated antihuman immunoglobulin G (0.1 ml) is added to each well, incubated at 37°C for 1 h, and then washed three times in PBS-Tween. Enzyme substrate is then added, and the plates are left at room temperature for 30 min, after which the reaction is terminated with 0.025 ml of 3 N NaOH. The plates are read visually.

Gastrointestinal tract infections

ETEC. Infections with ETEC result in both serum and secretory antibodies being produced against multiple antigens carried by these organisms, including the O antigen, the heat-labile enterotoxin, and the colonization factor antigens (12). Antibodies are not produced against the small-molecular-weight heat-stable enterotoxin. Since the ETEC are of many O serogroups, specific O antibodies cannot be easily identified. Also, since only a certain percentage of ETEC produce heat-labile enterotoxin or the recognized colonization factors, antibodies to these virulence factor antigens are not universally produced. Furthermore, the heat-labile enterotoxin is closely related immunologically to the enterotoxin of *Vibrio cholerae*, and therefore antibodies to these two enterotoxins have a high degree of cross-reactivity.

A serologic diagnosis of ETEC infection, although theoretically possible for certain strains of ETEC, can thus be made only retrospectively and is of limited usefulness.

Enteropathogenic *E. coli*. The enteropathogenic *E. coli*, or EPEC, are recognized only by their serotype (O and H antigens); other virulence factors have not been conclusively demonstrated. Since these organisms are of multiple serotypes (approximately 12 to 15, depending on the definition used), a single antibody assay is not possible. Furthermore, only a retrospective diagnosis would be possible by any antibody assay.

Shigella. Serum antibodies are formed during shigellosis against both somatic antigen (3) and the *Shigella* toxin (10). However, these tests are less than optimal in both specificity and sensitivity and would be useful only in retrospective diagnosis.

Nontyphoid *Salmonella*. Although antibodies are formed in response to infection with nontyphoid *Salmonella* spp. the large number of serotypes precludes any useful specific serologic diagnosis, even in a retrospective way, outside of a common-source outbreak situation involving a single serotype. Furthermore, there are many antigens common to multiple serotypes, making a specific serotype diagnosis difficult.

Systemic infections due to *Enterobacteriaceae*

Systemic infections with the *Enterobacteriaceae*, including urinary tract infections, often produce rises in serum antibodies to the somatic antigens of the infect-

ing strains. These are usually serotype specific, and diagnostic rises are seen only in convalescence, which, again, limits their use to retrospective diagnoses. In urinary tract infections, serum antibody titers do not differentiate between cystitis and pyelonephritis (16). Although the presence of antibody-coated bacteria in the urine was initially thought to signify the presence of an upper urinary tract infection (20), this test is now thought to be of only limited value in making this differentiation.

SUMMARY

Immunologic methods for the diagnosis of enterobacterial infections are only of clinical usefulness in two situations: (i) the identification of chronic typhoid carriers, and (ii) the diagnosis of acute typhoid fever in endemic areas in the developing world. Other enterobacterial infections with specific organisms, such as the ETEC, can be diagnosed serologically, but only in a retrospective manner.

LITERATURE CITED

1. **Barrett, T. J., P. A. Blake, S. L. Brown, K. Hoffman, J. Mateu Llort, and J. C. Feeley.** 1983. Enzyme-linked immunosorbent assay for detection of human antibodies to *Salmonella typhi* Vi antigen. J. Clin. Microbiol. **17:**625–627.

2. **Brodie, J.** 1977. Antibodies and the Aberdeen typhoid outbreak of 1964. I. The Widal reaction. J. Hyg. **79:**161–180.

3. **Caceres, A., and L. J. Mata.** 1974. Serologic response of patients with shiga dysentery. J. Infect. Dis **129:**439–443.

4. **Chau, P. Y., and R. S. W. Tsang.** 1982. Vi serology in screening of typhoid carriers: improved specificity by detection of Vi antibodies by counterimmunoelectrophoresis. J. Hyg. **89:**261–267.

5. **Engleberg, N. C., T. J. Barrett, H. Fisher, B. Porter, E. Hurtado, and J. M. Hughes.** 1983. Identification of a carrier by using Vi enzyme-linked immunosorbent assay serology in an outbreak of typhoid fever on an Indian reservation. J. Clin. Microbiol. **18:**1320–1322.

6. **Foote, S. C., and E. W. Hook.** 1979. *Salmonella* species (including typhoid fever), p. 1730–1750. *In* G. L. Mandell, R. G. Douglas, and J. E. Bennett (ed.), Principles and practices of infectious diseases. John Wiley and Sons, New York.

7. **Gilman, R. H., S. Islam, H. Rabbani, and H. Ghosh.** 1979. Identification of gallbladder typhoid carriers by a string device. Lancet **ii:**795–796.

8. **Guerra-Caceres, J. G., E. Gottuzzo-Herencia, E. Crosby-Dagnino, M. Miro-Quesda, and C. Carrillo-Parodi.** 1979. Diagnostic value of bone marrow culture in typhoid fever. Trans. R. Soc. Trop. Med. Hyg. **73:**680–683.

9. **Hoffman, T. A., C. J. Ruiz, G. W. Counts, J. M. Sachs, and J. L. Nitzkin.** 1975. Waterborne typhoid fever in Dade County, Florida. Clinical and therapeutic evaluation of 105 bacteremic patients. Am. J. Med. **59:**481–487.

10. **Keusch, G. T., M. Jacewicz, M. M. Levine, R. B. Hornick, and S. Kochwa.** 1976. Pathogenesis of shigella diarrhea. Serum anticytotoxin antibody response produced by toxigenic and non-toxigenic *Shigella dysenteriae* 1. J. Clin. Invest. **57:**194–202.

11. **Lanata, C. F., M. M. Levine, C. Ristori, R. E. Black, L. Jimenez, M. Salcedo, J. Garcia, and V. Sotomayor.** 1983. Vi serology in detection of chronic *Salmonella typhi* carriers in an endemic area. Lancet **ii:**441–443.

12. **Levine, M. M., D. R. Nalin, D. L. Hoover, E. J. Bergquist,**

R. B. Hornick, and C. R. Young. 1979. Immunity to enterotoxigenic *Escherichia coli*. Infect. Immun. **23:**729–736.

13. Mikhail, I. S., W. R. Sanborn, and J. E. Sippel. 1983. Rapid, economical diagnosis of enteric fever by a blood clot culture coagglutination procedure. J. Clin. Microbiol. **17:**564–565.

14. Nolan, C. M., J. C. Feeley, P. C. White, Jr., E. A. Hambie, S. L. Brown, and K.-H. Wong. 1980. Evaluation of a new assay for Vi antibody in chronic carriers of *Salmonella typhi*. J. Clin. Microbiol. **12:**22–26.

15. Pang, T., and S. D. Puthucheary. 1983. Significance and value of the Widal test in the diagnosis of typhoid fever in an endemic area. J. Clin. Pathol. **36:**471–475.

16. Sanford, B. A., V. L. Thomas, M. Forland, S. Carson, and A. Shelokov. 1978. Immune response in urinary tract infection determined by radioimmunoassay and immunofluorescence: serum antibody levels against infecting bacterium and *Enterobacteriaceae* common antigen. J. Clin. Microbiol. **8:**575–579.

17. Sangpetchsong, V., and S. Tharavanij. 1983. Diagnosis of typhoid fever by indirect hemagglutination with lyophilized cells. Southeast Asian J. Trop. Med. Public Health **14:**374–379.

18. Senewiratne, B., B. Chir, and K. Senewiratne. 1977. Reassessment of the Widal test in the diagnosis of typhoid. Gastroenterology **73:**233–236.

19. Taylor, J. P., W. X. Shandera, T. G. Betz, K. Schraitle, L. Chaffee, L. Lopez, R. Henley, C. N. Rothe, R. F. Bell, and P. A. Blake. 1984. Typhoid fever in San Antonio, Texas: an outbreak traced to a continuing source. J. Infect. Dis. **149:**553–557.

20. Thomas, V., A. Shelokov, and M. Forland. 1974. Antibody-coated bacteria in the urine and the site of urinary-tract infection. N. Engl. J. Med. **290:**588–590.

21. Widal, F. 1896. Serodiagnostic de la fièvre typhoide. Sem. Med. **16:**259.

22. Wong, K. H., and J. C. Feeley. 1972. Isolation of Vi antigen and a simple method for its measurement. Appl. Microbiol. **24:**628–633.

Chapter 55

Immune Response to *Vibrio cholerae*

CHARLES R. YOUNG, I. KAYE WACHSMUTH, ØRJAN OLSVIK, AND JOHN C. FEELEY

Several methods have been used to measure the immune response of humans to infection with *Vibrio cholerae*. Early literature on the subject has been reviewed extensively by Pollitzer (cited in reference 14); more recent work has been aptly summarized by Barua (cited in reference 14), Levine et al. (7), and Holmgren and Svennerholm (cited in reference 14). In the previous (2nd) edition of this manual, the reader will find more extensive reference citations and more detailed information for some of the traditional methods (14).

The most practical and easily performed methods involve the measurement of antibodies against somatic O antigens of *V. cholerae* by agglutination or vibriocidal antibody assays and the measurement of antibody ("antitoxin") against the heat-labile enterotoxin produced by *V. cholerae* (CT) (8, 14). Studies relevant to these procedures are discussed below.

Agglutination test

With the agglutination test, a variety of procedures and antigens have produced conflicting results. There is now almost universal agreement that O antibodies are best measured in an agglutination test with a suspension of living vibrios as the agglutinogen (14). Unlike the results with *Salmonella* spp., O agglutination with *V. cholerae* occurs rapidly, whereas H agglutination is a slowly developing reaction that is often difficult to detect and does not take place under the test conditions specified below (14). Furthermore, H antigens of *V. cholerae* are weak antigens and lack the specificity of O antigens, since *V. cholerae* serotypes O1 and non-O1 may share common H antigens (14). Boiled suspensions can be used to measure O agglutinations (14), but their agglutinability is greatly reduced. This reduction may reflect the loss of vibrio surface proteins, normally immunogenic for the patient.

When live antigens are used, a fourfold or greater rise in agglutination titer occurs approximately 90 to 95% of the time between acute- and convalescent-phase serum specimens obtained from persons with bacteriologically confirmed cases of cholera (1, 2, 5, 14). A variety of techniques have been used; the method used in these laboratories (see below) is a tube agglutination test, described previously (14). A microtiter agglutination test method amenable to assaying small-volume serum samples (e.g., finger-prick blood) has been described elsewhere (2). Our laboratories favor the vibriocidal procedure (see below) for the microtiter system because it is easier to read endpoints.

Vibriocidal test

Vibriocidal tests depend on the bactericidal effect of O antibody on *V. cholerae* in the presence of comple-

ment, and a number of techniques have been used. Dilutions of serum are allowed to react with a standardized inoculum of *V. cholerae* in the presence of excess guinea pig complement; after an incubation period to allow killing of the bacteria, the various dilutions of serum and appropriate controls are subcultured on agar (6, 14) or in broth (1, 5, 14) to assess the bactericidal effect. The procedure requires careful standardization and can be made extremely sensitive by using a small inoculum. The procedures in use in this laboratory are (i) a tube test that is a modification of the broth assay system of Muschel and Treffers (cited in reference 14) and (ii) a microtiter test nearly identical to that described by Benenson et al. (1) which is based on the tube test procedure (14) with volumes reduced to microtiter amounts.

Similar to the agglutination test, the vibriocidal test can be expected to demonstrate a rise in antibody in sera from 90 to 95% of patients with bacteriologically confirmed cases of cholera (1, 5, 14). Authors who have made such a comparison have found a very high, in fact nearly perfect, correlation between the results of living-vibrio agglutination tests and those of vibriocidal tests in detecting diagnostic rises in antibody levels with paired acute-convalescent sera (5, 14). The vibriocidal test is significantly more sensitive than the agglutination test; therefore, it detects a greater background of antibody levels in normal or acute-phase sera and gives higher titers with convalescent-phase sera (5, 14).

The vibriocidal antibody test has been extensively used for serological surveys, and the acquisition of significant levels of antibody, either through natural exposure or as a result of vaccine, has been correlated with apparent immunity to cholera on a population basis and in volunteer challenge studies (7, 14).

Other tests for antibodies against somatic antigens of *V. cholerae*

Indirect hemagglutination tests with *V. cholerae* have been examined by several workers in the past. In general these tests have not been found to have advantages over vibriocidal or agglutination tests. We have confirmed the observations of others who found that the indirect hemagglutination test is less sensitive than the vibrio agglutination test which uses live antigens (14).

Holmgren and Svennerholm have described an enzyme-linked immunosorbent assay (ELISA) measuring antibody in human sera, jejunal fluids, and colostrum to lipopolysaccharide extracted by hot phenol and water from *V. cholerae* serotype Inaba (12). Our laboratory has been able to measure antibodies to both Ogawa and Inaba serotype lipopolysaccharide, but, in our hands, the anti-lipopolysaccharide ELISA is much less sensitive than the vibriocidal test (unpublished data). This fact suggests that other antigens, such as outer membrane protein and cell-bound hemagglutinins, are also important immunogenic agents. Therefore, we still prefer to assay antibacterial antibodies by the vibriocidal test.

Antitoxin antibody

V. cholerae elaborates a well-characterized heat-labile enterotoxin (CT) which is antigenic and elicits an antibody or "antitoxin" response in most patients who are convalescing from the disease. This enterotoxin is structurally, biologically, and antigenically similar to the heat-labile enterotoxin of *Escherichia coli* (LT; 14). Cross-reactions between CT and LT must be considered in any antitoxin assay measuring either immunological reaction or neutralization of toxic activity (14).

Antitoxin levels may be assayed by in vivo toxin neutralization assays such as the ligated rabbit ileal loop, the infant rabbit model (14), or the rabbit skin permeability factor (PF) test. In vitro neutralization tests using the Y-1 strain of mouse adrenal cell cultures (Y-1) or Chinese hamster ovary cell cultures (CHO) are also feasible. The best standardized in vivo procedures are the skin PF assay and the much more laborious ileal loop assay. References for these methods are cited in the previous edition of this manual (14). A standard antitoxin unit has been proposed by Craig (cited in reference 14), and standard antitoxins calibrated according to Craig unitage are available from the Microbiology and Infectious Diseases Programs, National Institute of Allergy and Infectious Diseases, and the Bureau of Biologics, Food and Drug Administration. The in vitro cell culture systems are sensitive and reproducible assays for CT and have been standardized with cholera antitoxin (14).

Antitoxin levels may also be measured in vitro by passive hemagglutination tests. Good correlations with toxin neutralization assays have been obtained; stable, preserved, sensitized erythrocytes can be used in the test, and it can be performed in microtiter configuration (14). Table 1 compares the neutralization and hemagglutination tests for antitoxin and demonstrates the close correlation of results from several different laboratories.

TABLE 1. Summary of antitoxin titer of goat anticholera toxin (NIH lot 1)[a]

Method	Investigator	Antitoxin (U/ml)
PF	J. P. Craig	4,700
Rabbit ileal loop	N. F. Pierce	5,594
Cell culture		
Y-1	A. S. Benenson	5,750
	R. B. Sack	5,016
	I. K. Wachsmuth	4,470
CHO	R. L. Guerrant	4,470
	I. K. Wachsmuth	4,470
Mouse-IV	J. P. Craig	4,470
Hemagglutination	J. W. Peterson	4,470

[a] Available from Office of Biologics Research and Review, Food and Drug Administration, Bethesda, Md. Suitable for calibration of human working standard for ELISA by toxin neutralization tests.

The most recent, and perhaps most promising, methods for detection of enterotoxin and antitoxin are based on the ELISA with specific and readily available reagents. These methods are based on antigen-antibody complexes as well as the natural-receptor binding of CT and LT with G_{M1} ganglioside (14). This methodology can measure blocking or binding in the indirect toxin assay, or it can directly measure the serum antibody by using conjugated anti-human immunglobulin G (IgG) (15). By screening sera against LT purified from a human strain of *E. coli* (LTh) as well as against CT, the ELISA provides the easiest and most direct means of differentiating the two types of antitoxin responses (8).

A significant antitoxin response was detected in the ileal loop model and the PF test with sera from convalescent patients with bacteriologically confirmed cases of cholera (14). In a study of 16 patients by the ileal loop method, Pierce et al. (cited in reference 14) found the antitoxin response to be variable and frequently of small magnitude, but persisting at elevated levels for 12 to 18 months. Unlike the vibriocidal antibody response, the antitoxin response was diminished by prompt antimicrobial therapy. Benenson et al. (cited in reference 14) reported a diagnostic rise in antitoxin in 73% of bacteriologically proven cases by the PF test. Hochstein et al. (6), using a hemagglutination test, found a response in 9 of 15 cholera patients for whom paired sera were available.

The ELISA for antitoxin has detected a seroconversion in 58 (88%) of 66 volunteers excreting *V. cholerae*, including 50 (93%) of 54 patients with clinical cholera (M. M. Levine, personal communication). With both the Y-1 and the CHO cell culture assays for antitoxin, specimens from three of eight culture-negative diarrheal patients demonstrated a significant anti-LT rise during an outbreak due to an enterotoxigenic *E. coli* strain, whereas specimens from four of six culture-positive patients failed to show a rise in titer (14). In volunteer studies with enterotoxigenic *E. coli*, however, sera from 89% of culture-positive patients did show a rise in antitoxin as well as in antisomatic antibody (14). Measurement of antitoxin response would appear, therefore, somewhat less sensitive than the agglutination or vibriocidal tests for *V. cholerae*. In addition, since it has been observed that nontoxigenic strains of *V. cholerae* possessing the O1 antigen can induce diarrhea in humans, a lack of antibody to toxin does not necessarily rule out a cholera infection (10). However, in some cases, measurement of antitoxin may offer certain diagnostic advantages since, unlike vibriocidal or agglutinating antibody, antitoxin is not stimulated by most currently available cholera vaccines (14). It may also offer an additional diagnostic tool for enterotoxigenic *E. coli*, which poses a very difficult isolation problem even for well-equipped laboratories using toxin detection assays (14).

On the basis of our experience, we recommend the rabbit skin PF test (14), the indirect hemagglutination test (6), and the ELISA described below (8) as the most suitable and most easily standardized in vivo and in vitro antitoxin procedures available at this time. Because the first two tests require special technical experience or reagents not generally available or both, detailed test procedures are given only for the simpler micro-ELISA method.

ANTISOMATIC REAGENTS

Only the macroscopic tube agglutination and microtiter vibriocidal assay are described below. Either procedure is an acceptable method when acute- and convalescent-phase sera are used for a retrospective serodiagnosis of cholera.

V. cholerae (either classical or El Tor biotype) occurs mainly as two serotypes: Ogawa (O antigen formula, AB) and Inaba (O antigen formula, AC). A third and very rare serotype, Hikojima (ABC), also occurs.

Because of differences in type-specific antigens B and C, it has been the practice of most laboratories, including ours, to use both serotypes as test antigens. Antibodies with anti-A, anti-B, and anti-C specificities operate in both tests. Since the dominant antibody response generally is group specific (anti-A), experience indicates that it is not necessary to use both serotypes except in very rare cases. When a single antigen is used, the Ogawa serotype is preferred for two reasons: (i) it often gives greater cross-reactivity with anti-Inaba sera than Inaba antigen gives with anti-Ogawa sera (J. C. Feeley, unpublished data), and (ii) the Ogawa serotype shows a lower level of cross-reactivity with *Brucella* and *Citrobacter* species and *Yersinia enterocolitica*.

Antigens

Stock cultures of *V. cholerae* serotypes Ogawa (strain VC12) and Inaba (strain VC13) are maintained in the freeze-dried state. After reconstitution and purity checks, the cultures are maintained on Trypticase agar (Trypticase [BBL Microbiology Systems, Cockeysville, Md.], 1%; NaCl, 1%; agar, 1.5%) slants at 4°C with monthly transfers. It is our practice to make no more than three transfers before opening a new freeze-dried culture. These cultures are used for both vibriocidal and agglutination tests.

VBS

Veronal-buffered saline (VBS) is prepared by dissolving 83.0 g of NaCl and 10.19 g of sodium 5,5-diethylbarbiturate in 1,500 ml of distilled water in a 2,000-ml volumetric flask. Then 34.58 ml of 1 N HCl is added, and the volume is brought up to 2,000 ml. The solution is stored in a refrigerator and discarded after 2 weeks. For use in the test, a fivefold dilution is made in sterile distilled water (pH should be 7.3), and the unused portion is discarded daily. The addition of Mg^{2+} (14) is not necessary because of the high concentration of guinea pig serum in the test.

Complement

Pooled nonvibriocidal guinea pig serum is used as complement. Individual guinea pig sera are pretested for naturally occurring vibriocidal activity against *V. cholerae* at the same concentration used in the tests; then 25 to 30 nonvibriocidal sera are pooled, distributed in 5- to 10-ml amounts, and stored at −70°C. Activity is retained for at least 6 months. In our experience, approximately 5% of normal guinea pig sera have natural vibriocidal activity, although this percentage may vary with different animal colonies. Commercial freeze-dried guinea pig complement may

be used. In this case, the diluent supplied by the manufacturer should not be used since it contains a preservative; VBS (pH 7.3) should be used instead. Each new lot of complement should be pretested as described above. Other animal sources of complement have been unsatisfactory.

A reference preparation of cholera convalescent-phase human serum (catalog no. G-005-501-572) can be obtained from the Research Resources Branch, National Institute of Allergy and Infectious Diseases, Bethesda, MD 20014. This serum has been subjected to collaborative vibriocidal assays by several laboratories, including the Centers for Disease Control, which have used this test, and the serum has been found useful for standardization of the procedure.

Normal rabbit or human serum can be used as a negative control. However, many healthy human subjects but only a few normal rabbits can be expected to have detectable levels of naturally occurring antibody by the vibriocidal test.

All other reagents, media, and materials are available from commercial sources.

ELISA ANTITOXIN REAGENTS

The ELISA method outlined below is that described by Levine et al. (8). Sera are tested at a single dilution against both purified CT and LTh. The resulting net optical densities (net ODs) are compared by ratio. In this way the two immune responses can be differentiated.

The procedure is applicable in most laboratories since both protein toxins have been characterized and purified. Cholera enterotoxin is available commercially, while reliable methods for purification of LTh have been published (3, 14). In addition, microtiter equipment, including plates, lids, dispensers, spectrophotometers, and other materials, are available from several commercial sources; when relevant, the manufacturer will be given in the test protocols.

Antigens

Purified CT can be purchased from Schwarz/Mann, Cambridge, MA 02142-007, or List Biological Laboratories, Inc., Campbell, CA 95008. Both sources supply the toxin in 1- and 5-mg lyophilized samples. LTh can be purified by the methods previously referred to. The purified toxins are dissolved and stored in phosphate-buffered saline (PBS; pH 7.2) at −70°C in samples containing 200 μg of protein per ml. Normally samples are thawed rapidly for single use, although several freeze-thaw procedures can be tolerated without adverse effects.

Enzyme-conjugated antibody

Goat antisera to human class-specific immunoglobulins coupled with alkaline phosphatase are available from a wide variety of commercial sources (e.g., Kirkegaard & Perry Laboratories, Gaithersburg, Md.). These commercial reagents are usually prepared as described by Voller et al. (13), chromatographically purified, and tested for specificity and sensitivity. They can be used in very dilute working solutions and are relatively inexpensive. Conjugates are sold in liquid or lyophilized form and are stored either at 4 to 8°C or frozen, as recommended by the manufacturer.

Substrate

The alkaline phosphatase substrate is disodium *p*-nitrophenyl phosphate. It is available commercially as "Sigma 104" in 5-mg tablets (Sigma Chemical Co., St. Louis, Mo.). One tablet is dissolved immediately before use in 5 ml of fresh (up to 2-week-old) 10% diethanolamine buffer to give a final concentration of 1 mg/ml. Recently a phosphatase substrate kit, containing buffer concentrate and 5-mg tablets, has been made available by Kirkegaard & Perry. The kit eliminates the need for making 10% diethanolamine buffer and can be stored for at least 6 months.

Buffers

Coating buffer PBS, PBS with 0.05% Tween 20, diethanolamine buffer, and 3 M sodium hydroxide are described by Voller et al. (13).

Control sera

Prechallenge adult volunteer or unexposed healthy adult sera are pooled for a negative reference control. Sera from postchallenge adult volunteers or from adults with known infection are pooled for a positive reference control. All controls should be confirmed by testing in one of the neutralization assays.

A positive human reference serum of known cholera antitoxin unitage by the PF assay has been supplied by M. M. Levine, University of Maryland, and is available through the Division of Bacterial Diseases, Centers for Disease Control, Atlanta, Ga.

TEST PROCEDURES

Tube agglutination test

Serum preparation. Serum with or without inactivation at 56°C for 30 min may be tested with no detectable difference, although some slight lysis of the live antigen suspension may be noted in low dilutions with inactivated sera having high titers of complement. Serum should not contain a preservative, since it might cause lysis of the rather light antigen preparation.

Antigen preparation. One loopful of growth from a 16- to 18-h (overnight) culture of the test strains (Ogawa only or Ogawa and Inaba) on Trypticase agar is inoculated into 100 ml of Trypticase broth (Trypticase, 1%; NaCl, 1%) in a 250-ml Erlenmeyer flask. Then the test strains are incubated at 35°C without shaking for 4 to 6 h or until a turbidity of 1 opacity unit of the U.S. Opacity Standard (obtained from Bureau of Biologics, Food and Drug Administration, Bethesda, MD 20014) is achieved or exceeded. If the culture is too turbid, it should be diluted in sterile Trypticase broth until the turbidity level is the same as that of the opacity standard by visual comparison. At this point, the antigen suspension may be used immediately or placed in an ice-water bath for up to 4 h.

Test protocol

1. For each serum (unknown or control) to be tested, set up a row of six to eight 13- by 100-mm tubes for each serotype antigen to be used.

2. Add 0.9 ml of 0.85% NaCl to the first tube and 0.5 ml of 0.85% NaCl to the remaining tubes.

3. Add 0.1 ml of serum to the first tube, mix, and serially transfer 0.5-ml volumes to successive tubes in the row, discarding 0.5 ml from the last tube.

4. Add 0.5 ml of each antigen to each tube containing serum dilutions and to an antigen control tube containing 0.5 ml of saline.

5. Shake the rack and incubate the tubes in a 37°C water bath for 1 h. Tests may be read at this time or, preferably, after overnight refrigeration at 4°C. Agglutination is easier to read after overnight refrigeration, and endpoints will often be 1 dilution higher.

6. After the tubes warm to room temperature (to allow condensation film to evaporate), tap each tube gently and observe for agglutination. A black background attached behind the hood of a fluorescent lamp is useful.

7. Record the titer as the dilution factor of the highest final dilution (after antigen is added, the first tube dilution is 1:20) showing definite agglutination. Antigen control and negative serum control should show no agglutination, and the positive control serum should react within ±1 dilution of its expected titer.

Microtiter vibriocidal antibody test

Serum preparation. Sterile serum is preferred, but not absolutely essential. Visibly contaminated sera are unsatisfactory. Sera are not inactivated, but inactivation at 56°C for 30 min rarely affects the titer except for that of low levels of naturally occurring antibody in certain normal sera. Since an excess of complement is used in the system, inactivation of complement in the test serum is not an important consideration.

Antigen preparation. The afternoon before the test, the test strain(s) should be inoculated onto heart infusion agar slants and incubated at 35°C. Uninoculated heart infusion agar slants should be placed in the incubator to prewarm. After 16 to 18 h of incubation, the prewarmed slants should be inoculated with 1 loopful from the overnight culture and then incubated for 4 h at 35°C. Chilled VBS (pH 7.3) is used to wash growth from slants, and the turbidity is photometrically adjusted to the equivalent of 10 opacity units/ml (U.S. Opacity Standard). To prepare a suspension of 1 opacity unit/ml, the standardized suspension is diluted 1:10 in chilled VBS. The suspension should be promptly mixed with complement, as described below.

Complement. Guinea pig complement should be diluted 1:5 in chilled VBS. Equal volumes of complement and of bacterial suspension (1 opacity unit/ml) are mixed. The mixture should be maintained in an ice-water bath and used within 30 min.

Test protocol

1. Use round-bottom microtiter plates. Prepare an initial 1:5 dilution of each serum in microtiter wells by placing 1 loopful (0.025 ml) of each serum in 0.1 ml (4 0.025-ml drops) of VBS.

2. For each serum to be tested (unknown and control), allow a row of 8 to 10 wells for each antigen used. Add 0.025 ml (1 drop) of VBS to each of these wells.

3. Add 1 loopful (0.025 ml) of serum diluted 1:5 (step 1) to the first well, rotate the loops, and serially transfer serum to successive wells in the row, discarding 1 loopful from the last well.

4. Set up two complement controls for each test culture in 13- by 100-mm tubes to be used to monitor growth photometrically. Add 0.5 ml of VBS to each tube. For each culture, also include a complement control well containing 0.025 ml of VBS (to be used for visual grading of growth).

5. Add 1 drop (0.025 ml) of complement-bacteria mixture to each well as appropriate, and add 0.5 ml of the mixture to the complement-photometer control tubes.

6. Seal the plates with sealing tape, and incubate the plates and complement control tubes in a 37°C water bath for 1 h.

7. After incubation, add 0.15 ml of brain heart infusion broth to plate wells, and add 3.0 ml of the broth to complement-photometer tubes. Reseal the plates, and return them to the water bath along with one complement control tube for each culture. Place the other complement control tubes in an ice bath (this will be used as a photometer blank).

8. Allow growth to proceed until the OD of the complement control tube reaches 0.15 at 580 nm in a Coleman Junior spectrophotometer in which the refrigerated tube is used as a blank. This reading is near the end of, but still within, the logarithmic phase of growth and usually requires 2 to 2.5 h to attain. (It is advisable to determine a growth curve for the particular conditions [media, complement, etc.] prevailing in the laboratory.) Growth should not be continued beyond this point.

9. Read the plates by placing them on a test-reading mirror with transmitted light against a black background. Crystal-clear yellowish wells (growth inhibited) are readily distinguished from turbid wells in which growth has occurred. The titer is recorded as the dilution factor of the highest dilution (after bacteria-complement mixture is added; the first well is diluted 1:20) in which growth was visibly inhibited compared with the complement control well. This comparison can best be made after overnight refrigeration, because then both turbidity and buttons of sedimented bacteria are readily visible. The positive control serum should react within ±1 dilution of its expected titer. The negative control should show no bactericidal effect.

Note. If desired, an anticomplementary control in which hemolysin-sensitized sheep erythrocytes are used to detect anticomplementary sera can be included. In hundreds of sera tested, an anticomplementary reaction was never encountered, and the procedure was eliminated, as described by Benenson et al. (1). Because of the excess complement in the system and the high dilutions of sera of which endpoints are detected, an anticomplementary reaction is not likely to be a problem.

ELISA for antitoxin

Serum preparation. Sera do not require sterilization or inactivation at 56°C for 30 min. Although preservatives which most often affect tissue culture do not interfere with the ELISA, most sera can be collect-ed and stored at −70°C without loss of titer and without growth of possible contaminants.

In the following test protocols, the outside wells of vertical and horizontal rows in each microtiter plate are disregarded so that 60 of the 96 wells are used for assay. Microtiter plates are usually incubated with plastic lids, and the outside wells are filled with 0.1 ml per well of the washing buffer to ensure a constant temperature for all wells during the incubation steps.

Standardization procedures. (i) Specificity and sensitivity of conjugate. It is necessary to test the specificity and sensitivity of each new lot of conjugate by assaying activity to its heterologous classes as well as to its homologous immunoglobulin class.

1. The wells of a polystyrene microtiter plate (Dynatech Laboratories, Inc., Alexandria, Va.) are coated with 0.1 ml of 10-fold dilutions (1 to 1,000 ng/ml) of purified class-specific immunoglobulins in coating buffer for 1 h at 37°C. A background control row of coating buffer only is included (plates may also be coated overnight at 4°C in a humidity chamber.)

2. The wells are emptied and washed three times (3 min each) with PBS, pH 7.2. Remaining unbound plastic sites of each well are blocked for 1 h at 37°C with 0.1 ml of 5% heat-inactivated fetal bovine serum (or bovine serum albumin) diluted in PBS.

3. The wells are emptied and washed as described in step 2 with PBS containing 0.05% Tween 20 (polyoxyethylene sorbitan monolaurate; J. T. Baker Chemical Co., Phillipsburg, N.J.) and 1% heat-inactivated fetal bovine serum (washing buffer).

4. The conjugate stock preparation is diluted in washing buffer or PBS, according to the instructions of the manufacturer, and 0.1 ml of each dilution is incubated for 1 h at 37°C in wells coated with each concentration of the immunoglobulin. Each dilution is also incubated in a background control well.

5. The wells are emptied and washed as described in step 3, after which 0.1 ml of *p*-nitrophenyl phosphate solution (1 mg/ml) is reacted in all wells for 30 min at 37°C.

6. The reaction is stopped by adding 25 µl of 3 M NaOH to each well.

7. The OD of each well is read at the 405-nm wavelength of light. Microplate spectrophotometers are available from Flow Laboratories, Inc., McLean, Va.; Dynatech; Gilford Instruments, Inc., Oberlin, Ohio; and Litton Bionetic Laboratory Products, Charleston, SC 29405.

8. The net OD of each dilution is calculated by subtracting the OD of the background control well from the OD of its corresponding test well.

9. The greatest dilution of conjugate reacting visibly (OD of 0.10) with the lowest concentration of purified immunoglobulin is selected as the working dilution. It is important that this reaction is specific for the immunoglobulin class to be measured.

(ii) Antigen concentration. Repeat the following procedure for each new lot of antigen.

1. The wells of a polystyrene plate are coated with 0.1 ml of various concentrations of CT or LTh in PBS (0.25, 0.5, 1, 5, and 10 µg/ml) for 1 h at 37°C. A row of background control wells is also included.

2. The wells are emptied and washed with PBS, and the unbound plastic sites are blocked as described in

TABLE 2. Distribution of anti-Ogawa titers in sera of healthy individuals in the United States

Test	Yr of collection	No. of sera with titers of:							
		<20	20	40	80	160	320	640	>640
Agglutination[a]	1962	113	9	6	1	3	0	1	0
Vibriocidal[b]	1967–1968	309		95[c]		16	10	7	4

[a] J. C. Feeley, unpublished data.

[b] Based on Gangarosa et al. (cited in reference 14).

[c] Includes 20 to 80 range.

step 2 (above) of the standardization procedure for specificity and sensitivity.

3. After being washed as described in step 3 above, the known positive control serum is diluted 10-fold (1:10 to 1:1,000) in washing buffer, and 0.1 ml of each dilution is incubated for 1 h at 37°C with each concentration of antigen. Each dilution is also incubated in the appropriate background control well.

4. The ELISA is completed sequentially by the addition of appropriately diluted conjugate for 1 h at 37°C followed by substrate for 30 min at 37°C. The reaction is stopped with 3 M NaOH. Net ODs for each test well are calculated.

5. The net ODs for each dilution are plotted against the antigen concentrations. The lowest concentration of antigen at which all sera dilutions reach a plateau is considered optimal. We have determined this concentration to be 1 µg/ml for both LTh and CT.

Test protocol

1. The wells of a polystyrene microtiter plate are coated with 0.1 ml of CT or LTh (1 µg/ml) in PBS, pH 7.2, for 1 h at 37°C. A background control well of PBS only is included for each antigen well. Plates should be coated so that each specimen is assayed for anti-CT and anti-LTh on the same plate.

2. After incubation the wells are emptied and washed three times (3 min each) with PBS, and the unbound plastic sites are blocked as described in step 2 of the procedure for standardizing specificity and sensitivity.

3. Specimens diluted 1:50 in washing buffer are incubated in the appropriate wells for 1 h at 37°C.

4. The wells are emptied and washed, and the ELISA is completed sequentially with appropriately diluted conjugate for 1 h at 37°C followed by substrate for 30 min at 37°C. The reaction is stopped with 3 M NaOH. Net ODs are calculated.

5. For paired sera, a difference between the net ODs of acute- and convalescent-phase sera of 0.2 or greater is considered significant.

6. For any serum with a net OD of ≥0.30 for each toxin, the net OD of anti-CT is divided by the net OD of anti-LTh. This ratio can be used to differentiate which of the two infections is represented by the response. A ratio of >0.7 indicates a cholera infection, whereas a ratio of ≤0.7 indicates a recent LTh infection (see below, under Interpretation and Clinical Indications).

INTERPRETATION

Some concept of the normal range of agglutination and vibriocidal titers experienced in the normal population of healthy individuals in the United States is given in Table 2. A more extensive treatment of the problem of naturally acquired antibody has been presented by Gangarosa et al. (cited in reference 14). Data illustrative of the agglutinating and vibriocidal antibody responses of cholera patients are shown in Table 3. In the micro-ELISA assay, an increase in the net OD from the acute- to the convalescent-phase serum of 0.2 or greater indicates a significant antitoxin response.

Studies measuring antitoxin neutralization for both LT and CT have demonstrated that in the United States there is little background-level antitoxin activity. The higher base-line levels in the populations of areas in which cholera is endemic indicate a previous exposure to toxin and a probable anamnestic response when compared with the lower rises in convalescent-phase titer in the population of the United States (14).

Paired or serial sera are preferable for the establishment of a retrospective diagnosis of cholera, particularly in areas in which cholera is endemic. A single specimen tested by both the vibriocidal and ELISA methods, however, can provide reasonably secure evidence for diagnosis. The absence of vibriocidal antibody and ELISA antitoxin 10 to 28 days after illness virtually excludes a diagnosis of cholera. The presence of antibody in either assay system supposes cholera infection. However, these data must be qualified. Since in some instances vibriocidal antibody can remain elevated for 6 months to 1 year (4) and antitoxin levels can remain elevated for up to 2 years (9), the possibility of false-positive results must be minimized. Several investigators have successfully resolved this problem by using elevated cut-off antibody levels in the interpretation of their data. Vibriocidal titers of ≥1:320 and ≥1:1,280 have been suggested (4, 11), while an ELISA antitoxin net OD of ≥0.30 has been used (11). In areas in which enterotoxigenic E. coli is endemic, the possibility of a false-positive result is further minimized by screening the sera for both anti-CT and anti-LTh. A specimen having a net OD of ≥0.30 for each toxin and an anti-CT/anti-LTh ratio greater than 0.7 indicates cholera infection.

TABLE 3. Antibody response of cholera patients as measured by agglutination and vibriocidal tests[a]

Day of disease	No. of sera tested	Agglutination		Vibriocidal	
		GMAT[b]	Range	GMAT	Range
1–4	39	23	<32–512	362	<32–16,380
5–10	24	223	<32–4,096	11,590	512–262,144
11–22	27	178	32–2,048	23,170	512–131,072

[a] Adapted from Feeley (cited in reference 14).

[b] GMAT, Geometric mean antibody titer. For purposes of calculations, titers of <32 were arbitrarily assumed to be 16.

CLINICAL INDICATIONS

The cholera serological methods described here can be useful seroepidemiological tools in investigations of cholera outbreaks. When these methods are used in conjunction with one another, retrospective diagnoses of illness due to *V. cholerae* can be made with confidence over time. By using a combination of vibriocidal antibody and ELISA antitoxin assays, it is possible to base a diagnosis on either paired acute- and convalescent-phase sera or a single specimen.

On the basis of volunteer studies and natural infections with *V. cholerae*, diarrheal illness correlates better with a rise in antisomatic antibody than with an antitoxin response (1, 7, 14). Thus a retrospective diagnosis can be established with a high degree of certainty by titration of paired acute- and convalescent-phase sera in the vibrio agglutination or vibriocidal tests. Acute-phase sera should be collected 0 to 3 days after onset of illness, and convalescent-phase sera should be collected 10 to 21 days after onset. Demonstration of a fourfold or greater rise in titer is diagnostic, provided recent cholera immunization can be ruled out.

Vibriocidal titration of a single convalescent serum is usually not worthwhile. Vibriocidal antibody is relatively short lived; titers peak within 1 to 6 months. In addition, elevated levels of vibriocidal antibodies are found in many adults in the United States (14), and in Bangladesh increasing levels of vibriocidal antibodies develop with advancing age, even in the absence of known or suspected cholera infection (14). However, the prevalence and levels found in adults in the United States are much lower than those found in individuals living in areas in which cholera is endemic (9, 14). To minimize the possibility of a false diagnosis of cholera infection, researchers surveying populations in North America have found it necessary to use vibriocidal titers of $\geq$1:320 (11) and $\geq$1:1,280 (14) as reference levels of antibody. A titer of 1:640 would seem reasonable (Table 2).

Antigenic cross-reactions detectable by agglutination or vibriocidal tests are reported to occur with *Brucella* sp., *Y. enterocolitica* serotype 9, *Citrobacter* sp., and possibly other enteric organisms. Except in known areas in which cholera is endemic, one must assume that these elevated levels of antibodies are due to antigens other than *V. cholerae*.

Thus in a single serum sample the absence of vibriocidal or agglutinating antibody 10 to 28 days after illness would raise serious doubts about the likelihood of a cholera infection, but a single sample with a titer between 1:20 and 1:1,280 would reveal little about the source of infection.

The ELISA IgG antitoxin assay permits both a retrospective diagnosis based on paired acute- and convalescent-phase sera and the identification of "old" infections based on a single serum specimen. A rise in net OD of 0.2 or greater between the acute- and convalescent-phase sera indicates cholera infection. Since IgG antitoxin peaks between days 21 and 28, the acute-phase serum should be collected 0 to 3 days after onset of illness, and the convalescent-phase serum should be collected 21 to 28 days after onset. Identification of previous exposure to *V. cholerae* based on a single sample is more problematic.

In contrast to vibriocidal antibodies, antitoxin antibodies are long lived. Snyder et al. have reported elevated antitoxin levels 9 months after illness (11), while Levine et al., using healthy North American volunteers in challenge studies, have demonstrated elevated levels for up to 2 years postchallenge (9). However, the interpretation of elevated antitoxin levels can be difficult since many strains of *E. coli* produce an LT immunologically similar to the enterotoxin of *V. cholerae* (14). In many instances, known cholera antisera when tested against LTh give greater net ODs than when tested against CT, although the net ODs for both toxins are always close in range (8). Therefore, in areas in which LTh infections are endemic, it is imperative to distinguish between CT and LTh antitoxin responses.

Levine et al. (8) have shown that although cholera antisera often give higher net ODs to LTh than to CT, LTh antisera always give lower net ODs to CT than to LTh. Using this information, they have developed a minimum ratio (net OD response to CT divided by net OD response to LTh) of 0.7 as a way of distinguishing CT antitoxin response from LTh antitoxin response. When they applied this criterion to data from healthy North Americans challenged with *V. cholerae* and to data from children and teenagers from the United States, Chile, and Bangladesh, this value was confirmed. Only in sera from postchallenge North Americans secreting *V. cholerae* and in sera from Bangladesh, an area in which cholera is endemic, was the ratio above 0.7. This result indicates that a ratio above 0.7 is specific for past cholera infection. To minimize the chances of false diagnosis based on a single sample in areas in which cholera is endemic, both Synder et al. (11) and Levine et al. (8) use a net OD of $\geq$0.30 as indicative of significant antitoxin activity.

If a specimen cannot be screened for both CT and LTh antitoxin activity, a confident identification of infection can still be made on a single sample if the sample is assayed for vibriocidal antibodies and ELISA IgG antitoxin to CT. A serum with a vibriocidal titer of $\geq$1:640 and an ELISA net OD of $\geq$0.30 would be evidence of a past cholera infection.

The serological methods reported above can be used individually or in combination with one another to make retrospective diagnoses based on data from paired acute- and convalescent-phase sera or to identify past infection with the data from a single serum sample. The versatility and dependability of these assays should prove useful in epidemiological investigations of cholera infections in environments in which cholera is endemic as well as in those in which it is not endemic.

LITERATURE CITED

1. **Benenson, A. S., A. Saad, and W. H. Mosley.** 1968. Serological studies in cholera. 2. The vibriocidal antibody response of cholera patients determined by a microtechnique. Bull. W.H.O. **38:**277–285.
2. **Benenson, A. S., A. Saad, and M. Paul.** 1968. Serological studies in cholera. 1. Vibrio agglutinin response of cholera patients determined by a microtechnique. Bull. W.H.O. **38:**267–276.
3. **Clements, J. D., and R. A. Finkelstein.** 1979. Isolation and characterization of homogeneous heat-labile enterotoxins with high specific activity from *Escherichia coli*

cultures. Infect. Immun. **24**:760–769.

4. **Clements, M. L., M. M. Levine, C. R. Young, R. E. Black, Y. L. Lim, R. M. Robins-Browne, and J. P. Craig.** 1982. Magnitude, kinetics and duration of vibriocidal antibody responses in North Americans after infection of *Vibrio cholerae.* J. Infect. Dis. **145**:465–473.

5. **Feeley, J. C.** 1965. Comparison of vibriocidal and agglutinating antibody responses in cholera patients, p. 220–222. *In* Proceedings. Cholera Research Symposium. U.S. Public Health Service Publication no. 1328. U.S. Public Health Service, Washington, D.C.

6. **Hochstein, H. D., J. C. Feeley, and W. E. DeWitt.** 1970. Titration of cholera antitoxin in human sera in microhemagglutination with formalinized erythrocytes. Appl. Microbiol. **19**:742–745.

7. **Levine, M. M., D. R. Nalin, J. P. Craig, D. Hoover, E. J. Berquist, D. Waterman, H. Preston, R. B. Hornick, N. P. Pierce, and J. P. Libonati.** 1979. Immunity to cholera in man: relative role of antibacterial versus antitoxic immunity. Trans. R. Soc. Trop. Med. Hyg. **73**:3–9.

8. **Levine, M. M., C. R., Young, R. E. Black, Y. Takeda, and R. A. Finkelstein.** 1985. Enzyme-linked immunosorbent assay to measure antibodies to purified heat-labile enterotoxins from human and porcine strains of *Escherichia coli* and to cholera toxin: application in serodiagnosis and seroepidemiology. J. Clin. Microbiol. **21**:174–179.

9. **Levine, M. M., C. R. Young, T. P. Hughes, S. O'Donnell, R. E. Black, M. L. Clements, R. Robins-Browne, and Y. L. Lim.** 1981. Duration of serum antitoxin response following *Vibrio cholerae* infection in North Americans: relevance for seroepidemiology. Am. J. Epidemiol. **114**:348–354.

10. **Morris, J. G., Jr., J. L. Picardi, S. Lieb, J. V. Lee, A. Roberts, M. Hood, R. A. Gunn, and P. A. Blake.** 1984. Isolation of nontoxigenic *Vibrio cholerae* O group 1 from a patient with severe gastrointestinal disease. J. Clin. Microbiol. **19**:296–297.

11. **Snyder, J. D., D. T. Allegra, M. M. Levine, J. P. Craig, J. C. Feeley, W. E. DeWitt, and P. A. Blake.** 1981. Serologic studies of naturally acquired infection with *Vibrio cholerae* serogroup O1 in the United States. J. Infect. Dis. **143**:182–187.

12. **Svennerholm, A. M., M. Jertborn, L. Gothefors, A. M. M. M. Karim, D. A. Sack, and J. Holmgren.** 1984. Mucosal antitoxic and antibacterial immunity after cholera disease and after immunization with a combined B subunit-whole cell vaccine. J. Infect. Dis. **149**:884–893.

13. **Voller, A., D. Bidwell, and A. Bartlett.** 1976. Microplate enzyme immunoassays for the immunodiagnosis of virus infections, p. 506–512. *In* N. R. Rose and H. Friedman (ed.), Manual of clinical immunology. American Society for Microbiology, Washington, D.C.

14. **Wachsmuth, I. K., J. C. Feeley, W. E. DeWitt, and C. R. Young.** 1980. Immune response to *Vibrio cholerae*, p. 464–473. *In* N. R. Rose and H. Friedman (ed.), Manual of clinical immunology, 2nd ed. American Society for Microbiology, Washington, D.C.

15. **Young, C. R., M. M. Levine, J. P. Craig, and R. Robins-Browne.** 1980. Microtiter enzyme-linked immunosorbent assay for immunoglobulin G cholera antitoxin in humans: method and correlation with rabbit skin vascular permeability factor technique. Infect. Immun. **27**:492–496.

Chapter 56

Immunology of Yersiniae†

JANET M. FOWLER AND ROBERT R. BRUBAKER

The genus *Yersinia* was constructed to accommodate those pasteurellae found to share physiological properties and exhibit DNA homology with enteric bacteria. Placed in the family *Enterobacteriaceae*, this genus now contains the mammalian pathogens *Y. pestis*, *Y. pseudotuberculosis*, and *Y. enterocolitica*, plus *Y. ruckeri*, the causative agent of red mouth disease of salmon and trout. Also included are the opportunistic pathogens *Y. intermedia*, *Y. frederiksenii*, and *Y. kristensenii*, which are often encountered as evident commensals or as part of the normal flora of natural environments (6).

All species of medical importance are facultative intracellular parasites. Their ability to penetrate and grow within a variety of host cells undoubtedly accounts for the characteristic inflammation of lymphatic tissue observed throughout the course of disease. This symptom is especially pronounced in the case of plague caused by *Y. pestis*, in which regional lymph nodes can become grossly enlarged as "buboes." Intracellular proliferation of yersiniae does not, however, preclude their isolation from extracellular spaces or fluids, nor does it prevent the expression of diagnostic immunological responses (2, 3, 6).

DISEASE SYMPTOMS

Y. pestis

Bubonic plague presents a distinct clinical picture which is easily recognized by physicians already alerted to the epidemic presence of *Y. pestis*. More difficult is correct diagnosis of the first case of an endemic outbreak in sufficient time to permit effective antibiotic therapy. Typical symptoms consist of sudden fever, chills, weakness, and headache occurring 2 to 8 days after infection by flea bite. Concomitantly or shortly thereafter, the presence of a bubo in the groin, axilla, or neck becomes painfully evident to the patient, although the more distal portal of entry often remains uninflamed. If appropriate treatment with antibiotics is not initiated at this time, further invasion of organs occurs, with widespread destruction of reticuloendothelial cells accompanied by septicemia. The mortality in typical untreated cases of human plague ranges from 50 to 90%. In septicemic plague, in which organisms gain immediate access to fixed macrophages of liver and spleen without formation of buboes, or pneumonic plague, the mortality rate is generally higher (3, 6).

Y. pseudotuberculosis

In contrast to closely related *Y. pestis*, cells of *Y. pseudotuberculosis* typically gain access to the mam-

†Article no. 11422 of the Michigan Agricultural Experiment Station.

malian host via the oral route. The resulting disease can be extremely severe in certain experimental animals, especially the guinea pig, in which a rapid fulminating septicemia or prolonged wasting disease with formation of buboes is typically observed. Pseudotuberculosis in humans generally reflects an acute mesenteric lymphadenitis signaled by abdominal pain and fever but not diarrhea. This syndrome has frequently been confused with appendicitis, but the organisms are typically present within the mesentery rather than the appendix. Human pseudotuberculosis may also rarely occur as severe septicemia (6).

Y. enterocolitica

Also acquired by the oral route, *Y. enterocolitica* usually causes a terminal ileitis in humans. Lower-right-quadrant abdominal pain may also occur, which, as with *Y. pseudotuberculosis*, is often mistaken for appendicitis. However, unlike pseudotuberculosis, yersiniosis caused by *Y. enterocolitica* is frequently accompanied by diarrhea. Erythema nodosum and arthritis can occur as delayed immunological reactions. The differences in symptoms between pseudotuberculosis and yersiniosis in humans are summarized in Table 1. The severity of disease expressed by *Y. enterocolitica* in experimental animals is related to the serotype. Highly virulent serotype 08 organisms exhibit patterns of growth in organs and blood indistinguishable from those of *Y. pseudotuberculosis* and *Y. pestis*, whereas isolates of other serotypes are generally avirulent in mice, rats, and guinea pigs (2, 6).

ISOLATION

Y. pestis

Attempts to isolate *Y. pestis*, a dangerous organism, should be undertaken only in laboratories equipped with special safety facilities. Unfortunately, in practice it may become necessary to identify the bacteria in clinical material. Every precaution should be taken in such cases to utilize antiseptic techniques and practice responsible methods of disposal.

In typical cases of plague, the organisms are obtained by aspiration of the bubo. In the early course of disease it may be necessary to inject and then withdraw a small volume of saline to obtain sufficient fluid for examination. This aspirate will generally contain enough bacteria to permit ready detection by direct microscopy. The organisms may also be observed in the sputum and blood of patients with pneumonic and septicemic plague, respectively, but high numbers in these fluids indicate an unfavorable prognosis. Plague bacilli can readily be cultivated from such fluids or from bubo aspirates by streaking on a variety of enriched solid media followed by incubation for 2

TABLE 1. Contrasting clinical and pathological features of infections caused by *Y. enterocolitica* and *Y. pseudotuberculosis*[a]

Feature	Characteristic of:	
	Y. enterocolitica	*Y. pseudotuberculosis*
Clinical	Diarrhea common	Diarrhea rare
Stool culture	Usually positive	Usually negative
Intestinal pathology	Terminal ileitis common; appendix usually normal but occasionally inflamed with microabscesses and necrosis	Ileum usually normal; appendix may show mild inflammation
Mesenteric lymph nodes	Inflamed, with necrosis and histiocytic inflammatory response	Inflamed, with reticular cell proliferation and granulocytic cell response

[a] From Butler (6).

days at room temperature. Tryptose blood agar (Difco Laboratories, Detroit, Mich.) is routinely used for this purpose (6).

Y. pseudotuberculosis

Primary isolates of *Y. pseudotuberculosis* may be difficult to obtain from human sources despite the occurrence of overt symptoms of disease. In typical severe lymphadenitis, it is often possible to culture the bacteria from a section of mesenteric lymph node removed during surgery for putative appendicitis. The organisms are infrequently recovered directly from fecal material obtained from patients with this form of pseudotuberculosis. Bacteria can readily be cultured from the blood of patients with rare septicemic pseudotuberculosis or from a variety of tissues or blood obtained from infected experimental animals. Of the latter, the guinea pig is acutely sensitive to *Y. pseudotuberculosis* and has frequently been used for enrichment, with 1-ml samples suspected of containing the organisms being injected intraperitoneally. Overt symptoms of disease occur in 1 to 2 weeks. The bacteria can also be recovered by cold enrichment, with samples in phosphate-buffered saline (pH 7.8) or nutrient broth being incubated for up to 2 weeks at 4°C. Since shifts in population resulting in avirulence can occur upon incubation in vitro at 37°C, it is preferable to undertake primary isolations on solid media at room temperature. At 26°C, the organisms form visible colonies from single cells on tryptose blood agar in 1 day. Growth on media containing bile-salts such as MacConkey agar may occur somewhat more slowly (6).

Y. enterocolitica

Since *Y. enterocolitica*, unlike *Y. pseudotuberculosis*, frequently causes diarrhea, it is often encountered during attempts to isolate salmonellae, enterotoxigenic *Escherichia coli*, or other enteric bacteria from fecal samples. Isolation of typical strains is often facilitated by the use of cold enrichment and selective media, with incubation at room temperature as noted

TABLE 2. Distinguishing features of members of the genus *Yersinia*[a]

Property	Response of:		
	Y. pestis	*Y. pseudo-tuberculosis*	*Y. entero-colitica*
Oxidase	−	−	−
Nitrate reduction	+/−	+	+
Fermentation of:			
Rhamnose	−	+	−
Glycerol	+/−	+	+
Glucose	+	+	+
Melibiose	−	+	−
Sucrose	−	−	+
Christensen urea	−	+	+
Ornithine decarboxylase	−	+	−
Citrate utilization	−	−	−
Motility at:			
26°C	−	+	+
37°C	−	−	−
Triple sugar-iron			
Slant	Alkaline	Alkaline	Acid
Butt	Acid	Acid	Acid
Gas or H_2S	None	None	None

[a] Adapted from Butler (6).

for *Y. pseudotuberculosis*. As with other yersiniae, cultivation at 37°C can result in population shifts resulting in avirulence (2, 6).

DETERMINATIVE BACTERIOLOGY

Yersiniae can easily be distinguished by standard bacteriological tests after isolation in pure culture. Some reactions sufficient to permit identification of typical strains are shown in Table 2. A few additional fermentations allow determination of *Y. ruckeri* and environmental species (Table 3).

Since *Y. pestis* grows slowly on many diagnostic media, a number of alternative procedures have been devised to permit rapid identification when serological reagents are not available (10). A recently devised valuable addition to this type of test is determination of the unique constitutive isocitrate lyase activity of the organism (8). Bacteria are grown for 24 h at 26°C on tryptose blood agar, and a loopful of bacteria is suspended in a Wasserman tube containing 0.1 ml of MOPS-Triton buffer (0.1 M MOPS [morpholinepropanesulfonic acid] at pH 7.7, 5 mM $MgCl_2$, 1 mM Na_2Ca-EDTA, and 0.2% Triton X-100). Add 0.1 ml of DL-isocitrate (8 μM) in MOPS-Triton buffer, incubate

TABLE 3. *Y. enterocolitica* and *Y. enterocolitica*-like organisms showing DNA relatedness[a]

Property	Response of:			
	Y. entero-colitica	*Y. inter-media*	*Y. frederik-senii*	*Y. kristen-senii*
Sucrose	+[b]	+	+	−
Rhamnose	−	+	+	−
Raffinose	−	+	−	−
Melibiose	−	+	−	−
α-Methylglucoside	−	+	−	−

[a] From Butler (6).
[b] +, Fermentation of carbohydrate.

for 15 min at room temperature, and then add 0.05 ml of 5.0% phenylhydrazine hydrochloride in 0.4 mM oxalic acid. Heat to a boil, and then immediately place the tube in an ice-water bath. Add 0.1 ml of 12 N HCl, mix, and then add 0.05 ml of aqueous 5% potassium ferricyanide. A positive result is indicated by the formation of a red precipitate, whereas a negative reaction remains yellow.

DETERMINANTS OF VIRULENCE

Y. pestis, *Y. pseudotuberculosis*, and *Y. enterocolitica* all possess a plasmid of approximately 45 megadaltons which mediates an in vitro nutritional requirement for Ca^{2+} at 37 but not at 26°C. The physiological significance of this requirement is unknown, but the phenomenon provides a general mechanism for identification of wild-type yersiniae by virtue of their inability to form colonies on oxalated solid medium (7). The medium is prepared by the addition of 40 ml of 0.25 M $MgCl_2$ and 40 ml of 0.25 M sodium oxalate to 40 g of tryptose blood agar (Difco) in 920 ml of water; all ingredients are autoclaved separately. Note that avirulent mutants lacking the plasmid in question will form colonies on this medium at 37°C and that some wild-type isolates may also form colonies of reduced size. Nevertheless, demonstration of differential colony number or size on this magnesium oxalate agar provides strong evidence for the presence of wild-type yersiniae (3–5).

Y. pestis contains two additional plasmids, which probably encode invasive and toxic activities, accounting for the symptoms of plague as opposed to the considerably milder diseases caused by *Y. pseudotuberculosis* and *Y. enterocolitica* (3–5). No other major mechanisms of pathogenesis have been defined in *Y. pseudotuberculosis*, for which wild-type strains of all known serotypes are of equal virulence. In contrast, the majority of *Y. enterocolitica* isolates are unable to undergo dissemination in experimental animals. As already noted, a notable exception is the 08 serotype, endemic in rural portions of the northeastern United States, which can cause a systemic disease in mice as severe as plague or pseudotuberculosis (11). No explanation presently exists for the high virulence of serotype 08 isolates.

SEROLOGICAL DIAGNOSIS

Y. pestis

Serological tests for *Y. pestis* are generally based on the expression of capsular or fraction I antigen. The most widely used procedure is a passive hemagglutiation assay useful for diagnostic confirmation of human cases and detection of sylvatic or enzootic plague in animal reservoirs. Fraction IA, extracted by the method of Baker et al. (1), and sheep erythrocytes, sensitized by the procedure described by the World Health Organization Expert Committee on Plague (12), are utilized in this widely used technique. The method involves the addition of 0.025 ml of normal rabbit serum (diluted 1:100 in 0.9% NaCl) to each well of a microtiter plate, which constitutes the passive hemagglutination (PHA) portion of the assay. At the same time, each well of a second microtiter plate,

representing a parallel passive hemagglutination inhibition (PHI) assay, receives 0.025 ml of normal rabbit serum containing fraction IA (serum diluted 1:100 in 0.9% NaCl containing 100 µg of antigen per ml). Test and normal control sera (0.025 ml) are then added to the first wells of rows 1 and 2, respectively. Eleven twofold dilutions are made across the row with a microdiluter set at 0.025 ml, and then 0.025 ml of sensitized sheep erythrocytes (0.5% by volume in normal rabbit serum diluted 1:250 in 0.9% NaCl) are added to all of the wells. After gentle swirling, the plates are covered and incubated overnight at 4°C. PHA titers are recorded and compared with PHI titers. Sera are termed positive when repeated tests yield PHA titers of ≥1:16 with an 8-fold or greater reduction in PHI titers. This assay requires considerable time to perform and, as already noted, is used primarily for confirmation rather than primary diagnosis.

Rapid diagnosis of plague can be made by staining the bacteria in bubo aspirates, sputum, or blood with fluorescent antibody to fraction I. The successful primary diagnosis by this method is dependent upon immediate access to conjugated antibody.

Y. pseudotuberculosis

Serospecificity of *Y. pseudotuberculosis* is dependent upon the presence of immunodominant 3,6-dideoxyhexoses on O groups of the 10 recognized serotypes. (An exception is the rough serotype VB, which lacks ascarylose [9].) The majority of human infections are caused by organisms of serotypes IA and IB; however, those infections caused by serotype III isolates often seem more severe (due, perhaps, to the existence in these bacteria of a unique exotoxin). Serotypes II and IV exhibit cross-antigenicity with group B and D salmonellae, respectively, and serotype VI contains the 3,6-dideoxysugar colitose and thus may cross-react with certain pathogenic *E. coli* (9).

Serological diagnosis is traditionally performed in tubes as a Widal agglutination assay with Formalin-killed *Y. pseudotuberculosis* of serotype IA grown on solid medium at room temperature. Dilutions of patient serum ranging from 1:5 to 1:5, 120 are used, with inclusion of known positive and negative sera. A test serum titer of ≥1:160 suggests the occurrence of infection. A number of additional procedures, including an enzyme-linked immunosorbent assay and solid-phase radioimmunoassay, have been described by various authors. These methods may prove to be more accurate in permitting early diagnosis of *Y. pseudotuberculosis*, which, as already noted, is not easily isolated during the course of human disease (see reference 6).

Y. enterocolitica

Serotypes of *Y. enterocolitica* involved in human disease are primarily 03, 08, and 09 (serotype 08 is common only in North America). Only these organisms, therefore, need to be used for serodiagnostic assay. As with *Y. pseudotuberculosis*, serodiagnosis is undertaken by a Widal-type agglutination assay with a standard isolate of human origin. The bacteria are grown at 26°C, washed, and suspended in 0.9% NaCl before being autoclaved for 2.5 h. After two additional washes and final suspension in saline, the organisms are used as test antigens. Unknown sera are diluted in saline and allowed to react overnight at 37°C with the prepared antigen. An agglutination titer of 1:160 is suggestive of infection, whereas a titer of $\geq$1:1,280 indicates acute disease. Low titers of 1:40 to 1:80 may persist for a year or longer and should be interpreted with caution (since they may reflect antibody directed against an antigen common to brucellae and serotype 09 *Y. enterocolitica* or an undefined activity present in patients with thyroid disease).

A number of additional serodiagnostic assays for *Y. enterocolitica* have recently been described, including PHI, enzyme-linked immunosorbent assay, and solid-phase radioimmunoassay (see reference 6). These methods utilize reagents requiring considerable time to prepare, and thus they may be efficient only in laboratories routinely occupied with diagnosis of yersiniae. Furthermore, modifications of these newer procedures may be required to avoid false-positive reactions caused by cross-reactivity to common antigens (6). The nature of these reactions should become evident with further analyses of lipopolysaccharide chemotypes.

ADDITIONAL READING

The recent book, *Plague and Other Yersinia Infections*, by Thomas Butler (6), provides an excellent overview of the yersiniae and their diagnosis. Special aspects of disease caused by *Y. enterocolitica* and its diagnosis have been considered by Bottone (2). Virulence mechanisms have also been reviewed (3–5).

LITERATURE CITED

1. **Baker, E. E., H. Sommer, L. E. Foster, E. Meyer, and K. F. Meyer.** 1952. Studies on immunization against plague. I. The isolation and characterization of the soluble antigen of *Pasteurella pestis*. J. Immunol. **68:**131–145.
2. **Bottone, E. J. (ed.).** 1981. *Yersinia enterocolitica*. CRC Press, Boca Raton, Fla.
3. **Brubaker, R. R.** 1972. The genus *Yersinia*: biochemistry and genetics of virulence. Curr. Top. Microbiol. **57:**111–158.
4. **Brubaker, R. R.** 1979. Expression of virulence in yersiniae, p. 168–171. *In* D. Schlessinger (ed.), Microbiology—1979. American Society for Microbiology, Washington, D.C.
5. **Brubaker, R. R.** 1983. The Vwa$^+$ virulence factor of yersiniae: molecular basis of the attendant nutritional requirement for Ca^{2+}. Rev. Infect. Dis. **5**(Suppl. 4):S748–S758.
6. **Butler, T.** 1983. Plague and other *Yersinia* infections. Plenum Publishing Corp., New York.
7. **Higuchi, K., and J. L. Smith.** 1961. Studies on the nutrition and physiology of *Pasteurella pestis*. VI. A differential plating medium for the estimation of the mutation rate to avirulence. J. Bacteriol. **81:**605–608.
8. **Quan, T. J., J. J. Vanderlinden, and K. R. Tsuchiya.** 1982. Evaluation of a qualitative isocitrate lyase assay for rapid presumptive identification of *Yersinia pestis* cultures. J. Clin. Microbiol. **15:**1178–1179.
9. **Samuelsson, K., B. Lindberg, and R. R. Brubaker.** 1974. Structure of O-specific side chains of lipopolysaccharides from *Yersinia pseudotuberculosis*. J. Bacteriol. **117:**1010–1016.
10. **Surgalla, M. J., E. D. Beesley, and J. M. Albizo.** 1970. Practical applications of new laboratory methods for plague investigation. Bull. W.H.O. **42:**993–997.
11. **Une, T., and R. R. Brubaker.** 1984. In vivo comparison of avirulent Vwa$^-$ and Pgm$^-$ or Pst^r phenotypes of yersiniae. Infect. Immun. **43:**895–900.
12. **World Health Organization Expert Committee on Plague.** 1970. Fourth report. W.H.O. Tech. Rep. Ser. **447:**23–25.

Chapter 57

Pasteurellae

PHILIP B. CARTER

The current edition of *Bergey's Manual of Systematic Bacteriology* (4) recognizes six species in the genus *Pasteurella*: *P. multocida* (type species), *P. haemolytica*, *P. pneumotropica*, *P. ureae*, *P. aerogenes*, and *P. gallinarum*. Of these, only *P. multocida* is important as a human pathogen; this organism is a prominent cause of respiratory infections and septicemias in a large variety of animal species (hence its name). *P. haemolytica* is an important cause of respiratory disease in ruminants, and *P. pneumotropica* is a threat to the health of laboratory animals. The remaining three species are considered members of the mucosal flora of animals and have a very low capacity for causing disease. *P. multocida* was one of the earliest bacterial pathogens studied; it was known initially as the cause of fowl cholera and was used by Pasteur in his earliest demonstrations of the efficacy of immunization in the prevention of disease. This microorganism has remained important in animal health and disease and has continued to be the object of much investigation over the decades. For this reason the majority of work on *Pasteurella* serotyping has been performed with *P. multocida*. *P. haemolytica* has rather recently been recognized as an important respiratory pathogen in ruminants and is known to be a cause of "shipping fever" in cattle; its serology has essentially followed the scheme developed for *P. multocida*.

The pioneering work of Gordon R. Carter (3) on the serological differentiation of *P. multocida* by using capsular antigen differences is still valid today. By using capsular differences, combined with the 11 somatic antigen differences originally described by Namioka and Murata (9) and later refined by Heddleston et al. (7), it is possible to differentiate *P. multocida* into 15 serotypes. The capsular antigens are designated by letters A, B, D, and E (the original description listed capsular antigens A through D, but type C was later judged invalid and a new antigen was designated E). Somatic antigens are designated by arabic numeral, and the presently accepted serotype designations for *P. multocida* are combinations of a letter and a numeral (e.g., serotype 5:A). A similar method of differentiation has been developed by Biberstein et al. (1) for *P. haemolytica*. In this species, 15 capsular serotypes have been described and have been found to be more dependable than somatic antigens for serological differentiation. Unfortunately, the convention has developed of designating capsular serotypes of *P. haemolytica* by numeral, omitting somatic designations, and indicating biotype (differentiated by whether an isolate ferments arabinose [A] or trehalose [T]). This has led to the confusing situation in which the numeral represents the somatic serotype for *P. multocida* and the capsular serotype for *P. haemolytica*. Thus, the serotype A5 designation for *P. haemolytica* means biotype A, capsular serotype 5.

Several serological typing schemes for pasteurellae have been developed by using a variety of techniques, including slide (plate) and tube agglutination, indirect or passive hemagglutination, agar gel diffusion, passive protection, hyaluronidase decapsulation, and acriflavine flocculation. However, a comparison of the various published schemes for the serological differentiation of *P. multocida* revealed considerable overlap and lack of correlation among systems (2). Although the dependability of *P. multocida* capsular serodifferentiation has been questioned (2, 8) and there has been increased reliance on the nonserological differentiation scheme using hyaluronidase (serotype A) and acriflavine (serotype D) developed by Carter and Rundle (5), the capsular antigens are authentic (K. A. Brogden, personal communication) and the recommended system is that of a combination of Carter's capsular scheme and the somatic designations of Heddleston et al. on agar gel immunodiffusion (7). In actual practice, the capsular designation does not pose a real problem since there are geographic and species limitations; capsular types A and D are found only in North America, the former predominantly in fowl, while types B and E are associated with infections in Asia, Australia, and Africa. The agar gel immunodiffusion test has proven reliable and avoids problems in the indirect hemagglutination (IHA) assay that are associated with direct agglutination of erythrocytes by some *P. multocida* serotypes (10).

The presently accepted method of serotyping *P. haemolytica* is the IHA test developed by Biberstein et al. (1) and its modifications which dependably type 90% of isolates. Strains untypable by IHA most often belong to the A biotype and can be differentiated into as many as nine recognized serotypes, which do not cross-react with IHA-positive serotypes, through the use of countercurrent immunoelectrophoresis (6).

It is uncommon for regional diagnostic laboratories to perform *Pasteurella* serotyping. Isolates usually are sent to national laboratories.

REAGENTS

P. multocida

Capsular antigens are prepared by heating isolates harvested from nutrient agar plates at 56°C for 30 min. The bacterial cells are pelleted, and the supernatant is used to coat erythrocytes. Antisera to capsular antigens are prepared by immunizing rabbits with Formalin-killed *P. multocida*.

Somatic antigens for the agar gel immunodiffusion test are prepared by suspending cells, cultured on glucose starch agar for 24 h at 37°C, in 0.3% neutral Formalin diluted in 0.85% phosphate-buffered saline. The suspension of cells is heated at 100°C for 1 h and centrifuged, and the supernatant is collected for use in the gel diffusion precipitin test.

Reference antisera may be obtained from the National Animal Disease Center, Ames, Iowa, or may be prepared by immunizing chickens with reference strains obtainable from the National Animal Disease Center. Antisera are prepared in 12- to 16-week-old male chickens immunized subcutaneously in the neck with a Formalin-killed bacterin of *P. multocida* suspended in Freund incomplete adjuvant. The animals are boosted intramuscularly in the breast 3 weeks later and bled 7 days after being boosted. Sera are collected, preserved with 0.01% Merthiolate and 0.06% phenol, and tested for specificity. Sera used in the IHA assay should be inactivated by heating at 56°C for 30 min.

P. haemolytica

Capsular antigens for use in the IHA assay of Biberstein et al. (1) are prepared as described above, although it is possible to sensitize erythrocytes without prior sedimenting of the bacterial cells.

Reference strains and antisera may be obtained from the National Animal Disease Center, or antisera may be prepared by immunizing rabbits with reference strains.

TEST PROCEDURE

IHA

P. multocida. Human group O erythrocytes are washed three times in phosphate-buffered saline and coated with the capsular antigen (prepared as described above) by adding 3 ml of bacterial extract to 0.2 ml of packed erythrocytes and incubating at 37°C for 2 h. The erythrocytes are washed in saline and used in a standard hemagglutination assay performed in tubes or microtiter plates.

P. haemolytica. Fresh or glutaraldehyde-fixed bovine erythrocytes are washed and coated with capsular material, prepared as described above, for 30 to 60 min at 37°C. The coated erythrocytes are washed three times and used in the standard hemagglutination assay.

Gel diffusion precipitin test (National Animal Disease Center modification of the method of Heddleston et al. [7])

Gel diffusion agar is prepared by flooding standard microscope slides (25 by 75 mm) with 5 ml of warm 0.9% Noble agar in 8.5% NaCl; the slides are held at room temperature in a moist chamber until used. Six peripheral wells and one central well, each 3.5 mm in diameter, are cut in the agar 5.5 mm from center to center; antiserum is placed in the center well, and the test antigens are placed in the peripheral wells. The slides are incubated overnight at 37°C, and precipitin lines are read.

Nonserologic determinations of *P. multocida* capsular types A and D

Serotypes A and D, the only ones associated with human disease, may be determined by nonserologic methods. The capsule of *P. multocida* type A is composed of hyaluronic acid. Colonies of this serotype ordinarily appear mucoid and flowing on agar but grow as minute colonies in the presence of hyaluronidase; the growth of other capsular serotypes is unaffected by the presence of hyaluronidase. Type D organisms flocculate when suspended in a 0.01% solution of acriflavine.

LITERATURE CITED

1. **Biberstein, E. L., M. Gills, and H. Knight.** 1960. Serological types of *Pasteurella haemolytica*. Cornell Vet. **50**: 283–300.
2. **Brogden, K. A., and R. A. Packer.** 1979. Comparison of *Pasteurella multocida* serotyping systems. Am. J. Vet. Res. **40**:1332–1335.
3. **Carter, G. R.** 1955. Studies on *Pasteurella multocida*. I. A hemagglutination test for identification of serological types. Am. J. Vet. Res. **16**:481–484.
4. **Carter, G. R.** 1984. Genus I. *Pasteurella* Trevisan 1887, 94[AL], p. 552–558. *In* N. R. Krieg and J. G. Holt (ed.), Bergey's manual of systematic bacteriology, vol. 1. The Williams & Wilkins Co., Baltimore.
5. **Carter, G. R., and S. W. Rundle.** 1975. Identification of type A strains of *Pasteurella multocida* using staphylococcal hyaluronidase. Vet. Rec. **96**:343.
6. **Donachie, W., J. Fraser, M. Quirie, and N. J. L. Gilmour.** 1984. Studies on strains of *Pasteurella haemolytica* not typable by the indirect haemagglutination test. Res. Vet. Sci. **37**:188–193.
7. **Heddleston, K. L., J. E. Gallagher, and P. A. Rebers.** 1972. Fowl cholera: gel diffusion precipitin test for serotyping *Pasteurella multocida* from avian species. Avian Dis. **16**:925–936.
8. **Manning, P. J.** 1982. Serology of *Pasteurella multocida* in laboratory rabbits: a review. Lab. Anim. Sci. **32**:666–671.
9. **Namioka, S., and M. Murata.** 1961. Serological studies on *Pasteurella multocida*. II. Characteristics of somatic (O) antigen of the organism. Cornell Vet. **51**:507–521.
10. **Rimler, R. B., P. A. Rebers, and M. Phillips.** 1984. Lipopolysaccharides of the Heddleston serotypes of *Pasteurella multocida*. Am. J. Vet. Res. **45**:759–763.

Chapter 58

Immune Response to *Francisella tularensis*

MERRILL J. SNYDER

The difficulty and hazards of cultivating *Francisella tularensis* in the routine laboratory have influenced the use of serological testing for conventional laboratory confirmation of tularemic infection. Since bacteriological methods are essentially unavailable, serological results assume greater importance. The bacterial agglutination test in which formalinized whole cells are used has had wide and long application in the clinical diagnostic laboratory (7). However, other immunological techniques have been evaluated and, in special laboratories, can be employed in the study of the immune response to this organism. These techniques include microagglutination (2), enzyme-linked immunosorbent assay (ELISA; 4, 15), radioimmune assay (8), and skin test (3). Many other tests have been described. The last, in conjunction with the agglutination test, has been used extensively in epidemiological surveys.

The intracellular fate of *F. tularensis* has been studied, and attempts have been made to explain the resistance to intracellular killing of virulent strains compared with the attenuated vaccine strain (10).

The emphasis upon humoral antibody in the immunological approach to diagnosis is in conflict with the demonstrations that cell-associated immune factors have major importance in the acquired resistance to this obligate intracellular parasite. Passively transferred spleen cells of mice immunized with living attenuated tularemia vaccine enabled nonimmune syngeneic recipients to survive a virulent *F. tularensis* challenge which would otherwise have been fatal (5). After immunization of humans, specifically committed T cells stimulated by tularemia antigens to form blast cells and to synthesize DNA have been shown to increase (13). When lymphocytes from individuals with delayed skin test hypersensitivity to tularemia are exposed to the bacillus or its antigens, active rosette-forming cells are produced (6). These techniques have been used to characterize the lymphocytic response in humans after natural infection and after vaccination (14). Cell-mediated immunity and humoral immunity both were demonstrated early, reached respectable titers, and persisted for several years (9, 11). These host cell-*F. tularensis* interrelationships give new insights into the immunopathogenesis of tularemia and provide a model for the study of immunological responses at the cellular level.

CLINICAL INDICATIONS

The ELISA has replaced agglutination as the test of choice in those laboratories having the facilities for this test as well as the tularemia antigens with which to coat the plates. No commercial source of this test is available, perhaps because of the infrequent call for tularemia testing in the routine clinical laboratory. Therefore agglutination remains the mainstay in these laboratories.

A serum specimen should be taken for agglutination of ELISA as soon as and whenever the clinical diagnosis of tularemia is considered. The most common clinical presentation of tularemia infection is ulceroglandular disease. Patients with pulmonic and typhoidal tularemia have rare and frequently unsuspected infections. The history of tick bite or exposure to rabbits and other sick-looking animals should alert the physician to the possibility of *F. tularensis* infection. Very small numbers of virulent organisms (<50) can cause either the ulceroglandular or pulmonic form of the disease. The serological results can be used to support and, under the proper circumstances, confirm the diagnosis. Uncommon cross-reactions with *Brucella* spp. and *Proteus vulgaris* OX19 antibodies have been reported, but, almost invariably, homologous titers exceed heterologous. Treatment of serum with dithiothreitol has been used to eliminate this cross-reactivity (1). As stated above, *F. tularensis* agglutinins remain elevated for years after exposure, and a single positive finding may be the consequence of a past infection rather than the present illness. A rising titer in subsequent serum specimens, as always, aids interpretation.

AGGLUTINATION PROCEDURE

Dilutions of serum, usually 1:10 to 1:2,560, are made in 0.5 ml of physiological saline by the twofold serological dilution technique in 12- by 75-mm test tubes. An equal quantity of tularemia antigen containing 3×10^9 formalinized *F. tularensis* cells, usually avirulent strain B38 of Francis, is added to each tube and mixed by shaking. The tubes are incubated at 37°C for 2 h and then placed in a refrigerator at approximately 4°C overnight (18 h). The tubes are read with a suitable light source without magnification by gently shaking or flipping and observing for agglutination. Readings are recorded as "complete" agglutination when the background liquid is clear, "partial" when clearly visible agglutinated particles are suspended in a cloudy fluid, "questionable" when one is uncertain of the presence of particles, and "negative" when a homogeneous cloudy suspension without clumps is seen. Readings of finer gradation or based upon the size of the clumps are unwarranted. The titer is reported as the greatest final dilution of serum showing definite and unquestionable agglutination of the antigen.

Suitable positive low-titered (<1:160) and high-titered (>1:160) human sera as well as negative serum should be included with each test.

Antigen is usually prepared from *F. tularensis* B38 of Francis (ATCC 6223) grown on glucose-cysteine-blood agar at 37°C for 24 h. Growth is harvested with physiological saline containing 0.5% formaldehyde (1.35% Formalin), washed four times by centrifugation and suspension in fresh 0.5% formaldehyde-saline solution, and finally suspended for use at a turbidity representing 3×10^9 cells per ml.

Strain B38 is avirulent and therefore is recommended for use, although antigens prepared from virulent strains such as Schu S-4 give a somewhat greater sensitivity to the test. The use of phenol instead of formaldehyde reduces the sensitivity of the antigen. Not all commercial antigens are of equal sensitivity, although they are prepared in accord with recommendations of the National Institutes of Health (circular E-677, revised). Recently, several investigators have used the vaccine strain LVS as antigen, but comparisons of the sensitivity and reactivity of antigens prepared from this strain to those of standard antigens have not been reported.

Satisfactory antigens are available commercially from many sources including Difco Laboratories, Detroit, Mich., and BBL Microbiology Systems, Cockeysville, Md. Reference serum can be obtained from the Centers for Disease Control, Atlanta, Ga.

ELISA PROCEDURE

Suitable antigens for the coating of tubes or plates have been prepared with *F. tularensis* LVS. Either the phenol-water-extracted lipopolysaccharide (4) or the protein supernatant of sonically disrupted cells (15) has been used. The basic test procedure for ELISA was essentially followed. Results with both antigens were specific and highly sensitive for antibodies to *F. tularensis* and correlated with each other and with the results of bacterial agglutination. Not unexpectedly, some cross-reaction with other bacterial infections was obtained with the lipopolysaccharide antigen, but this cross-reactivity was low in titer. Since these titers did not approximate the specific titers obtained, they present no problem to interpretation.

INTERPRETATION

The broad experience with tularemia in volunteers infected by the intracutaneous and respiratory routes has furnished valuable information about antibody response in individuals in whom both dose and time of infection are known (12). Similar experience has not been reported with the use of ELISA. Persons without previous experience with tularemia or tularemia vaccine demonstrate circulating antibody by agglutination in 3 weeks (range, 14 to 31 days) and by hemagglutination in 2 weeks (range, 10 to 21 days) after infection. Limited data indicate that antibodies demonstrable by ELISA can be demonstrated this early, with titers in this test some 10-fold higher than those obtained by agglutination. The mean peak agglutination titer of 1:640 (maximum titer, 1:2,560) is reached by week 5 after inoculation, whereas the mean peak hemagglutination titer of 1:10,240 (maximum titer, 1:80,000) is attained by week 4 postinfection. Responses to pulmonary and intradermal challenges are similar.

Agglutination titers greater than 1:40 to 1:80 are of diagnostic significance, as are ELISA titers greater than 1:500, but both may be an indication of previous infection; antibodies are demonstrable years after infection. Since peak antibody titer may not be reached until at least 1 month into the disease, dem-

onstration of a rise in titer in serially obtained specimens at 7- to 10-day intervals provides the clinician with additional diagnostic assurance. Partitioning immunoglobulin G and M antibodies in the ELISA procedure may also be helpful. Difficulties infrequently occasioned by cross-reactions with *Brucella* spp. and *P. vulgaris* OX19 can be eliminated by parallel testing with these antigens whenever serum is tested for tularemia agglutinins or by treatment of the serum with dithiothreitol before testing.

LITERATURE CITED

1. **Behan, K. A., and G. C. Klein.** 1982. Reduction of *Brucella* species and *Francisella tularensis* cross-reacting agglutinins by dithiothreitol. J. Clin. Microbiol. **16:**756–757.
2. **Brown, S. L., F. T. McKinney, G. C. Klein, and W. L. Jones.** 1980. Evaluation of a safranin-O-stained antigen microagglutination test for *Francisella tularensis* antibodies. J. Clin. Microbiol. **11:**146–148.
3. **Buchanan, T. M., G. F. Brooks, and P. S. Brachman.** 1971. The tularemia skin test. Three hundred and twenty-five skin tests in 210 persons: serologic correlation and review of the literature. Ann. Intern. Med. **74:**336–343.
4. **Carlsson, H. E., A. A. Lindberg, G. Lindberg, B. Hederstedt, K.-A. Karlsson, and B. O. Agell.** 1979. Enzyme-linked immunosorbent assay for immunological diagnosis of human tularemia. J. Clin. Microbiol. **10:**615–621.
5. **Eigelsbach, H. T., D. H. Hunter, W. A. Janssen, H. G. Dangerfield, and S. G. Rabinowitz.** 1975. Murine model for study of cell-mediated immunity: protection against death from fully virulent *Francisella tularensis* infection. Infect. Immun. **12:**999–1005.
6. **Felsburg, P. J., and R. Edelman.** 1977. The active E-rosette test: a sensitive *in vitro* correlate for human delayed-type hypersensitivity. J. Immunol. **118:**62–66.
7. **Francis, E., and A. C. Evans.** 1926. Agglutination, cross-agglutination and agglutinin absorption in tularemia. Public Health Rep. **41:**1273–1295.
8. **Hambleton, P., and R. E. Strange.** 1977. Determination of antibacterial antibodies in serum by immunoradiometric assays. J. Med. Microbiol. **10:**151–160.
9. **Koskela, P., and E. Herva.** 1980. Cell-mediated immunity against *Francisella tularensis* after natural infection. Scand. J. Infect. Dis. **12:**281–287.
10. **Löfgren, S., A. Tärnvik, G. D. Bloom, and W. Sjöberg.** 1983. Phagocytosis and killing of *Francisella tularensis* by human polymorphonuclear leukocytes. Infect. Immun. **39:**715–720.
11. **Sandström, G., A. Tärnvik, H. Wolf-Watz, and S. Löfgren.** 1984. Antigen from *Francisella tularensis:* nonidentity between determinants participating in cell-mediated and humoral reactions. Infect. Immun. **45:**101–106.
12. **Saslaw, S., and S. Carhart.** 1961. Studies with tularemia vaccines in volunteers. III. Serologic aspects following intracutaneous or respiratory challenge in both vaccinated and nonvaccinated volunteers. Am. J. Med. Sci. **241:**689–699.
13. **Tärnvik, A., and S. E. Holm.** 1978. Stimulation of subpopulations of human lymphocytes by a vaccine strain of *Francisella tularensis.* Infect. Immun. **20:**698–704.
14. **Tärnvik, A., G. Sandström, and S. Löfgren.** 1979. Time of lymphocyte response after onset of tularemia and after tularemia vaccination. J. Clin. Microbiol. **10:**854–860.
15. **Viljanen, M. K., T. Nurmi, and A. Salminen.** 1983. Enzyme-linked immunosorbent assay (ELISA) with bacterial sonicate antigen of IgM, IgA, and IgG antibodies to *Francisella tularensis:* comparison with bacterial agglutination test and ELISA with lipopolysaccharide antigen. J. Infect. Dis. **148:**715–720.

Chapter 59

Haemophilus influenzae Type b: Assays for the Capsular Polysaccharide and for Antipolysaccharide Antibody

RICHARD INSEL AND PORTER ANDERSON

Haemophilus influenzae has at least three kinds of surface components immunogenic for humans, i.e., a polysaccharide capsule, outer membrane proteins, and lipopolysaccharide. The capsule is the basis for the standard antigenic typing of encapsulated strains; there are six types, designated a through f. *H. influenzae* type b is responsible for almost all invasive diseases caused by this species. Its capsule is composed of a linear polymer of ribose, ribitol, and phosphate [(–3)β-D-ribose(1→1)ribitol(5-phosphate–)] abbreviated PRP.

The most frequent serious disease caused by *H. influenzae* type b is meningitis; other diseases caused by this organism are pneumonia, epiglottitis, cellulitis, arthritis, osteomyelitis, and pericarditis. *H. influenzae* type b is the most common cause of bacterial meningitis in this country. Most infections occur in persons less than 6 years of age, with a peak incidence of meningitis at age 3 to 12 months.

The polysaccharide capsule is released from the bacteria during growth and in stationary phase. Several immunologic assays have been developed to detect the capsular antigen in body fluids as an aid in the diagnosis of clinical infection. These assays include latex agglutination, *Staphylococcus aureus* coagglutination, counterimmunoelectrophoresis (CIE), enzyme-linked immunosorbent assays (ELISA) and radioactive antigen-binding inhibition assays. The first assay will be described in detail because it is one of the most sensitive and widely performed assays.

Humans exposed to *H. influenzae* type b may respond with serum antibody production to all three kinds of surface components. The lipopolysaccharide and the outer membrane proteins of these bacteria are incompletely characterized. Antibodies to these complex components are under active investigation, but their role in host defense is incompletely defined at present. This article will deal further only with serum antibody to PRP, which has been extensively studied and is an important component of immunity to *H. influenzae* type b.

Several assays have been developed to measure antibody to the polysaccharide capsular antigen. Serum bactericidal activity against *H. influenzae* type b can be used to detect complement-fixing anti-PRP antibodies; the assay is tedious to perform and also detects antibodies directed to other surface antigens of *H. influenzae* type b. Passive hemagglutination, with PRP-sensitized erythrocytes, is rapid and inexpensive and does not require the use of radioactive reagents. It is suitably sensitive for the detection of antibodies in human adults and older children, but insufficiently sensitive for the detection of antibody in human infants. At 37 or 25°C passive hemagglutination is much more sensitive to immunoglobulin M (IgM) than to IgG human antibodies; however, at 4°C the sensitivity to IgG increases. For antibody measurements of infant sera, a more sensitive assay is required. Radioactive antigen-binding assays and ELISA are sensitive, reproducible, and simple to perform. Protective antibody titers, as discussed below, have been estimated with the radioantigen-binding assay. Because of the difficulty, instability, and expense of making the pure radioantigen, the radioantigen-binding assay is not practical or economical to establish unless large numbers of samples are being studied.

CLINICAL INDICATIONS AND INTERPRETATION

Antigen detection assays

Clinical indications for detection of antigen include (i) rapid confirmatory specific diagnosis of suspected *H. influenzae* type b infection; (ii) diagnosis when Gram stains and culture do not reveal infection, e.g., after antibiotic treatment; and (iii) assessment of efficacy of treatment of *Haemophilus* disease and prediction of increased complication from infection. Rapid diagnosis is only an adjunct to diagnosis and should not replace culture and Gram stains.

The polysaccharide capsule of the bacterium has been detected in serum, cerebrospinal fluid (CSF), urine, nasopharyngeal secretions, tears, and synovial, pleural, and pericardial fluids. Antigen detection techniques may be more reliable than Gram stain when the latter is performed by an inexperienced individual. Most patients with *H. influenzae* type b meningitis will have detectable antigen in the CSF, serum, or urine. Higher levels of antigen are found in CSF more often than in serum early in meningitis. Levels of serum antigen detected in patients with pneumonia, cellulitis, or epiglottitis are less than those detected in patients with meningitis. Urine may be the only body fluid in which antigen can be detected.

The concentration of antigen in a body fluid will depend on many variables, including the number of bacteria in the host, the duration of infection, and the rapidity of antibody production, which prevents antigen detection and rapidly clears the antigen. Antibiotic treatment before diagnosis of infection by *H. influenzae* type b does not necessarily negate detection of PRP. Antigen may persist in the serum of patients with meningitis for several weeks despite adequate antimicrobial therapy, but the high levels of antigen in CSF usually clear within several days with adequate therapy. Correlation between the initial CSF or serum antigen level in meningitis patients and the severity of symptoms or complications from the disease has been described, but is controversial. Prolonged detection of high levels of serum antigen in meningitis patients is associated with increased complications from the disease.

Several assays have been developed to detect antigen (5). The ideal assay would be simple, rapid, inexpensive, sensitive, and specific. The latex and *S. aureus* agglutination assays, which use antibody-coated latex beads or killed *S. aureus*, best fulfill these criteria. Electrophoresis equipment is not required to perform these assays, and several commercial kits are available in the United States. CIE is still widely performed but requires an electrophoresis apparatus and is not as sensitive as agglutination assays. Commercial sources of antisera are available for performing CIE. The radioantigen-binding inhibition assay and ELISA to detect antigen are quite sensitive, but they are restricted to laboratories performing the antibody assay and require a longer time to perform than several of the other assays.

Pitfalls of antigen detection assays include false-positives produced by rheumatoid factors in serum samples or by cross-reactive antigens on other bacteria in a body fluid. Controls should be routinely performed to avoid the former, and to avoid the latter, body fluids should be routinely cultured to confirm a presumptive diagnosis based on antigen detection. False-negatives may occur when antigen concentrations in a body fluid are below the levels of detection. Body fluid samples can be concentrated to increase the sensitivity of the assays.

Antibody assays

Anti-PRP antibody assays have been used primarily in experimental studies of the relationship between antibody and immunity to disease and in the evaluation of the immunogenicity of capsular polysaccharide vaccines. Presently there are few indications for measuring the antibody in a general clinical immunology laboratory.

Antibody to PRP may be acquired by the transplacental route and actively produced upon exposure to *H. influenzae* type b or cross-reactive organisms. Antibody declines after birth to a nadir at age 3 to 9 months and then increases gradually with age, reaching adult levels at about 6 years of age. Levels are extremely variable among individuals and depend upon a number of factors, including the duration since the last antigenic exposure. Thus, defining a "normal" titer expected for an individual is problematic. Serum antibody is thought to mediate protection by both opsonic and bacteriolytic mechanisms. Estimates of a protective anti-PRP antibody titer (0.1 to 0.15 µg/ml) have been based on quantitation of antibody to PRP of (i) patients with agammaglobulinemia treated and seemingly protected with immune serum globulin, (ii) newborns, who appear to be protected by passively obtained maternal antibody, and (iii) normal children immunized with PRP in a protective trial (7, 8, 10). It is difficult, however, to define a protective titer. The estimates have not included the possible role of mucosal antibody in normal individuals, the possible protection afforded by antibody to noncapsular bacterial surface antigens, or the heightened responsiveness of immunized individuals to bacterial exposure, which may not be reflected in the antibody titer. Moreover, all serum antibody classes may not mediate protection, and the protective level may be different for antibody classes and subclasses.

A purified capsular polysaccharide vaccine has recently been licensed by the U.S. Food and Drug Administration for childhood immunization. The postimmunization antibody level is age dependent (4, 7, 8, 10). Although adultlike responses are not produced until after about 6 years of age, protection against invasive disease appeared to be induced sometime after age 18 months (7). Adults respond to immunization with levels of antibody ranging from 1 to 100 µg/ml, and the antibody persists at high levels for years. The majority of postimmunization antibody in adults is IgG, although IgA and IgM antibodies are detected (4).

Detection of antibody responses to PRP after clinical infection requires a very sensitive assay. The postinfection antibody response of young infants may be low and delayed several months. Infants with a poor response may be subject to a second *H. influenzae* type b infection. It may be difficult to interpret results of antibody levels after infection also because of the variable amount of antigenic exposure, the persistence of circulating PRP, and the possibility of a genetic control of predisposition to disease and of antibody response. Thus, attempting serodiagnosis by antibody assay might give a false-negative conclusion. Whether the antibody level at a given interval after infection would have value in predicting susceptibility to a recurrence is uncertain and requires further investigation. If a second infection by *H. influenzae* type b does occur, the assay may be a useful adjunct to a general immunologic evaluation of the patient. Titers of anti-PRP antibody of healthy infants at different ages before and after immunization have been described previously (1, 7, 8, 10). Recurrence of disease might be associated with a rather specific inability to produce anti-PRP antibody as observed in the Wiskott-Aldrich syndrome or IgG2 subclass deficiency. In contrast, patients with a generalized antibody immunodeficiency disease will have abnormal antibody responses to protein as well as polysaccharide antigens and low immunoglobulin levels.

Some patients with antibody deficiency are managed with immune serum globulin or plasma to prevent pyogenic infections such as those from *H. influenzae* type b. The antibody assay may be useful in selecting a plasma donor who has a high anti-PRP antibody level, which would provide a higher level of antibody in the recipient.

Sensitive assays to quantify antibody to PRP have included both radioactive antigen-binding assays and ELISA. In the radioantigen-binding assay, serum is equilibrated with radiolabeled PRP, after which the PRP bound to antibody is separated from unbound PRP by precipitating the antigen-antibody complex with antiglobulin, half-saturated ammonium sulfate (the Farr technique), or polyethylene glycol (6). The percentage of radioactive polysaccharide antigen bound by an experimental serum may be compared with binding values of dilutions of a standard reference serum in which the antibody concentration has been established. The test serum may thus be assigned an antibody concentration equal to that of the reference serum diluted to equivalent binding. This value is only an estimate of antibody content of the test serum because antigen binding is dependent on both the antibody affinity and amount. The binding must be determined in antigen excess. If a serum is in antibody excess, then either it is further diluted or the antigen concentration is increased.

The assay requires PRP to be radiolabeled. Commonly, labeling has been done either intrinsically with ^{3}H, by growing the bacteria in ^{3}H-labeled glucose or ribose, or extrinsically with ^{125}I, by the coupling of tyramine to PRP before the PRP is radiolabeled (8). In a refined version of the assay, a second isotope unaffected by antibody has been employed as a fluid volume marker (3). The second isotope obviates the necessity of either washing the antigen-antibody precipitate or accurately removing a precise volume of supernatant for counting. However, in this chapter only [^{125}I]PRP, the single label technique, and ammonium sulfate precipitation will be described, because [^{125}I]PRP is easier to prepare reproducibly than [^{3}H]PRP, the calculation of results is simpler, and the ammonium sulfate technique was used in assays in which protective titers were estimated. The antibody assay described below is that developed by John Robbins and Rachel Schneerson of the National Institutes of Health. A workshop will be convened at the National Institutes of Health in 1985 to standardize the antibody assay so that results from different laboratories will be comparable.

ELISA techniques for antibody have been performed by binding PRP directly to some types of microtiter plates, by binding PRP to poly-L-lysine-coated microtiter wells, or by coupling PRP to a ligand that allows reproducible binding to the plates. Ligands that have been employed include protein carriers, biotin (which will then allow binding to avidin-coated wells), and tyramine. The last technique, which will be described below, produces an antigen that is stable for over a year and generates a sensitive and specific assay.

TEST PROCEDURES AND REAGENTS

A detailed description of the latex agglutination assay is provided because of its sensitivity (as low as 0.2 to 0.5 ng of PRP per ml, which is approximately 10- to 50-fold lower than that of CIE), wide acceptance, and similarity in sensitivity and assay technique to the coagglutination assay (2, 9). The basis of the assay is that PRP in body fluids causes visible agglutination of latex particles coated with antibody to PRP. Commercial kits for latex and *S. aureus* agglutination assays are available.

Reagents for latex agglutination antigen assay

Polystyrene latex particles. Use 0.81-μm beads.

Antiserum to *H. influenzae* type b. Rabbit, burro, and equine antisera as well as monoclonal antibody to PRP have been used. Commercial rabbit antiserum has been employed in the assay. A suitable antiserum must have a high titer of antibody to PRP. Other bacterial polysaccharides have cross-reactive deter-

minants that may bind to the antibody. This cross-reactivity varies with the animal species and with individual animals in which the antisera are produced. The cross-reactive antigens include pneumococcal polysaccharide types 6A, 6B, 15, 29, and 35, *Escherichia coli* K-100 polysaccharide, and antigens of certain gram-positive organisms. This potential cross-reactivity may have clinical relevance and must be considered; e.g., pneumococcal type 6 is an invasive pathogen for humans. Serologic cross-reactivity can be evaluated by testing the anti-PRP serum in the assay with supernatants of the broth cultures of these bacteria (available from American Tissue Type Culture Collection, Rockville, Md.). If there is reactivity with these polysaccharides, then the antiserum must be absorbed with the corresponding bacteria.

Dilute the antiserum in glycine-buffered saline (GBS) in serial dilutions to determine the optimal dilution to be used for sensitization of the latex particles. Either the whole antiserum or the gamma globulin fraction has been used to sensitize the latex particles. The use of the globulin fraction may provide a more sensitive assay. Normal animal serum without anti-PRP activity is used as a control for the assay.

GBS. Mix 7.3 g of glycine, 10.0 g of sodium chloride, and 1.0 g of sodium azide. Dissolve in 900 ml of distilled water. Adjust the pH to 8.2 with 1 M NaOH. Add distilled water to make 1 liter.

Latex wash solution (GBS + 0.1% bovine serum albumin). Add 0.1 g of bovine serum albumin (BSA) to 100 ml of GBS.

Latex diluent (10×). Mix 7.5 ml of GBS and 2.5 ml of normal serum (rabbit or burro) without anti-PRP antibody.

Sensitized latex particles (0.125%) (antibody positive and control). To an Eppendorf tube (1.5 ml, conical polypropylene; catalog no. 690, Walter Sarstedt, Inc., Princeton, N.J.), add 25 μl of anti-*H. influenzae* type b or normal serum, 525 μl of GBS, and 50 μl of 1.5% suspension of latex. Incubate for 1 h at room temperature with intermittent mixing. Centrifuge at 8,000 × g for 5 min. Aspirate the supernatant. Wash the latex twice in latex wash solution by thorough suspension and centrifugation; suspend in 0.54 ml of latex wash solution, and add 0.06 ml of 10× latex diluent. Store at 4°C. This is enough latex for about 60 assays; larger amounts can be prepared. Gently vortex the latex suspension before it is used, and then centrifuge the latex suspension at 200 × g for 2 to 3 min to pellet any large aggregates. Use the supernatant suspension in the assay. The sensitized latex is stable for at least 4 months.

PRP standards. PRP is stored in water at concentrations of at least 10 μg/ml. Dilute in serial twofold dilutions from 8 ng/ml to 0.0625 ng/ml in fetal bovine serum (FBS) without anti-PRP antibody; FBS is used as a negative control.

Body fluid specimens and dilutions. Body fluid specimens should be clarified by centrifugation. Urine should also be passed through a filter (0.45-μm pore size) if inconclusive results in the assay occur. Plasma should not be used. Lipemic or turbid samples may produce inconclusive results. An undiluted specimen and a fivefold dilution should be examined initially. If the specimen has detectable antigen, then it should be diluted in serial two- to fivefold dilutions to estimate the concentration of antigen. Dilutions are performed with the latex wash solution.

Reducing agent. Rheumatoid factors in serum may bind to the control latex and produce inconclusive results. If this occurs, the serum is heat-inactivated at 56°C for 30 min and then made to 0.0026 M in dithiothreitol (DTT) with 0.026 M DTT in GBS and incubated for 1 h at room temperature. The treated serum is immediately tested undiluted and diluted in latex wash solution. The PRP standards should be incubated with DTT in a similar manner, because DTT may reduce the sensitivity of the assay.

Assay method for latex agglutination assay

1. Add 50 μl of specimen, PRP standard, or FBS (as a negative control) to 10 μl of both the positive and the control sensitized latex particles (0.125%) on a clean serologic ring slide. Mix. All reagents should be at room temperature before they are used.

2. The reaction mixture must be maintained in suspension without evaporation. It has proved satisfactory to oscillate the slide at 140 to 180 rpm within a humidified chamber attached to a platform shaker at room temperature.

3. Agglutination is assessed initially at 10 and then at 45 min with indirect lighting above a black background.

4. The specimens are compared with both positive and negative controls. Agglutination is considered positive if increased granularity or clumping of the latex is observed. The negative control must produce no agglutination of the control or antibody-positive latex particles. If agglutination occurs spontaneously in this diluent control, then the latex must be vortexed and respun to eliminate aggregates. The test specimen must show no agglutination of the control latex. An endpoint of agglutination is determined for the sample and for the PRP standards. The PRP concentration in the test sample is equal to the minimal detectable concentration of PRP times the reciprocal of the highest sample dilution with positive agglutination.

5. If a urine sample produces agglutination of control beads, the sample should be filtered as described above. Agglutination of serum samples may occur with the control latex particles due to binding of human antibody to the animal serum on the latex particle. If this occurs, then the specimen should be treated with the reducing agent and retested. If the results are still inconclusive, the sample should be retested after incubation in a boiling-water bath for 2 min.

Reagents for radioantigen-binding antibody assay

Phosphate-buffered saline with Merthiolate (PBS-M). Mix 28 ml of 0.1 M NaH_2PO_4, 72 ml of 0.1 M Na_2HPO_4, 8.5 g of NaCl, and 850 ml of water. Check the pH and adjust it to pH 7.4. Add water to 1 liter and autoclave. Add 0.1 g of thimerosal per liter.

PBS-M-BSA. Dissolve 0.1 g of BSA in 100 ml of PBS-M.

[125I]PRP. For preparation, see below.

[125I]PRP assay solution. It may be appropriate to dilute radioactive PRP in PBS-M-BSA to approximately 0.5 μCi/ml to use 10 μl of each sample or

reference serum dilution. The ideal dilution and volume of PRP, however, will be based on the specific activity of the antigen and the range in which antibody is to be detected.

Serum diluent. Use FBS without PRP-binding activity. It is heat-inactivated at 56°C for 30 min. Each lot of FBS must be examined to ascertain the absence of antibodies. FBS is the diluent for the reference serum and the test sera in antibody excess.

Reference serum. The antibody concentration of a designated reference serum is quantified by precipitin analysis and is available through the Office of Biologics, U.S. Food and Drug Administration. Dilute the reference serum serially, twofold, through the range of 3 to 90% binding.

Saturated ammonium sulfate. Dissolve 90 g of ammonium sulfate in 100 ml of distilled water with heating. Cool and store at 4°C (crystals of excess salt should form).

Assay method for radioantigen-binding assay

1. Add 50 μl of the radioactive PRP solution to an Eppendorf tube.

2. Add 25 μl of (undiluted or diluted) serum. Vortex gently to mix the solutions. Incubate at 4°C overnight.

3. Add 75 μl of saturated ammonium sulfate. Vortex and incubate for 1 h at 4°C.

4. Centrifuge at 8,000 × g for 5 min.

5. Without disturbing the precipitate, precisely remove 75 μl of the supernatant, and count in a gamma spectrometer.

6. The following standards need to be counted with each assay.
   a. Total antigen. Mix 50 μl of PRP solution with 25 μl of the serum diluent. Process as in steps 3, 4, and 5.
   b. Background. Mix 50 μl of water with 25 μl of serum diluent. Process as in steps 3, 4, and 5.

7. Correct the counts for the background, and calculate the percentage of antigen bound as follows:

$$\% \, [^{125}I]PRP \text{ bound} = 100[1 - (\text{cpm in sample/cpm in total antigen})]$$

8. Determine the binding of the reference serum at various dilutions. Plot the percentage of antigen bound (linear scale) versus the antibody concentration (logarithmic scale). Use this calibration curve to estimate the antibody concentration of the sample serum. The calibration curve must be determined regularly due to degradation of the radioactive PRP over time because of radiodecomposition. The volume of serum used in the assay may be increased to increase the sensitivity of the assay. This will necessitate increasing the volume of saturated ammonium sulfate. If the binding of a sample serum exceeds 90%, then it must be further diluted for an accurate determination of its binding activity.

Reagents for ELISA antibody assay

PRP ELISA antigen. See below (preparation of PRP for antigen and antibody assays).

Anti-immunoglobulin-enzyme conjugates and buffers. See chapter 17.

Assay method for ELISA

1. The optimum coating concentration of antigen should be determined by coating microtiter wells for 90 min at 37°C with 0.01 to 10 µg of derivatized PRP per ml of PBS.

2. The plates are then washed three times with PBS–0.05% Tween and incubated overnight at 20°C with serial serum dilutions, followed by incubation for another day with anti-immunoglobulin-enzyme conjugates diluted in PBS–0.05% Tween. After being washed, the enzyme substrate is added. The details of the performance of the ELISA are provided in chapter 17.

3. The assay should be standardized with reference serum, which can be obtained from the Office of Biologics, U.S. Food and Drug Administration. Negative and positive controls should be performed with each assay.

Preparation of PRP for antigen and antibody assays

PRP is used as a standard in antigen detection assays and is tyraminated for the radioantigen-binding assay and ELISA and iodinated for use in the former. It is isolated and purified from the culture supernatant after growth of *H. influenzae* type b to late stationary phase (see below).

Isolation of PRP

1. Centrifuge the 6 liters of culture at 10,000 × g for 15 min, and collect the supernatant. Do not use polycarbonate vessels. Recentrifuge the supernatant to further clarify.

2. Add hexadecyltrimethylammonium bromide (Cetavlon, Eastman Organic Chemicals, Rochester, N.Y.) to the supernatant to a concentration of 0.01 M, and incubate at 4°C for 30 min. Perform all further steps at 0 to 4°C unless otherwise specified.

3. Centrifuge at 10,000 × g for 10 min, and retain the gummy, brown precipitate.

4. Extract the precipitate vigorously with 1 liter of 0.1 M NaCl, and centrifuge at 10,000 × g for 10 min. Discard the supernatant. Extract the residual precipitate with 0.25 liter of 0.25 M NaCl. Centrifuge as described previously, but retain the supernatant. Discard the precipitate.

5. Add 2 volumes of cold absolute ethanol, and incubate at −20°C overnight.

6. Centrifuge at 10,000 × g at 4°C for 30 min.

7. Discard the supernatant; dissolve the precipitate in 1 liter of sodium phosphate buffer, pH 7. Repeat steps 2 through 6.

8. Discard the supernatant; dissolve the precipitate in 0.25 liter of distilled water, and transfer it to a 1-liter glass-stoppered bottle.

9. Add an equal volume of 90% freshly distilled phenol and vigorously agitate for 30 min at room temperature. Centrifuge at 10,000 × g at 4°C in glass for 10 min, and retain the aqueous phase. The phenol extraction should be repeated until the interface is clear.

10. Precipitate PRP from the aqueous phase by adding NaCl to 0.1 M and then adding 2 volumes of ethanol; centrifuge and dissolve as described in steps 6 and 8. Repeat until A_{260} falls to a plateau, indicating the removal of residual phenol.

11. Dissolve the precipitate in 0.5 M NaCl and fractionate on a column of Sepharose 2B equilibrated with 0.5 M NaCl. Assay the fractions for protein with the Folin phenol reagent and BSA as standard and for ribose with the orcinol reaction and D-ribose as standard. Retain and pool the fractions with a protein-to-ribose ratio of less than 0.02. (The void volume fractions may have a high ratio.) Precipitate as described in steps 5 and 6, dissolve and dialyze in water, and lyophilize. PRP in sodium salt form is approximately 39% ribose, 5% Na, and 9% P. A_{260} and A_{280} indicate the degree of contamination with nucleic acids and proteins.

Tyramination of PRP for radioantigen-binding assay

1. Add 5 mg of PRP in 1 ml of water to a screw-capped vial containing a small magnetic stirring bar. Adjust the pH to 10.5 with 0.1 M NaOH.

2. Immediately add 1.2 mg of CNBr (freshly dissolved in water at 100 mg/ml; note the biohazard). Maintain the pH at 10.2 to 10.5 with 0.1 M NaOH for 6 min.

3. Immediately add 5 mg of tyramine dissolved in 0.2 ml of 0.5 M $NaHCO_3$. Seal and mix at room temperature for 2 h and then at 4°C overnight.

4. Dialyze the mixture or fractionate it on a column of Bio-Gel P-10 equilibrated with 0.01 M phosphate buffer, pH 7.5. Assay samples of fractions for ribose colorimetrically by the orcinol assay. The tyramine-PRP (along with unconjugated PRP) should elute in the void volume. Retain and store frozen.

Iodination of tyramine-PRP

1. Iodinate the antigen by the chloramine T method as follows. Add 50 µl of tyramine-PRP at 1 mg of PRP per ml in 0.5 M sodium phosphate buffer (pH 7.5) to 1 mCi of ^{125}I at 300 to 400 mCi/ml. Add 10 µl of chloramine T at 5 mg/ml, and mix. After 60 s, add 25 µl of sodium metabisulfite at 5 mg/ml, and then add 50 µl of KI at 10 mg/ml.

2. Immediately fractionate on a Sepharose column equilibrated with 0.01 M phosphate buffer, and determine and retain the radioactive fractions. Add BSA to 1%. Pool the fractions meeting criteria 3 and 4 below, freeze small samples quickly with dry ice and acetone, and store at −70°C.

3. The radioactive PRP antigen should not be precipitable with half-saturated ammonium sulfate. Incubate a sample of the radioactive antigen with an equal volume of either saturated ammonium sulfate or distilled water for 4°C for 1 h. Centrifuge at 8,000 × g for 2 min at 4°C, and count a sample of the supernatants. If a significant percentage of the antigen is precipitable, then incubate the radioactive antigen pool with an equal volume of saturated ammonium sulfate for 1 h at 4°C. Centrifuge, retain the nonprecipitable supernatant, and dialyze in 0.01 M phosphate to remove ammonium sulfate. Freeze small samples quickly with dry ice and acetone, and store at −70°C.

4. All of the radioactivity should be bound by a serum containing anti-PRP antibody, and this binding should be completely blocked by the addition of excess nonradioactive PRP. The specific activity of the

labeled PRP can be determined by comparing the degree of inhibition produced by unlabeled PRP of the same size with that produced by the labeled PRP in the radioantigen-binding assay.

Tyramination of PRP for ELISA

1. Add 1 mg of PRP to 1 ml of 0.1 M $NaHCO_3$, and adjust the pH to 10.5 with 0.1 M NaOH.

2. Add 50 mg of CNBr (freshly dissolved in distilled water at 150 mg/ml; note the biohazard). Maintain the pH at 10.2 to 10.5 with 0.1 M NaOH for 6 min. This high ratio (50:1) of CNBr to PRP, which is greater than that used in the preparation of PRP for radioiodination, is required to allow PRP to bind to polystyrene and will produce a high-molecular-weight PRP that is heavily tyraminated. Approximately 10 times as much tyramine will be incorporated into PRP as in the preparation for the iodination protocol described above.

3. Immediately add 0.4 mg of tyramine dissolved in 0.1 M $NaHCO_3$. Seal and mix at 20°C for 10 min, and then adjust the pH to 8.6 with 0.1 M NaOH. Stir for 1 h at 20°C and then overnight at 4°C.

4. Dialyze against three changes of PBS-M. Store at 4°C.

5. Assay at 0.01 to 10 μg of PRP per ml on ELISA plates to determine optimal working concentration.

Cultures of *H. influenzae* type b

1. Add to dialysis bags 61 g of tryptone (Difco Laboratories, Detroit, Mich.) and 30.5 g of yeast extract (Difco). Dialyze against 4 liters of water containing 2 g of NaCl and 5 ml of chloroform for 40 h at 4°C.

2. Discard the bags. Add 30.5 g of glucose to the dialysate. Adjust the volume to at least 3,660 ml. Dispense 60 ml of the dialysate and glucose (dTYED) to a 500-ml culture flask (starter), and add 20 ml of distilled water. Dispense 300 ml of dTYED to each of 12 baffled 2-liter flasks, and add 100 ml of distilled water.

3. Dissolve 72 g of Na_2HPO_4 and 9 g of $NaH_2PO_4 \cdot H_2O$ in water up to a volume of 1,220 ml. Add 20 ml of this phosphate buffer to one bottle and 100 ml of the remainder to each of 12 bottles. Autoclave the phosphate buffer and the dTYED (separately!) at 15 lb/in² for 15 min.

4. Dissolve 6 mg of hemin (Eastman) with 1 ml of 1 M NH_4OH in a sterile tube. Add 1 ml of 99% ethanol. Incubate for at least 1 h at 37°C. Add 4 ml of sterile water. Streak onto a blood agar plate to check sterility.

5. Dissolve 6 mg of NAD (grade III, Sigma Chemical Co., St. Louis, Mo.) in 6 ml of water, and sterilize by passing through a filter (0.22-μm pore size).

6. For starter culture, combine 20 ml of phosphate buffer with 80 ml of dTYED. Add 0.1 ml each of the hemin and NAD solutions. Heavily inoculate with *H.*

influenzae type b grown overnight on chocolate agar or other suitable solid medium. Incubate with shaking at 37°C until a distinct increase in turbidity has occurred. Add the remaining hemin and NAD solutions.

7. For 0.5-liter cultures, add 100 ml of phosphate buffer to 400 ml of dTYED in the baffled 2-liter flasks. Add 9 ml of the starter mixture. Incubate with shaking at 37°C for 18 h. Examine for purity by Gram stain; also streak onto blood agar (nonpermissive for *H. influenzae* type b) as a check for low-level contamination. Add phenol to 0.1% to kill the bacteria.

We thank Rachel Schneerson for a helpful critique of the radioantigen-binding antibody assays.

This work was supported in part by contract AI 12673 and grant AI 17217 from the National Institute of Allergy and Infectious Diseases.

LITERATURE CITED

1. **Anderson, P. W., D. H. Smith, D. L. Ingram, J. Wilkins, P. F. Wehrle, and V. M. Howie.** 1977. Antibody to polyribophosphate of *Haemophilus influenzae* type b in infants and children: effect of immunization with polyribophosphate. J. Infect. Dis. **136**(Suppl.):S57–S62.

2. **Collins, J. K., and M. T. Kelly.** 1983. Comparison of Phadebact coagglutination, Bactogen latex agglutination, and counterimmunoelectrophoresis for detection of *Haemophilus influenzae* type b antigens in cerebrospinal fluid. J. Clin. Microbiol. **17**:1005–1008.

3. **Gotschlich, E. C.** 1971. A simplification of the radioactive antigen-binding test by a double label technique. J. Immunol. **107**:910–911.

4. **Insel, R. A., P. Anderson, M. E. Pichichero, M. E. Amstey, G. Ekborg, and D. H. Smith.** 1982. Anticapsular antibody to *Haemophilus influenzae* type b, p. 155–168. *In* S. H. Sell, and P. F. Wright, (ed.), *Hemophilus influenzae* epidemiology, immunology, and prevention of disease. Elsevier Biomedical Press, New York.

5. **Kaplan, S. L., and R. D. Feigin.** 1980. Rapid identification of the invading microorganism. Pediatr. Clin. N. Am. **27**:783–803.

6. **Kuo, J. S. C., N. Monji, R. S. Schwalbe, and D. McCoy.** 1981. A radioactive antigen-binding assay for the measurement of antibody to *Haemophilus influenzae* type b capsular polysaccharide. J. Immunol. Methods **43**:35–47.

7. **Peltola, H., H. Kayhty, A. Sivonen, and P. H. Makela.** 1977. *Haemophilus influenzae* type b capsular polysaccharide vaccine in children: a double-blind field study of 100,000 vaccinees 3 months to 5 years of age in Finland. Pediatrics **60**:730–737.

8. **Robbins, J. B., J. C. Parke, Jr., R. Schneerson, and J. K. Whisnant.** 1973. Quantitative measurement of "natural" and immunization-induced *Haemophilus influenzae* type b capsular polysaccharide antibodies. Pediatr. Res. **7**:103–110.

9. **Scheifele, D. W., J. I. Ward, and G. R. Siber.** 1981. Advantage of latex agglutination over countercurrent immunoelectrophoresis in the detection of *Haemophilus influenzae* type b antigen in serum. Pediatrics **68**:888–891.

10. **Smith, D. H., G. Peter, D. L. Ingram, A. L. Harding, and P. Anderson.** 1973. Responses of children immunized with the capsular polysaccharide of *Haemophilus influenzae* type b. Pediatrics **52**:637–644.

Chapter 60

Immune Response to Brucellae

MARGARET E. MEYER

The host immune response to infection with *Brucella* organisms is both humoral and cell-mediated, with the latter response accompanied by delayed-type hypersensitivity. The cell-mediated immune response governs the course and outcome of the disease. The humoral antibodies are predominantly of the classes immunoglobulin M (IgM), IgG, and IgA, and since the levels of the antibodies change during the course of the disease, they can serve as useful indices of the status of infection. The first immunoglobulin to appear is IgM, and for the first several days, it is the only one present. As the disease progresses, IgM recedes quantitatively and IgG becomes predominant. In chronic brucellosis, IgG may be produced for an extended period.

There are a variety of serologic tests that detect and measure the humoral antibodies. The four tests that most adequately cover the quantitative changes in the immunoglobulin patterns of acute, subacute, and chronic brucellosis are the standard tube and mercaptoethanol agglutination tests, the Coombs anti-human globulin test, and the complement fixation (CF) test. There are many other serologic tests, as well as skin tests, that may be useful either under special circumstances or for survey purposes (Table 1).

CLINICAL INDICATIONS

Acute brucellosis ordinarily should not be difficult to recognize and diagnose, once it is included on a suspect list in a differential diagnosis. With the relatively few cases that now occur annually in the United States, physicians are apt either to be unfamiliar with this disease or to believe it "can't happen here" and omit it from consideration. Brucellosis should be included as a possibilty in a differential diagnosis when a patient has symptoms resembling those of influenza, such as headaches, tiredness, night sweats, muscle soreness, and a rising and falling temperature, and when these symptoms persist for more than 7 to 10 days. Also, in contrast to patients with influenza, patients with brucellosis should reveal in response to careful questioning that they either have been near a probable source of infection or have traveled, especially in southern Europe or the developing countries.

Chronic brucellosis is more difficult to recognize and frequently is elusive to confirm by laboratory tests. Chronic brucellosis can be described as a state of essentially ill health that follows an acute or subacute case of brucellosis, although it may also develop insidiously in the absence of an acute attack of the disease. Symptoms of chronic brucellosis usually include tiredness, depression, headache, muscular and articular pain, anorexia, weight loss, and low-grade fever. Sometimes the symptoms are vague or bizarre. Occasionally, they can be accounted for by specific lesions.

INTERPRETATION

When the clinical picture points to a possibility of brucellosis, the first serologic test should be the standard tube agglutination test. The minimum titer indicative of the possibility of active infection is considered to be 1:160, with a second test 7 to 14 days later showing a rising titer, frequently fourfold that of the first sample. At the peak of the acute stage of the disease, a serum antibody titer of 1:1,250 or even 1:5,120 is not uncommon. However, the serologic tests serve only to help substantiate a presumptive clinical diagnosis. Final diagnostic confirmation depends upon isolation of the causal organism. Therefore, at the time blood is drawn for the first serologic test, a sufficient amount should be obtained for culture. Blood for culture is best drawn at the time of the rising temperature and before the administration of antibiotics. Techniques of organism isolation and identification are described in references 1 and 2.

As a general rule, patients with acute brucellosis will have serum antibodies that are detectable by the standard tube agglutination test. If this test is completely negative, there remains only a remote possibility that the individual has brucellosis.

If the history and clinical indications still suggest the possibility of brucellosis, the sequence of events for further testing should be (i) additional and repeated attempts at blood culture, (ii) the mercaptoethanol agglutination test, (iii) the Coombs antiglobulin test, and (iv) the CF test.

As with the standard tube agglutination test, a titer of 1:160 by the mercaptoethanol agglutination test indicates active infection (persistent IgG agglutinins).

Some human sera contain blocking antibodies that interfere with the agglutination reaction between *Brucella* antigen and antibody. The Coombs anti-human globulin test removes the intereference of the blocking antibodies. This test is considered positive when there is a rising antiglobulin titer or at least a fourfold increase in the agglutination titer after the addition of anti-human globulin to the test system.

Among these four tests more or less routinely used in the serologic diagnosis of brucellosis, the CF test is usually the test of last resort. It is more useful in diagnosing chronic rather than early, acute brucellosis. A CF titer of 1:16 is considered indicative of infection. For a complete description of the CF test for brucellosis, see references 1 and 2.

REAGENTS

The six species of organisms in the genus *Brucella* are *B. abortus*, *B. suis*, *B. melitensis*, *B. canis*, *B. ovis*, and *B. neotomae*. For detecting infections caused by *B. abortus*, *B. suis*, and *B. melitensis*, *B. abortus* antigen can be used, as it reacts equally well with antibodies induced by each of these three species.

TABLE 1. Serologic tests for *Brucella* antibodies

Test	Advantages	Disadvantages
Standard tube agglutination	Simple to perform Easy to read Standardized antigen available Detects disease in early stages Detects IgM	Does not detect nonagglutinating antibody; therefore false-negatives can occur
Mercaptoethanol agglutination	Persistent IgG agglutination indicates continuing infection that requires treatment Important in diagnosis in humans and should be performed in all suspected cases	False-negatives if nonagglutinating antibodies are present
Coombs anti-human globulin	Demonstrates presence of incomplete antibodies, particularly IgG and IgA	Laborious to perform
Complement fixation	Useful in detecting chronic brucellosis Detects IgG, but not IgM	Often negative in early stages of disease
Radioimmune assay test (5)	Detects IgG, IgM, and IgA Insensitive to IgM, so more sensitive than agglutination test	Requires facilities for working with radiolabeled chemicals
Conglutinating CF test (3)	Useful in early stages of diseases when conventional tests are negative	The usual complexities of a CF test
Rose bengal plate agglutination test (6)	Valuable for diagnosis in areas with no laboratory facilities Good screening test in areas with laboratory facilities	Possibly too sensitive

B. canis can cause brucellosis in humans, but infections due to this species are rare. There have been only some 30 confirmed cases in the United States in the last 20 years, and most of these cases have occurred when there has been either massive or repeated exposures, i.e., in laboratory personnel and kennel attendants. A few cases have occurred from contact with an infected pet dog, usually an aborting female.

B. canis is of nonsmooth (mucoid) colonial morphology, and the serologic detection of *B. canis* antibodies requires homologous antigen.

B. ovis and *B. neotomae* have not been incriminated as causes of infection in humans.

For the preparation of *B. abortus* antigen, it is critical that the culture be of absolutely smooth colonial morphology. Most *Brucella* strains show considerable variation from smooth to rough, and it requires special lighting and a trained and experienced eye to detect the initial and subtle changes in colonial morphology as a culture becomes rough. The strain of *B. abortus* used essentially throughout the western world for antigen production, *B. abortus* 1119, was selected for this use because of its relatively high degree of morphologic stability. Nonetheless, its morphology can drift toward rough. Since standardized, reliable, relatively inexpensive *B. abortus* antigen is commercially available, it is neither necessary nor advisable for individual laboratories to make their own *B. abortus* antigen.

B. abortus antigen and control antiserum, produced by Difco Laboratories and BBL Microbiology Systems, can be purchased through Van Waters and Rogers and American Scientific Products.

Hyland Diagnostics, Division of Travenol Laboratories, Inc., Deerfield, Ill., produces and also distributes *B. abortus* antigen and antisera.

From each of these vendors, *B. abortus* antigen can be purchased singly or as a member antigen in the Febrile Antigen Set.

If for some reason it is necessary for a laboratory to make its own antigen, a subculture of *B. abortus* 1119 can be obtained from the Communicable Diseases Center, Atlanta, Ga., or from National Animal Diseases Center, Ames, Iowa. Directions for making the antigen can be found in reference 4.

Since there has been so little demand for *B. canis* antigen for the diagnosis of human infection, it is not available commercially. It is not advisable for individual laboratories to make this antigen either. *B. canis* is of stable mucoid colonial morphology, and it is difficult to prepare a standardized antigen from it. Clinicians needing specimens examined for *B. canis* antibodies can send serum to Medical Center Clinical Laboratories, Russell Ambulatory Clinic, Birmingham, AL 35294. This laboratory will do a microtiter agglutination screening test and a mercaptoethanol tube test if the screening test is positive. The fee is $11.50.

For laboratories needing to make *B. canis* antigen, a subculture of *B. canis* can be obtained from the National Animal Diseases Center, U.S. Department of Agriculture, Ames, IA 50010. For details on making the antigen and performing the mercaptoethanol tube agglutination test, see references 1 and 2.

TEST PROCEDURES

Standard tube agglutination test

1. Do not inactivate the serum.
2. Dilute *B. abortus* antigen 1:20 (or according to the instructions of the manufacturer) with phenolized saline (0.85% NaCl containing 0.4% phenol).

TABLE 2. Contents of test tubes for standard tube agglutination test[a]

Ingredient	Tube no.									
	1	2	3	4	5	6	7	8	9	10
0.85% saline (ml)	0.9	0.5	0.5	0.5	0.5	0.5	0.5	0.5	0.5	0.5
Serum (ml)	0.1	Transfer 0.5 ml from tube 1 to tube 2 and continue serial dilution through tube 9. Discard 0.5 ml from tube 9.								—
Antigen (ml)	0.5	0.5	0.5	0.5	0.5	0.5	0.5	0.5	0.5	0.5
Final serum dilution	20	40	80	160	320	640	1,280	2,560	5,120	NA

[a] Symbols: —, no serum added; NA, not applicable.

3. Set up 10 test tubes (12 by 50 mm, with round bottoms) as shown in Table 2.

4. Set up test tubes as described in step 3, with known positive serum with a titer of at least 1:160 (minimum diagnostic titer).

5. Mix thoroughly by shaking. Incubate at 37°C for 48 h.

6. Titer is recorded as the highest dilution of serum showing complete clumping of antigen with a clear supernatant. Dilutions showing partial agglutination are recorded as I (incomplete agglutination) or Tr (trace).

Mercaptoethanol agglutination test

1. This test is performed at the same dilutions and read in the same manner as the standard tube agglutination test.

2. Serum is diluted with 0.85% NaCl containing 0.1 ml of 2-mercaptoethanol (rather than with phenolized saline). Dithiothreitol (0.005 ml in 0.85% NaCl), which does not have an offensive odor, can be used in place of the mercaptoethanol.

3. Do antigen and serum controls.

Coombs anti-human globulin test

1. Serum dilutions, prepared in phosphate-buffered saline (PBS) at pH 7.2, are the same as in the standard tube agglutination test (0.5-ml volumes).

2. Dilute B. abortus antigen 1:100, and add 0.5 ml to each tube.

3. Incubate at 37°C for 24 h.

4. Record the results, and remove tubes with serum dilutions showing either complete or partial agglutination.

5. Centrifuge the remaining tubes for 15 min at 2,000 × g.

6. Discard the supernatant, and resuspend the deposit in 0.5 ml of PBS.

7. Repeat step 6 three times.

8. Suspend the cells in 0.9 ml of PBS and add 0.1 ml of anti-human globulin. The final dilution of anti-human globulin is as recommended by the manufacturers.

9. The test is positive when at least a fourfold rise in agglutination titers occurs after treatment with anti-human globulin.

LITERATURE CITED

1. **Alton, G. G., L. M. Jones, and D. Peitz.** 1975. Laboratory techniques in brucellosis, 2nd ed. World Health Organization Monograph Series no. 55. World Health Organization, Geneva.

2. **Elberg, S. S. (ed.).** 1981. A guide to diagnosis, treatment, and prevention of human brucellosis. World Health Organization Veterinary Public Health document 81.31. World Health Organization, Geneva.

3. **Farrell, I. D., P. M. Hinchliffe, and L. Robertson.** 1975. The use of the conglutinating complement fixation test in the diagnosis of human brucellosis. J. Hyg. 74:29–33.

4. **McCullough, N. B.** 1976. Immune response to *Brucella*, p. 304–311. *In* N. R. Rose and H. Friedman (ed.), Manual of clinical immunology. American Society for Microbiology, Washington, D.C.

5. **Parrat, D., K. H. Nielsen, and R. G. White.** 1977. Radioimmunoassay of IgM, IgG, and IgA *Brucella* antibodies. Lancet i:1075–1078.

6. **Russel, A. O., C. M. Patton, and A. F. Kaufmann.** 1978. Evaluation of the card test for diagnosis of human brucellosis. J. Clin. Microbiol. 7:454–458.

Chapter 61

Serological Response to *Bordetella pertussis*

CHARLES R. MANCLARK, BRUCE D. MEADE, AND DON G. BURSTYN

The serological response following pertussis disease or immunization with pertussis vaccine has been measured with agglutination assays (13, 14, 19), precipitins (2), bactericidal assays (1), complement fixation (5, 26), and enzyme-linked immunosorbent assay (ELISA) (4, 7, 11, 12, 29, 34, 35). To date, no specific serologic procedure is available that has been proved to be a direct measure of the host's immunity to infection or disease (18). Most methods have employed either whole cells or crude extracts as the diagnostic antigen. Recently, however, highly purified components of *Bordetella pertussis* have become available, and new methods have been developed to measure the immune responses after infection or injection.

Historically the most widely used assays have been those which measure the agglutination of whole cells. The agglutination procedure is simple, inexpensive, and the assay for which the clinical significance is best understood. The newer ELISA procedures, which employ highly purified antigens from *B. pertussis*, have been designed to measure isotype-specific responses following disease and immunization with classical whole-cell or the experimental acellular pertussis vaccines.

AGGLUTINATION

Clinical Indications and Applications

The efficacy of pertussis vaccine for the prevention of whooping cough was demonstrated by the British Medical Research Council (20–22). These studies established the value of the mouse potency test for measuring vaccine potency and showed that serum agglutinin titers correlated with clinical protection. Immunization with pertussis vaccine or recovery from pertussis disease may not always result in the production of agglutinins, and immunity may exist in the absence of demonstrable agglutinins; however, disease does not occur in the presence of agglutinins of high titer (13, 25, 30). Agglutinin responses to disease were lower and more irregular than responses to immunization with whole-cell vaccine (24, 37). The production or presence of agglutinins in vaccinees is indirect evidence of vaccine potency and has been shown to be related to the protective power of a vaccine (10). Agglutination tests are of value in epidemiological studies to evaluate the immunological experience of a survey population with *B. pertussis* infection or vaccine, but they are of limited utility in the evaluation of individual clinical cases.

A variety of methods for performing agglutination tests on pertussis antisera have been proposed (10, 14, 16, 24, 36). Although the tests differ in their specifics, they have certain common characteristics. Nearly all of the methods employ a variety of expedients to ensure maximal contact of antigen and antibody. Techniques such as using concentrated reactants, shaking, water bath convection, or prolonged incubation are useful.

Since assays for pertussis antibody have their greatest application in epidemiological studies of pediatric populations, the recommended method requires small serum volumes and a minimum of manipulative procedures and demands no critically timed steps to determine accurate titration endpoints.

The choice of the diagnostic antigen is important. Most methods recommend that the antigen be prepared from a young, actively growing phase 1 culture of a *B. pertussis* strain of representative or broad antigenic coverage. In evaluating the response to vaccine, it is possible and practical to use the vaccine strain as a diagnostic agglutinating antigen, provided it is shown to be both typical and antigenically stable. For evaluations of exposure to natural infection or response to vaccines for which the origins and antigenic content are unknown, mixtures of *B. pertussis* strains to ensure broad antigenic coverage have been used, but recent experience in our laboratory has shown that diagnostic antigens prepared from a single strain and preserved by freeze-drying are stable and give results comparable to those obtained with the antigen (a mixture of *B. pertussis* strains 134 and 165) previously recommended (19).

Comparisons of results obtained by different test methods are difficult because diagnostic antigens differ qualitatively and quantitatively, as do test methods, incubation times, and endpoint determinations. The reproducibility obtained by an individual method is best controlled by use of a reference antiserum of known titer. Unless titrations are comparable and reproducible, meaningful comparisons of test results cannot be made, and the concept of using significant increases in titer (e.g., fourfold) as a measure of vaccine or disease experience is of no value (28).

The procedure outlined below is a microagglutination test requiring 0.1 ml of the patient's serum. It has been used in epidemiological studies involving large numbers of serum specimens and has been useful for titrating both pertussis immune globulin (human) and sera from individual patients. Reproducibility has been improved by using as antigen a freshly reconstituted freeze-dried suspension of a single *B. pertussis* strain of demonstrated stability, specificity, and broad antigenic coverage. Reproducibility is further controlled by use of a standard antipertussis serum. A detailed laboratory procedure is available upon request from the authors.

Test Procedure

Twofold serial dilutions of the antisera to be tested (paired sera should be tested simultaneously) are made in microagglutination plates with eight rows of 12 round-bottom wells (U plates). Saline is delivered with 0.05-ml pipettes, and the sera are diluted with 0.05-ml calibrated diluters. Place 0.05 ml of saline (0.15 M NaCl) diluent in all except the first well of each row. Add 0.1

ml of the test antiserum (inactivated at 56°C for 30 min) to the first well of each row. Using the diluter, remove 0.05 ml from the first well to the second of that row and mix; then remove 0.05 ml from the second to the third well (using same diluter), and repeat to the 11th well; then discard 0.05 ml. Repeat for each antiserum to be tested, using one row per antiserum. The 12th well contains only saline and antigen and serves as the antigen control. In addition, a titration is done with a reference or standard antiserum of known titer.

After all antiserum dilutions have been made, 0.05 ml of working antigen is added to each well. The plates are covered with plastic seals, mixed (vigorous and complete mixing by hand or with a Vortex, microshaker, or other suitable device is necessary), and incubated overnight at 35°C. Results are read with obliquely transmitted light at 5 to 10 diameters magnification or with a test-reading mirror. A negative test will appear as a thick button of cells. Complete agglutination or a 4+ reaction appears as a folded sheet of cells covering the bottom of the well. A 1+ reaction is defined as a thin sheet of cells with slight button formation and is taken as the titration endpoint. An assay is considered valid if the measured titer of the reference serum does not differ by more than one dilution from its previously established value.

Reagents

B. pertussis 460 was obtained as strain 3838 from J. Nagel of the Rijks Instituut voor de Volksgezondheid, Bilthoven, The Netherlands. Typical *B. pertussis* 460 (serotype 1.2.3.4.6), shown to be stable in saline and to meet the criteria for phase 1 organisms (15), is grown in 2,800-ml baffled Fernbach flasks containing 1,300 ml of modified Stainer-Scholte medium (33) on a platform shaker (105 rpm, 2.5-cm orbit) at 35°C for 36 to 40 h. Cells are harvested by centrifugation, and a stock cell suspension containing 1.80 mg of total Kjeldahl nitrogen per ml (equal to ca. 400 U.S. opacity units per ml) is prepared in saline containing 0.02% thimerosal and stored at 2 to 8°C. Working suspensions of cells at 0.09 mg of total Kjeldahl nitrogen per ml are made fresh each day.

Alternatively, the antigen may be preserved by freeze-drying in 3% (wt/vol) dextran (average molecular weight, 70,000). An equal volume of the stock cell suspension (containing 1.80 mg of total Kjeldahl nitrogen per ml) is mixed with an equal volume at 6% (wt/vol) dextran-saline. One milliter of the suspension is distributed to each vial, the contents are freeze-dried, and the vials are sealed under negative pressure. Reconstitution with 10 ml of saline on the day of use provides the working suspension of the antigen.

Modified Stainer and Scholte liquid medium (33)

Basal medium

L-Glutamate (monosodium salt)	10.72 g
L-Proline	0.24 g
Sodium chloride	2.50 g
Potassium phosphate (monobasic)	0.50 g
Magnesium chloride (hexahydrate)	0.10 g
Calcium chloride	0.02 g
Tris	1.52 g
Distilled water to	1,000 ml

Dissolve ingredients and adjust to pH 7.6 with concentrated hydrochloric acid. Sterilize at 121.6°C for 15 min. The medium can be stored at 2 to 8°C or at room temperature.

Supplement

L-Cystine	4.00 g
Ferrous sulfate (heptahydrate)	1.00 g
Ascorbic acid	2.00 g
Niacin	0.40 g
Glutathione (reduced)	10.00 g

Dissolve L-cystine in 120 ml of 1 N hydrochloric acid and bring to 1,000 ml with distilled water. Dissolve remaining ingredients without heating. Sterilize by membrane filtration. Store at 2 to 8°C. After basal medium has cooled, but just before use, add 10 ml of freshly prepared supplement per liter of basal medium. The addition of 1 g of Dowex 1-X8 (20 to 50 mesh) anion-exchange resin to each liter of complete medium enhances growth from small inocula.

Other materials

The following materials can be obtained from Dynatech Laboratories, Inc., Alexandria, Va.; Fisher Scientific Co., Pittsburgh, Pa.; or American Scientific Products, McGraw Park, Ill.: disposable U plates (Dynatech no. 001-010-2201); disposable pipettes, 0.05 ml (Dynatech no. 001-010-3901); calibrated diluter, 0.05 ml (Dynatech no. 001-010-1004); plate sealers, clear pressure-sensitive film (Dynatech no. 001-010- 3501); test-reading mirror (Dynatech no. 001-010-4900); microshaker (Dynatech no. 002-963-0090). (This listing is provided to show the availability of materials and does not constitute a recommendation.)

Interpretation

We have found the recommended microagglutination assay to be uncomplicated with easily determined and reproduced titration endpoints. The method employs a stable antigen of known composition and reactivity and is monitored with a reference antiserum control. Little nonspecific agglutination occurs with samples that have been inactivated at 56°C for 30 min. In the absence of recent vaccination, a significant increase in antibody titer (fourfold or greater) is supportive, but not diagnostic, of pertussis infection.

High agglutinin titers have been correlated with protection from disease (21, 25, 27, 30); in two studies, titers of 1:320 or greater were shown to be protective (25, 30). Conversely, it has been reported that protection may occur in infants with low agglutinin responses (8, 25, 30). However, these studies used a variety of agglutination methods and cannot be related quantitatively to the current procedure. No definitive study has been done to relate agglutinin titers obtained by the current method to clinical protection from pertussis. Until such a study is done, it would seem reasonable to accept the demonstration of a fourfold or greater increase in titer in at least 80% of vaccinees as acceptable evidence of potency for whole-cell vaccines.

ELISA

Clinical Indications and Applications

Filamentous hemagglutinin (FHA), lymphocytosis promoting factor (LPF), and the agglutinogens have been proposed as important protective antigens (18). Recently, two antigenically distinct types of fimbriae have been purified from *B. pertussis* and have been shown to represent at least two of the serotype-specific agglutinogens (3, 38; J. L. Cowell, unpublished data). The ELISA procedure has been used to quantitate FHA and LPF, and highly purified FHA, LPF, and fimbrial agglutinogens have been employed to measure antibodies to these antigens (3, 4, 7, 12).

Using whole *B. pertussis* cells as the antigen in an ELISA, Ruuskanen et al. (29) reported an immunoglobulin G (IgG) response but low or undetectable IgM and IgA responses in sera from vaccinees. The same ELISA method and antigen were used by Viljanen et al. (34), who demonstrated IgG, IgM, and IgA responses in sera from pertussis patients and proposed that the presence of an IgM or IgG response was evidence of recent disease (23). Goodman et al. (11) used the ELISA to detect secretory IgA in nasopharyngeal secretions during and after natural infection, but they were not able to detect IgA after vaccination.

Granström and associates (12) reported increases in IgG anti-FHA titers during pertussis and proposed that high IgG and positive IgM titers to FHA were presumptive evidence of recent infection although some patients did not manifest an IgM response. They were unable to relate IgA responses to infection.

Burstyn and colleagues (7) studied the immune response of vaccinees and patients with an ELISA procedure that used highly purified FHA and LPF and showed that children vaccinated with DTP (diphtheria and tetanus toxoids and pertussis vaccine) generally developed IgG and IgM antibodies to both antigens. An exception to this was that infants with high cord-blood IgG anti-LPF titers did not produce IgG anti-LPF when immunized with whole-cell pertussis vaccine, whereas children with low cord-blood IgG anti-LPF titers gave a good anti-LPF response (7). An IgA response was seldom detected in infants, children, adolescents, or adults after vaccination with whole-cell vaccine, whereas an IgA anti-FHA response was detected in sera from patients with disease (4, 7, 35).

Test Procedure

The principles and procedures for the ELISA are similar to the indirect method for assaying antibody described by Voller and Bidwell in chapter 17 of this volume. Antibodies to *B. pertussis* may be measured by the following method. A detailed laboratory procedure is available upon request from the authors.

1. Optimal concentrations (Appendix) or 5 μg of antigen (FHA, LPF, or fimbrial agglutinogen) per ml is diluted in coating buffer, and 50 μl is placed in wells of polystyrene microtiter plates. Plates are covered with plastic seals, and adsorption of the antigen onto the plates is allowed to proceed overnight at 28°C, preferably in a constant-temperature incubator.

2. Washing requires several cycles of adding and aspirating or removing the wash solution. The number of washes and the length of time wash solution is allowed to remain in wells depend on the efficiency of the particular washing system used. If there is excessive background in the assays, increase the number of wash cycles used.

3. Serially dilute the test serum and a positive reference serum in phosphate-buffered saline (PBS)-Brij (see below) in a second uncoated plate. Start with a 1:20 dilution, followed by eight twofold serial dilutions of the reference serum. For the test serum, four threefold dilutions starting with a 1:30 dilution are used. Transfer 50 μl of diluted serum or PBS-Brij controls to wells. Plates are sealed and incubated at 28°C for 3 h.

4. Plates are washed as described in step 2.

5. Dilute alkaline phosphatase-conjugated anti-immunoglobulin to the working dilution in PBS-Brij (Appendix). Add 50 μl to each well. Seal plates and incubate for 3 to 18 h at 28°C.

6. Wash plates as described in step 2.

7. Immediately before use, prepare a 1-mg/ml phosphatase substrate solution in substrate buffer. Add 100 μl to each well. Read absorbance at 405 nm 30 min after the addition of substrate. If necessary, the colorimetric reaction can be terminated by the addition of 10 μl of 5 M NaOH.

Calculation of ELISA Unitage

ELISA antibody units for the test sample are determined relative to the reference serum. Data for each test sample and the reference serum are plotted as log_{10} dilution versus the optical density (OD) at 405 nm (OD_{450}) (Fig. 1).

The unitage of the test serum relative to the reference serum is calculated with a parallel-line bioassay by determining the antilog difference between the x-intercepts of the reference serum and the test serum curves redrawn with parallel slopes (6). Each line is redrawn before analysis, using a calculated common slope. The unitage of the test serum is determined by multiplying its relative titer by the assigned unitage of the reference serum.

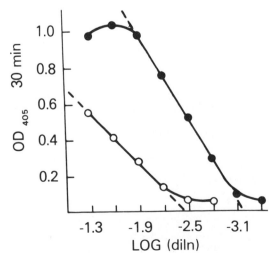

FIG. 1. Typical example of reference (●) and test (○) serum data plotted as OD_{405} versus log of serum dilution.

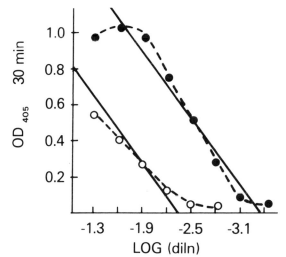

FIG. 2. The same data as in Fig. 1, with the linear position of each curve replotted according to the calculated common slope (solid line). The x-intercepts of the redrawn lines are used to calculate unitage.

The following calculations are made using only points in the linear region of each dose-response curve:

(i) Mean OD = $\bar{X}$ = $\Sigma(Xi)/n$ (n = number of points used)

Mean log dilution = $\bar{Y}$ = $(\Sigma Yi)/n$

(ii) $A_1 = \Sigma(Xi - \bar{X})^2$

$A_2 = \Sigma(Yi - \bar{Y})^2$

$A_3 = \Sigma(Xi - \bar{X})(Yi - \bar{Y})$

(iii) Slope = $M = A_3/A_1$

(iv) Correlation coefficients = $R = \dfrac{A_3}{\sqrt{A_1 A_2}}$

(v) Variance = $V = (A_2 - M^2 A_1)/(n - 2)$

Data for reference *(r)* and a test sample *(t)* are pooled, and the following calculations are made:

(i) Pooled variance = $V_p = [(n_r - 2)V_r + (n_t - 2)V_t]/(n_r + n_t - 4)$

(ii) $C = 1/(A_1)_r + 1/(A_1)_t$

(iii) $E = \sqrt{VC}$

(iv) $T = (M_r - M_t)/E$ df = $n_r + n_t - 4$

Calculated values must meet the following criteria:

(i) Correlation coefficients *(R)* ≥ 0.8

(ii) T < tabulated t values at $P = 0.1$ (consult standard statistical text for values)

(iii) Slope (M_t) > 0.01

If all criteria are met, unitage is calculated by the parallel-line bioassay method, as follows.

Parallel-line bioassay method

The linear portions of the reference and test sera dose-response curves are redrawn using a common, pooled slope (Fig. 2).

Pooled slope = $M_p = [(A_3)_r + (A_3)_t]/[(A_1)_r + (A_1)_t]$

New intercepts = B:

$B_{yr} = \bar{Y}_r - M_p\bar{X}_r$ $B_{yt} = \bar{Y}_t - M_p\bar{X}_t$

$B_{xr} = -B_{yr}/M_p$ $B_{xt} = -B_{yt}/M_p$

Log_{10} (relative potency) = $W = B_{xr} - B_{xt}$

Relative potency = 10^W

Potency = (relative potency) × (units contained in reference serum)

Parallel line: single-point method

If the test sample is either very high or low in potency relative to the reference (Fig. 3), and any of the criteria for the use of the parallel-line bioassay method have not been satisfied, the single-point method can be used. Sera with high unitage can also be reassayed at higher dilutions.

The values calculated above for the reference are used to calculate x- and y-intercepts.

$B_{yr} = \bar{Y}_r - M_r\bar{X}_r$

$B_{xr} = -B_{yr}/M_r$

For samples of low potency, the absorbance (OD_t) of the initial dilution is used to calculate potency. For samples of high potency, the OD_t of the last dilution is used to calculate potency. The x- and y-intercepts for the test samples are calculated as follows:

$B_{yt} = OD_t - M_r [\log (\text{diln})_t]$

$B_{xt} = B_{yt}/M_r$

Log_{10} (relative potency) = $W = (B_{xr} - B_{xt})$

Relative potency = 10^W

Potency = (relative potency) × (units contained in reference serum)

Equipment and Materials

Buffers

0.1 M Carbonate buffer, pH 9.6 (coating buffer)

Na_2CO_3	1.59 g
$NaHCO_3$	2.93 g
Distilled water to	1,000 ml

0.1 M PBS, pH 7.4 (10× PBS)

NaCl	85.00 g
Na_2HPO_4	11.93 g
Distilled water to	1,000 ml

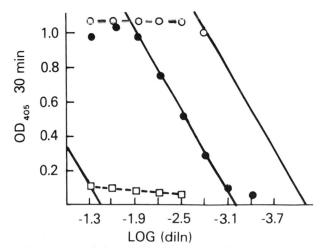

FIG. 3. Use of the single-point parallel-line method to calculate ELISA unitage of samples where there is evidence of lack of parallelism between the slopes of the linear portion of the reference serum (●) and a test serum. For sera of low unitage (□) the OD_{405} at the least dilute sample is used. For sera of high unitage (○) the OD_{405} at the most dilute sample is used.

0.01 M PBS, pH 7.4

Dilute 10× PBS 1:10 in distilled water.

10× PBS + 1% Brij 35 (10× PBS-Brij)

10× PBS	96.7 ml
Brij 35 (Sigma; 30%, wt/vol)	3.3 ml

PBS + 0.1% Brij 35 (PBS-Brij)

10× PBS	200 ml
Distilled water	1,800 ml
Brij 35 (30%, wt/vol)	6.7 ml

0.1 M Sodium phosphate, pH 6.8 (0.1 M Na_2HPO_4)

Na_2HPO_4	14.2 g
Distilled water	800 ml

Adjust pH to 6.8 with 6 N HCl.

Distilled water to	1,000 ml

1 M Tris + 0.3 mM $MgCl_2$, pH 9.8 (substrate buffer)

Tris	121.1 g
Distilled water	700 ml
$MgCl_2$ (1 M)	0.3 ml

Adjust pH to 9.8 with 6 N HCl.

Distilled water to	1,000 ml

Solutions

10% (wt/vol) Bovine serum albumin

Bovine serum albumin, Sigma fraction V	2 g
PBS to	20 ml

Note: Make fresh daily.

2% Glutaraldehyde

Glutaraldehyde, 25%, electron microscopy grade	1.0 ml
0.1 M Na_2HPO_4	11.5 ml

Note: Make fresh daily. Keep in ice bath.

1 M Magnesium chloride (1 M $MgCl_2$)

$MgCl_2 \cdot 6H_2O$	20.33 g
Distilled water to	100 ml

0.85% Saline + Brij 35 (washing solution)

NaCl	17 g
Distilled water to	2,000 ml
Brij 35 (30%, wt/vol)	6.7 m

Note: Tween 20 may be substituted for Brij 35.

60% Saturated ammonium sulfate

$(NH_4)SO_4$	39 g
Distilled water	100 ml

90% Saturated ammonium sulfate

$(NH_4)_2SO_4$	66.2 g
Distilled water	100 ml

2% Sodium azide (2% NaN_3)

NaN_3	2 g
Distilled water to	100 ml

Chemicals and Reagents

6 N HCl
0.1 N NaOH
Ready-made conjugates may be obtained from numerous commercial sources or prepared as outlined in chapter 17.
Sigma 104 phosphatase substrate (*p*-nitrophenyl phosphate)
Alkaline phosphatase, Sigma type VII-T
Class-specific antiserum (e.g., goat anti-human IgA, goat anti-mouse IgG)
ELISA reference serum can be obtained from the authors.
Methods for the preparation of filamentous hemagglutinin and lymphocytosis promoting factor and criteria for purity are provided by Cowell et al. (9), Sato et al. (31), and Sekura et al. (32).

Equipment

96-Well polystyrene microtiter plates (e.g., Immulon, Dynatech Labs) or 3-ml polystyrene tubes or disposable polystyrene cuvettes (Starstedt)
Collodion bag apparatus
Collodion bag (dialysis tubing can be used instead)
Centrifuge (microcentrifuge if available)
Spectrophotometer or microtiter plate reader if using microtiter plates

Sources

The following companies supply equipment and materials for ELISA: Dynatech Laboratories, Inc., Alexandria, Va.; Falcon Plastics, Becton Dickinson and Co., Oxnard, Calif.; Schleicher & Schuell, Inc., Keene, N.H.; Sigma Chemical Co., St. Louis, Mo.; and Starstedt, Inc., Princeton, N.J. (This listing is provided to show the availability of materials and does not constitute a recommendation.)

Interpretation

The ELISA has been used to assess the immune response to infection with *B. pertussis* or injection with pertussis vaccine.

During clinical pertussis, IgG, IgM, and IgA serum anti-*B. pertussis* titers increase, although there may not be a coincidental increase in all three isotypes. A rise in IgM antibody titer is indicative of recent exposure to antigen and is observed in vaccinees and in individuals exposed to infection or with symptoms of disease (17). IgG titers also rise after vaccination, in those with pertussis, and in those who have been exposed to disease but have no overt clinical symptoms (35). IgA titers are associated with disease. IgA titers seldom rise above background levels after vaccination or in those without symptoms of pertussis.

Base-line ELISA titers probably vary with age, vaccination history, and the epidemiologic patterns of a region. Anti-FHA IgG and IgM and anti-LPF IgG and IgM titers may rise after each dose of vaccine. IgG antibodies found in infants' sera before vaccination are usually due to passively transferred maternal antibodies.

Comparisons of the results of ELISAs done in different laboratories have been hampered by the lack of standardization of reference sera, test protocols, and the methods of calculating results. The procedure described here utilizes highly purified reagents, a defined assay protocol, a single reference serum, and a standardized method for calculating results and provides reproducible estimates of the serological response to *B. pertussis* (4, 7).

APPENDIX
ELISA

Determination of optimal antigen concentrations for coating

Run ELISA with the following modifications.

Adsorption. Make six twofold serial dilutions of coating antigen in coating buffer. The initial dilution should result in a protein concentration of 10 µg/ml. Coat duplicate wells with each dilution.

Addition of sample. Add positive reference serum to all wells at a 1:100 dilution in PBS-Brij.

Addition of conjugate. Use optimal dilution of conjugate found below.

Addition of substrate. Read after 30 min. Graph OD versus log (antigen concentration). The antigen concentration giving an OD of 1.0 is the "working antigen concentration."

Determination of optimal conjugate dilution

Run ELISA with the following modifications.

Adsorption. Coat plate with antigen at optimal concentration if known, or at 5 µg/ml if unknown.

Addition of sample. Add positive reference serum to all wells at a 1:100 dilution in PBS-Brij.

Addition of conjugate. Make six twofold serial dilutions of conjugate in PBS-Brij. The initial dilution of conjugate should be 1:50. Add samples to duplicate wells. Incubate for 3 h and wash as usual.

Addition of substrate. Read absorbance after 30 min. Graph OD versus log of conjugate dilution. The conjugate dilution giving an OD of 1.0 is the "working dilution of conjugate."

LITERATURE CITED

1. **Ackers, J. P., and J. M. Dolby.** 1972. The antigen of *Bordetella pertussis* that induces bactericidal antibody and its relationship to protection of mice. J. Gen. Microbiol. **70:**371–382.
2. **Aftandelians, R., and J. D. Conner.** 1973. Immunologic studies of pertussis. Development of precipitins. J. Pediatr. **83:**206–214.
3. **Ashworth, L. A. E., A. Robinson, L. I. Irons, C. P. Morgan, and D. Isaacs.** 1983. Antigens in whooping cough vaccine and antibody levels induced by vaccination of children. Lancet **ii:**878–881.
4. **Baraff, L. J., R. D. Leake, D. G. Burstyn, T. Payne, C. L. Cody, C. R. Manclark, and J. W. St. Geme, Jr.** 1983.

Immunologic response to early and routine DTP immunization in infants. Pediatrics **73:**37–42.
5. **Bradstreet, C. M. P., A. J. Tannahill, J. M. B. Edwards, and P. F. Benson.** 1972. Detection of *Bordetella pertussis* antibodies in human sera by complement-fixation and immunofluorescence. J. Hyg. **70:**75–83.
6. **Brownlee, K. A.** 1965. Statistical theory and methodology in science and engineering, 2nd ed. p. 334–396. John Wiley & Sons, Inc., New York.
7. **Burstyn, D. G., L. J. Baraff, M. S. Peppler, R. D. Leake, J. St. Geme, Jr., and C. R. Manclark.** 1983. Serological response to filamentous hemagglutinin and lymphocytosis-promoting toxin of *Bordetella pertussis*. Infect. Immun. **41:**1150–1156.
8. **Butler, N. R., B. D. R. Wilson, P. F. Bensen, J. A. Dudgeon, J. Ungar, and A. J. Beale.** 1962. Response of infants to pertussis vaccine at one week and to poliomyelitis, diphtheria, and tetanus vaccine at six months. Lancet **ii:**112–114.
9. **Cowell, J. L., Y. Sato, H. Sato, B. An der Lan, and C. R. Manclark.** 1982. Separation, purification, and properties of the filamentous hemagglutinin and leukocytosis promoting factor-hemagglutinin from *Bordetella pertussis*. Semin. Infect. Dis. **4:**371–397.
10. **Evans, D. G., and F. T. Perkins.** 1953. An agglutinin-production test in the study of pertussis vaccine. J. Pathol. Bacteriol. **66:**479–488.
11. **Goodman, Y. E., A. J. Wort, and F. L. Jackson.** 1981. Enzyme-linked immunosorbent assay for detection of pertussis immunoglobulin A in nasopharyngeal secretions as an indicator of recent infection. J. Clin. Microbiol. **13:**286–292.
12. **Granström, M., A. A. Lindberg, P. Askelöf, and B. Hederstedt.** 1982. Detection of antibodies in human serum against the fimbrial haemagglutinin of *Bordetella pertussis* by enzyme-linked immunosorbent assay. J. Med. Microbiol. **15:**85–96.
13. **Kendrick, P. L., R. Y. Gottshall, H. D. Anderson, V. K. Volk, W. E. Bunney, and F. H. Top.** 1969. Pertussis agglutinins in adults. Public Health Rep. **84:**9–15.
14. **Kendrick, P.** 1933. Rapid agglutination technique applied to *H. pertussis* agglutination. Am. J. Public Health **23:**1310–1312.
15. **Kloos, W. E., W. J. Dobrogosz, J. W. Ezzell, B. R. Kimbro, and C. R. Manclark.** 1979. DNA-DNA hybridization, plasmids, and genetic exchange in the genus *Bordetella*, p 70–80. *In* C. R. Manclark and J. C. Hill (ed.), International symposium on pertussis. DHEW (NIH) 79-1830. U.S. Government Printing Office, Washington, D.C.
16. **Macaulay, M.** 1979. The serological diagnosis of whooping cough. J. Hyg. **83:**95–102.
17. **Macaulay, M. E.** 1981. The IgM and IgG response to *Bordetella pertussis* vaccination and infection. J. Med. Microbiol. **14:**1–7.
18. **Manclark, C. R., and J. L. Cowell.** 1984. Pertussis, p. 69–106. *In* R. Germanier (ed.), Bacterial vaccines. Academic Press, Inc., New York.
19. **Manclark, C. R., and B. D. Meade.** 1980. Serological response to *Bordetella pertussis*, p. 496–499. *In* N. R. Rose and H. Friedman (ed.), Manual of clinical immunology, 2nd ed. American Society for Microbiology, Washington, D.C.
20. **Medical Research Council.** 1951. Prevention of whooping cough by vaccination. Br. Med. J. **1:**1463–1471.
21. **Medical Research Council.** 1956. Vaccination against whooping cough: relation between protection in children and results of laboratory tests. Br. Med. J. **2:**454–462.
22. **Medical Research Council.** 1959. Vaccination against whooping cough: final report to Whooping Cough Immunization Committee. Br. Med. J. **1:**994–1000.

23. **Mertsola, J., O. Ruuskanen, T. Kuronen, and M. D. Viljanen.** 1983. Serologic diagnosis of pertussis: comparison of enzyme-linked immunosorbent assay and bacterial agglutination. J. Infect. Dis. **147:**252–257.

24. **Miller, J. J., and R. J. Silverberg.** 1939. The agglutinative reaction in relation to pertussis and prophylactic vaccination against pertussis with description of a new technique. J. Immunol. **37:**207–221.

25. **Miller, J. J., R. J. Silverberg, T. M. Saito, and J. B. Humber.** 1943. An agglutinative reaction for *Haemophilus pertussis*. II. Its relation to clinical immunity. J. Pediatr. **22:**644–651.

26. **Mishulow, L., M. Siegel, M. Leifer, and S. Kerkey.** 1942. A study of pertussis antibodies. Am. J. Dis. Child. **63:**875–880.

27. **Preston, N. W.** 1970. Pertussis agglutinins in the child. International Symposium on Pertussis, Bilthoven, 1969. Symp. Ser. Immunbiol. Stand. **13:**121–125.

28. **Preston, N. W., and T. N. Stanbridge.** 1975. Whooping cough vaccination. Lancet **i:**1089.

29. **Ruuskanen, O., M. K. Viljanen, T. T. Salmi, O. P. Lehtonen, K. Kouvalainen, and T. Peltonen.** 1980. DTP and DTP-inactivated polio vaccines: comparison of adverse reactions and IgG, IgM and IgA antibody responses to DTP. Acta Paediatr. Scand. **69:**177–182.

30. **Sako, W.** 1947. Studies on pertussis immunization. J. Pediatr. **30:**29–40.

31. **Sato, Y., J. L. Cowell, H. Sato, D. G. Burstyn, and C. R. Manclark.** 1983. Separation and purification of hemagglutinins from *Bordetella pertussis*. Infect. Immun. **41:**313–320.

32. **Sekura, R. D., F. Fish, C. R. Manclark, B. Meade, and Y. Zhang.** 1983. Pertussis toxin: affinity purification of a new ADP-ribosyltransferase. J. Biol. Chem. **258:**14647–14651.

33. **Stainer, D. W., and M. J. Scholte.** 1970. A simple chemically defined medium for the production of phase I *Bordetella pertussis*. J. Gen. Microbiol. **63:**211–220.

34. **Viljanen, M. K., O. Ruuskanen, C. Granberg, and T. T. Salmi.** 1982. Serological diagnosis of pertussis: IgM, IgA and IgG antibodies against *Bordetella pertussis* measured by enzyme-linked immunosorbent assay (ELISA). Scand. J. Infect. Dis. **14:**117–122.

35. **Wassilak, S., G. Smith, P. Garbe, D. Burstyn, C. Manclark, and W. Orenstein.** 1983. Pertussis outbreak in Colorado: use of a newly-developed diagnostic test, p. 37–41. *In* R. F. Campolucci (ed.), 18th Immunization Conference proceedings. Centers for Disease Control, Atlanta.

36. **Wilkins, J., F. F. Williams, P. F. Wherle, and B. Portnoy.** 1971. Agglutinin response to pertussis vaccine. I. Effect of dosage and interval. J. Pediatr. **79:**197–202.

37. **Winter, J. L.** Development of antibodies in children convalescent from whooping cough. Proc. Soc. Exp. Biol. Med. **83:**866–870.

38. **Zhang, J. M., J. L. Cowell, A. C. Steven, P. H. Carter, P. P. McGrath, and C. R. Manclark.** 1985. Purification and characterization of fimbriae isolated from *Bordetella pertussis*. Infect. Immun. **48:**422–427.

Chapter 62

Serodiagnosis of *Legionella pneumophila* Disease

HAZEL W. WILKINSON

The indirect immunofluorescence assay (IFA) has been used to detect the immune response to *Legionella pneumophila* and, therefore, to provide serologic evidence of legionellosis since 1977, when the etiologic agent of Legionnaires disease was first described (1, 9). For several years this test was the most often used laboratory test for legionellosis because of the inability of the organism to compete with normal flora when it was cultured on artificial media and because of the invasive techniques often required to obtain a specimen suitable for direct immunofluorescence staining or to obtain an uncontaminated specimen for culturing. Subsequent improvement of selective enrichment media and their commercial availability have somewhat lessened the dependence on serologic testing, but it is still useful when tissue specimens or body fluids other than serum are unavailable for demonstration of the bacteria or their soluble antigens.

The humoral immune response to *Legionella* infection is multiple (8). Sera from patients can have various combinations of antibodies that are serogroup specific, *Legionella* common antigen specific, and nonspecific (8). The nonspecific antibodies react with a variety of gram-negative bacteria but do not lower the specificity of the test at the recommended cutoff levels when sera from patients with pneumonia are tested (7). Both specific and nonspecific IFA titers can be the result of immunoglobulin G (IgG), IgM, and IgA responses, either singly or combined. Therefore, serologic tests for legionellosis must detect all immunoglobulin classes for optimal test sensitivity. It is not necessary to distinguish IgM from IgG titers, as both immunoglobulin classes reach detectable levels concurrently, and both can remain elevated in sera from convalescent patients for months or even several years after the initial episode of pneumonia (4). The IFA remains the reference test of choice because it can detect all antibody classes, and, perhaps more importantly, it is the only serologic test for antibody that has been adequately standardized (7). Enzyme-linked immunosorbent assays and the FIAX test compare favorably with the IFA (3, 4) and are suitable alternatives for laboratories equipped to perform them. Agglutination tests measure primarily IgM antibody; therefore, they may lack sufficient sensitivity for immunodiagnostic assays.

CLINICAL INDICATIONS

Patients with suspected Legionnaires disease

Several tests are available for the laboratory diagnosis of legionellosis. Serologic tests should be used only if specimens are unavailable for culturing or for identifying the bacteria in situ, or if the latter tests give negative results for *Legionella* species and other common causes of pneumonia. Serology is the last method of choice because it furnishes data only retrospectively, weeks past the acute stage of illness. Furthermore, titers cannot be used to determine the serogroup or species of the infecting *Legionella* strain because common surface antigens are shared by multiple species. The primary value of serologic testing is to provide a confirmatory diagnosis of legionellosis during the patient's convalescence when other tests have failed to do so earlier. For these patients, acute- and convalescent-phase sera should be drawn 3 to 6 weeks apart and should be tested simultaneously with the IFA or with an alternative test that has been standardized or that gives test results comparable to those obtained with the reference IFA. Seroconversion to an IFA titer of at least 128 is considered evidence of recent Legionnaires disease (see below). For patients with pneumonia, the specificity and reproducibility of the test were estimated to be 99 and 98%, respectively (7). For patients with other clinical manifestations, the specificity of the test is unknown. Sensitivity has been estimated for serology, direct immunofluorescence, culture, and antigen detection tests, but these estimates are relative to sample selection based on the same tests being evaluated. The state of the art of these tests and the expertise of the laboratories at the time of the evaluations may have also been pertinent factors. Predictive values have been difficult to estimate for the same reasons.

Surveys in epidemic investigations or normal populations

The IFA can be a valuable adjunct to epidemiologic investigation of possible outbreaks of Legionnaires disease. The same criteria can be used to confirm epidemic and sporadic cases: seroconversion to a titer of ≥128 for patients with pneumonia. In addition, single or standing titers of ≥256 are often used to define possible cases if paired sera or appropriately timed sera are unavailable. The significance of these titers must be determined with the appropriate epidemiologic controls, which are especially important if antigens have not been standardized or if sera are from individuals who do not have pneumonia, e.g., those with flulike symptoms described as Pontiac fever by epidemiologic criteria. The etiology of Pontiac fever has never been documented by culture or by direct immunofluorescence from patient specimens, and the possibility remains that IFA titers in the sera of these patients are the result of polyclonal activation of the immune response by unrelated organisms (especially for those with low titers) or the result of antibodies to cross-reactive antigens.

Serosurveys of "normal" populations to determine past exposure to or infection with *Legionella* species are impractical and are not likely to yield useful or new information. The bacteria are ubiquitous in fresh water, both in natural reservoirs and in heat dissemination systems. The prevalence of IFA titers of ≥128 against the *L. pneumophila* serogroup 1 antigen has varied from 0.1 to 20.0% in well populations in the United States and Europe (5). Whether this variance is because of differences in exposure cannot be determined with available data. Twelve percent of a sample of sera from the United States had IFA titers of ≥256 against one or more antigens prepared with multiple *Legionella* species (10). At least some of the titers may have been the result of antibodies against nonspecific antigens, as the organisms share surface antigens with other gram-negative bacteria.

Legionella species and serogroups

Results of testing reference specimens by direct immunofluorescence assay suggest that *L. pneumophila* serogroup 1 is the most prevalent cause of *Legionella* pneumonia (5). Eight additional serogroups of *L. pneumophila* and 10 additional *Legionella* species have been described, with two serogroups each within *L. bozemanii* and *L. longbeachae*. Multiple serogroups have not yet been described for *L. dumoffii*, *L. gormanii*, *L. micdadei*, *L. jordanis*, *L. oakridgensis*, *L. wadsworthii*, *L. feeleii*, or *L. sainthelensi*. Additional subtypes within *L. pneumophila* serogroup 1 have been defined with monoclonal antibodies (2). Because of the multiple antibody response in humans to serogroup, serotype, and species antigens of this expanding list of legionellae, different serogroup antigens, different strains within the same serogroup, different methods of preparing the antigen, and differences in conjugate specificity can cause discrepant serologic test results (6).

INTERPRETATION

A fourfold or greater increase in titer to ≥128 against a heat-killed antigen of *L. pneumophila* serogroup 1 in sera obtained in the acute (onset date ± 1 week) and the convalescent (3 to 6 weeks after onset) phases of pneumonia provides serologic evidence of Legionnaires disease. A single or standing titer of ≥256 has generally been accepted as presumptive evidence of infection at an undetermined time, but even this cautious definition is not very useful because of high background levels of antibody in some population groups. Even if the antibody level in an indigenous population is known, the significance of a single titer is tenuous because of the persistence of antibody in many patients for months or years after onset.

Data supporting the validity of this interpretation were obtained with *L. pneumophila* serogroup 1 antigens, including the Philadelphia 1 strain used in the IFA. The same interpretation may be valid for determining the immunologic response to disease caused by other serogroups and species of *Legionella*, because titers of a similar magnitude against the other *Legionella* antigens are measured occasionally in sera from patients with suspected legionellosis. Insufficient numbers of sera have been available from patients with proven legionellosis due to these organisms to validate this assumption.

When tests are performed and interpreted in nonreference laboratories (e.g., commercial laboratories), the submitter should ask for sufficient documentation of the performance of the test relative to a standardized test and should be especially suspicious when laboratories claim a "positive" test result for any of the following: titers obtained against non-*L. pneumophila* antigens, single or standing titers in the absence of seroconversion, seroconversions to levels of <128, and seroconversions claimed for paired sera not tested at the same time and with the same reagents.

REAGENTS

Bacterial antigen

Any work with the live organism that may generate aerosols should be done in a biological safety cabinet. The reference IFA strain for *L. pneumophila* serogroup 1 is strain Philadelphia 1 (ATCC 33152).

1. Inoculate the organism heavily onto a slant of buffered charcoal-yeast extract agar (screw-capped test tube [20 by 150 mm] containing 10 ml of medium). Incubate the loosely capped agar tube at 35°C until good growth occurs (approximately 2 days).

2. Add 2 ml of sterile distilled water to the tube. Gently rub the growth off the slant with a Pasteur pipette, and transfer the suspension to a screw-capped test tube.

3. Place the tube containing the cell suspension in a boiling-water bath for 15 min to kill the cells.

4. Streak a buffered charcoal-yeast extract agar plate to confirm cell death. Use 0.1 ml of the cell suspension and the same medium and incubation conditions as in step 1. Observe for growth for at least 10 days to assure that the antigen is sterile, but proceed immediately to step 5.

5. Pack the cells by centrifugation (2,000 × *g* for about 5 min in a tabletop clinical centrifuge). Discard the supernatant fluid. Resuspend the bacterial sediment in 2 ml of sterile distilled water (concentrated antigen suspension).

6. Make working dilutions of the concentrated antigen suspension in 0.5% normal chicken yolk sac in sterile distilled water. It is generally best to try several antigen dilutions in the 1:20-to-1:80 range in the IFA. High concentrations of bacterial cells can reduce titers because proportionally fewer antibody molecules are bound per bacterial cell, and low concentrations make slide reading difficult because there are too few fields of cells and too few cells per field. Most antigens are dispersed optimally at a dilution of 1:50 (optical density 0.08 to 0.10 at 660 nm with a 1-cm light path, or approximately 500 to 600 organisms per microscopic field at a magnification of ×315).

7. Add the preservative sodium azide (NaN_3), to a concentration of 0.05%.

8. Store antigens at 4°C. They are stable for at least 2 months.

Glycerol mounting medium

Combine 1 part of 0.5 M carbonate-bicarbonate buffer (pH 9.0) and 9 parts of neutral glycerol (reagent grade), and mix by stirring (do not shake). Check the pH often. Oxidation of glycerol causes a drop in pH which quenches fluorescein isothiocyanate fluorescence.

Carbonate-bicarbonate buffer, pH 9.0, 0.5 M

Stock solutions: (A) 5.3 g of Na_2CO_3 per 100 ml of distilled water; (B) 4.2 g of $NaHCO_3$ per 100 ml of distilled water.

Working solution: combine 4.4 ml of stock solution A and 100.0 ml of stock solution B; if the pH is below 9.0, continue to add solution A until the working solution is pH 9.0.

Phosphate-buffered saline, pH 7.6, 0.01 M

Stock solution: 12.4 g of Na_2HPO_4, 1.8 g of $NaH_2PO_4 \cdot H_2O$, and 85.0 g of NaCl per liter of distilled water.

Working solution: dilute stock solution 1:10 in distilled water, and adjust the pH to 7.6, if necessary.

Buffered chicken yolk sac suspension, 3%

Mix equal volumes of yolk sacs (from 12- to 14-day embryonated eggs, approximately 4 g of yolk sac per egg, separated as much as possible from yolk material) and phosphate-buffered saline (PBS; pH 7.6, 0.02 M) containing 0.05% sodium azide. Homogenize in an Omnimixer or Waring blender. Filter the suspension through two layers of sterile gauze, and then dilute with PBS containing azide to 0.5% for antigen preparation or to 3% for serum diluent.

Commercial availability

Several manufacturers have begun selling *Legionella* IFA reagents, some of which have been evaluated and found to be satisfactory by the Centers for Disease Control. For current information on commercial reagents that meet Centers for Disease Control specifications, contact: Chief, Evaluation Branch, Biological Products Program, Center for Infectious Diseases, Centers for Disease Control, Altanta, GA 30333.

IFA

Preparation of antigen slides

1. Mix thoroughly the working dilution of the heat-killed antigen suspension. With a Pasteur pipette, apply enough antigen to each well of a microscope slide to cover the well with the antigen; remove the excess liquid with the same pipette (e.g., acetone-resistant glass slide [25 by 75 mm] with 12 staggered wells 5 mm in diameter; Cel-Line Associates, Inc., Newfield, N.J.).
2. Allow the slide to air dry (may take up to 30 min).
3. Fix the antigen smears to the slide by placing the slide in an acetone bath for 15 min.
4. Allow the slide to air dry.
5. If the slide is to be stored for future use, place it in a freezer at $-20°C$. Frozen slides are stable for at least 2 months.

Titration of sera

1. Prepare a 1:16 dilution of the serum in 3.0% normal chicken yolk sac suspended in PBS (pH 7.6, 0.01 M). Make subsequent doubling dilutions through

1:2,048 in PBS. Large numbers of sera can be diluted expeditiously by using rigid polystyrene U-bottomed microtitration trays (Linbro Div., Flow Laboratories, Inc., Hamden, Conn.; Dynatech Laboratories, Inc., Alexandria, Va.) and an automatic diluter (Dynatech). Place 0.01 ml of serum in a test tube containing 0.15 ml of normal chicken yolk sac suspension, and make subsequent twofold dilutions in wells on the microtitration tray, using PBS and 0.05-ml volumes. Alternatively, replace the automatic diluter with hand diluters, or make all dilutions in test tubes.
2. Using a Pasteur pipette, place a drop of each serum dilution from 1:64 to 1:2,048 (or to 1:256 if sera are being screened first) in its well of fixed antigen on a slide. Incubate the slide in a moist chamber (e.g., a petri dish containing moist filter paper) at 37°C for 30 min.
3. Rinse the slide quickly with PBS and place it in a PBS bath for 10 min. Remove the slide from the bath and either air dry or very gently blot dry.
4. Place a drop (approximately 20 µl) of fluorescein isothiocyanate-labeled anti-human immunoglobulin (conjugate) in each well. The conjugate must have reactivity with IgG, IgM, and IgA. Incubate as described above for 30 min.
5. Rinse the slide quickly with PBS, place it in a PBS bath for 10 min, rinse it quickly with water, and air dry or very gently blot dry.
6. Add several drops of buffered glycerol to the slide and mount with a cover slip (no 1; 24 by 60 mm). (Check the pH of the buffered glycerol mounting fluid frequently; the fluid should not be used if the pH is below 8.)
7. Read the slides on a fluorescence microscope.
8. The titer is recorded as the reciprocal of the highest dilution of serum that gives 1+ fluorescence intensity.

Controls

1. Human or simian serum having a specified titer of ≥256 should be used as a control for IFA. For the test to be considered valid, the titer obtained with the control serum should not vary more than twofold from the titer specified for that serum.
2. To test for nonspecific binding of the conjugate, substitute PBS for serum. If bacterial cells are visible, the fluorescence intensity must be <1+ (see below).
3. To test for autofluorescence of the bacteria (visible with some filter systems), substitute PBS for serum but with no added conjugate.

Fluorescence microscopy

Scoring of fluorescence intensities. Fluorescence intensities are scored as follows: 4+ = brilliant yellow-green staining of bacterial cells; 3+ = bright yellow-green staining; 2+ = definite but dim staining; 1+ = barely visible staining; − = no staining. Disregard staining of filamentous cells and of cells on or adjacent to fluorescent yolk sac material. The dim autofluorescence of the cells that can occur with some filter systems should not be interpreted as specific staining. The PBS control without conjugate can be used as a guide.

Microscope assemblies. A fluorescence microscope, preferably with epi-illumination, equipped for fluorescein isothiocyanate excitation should be used. Example: Leitz Dialux 20 fluorescence microscope equipped with an HBO-100 mercury incident light source; the Leitz I-cube filter system (2 × KP490 and a 1-mm GG 455 primary filter, TK510 dichroic beam-splitting mirror, and K515 secondary filter), ×40 dry objective, and ×6.3 eyepieces (magnification, ×315) (Leitz/Opto-Metric Div. of E. Leitz Inc., Rockleigh, N.J.). Titers can vary with different microscopes, but the variation can often be compensated for by changing the magnification, light source, or filters.

Quality assurance

If titers of control sera vary from the expected by more than twofold, check and correct the following.
1. Fluorescence microscope lamp. Mercury arc lamps can "fade out" toward the end of their expected number of useful hours.
2. pH of the buffered glycerol mounting medium, buffer, conjugate, normal chicken yolk sac, and distilled water. An acid pH causes quenching of fluorescein isothiocyanate fluorescence.
3. Clarity of conjugate and sera. Contaminants can degrade immunoglobulins.
4. Freezers and refrigerators used to store sera and reagents. Repeated fluctuations in temperature can denature proteins.
5. Fluorescence microscope lamp mount flexible current lead. Excessive heat buildup can eventually fray and then break the bundle of wires. When the wires are frayed but not yet separated completely, the diminished light intensity can cause perceived lower serum titers.
6. Control serum. If a different control serum gives its expected titer, the first control may no longer be satisfactory.

Present status of standardization

The *Legionella* IFA has been standardized as a diagnostic test only for patients with *L. pneumophila* serogroup 1 pneumonia (i.e., Legionnaires disease), as insufficient numbers of sera have been available from patients with well-documented infections due to other serogroups or species, or with clinical manifestations other than pneumonia. The antigens that have been standardized for this purpose are the *L. pneumophila* serogroup 1 strain, Philadelphia 1, and a polyvalent antigen containing serogroups 1 through 4.

ADDENDUM IN PROOF

Since this chapter was written, 11 additional *Legionella* species have been described, for a total of 22 species comprising 33 serogroups (W. L. Thacker, B. B. Plikaytis, and H. W. Wilkinson, J. Clin. Microbiol. **21**:779–782, 1985).

LITERATURE CITED

1. **McDade, J. E., C. C. Shepard, D. W. Fraser, T. R. Tsai, M. A. Redus, W. R. Dowdle, and the Laboratory Investigation Team.** 1977. Legionnaires' disease. Isolation of a bacterium and demonstration of its role in other respiratory disease. N. Engl. J. Med. **297**:1197–1203.
2. **McKinney, R. M., W. L. Thacker, D. E. Wells, M. C. Wong, W. J. Jones, and W. F. Bibb.** 1983. Monoclonal antibodies to *Legionella pneumophila* serogroup 1: possible applications in diagnostic tests and epidemiologic studies. Zentralbl. Bakteriol. Parasitenkd. Infektionskr. Hyg. Abt. I Orig. Reihe A **255**:91–95.
3. **Sampson, J. S., H. W. Wilkinson, V. C. W. Tsang, and B. J. Brake.** 1983. Kinetic-dependent enzyme-linked immunosorbent assay for detection of antibodies to *Legionella pneumophila*. J. Clin. Microbiol. **18**:1340–1344.
4. **Wilkinson, H. W.** 1982. Serologic diagnosis of legionellosis. Lab. Med. **13**:151–157.
5. **Wilkinson, H. W.** 1983. Status of serologic tests for *Legionella* antigen and antibody at the Centers for Disease Control. Zentralbl. Bakteriol. Parasitenkd. Infektionskr. Hyg. Abt. I Orig. Reihe A **255**:3–7.
6. **Wilkinson, H. W., and B. J. Brake.** 1982. Formalin-killed versus heat-killed *Legionella pneumophila* serogroup 1 antigen in the indirect immunofluorescence assay for legionellosis. J. Clin. Microbiol. **16**:979–981.
7. **Wilkinson, H. W., D. D. Cruce, and C. V. Broome.** 1981. Validation of *Legionella pneumophila* indirect immunofluorescence assay with epidemic sera. J. Clin. Microbiol. **13**:139–146.
8. **Wilkinson, H. W., C. E. Farshy, B. J. Fikes, D. D. Cruce, and L. P. Yealy.** 1979. Measure of immunoglobulin G-, M-, and A-specific titers against nonspecific, gram-negative bacterial antigens in the indirect immunofluorescence test for legionellosis. J. Clin. Microbiol. **10**:685–689.
9. **Wilkinson, H. W., B. J. Fikes, and D. D. Cruce.** 1979. Indirect immunofluorescence test for serodiagnosis of Legionnaires disease: evidence for serogroup diversity of Legionnaires disease bacterial antigens and for multiple specificity of human antibodies. J. Clin. Microbiol. **9**:379–383.
10. **Wilkinson, H. W., A. L. Reingold, B. J. Brake, D. L. McGiboney, G. W. Gorman, and C. V. Broome.** 1983. Reactivity of serum from patients with suspected legionellosis against 29 antigens of legionellaceae and *Legionella*-like organisms by indirect immunofluorescence assay. J. Infect. Dis. **147**:23–31.

Chapter 63

Serotypes and Immune Responses to *Pseudomonas aeruginosa*

GERALD B. PIER AND RICHARD B. MARKHAM

The genus *Pseudomonas* consists of 160 species of motile, aerobic, gram-negative rods which are ubiquitous. Only a few of these species assume medical importance, *P. aeruginosa* being primary among them. While not particularly invasive in the normal host, *P. aeruginosa* can produce life-threatening infections in immunocompromised patients, especially granulocytopenic patients and extensively burned patients. In addition, patients with cystic fibrosis (CF) have persistent colonization of their respiratory tract with these bacteria, and this colonization has been associated with worsening of the respiratory function of these patients. The relative resistance of *P. aeruginosa* to the commonly used antimicrobial agents has rendered it a continuing source of nosocomial infection.

Immune resistance to infection with *P. aeruginosa* appears to be multifactorial. The importance of polymorphonuclear leukocytes and opsonizing antibodies in the resolution or prevention of bacteremia has been stressed by many investigators. Epidemiologic studies have shown that patients surviving *P. aeruginosa* infections make a brisk antibody response to the bacterial antigens (5) and that high levels of antibody, if present in a patient's serum at the onset of bacteremia, are associated with survival (10). However, a protective level or titer of antibody has not been established. On the other hand, high levels of opsonizing antibody do not appear to protect CF patients from exacerbations of the lung disease which is apparently associated with increased *Pseudomonas* colonization (8). Recent reports have suggested that T lymphocytes can also play a role in resistance to infection with these bacteria (7), whereas, somewhat paradoxically, other studies have suggested that *P. aeruginosa* may interfere with the expression of cell-mediated immunity.

Numerous interacting virulence factors produced by *P. aeruginosa*, including exotoxins, exoproteases, endotoxin, flagellation, and antibiotic resistance, are likely involved in pathogenesis. More than 90% of clinical isolates of *P. aeruginosa* make exotoxin A, a potent toxin whose enzymatic activity, ADP ribosylation of the elongation factor 2 protein of ribosomes, is identical to that of diphtheria toxin. The majority of strains also make elastase, alkaline phosphatase, lipase, hemolysins, a leukocidin or cytotoxin, and a newly described exotoxin called exoenzyme S. The presence of flagella for mobility has also been shown to be an important virulence factor, and typing schemes based on heat-labile flagellar antigens have been proposed (2). Therefore, there are numerous antigens made by *P. aeruginosa* which could potentially provide information about the relatedness of strains. In addition, information about the role of immunity to these antigens in protecting an at-risk host from *P. aeruginosa* infections could be helpful in the choice of an appropriate immunotherapeutic modality.

Although typing and analysis of patients' responses to the multitude of virulence factors presented by *P. aeruginosa* would be informative, they would also be prohibitively complex and expensive. Brokopp and Farmer (4) have described methods for typing *P. aeruginosa* by biotype, antibiogram, serotype of heat-stable O antigens, bacteriocin (pyocine), and bacteriophage systems. They recommended that serological typing should be used as the first definitive method.

At least nine different typing schemes for heat-stable O antigens have been proposed. All of these systems overlap; i.e., they are based on the same or closely related antigenic determinants. Some systems contain more strains than others. A commonly used system in the United States, the Fisher-Devlin-Gnabasik immunotyping scheme, comprises seven types which account for 80 to 98% of all clinical isolates. The other commonly used system is the International Antigenic Typing Scheme (IATS), composed of 17 *P. aeruginosa* serotypes. The IATS system is composed of 7 strains serologically identical to the Fisher immunotype strains, plus 10 additional strains. Because of the availability from Difco Laboratories of a set of sera and antigens comprising the 17 IATS strains, serological typing of *P. aeruginosa* is the method of choice for differentiation of isolates. Serotypes of *P. aeruginosa* are based on the heat-stable O antigen located in the polysaccharide portion of the lipopolysaccharide (LPS). Serotyping can easily be performed on live suspensions of bacteria grown overnight on a plate of Mueller-Hinton agar (3). Furthermore, it is antibody to the O-serotype antigen that has been best correlated with protective immunity (10).

Mucoid-appearing strains of *P. aeruginosa* are often isolated from sputum cultures of CF patients. These strains elaborate an extracellular mucoid exopolysaccharide that is antigenically distinct from the serotype determinants. Patients with CF who are colonized with mucoid *P. aeruginosa* make high-titered antibody responses to mucoid exopolysaccharide (8). However, this antibody is clearly ineffective in mediating clearance of *P. aeruginosa* from the respiratory tract. Some strains of mucoid *P. aeruginosa* express conventional serotype antigens, and these strains can be typed by the IATS system. Recent reports indicate that up to 80% of mucoid *P. aeruginosa* strains cannot be serotyped and, in fact, are deficient in their production of O-polysaccharide side chains (6).

Other *Pseudomonas* species may be encountered in the laboratory. *P. cepacia* can survive in chemical solutions used to sterilize the tops of blood culture bottles. The result can be pseudobacteremia due to contamination. *P. cepacia* is also being isolated with increasing frequency from CF patients and immunocompromised hosts. *P. cepacia* does not react with *P. aeruginosa* typing sera. *P. pseudomallei* causes melioidosis. This disease is endemic to Southeast Asia. The use of an indirect hemagglutination assay for the detection of antibodies to *P. pseudomallei* can aid in the diagnosis of this infection (1).

CLINICAL INDICATIONS

Neither serotyping of *P. aeruginosa* strains nor determination of antibody levels is routinely required for diagnosis or treatment of *P. aeruginosa* infections. However, when there is a suspicion of either a local outbreak or a point source of infection, serotyping of strains could provide important information. Serotyping is generally reliable and reproducible and most often will correctly identify multiple isolates from the same source (3, 4). In addition, because of the multiple colonial morphologies that a given isolate of *P. aeruginosa* will express on laboratory media, serotyping may be important to show that these morphologically distinct colonies are, in fact, the same strain of *P. aeruginosa*. When serotype data are combined with the antibiograms routinely obtained in the clinical laboratory, a case for the similarity or difference of *P. aeruginosa* isolates can be made. However, antibiotic resistance in *P. aeruginosa* can change rapidly under different environmental conditions or selective pressures. Therefore, the use of an additional typing scheme such as pyocin or phage typing may be indicated to differentiate strains of the same serotype. These methods require that a laboratory have the pyocin producer and indicator strains, or phage stocks, and the capability of performing these tests. Since most clinical laboratories lack this capability, it is generally assumed that isolates of the same serotype are identical.

INTERPRETATION

Performance of the agglutination test for serotyping *P. aeruginosa* strains either as recommended by the manufacturer of the antiserum set or by an alternative means (3, 4) will yield one of five possible results. (i) The isolate will agglutinate monospecifically in a single typing serum. This indicates the serotype of that isolate. (ii) The strain will agglutinate in two sera. If the serotypes are closely related (such as 7 and 8) or have been previously reported as having a common reaction (such as 2 and 5, 5 and 16, or 6 and 10), then the agglutination in two sera is considered a positive reaction for a dual or bitypable strain. (iii) A strain will agglutinate in three or more typing sera (polyagglutinate). This reaction usually means that these strains are rough isolates, producing little to no serotype antigen on the LPS (6). (iv) A strain may not agglutinate in any sera (nonagglutinable). Like the polyagglutinable strains, these strains are also likely to be LPS rough. (v) A strain may agglutinate in a control well containing either normal serum or saline (autoagglutinable). This property can sometimes be overcome by passing the bacterial suspension through a syringe with a 27-gauge needle attached. To deter-

mine if polyagglutinable, nonagglutinable, or autoagglutinable strains are, in fact, serum-sensitive strains, a simple serum sensitivity test can be performed (6). This test is described below. If an isolate recovered from a sputum culture is found untypable and serum sensitive, then it is a typical strain from a CF patient, even if the isolate does not express the classic mucoid morphology of CF strains. Occasional reports are seen in which a diagnosis of CF is initially suspected because of a positive sputum culture containing *P. aeruginosa*.

REAGENTS

For serotyping

Pseudomonas aeruginosa antisera kit (Difco)
Pseudomonas aeruginosa antigen kit (Difco)
Mueller-Hinton agar
Sterile saline
Glass tubes (12 × 75 mm)
Spectrophotometer or a turbidity standard (0.05 ml of 0.048 M of barium chloride added to 99.5 ml of 0.36 N sulfuric acid)
Micropipette
Microtiter plate or a glass plate marked into squares with a wax marking pencil
Viewing mirror
Light source
Sterile swabs
Normal rabbit serum
If desired, but not necessary, *P. aeruginosa* serotype strains 1 through 17, no. 33348 through 33364, American Type Culture Collection, 15th catalog, p. 171

For serum sensitivity testing

Human complement source, either fresh or from serum stored at −70°C
1% Proteose peptone in saline
Screw cap tubes (16 by 125 mm)
Sterile glass tubes (12 by 75 mm) with tops
Pipettes
37°C incubator
Spectrophotometer (visible light)

TEST PROCEDURES

Standardization of antisera

The manufacturer recommends rehydrating the lyophilized vial of antisera with 1 ml of sterile distilled water and then making a 1:10 dilution for use. Because of lot-to-lot variation in the potency of a given serum, we recommend determining the titers of each vial against its homologous antigen as follows.

1. On a microtiter plate, add 15 μl of sterile saline to each of seven wells for each serum to be tested.

2. To well 1 add 15 μl of undiluted serum.

3. Make serial twofold dilutions out to well 6. This procedure will give dilutions of 1:2 to 1:64. Well 7 is a control.

4. Add 15 μl of the homologous test antigen (either *Pseudomonas aeruginosa* antigen [Difco] or a suspension of the homologous serotype organism, obtained

from the American Type Culture Collection [and prepared as described below]) to all seven wells.

5. Mix by shaking, but be careful not to spill.

6. Place the microtiter plate on the viewing mirror, with a light source above the plate.

7. In 5 to 30 min, score for positive agglutination (formation of a speckled appearance of the bacteria), and record the highest dilution of serum that gives positive agglutination. This is the serum's titer.

8. For each individual serum, make dilutions in saline containing a preservative (1:10,000 Merthiolate, for example) to yield the previously determined titer.

9. Test each serum dilution against all 17 strains. Record cross-reactions. Cross-reactions can be eliminated by adsorption of the cross-reacting serum with the cross-reacting bacteria.

10. As a means of conserving sera, pools of 5 or 6 individual sera can be made if one is careful to make the pools so that each individual serum is at or above its titer. Strains can be screened with the pools and then serotyped, using only the individual components of the pool.

Serotyping test strains with live cells

The following is a modification of the manufacturer's recommended procedure.

1. Grow the *P. aeruginosa* strain on Mueller-Hinton agar overnight.

2. Using a sterile swab, suspend the culture in sterile saline in a tube (12 by 75 mm) to a density close to that of the turbidity standard. Alternatively, suspend the bacteria to an optical density at 650 nm of ≥ 2.0 in a spectrophotometer. This is a critical concentration.

3. Add 15 μl of each test serum (or pool) to either a microtiter well or a square on a glass slide marked with a wax pencil. For each strain also have a well with 15 μl of normal rabbit serum.

4. Add 15 μl of the bacterial suspension of each serum.

5. Mix by shaking or rocking. Inspect in 5 to 30 min for agglutination.

6. Report the serotype as that corresponding to the serum or sera in which you see positive agglutination.

7. If the strain agglutinates in three or more sera (polyagglutinable), does not agglutinate in any sera (nonagglutinable), or agglutinates in all sera including the normal sera (autoagglutinable), perform the following assay if desired.

Serum sensitivity test

1. Add 0.5 ml of 1% proteose peptone in saline to seven tubes (12 by 75 mm).

2. To tube 1 add 0.5 ml of human serum prepared to keep the complement pathway intact (animal complement cannot be used). Also add 0.5 ml of human complement to tube 2.

3. Make twofold serial dilutions of the complement in tubes 3 through 7. Tube 8 is the control without complement.

4. Suspend the bacteria from the plate in 1% proteose peptone to an optical density at 650 nm of 0.4 in a glass tube with a 125-mm path length (16- by 125-mm screw cap tubes are used for this).

5. Make a 1:10,000 dilution of the bacterial suspension in 1% proteose peptone.

6. Add 0.5 ml of the bacterial suspension to each tube, including tube 8 (no complement).

7. Incubate at 37°C overnight.

8. Score each tube as positive (cloudy) or negative (clear) for growth.

9. If a bacterial strain does not grow in tubes containing 6.25% or less complement (tubes 4 through 7), the strain is considered serum sensitive and LPS rough. If the strain grows in any of tubes 1 through 3 (12.5 to 50% complement), it is probably serum resistant.

10. If a strain is not typable and is serum resistant, repeat the serotyping with heated cells as described by the manufacturer of the typing sera. If a strain is still not typable, recheck to ascertain that it is *P. aeruginosa* rather than another *Pseudomonas* species.

LITERATURE CITED

1. **Alexander, A. D., D. L. Huxsoll, A. R. Warner, Jr., V. Shepler, and A. Dorsey.** 1970. Serological diagnosis of human melioidosis with indirect hemagglutination and complement fixation tests. Appl. Microbiol. **20**:825–833.

2. **Ansorg, R.** 1978. Flagella specific II antigenic schema of *Pseudomonas aeruginosa*. Zentralbl. Bakteriol. Parasitenkd. Infektionskr. Hyg. Abt. I Orig. Reihe A **242**:228–238.

3. **Bergan, T.** 1973. Epidemiological markers for *Pseudomonas aeruginosa*. I. Serogrouping, pyocine typing and their interrelations. Acta Pathol. Microbiol. Scand. Sect. B **81**:70–80.

4. **Brokopp, C. D., and J. J. Farmer.** 1979. Typing methods for *Pseudomonas aeruginosa*, p. 90–134. *In* R. G. Doggett (ed.), *Pseudomonas aeruginosa:* clinical manifestations of infection and current therapy. Academic Press, Inc., New York.

5. **Crowder, J. G., M. W. Fisher, and A. White.** 1972. Type specific immunity in *Pseudomonas* diseases. J. Lab. Clin. Med. **79**:47–54.

6. **Hancock, R. E. W., L. M. Mutharia, L. Chan, R. P. Darveau, D. P. Speert, and G. B. Pier.** 1983. *Pseudomonas aeruginosa* isolates from patients with cystic fibrosis: a class of serum-sensitive, nontypable strains deficient in lipopolysaccharide O side chains. Infect. Immun. **42**:170–177.

7. **Pier, G. B., and R. B. Markham.** 1982. Induction in mice of cell-mediated immunity to *Pseudomonas aeruginosa* by high-molecular-weight polysaccharide and vinblastine. J. Immunol. **128**:2121–2125.

8. **Pier, G. B., W. J. Matthews, Jr., and D. D. Eardley.** 1983. Immunochemical characterization of the mucoid exopolysaccharide from *Pseudomonas aeruginosa*. J. Infect. Dis. **147**:494–503.

9. **Pier, G. B., and D. M. Thomas.** 1983. Characterization of the human immune response to a polysaccharide vaccine from *Pseudomonas aeruginosa*. J. Infect. Dis. **148**:206–213.

10. **Pollack, M., and L. S. Young.** 1979. Protective activity of antibodies to exotoxin A and lipopolysaccharide at the onset of *Pseudomonas aeruginosa* septicemia in man. J. Clin. Invest. **63**:276–286.

Chapter 64

Immune Response to *Listeria monocytogenes*

THOMAS B. ISSEKUTZ, SPENCER H. S. LEE, AND ROBERT BORTOLUSSI

Listeria monocytogenes is a short, motile, gram-positive rod that has been associated with a wide variety of clinical diseases in humans. The organism is a facultative anaerobe, produces catalase, and can grow over a wide temperature range on ordinary media, producing a narrow zone of beta-hemolysis on agar containing 5% sheep blood. A typing system for the organism is available, based on agglutination patterns to somatic (O) or flagellar (H) antigens on the organism. Since serotypes 1a, 1b, and 4b account for over 90% of all human isolates, the system has only limited practical application for epidemiological purposes. However, a phage typing system is currently under investigation for international use (A. Audurier, Laboratoire de Microbiologie, Hopital Trousseau, CHR de Tours, 37044 Tours-Cedex, France).

The immune response to infections with *L. monocytogenes* includes both humoral and cell-mediated components (3b); however, the role(s) of each component in immunity to infection in humans is poorly defined. Virulence of the organism appears to be related to its ability to survive within phagocytic cells for several days after being ingested by cells in the reticuloendothelial system. Three to four days after phagocytosis, macrophage activation occurs in an immunocompetent host, and intracellular killing of the bacteria also occurs. Subjects with ineffective T-cell or macrophage function are particularly at risk of developing severe clinical disease.

Most of the studies on humoral immunity to listeria suggest that antibody is largely in the immunoglobulin M (IgM) class (3a, 4). Humoral immunity does not appear to be a major contributing factor for disease, with the possible exception of disease in neonates. Humans with defects solely in their humoral immune system do not have an increased risk of infection; moreover, animals given immune serum are not protected against clinical illness.

A number of serological tests have been developed and proposed for clinical use to aid in establishing a diagnosis of listeriosis. These include precipitation (2), antihemolysin (3), hemagglutination (1), and enzyme-linked immunosorbent assay (3a, 6) techniques. In 1972, Larsen and Jones (4, 5) used a modification of the method described by Osebold and Sawyer (7) to test a number of sera. Since that time, the agglutination test described below has been offered as a diagnostic service by the Centers for Disease Control.

CLINICAL INDICATIONS

Listeria infection in humans can produce a variety of clinical diseases which may manifest as spontaneous abortions, stillbirths, meningitis, pneumonitis, septicemia, endocarditis, or a flulike illness in pregnant women. Although most listeria infections occur in neonates, pregnant women, immunocompromised patients, and the elderly, occasional cases have been reported in apparently healthy subjects. Moreover, despite antibiotic therapy, neonate mortality from listeria meningitis is still 30 to 50%.

A serological diagnosis of listeria infection is best made, as are most serological diagnoses, on the basis of a rise in specific antibody titer between an acute and a convalescent serum collected at a 2- to 3-week interval. Even when such serum samples are available, serology is unreliable in newborns and immunocompromised patients, both of whom may show no evidence of a rise in their antibody titers. The serological tests are primarily useful in epidemiological studies of listeria infections in the community and are of particular value in the study of epidemic outbreaks of listeriosis. In addition, both serology and the in vitro listeria-stimulated blastogenic response are useful measurements for research purposes. In particular, because of the demonstrated importance of T cells in resistance to listeria infections, the latter assay is biologically relevant.

The standard serological procedure for listeria antibody has been the agglutination assay described below. A recent study has demonstrated the superiority of the complement fixation assay over microagglutination and enzyme-linked immunosorbent assays in an outbreak of listeria type 4b (3a). An additional advantage is that the reagents for the complement fixation test are commercially available; therefore, this test is also described below.

All of the tests for antibody and T-cell blastogenesis have many pitfalls. First, *L. monocytogenes* has several antigens which strongly cross-react with those of *Staphylococcus aureus* and *Streptococcus faecalis*, as well as possibly with antigens of some other bacteria (3a). Thus, probably due to previous exposure to cross-reacting antigens, substantial listeria agglutination titers are found in some patients with no known exposure to this bacterium. Absorption of serum from these patients with *S. aureus* decreases but does not totally remove all of the cross-reactive antibody. Similarly, trypsin treatment of *L. monocytogenes* before it is used in the agglutination assay does not obviate this cross-reacting antibody. Second, the predominant portion of the antibody response to listeria after infection does not switch from the IgM to the IgG isotype but remains as IgM (3a). Therefore, the presence of antilisteria IgM cannot be taken to indicate recent infection. Finally, both tests of specific antibody and tests of T-cell blastogenic activity have demonstrated that newborns and immunocompromised patients with listeriosis may not mount a specific immune response to this organism. Thus, among these patients, immunological assessment for evidence of listeria infection must be considered unreliable.

AGGLUTINATION TEST

Reagents

Three test antigens and one absorption antigen are needed for the performance of the agglutination test. The two *L. monocytogenes* strains that are used for listeria antigen preparation are serotype 1a, NCTC 7973, H. P. R. Seeliger, ATCC 19111, and serotype 4b, CDC KC683 or 1709. These strains are found in the majority of clinical isolates from patients in North America and may be obtained from the Division of Bacterial Diseases, Centers for Disease Control, Atlanta, Ga. The two *S. aureus* strains necessary for absorption and antigen are CDC 1641y, and CDC 4282. Either of the *S. aureus* strains can be used in serum absorption provided that the other strain is used as the test antigen.

Sorensen phosphate-buffered saline (PBS), pH 7.3, is prepared by mixing 23.0 ml of a solution of 0.2 M monobasic sodium phosphate (27.8 g in 1,000 ml of 0.85% saline) with 77.0 ml of 0.2 M dibasic sodium phosphate (53.65 g of $Na_2HPO_4 \cdot 7H_2O$ in 1,000 ml of 0.85% saline) and then diluting to 200 ml with 0.85% saline. Final adjustment of pH may be done with either solution. Tryptose broth, tryptose agar, and Trypsin 1-300 are available from Difco Laboratories, Detroit, Mich. Thimerosal is available as ethylmercurithiosalicylic acid sodium salt from Fisher Scientific Co., Pittsburgh, Pa.

Antigen preparation

A stock suspension of *L. monocytogenes* and *S. aureus* is prepared as described by Larsen and Jones (5).

Cultures of listeria and *S. aureus* in 5 ml of tryptose broth are incubated overnight at 35°C. These cultures are used to seed 10 to 20 tryptose agar petri dishes which are then incubated for 48 h at 35°C. Bacteria are harvested from the agar surface in a minimal amount of 0.15 M NaCl (0.85% saline), steamed for 1 h at 100°C, and then washed twice in PBS. After the second wash, bacteria are suspended in PBS to a concentration that, when diluted 1:20, will read 50 to 53% optical transmission (T) at 430 nm on a Coleman Junior spectrophotometer. The concentrated suspensions are treated with crude trypsin for 15 min at 35°C by adding 1 part 1% trypsin in pH 7.3 PBS to 9 parts suspension. The organisms are washed twice in saline and suspended to their original standardized concentration. Suspensions may be preserved with thimerosal (Merthiolate) at a final concentration of 1:10,000.

Sera preparation

L. monocytogenes antiserum can be produced in rabbits or purchased from Difco. Human sera should be absorbed with either of the *S. aureus* antigens to remove cross-reactive agglutinins (5).

Test procedure

Since each serum must be tested with three antigens, three rows of six tubes (12 by 75 mm) each are necessary.

1. Add 0.5 ml of absorbed serum to tube 1 in each row.
2. Add 0.25 ml of 0.85% saline to tubes 2 through 6.
3. Transfer 0.25 ml of serum from tube 1 to tube 2, mix thoroughly, and continue serial dilutions through tube 6, discarding the last 0.25 ml from each row.
4. Dilute stock antigens in saline to read 50 to 53% T on a Coleman Junior spectrophotometer at 430 nm (usually 1:20 dilution of stock).
5. Add 0.25 ml of diluted antigen to each tube, e.g., row 1, *L. monocytogenes* serotype 1a; row 2, *L. monocytogenes* serotype 4b; and row 3, *S. aureus* (the strain not used for absorption).
6. Shake the rack and incubate it in a 50°C water bath for 2 h.
7. Refrigerate the rack of tubes overnight.
8. After the tubes have warmed to room temperature, tap each tube and read recording titers as the highest dilution with a strong agglutination.

Controls

Sera from bacteriologically confirmed and serotyped cases of human listeriosis are particularly helpful in establishing antigen titers, but rabbit immune sera for each of the two *L. monocytogenes* antigens can be successfully substituted for human sera. A negative control for the antigen containing only antigen and diluent is also prepared. Controls should be run each time the test is performed. If there is a drop in the endpoint titer, recheck the T percentage of the diluted antigen. A lower T percentage indicates autolysis of the antigen, and the concentration of the diluted antigen should be readjusted.

Interpretation

Table 1 shows the distribution of the geometric mean agglutination titers (GMAT) for sera of convalescent patients from whom *L. monocytogenes* was isolated, as well as for a control group of persons with no evidence of having had listeriosis. All sera were examined according to the procedure described above, including absorption with *S. aureus*.

Sera from neonates from whom *L. monocytogenes* had been isolated and sera from normal neonates were negative with all of the antigens at the first dilution tested. Mothers of neonates from whom the organism had been isolated had GMAT which were significantly higher than the GMAT of sera from control mothers. Significant differences were seen when the serum titers of listeria 4b isolates from nonimmunosuppressed patients were compared with serum titers of normal controls of the same age. However, in confirmed cases of listeriosis among immunosuppressed patients, the titers did not rise above 1:25.

Although there are significant differences in the GMAT of the patient and control groups, the ranges of titers within the two groups overlap considerably. Therefore, a high-titered single serum in certain select groups (mothers of neonates and elderly patients with symptoms indicative of listeriosis) may be suggestive, and a fourfold or greater rise in titer may be considered presumptive for listeriosis; however, a confident diagnosis of listeriosis requires isolation of the organism.

TABLE 1. GMAT for sera from controls and from patients with *L. monocytogenes* isolates[a]

Type of serum and group identification	No. of sera in group	GMAT for *L. monocytogenes*[b]	
		Serotype 1a	Serotype 4b
Neonate			
1a-1b or 4b infection	14	12.5	12.5
Control	29	12.5	12.5
Mother of neonate:			
With 1a-1b isolate	9	147.0[c]	39.7
With 4b isolate	8	70.7	70.7[d]
Control	25	67.8	27.2
Nonimmunosuppressed patient, 1–60 yr old			
1a-1b isolate	6	56.1	31.5
4b isolate	14	78.0	60.9[e]
Control	222	64.0	16.0
Nonimmunosuppressed patient, over 61 yr old			
1a-1b isolate	5	57.4[f]	19.9
4b isolate	3	79.3	50.0[g]
Control	25	18.9	12.5
Immunosuppressed adult			
1a-1b or 4b	16	12.5	12.5

[a] Modified from a report by Larsen, Wiggins, and Albritton, as originally presented in the 2nd edition of this manual.

[b] For calculations, log of 6.25 was used for titers less than 12.5 and log of 12.5 was used for titers less than 25 when starting dilution was 1:25.

[c] For mothers of neonates with 1a or 1b isolates versus control mothers, $P < 0.02$.

[d] For mothers of neonates with 4b isolates versus control mothers, $P < 0.005$.

[e] For patients with 4b sepsis versus controls of the same age, $P < 0.001$.

[f] For patients with 1a or 1b sepsis versus controls of the same age, $P < 0.02$.

[g] For patients with 4b sepsis versus controls of the same age, $P < 0.01$.

COMPLEMENT FIXATION TEST

The complement fixation test is performed by a standard microtiter method. All of the necessary reagents and their preparations as well as the equipment required for performing a complement fixation test are described in chapter 10 of this manual. Also included in the same chapter are techniques for determining proper concentrations of test components, such as the hemolytic system, and complement unitage.

The test antigen is a pool of *L. monocytogenes* types 1a and 4b available commercially in lyophilized form from H. D. Supplies, United Kingdom. In Canada, it is distributed through NCS Diagnostics, Inc., Mississauga, Ontario L4X 2E2 (catalog no. CFL-2). For use, the antigen is reconstituted with distilled water and may be stored at 4°C for up to 1 year.

Listeria positive and negative control sera, which can be obtained from the same manufacturer and supplier as the antigen, are included in each series of tests. Test sera are collected in sterile plastic tubes and can be stored at −20°C.

Antigen preparation

For use in the test, the antigen is standardized by performing a block titration with known positive serum in a microtiter plate according to a previously described procedure (8). Briefly, serial twofold dilutions of antigen are allowed to react against serial twofold dilutions of a listeria positive control serum. An optimal dilution of the antigen giving a positive result is obtained at the concentration of antigen used in the test. Likewise, the titer of the positive control serum is established as a reference for all subsequent tests.

Serum preparation

Before being tested, all sera must be heat inactivated for 30 min in a 56°C water bath. Previously heated sera should be reheated for 15 min at 56°C on the day of testing.

Test procedure

Veronal buffer diluent (VBD) is used for all dilutions and as a substitute for the antigen in the wells that serve as control for anticomplementary activity in the sera. The micromethod is performed with 5 50% hemolytic (CH_{50}) U of complement and a 1.4% suspension of optimally sensitized sheep erythrocytes.

The procedure for the complement fixation test is as follows.

1. Place appropriately labeled, disposable, U-well, plastic microtiter plates on damp underpads to act as a static charge eliminator. For each test serum, use one row for antigen (designated as test row) and one row for test serum control.

2. Set up a control plate with one row for known positive control serum and one row for known negative control serum. In addition, one well is used for each of the following reagent controls:

Sheep erythrocyte control . . . . add 0.1 ml of VBD

Complement control

    5   CH_{50} U. . . . . add 0.05 ml of VBD
    2.5 CH_{50} U. . . . . add 0.05 ml of VBD
    1.25 CH_{50} U. . . . . add 0.05 ml of VBD

Antigen and complement control

    5   CH_{50} U. . . . . add 0.025 ml of VBD
    2.5 CH_{50} U. . . . . add 0.025 ml of VBD
    1.25 CH_{50} U. . . . . add 0.025 ml of VBD

3. Dispense 0.075 ml of VBD into the first well in each row of the test plate as well as into each of the positive and negative control serum rows on the control plate; with a 0.025-ml dropper, add 0.025 ml of VBD to the remaining wells of each row.

4. Place 0.025-ml microdiluters in a beaker with just enough VBD to cover the tips. Blot the diluters dry before picking up serum.

5. Pick up 0.025 ml of serum with a microdiluter, and prepare serial twofold dilutions, thus giving dilu-

tions of 1:4 to 1:512. Twirl the microdiluters rapidly 15 times for every well.

6. With a 0.025-ml dropper, add 0.025 ml of antigen (diluted according to the result of block titration) to the test rows on the test plate, the positive and negative serum control rows, and the three antigen and complement control wells on the control plate. Only wells containing 1:8 to 1:512 serum dilutions receive the test antigen.

7. Add 0.025 ml of VBD to the test serum control rows in the same manner as serum was added to the test plate. Mix each plate on a plate mixer (Micro-Shaker, Dynatech Laboratories, Inc., Alexandria, Va.). Cover the plates and incubate them at 4°C for 20 min.

8. Prepare an optimal dilution of complement as determined in the complement titration to give a concentration of 5 CH_{50} U in 0.05 ml, and let this dilution sit on ice for 20 min.

9. After 20 min of incubation, use a 0.05-ml dropper to add 0.05 ml of complement to each well (except sheep erythrocyte control wells and wells to received 2.5 and 1.25 CH_{50} U), and mix.

10. Dilute 5 CH_{50} U of complement to 1:2 and 1:4 with VBD to give 2.5 and 1.25 CH_{50} U of complement, respectively. Add 0.05 ml of these diluted complements to the remaining complement as well as to the antigen and complement control wells on the control plate, and mix.

11. Cover the plates and incubate them at 4°C for 14 to 18 h.

12. Warm the plates to room temperature for approximately 20 min.

13. Sensitize the 2.8% sheep erythrocyte suspension with an equal volume of an optimally predetermined concentration of hemolysin by slowly adding hemolysin to the erythrocytes while swirling the flask. Incubate in a 37°C water bath for 15 min.

14. Add 0.025 ml of sensitized sheep erythrocytes to all wells in each plate, mixing each plate on a plate mixer after the cells are added.

15. Incubate the plates at 37°C for 30 min.

16. After incubation, centrifuge the plates at 1,200 rpm for 3 min, and read the test results.

17. Reading and recording test results
   a. Before reading and recording test results, examine the reagent control results to see whether they are acceptable. They should read as follows:
      Complement control
         at 5 CH_{50} U—complete lysis
         at 2.5 CH_{50} U—partial to complete lysis
         at 1.25 CH_{50} U—no lysis to partial lysis
      Sheep erythrocyte control, no lysis
      Antigen and complement control
         at 5 CH_{50} U—complete lysis
         at 2.5 CH_{50} U—partial to complete lysis
         at 1.25 CH_{50} U—no lysis to partial lysis
      If the control results are not acceptable, disregard the test results and repeat the test.
   b. Read and record the positive and negative serum results. The titers of the control sera with the test antigen must be within one twofold dilution of the titer obtained from block titration. Otherwise, disregard the test results and repeat the test.
   c. Read and record the test results. The titer of the test serum with the test antigen is the highest

dilution producing no hemolysis. The test serum control row should show complete hemolysis. This result ensures that the serum itself does not fix complement (i.e., it is anticomplementary), an activity which would give false-positive readings in the test. In the absence of anticomplementary activity, sera having a positive reaction (no hemolysis) at a 1:8 dilution or above are considered positive for complement-fixing *L. monocytogenes* antibodies.

Interpretation

In general, serological proof of listeria infection can be based on a demonstration of rising anti-complement-fixing antibody titers (a greater than fourfold difference in paired acute and convalescent sera). However, information concerning this aspect of the serological response in listeria infection is lacking. In a recent study of listeriosis caused by *L. monocytogenes* serotype 4b in the Canadian Maritime provinces, several serological methods for the diagnosis of this infection (4) were compared. In this study, paired sera were not available, and single convalescent sera were tested. The results in Table 2 show a significant difference between cases and controls ($P < 0.0005$). The specificity of the test was 91% and the sensitivity was 78%. The test had a positive predictive value of 75% and a negative predictive value of 92%.

LYMPHOCYTE BLASTOGENIC ASSAY

Reagents

The two *L. monocytogenes* strains 1a and 4b and one of the *S. aureus* strains described above in the agglutination assay section may be used. Ficoll-Paque can be obtained from Pharmacia Fine Chemicals, Inc., Piscataway, N.J. Hanks balanced salt solution (HBSS), RPMI 1640 medium, human AB serum, penicillin-streptomycin, 96-well microculture plates, and a MASH harvester can all be obtained from Flow Laboratories, Mississauga, Ontario, Canada. Phytohemagglutinin (PHA) is available from Difco, and [³H]thymidine (6.7 Ci/mmol) and Econofluor can be purchased from New England Nuclear Corp., Lachine, Quebec, Canada.

Antigen preparation

The bacteria are grown overnight at 37°C in 50 ml of tryptose broth. The bacteria are pelleted by centrifugation, the broth is discarded, and the bacteria are

TABLE 2. Distribution of titers of complement-fixing antibody to *L. monocytogenes* types 1a and 4b antigens among control and listeria-infected cases

Titer	% Serum samples	
	Control ($n = 75$)	Listeria-infected cases ($n = 27$)
<1:8	91	22
1:8	5	30
1:16	3	6
1:32	1	23
1:64	0	18

washed in PBS and then suspended to 0.5% in PBS (vol/vol). Formalin is added to a concentration of 0.5%, and the bacteria are incubated for 1 h at room temperature. The Formalin-killed bacteria are then washed three times and suspended in PBS at a volume of 1% (vol/vol). These stock bacteria are stored frozen in aliquots at −70°C for up to 3 months.

Test procedure

1. Heparinized blood (5 ml) is carefully layered onto 3 ml of Ficoll-Paque and centrifuged at room temperature for 20 min at 400 × g.

2. The mononuclear cells at the interface between the plasma (top layer) and Ficoll-Paque (second layer) are removed and diluted in three volumes of HBSS, and the cells are pelleted by centrifugation at 400 × g for 10 min. The supernatant is discarded, and the cells are suspended in 10 ml of HBSS and centrifuged at 300 × g for 10 min. This cell washing procedure is repeated once.

3. The cells are suspended in RPMI 1640 culture medium supplemented with 10% heat-inactivated human AB serum and penicillin-streptomycin at a concentration of 10^6 cells per ml.

4. Cultures are prepared by adding 0.2 ml of the cell suspension to each of 18 wells on a flat-bottom, 96-well microculture plate.

5. Triplicate cultures are then set up as follows. The first three wells receive no additional stimulus. The second three wells receive 20 μl each of Formalin-killed L. monocytogenes diluted to a concentration of 0.1% in culture medium. The third set of wells receives 20 μl per well of Formalin-killed L. monocytogenes diluted to a concentration of 0.01% in medium. The fourth set receives 20 μl per well of killed 0.1% S. aureus. The fifth set receives 20 μl per well of 0.01% S. aureus. The sixth set of microcultures receives 20 μl per well of 10% PHA diluted in medium.

6. Microculture plates are then incubated for 6 days at 37°C in an atmosphere of humidified 5% CO_2 in air.

7. On day 6, 0.5 μCi of [³H]thymidine is added to each well, and cultures are incubated overnight.

8. The next day, the cells are harvested on a MASH harvester, and the incorporation of [³H]thymidine by the cells is determined by liquid scintillation counting of the filter papers in 3 ml of Econofluor.

Controls

Simultaneously with each test blood sample, a blood sample from a normal donor should be tested. Both the patient and the normal control should demonstrate a greatly increased [³H]thymidine uptake for the cells stimulated with PHA compared with the unstimulated cells in the first set of wells. With repeated assays, the normal range for the response to PHA, usually 50,000 to 150,000 cpm, can be readily determined for each laboratory. Similarly, both normal and patient samples exhibit a strong proliferative response in the presence of S. aureus, with a 5- to 20-fold increase in [³H]thymidine incorporation over unstimulated cells. The optimal response of L. monocytogenes usually occurs at a concentration of 0.01%, but the concentration which gives the best reproduc-

TABLE 3. Lymphocyte blastogenic response to L. monocytogenes, S. aureus, and PHA

Subject (n)	Tritiated thymidine incorporation (cpm per culture)			
	Medium	PHA	S. aureus	L. monocytogenes
Infected mothers (7)	1,608[a]	73,842	14,033	16,853[b]
Control mothers (4)	646	54,899	21,864	3,684

[a] Mean.
[b] Infected mothers > control mothers, P = 0.012.

ibility and strongest response in any given laboratory should be used.

Interpretation

Table 3 shows the results of lymphocyte blastogenic assays on a group of women 1 year after natural infection with listeria during pregnancy and on a matched control population (3b). Both groups demonstrated strong, consistent responses to PHA and S. aureus. The control group also exhibited a weak but definite response in the presence of L. monocytogenes, due possibly to antigenic cross-reactivity. The pregnant women with previous listeriosis had a strong response, which was significantly (P = 0.012) greater than that of the controls, to this stimulus. There was some overlap of the response to listeria between the normal and infected subjects. Listeria-infected infants of these mothers showed no blastogenic response to L. monocytogenes (data not shown).

The lymphocyte blastogenic assay can yield useful information on the cell-mediated response to listeria infection, but it should not be employed as a basis for the diagnosis of listeriosis.

LITERATURE CITED

1. **Antonissen, C. J. M., K. P. M. Van Kassel, H. Van Dijk, and J. M. N. Willers.** 1981. Development of a simple passive hemagglutination inhibition assay for Listeria monocytogenes lipoteichoic acid. J. Immunol. Methods **44**:351–357.

2. **Delvallez, M., Y. Carlier, D. Bout, A. Capron, and G. R. Martin.** 1979. Purification of a surface-specific soluble antigen from Listeria monocytogenes. Infect. Immun. **25**:971–977.

3. **Girard, K. F., A. J. Sbarra, and W. A. Bardawil.** 1963. Serology of Listeria monocytogenes. I. Characteristics of the soluble hemolysin. J. Bacteriol. **85**:349–355.

3a.**Hudak, A. P., S. H. Lee, A. C. Issekutz, and R. Bortolussi.** 1984. Comparison of three serological methods—enzyme-linked immunosorbent assay, complement fixation and microagglutination in the diagnosis of human perinatal Listeria monocytogens infection. Clin. Invest. Med. **7**:349–354.

3b.**Issekutz, T. B., J. Evans, and R. Bortolussi.** 1984. The immune response of human neonates to Listeria monocytogenes infection. Clin. Invest. Med. **7**:281–286.

4. **Larsen, S. A., J. C. Feeley, and W. L. Jones.** 1974. Immune response to Listeria monocytogenes in rabbits and humans. Appl. Microbiol. **27**:1005–1013.

5. **Larsen, S. A., and W. L. Jones.** 1972. Evaluation and standardization of an agglutination test for human listeriosis. Appl. Microbiol. **24**:101–107.

6. **Meyer, S., and H. Brunner.** 1981. Enzym-Immunoassay bei Listeriose: Antikorper- und Antigen-nachweis-Vorlaufige Mitteilung. Zentralbl. Bakteriol. Parasitenkd. Infektionskr. Hyg. Abt. 1 Orig. Reihe A **248:**469–478.

7. **Osebold, J. W., and M. T. Sawyer.** 1955. Agglutinating antibodies for *Listeria monocytogenes* in human serum. J. Bacteriol. **70:**350–351.

8. **U.S. Public Health Service.** 1981. Standardized diagnostic complement fixation method and adaptation to microtest. Department of Health, Education, and Welfare, U.S. Public Health Service publication. Washington, D.C.

Chapter 65

Immune Response to *Corynebacterium diphtheriae* and *Clostridium tetani*

JOHN P. CRAIG

The exotoxins of *Corynebacterium diphtheriae* and *Clostridium tetani* are highly antigenic proteins. Parenteral injection of toxoids prepared from these toxins regularly evokes neutralizing antitoxins which are highly protective against the risk of disease in humans. These two toxoids are among the most effective prophylactic immunogens in general use today. Moreover, good methods for the assay of these antitoxins have existed for decades. The measurement of the immune response during the natural course of disease in the individual patient, however, has played no role in the diagnosis or management of these infections. Regular clinical laboratories seldom maintain the capability of titrating diphtheria or tetanus antitoxin levels; these methods have been used almost exclusively as research tools for epidemiologic investigations or for the study of immunogenicity of toxoids. There are four reasons for this: (i) the pathogenesis of these two toxinoses demands that an immediate decision for or against specific immunotherapy be made on clinical grounds or, in the case of diphtheria, with the assistance of direct bacteriologic examination; (ii) the assay methods now available are too time-consuming to be used as admission procedures to aid the clinician in deciding on the need for immunotherapy; (iii) in all cases in which there are reasonably good clinical grounds for suspecting either of these diseases, specific immunotherapy is begun at once, rendering convalescent determinations of little value; and (iv) with tetanus, and also in some individuals with diphtheria, the pathogenic dose of toxin is less than the immunogenic dose, and therefore, even in untreated cases, determination of serum antitoxin levels during convalescence would not be a reliable retrospective diagnostic tool. For these reasons, there are also almost no data on the immune response in untreated patients, and the natural sequence of immunologic events in these diseases in virtually unknown. In communities in which laboratories capable of titrating antitoxins exist, virtually all patients with recognized cases of tetanus and diphtheria receive therapeutic antitoxin.

DIPHTHERIA

The best evidence concerning the immune response to infection with diphtheria bacilli was derived from epidemiologic studies carried out before the introduction of toxoid. These studies employed the Shick test, which was the earliest method of estimating diphtheria antitoxin levels on a routine basis. The majority of children in two American cities in the 1920s had experienced immunizing infections with diphtheria by the age of 15 (Fig. 1). Since few of these children had clinical disease, Frost (4) reached the inevitable conclusion that in most individuals enough toxin is liberated during inapparent infection to evoke an immune response. This is especially interesting in view of the fact that some individuals with clinically manifest disease may not develop detectable antitoxin. It is also generally accepted that diphtheria almost never occurs in individuals with preexisting antitoxin levels of ≥ 0.01 antitoxin unit (AU) per ml.

A number of methods are now available for the determination of diphtheria antitoxin levels in body fluids. The Schick test, although not a laboratory procedure, remains a reliable, roughly quantitative measure of antitoxic immunity (see below). Several in vitro methods have been developed, and some of these have been successfully used in epidemiologic surveys in which it was necessary to estimate antitoxin levels in large numbers of sera (see below). The reference method, however, against which all other methods continue to be compared, is the in vivo toxin neutralization assay which depends on neutralization of the effect of diphtheria toxin in guinea pig or rabbit skin. The method first described by Jensen (6) is detailed below. This is recommended as the method least fraught with problems of technique, interpretation, and reproducibility. Moreover, the materials required are inexpensive and almost universally available. No specialized equipment or reagents are needed.

Passive hemagglutination (PHA) of toxin-coated erythrocytes is now widely used for the detection of diphtheria antitoxin in sera (8). Diphtheria toxin is adsorbed to formalinized and tannic acid-treated sheep or horse erythrocytes. These cells are then agglutinated by specific diphtheria antitoxin. The tanned cells may be treated with bis-diazobenzidine to improve adsorption of toxin. There is a good statistical correlation between titers obtained by the PHA method and those obtained by toxin neutralization in rabbit skin, indicating that the PHA test primarily is detecting specific antitoxin (8). However, most workers agree that in individual sera there may be marked discrepancies, up to eightfold, which render the interpretation of the PHA test very risky in the individual patient (8). Kameyama et al. (7) showed that the ratio of PHA to neutralizing antibody titers rose with repeated booster immunizations and that the high PHA values were associated with the appearance of antibody against fragment A of the diphtheria toxin molecule. Anti-fragment A was detectable in the binding (PHA) assay but had poor toxin-neutralizing capacity. These observations emphasize the fact that PHA is a binding assay which does not measure neutralization of the biologic effect of toxin. Therefore, if an accurate measure of antitoxic activity of an individual body fluid is desired, an in vivo test is recommended. Moreover, the use of an animal as an indicator system obviates many of the technical variables inherent in an in vitro technique. For these reasons, we have

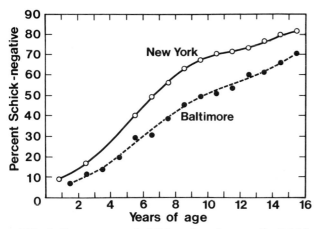

FIG. 1. Percentages of children found naturally Schick negative in New York (1923) and Baltimore (1922 through 1925). After Frost (4) and Zingher (15).

selected the rabbit intracutaneous method as the method of choice.

A radioimmunoassay has been developed for the detection of diphtheria antitoxin in human sera (11). In a limited comparative study the correlation with the intradermal neutralization test was good, but as in the case of PHA, a significant number of discrepancies were reported. These discrepancies were probably due to the fact that radioimmunoassay detected nonneutralizing or nonavid antibody. Radioimmunoassay may be useful for epidemiologic surveys, but great reliance should not be placed on individual values. A microlatex test has also been described (9), but comparison with the in vivo assay has not been reported. Precipitation inhibition counterimmunoelectrophoresis has also been described (13). The sensitivity of this method was about 40 times that of conventional counterimmunoelectrophoresis, but was still far below that which can be achieved with the intradermal neutralization assay.

Tissue culture methods have also been used extensively in the titration of diphtheria antitoxin. These methods are based on the fact that diphtheria toxin causes readily observable changes in several cell lines as a result of its inhibitory effect on protein synthesis. Specific antitoxin neutralizes this effect. As one might expect, tissue culture methods show closer agreement with the rabbit skin neutralization method than does PHA, since both tissue culture and skin methods depend on neutralization of the biologic activity of the toxin. The technique described by Miyamura et al. (12), employing VERO cells and depending on color change as the endpoint, is the simplest and most satisfactory tissue culture method available. The establishment of a tissue culture system for a procedure which is rarely done in a clinical laboratory seems to be inadvisable, however, and the rabbit skin method probably has fewer problems.

TETANUS

As for diphtheria, the most reliable and relevant method of tetanus antitoxin determination involves in vivo neutralization of toxin, in which only antibodies

of the immunoglobulin G class seem to be effective. In this case, the mouse neutralization assay is the most widely used (1). The method is described in detail below.

Tetanus PHA has been used extensively in serologic surveys as well as in studies on the antigenicity of toxoids (5). The same problems apply here as in the case of diphtheria PHA. The test is highly sensitive and probably better correlated with neutralization titers than is diphtheria PHA. However, discrepancies between neutralization and PHA titers in individual sera are frequent (5). Treatment of sera with 2-mercaptoethanol may reduce the discrepancies between PHA and neutralization assays.

An enzyme-linked immunosorbent assay (ELISA) can be used for the determination of serum tetanus antitoxin levels (10). ELISA is simple and relatively inexpensive and can detect antitoxin of specific immunoglublin types. Titers may be higher with ELISA than with neutralization assays, especially in recently immunized people, suggesting the presence of low-avidity antibodies.

ELISA has in some hands proven to be as sensitive as the neutralization test for the detection of antitoxin (10), but problems in reproducibility remain, probably due to differences in materials used in the manufacture of microtiter plates. In spite of the ability of ELISA to detect immunoglobulin G antitoxin, which presumably contains all of the toxin-neutralizing activity, differences in binding activity and neutralization continue to appear.

Counterimmunoelectrophoresis can be used for the detection of tetanus antitoxin (14), but because of its insensitivity this method is useful only in screening sera containing relatively high levels (>7.0 IU/ml) of antitoxin. A solid-phase radioimmunoassay has also been described for the detection of tetanus antitoxin (3), but no comparisons with in vivo neutralization tests have yet been reported.

For the reasons stated above, it is recommended that in a clinical laboratory, where values in individual patients are important, the more reliable mouse neutralization test be employed. There is no tissue culture method available for the titration of tetanus toxin or antitoxin.

CLINICAL INDICATIONS

There are few indications for the determination of diphtheria or tetanus antitoxin levels in a clinical laboratory.

Probably the most frequent need for these assays today is in connection with studies of immunocompetence. The response to diphtheria or tetanus toxoid in individuals suspected of immunodeficiency disorders is gaining wider use. Although the Schick test has been used for this purpose, it is only roughly quantitative and has the disadvantage of requiring injections and repeated observations of the patient. The rabbit intracutaneous assay for diphtheria antitoxin and the mouse neutralization test for tetanus antitoxin are the assays of choice. With these assays, the actual neutralizing capacity of the antibody can be measured as precisely as desired.

The measurement of diphtheria antitoxin by a rapid PHA method on admission may provide the clinician with information which may be helpful in deciding whether to give antitoxin. If the clinical diagnosis is in doubt, the presence of high levels of diphtheria antitoxin would militate against a diagnosis of diphtheria and obviate the need for immunotherapy. This approach could be of value in reducing unnecessary cases of serum sickness and deserves further study. It is not clear what level of antitoxin should be considered high enough to eliminate the need for antitoxin treatment. A value of ≥ 0.4 AU/ml has been suggested (13a). The fact that individual discrepancies between PHA and neutralizing antibody titers are not rare, however, makes one worry about basing the decision to give or withhold antitoxin on a single PHA assay. At present there is no known assay system which can provide evidence of neutralizing diphtheria antitoxin in less than 2 or 3 days.

PROCEDURES

Shick test

Although the Schick test is not a laboratory procedure, it must be considered along with other indicators of the immune response to diphtheria toxin antigen. The Schick test is capable of dividing the population into two broad categories, designated Schick positive and Schick negative, based on their response to approximately 1/50 of a guinea pig minimal lethal dose of diphtheria toxin (roughly 0.5 ng). It is generally agreed that most persons who are Schick positive possess a serum antitoxin level of <0.01 AU/ml, while most persons who are Schick negative possess levels of ≥ 0.01 AU/ml. Although this generalization can be applied to epidemiologic studies involving large groups, many individual exceptions are found when serum antitoxin titers as determined by the rabbit intracutaneous method are compared with Schick test results (2).

The Schick test is of no value in determining the need for diphtheria antitoxin in the treatment of diphtheria. The results of the test are available no earlier than 18 to 24 h after application of the test, and the decision regarding specific immunotherapy must be made as soon as the diagnosis of diphtheria is considered.

Schick test reagents must be obtained from laboratories which are licensed to produce biologic materials for human use. Under no circumstances should materials prepared in an unlicensed laboratory be used for testing in humans.

The Schick test is performed by injecting 0.1 ml of the appropriate dilution of diphtheria toxin (approximately 1/5 guinea pig minimal lethal dose per ml) intracutaneously on the flexor surface of one arm and 0.1 ml of the same material which has been heated for 30 min at 70°C on the other arm. Some suppliers of Schick test materials provide a dilution of fluid diphtheria toxoid as control material instead of heated toxin. In such cases, the dose of control toxoid often contains much more toxin-derived antigen than does the Shick toxin. This has the advantage of providing the subject with a small booster dose of diphtheria toxoid, but the disadvantage of not being a true control.

The importance of including a control injection needs to be stressed. Most toxins used in the preparation of Schick test reagents are not highly purified. They may contain a variety of corynebacterial antigens immunologically unrelated to the toxin; these antigens may evoke skin responses which are usually delayed and which may be confused with the skin response to diphtheria toxin. A smaller number of individuals develop immediate-type wheal and flare reactions to either or both toxin and control materials, but these reactions disappear within a few hours. Therefore, they pose no problem in interpretation of the Schick test. To gain the most information from a Schick test, the reactions should be examined daily and the diameter of redness and the diameter and intensity of induration should be recorded. The findings in the four categories of responses are shown in Table 1. Certain qualitative differences in response are important and can be recognized by the careful observer, but cannot be presented in a table. These differences are described below.

Typically, the redness produced by the toxin in a nonimmune person appears at about 18 h as a rosy blush 8 to 12 mm in diameter, growing more intensely red and reaching a maximum size of 10 to 25 mm in 3 to 5 days. A central blanched area of necrosis may develop. The redness fades very slowly, often leaving an area of increased pigmentation for a year or more. Although the positive Schick test may be accompanied by slight to moderate edema, the marked induration of a typical reaction of delayed-type hypersensitivity does not appear, and redness alone is the major feature.

In the typical pseudoreaction, the redness and induration appear on both arms. These pseudoreactions usually resemble positive tuberculin reactions, and they wax and wane with identical time courses. The peak of the reaction is at 48 to 72 h. However, if the control material contains more antigen than does the toxin, the reaction size will be greater at the control site.

In individuals with adequate circulating and tissue antitoxin but with no sensitivity to other corynebacterial antigens, no reaction whatsoever will be seen on either arm from day 2 on. It is important to recognize that the in vivo combination of toxin and antitoxin does not give rise to a visible skin response, except for the occasional immediate reaction which may occur during the first few hours after administration. Such reactions are spent within day 1 and do not interfere with the interpretation of the Schick test.

Combined reactions are the most difficult to interpret, and indeed, a clear-cut determination of the

TABLE 1. Schick test responses

Schick reaction	Reaction with:				Interpretation	
	Toxin		Control		Circulating antitoxin	Sensitivity to bacterial antigens
	36 h	120 h	36 h	120 h		
Positive	±	+	0	0	0	0
Negative	0	0	0	0	+	0
Pseudo-reaction	+	0	+	0	+	+
Combined reaction	+	+	+	0	0	+

status of antitoxin immunity cannot be made in some individuals. A very marked reaction of delayed-type hypersensitivity to nontoxin antigens may persist for more than a week and mask the reaction to toxin. Usually a decision can be made at 2 to 3 weeks. In a true pseudoreaction both lesions will have faded at the same rate. In a combined reaction, evidence of toxin-mediated necrosis will persist longer than the lesion of delayed-type hypersensitivity.

The amount of antigen in the usual Schick test materials will exert a substantial booster effect in individuals possessing low levels of antitoxin and even in some Schick-positive individuals who had been previously primed with toxin or toxoid. Individuals who possess detectable antitoxin levels (≥ 0.001 AU/ml) at the time of Schick testing develop, on the average, 10-fold rises in circulating antitoxin titer in response to the Schick test, even when the control material contains only the same amount of toxin antigen as does the test toxin (unpublished data).

Rabbit intracutaneous method for titration of diphtheria antitoxin

The rabbit intracutaneous method first described by Jensen (6) is probably the simplest and most reliable. The backs of two adult white rabbits are clipped as closely as possible with an electric clipper fitted with a head designed for clipping rabbit fur. The small animal clipper with Angra head (Sunbeam-Oster Co., Milwaukee, Wis.) is satisfactory. During moulting, many rabbits are found to have irregular, patchy areas of dense and rapid hair growth. If during clipping it is found that a rabbit has more than a few such patches, it is best to reject that animal and select another because these areas are unsuitable for injection. The margins of such patches are indurated and reddened. During clipping, it is necessary to restrain the rabbit on an operating board with all four legs held sufficiently taut to prevent struggling. Mark off the clipped area in approximately 15-mm squares in a grid, using a black felt pen. Sixty to 100 squares can easily be accommodated on the back of a 2.5- to 4-kg rabbit. Depilation is undesirable because it causes generalized erythema and dryness and cracking of rabbit skin, which makes the reading of the lesions produced by diphtheria toxin more difficult. If rabbits free of areas of heavy hair growth are selected, the amount of growth at 3 days will be slight and can be removed by a light clipping just before reading.

Potencies of antitoxins are expressed in units. It is therefore necessary to determine the proper test dose of the sample of diphtheria toxin selected by titrating it against a sample of standard antitoxin. The most satisfactory toxin dose for this type of antitoxin titration is the Lr/20,000 dose. An Lr (limit of redness) dose of diphtheria toxin is defined as that amount of toxin which when mixed with 1 AU of diphtheria antitoxin and injected intracutaneously will elicit a minimal area of redness. The Lr/20,000 is the amount of toxin which will elicit the same minimal area of redness in the presence of 1/20,000 AU. The fixed reference point in all these assays is the AU, which was originally arbitrarily assigned to an antitoxic serum and against which all subsequent antitoxins have been calibrated. The toxin, which is much more labile than antibody, is always measured by titration against antitoxin.

Diphtheria toxin batches vary so greatly in potency that no guide can be offered for initial titration. Crude culture filtrates or partially purified preparations are as satisfactory as highly purified toxins for antitoxin titrations. One Lf (limit of flocculation) dose of toxin is roughly equal to 1 Lr dose. Therefore, if the Lf potency of the toxin is provided, the general magnitude of toxic potency can be predicted. In any case, when the assay is being newly established in a laboratory it will be necessary to carry out preliminary screening titrations to establish the approximate potency of the toxin to be used.

Use borate-buffered saline (pH 7.5) containing 0.1% gelatin as the diluent for both toxin and antitoxin as well as for the sera to be tested. Diphtheria toxin is heat labile, and although it is not rapidly deactivated at room temperature, it is best to carry out all procedures in ice baths to maintain constant conditions. A convenient procedure is to keep in the freezing compartment of the refrigerator a supply of pans 4 to 5 in. (ca. 10 to 13 cm) deep containing 1 in. (ca. 2.5 cm) of water. By adding another inch of water, an ice bath for test tube racks is quickly produced, obviating the need for a supply of crushed ice. Test tube racks containing toxin-antitoxin mixtures can be returned to these ice trays after incubation at 37°C, and the mixtures can be kept at 0 to 4°C throughout the injection period.

For the screening test, prepare 10 serial three- to fivefold dilutions of toxin encompassing the expected Lr/20,000 endpoint. To a series of 10 test tubes (13 by 100 mm) add 0.5 ml of standard diphtheria antitoxin containing 0.001 AU/ml. To these tubes add 0.5 ml of each appropriate toxin dilution. Mix by gentle shaking and incubate at 37°C for 1 h; then transfer the tubes to an ice bath. Inject each of the toxin-antitoxin mixtures in 0.1-ml volumes intracutaneously in duplicate on the backs of each of two rabbits. Each injection site will thus receive 1/20,000 AU. If strict objectivity is desired, a randomized pattern should be prepared on paper, and the mixtures should be injected accordingly. Use disposable 26-gauge, 3/8-in. (ca. 1-cm), intradermal bevel needles on glass tuberculin syringes. Inject with the bevel downward. Plastic syringes may be used, but the removal of air bubbles during filling may be troublesome. Failure to expel all air from syringes and needle hilts leads to inaccurate injection volumes.

Read the reactions at 3 days. Only slight differences will be noted if the reading is done at 2 or 4 days. Record the diameter of redness to the nearest millimeter.

Determine the mean erythema diameter for each mixture. On graph paper plot diameters on the ordinate against the log of the toxin dose on the abscissa. The amount of toxin which yields a mean erythema diameter of 8 mm can be considered the preliminary Lr/20,000 dose. If the proper range of toxin doses has been chosen, diameters of erythema should range from 0 to ≥ 20 mm. If complete neutralization has not been achieved with a lower toxin dose, or if lesions at least 15 mm in diameter have not been achieved with higher doses, repeat the screening test after raising or lowering the range. Diphtheria toxin evokes palpable swelling as well as redness, but the diameter of induration or edema is difficult to estimate, whereas the margin of erythema is usually discrete and easily measurable.

After the Lr/20,000 screening test has been completed, repeat the test using 0.10-log increments of toxin instead of the three- to fivefold increments. The amount of toxin yielding a mean erythema diameter of 8 mm in this test can be considered the final Lr/20,000 dose to be used for antitoxin titrations. Once this value has been determined for a given batch of properly aged toxin, it will remain stable as long as the undiluted toxin sample is kept refrigerated. Fresh dilutions should be made from the neat stock once a week because diluted toxin samples are not stable. Newly prepared toxin usually loses potency more rapidly during the first few months due to spontaneous toxoiding.

All human and animal sera to be injected in rabbit skin should be inactivated at 56°C for 30 min. Some human sera contain components which produce redness and induration which may resemble the lesion elicited by diphtheria toxin. These components are usually, but not always, destroyed by inactivation. Therefore, a serum control of the highest concentration of the serum tested should be included in each test. When the Lr/20,000 dose of toxin is used, any serum dilution which yields a lesion of <8 mm in diameter can be considered to contain >0.001 AU/ml, and dilutions which yield lesions of >8 mm in diameter can be considered to contain <0.001 AU/ml. The accuracy desired will determine the serum dilution increments employed. For survey purposes, 10-fold serum dilutions are usually employed, and all persons possessing >0.01 AU/ml are considered the equivalent of Schick negative. In the rare clinical situations in which the determination of diphtheria antitoxin levels is critical, twofold serum dilutions would probably be required.

Prepare the desired serial dilutions of inactivated test sera in borate-gelatin buffer, and dispense 0.3 to 0.4 ml of each dilution into chilled test tubes. Dispense an extra tube of the highest serum concentration. To the serum control tube add an equal volume of diluent. To all other tubes add an equal volume of diphtheria toxin containing 20 Lr/20,000 doses per ml. (This is the Lr/20,000 concentration determined above; 0.05 ml of this material will contain 1 Lr/20,000 dose.) Include an Lr/20,000 titration in each rabbit test in order to ensure that the test dose on that day is actually at or near the Lr/20,000 level. Also include a toxin control containing equal volumes of the test dose of toxin and diluent. The Lr/20,000 titration of that day will determine the actual endpoint in that day's test. For example, if the test dose which was assumed to be 1 Lr/20,000 actually yielded a 6-mm lesion in the Lr/20,000 titration, then 6 mm should be the cutoff value in the antitoxin titrations.

Since all determinations are done on each of two rabbits, the diameters elicited by a given toxin-serum mixture can be averaged. The antitoxin content of an unknown serum is expressed as a range. For example, if a serum dilution of 1:2 completely neutralized the Lr/20,000 dose of toxin, a dilution of 1:4 yielded redness 10 mm in diameter, and the test dose that day

evoked a lesion 8 mm in diameter in the presence of 1/20,000 AU of standard antitoxin, then the antitoxin titer of that serum would be >1/500 but <1/250 AU/ml (>1/10,000 but <1/5,000 AU/0.05 ml).

It is important to titrate all the sera from a single patient on the same set of rabbits. In spite of adequate serum and toxin controls, rabbits may differ markedly in their susceptibility to diphtheria toxin; this can be reflected in differences in endpoints.

The rabbit intracutaneous test may be useful in estimating immunocompetence by determining serum antitoxin levels after the parenteral administration of diphtheria toxoid. The antitoxin response to protein antigens such as diphtheria toxoid is a measure of the competence of the T-cell-dependent B-cell-antibody-synthesizing system. Although Schick tests are sometimes used for this purpose, the rabbit skin test is superior because it allows for more precise measurement of the antitoxin level. Moreover, the Schick test is designed to detect very low levels of diphtheria antitoxin (0.01 AU/ml). To properly assess immunocompetence, one must be able to recognize a higher range of titers.

Titration of tetanus antitoxin by the mouse toxin neutralization test

The procedure for titration of tetanus antitoxin is based upon the capacity of tetanus antitoxin to protect mice from death after the subcutaneous injection of tetanus toxin. The following procedure is based on the method of Barile et al. (1).

The sample of tetanus toxin to be used must first be titrated against a standard tetanus antitoxin to determine the L+/1,000 toxin dose. The L+/1,000 dose is the least amount of tetanus toxin which when mixed with 1/1,000 AU of antitoxin and injected subcutaneously in mice in a volume of 0.5 ml causes the death of all mice by 96 h.

Use female 15- to 18-g mice; males tend to fight. Any strain may be used, but strain and source should not be changed once the titration procedure has been established. Preliminary estimation of the L+/1,000 dose of toxin can be made in groups of four to six mice. In all mouse tests, pool all mice needed for the test, including all controls, and distribute randomly into the groups required.

Phosphate-buffered saline (0.067 M, pH 7.4) containing 0.2% gelatin is used as the diluent for all reagents.

For the initial screening test to estimate the L+/1,000 dose of toxin, add constant volumes of standard antitoxin containing 0.004 AU/ml to a series of 8 to 10 tubes. Prepare a series of three- to fivefold dilutions of tetanus toxin, and add an equal volume to each tube of antitoxin. Shake gently, incubate for 1 h at 37°C, and then keep the mixtures at 4 to 8°C until the time of injection.

Inject 0.5 ml of each toxin-antitoxin mixture subcutaneously in the right inguinal fold of 4 to 10 mice per dose, using 26-gauge, 3/8-in. needles. Each injection contains 0.001 AU. Observe for 96 h and record the number of deaths. The smallest dose of toxin which kills all mice is the approximate L+/1,000 dose. (The corresponding toxin dilution contained 4 L+/1,000 doses per ml.)

To ascertain a more precise L+/1,000 dose, repeat

the test using narrower increments of toxin and 4 to 10 mice per toxin dose. Since tetanus toxin produces very precise and reproducible results in mice, good results may be obtained by using a very narrow range of doses. Increments of 5% over a twofold range can usually be used successfully. For example, the following progression (in micrograms of toxin per mouse) has been used: 16, 17, 18, 19, 20, 20.5, 21, 21.5, 22, 22.5, 23, 23.5, 24.

For serum titrations, test sera should be inactivated at 56°C for 30 min. Constant volumes of 2- to 10-fold dilutions of serum are dispensed into test tubes (13 by 100 mm). To each tube add an equal volume of toxin containing 1 L+/1,000 dose per ml. Each mouse thus receives 1 L+/4,000 dose of toxin per injection volume of 0.5 ml (one-fourth of an L+/1,000 dose). Run a concurrent L+/1,000 titration of the toxin against standard antitoxin as described above, using the same pool of mice. One group of mice should also receive the toxin test dose (1 L+/1,000 dose per ml) mixed with an equal volume of diluent. For serum titrations, groups of two to four mice per serum dilution give satisfactory results. The test is considered satisfactory if the concurrent L+/1,000 dose of toxin is within 25% of the test dose.

The results are interpreted as follows: if all mice are protected by undiluted serum but all die at 1:10 dilution, then 0.25 ml of the undiluted serum contained >0.00025 AU and 0.25 ml of the 1:10 dilution contained <0.00025 AU. Thus, the serum contained >0.001 but <0.01 AU/ml. For purposes of calculation such a serum can be assigned a value equal to the logarithmic mean of the values, or 0.003 AU/ml. For more precise titration, narrower increments of test sera can be used. Also, the level of testing can be shifted by using multiples or fractions of the L+/1,000 dose of toxin.

As in the case of diphtheria antitoxin, determination of serum tetanus antitoxin is of no value in determining the need for prophylactic or therapeutic antitoxin in the management of tetanus. This decision must be made on clinical grounds and certainly cannot await the outcome of a 4-day mouse test.

The determination of antitoxin level in serum collected before antitoxin therapy may be of retrospective academic interest in situations in which the diagnosis of tetanus was in doubt but in which antitoxin was administered. A pretreatment antitoxin titer of >0.01 AU/ml would indicate strongly against a diagnosis of tetanus. On the other hand, tetanus is usually considered a nonimmunizing disease because the pathogenic dose is much less than the immunogenic dose of this antigen. Therefore, the absence of antitoxin in serum collected after recovery from an illness in an untreated individual does not rule out the possibility that the illness was tetanus.

REAGENTS

Toxins

Diphtheria toxin can be purchased from List Biological Laboratories, Campbell, Calif. Tetanus toxin is not available commercially. Samples of both toxins can sometimes be obtained upon request from phar-maceutical companies which are engaged in the manufacture of diphtheria and tetanus toxoids.

Standard antitoxins

Samples of international standard diphtheria and tetanus antitoxins are supplied to qualified laboratories by the Bureau of Biologics, Food and Drug Administration, Rockville, Md. The Bureau supplies a single small vial containing low-titer antitoxin preserved in glycerol. This sample is to be used by the receiving laboratory in preparing and substandardizing its own stock. Therefore, it is necessary to purchase antitoxins from pharmaceutical houses or state laboratories which prepare diphtheria and tetanus antitoxins for prophylactic or therapeutic use. The approximate potency of these antitoxins is indicated on the label, but they must be precisely substandardized against the official standard preparation before they can be used as a reference reagent. Tetanus immune globulin (TIG) of human origin can be purchased from several pharmaceutical companies and then substandardized against the standard reagent.

Schick test materials

It is regrettable that there is no longer a commercial source of Schick toxin available in the United States. Until recently, Schick test outfits were prepared by the Biologic Laboratories of the Department of Public Health of the Commonwealth of Massachusetts, Jamaica Plain. However, they have recently discontinued production. There is therefore no licensed Schick testing material in the United States at present.

Borate-gelatin buffer

0.5 M H_3BO_3	100 ml
1.5 M NaCl	80 ml
5% Gelatin	20 ml
1 N NaOH to	pH 7.5
Water to	1,000 ml

LITERATURE CITED

1. **Barile, M. F., M. C. Hardegree, and M. Pittman.** 1970. Immunization against neonatal tetanus in New Guinea. 3. The toxin-neutralization test and the response of guinea pigs to the toxoids as used in the immunization schedules in New Guinea. Bull. W.H.O. **43**:453–459.
2. **Craig, J. P.** 1962. Diphtheria: prevalence of inapparent infection in a nonepidemic period. Am. J. Public Health **52**:1444–1452.
3. **Dow, B. C., A. Barr, R. J. Crawford, and R. Mitchell.** 1983. A solid-phase radioimmunoassay for detection of tetanus antibody. Med. Lab. Sci. **40**:73–74.
4. **Frost, W. H.** 1928. Infection, immunity and disease in the epidemiology of diphtheria with special reference to studies in Baltimore. J. Prev. Med. **2**:325.
5. **Gupta, R. A., S. C. Maheshwari, and H. Singh.** 1984. The titration of tetanus antitoxin. III. A comparative evaluation of indirect haemagglutination and toxin neutralization titres of human sera. J. Biol. Stand. **12**:145–149.
6. **Jensen, C.** 1933. Die intrakutane Kaninchen Methode zur Auswertung von Diphtherie Toxin und Antitoxin. Acta Pathol. Microbiol. Scand. **10**(Suppl. 14).
7. **Kameyama, S., K. Yamauchi, S. Yasuda, and S. Kondo.** 1980. Influence of anti-fragment A of diphtheria toxin on

passive hemagglutination with antitoxin. Jpn. J. Med. Sci. Biol. **33:**67–80.

8. **Landy, M., R. J. Trapani, R. Formal, and I. Klugler.** 1955. Comparison of hemagglutination procedure and the rabbit intradermal neutralization test for the assay of diphtheria antitoxin in human sera. Am. J. Hyg. **61:**143–154.

9. **Lee, C. C.** 1982. Microlatex test for diphtheria antitoxin. Chin. J. Microbiol. Immunol. (Beijing) **15:**131–136.

10. **Melville-Smith, M. E., V. A. Seagroatt, and J. T. Watkins.** 1983. A comparison of enzyme-linked immunosorbent assay (ELISA) with the toxin neutralization test in mice as a method for the estimation of tetanus antitoxin in human sera. J. Biol. Stand. **11:**137–144.

11. **Menser, M. A., and J. R. Hudson.** 1984. Population studies of diphtheria immunity using antitoxin radioimmunoassay. J. Hyg. **92:**1–7.

12. **Miyamura, K., S. Nishi, A. Ito, R. Murata, and R. Kono.** 1974. Micro cell culture method for determination of diphtheria toxin and antitoxin titres using VERO cells. I. Studies on factors affecting the toxin and antitoxin titration. J. Biol. Stand. **2:**189–201.

13. **Moyner, K.** 1981. Precipitation inhibition counter immunoelectrophoresis (PICI) for the quantification of diphtheria antitoxin. J. Biol. Stand. **9:**131–136.

13a. **Nyerges, G., G. Nyerges, M. Surjan, J. Budai, and J. Csapo.** 1963. A method for the rapid determination of diphtheria antitoxin in clinical practice. Acta Pediatr. Acad. Sci. Hung. **4:**399–409.

14. **Winsnes, R., and G. Christiansen.** 1979. Quantification of tetanus antitoxin in human sera. II. Comparison of counterimmunoelectrophoresis and passive hemagglutination with toxin neutralization in mice. Acta Pathol. Microbiol. Scand. Sect. B **87:**197–200.

15. **Zingher, A.** 1923. The Schick test performed on more than 150,000 children in public and parochial schools in New York (Manhattan and the Bronx). Am. J. Dis. Child. **25:**392–405.

Chapter 66

Immune Response to Mycobacteria

M. J. LEFFORD

The immune response to mycobacterial infections is characterized by both cell-mediated immunity (CMI) and humoral manifestations, and tests have been developed to measure both types of reactivity. The classical method of detecting infection with *Mycobacterium tuberculosis* is the dermal delayed-hypersensitivity (DH) test, using culture filtrate components as antigens. This test is still useful both for the diagnosis of disease in individuals and for epidemiological studies. Serological tests using culture filtrate antigens also have a long, if less distinguished, history but have been applied less widely and are regarded as less useful. Indeed, the previous edition of this manual fairly summarized their status in the statement that "tests for serum antibodies are not at present suitable for use in the diagnostic laboratory" (7). This statement is still valid, but there has been renewed activity in this area which merits fuller recognition in this edition. Finally, the previous edition made no mention of leprosy, an omission that is remedied here. The first section of this chapter deals with infections caused by *M. tuberculosis* complex (which includes *M. bovis*) and other cultivable human pathogens; a separate section on leprosy follows.

TUBERCULOSIS

Tuberculin test

Tuberculin (3). The standard diagnostic test for tuberculosis and related mycobacterial infections is the tuberculin test, for which at least two types of antigen preparation and several testing procedures are extant. The original tuberculin, old tuberculin (OT), is made by cultivating a virulent strain of *M. tuberculosis* as a pellicle on liquid medium for several months, at which time the once colorless medium resembles a dark brown, cloudy soup. This culture medium contains bacterial secretory products in various stages of degradation, plus numerous nonsecreted constitutive bacterial products which result from the physical breakdown of dead bacterial cells. This material is autoclaved, filtered, and concentrated 10-fold. The resulting material (OT) contains a heterogeneous mixture of proteins, polysaccharides, lipids, and nucleic acids, some of which are in a state of partial or total denaturation. Since the proteins comprise the major, if not exclusive, antigenic moiety for skin testing, the other components are redundant at best and exert nonspecific inflammatory effects at worst. Consequently, OT is not used for definitive diagnostic tuberculin testing of adults but is still employed for epidemiological and survey studies, particularly in children (see below). In 1934, Seibert (10) developed an improved product designated purified protein derivative (PPD) that consisted of a trichloroacetic acid precipitate of OT. In the United Kingdom, PPD is still made in the same way, but in the United States ammonium sulfate is now used instead of trichloroacetic acid. These PPD preparations are depleted but not completely free of nonprotein components. The trichloroacetic acid preparations, in particular, contain substantial quantities of nucleic acids. PPD is a very crude product that can be considered purified only in comparison to OT. PPD contains numerous protein molecular species, many of which have been denatured during the long period of mycobacterial cultivation and subsequent autoclaving. It is also notable that no two batches of PPD are chemically and antigenically identical. For that reason PPD is standardized by biological assay, and its potency is expressed in tuberculin units (TU) by standardization against PPD-S, a reference tuberculin that was prepared by Seibert (10). The protein content of 5 TU is variously stated as approximately 0.1 or 0.2 μg. The former value represents the strict chemical equivalence and the latter the biological equivalence, taking into account the unavoidable loss of protein due to adherence to the glass or plastic of the vials and syringes.

PPD prepared from *M. tuberculosis* is designated tuberculin PPD to distinguish it from tuberculins that are prepared in similar fashion from culture filtrates of other mycobacterial species (Table 1). Tuberculin PPD and OT are the only materials licensed in the United States for use in humans, but other non-tuberculosis mycobacterial tuberculins, sometimes called sensitins, are available in Canada and elsewhere. Other products, such as disrupted mycobacterial cells and their constituents as well as components isolated from PPD, have been used in experimental animal research and for serological studies in humans.

Dosage. Historically, PPD was available in several strengths, allowing physicians to select a dose that they deemed appropriate. The chosen initial dose was often 1 TU. If the test result was negative at this dose, sequential testing with doses increasing to 250 TU was common. In 1971, a committee of the American Thoracic Society (ATS), convened to address the problem of tuberculin testing, suggested that only a 5-TU dose be used (6). Only this dose is in common use, but 1- and 250-TU presentations are commercially available. Commercial PPD is marketed as a lyophilized powder that is dissolved in accompanying sterile phosphate buffer solution to a strength of 5 TU/0.1 ml. This buffer ensures optimum stability of the PPD in solution and also contains 0.05% Tween 80, a wetting agent that minimizes the adsorption of PPD to its glass vial container and to the walls of the glass or plastic hypodermic syringe that is used to deliver the antigen. The rationale for the 5-TU dose is that it is sufficient to detect significant specific tuberculin DH, yet small enough to minimize positive cross-reactions attributable to sensitization with other mycobacterial species that may be present in the normal environ-

TABLE 1. Mycobacterial tuberculin-testing reagents[a]

Mycobacterial species	Tuberculin
M. tuberculosis complex	Tuberculin PPD[b]
M. avium/M. intracellulare	PPD-B
M. kansasii	PPD-Y
M. scrofulaceum	PPD-G
M. fortuitum	PPD-F
M. ulcerans	Burulin
M. marinum	PPD-Platy
M. chelonei	PPD-Glaze
M. leprae	Lepromin[c]

[a] The list is not comprehensive but includes the major species and their tuberculins.
[b] Licensed in the United States for use in humans.
[c] A bacterial suspension rather than a culture filtrate.

ment. In retrospect, the adoption of a single test dose was beneficial, if only for the reason that the data obtained by different investigators can now be validly compared. A problem with the older literature is that disparate doses of tuberculin were used, with or without Tween 80.

Antigen injection. The Mantoux test is the method of choice for diagnostic purposes in that an accurately measured quantity of antigen is injected intradermally. This test has severe disadvantages for survey work, since a separate needle and 1-ml hypodermic (tuberculin) syringe should be used for each patient and skill is required to perform an intradermal injection, particularly in elderly subjects with atrophic skin and in children. Because the test is so individualized, it is time-consuming, particularly when administered on a large scale. Two other types of test have been devised to circumvent these problems. There is a group of tests (tine, Mono-Vacc, and Heaf/Sterneedle) that depend on the introduction into the skin of an imprecise quantity of antigen by a multiple-puncture disposable device. In the tine test, the prongs of the tine are covered with dried OT. Use of the other devices requires the application of antigen solution (OT or PPD) to the epidermis, which is then punctured, analogous to the now defunct vaccination method for smallpox. The results of such tests are more difficult to read than the Mantoux test. They are also more difficult to interpret because extensive epidemiological studies of the type obtained by Mantoux testing are lacking. A seemingly better alternative is the jet-gun test, in which a precise volume of tuberculin PPD (0.1 ml) containing 5 TU can be injected intradermally without breaking the surface of the skin, raising a bleb 6 to 10 mm in diameter. In practice, a suboptimal dose can easily be injected by applying the device to the skin with insufficient pressure. All of these substitutes for the Mantoux test have been used in epidemiological studies, particularly of school children. However, all subjects who develop positive or doubtfully positive reactions should be retested using the Mantoux test.

The mechanics of the Mantoux test are as follows. The manufacturer's diluent is added aseptically as directed to the vial of lyophilized tuberculin PPD that dissolves easily. For each individual patient, the tuberculin solution is drawn into a sterile 1-ml hypodermic syringe mounted with a 26- or 27-gauge needle with a short bevel to contain 0.1 ml. The needle is inserted, bevel upward, into the cleaned and dried skin of the volar aspect of the forearm, and the 0.1-ml dose is injected intradermally, raising a bleb 6 to 10 mm in diameter. The test is read 48 to 72 h later as described below. It is not necessary to inject buffer into the skin of the contralateral arm as a control. Should there be a mishap with the injection, such as subcutaneous instead of intradermal injection, the patient can be immediately reinjected either in the other arm or at a distance of several centimeters in the same arm.

Reading of test. The time at which the reaction is read has undergone changes. Formerly, the test was read 24 h after injection, but such readings were sometimes vitiated by the occurrence of acute nonspecific or acute antibody-mediated inflammatory reactions, or both, that had not completely subsided in 24 h. Consequently, a 48-h reading was adopted which has, in turn, been replaced by a 72-h reading. Any reaction that is positive at 48 h need not be reexamined, but some patients generate slowly developing reactions that are not positive until 72 h postinjection. The criterion of a positive reaction is the presence of induration at the injection site. The limits of induration are determined by palpation and marked on the skin with a pen. The diameter of induration is measured transverse to the long axis of the forearm and recorded in millimeters. Erythema is of no significance and should be disregarded. Some reactions may proceed to necrosis and ulceration, indicating very high sensitivity.

Interpretation. The major problem of the tuberculin test is establishing the minimum diameter of induration that represents true DH. The aforementioned ATS committee proposed criteria for nonsensitivity (0 to 4 mm induration), doubtful sensitivity (5 to 9 mm induration), and positivity ($\geq$10 mm induration). More recently, another ATS committee has grappled with this problem (5). The data upon which their conclusions are based are drawn largely from studies of U.S. Navy recruits who were predominantly young male Caucasians, so these conclusions may not be applicable to other populations. The three basic observations were as follows.

(i) A large population of patients with bacteriologically proven tuberculosis was tested with 5 TU of tuberculin PPD. The resulting reactions ranged from 0 to 26 mm in diameter, and the frequency distribution of reaction sizes conformed to a unimodal normal curve with a mean of 16 to 17 mm. Similar results have been obtained in many studies of tuberculosis patients around the world.

(ii) Testing of healthy U.S. Navy personnel with a history of tuberculosis household contacts yielded an entirely different distribution. The single largest group (70%) had reactions 0 to 2 mm in diameter and were unambiguously tuberculin negative. The remaining reactions form a normal frequency distribution curve with a mean of approximately 16 mm. This bimodal distribution displays a distinct valley between the two peaks, favoring the adoption of a 5-mm reaction size demarcation, above which subjects may be considered to be tuberculin positive.

(iii) Testing of healthy personnel with no history of tuberculosis contact yielded a distribution resembling the right-hand side of a normal distribution with a positive skew. A few subjects had reactions ≥16 mm in diameter, but since there is a steady gradation of reaction sizes from zero on up, there is no clear point of demarcation between low, intermediate, and high reactors. The low reactors are presumed to be tuberculin negative and the high reactors tuberculin positive. The intermediate reactors comprise a mixture of negative and positive reactors derived from the upper tail of the negative-reactors distribution and the lower tail of the positive-reactors distribution, respectively. The intermediate reactors also include a group of subjects who have not been sensitized by *M. tuberculosis* but who exhibit cross-reactivity to tuberculin PPD by being sensitized to an environmental mycobacterial species. The frequency of nontuberculosis sensitization and the identity of the sensitizing species will vary with geographic location. For example, the prevalence of nontuberculosis sensitization is relatively high in the southeastern United States, and the causative organism is *M. intracellulare*.

Given this complex situation, there is no universally applicable criterion of positivity. If one accepts 5 mm as the criterion, then very few subjects who are truly infected with *M. tuberculosis* will be misdiagnosed as tuberculin negative. On the other hand, many subjects who have never been infected by *M. tuberculosis* would be misclassified as positive and subjected to the expense, inconvenience, and hazard of radiological and other tests. By moving the criterion of positivity to a 10-mm diameter, the properly tuberculin-negative subjects are correctly classified, but some tuberculosis subjects are missed. Shifting the criterion of positivity up and down the scale of reaction sizes generates a spectrum of similar compromises.

A reaction size of 10 mm or more is a good standard working criterion for a positive reaction. But that criterion must not be regarded as absolute and should be used with flexibility, depending on the clinical situation. Three hypothetical examples are described below.

(i) A patient who lives in a geographic area where the prevalence of tuberculosis is high and the prevalence of environmental mycobacterial sensitization is low is suspected of having tuberculosis. The 10-mm criterion of positivity is adequate, but given the high probability of tuberculosis infection and the low probability of other mycobacterial infection, reaction sizes of 5 mm or greater might be considered positive.

(ii) A student develops tuberculosis while residing at a small rural college. The regional prevalence of both tuberculosis and nontuberculosis mycobacterial infections is low. The other students at the college are to be tuberculin tested. Once again, the 10-mm criterion is adequate and might be shaded toward 5 mm, given the high probability of infection from the initial case.

(iii) If example ii occurs in a geographic region of relatively high prevalence of nontuberculosis mycobacterial infection, then reactions less than 10 mm in size are probably not indicative of tuberculosis infection, and even some 10-mm reactions may be attributable to the environmental species.

Obviously, such tuberculin reactions are not interpreted in a clinical vacuum. The physician should acquire other clinical, laboratory, and radiological evidence to assist with the interpretation of the tuberculin test.

The various multiple-puncture tuberculin tests are interpreted as follows. If the reaction consists of discrete papules, the diameter of the largest papule is measured. If papules are confluent, the diameter of the entire reaction is measured. The reaction sizes are interpreted by the same criteria as the Mantoux test. Vesiculation of a multiple-puncture test is considered indicative of tuberculin positivity. Any positive or doubtful multiple-puncture test should be reconfirmed by Mantoux test. It is good practice not to record a tuberculin test result simply as negative, positive, or doubtful. The reaction diameter should be recorded for later reference should the test be repeated or the patient's clinical condition require reinterpretation of the reaction.

Clinical indications. In clinical practice only the Mantoux test is indicated, since only this test provides for the injection of an accurately measured dose of PPD, and the interpretation of the test is based on a large body of evidence. The indications for the tuberculin test are suspected tuberculosis, the evaluation of contacts of tuberculosis patients, and to exclude tuberculosis. In practice, the test is also performed for the record on patients with known tuberculosis. The test is most useful in patients with extrapulmonary tuberculosis in which radiological examination yields ambiguous results and adequate bacteriological specimens are difficult to obtain. It should be emphasized that a positive test does not necessarily signify active tuberculosis, but may be obtained in three circumstances as follows: (i) prior mycobacterial infection, clinical or subclinical, that is now inactive or cured; (ii) clinical or subclinical active mycobacterial infection; and (iii) vaccination with *M. bovis* BCG.

Since the most common mycobacterial disease in the United States is still tuberculosis, *M. tuberculosis* can be presumed to be the cause of sensitization unless other infections are specifically indicated. By the same token, few people in this country have been vaccinated with BCG. In any case, this agent induces low levels of hypersensitivity that decrease progressively with time and is rarely the cause of a strong, unambiguous reaction.

Reliability. The tuberculin test is reliable provided a minimum of attention and skill is devoted to it. The minimum of attention involves the solution of the dried PPD in the proper volume of appropriate buffer using standard aseptic technique, the injection of the correct volume of antigen solution, and the avoidance of old solutions of antigen that may be immunologically inactive, or infected, or both. These requirements are not exacting for any trained professional. The elements of skill involve the ability to give an intradermal injection and accurately measure the diameter of induration. The latter is probably the most important variable affecting the reliability of the test. Considerable variation between observers has been established, and even a given observer may not accurately reproduce measurements to within 1 to 2 mm. This consideration alone should caution against strict adherence to criteria of positivity. For example, if a reaction is 9 mm in diameter, it should be appreciated that the reaction size might easily be remeasured by the same observer or another observer as 7 or 11 mm. Reliable, consistent measurements depend more upon experience than any other faculty.

The average physician or nurse who practices outside a specialist tuberculosis clinic has little opportunity to gather the required experience. For this reason, some nurses and physicians feel uncomfortable when required to perform tuberculin tests and tend to project that discomfort against the test itself, impugning it with an undeserved reputation for unreliability. There are other more substantive reasons for dissatisfaction. The test often requires personal attention by the physician, sometimes at inconvenient times, and the 72-h interval between antigen injection and reading may impose inconvenience on both patient and physician.

Specificity. The specificity of the test for the genus *Mycobacterium* is high, so a positive result provides compelling evidence of past or present mycobacterial infection. However, because of extensive sharing of antigenic determinants within the genus, there is corresponding cross-reactivity between mycobacterial species at both the T-cell (tuberculin DH) and B-cell (antibody) levels. In general, however, species-specific DH reactions are much stronger than those caused by cross-reactive DH. Consequently, the relatively small eliciting dose of 5 TU is much less prone to detect sensitization to heterologous mycobacterial species than are the much higher doses (250 TU) that were sometimes used in the past. Accordingly, a patient infected with *M. intracellulare* will likely develop a stronger reaction to PPD-B than to tuberculin PPD. The opposite would be true for a patient infected with *M. tuberculosis*. It follows that there is a place in clinical practice for the diagnostic use of species-specific mycobacterial tuberculins. At one time these reagents were available from the Centers for Disease Control, but their distribution has since been rescinded due to problems of standardization. At present, no tuberculins other than tuberculin PPD are licensed in the United States for use in humans, but they are available in Canada and elsewhere so their use is described here.

The rational use of these reagents requires that there be evidence, or at least strong suspicion, that a particular mycobacterial species, e.g., *M. fortuitum*, is the infecting agent. Testing should then proceed with the homologous sensitin (e.g., PPD-F) in parallel with tuberculin PPD, each reagent being injected into a different arm. Specific nontuberculosis infection is denoted by a diameter of induration that is either twice as long as, or exceeds by 5 mm, the diameter of induration caused by tuberculin PPD. The various species-specific tuberculins should not be used for multiple tuberculin testing of patients with obscure symptomatology or fever of unknown origin in the hope that something will turn up. As a rule of thumb, the more tuberculins that are used for testing, the more difficult the interpretation.

False results. Misleading results can be either false-positive or false-negative. Given that the tuberculin test is genus specific, all false-positive results, which are rare, are attributable to technical errors. These include the use of nonsterile equipment and contaminated tuberculins and the injection of an incorrect dose. False-negative results are more common and may also be technical in nature. The tuberculin may be old, overdiluted, or misinjected (too small a dose or injected subcutaneously). Intradermal injection may be particularly difficult in elderly subjects with thin, atrophic skin. The failure of such subjects to develop a positive reaction due to misinjection may be misinterpreted as either tuberculin negativity or immunodeficiency.

The technical causes of false-negative results are real enough, but there are more substantive causes of unreactivity, which is termed anergy. The causes of anergy are legion, and only major ones will be mentioned here. More comprehensive treatment of this topic may be found in textbooks of internal medicine and similar texts that deal with clinical tuberculosis.

Anergy may be transient or persistent. Transient anergy may be associated with the viral exanthemata (particularly measles), pertussis, influenza, pneumonia, and following immunization with live-virus vaccines and treatment with immunosuppressive drugs, particularly corticosteroids. Transient anergy may also be present in some forms of tuberculosis. Patients with early tuberculosis who are tested before the development of DH may give misleadingly negative results. On the other hand, patients with very extensive pulmonary tuberculosis or miliary tuberculosis may be anergic. Such anergy frequently disappears as the patient responds to appropriate chemotherapy.

Persistent anergy is associated with immunosuppressive diseases such as lymphomas and chronic debilitating diseases such as cancer, hypothyroidism, chronic substance abuse, and advanced progressive tuberculosis. Tuberculosis contacts who are treated with prophylactic antituberculosis chemotherapy often become tuberculin negative. Such reversion is unusual in patients with active disease who have been treated successfully. There is a small group of proven tuberculosis patients who are apparently normal in other respects, yet fail to generate positive tuberculin reactions, presumably because they are genetically determined low responders.

Retesting. In cases of doubtful tuberculin sensitivity, the test should be repeated. The most common reason for repeating a test is that the result of the first test is ambiguous, giving a reaction size 5 to 9 mm in diameter. The other major reason for retesting is an initial test result that is incompatible with the patient's condition, such as a negative result in a patient with proven tuberculosis. In such cases, the tuberculin test should be repeated 1 week after the first test, using either the opposite arm or a site on the same arm at least 5 cm from the first injection. The retest should be performed precisely as though it were a first test, using 5 TU. There is no valid reason to use increasingly large doses of tuberculin. Repeat tests can also be used to monitor the recovery of a patient from transient anergy or to establish that anergy is persistent. Repeated testing is particularly useful in patients whose once high DH has diminished with age. One or two repeat tests, at weekly intervals, may raise a doubtful reaction, or even a negative reaction, to a positive one. There is no risk of inducing tuberculin positivity in tuberculin-negative subjects by repeated testing, such as occurs with brucellin tests. Repeat tests are contraindicated in patients with high levels of hypersensitivity, who may suffer discomfort from the intensity of a severe reaction, which may in turn proceed to necrosis, ulceration, and scarring.

In vitro tests of CMI

Two in vitro analogs of the tuberculin skin test have been used in numerous small studies: lymphocyte transformation (LT) and production of migration inhibitory factor in response to PPD. For the latter type of test both unseparated blood leukocyte preparations and purified mononuclear cells have been used. These tests are normally performed on peripheral blood leukocytes, but lymph node and pleural fluid cells can also be used. In general, there is a close statistical association between positive tuberculin skin tests and the in vitro analogs, but, inevitably, there are discrepancies. In some studies one or the other of these in vitro tests has been superior to the skin test, while the reverse has also been observed. The essence of this problem is that while the tuberculin test is standardized, the method of performing and interpreting the in vitro tests is left to the whim of the investigator. Consequently, every conceivable variation of blood cell preparation, in vitro culture conditions, type and concentration of tuberculin, and evaluation of result can be found in the literature. It is therefore impossible to validly compare the accuracy of the skin and in vitro tests. Accordingly, the tuberculin skin test remains the standard of sensitization with *M. tuberculosis*, and the in vitro tests are reserved for research investigations.

Serological tests

The substantive shortcomings of the tuberculin skin test are concerned with its sensitivity and specificity. The problem of sensitivity is due to the inability of the test to distinguish between inactive and active tuberculosis; the distinction between unsensitized and sensitized individuals is satisfactory. The problem of specificity is manifest as the difficulty in distinguishing between sensitization by *M. tuberculosis* and other mycobacterial species. The specificity problem is not intrinsic to the tuberculin test as such, but is an expression of the nonspecificity of tuberculin PPD. The use of the same type of antigen in serological tests detracts from their specificity, yet the hope of increased sensitivity remains a possibility.

The history of serological tests, the first of which dates from 1904, reflects the history of immunological methods (9). Thus, in chronological order, serological tests were based on bacterial agglutination, precipitation in liquid, complement fixation, passive agglutination (erythrocytes and inert carriers), precipitation in gel, immunofluorescence, radioimmunoassay, and enzyme-linked immunosorbent assay (ELISA). Each type of test enjoyed initial success, but with increasing use disillusion has set in, and finally the test has been discarded. To what factors can this be attributed? Reference has already been made to the unsatisfactory nature of the antigens. Some methods were of low intrinsic sensitivity or were dependent on secondary antibody-antigen reactions that were in turn dependent on particular antibody isotypes. These technical problems have been overcome by the introduction of the radioimmunoassay and ELISA techniques. Some encouraging results have been reported by investigators using conventional tuberculin PPD, but the use of purified antigens is more promising. One antigen of note is antigen 5 of *M. tuberculosis*, which is thought to be more specific for that mycobacterial species than tuberculin PPD. The published data obtained by ELISA show that antigen 5 is superior to tuberculin PPD. The specificity of both tests is high, but the sensitivity of the antigen 5 assay is superior to that of the PPD assay (1). However, as with the tuberculin skin test, the accuracy of a serological assay varies with the prevalence of tuberculosis in the population being studied. In the aforementioned antigen 5 study, the patients were drawn from a tuberculosis hospital population in which the prevalence of tuberculosis was high and the prevalence of environmental mycobacteria was low. As the prevalence of tuberculosis decreases, so does the accuracy of the assay; an increasing prevalence of environmental mycobacteria would further vitiate its accuracy. In any case, the success of the antigen 5 study is clouded by two issues. First, the investigation was initiated by the protagonist of antigen 5, and such studies have historically enjoyed the greatest success. Second, antigen 5 is not available for general distribution and evaluation.

Further hopes for a satisfactory serological test rest on the production of species-specific monoclonal antibodies, some of which have already been described. The presumption is that such specific probes will allow the development of highly specific tests, based on competitive-binding assays. Yet one of the fundamental aspects of the immunobiology of tuberculosis is that CMI is usually strong and conspicuous, whereas antibody levels are unimpressively weak. Antimycobacterial antibody levels are substantially raised predominantly in patients with large bacterial loads denoting extensive disease. Such disease is just as easily and more definitively diagnosed by examination of sputum smears for acid-fast bacilli. Moreover, antibody titers are often highest, or first become positive, after the onset of antituberculosis chemotherapy. These considerations cast considerable doubt as to whether any serological test will fulfill the high expectations demanded of it.

LEPROSY

Lepromin test

As in tuberculosis, two types of immunological response, cell-mediated and humoral, have been harnessed for the diagnosis of leprosy. The provision of suitable antigens is a problem in leprosy because *M. leprae* cannot be grown on conventional bacteriological culture media or in tissue culture. Consequently, no *M. leprae* culture filtrate that is equivalent to tuberculin is available. Until recently, the major source of *M. leprae* was the tissue of leprosy patients, specifically those with lepromatous leprosy, in whom the load of bacilli is very high. That tissue was first autoclaved, then homogenized, filtered, preserved with phenol, and re-autoclaved. The final product, designated integral lepromin, consisted of leprosy bacilli, intact and in various stages of disintegration, and human tissue products. Lepromin was prepared in leprosaria for local use and for many years there was no standard of the type that applies to tuberculin PPD. Indeed, no standard for lepromin exists in the United States to this day, and lepromin is not licensed for human use in this country. The current international standard requires a density of 1.6×10^8 acid-fast bacilli per ml. In 1976, *M. leprae* was shown to infect the nine-banded armadillo *(Dasypus novemcintus)*, and tissues from such experimentally infected animals are now the major source of lepromin. Sufficient bacilli can be harvested from a single armadillo, or several animals, to yield a large batch of lepromin that is minimally contaminated with armadillo tissue. Armadillo-derived lepromin is designated lepromin-A to distinguish it from human-derived lepromin-H. The two sources of lepromin are immunologically indistinguishable.

The lepromin test is performed by injecting 0.1 ml of lepromin (1.6×10^7 bacilli) intradermally into the arm. Consequently, the lepromin test is prone to the same technical failures as the tuberculin test with respect to injection and reading. Two types of positive reaction may be elicited. The Fernandez reaction occurs 24 to 48 h after antigen injection; it closely resembles a positive tuberculin reaction and is measured in similar fashion. The epidemiology of Fernandez reactivity has not been as thoroughly studied as tuberculin reactivity, and the criterion of positivity has not been evaluated as rigorously. An area of induration 5 mm in diameter is generally accepted as positive, and even reactions as small as 3 mm are considered positive by some investigators. Intense, florid reactions of the type seen in individuals who are highly sensitive to tuberculin do not occur.

Unlike the tuberculin reaction, which is positive in a high proportion of subclinically infected contacts, the Fernandez reaction is less often positive. This lack of reactivity is often seen in household contacts who have a high probability of infection and is commonly observed even in patients with paucibacillary leprosy (tuberculoid and borderline tuberculoid). Such patients express strong CMI to *M. leprae* antigens in terms of lymphocyte transformation and tuberculoid granuloma formation. Because of its insensitivity, the Fernandez test is not widely used. The second type of positive reaction is the Mitsuda reaction. This reaction may be read 3 to 6 weeks after injection and also consists of an indurated lesion that may progress to superficial necrosis, ulceration, and scarring. Various criteria of positivity have been proposed, but an area of induration that is 5 mm in diameter is widely accepted. Nearly all normal, healthy individuals, including those who have never been exposed to *M. leprae*, develop a Mitsuda reaction, so a positive Mitsuda reaction is less an indicator of leprosy than it is a manifestation of immune competence. Consequently, a negative Mitsuda reaction has greater significance than a positive one. Negative reactions are obtained in patients with lepromatous leprosy, who do not express specific CMI to *M. leprae*. This anergy is very specific because such patients express positive reactions to tuberculin PPD.

LT

Because the Fernandez test is relatively insensitive in detecting subclinical and early leprosy, in vitro LT tests have been used instead. The usual antigen is integral lepromin or a bacterial disruption product derived from it. Such tests have proved useful for

TABLE 2. Skin test (Mitsuda reaction) and LT responses to lepromin[a]

Subjects	LT response	Mitsuda response
Normal	−	+++
Leprosy contact	+++	+++
Tuberculoid leprosy	+++	+++
Borderline leprosy	++	++
Lepromatous leprosy	−	−

[a] +++, Strongly positive response; ++, positive response; −, no response.

detecting subclinical infection and are also positive in patients with active leprosy of the tuberculoid to borderline types. *M. leprae*-specific LT is notably absent in lepromatous leprosy and is also negative in normal subjects who live in leprosy nonendemic areas. The combination of LT and Mitsuda tests efficiently discriminates between normal subjects and leprosy patients, as shown in Table 2. In practice, the usefulness of the LT test is limited because it has never been adequately standardized, it requires good laboratory facilities and highly trained personnel, and it is expensive. These requirements are difficult to fulfill in the countries where leprosy is most prevalent, so in practice the LT test is more a research tool than a practicable diagnostic test.

Serology

As for tuberculosis, serological tests for leprosy have a long but unimpressive history, and for similar reasons. The situation with leprosy is complicated by the fact that tuberculosis is a far more prevalent disease in countries where leprosy is endemic, so any serological test for leprosy must be able to distinguish between the antigens of *M. leprae* and *M. tuberculosis*. As noted above, the protein antigens within the genus *Mycobacterium* are highly cross-reactive, but much finer specificity can be found in the saccharide moieties of the cell wall glycolipids (2, 4). In particular, a phenolic glycolipid designated PGL-1 is present in the cell wall of *M. leprae* and appears to be secreted into the tissues of the infected host. Consequently, substantial quantities of this material can be recovered from *M. leprae*-infected armadillos. PGL-1 appears to be restricted to *M. leprae* and provides the basis for a specific serological test. Several groups of investigators have developed ELISAs to detect PGL-1 antibodies. There is a problem in handling PGL-1 as an antigen since it is a lipid and therefore insoluble in aqueous solution. It is possible to coat ELISA plates with PGL-1 in a fine oil-in-water emulsion, but it is easier to work with a water-soluble product. One such compound is deacylated PGL-1, which is sparingly soluble in water, but superior reagents have been developed by Brennan and his co-workers (8). They established that most of the antigenicity of PGL-1 resides in the terminal sugar of the trisaccharide moiety; they then synthesized the terminal disaccharide and linked it to a number of protein carriers such as bovine serum albumin, bovine gamma globulin, and human serum albumin. These reagents bind to ELISA plates, using standard procedures. The resulting antibody assays are highly sensitive and specific, but there are two limitations on their use. (i) The native and synthetic antigens are available on a very limited basis only through the National Institutes of Health for research purposes. (ii) Antibody-positive sera are found in a high proportion of patients with lepromatous leprosy, in a lower proportion of those with borderline leprosy, and in very few patients with tuberculoid leprosy. Unfortunately, lepromatous leprosy is easily diagnosed by other means, notably by examining slit-skin smears for acid-fast bacilli. Monoclonal antibodies to *M. leprae* have also been developed, but they have not yet been exploited for any practical purpose.

CONCLUSION

The fundamental deficiency in all diagnostic tests that depend on the measurement of antibodies or specific cellular hypersensitivity is that the immunological response lags behind the infectious disease process. Such tests often cannot distinguish between subclinical infection, active infection, and healed or cured active infection. The essence of the diagnosis of an active infection is the isolation of the infectious agent. Short of that ideal situation, which is often not realizable, the identification of a specific microbial product serves the same purpose. Immunological probes, both polyclonal and monoclonal, are already being used to detect mycobacterial antigens in patient specimens, and the preliminary data are encouraging. This approach will probably supersede the rather unsatisfactory antibody assays and may even dislodge the skin tests from their preeminent position.

Sources of materials

Tuberculin PPD (Parke, Davis & Co., Detroit, Mich.; Connaught Laboratories, Willowdale, Ontario, Canada)

Other tuberculins (Connaught Laboratories)

Lepromin (IMMLEP Program, World Health Organization, Geneva, Switzerland)

Multiple-puncture devices: four-tine device impregnated with OT (Lederle Laboratories, Pearl River, N.Y.) and with tuberculin PPD (Parke-Davis Co.)

and six-tine device (HEAF test) impregnated with tuberculin PPD (Connaught Laboratories)

LITERATURE CITED

1. **Balestrino, E. A., T. M. Daniel, M. D. S. de Latini, O. A. Latini, Y. Ma, and J. B. Scocozza.** 1984. Serodiagnosis of pulmonary tuberculosis in Argentina by enzyme-linked immunosorbent assay (ELISA) of IgG antibody to *Mycobacterium tuberculosis* antigen 5 and tuberculin purified protein derivative. Bull. W.H.O. **62:**755–761.
2. **Brennan, P. J.** 1983. The phthiocerol-containing surface lipids of *Mycobacterium leprae*—a perspective of past and present work. Int. J. Lepr. **51:**387–396.
3. **Chaparas, S. D.** 1984. Immunologically based diagnostic tests with tuberculin and other mycobacterial antigens. p. 195–200. *In* G. P. Kubica and L. G. Wayne (ed.), The mycobacteria: a sourcebook, vol. A. Marcel Dekker, Inc., New York.
4. **Cho, S.-N., D. L. Yanagihara, S. W. Hunter, R. H. Gelber, and P. J. Brennan.** 1983. Serological specificity of phenolic glycolipid I from *Mycobacterium leprae* and use in serodiagnosis of leprosy. Infect. Immun. **41:**1077–1083.
5. **Comstock, G. W., T. M. Daniel, D. E. Snider, P. Q. Edwards, P. C. Hopewell, and H. M. Vandiviere.** 1981. The tuberculin skin test. Am. Rev. Respir. Dis. **124:**356–363.
6. **Comstock, G. W., M. L. Furcolow, R. A. Greenberg, S. Grzybowski, R. A. Maclean, H. Baer, and P. Q. Edwards.** 1971. The tuberculin skin test. Am. Rev. Respir. Dis. **104:**769–775.
7. **David, H. L., and M. J. Selin.** 1980. Immune response to mycobacteria, p. 520–525. *In* N. R. Rose and H. Friedman (ed.), Manual of clinical immunology, 2nd ed. American Society for Microbiology, Washington, D.C.
8. **Fujiwara, T., S. W. Hunter, S.-N. Cho, G. O. Aspinall, and P. J. Brennan.** 1984. Chemical synthesis and serology of disaccharides and trisaccharides of phenolic glycolipid antigens from the leprosy bacillus and preparation of a disaccharide protein conjugate for serodiagnosis of leprosy. Infect. Immun. **43:**245–252.
9. **Lind, A., and M. Riddell.** 1984. Immunologically based diagnostic tests. Humoral antibody methods, p. 221–248. *In* G. P. Kubica and L. G. Wayne (ed.), The mycobacteria: a sourcebook, vol. A. Marcel Dekker, Inc., New York.
10. **Seibert, F. B.** 1934. The isolation and properties of the purified protein derivative of tuberculin. Am. Rev. Tuberc. **30:**713–725.

Chapter 67

Immunologic Responses to the Major Aerobic Actinomycete Pathogens

A. C. PIER

The major pathogens among the aerobic actinomycetes are found in the genera *Nocardia* and *Dermatophilus*, which contain the agents of nocardiosis and dermatophilosis, respectively. The diseases caused by these agents are widely divergent. Nocardiae are opportunistic pathogens contracted from the environment which cause acute to chronic systemic infections as well as localized granulomatous processes of subcutaneous tissues. *Dermatophilus congolensis* is an obligate parasite of the skin which causes an acute, contagious exudative dermatitis with rare involvement of deeper tissues.

CLINICAL INDICATIONS: NOCARDIOSIS

Nocardiosis is caused by three opportunistic soil-dwelling aerobic actinomycetes, namely, *Nocardia asteroides*, *N. brasiliensis*, and *N. caviae (N. otitidis-caviarum)*. There is a broad spectrum of clinical manifestations in nocardial infection, including pulmonary involvement in humans and dogs; granulomatous lesions of the subcutaneous tissues, lymph nodes, and often the bone in nearly all mammalian species; and a suppurative fibrotic mastitis in cattle. The propensity for nocardial infection to evoke erosive as well as proliferative tissue responses often results in extension of the infection to adjacent organs, development of sinus tracts from actinomycotic mycetoma, and systemic dissemination from vascular erosion or lymphatic drainage. The involvement of nearly all organ systems is possible with systemic nocardiosis, and invasions of the brain and bone are relatively frequent sequelae. The many possible clinical manifestations of nocardiosis are extensive and may resemble those of a variety of other infectious processes (e.g., actinomycosis, mycobacteriosis, and mycoses) from which they need to be differentiated for adequate therapy. Serologic and delayed cutaneous hypersensitivity (DCH) tests are helpful adjuncts to cultural isolation for determining the etiology of nocardiosis, particularly in the case of deep systemic or central nervous system infections.

Extracellular antigens of *N. asteroides* were developed in 1961 (5). They have been used diagnostically in bovine and human patients (9, 11) for detecting precipitins, complement-fixing (CF) antibodies, and DCH in affected individuals. Experimental infections in cattle indicate that precipitins appear in gel diffusion precipitin (GDP) tests 2 weeks after infection. After 3 to 4 weeks, CF antibodies are evident, and DCH can be elicited with intradermal injections. There is a high degree of specificity to these tests. Cross-reactions with CF or DCH tests in cattle with a variety of mycobacterioses were not encountered (9). In human sera, occasional apparent CF cross-reactions were observed in patients with leprosy (11). Additional utility of these antigens has been in their ability to subspecifically type strains of *N. asteroides*. Four distinct major antigenic types of *N. asteroides* have been identified by GDP techniques (6). This ability to subspecifically type *N. asteroides* isolates has permitted epidemiologic studies in infected groups from which different antigenic types were isolated (7, 12). Three additional antigenic types have been added to the original four by the use of antigen absorption techniques (2). Because of this antigenic complexity in *N. asteroides*, combined antigenic preparations, containing equal parts of all four basic antigens, are used in DCH and CF tests.

Interpretation of the GDP test is possible after 6 to 20 h of diffusion. A positive reaction is evidenced by the presence of one or two bands of precipitation depending on the antigenic type(s) of the infecting strain. Positive CF reaction is determined after overnight fixation at 4°C; titers of 1:16 are considered suspect, and titers of 1:32 or above are positive. Skin test responses are read 24 to 48 h after intradermal injection of 0.1 ml of combined antigen. Indurations 2.5 mm greater than the normal folded skin thickness are considered positive reactions. When mycobacterioses are cosuspects, comparative tests are recommended.

Reagents and procedures

For antigen preparation, a neopeptone dialysate medium containing 2% glucose is used. Neopeptone (240 g) is dissolved in 1 liter of distilled water. This solution is placed in dialysis tubing (Visking size 36; Visking Co., Div. of Union Carbide Corp., Chicago, Ill.) and dialyzed against 4 liters of distilled water for 6 h at 65 to 70°C and for 16 h at 4°C. Distilled water and glucose are added to produce final concentrations of 1.35 mg of nitrogen per ml and 2% glucose. The medium is dispensed in cotton-stoppered culture flasks and autoclaved for 30 min at 121°C. For production of standard diagnostic antigens, 500 ml of medium in 1-liter flasks is recommended. For typing isolates, 50 ml of medium in a 100-ml flask is adequate.

Inocula are prepared from each of the four type strains of *N. asteroides* in the following manner. The organism is grown on slants of brain heart infusion agar containing 5% bovine blood for 72 h at 36°C. The growth from several slants of the 72-h cultures is then suspended in sterile, phosphate-buffered saline (0.15 M, pH 7.4). A 1-ml volume of this suspension is used as inoculum for each 100 ml of medium.

Each flask is inoculated with a separate strain. The inoculated medium is incubated for 14 days at 37°C on a rotary shaker providing 160 oscillations per min. Cultures are inactivated by adding thimerosal to a final concentration of 1:10,000, and they are harvested by filtration 24 h later. For CF and DCH testing, equal parts of the antigenic preparation of each of the four antigenic type strains are combined. The combined antigen is used undiluted for DCH testing and is diluted 1:2 to 2:3 for use in the CF test to alleviate slight anticomplementary activity. For use in GDP tests, each antigenic type culture filtrate (or the filtrate of a strain to be typed) is processed separately and concentrated 10-fold by pervaporation in semipermeable membranes.

Gel diffusion medium contains 0.5 g of agarose and 0.01 g of thimerosal dissolved in 100 ml of barbiturate-buffered saline solution. The barbiturate-buffered saline solution (pH 7.3) is the same as that used in complement fixation tests with the nocardial antigen. It contains the following ingredients: 7.5 g of sodium 5,5-diethylbarbiturate, 11.5 g of 5,5-diethylbarbituric acid, 4.056 g of $MgSO_4 \cdot 7H_2O$, 170.0 g of NaCl, and 0.78 g of anhydrous $CaCl_2$ dissolved in distilled water to a final volume of 20 liters. A 3-ml volume of this medium (melted) is dispensed onto three-fourths of the surface of a standard microscope slide. After solidification, wells 3 mm in diameter are cut in the desired pattern, with 4 mm between antigen and serum wells. Micropipettes are used to fill the wells with unknowns and standard reagents, and then the gel diffusion slides are placed in a moist chamber (e.g., a closed petri dish containing a pledget of moist cotton), incubated for 20 h at room temperature, and read under a suitable light source and lens system.

ACTINOMYCOTIC MYCETOMA

Actinomycotic mycetoma is an ill-defined clinical condition that may be caused by several aerobic as well as anaerobic actinomycetes. Prominent among aerobic agents of the disease are members of the genera *Nocardia*, *Nocardiopis*, *Actinomadura*, and *Streptomyces*. With the exception of the extracellular culture filtrate antigens of *N. asteroides*, *N. brasiliensis*, and *N. caviae* (6, 9) and the polysaccharide cell wall-extracted antigens of *N. brasiliensis* (1), there are no generally accepted or widely applied serologic adjuncts to diagnosis of this group. Because the condition is heterogenous in origin and generally has sinus tracts which discharge microcolonies of the agent suitable for microscopic and cultural examination, immunologic adjuncts to diagnosis are less helpful than in systemic infections caused by *N. asteroides*. The application of serologic aids to the diagnosis of mycetomas in general has been reviewed elsewhere (3). A cell extract polysaccharide antigen of *N. brasiliensis* has been used effectively in DCH and GDP tests of patients with mycetoma of *N. brasiliensis* origin (1).

DERMATOPHILOSIS

Dermatophilosis is a clear-cut clinical entity caused by the obligate cutaneous parasite *D. congolensis*. The condition is a highly contagious exudative dermatitis that affects 28 or more species of domestic livestock, companion animals, wildlife, and humans. Dermatophilosis is considered a zoonotic disease. Diagnosis is customarily accomplished by examining Giemsa-stained smears of exudative crusts for the presence of

typical multidimensionally septate packets of zoospores. Cultural isolation of the easily overgrown organism is facilitated by streaking suspensions of emulsified crusts, filtered through a 1.2-μm-diameter syringe filter, over the surface of whole-blood agar or brain heart infusion blood agar. Typical sunken, adherent hemolytic colonies appear after 72 to 96 h of incubation at 37°C.

Immunologic adjuncts to diagnosis have been fluorescent-antibody staining of smears of old exudative crusts (8) and the use of serologic surveys to detect the prevalence and extent of infection among animal populations (4). *D. congolensis* appears to be an antigenically homogenous species (10). Killed whole-cell antigens and bacterins have been used to immunize cattle in regions in which the disease is endemic.

Serologic tests, including GDP and CF tests, have been conducted with antigens prepared from disintegrated washed cells (10).

Antigenic preparations for GDP tests or for raising specific antibody for the fluorescent antibody can be made easily from whole organisms. Serum broth cultures grown for 72 to 96 h at 37°C are inactivated (thimerosal to 1:10,000) and harvested by centrifugation. The cells are suspended in phosphate-buffered saline (0.15 M, pH 7.4) and broken by sonication or in a tissue disintegrator chamber with glass beads. The resulting disintegrated cell suspension is diluted to approximately 30% T at a wavelength of 540 nm. The antigenic suspension is preserved with thimerosal and used in a GDP test as described for *N. asteroides*.

A chloroform extract of *D. congolensis* cell walls has been used effectively in GDP and passive hemagglutination tests to detect antibodies in the serum and milk of cattle in regions in which dermatophilosis is endemic (4).

LITERATURE CITED

1. **Bojalil, L. F., and A. Zamora.** 1963. Precipitins and skin tests in the diagnosis of mycetoma due to *Nocardia brasiliensis*. Proc. Soc. Exp. Biol. Med. **113**:40–43.
2. **Kurup, V. P., and G. H. Scribner.** 1981. Antigenic relationships among *Nocardia asteroides* immunotypes. Microbios **31**:25–30.
3. **Mahgoub, E. S.** 1975. Serologic diagnosis of mycetoma. Pan Am. Health Organ. Sci. Publ. **204**:154–161.
4. **Makinde, A. A.** 1981. Detection of *Dermatophilus congolensis* antibody in the milk of streptothricosis infected cows. Res. Vet. Sci. **30**:374–375.
5. **Pier, A. C., and J. B. Enright.** 1961. *Nocardia asteroides* as a mammary pathogen of cattle. III. Immunologic reactions of infected animals. Am. J. Vet. Res. **23**:284–292.
6. **Pier, A. C., and R. E. Fichtner.** 1971. Serologic typing of *Nocardia asteroides* by immunodiffusion. Am. Rev. Respir. Dis. **103**:698–707.
7. **Pier, A. C., and R. E. Fichtner.** 1981. Distribution of serotypes of *Nocardia asteroides* from animal, human, and environmental sources. J. Clin. Microbiol. **13**:548–553.
8. **Pier, A. C., J. L. Richard, and E. F. Farrell.** 1964. Fluorescent antibody and cultural techniques in cutaneous streptothricosis. Am. J. Vet. Res. **25**:1014–1020.
9. **Pier, A. C., J. R. Thurston, and A. B. Larsen.** 1968. A diagnostic antigen for nocardiosis: comparative tests in cattle with nocardiosis and mycobacteriosis. Am. J. Vet. Res. **29**:397–403.
10. **Richard, J. L., J. R. Thurston, and A. C. Pier.** 1976. Com-

parison of antigens of *Dermatophilus congolensis* isolates and their use in serologic tests in experimental and natural infections, p. 216–227. *In* D. Lloyd and K. Sellers (ed.), Dermatophilus infection in animal and man. Academic Press, Inc., New York.

11. **Shainhouse, J. Z., A. C. Pier, and D. A. Stevens.** 1978. Complement fixation antibody test for human nocardiosis. J. Clin. Microbiol. **8:**516–519.

12. **Stevens, D. A., A. C. Pier, B. L. Beaman, P. A. Morozumi, I. S. Lovett, and E. T. Houang.** 1981. Laboratory evaluation of an outbreak of nocardiosis in immunocompromised hosts. Am. J. Med. **71:**928–934.

Chapter 68

Serodiagnosis of Syphilis

SANDRA A. LARSEN AND LYNDA L. BRADFORD

Background

Syphilis is one of a group of infections known as the treponematoses. *Treponema pallidum* is the causative agent of syphilis, and its variant Bosnia A is the causative agent of bejel, whereas yaws and pinta are caused by *T. pertenue* and *T. carateum*, respectively. These three treponemes are morphologically and antigenically quite similar and cannot be differentiated except by the nature of the lesion and the clinical course of the infection. None of the serologic tests for syphilis can be used to distinguish antibodies produced in response to *T. pallidum* from those produced in response to the other pathogenic treponemes. Although mass treatment campaigns from 1952 to 1969 were extremely successful in decreasing the prevalence of endemic treponematoses, yaws is still endemic in a number of areas of the world. Individuals who acquired infections before eradication of the disease from their area will, in all likelihood, still have antibodies that are reactive in the treponemal tests for syphilis.

Serologic tests for syphilis were first used in 1906 with the development of the nontreponemal complement fixation test by Wasserman. By 1935 approximately 19 different tests were available in the United States for the serodiagnosis of syphilis. Efforts to standardize the techniques began in that year. Currently there are 11 tests for syphilis for which reagents are commercially available and whose performance has met with standards set by the Centers for Disease Control (CDC) for syphilis serologic tests (Table 1).

Nontreponemal tests

With the many efforts to develop more sensitive and specific tests for syphilis, it seems ironic that the current screening tests, which are so critical to the diagnosis of the disease, are the biologically nonspecific nontreponemal tests. Antigens for these tests, traditionally termed cardiolipin or reagin tests, are basically modifications of the Venereal Disease Research Laboratory (VDRL) (9) antigen that contains cardiolipin, cholesterol, and lecithin. The nontreponemal tests measure both immunoglobulin G (IgG) and IgM antilipid antibodies formed by the host in response both to lipoidal material released from the damaged host cells early in infection and to lipid from the treponeme itself. Because of either the lipidic nature of the antigen or some unusual property of the antibody, the antigen-antibody reaction remains suspended, and flocculation occurs, rather than agglutination or precipitation as in most other serologic tests.

The nontreponemal tests are divided into two categories, i.e., microscopic and macroscopic (Table 1). Although the VDRL slide test is still the only test recommended for use with cerebrospinal fluid (CSF), its use as a screening test for syphilis has steadily declined over the past 10 years. Currently the most frequently used test is the macroscopic rapid plasma reagin (RPR) 18-mm-circle card test (9). The RPR card test has several advantages over the VDRL test: (i) it is a kit test, containing all needed reagents; (ii) unheated serum is used; (iii) the antigen is stabilized, and the remainder is not discarded at the end of each day; (iv) the reaction is read macroscopically; and (v) most materials are disposable.

Treponemal tests

Even though *T. pallidum* was identified in 1905 as the causative organism of syphilis, the first *T. pallidum*-specific test, the *Treponema pallidum* immobilization (TPI) test, was not developed until 1949 (6). Today the TPI is performed only in a few research laboratories in the United States. Other less expensive, more sensitive, and equally specific treponemal tests such as those listed in Table 1 have replaced the TPI as confirmatory tests for syphilis.

Dark-field microscopy (9) and its fluorescent counterpart, the direct fluorescent-antibody test for *T. pallidum* (DFA-TP) (1), although not actually serologic tests, are very useful in detecting *T. pallidum* in material collected from primary and secondary lesions or from regional lymph nodes during the secondary stage of the disease. The DFA-TP has certain advantages over dark-field microscopy: (i) smears can be mailed to a central laboratory; (ii) motile organisms are not required; (iii) pathogenic treponemes can be differentiated from nonpathogenic ones; and (iv) tissue sections from biopsy and autopsy material can be examined.

The choice of a serologic treponemal test for confirmation of syphilis has until recently been limited to either indirect fluorescent-antibody or hemagglutination techniques. Recently an enzyme-linked immunosorbent assay method has reached the commercial market; however, field experience, to date, is limited. Of the treponemal test techniques, the fluorescent-antibody-absorption (FTA-ABS) test (9) and its modification, the FTA-ABS double staining (DS) (4) test, are the most sensitive in all stages of syphilis. The FTA-ABS DS test, designed specifically for use with incident light microscopes, uses a *T. pallidum*-specific counterstain that eliminates the need for transmitted light to locate treponemes. The test is an improvement on the standard FTA-ABS test, since the possibility of improper alignment of the dark-field condenser is eliminated.

Although the field of syphilis serology is approximately 80 years old, the need for a serodiagnostic test for congenital syphilis still exists, as does the need for a more sensitive and specific test for neurosyphilis. Major breakthroughs are foreseen in the near future as a result of in vitro cultivation of the pathogenic

TABLE 1. Serologic tests for syphilis

Method and test	Reference	Type
Nontreponemal		
Venereal Disease Research Laboratory slide	9	Microscopic
Unheated serum reagin	7, 9	Microscopic
Rapid plasma reagin 18-mm-circle card	9	Macroscopic
Reagin Screen Test	5	Macroscopic
Automated reagin test	9	Automated macroscopic
Treponemal		
Direct fluorescent antibody for *T. pallidum*	1	Direct fluorescent antibody
Fluorescent treponema antibody-absorption	9	Indirect fluorescent antibody
Fluorescent treponema antibody-absorption double staining	4	Indirect fluorescent antibody
Microhemagglutination assay for antibodies to *T. pallidum*	8	Hemagglutination
Hemagglutination Treponemal Tests for Syphilis	10	Hemagglutination
Syphilis BioEnzabead (Litton Bionetics)		Enzyme-linked immunosorbent assay

treponemes, monoclonal antibody production, and recombinant DNA techniques.

CLINICAL INDICATIONS

Background

Because of its diverse clinical manifestations, syphilis may be considered both an acute and a chronic infection. The acute, symptomatic stages of primary and secondary syphilis are generally separated by a period of quiescence. The primary stage begins as a generalized bacteremia within hours of the organism entering the body. Preferential multiplication occurs at the site of entry, and as a result, a chancre develops, usually within 3 weeks. The secondary stage, which develops 6 weeks to 6 months after the infection, is characterized by disseminated lesions attributable to the systemic infection found at onset of the disease. Virtually every organ and tissue of the body is affected, including most body fluids. The early latent stage, syphilis of less than a 1-year duration, represents a conversion period to a chronic infection. The early latent stage is usually marked by at least one relapse to the secondary (acute) stage with cutaneous eruptions. As the duration of the latent stage increases, the frequency of relapse to an infectious stage decreases and the disease becomes asymptomatic. Latent syphilis, although not transmissible to sexual partners when asymptomatic, can still be transmitted to the fetus during pregnancy. The severity of the infection in congenital syphilis correlates with the stage of syphilis of the mother; that is, mothers with primary or secondary syphilis may deliver stillborns, whereas mothers with latent syphilis may deliver normal children. Late or tertiary syphilis occurs in 13 to 33% of patients 5 to 20 years after the initial infection and includes cardiovascular syphilis, neurosyphilis, and benign (gummatous) syphilis.

Congenital syphilis is the result of passage of *T. pallidum* across the placenta. Clinical manifestations may be present at birth but are more often seen at 3 weeks to 6 months of age. A primary stage does not occur in congenital syphilis, since the organism is inoculated directly into the fetal circulation. Signs of early congenital syphilis, i.e., before the age of 2 years, include skin rashes, mucous membrane lesions, anemia, and painful osteochondritis of the long bones. Late-onset congenital syphilis occurs after the age of

2. Clinical manifestations of late-onset congenital syphilis include blindness, deafness, deformed bones and teeth, and gummas.

A particular testing requirement exists for each stage of syphilis. A dark-field examination or DFA-TP should be performed on any lesion when primary, secondary, or congenital syphilis is a possibility. When specimens are properly collected, the dark-field methods are at least 95% sensitive. The dark-field and DFA-TP methods are useful for demonstration of *T. pallidum* in regional lymph nodes during secondary syphilis, and the DFA-TP can be used for the examination of autopsy, biopsy (3), or placental materials when necessary.

Nontreponemal tests

The nontreponemal tests are routinely used as screening tests and as a means of following the efficacy of treatment. In primary syphilis the nontreponemal tests may be nonreactive in up to 28% of the cases (Table 2). Reactivity in these tests does not develop until 1 to 4 weeks after the chancre first appears. For this reason, patients with suspect lesions and nonreactive nontreponemal tests should have repeat tests at 1 week, 1 month, and 3 months. Nonreactive tests during the 3-month period exclude the diagnosis of syphilis. The nontreponemal tests are reactive in secondary syphilis, almost without exception. Normally, patients with secondary syphilis will have nontreponemal test titers of 1:16 or greater, regardless of the test method used. Less than 2% of sera from these patients will exhibit a prozone. Nontreponemal test titers in early latent syphilis are similar to those in secondary syphilis. However, as the length of the latent stage increases, the titer decreases. Approximately 30% of the individuals with late latent syphilis will have nonreactive nontreponemal test results.

The CSF VDRL test is the only serologic test recognized as a standard test for the diagnosis of neurosyphilis. Asymptomatic neurosyphilis should not be diagnosed by a reactive CSF VDRL alone. Other diagnostic criteria for neurosyphilis include a reactive serum nontreponemal or treponemal test result, or both, five or more lymphocytes per mm^3 of CSF, and CSF total protein of $\geq$45 mg/dl. Symptomatic neurosyphilis is diagnosed by clinical symptoms supplemented with positive results in the diagnostic procedures described above.

TABLE 2. Sensitivity and specificity of nontreponemal tests

Test[a]	% Sensitivity by stage of untreated syphilis				Specificity[b]
	Primary	Secondary	Latent	Late	
VDRL	80 (74–87)[c]	100	96 (95–100)	71 (37–94)	98 (96–99)
RPR card	86 (81–100)	100	99 (95–100)	73	98 (93–99)
USR	80 (72–88)	100	95		99
RST	85[d]	100	97		97

[a] USR, Unheated serum reagin; RST, Reagin Screen Test.
[b] Based on CDC studies with clinic populations having nonsyphilis sexually transmitted disease.
[c] Range of sensitivity in CDC studies.
[d] Based solely on one study.

After treatment for syphilis, serial quantitative nontreponemal tests are used to measure the adequacy of therapy. Titers should be obtained at 3-month intervals for at least 1 year. After adequate treatment for primary and secondary syphilis, there should be at least a fourfold decline in titer by 3 months. For most patients, the titer continues to decline until little or no reaction is detected. Patients treated in the latent stage may show a more gradual decline in titer. Low titers will persist even after 2 years (2) in approximately 50% of patients treated for latent syphilis. The same nontreponemal test method should be used for all quantitative testing since up to fourfold (2 dilutions) and occasionally greater differences in titers may be obtained with certain sera in the various tests (Table 3).

A new diagnosis for syphilis may be established by a positive dark-field test or a fourfold increase in the quantitative nontreponemal test titer.

In congenital syphilis the role of the nontreponemal tests is to monitor the antibody titer. A rising titer in monthly serial bleedings from an infant over a 6-month period is diagnostic for congenital syphilis. By 3 months, if the infant was not infected in utero, passively transferred antibodies should no longer be detected in the nontreponemal tests.

All of the nontreponemal tests will occasionally give false-positive results. In general populations, the nonspecificity ranges between 1 and 2%. Acute false-positive reactions lasting less than 6 months usually occur after febrile diseases or immunizations or during pregnancy. However, rates of false-positive reactions during pregnancy are no greater than those seen in the general population, i.e., 1 to 2%. Chronic false-positive reactions are more often associated with

TABLE 3. Comparison of VDRL slide test titers with RPR card test and unheated serum reagin test titers

Test	Titer variation (dilution)	% of sera
VDRL = RPR		37.5
VDRL > RPR	1	7.2
	≥2	1.7
VDRL < RPR	1	30.0
	≥2	23.6
VDRL = USR[a]		50.4
VDRL > USR	1	12.1
	≥2	2.0
VDRL < USR	1	26.8
	≥2	8.7

[a] USR, Unheated serum reagin.

autoimmune diseases such as arthritis and lupus or with chronic infections. False-positive rates may exceed 20% in populations where the prevalence of intravenous drug use is high. When false-positive results occur, the titers are usually less than 1:8. Not all low titers are false-positive, since titers are low in latent syphilis. Similarly, not all high titers are true positives. In populations where intravenous drug use is prevalent, approximately 12% of the false-positive titers are 1:8 or greater.

Most of the potential problems with performance of the nontreponemal tests can be avoided if the instructions for test performance, reagent control, and general quality control are carefully followed. The use of plasma and cord sera may cause particular problems in the reading of test results, and testing with these specimens should be restricted to those times when a serum sample is absolutely unavailable.

Treponemal tests

The treponemal tests should be reserved for confirmatory testing when the clinical signs or history, or both, disagree with the reactive nontreponemal test results. The treponemal tests are qualitative procedures and therefore cannot be used to monitor the efficacy of treatment. When treatment is begun early in primary syphilis, however, about 10% of samples from these patients will be nonreactive within 2 years after treatment. Of the treponemal tests now available, the fluorescent-antibody procedures are the most sensitive in primary syphilis (Table 4). Like the nontreponemal tests, the treponemal tests are almost always reactive in secondary and latent syphilis. The sensitivity of the treponemal tests declines somewhat in the late stage of syphilis (Table 4), but in the majority of cases, once the treponemal tests are reactive, they remain reactive for the lifetime of the patient. In fact, in some patients with late syphilis, a reactive treponemal test may be the only means of confirming the suspected diagnosis. Currently, none of the treponemal tests are recommended for use with CSF.

In congenital syphilis, as in sexually acquired syphilis, the treponemal tests will be reactive. The reactivity in the treponemal tests may be either passively transferred to the fetus during pregnancy, as is the reactivity of the nontreponemal tests, or it may actually be due to infection. Passively transferred treponemal antibodies should be catabolized and become undetectable in the noninfected infant by the age of 6 months. This reactivity lasts for about 3 months longer than that for the nontreponemal tests.

TABLE 4. Sensitivity and specificity of treponemal tests

Test[a]	% Sensitivity by stage of untreated syphilis				% Specificity[b]
	Primary	Secondary	Latent	Late	
FTA-ABS	98 (70–100)[c]	100	100	96	98 (95–99)
FTA-ABS DS	90 (70–100)	100	100		99 (97–100)
MHA-TP	82 (69–90)	100	100	94	99 (98–100)
HATTS	85	100	100	94	99

[a] MHA-TP, Microhemagglutination assay for antibodies to *T. pallidum*; HATTS, hemagglutination treponemal tests for syphilis.

[b] Based on CDC studies in clinic populations having nonsyphilis sexually transmitted disease.

[c] Range of sensitivity in CDC studies.

The greatest value of the treponemal tests is to differentiate true-positive nontreponemal results from false-positive results. However, false-positive treponemal test results do occur with about the same frequency (1%) as false-positive nontreponemal test results (Table 4). Although some false-positive results in the treponemal tests are transient and their cause unknown, a definite association has been made between false-positive treponemal tests and the connective tissue diseases. When unexplained reactive results occur in elderly patients, attempts should be made to rule out acquired or congenital syphilis or infections with other treponemes before a diagnosis of false-positive serology is made.

Quality control is as essential for the treponemal tests as it is for the nontreponemal tests for reliable and reproducible results. Strict adherence to test procedures and the use of standardized reagents and controls are necessary to eliminate technical errors.

INTERPRETATION

The diagnosis of syphilis depends not only on the laboratory findings, but also on a carefully obtained history and a thorough physical examination. The most specific means of diagnosing syphilis is by dark-field microscopy or DFA-TP, providing such diseases as yaws, bejel, and pinta have been excluded. The demonstration of *T. pallidum* in lesion material in primary, secondary, early congenital, or infectious early latent stages constitutes a positive diagnosis. In contrast, negative dark-field or DFA-TP results do not exclude a diagnosis of ff;0syphilis, but may mean that organisms were not present in sufficient numbers in the specimen to be detected, that antitreponemal drugs were applied locally or taken systemically, or that the lesion has approached natural resolution or was of late syphilis.

Serologic tests must be interpreted according to disease stage, possible underlying disease conditions, and possibility of false-positive results. Ideally, all sera in suspected cases of syphilis should be tested first with a nontreponemal procedure, reactive results verified with a second specimen and quantitated, and cases in which clinical or epidemiologic evidence is counter to the diagnosis of syphilis confirmed with a treponemal test. With the proper use of the serologic tests, a reactive nontreponemal test with a reactive treponemal test gives a positive predictive value of approximately 97%, or only a 3% error factor. In contrast, if only one test is used, the positive predictive value, regardless of the method, is less than 50% in a low-prevalence disease such as syphilis.

Test misinterpretation for nontreponemal tests most often results from failure to (i) recognize the variation of plus or minus one dilution inherent in most serologic tests, (ii) establish the true positivity of test results, and (iii) recognize reactivity due to infection with nonvenereal treponematoses in serologic tests for syphilis. Syphilis serologic results in pregnancy are extremely difficult to interpret, especially in women who have histories of adequately treated syphilis. It is not uncommon to see an increase in a stable or previously nonreactive titer during pregnancy. However, treatment should be considered with any increase in titer, because of the serious consequence of failure to treat.

A major problem with interpretation of the FTA-ABS test has been eliminated with the new reporting system recommended by the CDC. When the treponemal test results and clinical opinion disagree, the treponemal test should be repeated. If disagreement persists, then the specimen should be sent to a reference laboratory for both immunofluorescence and hemagglutination tests. Nevertheless, the final diagnosis depends on clinical judgment.

TEST PROCEDURES

DFA-TP

See reference 1.

Principle

The DFA-TP is an immunofluorescent-antibody test in which an anti-*T. pallidum* globulin is labeled with a fluorochrome dye to identify the organism specifically. The test is a practical alternative to dark-field microscopy for smears which cannot be examined immediately and for the examination of oral lesions, where confusion of *T. pallidum* with other spiral organisms is often a problem. Lesion material can be collected in capillary tubes or directly on slides and mailed to a central laboratory for examination, since motile organisms are not required. The DFA-TP is applicable to the identification of *T. pallidum* in tissue sections as well (3).

Materials

1. Fluorescence microscope assembly
2. Slide board or holder
3. Moist chamber
4. Bibulous paper

5. Rubber bulbs, approximately 2-ml capacity
6. Loop, bacteriologic, standard 2 mm, 26 gauge, platinum
7. Microscope slides, 1 by 3 in. (ca. 2.5 by 7.6 cm), frosted end, approximately 1 mm thick
8. Cover slips, no. 1, 22 mm square
9. Disposable capillary pipettes, 5.75 in. (ca. 14.6 cm) long

Reagents

1. Sterile distilled water
2. Phosphate-buffered saline (PBS), pH 7.2
3. PBS, pH 7.2, with 2% Tween 80
4. Acetone, reagent grade; methanol, reagent grade
5. Mounting media consisting of 1 part buffered saline (pH 7.2) plus 9 parts glycerol (reagent quality)
6. Fluorescein isothiocyanate (FITC)-labeled anti-*T. pallidum* globulin that has been absorbed with the nonpathogenic *T. phagedenis* biotype Reiter treponeme and demonstrated to stain only *T. pallidum* after absorption. Lyophilized conjugate should be rehydrated with sterile distilled water and diluted with PBS with 2% Tween 80 according to the accompanying directions.

Preparation of specimens

1. Body fluids, lesion exudates, suspensions of macerated tissue, or other materials should be well mixed with a disposable pipette and rubber bulb to ensure even distribution of material.
2. If quantity allows, organisms in spinal fluids and aqueous humor fluids should be concentrated by centrifugation (12,000 to 16,000 rpm for 30 min). Supernatant fluid is carefully removed, and slides are made of the sediment for dark-field and fluorescent-antibody examination.
3. Lesion exudate may be collected in capillary tubes and sealed with plastic closure or putty for mailing to the laboratory. Store at 2 to 8°C until ready for shipment. Smears prepared in the clinic should be air dried and shipped to the laboratory without fixation.

Controls

Appropriate controls must be included in each test run.
1. **Positive control.** Smears made from FTA-ABS antigen or testicular impression smears made from *T. pallidum*-infected rabbits must be included.
2. **Negative control.** Smears made from washed nonpathogenic Reiter treponeme cultures, freshly obtained human mouth treponemes, or washed *T. denticola* biotype *microdentium* cultures may be included.

Identification of *T. pallidum* in fluids

1. Smear approximately 10 μl of test material within each circle or 1-cm area of a clean, grease-free slide, and allow the smear to air dry. If possible, four smears should be prepared for each specimen.
2. Fix the slides in acetone for 10 min or in 10% methanol for 20 min or air dry and gently heat fix. Fix all slides from an individual patient separately.

3. Cover each circle with approximately 30 μl of diluted conjugate or with a sufficient amount to cover the smear, and place the slides in a moist chamber at 35 to 37°C for 30 min.
4. Rinse the slides individually with PBS, and cover with PBS on a staining rack for a total of 10 min. Follow with a final rinse in distilled water. Reactive controls and nonreactive controls may be rinsed in the same staining dish. Process all unknown smears separately to prevent reactive treponemes from washing onto nonreactive smears.
5. Drain the slides to remove excess water. Blot areas outside of the smears with bibulous paper if necessary. Place a very small drop of mounting medium on each circle, and apply a cover slip. (The mounting medium should be dropped from a disposable capillary pipette. Discard any medium left in the pipette.)

Reading test results

1. A microscope equipped with UV and tungsten light sources is used for observations. When using an HBO-200 mercury bulb, a BG-12 exciter filter or a KP490 filter may be used in combination with an OG-1 barrier filter (K510 or K530).
2. A 45× high-dry objective is used for scanning the area and a 100×/1.25 oil immersion objective for verification. (For fluorescent-antibody testing with transmitted illumination, the oil immersion objective must be fitted with a funnel stop or equipped with a built-in iris diaphragm.)

Reporting test results

1. If FITC-stained treponemes are observed, report: "Treponemes, immunologically specific for *T. pallidum*, were observed by direct immunofluorescence."
2. If no treponemes were observed, report: "No treponemes were observed by direct immunofluorescence."

Precautions and potential problems

During the fixation and rinsing of smears, treponemes may be washed off the slides, particularly the control slides, and can adhere to other smears. Therefore, smears from patients must be handled individually to prevent *T. pallidum* organisms from adhering to nonreactive smears, resulting in a false-positive report. If staining dishes are used for controls, they must be cleaned after each use.

RPR 18-mm-Circle Card Test

See reference 9.

Principle

A stabilized suspension of standardized VDRL antigen and sized charcoal particles is used as the RPR card antigen. This antigen is added to the patient's serum, mixed on a mechanical rotator, and examined macroscopically for degree of flocculation. Any degree of reactivity obtained in the undiluted serum indicates a need to perform the quantitative test to determine the titer.

Kit

The RPR 18-mm-circle kit contains test antigen, disposable 20-gauge needle, antigen-dispensing bottle, plastic-coated test cards, disposable sampling straws-spreaders, and stirrers. Some kits also contain sera with specified reactivities of reactive, minimally reactive, and nonreactive.

Preliminary testing of antigen suspension

Before beginning the test, the RPR card antigen is transferred to the dispensing bottle, and the accuracy of the dispensing needle is checked. The needle should deliver 0.017 ml or 60 drops ± 2 drops per ml of antigen. To check the accuracy of the needle, place the needle on a 1-ml pipette, fill the pipette with RPR antigen suspension, and, holding the pipette in a vertical position, count the number of drops delivered in 0.5 ml. The needle is considered satisfactory if 30 drops ± 1 drop are obtained in 0.5 ml. A needle not meeting this specification should be replaced with another needle that does meet this specification.

Control sera are used to test the antigen suspension to confirm optimal reactivity before routine testing is performed. Control sera for nontreponemal tests are not used as reading standards. One must test the control serum of graded reactivity (reactive, minimally reactive, and nonreactive) each day, as described in the next section. Only RPR card antigen suspensions that produce the established reactivity pattern of the control sera should be used.

Equipment

1. Mechanical rotator with fixed speed or adjustable to 100 rpm ± 2 rpm circumscribing a circle 2 cm (3/4 in.) in diameter on a horizontal plane

2. Humidity cover. Any convenient cover containing a moistened blotter or sponge can be used to cover cards during rotation.

3. Safety pipetting device must deliver 0.05 ml (50 μl) of reagent for use in the quantitative test and may also be used for the qualitative test.

4. Light source for reading test results. A high-intensity lamp can be used.

Reagents

0.9% saline. Use 900 mg of dry sodium chloride (ACS) to each 100 ml of distilled water.

Diluent. A 1:50 dilution of serum nonreactive for syphilis prepared in 0.9% saline should be used in the quantitative procedure for making 1:32 and higher dilutions of serum specimens.

Antigen. Store antigen suspension in ampoules or in the antigen-dispensing bottle at 2 to 8°C. An unopened ampoule of antigen is stable until the expiration date. Antigen suspension in the plastic dispensing bottle (stored at 2 to 8°C) is stable for 3 months or until the expiration date, whichever comes first. Do not use the suspension beyond the expiration date. A new lot of antigen suspension should be tested in parallel with a reference reagent to verify that it is of standard reactivity before it is placed in routine use.

Collection, preparation, and storage of specimens

Collect blood obtained by venipuncture in dry tubes without anticoagulant, and allow the blood to clot. If necessary, centrifuge the specimen with sufficient force to sediment cellular elements from the serum. Generally, 1,500 to 2,000 rpm for 5 min is sufficient. Serum specimens may be retained in the original collection tube if the test is to be performed immediately. Store clear serum removed from the clot at refrigerator temperature (2 to 8°C) or frozen (−20°C) if a delay of more than 48 h is anticipated before testing. Avoid repeated freezing-thawing of specimens. Sera are tested without heating and must be at 23 to 29°C (73 to 85°F) at the time of testing.

Precaution. Human serum is a potential source of hepatitis B virus infection and acquired immunodeficiency syndrome (AIDS). Handle all specimens as though they were capable of transmitting these diseases. Do not mouth pipette. Decontaminate all materials before disposal.

RPR circle card test on serum: qualitative test

Note. Slide flocculation tests for syphilis are affected by room temperature. For reliable and reproducible results, control sera, RPR card test antigen suspension, and test specimens must be at room temperature, 23 to 29°C (73 to 85°F), when tests are performed.

1. With a dispensing or an automatic pipetting device that delivers 0.05 ml (50 μl), place 50 μl of unheated serum onto an 18-mm circle of the RPR test card.

2. With the reverse end of the dispensing device or with a toothpick, spread the specimen to fill the entire circle. Care should be taken not to allow the serum to spread beyond the confines of the circle. Use a clean spreader for each sample.

3. Gently resuspend the RPR antigen suspension. Hold the dispensing bottle in a vertical position, and add exactly 1 free-falling drop (1/60 ml) of suspension to each test area containing serum.

4. Place the card on a mechanical rotator under a humidity cover.

5. Rotate for 8 min at 100 rpm.

6. Read the test reactions in the wet state under a high-intensity light source immediately after removing the card from the rotator. Read the test without magnification. To better differentiate minimally reactive from nonreactive serum, immediately after rotation tilt the card to about 30° from horizontal and briefly rotate the card manually.

7. Report the results as follows:

Reactive—Characteristic clumping of the RPR card antigen from slight but definite (minimally reactive) to marked and intense (reactive)

Nonreactive—No clumping of RPR card antigen or only slight "roughness"

Note. Results are reported as reactive or nonreactive regardless of the degree of reactivity. Slight but definite flocculation should always be reported as reactive.

Specimens giving any degree of reactivity should be quantitated. Rough nonreactive results should also be quantitated to identify possible prozones.

8. Upon completion of the daily tests, remove the needle, rinse it with distilled or deionized water, and air dry. (Avoid wiping the needle because this removes the silicone coating.) Recap the dispensing bottle and store in the refrigerator.

RPR card test on serum: quantitative test

1. For each specimen to be tested, place 50 µl of 0.9% saline onto circles 2 through 5. Do not spread the saline.

2. Using a safety pipetting device, place 50 µl of serum specimen onto circles 1 and 2.

3. Mix the saline and the specimen in circle 2 by drawing the mixture up and down in the safety pipettor 5 or 6 times. Avoid the formation of bubbles.

4. Transfer 50 µl from circle 2 (1:2) to circle 3 (1:4), and mix.

5. Transfer 50 µl from circle 3 (1:4) to circle 4 (1:8), and mix.

6. Transfer 50 µl from circle 4 (1:8) to circle 5 (1:6), mix, and discard 0.05 ml.

7. Using a clear stirrer for each specimen, start at the highest dilution (1:16, circle 5), and with the broad end of the stirrer, spread the serum dilution within the confines of the circle. Repeat this action using the same sampling stirrer in circles 4, 3, 2, and 1.

8. Gently resuspend the RPR card antigen suspension in the dispensing bottle.

9. Holding the antigen suspension bottle in a vertical position, dispense 1 or 2 drops to clear the needle of air, and then place exactly 1 free-falling drop (1/60 ml) of antigen suspension onto each test area.

10. Place the card on the rotator under a humidity cover.

11. Rotate for 8 min at 100 rpm.

12. Read the test reactions as described in step 6 of the qualitative test (above).

13. Report results in terms of the highest dilution, giving any reactivity in accordance with the examples in Table 5.

14. If the highest dilution tested (1:16) is reactive, proceed as follows.

   a. Prepare a 1:50 dilution (2.0%) of nonreactive serum in 0.9% saline. (This is to be used for making 1:32 and higher dilutions of specimens to be quantitated.)

   b. Prepare a 1:16 dilution of the test specimen by adding 100 µl of the specimen to 1.5 ml of 0.9% saline. Mix thoroughly.

   c. Place 50 µl of the 1:50 nonreactive serum in circles 2, 3, 4, and 5 of an RPR card.

   d. Measure 50 µl of the 1:16 dilution of the test specimen to circles 1 and 2.

   e. Using the same pipettor, make serial twofold dilutions, and complete the test as described under steps 2 through 13 (RPR card quantitative test). Higher dilutions may be prepared, if necessary, in a similar manner.

Note. All dilutions may be made on the card if the 1:50 nonreactive serum is used as the diluent from circle 6 (1:32) on.

Reagent evaluation

It is the responsibility of the laboratory to ensure that reagents are of good quality and standard reactivity. To verify that each new lot is of standard reactivity, test each one in parallel with a reference reagent previously found to be satisfactory. Perform parallel testing on more than one testing day by using different specimens of graded reactivity for each test period. Obtain individual specimens of graded reactivity for parallel testing by selecting specimens from daily test runs and storing them in the freezer. Use fresh specimens from routine test runs for the nonreactive specimens. Perform tests in accordance with the techniques described and keep a permanent record of the results of all testing.

Control sera are used to test the antigen suspension to confirm optimal reactivity before routine testing, but they are not used as reading standards. Use only RPR card antigen suspensions that reproduce the established reactivity pattern of the control sera.

Criteria of acceptability for antigen

1. When tested with the nonreactive control serum, the antigen particles should be evenly dispersed and comparable with the reference antigen suspension in appearance.

2. Test results on controls and individual sera in qualitative tests should be comparable with those obtained with the reference antigen suspension.

3. The number of rough nonreactive results obtained with the new antigen suspension should not be greater than that obtained with the reference antigen suspension.

Procedure for testing antigen

1. Test the new lot of antigen suspension and the reference antigen suspension with control sera of graded reactivity.

2. If the established pattern of reactivity is obtained on the control sera with both new and reference antigen suspensions, compare the two antigen suspensions by qualitative testing of individual sera of various reactivities. Test at least 10 reactive, 15 intermediate (minimally reactive for RPR card test), and 25 nonreactive sera.

3. For all testing, arrange the specimens on cards so that the reactivity of the two antigen suspensions can be examined side by side.

4. Record the results of all testing, review the test results, and determine if the new antigen suspension meets the criteria of acceptability.

TABLE 5. Reporting results of the RPR card test on serum (quantitative test)[a]

| Reaction with undiluted serum (1:1) | Reaction at serum dilution of | | | | Report |
	1:2	1:4	1:8	1:16	
R_m	N	N	N	N	Reactive, 1:1 dilution or undiluted only
R	R	N	N	N	Reactive, 1:2 dilution
R	R	R_m	N	N	Reactive, 1:4 dilution
R	R	R	R	N	Reactive, 1:8 dilution

[a] N, Nonreactive; R, reactive; R_m, minimally reactive.

FTA-ABS DS Test

See reference 4.

Principle

The FTA-ABS DS test is a modification of the standard FTA-ABS test (9) developed specifically for use with microscopes with incident illumination. As with the standard test, the FTA-ABS DS is an indirect fluorescent-antibody procedure using *T. pallidum* as the antigen and sorbent prepared from nonpathogenic Reiter treponemes to increase specificity. The DS test employs a tetramethyl-rhodamine isothiocyanate (TMRITC)-labeled anti-human IgG globulin and a counterstain with FITC-labeled anti-*T. pallidum* conjugate which enables the technician to locate the organisms in a nonreactive test.

Equipment

Incubator adjustable to 35 to 37°C
Bibulous paper
Slide board or holder
Moist chamber. Place moistened paper inside a convenient cover fitting the slide board.
Loop, bacteriologic, standard 2 mm, 26 gauge, platinum
Oil, immersion, low fluorescence, nondrying, type A, Cargille code 1248
Safety pipetting devices
Water bath adjustable to 56°C

Microscope assembly

Lamp: HBO-50, HBO-100, or HBO-200
Oculars: 6×, 8×, or 10×
Objectives: 40×/1.30 oil, 63× oil, or 100×/1.25 oil
Filters: For FITC, use BG38, K480, 2KP490, TK510, and K515. For TMRITC, use BG-38, BG-36, KP560, K530, TK580, and K590.

Glassware

Microscope slides, 1 by 3 in., frosted end, approximately 1 mm thick, with two etched circles, 1-cm inside diameter
Cover slips, no. 1, 22 mm square
Dish, staining, glass or plastic, with removable slide carriers
Test tubes, 12 by 75 mm

Reagents

T. pallidum antigen. The antigen for the FTA-ABS test is a lyophilized suspension of *T. pallidum* (Nichols strain) extracted from rabbit testicular tissue and washed in PBS to remove rabbit globulin. The rehydrated suspension should adhere to the slide and yield sufficient treponemes for easy interpretation of staining. The antigen may be stored at 2 to 8°C for 1 week or placed on microscope slides, fixed in acetone, and frozen at −20°C or below. Discard the antigen suspension if it becomes bacterially contaminated or does not demonstrate the proper reactivity with control sera.

FTA-ABS test sorbent. Sorbent is a product prepared from cultures of Reiter treponemes and may be purchased in lyophilized or liquid state. The reagent is standardized by titration with a known serum containing high-titered nonspecific staining. Store sorbent, and rehydrate if lyophilized, according to accompanying directions.

Rhodamine-labeled anti-human IgG globulin (conjugate). The FTA-ABS DS anti-human IgG conjugate recognizes heavy-chain IgG. The conjugate should be evaluated in the FTA-ABS DS test to determine a satisfactory working titer and to verify that it meets the criteria concerning nonspecific staining and standard reactivity. Follow the directions of the manufacturer when using commercial reagents. Store lyophilized conjugate at 2 to 8°C. Dispense rehydrated conjugate in not less than 0.3-ml quantities, and store undiluted at −20°C or lower. Before being stored, a conjugate with a working titer of 1:1,000 or higher may be diluted 1:10 with sterile PBS containing 0.5% bovine serum albumin and 0.1% NaN₃. When conjugate is thawed for use, do not refreeze, but store at 2 to 8°C. Conjugate may be used as long as satisfactory reactivity is obtained with test controls. Discard conjugate if it becomes bacterially contaminated. Centrifuge before use if reagent is cloudy when thawed or becomes cloudy at 2 to 8°C. If a change in FTA-ABS DS test reactivity is noted in routine laboratory testing, the conjugate should be retitered to determine if it is the contributing factor.

Fluorescein-labeled anti-treponemal conjugate (counterstain). The conjugate should be of proven quality for the FTA-ABS DS test. Test each new lot of conjugate to determine its working dilution and to verify that it meets the criteria concerning standard reactivity for a counterstain. Store as described above for the rhodamine-labeled conjugate.

PBS, pH 7.2 ± 0.1. The formula (per liter) for PBS is:

NaCl .... 7.65 g
Na₂HPO₄ .... 0.724 g
KH₂PO₄ .... 0.21 g

Several liters may be prepared and stored in a large Pyrex (or equivalent) or polyethylene bottle. Determine the pH of each lot of PBS prepared for the FTA-ABS DS test. PBS outside the range of pH 7.2 ± 0.1 should be adjusted with 1 N NaOH. Discard bacterially contaminated PBS.

2.0% Tween 80 (polysorbate 80). To prepare PBS containing 2% Tween 80, heat the two reagents in a 56°C water bath. To 49 ml of sterile PBS, add 1 ml of Tween 80 by measuring from the bottom of a pipette, and rinse out the pipette. The 2% Tween 80 solution should have a pH of 7.0 to 7.2. Check the pH periodically because the solution may become acid. Discard if a precipitate develops or if the pH changes.

Mounting medium. The mounting medium is 1 part PBS (pH 7.2) plus 9 parts glycerol (reagent quality).

Other. Acetone (ACS).

Preparation of *T. pallidum* antigen smears

Mix the antigen suspension thoroughly by mixing on a vortex for 10 s or by drawing the suspension into a syringe with a 25-gauge needle and expelling it vigorously. Determine by dark-field examination that treponemes are adequately dispersed before slides are made for the FTA test. Additional mixing may be required. Wipe the slides with pre-etched circles with clean gauze to remove dust particles. *Note.* Unclean slides and slides of poor quality can affect the reactivity of the test. Slides should be cleaned by sonic vibration or alcohol wiping if treponemes are not clearly observed after staining. Prepare very thin *T. pallidum* antigen smears within each circle by using a standard 2-mm, 26-gauge, platinum wire loop. Generally, half a loop is sufficient antigen for two circles (1-cm inner diameter). Allow to air dry for at least 15 min. Two-circle slides are preferred for FTA-ABS DS tests to prevent serum runover when processing slides. (Multispot antigen slides are available commercially from several manufacturers. These slides must be sufficiently hydrophobic to prevent serum and conjugate runover during slide processing. Follow the recommendations of the manufacturer to be sure that serum and conjugate do not run between smears. If cross-contamination occurs, the test must be repeated. Reactivity from cross-contamination may occur in 30 s.) Fix the smears in acetone for 10 min, and allow them to air dry thoroughly. *Note.* Not more than 60 slides should be fixed with 200 ml of acetone. Store acetone-fixed smears at −20°C or below. Fixed, frozen smears are usable indefinitely, provided that satisfactory results are obtained with the control. Do not thaw and refreeze antigen smears.

Criteria of acceptability for antigen, sorbent, conjugate, and counterstain

An antigen is considered acceptable if (i) a sufficient number of organisms remain on the slides after staining so that tests may be read without difficulty; (ii) the antigen does not contain background material that stains to the extent that it interferes with the test reading; (iii) the number of organisms remains stable on antigen smears stored at −20°C; (iv) the antigen does not stain nonspecifically with a standard conjugate at its working titer; and (v) reportable test results on controls and individual sera are comparable to those obtained with an antigen previously found to be satisfactory. A sorbent is acceptable if it removes nonspecific reactivity of the nonspecific control serum and does not reduce the intensity of fluorescence of the reactive (4+) control serum to less than 3+ and if test results are comparable to those obtained with a previously satisfactory sorbent. An acceptable conjugate does not stain reference antigen nonspecifically at three doubling dilutions below the working titer of the conjugate, and test results on controls and individual sera are comparable to those obtained with a conjugate previously found to be satisfactory.

The counterstain is considered acceptable if it stains *T. pallidum* with 3+ to 4+ intensity when used at the working dilution recommended by the manufacturer. The minimal acceptable working dilution is 1:10.

Preparation of sera

Bacterial contamination or excessive hemolysis may render specimens unsatisfactory for testing. Heat the test and control sera at 56°C for 30 min before testing. Reheat previously heated test sera for 10 min at 56°C on the day of testing.

Controls

Store and use control sera from commercial sources according to accompanying directions. Include the following controls in each test run.

1. Reactive (4+) control. The reactive (4+) control is reactive serum or a dilution of reactive serum demonstrating strong (4+) fluorescence when diluted 1:5 in PBS and only slightly reduced fluorescence (a reduction of no more than 1+ fluorescence, i.e., 4+ changing to 3+) when diluted 1:5 in sorbent. Add 50 µl of reactive control serum to a tube containing 200 µl of PBS. Mix well at least eight times. (Tips may be left in the tube and used to dispense material to the slide.) Add 50 µl of reactive control serum to a tube containing 200 µl of sorbent. Mix well at least eight times.

2. Minimally reactive (1+) control. The minimally reactive (1+) control is a dilution of reactive serum demonstrating the minimal degree of fluorescence reported as reactive for use as a reading standard. The reactive (4+) control serum may be used for this control when diluted in PBS according to directions furnished by the manufacturer. This control is not further diluted in sorbent.

3. Nonspecific serum control. The nonspecific serum control is serum from a nonsyphilitic individual known to demonstrate 2+ or greater nonspecific reactivity in the FTA test at a 1:5 PBS dilution and essentially no staining when diluted 1:5 in sorbent. Add 50 µl of nonspecific control serum to a tube containing 200 µl of PBS. Mix well at least eight times. Add 50 µl of nonspecific control serum to a tube containing 200 µl of sorbent. Mix well at least eight times.

4. Nonspecific staining controls. Nonspecific staining controls are an antigen smear treated with 30 µl of PBS and another antigen smear treated with 30 µl of sorbent. Control patterns are shown in Table 6.

TABLE 6. Reactions with staining controls on the FTA-ABS DS test[a]

Control	Reaction[b]
Reactive control[c]	
1:5 PBS dilution	R4+
1:5 sorbent dilution	R(4+−3+)
Minimally reactive (1+) control[d]	R1+
Nonspecific serum control[c]	
1:5 PBS dilution	R(2+−4+)
1:5 sorbent dilution	N−±
Nonspecific staining control[c]	
Antigen, PBS, and conjugate	N
Antigen, sorbent, and conjugate	N

[a] If a gradual decrease of fluorescence in the reactive controls is observed over a period of time, this may indicate deterioration of control serums, reagents, or the light source. Test runs in which these results are not obtained are considered unsatisfactory and should not be reported.
[b] R, Reactive; N, nonreactive.
[c] Included to control reagents and test conditions.
[d] Included as a reading standard and equipment control.

Test procedure

1. Identify previously prepared slides by numbering the frosted end with a lead pencil.

2. Number the tubes to correspond to the sera and control sera being tested, and place in racks.

3. Prepare reactive (4+), minimally reactive (1+), and nonspecific control serum dilutions in sorbent or PBS, or both, according to the directions.

4. Pipette 200 μl of sorbent into a test tube for each test serum.

5. Add 50 μl of the heated test serum to the appropriate tube, and mix eight times.

6. Cover the appropriate antigen smears with 30 μl of the reactive (4+), minimally reactive (1+), or nonspecific control serum dilution.

7. Cover the appropriate antigen smears with 30 μl of the PBS and 30 μl of the sorbent for nonspecific staining controls.

8. Cover the appropriate antigen smears with 30 μl of the appropriate test serum dilution.

9. Prevent evaporation by placing slides within a moist chamber.

10. Place sides in an incubator at 35 to 37°C for 30 min.

11. Rinsing procedure.
    a. Place the slides in slide carriers, and rinse the slides with running PBS for approximately 5 s.
    b. Place the slides in a staining dish containing PBS for 5 min.
    c. Agitate the slides by dipping them in and out of the PBS at least 30 times.
    d. Using fresh PBS, repeat steps b and c.
    e. Rinse slides in running distilled water for approximately 5 s.

12. Gently blot the slides with bibulous paper to remove water drops.

13. Dilute TMRITC-labeled anti-human IgG globulin to its working titer in PBS containing 2% Tween 80.

14. Place approximately 30 μl of diluted conjugate on each smear.

15. Repeat steps 9 through 12.

16. Dilute FITC-labeled anti-treponemal globulin to its working titer in PBS containing 2% Tween 80.

17. Place approximately 30 μl of the diluted conjugate on each smear.

18. Repeat step 9.

19. Place the slides in an incubator at 35 to 37°C for 20 min.

20. Repeat steps 11 and 12.

21. Mount the slides immediately by placing a small drop of mounting medium on each smear and applying a cover glass.

22. Examine the slides as soon as possible. If a delay in reading is necessary, place the slides in a darkened room and read within 4 h.

23. Locate and focus treponemes with the FITC filter system.

24. After the treponemes have been located, dial in the TMRITC filters to read specific fluorescence.

25. Using the minimally reactive (1+) control slide as the reading standard, record the intensity of fluorescence of the treponemes according to Tables 7 and 8.

TABLE 8. Reporting system for FTA-ABS DS test

Initial test reading	Repeat test reading	Report
4+		Reactive
3+		Reactive
2+		Reactive
1+	>1+	Reactive
	1+	Reactive minimal[a]
	<1+	Nonreactive
<1+		Nonreactive
N–±		Nonreactive

[a] In the absence of historical or clinical evidence of treponemal infection, this test result should be considered equivocal. A second specimen should be submitted for serologic testing.

LITERATURE CITED

1. **Daniels, K. C., and H. S. Ferneyhough.** 1977. Specific direct fluorescent antibody detection of *Treponema pallidum.* Health Lab. Sci. **14:**164–171.

2. **Fiumara, N. J.** 1979. Serologic responses to treatment of 128 patients with late latent syphilis. Sex. Transm. Dis. **6:**243–246.

3. **Hunter, E. F., P. W. Greer, B. Swisher, K. R. Sulzer, C. E. Farshy, and J. Crawford.** 1984. Immunofluorescence staining of *Treponema* in tissues fixed with Formalin. Arch. Pathol. Lab. Med. **108:**878–880.

4. **Hunter, E. F., R. M. McKinney, S. E. Maddison, and D. D. Cruce.** 1979. Double-staining procedure for the fluorescent treponemal antibody-absorption (FTA-ABS) test. Br. J. Vener. Dis. **55:**105–108.

5. **March, R. W., and G. E. Stiles.** 1980. The reagin screen test: a new reagin card test for syphilis. Sex. Transm. Dis. **7:**66–70.

6. **Nelson, R. A., Jr., and M. M. Mayer.** 1949. Immobilization of *Treponema pallidum* in vitro by antibody produced in syphilitic infection. J. Exp. Med. **89:**369–393.

7. **Pettit, D. E., S. A. Larsen, V. Pope, M. W. Perryman, and M. R. Adams.** 1982. Unheated serum reagin test as a quantitative test for syphilis. J. Clin. Microbiol. **15:**238–242.

8. **Tomizawa, T., S. Kasamatsu, and S. Yamaya.** 1969. Usefulness of hemagglutination test using *Treponema pallidum* antigen (TPHA) for the serodiagnosis of syphilis. Jpn. J. Med. Sci. Biol. **22:**341–350.

9. **U.S. Department of Health, Education, and Welfare, National Communicable Disease Center, Venereal Disease Program.** 1969. Manual of tests of syphilis. Center for Disease Control, Atlanta.

10. **Wentworth, B. B., M. A. Thompson, C. R. Peter, R. E. Bawdon, and D. L. Wilson.** 1978. Comparison of a hemagglutination treponemal test for syphilis (HATTS) with other serologic methods for the diagnosis of syphilis. Sex. Transm. Dis. **5:**103–111.

TABLE 7. Intensity of fluorescence in FTA-ABS DS test

Reading	Intensity of fluorescence
2+ to 4+	Moderate to strong
1+	Equivalent to minimally reactive (1+) control
± to <1+	Visible staining, but less than 1+ control
–	None or vaguely visible, but without distinct fluorescence

Chapter 69

Serological Diagnosis of Leptospirosis

A. D. ALEXANDER

Leptospirosis is an acute, febrile, septicemic disease attributable to any one of a large number of serologically distinct members of the spirochetal species *Leptospira interrogans* (6). A second currently accepted species, *L. biflexa*, comprises the nonpathogenic leptospires commonly found in natural waters. In addition, organisms which are morphologically similar to leptospires have been isolated which resemble *L. biflexa* phenotypically but are genetically and antigenically distinct from members of either recognized species. They may represent a new species or genus (6). The various pathogenic leptospires are not readily distinguishable on the basis of morphological, biochemical, and cultural characteristics. They do, however, have distinct antigenic properties as disclosed in agglutination and agglutinin-adsorption tests. These properties are important for serological diagnosis and provide the basis for their classification by serovars (synonym: serotype), the basic taxon. Currently over 180 known pathogenic serovars have been arbitrarily assembled into 20 serogroups on the basis of common cross-reacting agglutinogens (6).

Leptospires occur naturally in a wide variety of feral and domestic mammals. In natural hosts, the spirochetes nest in the kidneys and are shed in the urine. Humans are accidental hosts. Infections are usually related to occupational or recreational activities which entail either direct contact with animal urine (e.g., abattoir workers, miners, sewer cleaners, or fish workers in rat-infested surroundings) or contact with natural waters and soils contaminated with animal urine (e.g., rice field workers, cane field workers, swimmers in ponds and streams about which livestock are pastured, etc.). The organisms invade hosts through abrasions in the skin or through mucosa of the nose, pharynx, eye, and esophagus.

The clinical manifestations of leptospirosis are variable and can include inapparent infections, flulike illnesses, "aseptic" meningitis, and, less frequently, an icteric-hemorrhagic form with severe liver and kidney involvement. Diagnosis is usually established in the laboratory by the demonstration of the organisms or by serological tests. The laboratory procedures for cultivation and identification of leptospires are described elsewhere (2). The onset of leptospirosis is usually abrupt, after an incubation period generally of 10 to 12 days (range, 3 to 30 days). Leptospiremia occurs at the time of disease onset and persists for about 1 week. Antibodies are usually detectable by the end of the first week of disease and reach maximal levels by the third or fourth week. Thereafter, antibody levels gradually recede but may be detectable for years.

MICROSCOPIC AGGLUTINATION TEST

The microscopic agglutination test is most often used and is generally accepted as the standard reference test for demonstration of leptospiral antibodies (1, 5). It has excellent sensitivity for the diagnosis of recent as well as past infections in humans and animals. However, the test has limitations because of its high serological specificity. Consequently, to ensure detection of antibodies which may be provoked by any of the large number of serovars, it is necessary to use a battery of different serovar antigens which cover most of the known cross-reactions of leptospires. The following 15 serovars have been recommended (1): *copenhageni, grippotyphosa, autumnalis, poi, wolffi, bratislava, canicola, borincana, pomona, castellonis, swajizak, tarassovi, pyrogenes, djatzi,* and *patoc*. Additional serovars recommended for supplementary tests are *shermani, panama, celledoni, djasiman, cynopteri,* and *louisiana*. *L. biflexa* serovar *patoc* is used because it frequently cross-reacts with leptospiral antibodies in human sera irrespective of the infecting serovar. The proposed list of antigens may be modified according to local experience and needs. Substitution of local isolates of the same or related type could provide a more sensitive test. In the continental United States, approximately 23 different pathogenic serovars have been disclosed in nonhuman animal hosts. However, relatively few serovars have been associated with infections in humans and domestic animals (7). Therefore, at this time the use of the following eight serovars as antigens would serve to detect all but rare cases of leptospirosis: *copenhageni, grippotyphosa, canicola, wolffi, pomona, djatzi, autumnalis,* and *patoc*. Sera that are found to be negative with the above eight antigens should be retested with the larger battery of antigens in those cases where leptospirosis is highly suspected on the basis of clinical and epidemiological findings. Extended testing is available at the Leptospirosis Reference Laboratory, Centers for Disease Control, Atlanta, Ga.

Preparation of antigen

Young cultures of leptospires in fluid medium are used as antigens. Organisms are grown in fluid medium containing rabbit serum (e.g., Stuart medium) or serum albumin plus fatty acid (EMJH medium). Formulas and commercial sources for media are given in the *Manual of Clinical Microbiology* (8). Media are inoculated with mature culture in amounts comprising 5 to 10% of the fresh culture volume and incubated at 30°C. Usually, suitable antigens are obtained after 4 to 7 days. Cultures for use as antigens are examined microscopically by dark-ground illumination for homogeneity, purity, and density. Some strains tend to form small clumps of cells or microcolonies, which can be confused with agglutination but which can often by avoided by frequent sequential transfers of cultures. If microcolonies are not too numerous, they may be removed from otherwise suitable cultures by centrifugation at 1,500 to 2,000 × *g* for 15 to 30 min. A culture density of approximately 2×10^8 organisms per ml is desirable. The density can be determined nephelometrically or by microscopic counts in a Petroff-Hausser chamber. Density can also be estimated by microscopic examination of a 0.01-ml drop under a cover slip (22 by 22 mm). A count of 100 to 200 leptospires per high dry field ($\times 450$ magnification) will provide an antigen of satisfactory density. Overly dense antigens may be diluted with medium or physiological salt solution.

Antigens may be used live or Formalin-treated. To prepare Formalin-fixed antigens, reagent-grade, neutral Formalin is added to a final concentration of 0.3% by volume to 4- to 7-day-old cultures previously checked for purity, density, and homogeneity. The Formalin-treated antigen is kept at room temperature for 1 to 2 h and then centrifuged for 10 min at 1,000 to 1,500 $\times g$ to remove clumped cells and extraneous material. Formalin-treated antigens are usually stable for 1 to 2 weeks if stored at 4°C. Stored antigen should be checked microscopically for appearance and homogeneity before each use. Fixed as well as live antigens may be tested for sensitivity by titration with standard homologous antisera.

Preparation of standard antisera

Antisera for most test serovars are available commercially (Difco Laboratories, Detroit, Mich.). Alternatively, antisera may be prepared in rabbits by injecting successive doses of 0.5, 1.0, 2.0, and 4 ml of live antigen into the marginal ear vein at 5- to 7-day intervals. Five- to seven-day cultures in Fletcher semisolid medium containing rabbit sera are used as a source of inoculum. Seven days after the last injection, homologous serum agglutinin titers are measured. If the titer is 1:6,400 or greater, blood is removed by cardiopuncture. Otherwise, an additional 4-ml antigen dose is administered. The separated serum is distributed into vials and can be stored in the frozen state (−20 to −30°C), in the freeze-dried state, or by the addition of glycerol (equal volume) or Merthiolate (1:10,000 concentration).

The use of live cultures has obvious potential infection hazards in the technical procedure as well as in the maintenance of infected rabbits which may become renal shedders of leptospires. For this reason many laboratories use as inocula cultures inactivated by Formalin or by heat (56°C for 30 min). Antisera prepared with killed antigens usually have lower titers than those elicited with viable organisms.

Agglutination test

Test sera are diluted with physiological salt solution or phosphate-buffered (pH 7.4) physiological salt solution. An initial serum dilution of 1:50 is prepared by adding 0.2 ml of serum to 9.8 ml of diluent; from this, serial fourfold dilutions to 1:3,200 are prepared. Each diluted serum is added in 0.2-ml amounts in a series of agglutination tubes or wells in plastic trays; an equal volume of antigen is then added to each tube or well in the serum dilution series, giving final dilutions of 1:100 to 1:6,400. The antigen-serum mixtures are shaken, incubated at room temperature for 2 to 3 h, shaken again, and examined for agglutination.

Small drops from the reaction mixtures are placed on a slide with a dropper or loop, spread to flatten, and examined microscopically ($10\times$ objective and $15\times$ ocular) by dark-ground illumination without the use of cover slips.

The microscopic agglutination test has been adapted for use with microtitration techniques (9). Twofold serum dilutions are prepared in microdilution plastic plates with flat-bottomed wells with the use of 0.05-ml microdiluters. Antigens are added in equivalent volume with disposable microliter pipettes. Plates are covered, gently shaken, kept at room temperature for 2 h, and then read after gentle shaking. Reactions in the well may be examined directly under a dark-field microscope by the use of a long-working-distance $10\times$ objective.

Two types of reactions are manifest with live antigens: agglutination and so-called "lysis." Agglutinated cell aggregates are generally spherical with occasional leptospires extruding from the surface. Some antigens may agglutinate along their longitudinal axis, giving a frayed-rope appearance. When "lysis" occurs, there are few or rare freely moving leptospires, and small refractile granules are seen. The granules are tightly packed, clumped cells.

"Lysis" does not occur when Formalin-fixed antigens are used. Agglutination is manifest as relatively large, irregularly outlined clumps which have a lacy appearance. Fixed antigens are less sensitive than live antigens and tend to react more broadly with diverse serovars.

Positive- and negative-control sera should be included in each test. Reference to reactions in controls is helpful in determining the degree of reaction and in distinguishing agglutinated clumps from microcolonies when the latter are present. Prozone phenomena may occur, especially with high-titer sera. Reactions are graded on the following basis: 4+ = 75% or more cells agglutinated; 3+ = 50 to 75% of cells agglutinated, many clumps present in each field; 2+ = 25 to 50% of cells agglutinated, at least one specific clump in each field; and 1+ = occasional small clump or small stellate aggregations.

The recommended end titer reaction (9) is defined as the highest final dilution of serum in the serum-antigen mixture in which 50% or more of the cells are agglutinated (3+ or 4+ reactions). Titers of 1:100 or greater are considered to be significant. Titers may range as high as 1:25,600 or greater. Since leptospiral agglutinins may persist for months and even years after infection, the presence of antibodies in a single serum sample may not necessarily reflect current illness but may have been incited at an earlier time. Generally, a titer of 1:1,600 or greater in a single specimen provides strong presumptive evidence of recent infection. Preferably, tests should be done on paired acute- and convalescent-phase serum samples. A demonstrable fourfold or greater rise in titer is significant.

The microscopic agglutination test has important drawbacks which limit its usefulness for the small diagnostic laboratory. It is laborious and time-consuming; it involves handling of live cultures with attendant risk to personnel and maintenance of a large number of serovars. A variety of alternative serological procedures have therefore been proposed (5, 11).

Procedures that have been adapted for routine use by various laboratories are the macroscopic (slide or plate) agglutination test with a battery of single or pooled Formalin-fixed antigens (9); three "genus-specific" tests in which *L. biflexa* antigens (e.g., strain Patoc) are used in macroscopic agglutination (5), hemolytic or indirect hemagglutination (4, 9), and complement fixation (11) tests; and an enzyme-linked immunosorbent assay (ELISA) (10).

MACROSCOPIC (SLIDE) AGGLUTINATION TEST

Slide test antigens consist of a standard suspension of Formalin-treated washed cells in a suitable buffer (9). Antigens are available commercially from Difco and from Fort Dodge Laboratories, Fort Dodge, Iowa. Those from Difco are prepared from 12 or more different serovars and are used singly or in pools of three. Antigens from Fort Dodge Laboratories are available only for 5 serovars and therefore have less serovar coverage than available pools of slide test antigens which incorporate at least 12 different serovars. The test is conducted on a glass slide or plate by mixing a drop of serum with a drop of antigen. The serum-antigen mixtures are shaken for a few minutes on a rotary shaker and then examined for agglutination by indirect light with a black background. Pooled antigens are usually stable for 9 months or longer. Older preparations may give nonspecific reactions. Nonspecific reactions resulting from clumpy antigens may frequently be eliminated by vigorous shaking of antigens before use. It is important to use positive- and negative-control sera in the performance of this test. The test is simple to perform and has good sensitivity and specificity for detecting antibodies in humans and animals with recent or current disease. It cross-reacts more broadly than the microscopic agglutination test but is less sensitive than the latter in detecting antibodies for retrospective studies, e.g., in serological surveys. Paired acute- and convalescent-phase sera can be tested with pooled or individual antigens to demonstrate titer conversions. Slide test titers are lower than microscopic agglutination test titers and generally range to 1:160.

MACROSCOPIC (SLIDE) AGGLUTINATION TEST WITH THERMORESISTANT *L. BIFLEXA* PATOC ANTIGEN

The thermoresistant *L. biflexa* Patoc antigen agglutination test is a simple, safe procedure that is used in various laboratories in France, England, and Italy. The antigen is not commercially available at present. It consists of a dense suspension of Formalin-treated, heated cells of *L. biflexa* strain Patoc. The antigen reacts broadly with antibodies to diverse pathogenic serovars. Antigen is prepared from a well-grown culture of strain Patoc in a fluid medium such as EMJH to which neutral Formalin is added to a final concentration of 0.2% by volume. The Formalin-treated culture is held at room temperature for 2 h, then centrifuged in the cold at 1,300 × g for 30 min to sediment the leptospires, which are suspended in phosphate-buffered salt solution (pH 7.2) and again collected by centrifugation and resuspended to a creamy consistency with phosphate-buffered salt solution by use of a 16- to 18-gauge needle or Pasteur pipette. The suspension is transferred to a bottle containing glass beads and held at 4°C for 24 h or longer with intermittent shaking. The bottle is then placed in a beaker containing cold water which is heated to boiling and held at 100°C for 30 min. After cooling, the density of the suspension is adjusted to twice that of the no. 10 McFarland standard. Gross particles and clumps of cells are removed by centrifugation at 1,000 to 1,500 × g for 5 min. The antigen is stored at 4°C and is reportedly stable for at least 1 year.

The test is conducted on a glass slide by mixing one drop each of serum and a 1:10 dilution thereof with an equal volume of antigen with the use of a toothpick. The slide is rotated on a shaker for a few minutes, and the mixtures are examined for agglutination by indirect light with a dark background. The test is principally used as a screening test but may be used to demonstrate antibody titer changes in paired acute- and convalescent-phase sera. Titers range up to 1:512. The sensitivity of the test in detecting antibodies in humans with current or recent infections is reportedly good, but it may have limitations for use in detecting antibodies in retrospect, months after infection. Its reliability for testing animal sera is equivocable; further observations are needed.

HEMOLYTIC AND INDIRECT HEMAGGLUTINATION TESTS

The hemolytic test (3) is conducted with one antigen consisting of a 50% ethyl alcohol-soluble, 95% ethyl alcohol-insoluble extract from leptospiral cells. The antigen is not available commercially at present. *L. biflexa* strains (e.g., serovar *codice*, *andamana*, or *patoc*) are commonly used as a source of the extracted antigen, which can be stored for years in the freeze-dried state without loss of activity. The antigen is very light. To prevent evacuation of antigen during freeze-drying, a binder, human albumin in a concentration of 2%, is added to stock solutions. The optimal antigen dilution for sensitizing sheep erythrocytes is predetermined by checkerboard titration with a standard reference antiserum; pooled rabbit antiserum from diverse serovars may be used as the standard reference serum. The antigen-sensitized cells are washed and resuspended to a concentration of 1% and are then added together with guinea pig complement to serial dilutions of sera. The reaction mixtures are incubated at 37°C for 1 h. A positive reaction is manifested by lysis of sensitized erythrocytes. Details on the preparation, standardization of antigens, and conduct of the test are given by Cox (3). Titers of 1:100 and greater are usually considered to be significant. In the extensive test series reported by Cox et al. (4), convalescent-phase serum titers were generally greater than 1:1,000 and ranged as high as 1:100,000. Microtiter techniques can be used for the hemolytic test.

The test can detect antibodies in human sera irrespective of the infecting serotypes, but it may lack sensitivity for detecting antibodies in animal sera, and its use for this purpose is not recommended. It has limited usefulness as a serological survey tool. The hemolytic test is particularly useful for diagnosis of cases in endemic areas of multiple leptospirosis and for testing large numbers of samples. It is relatively laborious for testing few samples and consequently has rarely been used in the United States. The test has been simplified by the use of sensitized erythrocytes which have been fixed with either glutaraldehyde or pyruvic aldehyde (9). The fixed antigens are used in an indirect hemagglutination procedure with sheep or human O erythrocytes. The indirect hemagglutination test has been extensively evaluated at the Centers for Disease Control, Atlanta, Ga. (9). To date, the test has been found to have excellent genus specificity and excellent sensitivity for detecting antibodies in the early stages of disease. Titers ranged from 1:100 to 1:51,200. The test may become negative a few weeks after convalescence. Its usefulness for detecting antibodies in animal sera has not been reported. The test would appear to be a promising tool for the small diagnostic laboratory if reagents become available.

ELISA

Laboratories equipped for ELISA tests may find the ELISA test of Terpstra et al. (10) useful. The antigen is broadly reactive with antibody of diverse serovars. It is not commercially available at present. It is prepared from a dense culture in EMJH medium of *L. interrogans* serovar *icterohaemorrhiae*, strain Wijnberg, or alternatively, *L. biflexa* strain Patoc. Formalin is first added to the culture to a final concentration of 0.5% by volume to kill cells. Then the culture is heated for 30 min in a water bath with boiling water, cooled to room temperature, and centrifuged for 30 min at $10,000 \times g$. The supernatant fluid is used as antigen, which is distributed into the wells of polystyrene microtiter plates in 100-μl amounts and allowed to dry at room temperature. The antigen in coated plates is stable for at least 6 months when plates are stored in a dry place at room temperature. Thereafter, when used, the usual procedures in ELISA tests are followed by the sequential additions between incubations and washes of (i) serial twofold diluted amounts of test serum, (ii) a predetermined amount of an optimum dilution of peroxidase-labeled anti-human immunoglobulin, and (iii) the peroxidase substrate (solution of 5-aminosalicylic acid containing H_2O_2). A positive reaction is indicated by a brown color. Details for the conduct of the test are given by Terpstra et al. (10). As described, positive reactions at serum dilutions of 1:40 and greater are considered to be significant. Titers may be as high as 1:20,480, with most falling in the range of 1:160 to 1:1,280. The sensitivity of the test for animal sera or for detecting antibodies in retrospect is not recorded.

COMPLEMENT FIXATION TEST WITH *L. BIFLEXA* ANTIGEN

The complement fixation test, like the hemolytic test, utilizes an *L. biflexa* antigen and has genus-specific activity (11). It has had favorable application in Romania and Great Britain. The antigen consists of a washed, Merthiolate-killed suspension of leptospires, concentrated to about 2% of the original culture volume in physiological saline. It is preserved by the addition of sodium azide (final concentration, 1:1,000) and is kept at 4°C. Turner (11) has found this test to be useful in detecting current and recent infections in humans. Titers in proved cases range from 1:128 to 1:5,120. The test is not suitable for testing animal sera.

The optimal dilution of antigen is predetermined by conventional checkerboard titration with a standard antiserum (e.g., pooled rabbit antiserum as in the hemolytic test). The complement fixation test antigen is not available commercially.

CLINICAL USEFULNESS

Serological tests for leptospirosis are used not only for diagnosis of cases in humans but even more frequently for diagnosis of cases in domestic animals, particularly dogs, cattle, and swine. Tests are also used for epidemiological investigations, which frequently entail retrospective determination of antibodies which may have been provoked many months previously. The microscopic agglutination test, when used with a judicious selection of antigens, serves all of these purposes. Moreover, the test frequently provides clues to the identity of the infecting serovar. It is stressed, however, that the determination of the infecting serovar can only be definitely established by isolation and typing of the organism. The identification of the infecting serovar is obviously important for epidemiological investigations, but it has little or no importance for the clinician in management and treatment of human cases. Consequently, a laboratory diagnosis of leptospirosis per se would serve the primary needs of the clinician and could be fulfilled by the use of the relatively simple slide test with pooled antigens or with a genus-specific test.

The slide test with Formalin-treated antigens could also serve the serological diagnostic needs in veterinary medicine. Its usefulness for seroepidemiological surveys has limitations because of test sensitivity in detecting antibodies of long duration. Nevertheless, the slide test can still be advantageously used for serological surveys if an index of the percentage of missed positives is derived by testing an appropriate portion of the negative sample population with the conventional microscopic agglutination test.

The genus-specific hemolytic, indirect hemagglutination, and complement fixation tests are not recommended for use with animal sera. The applicability of the thermoresistant *L. biflexa* Patoc antigen slide and ELISA tests for testing animal sera requires further study. When used for seroepidemiological surveys, the sensitivity of the various genus-specific tests should be monitored by parallel testing with the microscopic agglutination tests, as suggested above for slide test antigens. Unfortunately, the current serological procedures rarely establish a diagnosis before the first week of disease. There is still a critical need for a rapid, laboratory diagnostic test.

LITERATURE CITED

1. **Abdussalam, M., A. D. Alexander, B. Babudieri, K. Bogel, C. Borg-Peterson, S. Faine, E. Kmety, C. Lataste-Dorolle, and L. H. Turner.** 1972. Research needs in leptospirosis. Bull. W.H.O. **47:**113–122.
2. **Alexander, A. D.** 1985. *Leptospira*, p. 473–478. *In* E. H. Lennette, A. Balows, W. J. Hausler, Jr., and H. J. Shadomy (ed.), Manual of clinical microbiology, 4th ed.

American Society for Microbiology, Washington, D.C.

3. **Cox, C. D.** 1957. Standardization and stabilization of an extract from *Leptospira biflexa* and its use in the hemolytic test for leptospirosis. J. Infect. Dis. **101:**203–209.

4. **Cox, C. D., A. D. Alexander, and L. C. Murphy.** 1957. Evaluation of the hemolytic test in the serodiagnosis of human leptospirosis. J. Infect. Dis. **101:**210–218.

5. **Faine, S. (ed.).** 1982. Guidelines for the control of leptospirosis. W.H.O. Offset Publication no. 67. World Health Organization, Geneva.

6. **Johnson, R. C., and S. Faine.** 1984. Family II. *Leptospiraceae*, Hovind-Hougen, 1979, 245, p. 62–67. *In* N. R. Krieg, and J. G. Holt (ed.), Bergey's manual of systematic bacteriology, vol. 1. Williams & Wilkins, Baltimore.

7. **Kaufman, A. F.** 1976. Epidemiological trends of leptospirosis in the United States, 1965–1974, p. 177–189. *In* R. C. Johnson (ed.), The biology of parasitic spirochetes. Academic Press, Inc., New York.

8. **Phillips, B., and P. Nash.** 1985. Culture media, p. 1051–1092. *In* E. H. Lennette, A. Balows, W. J. Hausler, Jr., and H. J. Shadomy (ed.), Manual of clinical microbiology, 4th ed. American Society for Microbiology, Washington, D.C.

9. **Sulzer, C. R., and W. L. Jones.** 1976. Leptospirosis. Methods in laboratory diagnosis (revised edition). Department of Health, Education, and Welfare Publication no. (CDC) 76–8275.

10. **Terpstra, W. J., G. S. Ligthart, and G. S. Schoone.** 1980. Serodiagnosis of human leptospirosis by enzyme-linked-immunosorbent-assay (ELISA). Zentralbl. Bakteriol. Parasitenkd. Infektionskr. Hyg. Abt. I Orig. Reihe A **247:**400–405.

11. **Turner, L. H.** 1968. Leptospirosis. II. Serology. Trans. R. Soc. Trop. Med. Hyg. **62:**880–889.

Chapter 70

Serology of Mycoplasmal Infections

GEORGE E. KENNY

BIOLOGICAL CHARACTERISTICS OF THE ORDER *MYCOPLASMATALES*

The organisms classified in the order *Mycoplasmatales* are small organisms (0.3 to 0.5 μm) which are bounded by a unit membrane without evidence of a cell wall. The lack of a cell wall makes their immunology strikingly different from that of conventional bacteria because the immune response is directed at cell membrane components rather than toward cell wall and capsular materials found on bacteria. Furthermore, the organisms can be readily killed by antibodies directed against the membrane in contrast to the relative resistance of bacteria to antibody-mediated killing. The most important facet of their behavior in disease is the fact that they are surface parasites of animal cells.

TAXONOMY AND NOMENCLATURE

The order *Mycoplasmatales* contains some 70 species, of which 10 are found in humans (Table 1). Two genera, *Mycoplasma* and *Ureaplasma*, appear to be important in human infections (5, 30, 31). *Acholeplasma* spp. are found in sewage as well as in human specimen materials. The most important factor for human serological studies is that the species found in man are antigenically heterogeneous. These species can be divided into five antigenic groups. The five species which use arginine and do not ferment glucose make up serological group 7 (12). *Mycoplasma fermentans* utilizes both arginine and glucose and is the only representative of serogroup 6 in humans. Two glycolytic species, *M. pneumoniae* and *M. genitalium*, are serologically related and appear to share their lipid antigen specificities (15, 20). Consequently, *M. genitalium* is provisionally classified in group 4 with *M. pneumoniae*. The organisms also differ in classes of major antigens; *M. pneumoniae* and *M. genitalium* have major lipid antigens, whereas the major antigens of both *M. hominis* and *Ureaplasma urealyticum* appear to be proteins (11, 12). These differences in antigen class greatly complicate the development of serological tests for diagnosis of mycoplasmal infections since results from one organism cannot be extrapolated to other organisms.

PATHOGENESIS FOR HUMANS

M. pneumoniae is a major cause of primary atypical pneumonia, which accounts for 10 to 20% of total pneumonia cases (4, 5, 19). The other respiratory mycoplasmas, *M. orale*, *M. buccale*, and *M. faucium*, are not pathogens and are found in most human throats. *M. salivarium* is found only in humans with teeth and then in higher concentrations in diseased periodontal pockets than in normal pockets.

In the genital tract, the role of mycoplasmas in disease is much more complicated (31). Both *U. urealyticum* and *M. hominis* are found in normal persons without disease (e.g., some 70% of normal women carry *U. urealyticum*). When these organisms invade beyond their "normal habitat" (the urethra or vagina), they seem to be effective opportunists. *U. urealyticum* is involved in several diseases: (i) mild postpartum fever, (ii) upper urinary tract disease, (iii) neonatal infections, and (iv) prostatitis. *M. hominis* appears to be involved in some pelvic inflammatory diseases and has been isolated from joints and other sites distant from the genital tract. The role of either organism in nongonococcal urethritis or infertility is controversial. *M. genitalium* may be associated with pelvic inflammatory disease as judged by the fluorescent-antibody response of patients (21). *M. fermentans* is a rare isolate from the genital tract.

SEROLOGICAL TESTING

Interest has recently emerged in the detection of mycoplasmal infections, particularly infections associated with the genital tract. The technology for detecting antibodies to the genital mycoplasmas, however, is poorly developed, and only some provisional methods and general guidelines for the future can be given. Considerable emphasis will be placed on enzyme-linked immunosorbent assays (ELISAs) for the detection of mycoplasmal antibodies, but simple, reliable, and sensitive tests are not yet available. The situation for the diagnosis of *M. pneumoniae* infections is better because the conventional complement fixation test using lipid antigens gives satisfactory results when diagnosing respiratory infections.

Two general forms of tests have been widely used for the detection of mycoplasmal antibodies: the complement fixation test and the metabolic inhibition test. The metabolic inhibition test is unique to mycoplasmas and is based on the premise that the inhibition of the growth of the organism is reflected by the failure of the organism to make a metabolic product. The complement fixation test has the advantage that the methodology is well established but the disadvantage that large amounts of organisms are required. The metabolic inhibition test has the advantage that only small amounts of organisms are required but the disadvantages that the test requires live organisms and that the endpoint changes over time. The oldest serological test is the immunofluorescence test, which has the advantages of requiring only small amounts of antigen and detecting antibody class. The disadvantage of this test is its technical difficulty; however, many laboratories now have high technical competence in immunofluorescence testing.

TABLE 1. Characteristics, antigens, nomenclature, and habitats of *Mycoplasmatales* organisms found in humans

Organism	Serological group[a]	Lipid anitigen[b]	Metabolic markers[c]	Habitat
Mycoplasma pneumoniae	4	++++	G	Throat, lungs
Mycoplasma genitalium	4?	++++	G	Genital tract
Mycoplasma hominis	7	+	A	Genital tract, oral cavity
Mycoplasma salivarium	7	+	A	Periodontal crevices, oral cavity
Mycoplasma orale	7	+	A	Oral cavity
Mycoplasma faucium	7	+	A	Oral cavity
Mycoplasma buccale	7	+	A	Oral cavity
Mycoplasma fermentans	6	+++	AG	Genital tract
Ureaplasma urealyticum	8?	+	U	Genital tract (mouth, rarely)
Acholeplasma laidlawii	2	++	G	Skin, oral cavity, originally found in sewage

[a] Serological group as described previously (12).

[b] ++++, Major antigenic activity; ++, significant antigenic activity; +, trace activity. When carefully examined, all mycoplasmas indicate some activity in either their glycolipids (if present) or their phospholipids. For all organisms, protein antigens show major antigenic activity.

[c] G, Glycolytic; A, arginine utilizer; U, urea utilizing.

Preparation of antigens

For tests requiring concentrated organisms (complement fixation, ELISA, and immunoblotting), the organisms are cultivated in an appropriate broth medium (11, 13, 14) supplemented with 10% horse serum (or bovine serum as appropriate). Organisms are concentrated, washed three times with saline, and concentrated to at least 1 to 10 mg/ml. Antigens are stored at −20°C.

Complement fixation

The use of the lipid antigen for *M. pneumoniae* is preferred over the use of the whole organism because the antigen is less anticomplementary and gives greater differences in titer between acute and convalescent sera (17).

Preparation of lipid antigen. Five milliliters of 100-fold-concentrated organisms (approximately 10 mg of organism) are placed in a separatory funnel, and the following reagents are added in order, with vigorous shaking after each addition: 50 ml of methanol, 100 ml of chloroform, and 37.5 ml of 0.1 M KCl (17). This mixture is allowed to stand until two clear phases separate (separation of phases may be accelerated by chilling and then warming to room temperature). The lower phase (chloroform) is removed and evaporated to dryness (a rotary evaporator is useful but not indispensible since the chloroform phase will eventually evaporate in a hood). The antigen is solubilized in 5 ml of ethanol by scraping the drying container with a glass rod or a rubber policeman. Dissolving the lipids may be accelerated by placing the flask in a 56°C water bath. The ethanolic suspension appears turbid, and this turbidity increases upon storage in the cold (−20°C is recommended). This procedure is designed for simplicity and not as a definitive method for purifying lipids. The organic solvents are present in great excess and as much as 10 times the protein content of organisms could be fractionated without any danger of overloading the procedure, provided that the volume of antigen is not increased. The fractionation of the lipids is rapid and does not require shaking for more than several minutes at each step. Finally, the lipid antigen is extraordinarily stable; thus, its activity is not impaired by any of the recommended steps.

For use, the alcoholic extract is complexed with bovine albumin: 1 part of alcoholic extract is mixed with 3 parts of bovine albumin (fraction V or better grade) in the diluent used for complement fixation testing. Both reagents should be heated to 56°C before mixing in order to facilitate complexing. The complexed antigen should be stored at 4°C or frozen. At each use it should be heated to 56°C for 5 min to resolubilize the lipids.

Serological testing. The solubilized and complexed material can be titrated in any standard complement fixation test. In a standard checkerboard titration, the endpoint of the antigen titration is that amount of antigen which gives complete fixation against 4 U of antibody (block titrations of *M. pneumoniae* give reasonably "square" block titrations; i.e., neither excess antigen nor antibody markedly increases the titer of the other reagent). If human antisera cannot be obtained for initial testing, animal antisera may be used with the caution that the antigen titers, though similar within two- to fourfold, are not identical to those obtained with human antiserum. For routine testing, the control human serum should have a titer of ≥1:64 and should be used for antigen titrations and as a daily control for testing the sera. Once the antigen titer has been determined for a batch of complexed material, this titer will be stable either in a freezer or at 4°C (provided that the material is warmed briefly at 56°C before each use). The anticomplementary control must contain the same concentration of bovine albumin as the test antigen to guard against the test's measuring complement-fixing antibodies to bovine albumin. A daily antigen titration against four antibody units should be included with each test. Four antigen units are used in the test with two "full" complement units.

Metabolic inhibition testing

The metabolic inhibition test measures the ability of antibody to prevent the growth of the organisms as indicated by the failure of a culture of organisms to produce a normal end product (acid, ammonia, or reduction of tetrazolium, which is demonstrated as a color change in the pH or redox indicator in the

erum standards, normal human dissociated serum (negative control), and dissociated serum from a mannanemic rabbit (positive control). Cover the plate with another microtiter plate, and incubate it for 30 min at 4°C. Aspirate the contents of wells to avoid aerosols.

3. Wash the plate three times with PBS-T, and at the fourth wash, let the plate stand for 5 min as described above.

4. Add appropriately diluted peroxidase-labeled anti-*C. albicans* IgG conjugate, 0.2 ml per well, and incubate at 4°C for 30 min.

5. Wash the plate as described above.

6. Prepare the substrate solution for use by mixing the stock solution of *o*-phenylenediamine–3% H_2O_2–dH_2O in the proportions 0.5 ml:0.1 ml:50 ml. Add 200 μl to each well, and incubate for 1 h at room temperature in the dark.

7. Add 25 μl of 4 M H_2SO_4 per well to stop the reaction. (The eyes should be protected.)

8. Scan the plate on the microELISA reader at 490 nm.

9. Plot a graph for absorbance (*y*-axis, log scale) versus log concentration (*x*-axis). See Fig. 2 and 3.

10. Calculate nanograms of mannan per milliliter with respect to the standard curve.

Calculating mannan concentrations

1. Obtain the mean of triplicates for each mannan concentration for the normal human serum blanks and for the unknowns. Subtract the A_{490}, if any, of the blank from each mannan-containing sample and from the unknown.

2. Plot the standard curve for A_{490} versus mannan concentration on graph paper.

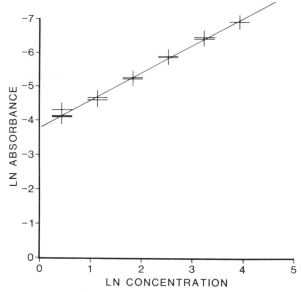

FIG. 3. Logarithmic transformation (ln-ln) of the standard curve shown in Fig. 2 generated by the Hewlett-Packard 86 computer.

3. Interpolate the value of the unknown with respect to the standard curve.

4. The significance of pertinent positive and negative controls for the EIA is reviewed as follows.

The wells receiving the normal human serum serve as blank controls for the background. Typically, these wells develop no color. The absorbance of mannan concentrations, "spiked" into serum, allows construction of a standard curve and controls for run-to-run variation. The in vivo mannanemia sample, obtained from infected rabbits, more closely represents mannan in patients' sera and provides another benchmark for run-to-run variations.

A computer program that prints the standard curve, calculates the concentration of mannan in unknown samples, and prints the results, including mean A_{490}, mannan in nanograms per milliliter, and the coefficient of variation, is available in a diskette (5.25 in. [ca. 13.3 cm]) for use with the Hewlett-Packard 86 computer, through the Division of Mycotic Diseases, CDC. A sample mannan determination is shown in Table 1, giving the A_{490} in each well. Table 2 shows how the computer program reduces the data and computes variation in the standard curve. Table 3 shows how the absorbance values of the standards and unknowns are converted into antigen concentrations in nanograms per milliliter with respect to the best-fit line through all points of the standard curve. These computations are determined by the computer program. Note that small deviations occur between the nominal mannan concentrations of standards spiked into sera and the values recorded with respect to the standard curve.

Interpretation. Heat-stable mannan-polysaccharide antigens have been detected by EIA in the sera of immunosuppressed rabbits infected with *C. albicans* (4) and in humans (5). The sensitivity of detection is 65 to 70% in human cancer patients. Specificity is 100%. Since mannan is not a normal serum constituent, concentrations greater than 2 ng/ml are presumptive

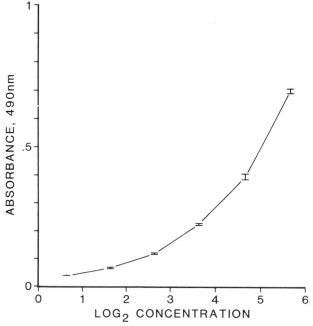

FIG. 2. Standard curve (semilog₂) of mannan in serum (1.56 to 50 ng/ml) in the EIA for antigenemia. Triplicates at each mannan concentration.

TABLE 1. A_{490} for mannan standards, normal human serum control, and unknowns[a] in the double-antibody sandwich EIA for antigenemia

Well		Mannan standards (ng/ml) [b]:						NHS[c]	Control[d]			
		1.56	3.13	6.25	12.5	25	50					
A	0.000	0.000	0.000	0.000	0.000	0.000	0.000	0.000	0.000	0.000	0.000	0.000
B	0.000	0.076	0.125	0.264	0.454	0.691	1.041	0.000	0.124	0.001	0.000	0.002
C	0.000	0.073	0.126	0.245	0.424	0.710	1.059	0.000	0.141	0.000	0.000	0.003
D	0.000	0.069	0.117	0.243	0.424	0.640	1.050	0.000	0.114	0.000	0.000	0.010
E	0.000	0.000	0.013	0.560	0.029	0.005	0.522	0.030	0.000	0.271	0.000	0.000
F	0.000	0.000	0.021	0.614	0.042	0.004	0.498	0.028	0.000	0.269	0.000	0.000
G	0.000	0.000	0.000	0.383	0.003	0.000	0.508	0.023	0.000	0.251	0.000	0.000
H	0.000	0.000	0.000	0.000	0.000	0.000	0.000	0.000	0.000	0.000	0.000	0.000

[a] Unknowns, wells E, F, and G in columns 4, 7, 8, and 10.
[b] Wells B, C, and D in columns 2 through 7.
[c] NHS, Normal human serum; wells B, C, and D in column 8.
[d] Positive mannanemic control (rabbit); wells B, C, and D, in column 9.

evidence of infection. The sensitivity limit of the mannanemia EIA is 1 ng/ml of serum. Mannans of *C. albicans* serotype A and *C. tropicalis* are detected. Mannanemia may be a transient event, and close monitoring of high-risk patients is warranted. Patients receiving systemic immunosuppressive drugs who are primarily granulocytopenic and have a fever of unknown origin despite broad-spectrum antibacterial therapy should be monitored twice weekly. At the same time, blood cultures should be drawn (4).

Coccidioidomycosis

The CF and tube precipitin (TP) tests are valuable aids in diagnosing and determining the prognosis of coccidioidomycosis. The two tests measure at least three different antigen-antibody systems. The antigen responsible for evoking IgM in the TP test has been identified as factor 2 of coccidioidin, a protein that is stable to heat (60°C, 30 min), alkali, and trypsin (3). The TP test is most effective in detecting early primary infection or an exacerbation of existing disease. It is most frequently used in areas in which the disease is endemic. The CF procedure is the most widely used serological test for coccidioidomycosis, and its reacting antibodies persist for longer periods than those reactive in the TP test. Smith et al. (24) found that the combination of CF and TP tests yielded positive results in over 90% of the primary symptomatic cases of coccidioidomycosis. Screening tests (10), such as the

latex particle agglutination (LPA) and ID tests, which yield results comparable to those of the TP and CF tests, respectively, can be used by those laboratories not in a position to perform the TP or CF tests. A variation of the ID test, with a heated toluene-induced lysate of mycelium as antigen, has also been shown to yield qualitative results that correlate with those obtained with the TP test. This test, referred to as the IDTP procedure, is recommended as a screen for detecting sera that may yield a positive TP test (10). The use of heated and unheated coccidioidin in ID tests readily permits the detection and distinction of precipitins and complement-fixing antibodies reactive with the F antigen. In addition, concentrating clinical specimens 8- to 10-fold appears to enhance the detection of these antibodies (20).

Clinical indications

Serologic tests for coccidioidomycosis should be considered whenever patients display symptoms of

TABLE 2. Statistical analysis of the standard curve[a] for determining mannan concentrations in serum

Mannan standard (ng/ml of serum)	A_{490}		
	Mean	SD[b]	CV (%)[c]
1.56	0.073	0.004	4.8
3.12	0.123	0.005	4.0
6.25	0.251	0.012	4.6
12.5	0.434	0.017	4.0
25.0	0.680	0.036	5.3
50.0	1.050	0.009	0.9

[a] Slope, 0.79; y intercept, −2.92; coefficient of determination, 0.9944.
[b] SD, Standard deviation.
[c] CV, Coefficient of variation.

TABLE 3. Mannanemia EIA interpolations of standards and unknowns with respect to the standard curve of mannan in serum

Specimen		A_{490}		
	Antigenemia (ng/ml)	Mean	SD[a]	CV (%)[b]
Mannan standard (ng/ml)				
1.56	1.46	0.073	0.004	4.8
3.13	2.86	0.123	0.005	4.0
6.25	7.1	0.251	0.012	4.6
12.5	14.3	0.434	0.017	3.9
25.0	25.3	0.680	0.036	5.3
50.0	44.1	1.050	0.009	0.8
Positive mannanemic control	2.97	0.126	0.014	10.8
Unknown[c]				
1	17.9	0.519	0.121	23.2
2	17.5	0.509	0.012	2.3
3	0.4	0.027	0.004	13.3
4	7.5	0.264	0.011	4.1

[a] SD, Standard deviation.
[b] CV, Coefficient of variation.
[c] Infected rabbits.

pulmonary or meningeal infections and have lived or traveled in areas in which *C. immitis* is endemic.

These tests should be used particularly when such patients demonstrate sensitivity to a coccidioidin or spherulin skin test.

Serum precipitins may be detected within 1 to 3 weeks after the onset of primary infections in a large percentage of cases in which CF tests have not yet become positive. These precipitins are diagnostic but not prognostic. Precipitins are rarely detected 6 months after infection, but they could reappear if the infection spreads or relapse occurs. Precipitins may persist in disseminated cases. They are rarely found in the CSF of patients with coccidioidal meningitis, so the TP test is of little value in analyzing CSF specimens. The CF test becomes positive later than the precipitin test and is most effective in determining disseminated disease. The CF titer results parallel the severity of the infection (10); titers rise as the disease progresses and decline as the patient improves.

Qualitative data similar to those obtained in the TP and CF tests may be obtained from the screening LPA and ID procedures, respectively.

Test 1. TP test.

The TP test is performed with two dilutions of coccidioidin and constant amounts of serum (10). The antigen dilutions are used to obviate the possible occurrence of a false-negative result due to inhibition of the precipitin reaction by excess antigen.

Reagents and equipment

1. Undiluted serum containing Merthiolate diluted 1:10,000

2. *C. immitis* precipitinogen (coccidioidin), undiluted and diluted 1:10. A final concentration of 1:10,000 Merthiolate is added as a preservative.

3. Saline buffered at pH 7.0 with 0.067 M phosphate buffer for use as diluent and control containing Merthiolate at a concentration of 1:10,000

4. Culture tubes, 7 by 70 to 75 mm

Procedure

1. Add 0.2 ml of test serum to each of three tubes.

2. Add 0.2 ml of undiluted antigen to the serum in tube 1, and add 0.2 ml of a 1:10 antigen dilution to the serum in tube 2.

3. Add 0.2 ml of control saline to the test specimen in tube 3.

4. Mix thoroughly.

5. Incubate at 37°C and read daily for 5 days by sharply flicking the bottom of the tube while holding the tube between thumb and forefinger.

6. A button or a flake of precipitate in either of the first two tubes is a positive test. The TP test may be applied to sera and pleural fluids.

Reagents. The antigens for both the TP and CF tests are filtrates of mycelial cultures of multiple or single isolates of *C. immitis*. Coccidioidin is prepared by a variety of procedures. In the most widely known procedure, filtrates are produced from cultures grown in a synthetic asparagine-glycerol-salts medium originally devised for tuberculin production. Preparing coccidioidin in this medium usually requires incubation for several weeks at room temperature. Coccidioidin antigens can be prepared within 1 week by a toluene lysis technique (10).

Heating coccidioidin at 60°C for 30 min destroys the F antigen responsible for the CF activity, but the precipitinogen associated with the TP reaction is retained (10).

The LPA test uses latex particles sensitized with coccidioidin heated at 60°C for 30 min. LPA kits may be obtained from Meridian. The LPA test should not be applied to CSF or to diluted sera, because false-positive reactions are likely. It is not known whether such difficulties would occur with pleural, joint, or ascitic fluids (10).

Interpretation. Early coccidioidomycosis is usually detected by the TP, IDTP, and LPA tests. A positive TP test, indicated by the appearance of a precipitated button or flake in any dilution, is considered diagnostic. In about 80% of all infections, the TP test becomes positive within 2 weeks of the onset of symptoms. It is diagnostic but not prognostic. Precipitins are infrequently detected 6 months after infection.

The IDTP test is more sensitive than the TP test but less sensitive than the LPA test. The LPA test, however, is not as specific as the IDTP and TP tests; approximately 6 to 10% false-positive reactions may occur with the LPA test. The LPA test, however, may become positive before the TP test. A positive LPA reaction must be confirmed by a TP or CF test. The LPA results can be obtained in 4 min (10).

Test 2. CF test.

The standardized LBCF test with coccidioidin is recommended for the titration of sera from patients with suspected coccidioidomycosis. Details for performing the test have been previously published (19). In addition, the blastomycosis tests are described above. The microadaptation of the CF test for coccidioidomycosis gives results comparable to those of the macrotest (10). The CF tests may be performed on serum, CSF, plasma, and pleural and joint fluids.

Coccidioidin is prepared as described above for the TP test. Since the CF antigen is destroyed by heating at 60°C for 30 min, this antigen should not be heated. The CF antigen may be purchased from Immuno-Mycologics, M. A. Bioproducts, or Meridian.

The qualitative ID test with unheated coccidioidin yields results which compare with those obtained with the CF test. Concentration of sera before testing by ID and CF tests can be useful in detecting chronic-case specimens which might ordinarily be missed in such tests (20). Recent studies suggest that titers similar to those obtained in CF tests may also be obtained in quantitative tests (28).

Spherulin, an extract of in vivo-produced spherules of *C. immitis*, appears to be as sensitive as coccidioidin in the CF test, but less specific (10).

Interpretation. Any CF titer with coccidioidin should be considered presumptive evidence for *C. immitis* infection. The ID test with a filtrate antigen (10) gives results that correlate with those observed with the CF test. The ID test with reference reagents is highly specific. Titers of 1:2 and 1:4 in the CF test usually indicate early, residual, or meningeal coccidioidomycosis. However, sera demonstrating such titers have also been obtained from patients not known to have coccidioidomycosis. The parallel use of CF and ID tests is an effective means of specifically diagnosing coccidioidomycosis in patients with low levels of complement-fixing antibodies. Studies indicate that sera positive in the CF test in the 1:2 to 1:8 range and also positive in the ID test reflect active or recent *C. immitis* infections (10). Obviously, when low titers are obtained, a diagnosis of coccidioidomycosis must be based on subsequent serologic tests and preferably on clinical and mycologic studies. Generally, CF titers greater than 1:16 indicate disseminating disease. Negative serologic test results do not exclude a diagnosis of coccidioidomycosis. About 5% of all CSF specimens from patients with coccidioidal meningitis are negative in the CF test, and serum samples from many patients with chronic cavitary coccidioidomycosis are negative.

The coccidioidin skin test is considered a valuable screen for serologic testing. Conversion from a negative to a positive skin test reaction is pathognomic and is usually the earliest immunologic response to infection. Studies have indicated that there is a strong positive correlation in patients with primary coccidioidomycosis (without impending or concomitant disseminating disease) between serologic positivity and a positive coccidioidin skin test. Unlike the serologic reactions sometimes noted after the histoplasmin skin test, coccidioidin and spherulin skin tests do not elicit an antibody response to coccidioidin in previously sensitized persons (10).

Cryptococcosis

Conventional methodology for the diagnosis of cryptococcosis is time consuming and, in many cases, inadequate. Until recently, persons suffering from cryptococcosis were considered essentially immunologically inert. Previous immunologic tests had only limited applications (10), and even then results were difficult to interpret. During the last 2 decades, work on serologic procedures for cryptococcosis has resulted in the development of diagnostically and prognostically useful tests. These procedures are an indirect fluorescent-antibody (IFA) technique, an EIA, and a tube agglutination (TA) test for cryptococcal antibodies and a LA test and an EIA for cryptococcal antigen (10, 11). The antibody tests are of value in detecting early or localized cryptococcosis and in determining a prognosis. They are, however, less specific than the LA test. More recently, an EIA with *Cryptococcus neoformans* galactoxylomannan antigen was evaluated for its ability to detect IgM antibody. Such antibodies were found in approximately 22% of 55 cryptococcosis patients examined (21). Cross-reactions similar to those noted with IgG antibodies with IFA, although markedly reduced, were still evident.

The EIA has the potential of detecting cryptococcal antigen earlier and at lower concentrations than LA. It is also not subject to prozone reactions. Preliminary EIA tests for cryptococcal antigens detected 6 ng of the major viscous capsular polysaccharide per ml in contrast to 35 ng/ml detectable by LA. The test, however, requires a few hours to perform, in contrast to the few minutes needed for the simple LA test (11). Because the LA test is very specific, has both diagnostic and prognostic value, is simple to perform, and is widely used, this procedure is herein described in detail.

Clinical indications

Serologic tests for *C. neoformans* antigens or antibodies or both should be considered with patients who have symptoms of pulmonary or meningeal infection. Cutaneous, skeletal, and visceral involvement occurs as the result of dissemination. The disease may be primary, but many cases are associated with various debilitating diseases, such as Hodgkin's disease, acquired immunodeficiency syndrome (AIDS), leukemia, or diabetes.

It is interesting to note that the CDC AIDS Task Force has demonstrated 5,091 cases of AIDS as of July 1984. Of these cases, 333 (6.5%) demonstrated complications from cryptococcal infection, mainly of the meningeal form (Richard Selik, personal communication).

The IFA and TA antibody tests are reactive with about 50% of the sera from patients with active cases of extrameningeal cryptococcosis. The IFA test has a specificity of about 77%, whereas the TA test has a specificity of about 89% (10). Although the IFA test is not entirely specific, it is valuable in diagnosing those cases of cryptococcosis that are negative for *C. neoformans* agglutinins and antigens. The TA test for cryptococcal antibodies has been found to be diagnostically reliable. Agglutinins were detected in the early stages of central nervous system infection and in infections with no central nervous system involvement (10).

The LA test has been successfully used for the specific detection of cryptococcal antigen in sera and CSF from persons with proven cryptococcosis. The test is valuable in diagnosing active nonmeningeal and meningeal cryptococcosis, particularly the latter. Of 330 patients recently studied with proven meningeal cryptococcosis, 328 (99%) had CSF positive for cryptococcal antigen by the LA test (10). The test is also more sensitive in diagnosing cryptococcal meningitis than the India ink preparation, which has a sensitivity of <50%, for detecting *C. neoformans* yeast cells in the CSF (11).

LA titers of 1:8 or greater are considered strong evidence of active infection. Titers of 1:4 or less, although diagnostic in many instances, have been demonstrated in sera and CSF specimens of symptomatic patients without corroborating culture or histologic evidence of cryptococcosis (10). False-positive serum reactions are uncommon and occur mainly with sera from some patients with severe rheumatoid arthritis. These specimens may be recognized by their reactivity with latex sensitized with normal globulins or by their inactivation after treatment with 0.003 M dithiothreitol (10). Nonspecific agglutination has also been noted in CSF (10) and sera from patients without rheumatoid arthritis. False-positives due to rheumatoid factor or other interfering proteins in sera may be eliminated by boiling the specimens with disodium EDTA (11) or by treating the specimens with a final concentration of 5 mg of pronase per ml (25).

Cryptococcosis is best diagnosed serologically through the concurrent use of three tests, i.e., the LA test for antigen and the IFA and TA tests for *C. neoformans* antibodies (10).

Test 1. LA test for cryptococcal antigen

Equipment and reagents

1. GBS–0.1% BSA, pH 8.4
2. Polystyrene latex particle suspension, 0.81-μm-diameter polystyrene spheres (Difco and Dow)
3. Latex particles optimally sensitized with rabbit anti-*C. neoformans* globulin (LI)
4. Latex sensitized with rabbit normal (preimmune) globulin (LN)
5. Sera
   a. Reference serum positive for human cryptococcosis, with a known antigen titer (expressed as the highest dilution demonstrating 2+ agglutination)
   b. Negative control human serum
   c. Human serum positive for rheumatoid factor (negative for *C. neoformans* antigen)
   d. Patient's serum, CSF, or urine specimen
6. Water bath, 56°C
7. Rotary shaker
8. Glass slides, 50 by 75 mm (marked with 12 circles, each 1.5 cm in diameter)
9. Microtitration droppers or microliter pipettes, 0.025 and 0.05 ml

Procedure

1. Inactivate the sera and CSF specimens at 56°C for 30 min. Urine specimens should be inactivated by heating them in a boiling-water bath for 10 min. CSF specimens may be similarly treated, if necessary, and then retested.
2. Place positive and negative control sera and the patient's specimen in a test tube rack in the order to be tested.
3. Add a 0.025-ml drop of LI reagent to each of the circles on a slide.
4. Add 0.05-ml drops of positive and negative control sera and up to 10 patients' undiluted specimens to the drops of the LI reagent in separate circles. Mix the drops.
5. Place the slide on a rotary shaker, and rotate it at 125 ± 25 rpm for 5 min.
6. Read the test immediately for macroscopic agglutination by visual inspection over a dark background. The positive control must show 2+ agglutination (small but definite clumps with a slightly cloudy background); the negative control must show no agglutination. Check the reactions of the patient's specimens and record as positive all those showing agglutinations equal to or greater than the 2+ positive control serum.
7. Test all serum and CSF specimens that are positive in the screening test with the LN control reagent to rule out false-positive reactions due to rheumatoid factor or other interfering proteins. Include the rheumatoid factor-positive serum as a control.
8. Serially dilute all specimens positive with LI reagent and negative with LN reagent to make 1:2, 1:4, and 1:8 dilutions, etc. Prepare dilutions in GBS-BSA. Titer until the 2+ endpoint is attained.
9. Record the titer of each specimen as the highest dilution that gives a 2+ agglutination.
10. Consider as equivocal the results of tests in which sera react with both the LI and LN reagents. Then proceed to treat the specimen to eliminate any interfering protein, and retest for the presence of antigen.

Controls. A positive control serum showing 2+ agglutination (small but definite clumps with a slightly cloudy background) and a negative control serum must be included each time the test is performed. Rheumatoid factor in a patient's serum may interfere with the test. To avoid false-positive results due to rheumatoid factor or other interfering proteins, sera positive with the LI reagent should always be tested with the LN reagent.

Reagents. A properly standardized suspension of latex particles, with an absorbance of 0.30 ± 0.02 when diluted 1:100, is sensitized with an optimal dilution of 4% rabbit anti-*C. neoformans* globulins. Similarly, such a standardized suspension is sensitized with a dilution (same as for LI) of preimmune 4% rabbit globulin obtained from the rabbit(s) later used to produce the LI.

Kits for detecting *C. neoformans* antigen in clinical specimens are available from American Scientific Products, McGaw Park, Ill., M. A. Bioproducts, Meridian, and Wampole Laboratories, Inc., Cranbury, N.J.

Interpretation. The LA test for *C. neoformans* antigens has both diagnostic and prognostic value. A positive reaction in serum or CSF of an untreated patient at titers of 1:4 or less is highly suggestive of cryptococcal infection. LA titers of 1:8 or greater usually indicate active cryptococcosis. The antigen titer is usually proportional to the extent of infection, with increasing titers reflecting progressive infection and a poor prognosis indicating response to chemotherapy and progressive recovery. Failure of the titer to fall during therapy suggests inadequate treatment (10).

LA tests in which sera react with both LI and LN reagents should be considered equivocal. Since cryptococcosis and arthritic conditions may occur concomitantly, tests with both LI and LN reagents should be performed. A fourfold or greater titer with the LI reagent suggests cryptococcosis, but additional specimens taken subsequently should be examined for titer change.

The controlled LA test appears to be highly specific. Some researchers, however, have reported occasional false-positive reactions at low dilutions, particularly in CSF (10). A negative reaction should not exclude a diagnosis of cryptococcosis, especially when only one specimen has been tested and the patient shows symptoms consistent with those of cryptococcosis. False-negative reactions are uncommon. The few that have occurred were associated with a prozone occurring in specimens demonstrating high antigen titers, specimens from patients infected with nonencapsulated or dry variants of *C. neoformans*, and specimens obtained in the very early stages of infection. Weakly reactive undiluted sera (±, +) should be checked for prozone reactivity by testing higher dilutions of sera. Specimens may also be negative due to immune complex formation. Dissociation of such complexes with pronase will free antigen so that it can be detected by antibody-coated latex particles (Glenn Roberts, personal communication).

Test 2. IFA test for *C. neoformans* antibody

Heat-killed *C. neoformans* serotype A cells are heat fixed to a slide and covered with a 1:16 dilution of the heat-inactivated serum. After incubation, the preparation is washed, air dried, and treated with anti-human immunoglobulin conjugated to fluorescein isothiocyanate. A positive reaction is indicated by the cells staining to an intensity of 2+ or greater.

Test 3. TA test for *C. neoformans* antibody

Formalin-killed whole yeast cells heated at 56°C for 30 min are used in the agglutination test (10). The cells are adjusted to a concentration of 7.5×10^6 cells per ml, and 0.25-ml volumes of serial twofold dilutions of serum (inactivated at 56°C for 30 min) are mixed with equal volumes of yeast cells. The mixtures are placed on a rotary shaker for 2 min, incubated at 37°C for 2 h, and then refrigerated at 4°C for 72 h, during which time readings are taken at 24-h intervals. The serum titer is the highest dilution that shows any degree of agglutination. The antibody tests are performed only on serum. Positive and negative controls must always be included in each run.

Reagents for the antibody test are not commercially available.

Interpretation. A positive antibody test suggests infection by *C. neoformans* and could also reflect a past infection or a cross-reaction. Antibodies may be detected in the early course of the disease and in localized infections. As the disease progresses, abundant antigens may be produced and detected with concurrent exclusion of antibody. The antibody test may have prognostic value. With effective chemotherapy, the antigen titer declines, and antibody may become demonstrable by one or both tests.

Histoplasmosis

Serologic evidence is often the prime factor responsible for a definitive diagnosis of histoplasmosis. Such evidence can be obtained through CF, ID, and LA tests, used singly or in some combination. Of these procedures, the most widely used is the CF test. Properly performed, either as a tube or a microtitration procedure (10), the CF test can yield information of diagnostic and prognostic value. Over 90% of the culturally proven cases of histoplasmosis may be positive by the CF test if the patient's illness is monitored by testing sera collected at 2- to 3-week intervals (10). Unfortunately, CF tests are relatively complex and expensive and should be performed only by highly trained personnel.

Clinical indications

Serologic tests for histoplasmosis should be applied to clinical specimens (serum, plasma, peritoneal fluid, or CSF) from patients with respiratory illness, hepatosplenomegaly, signs of extrapulmonary systemic infection, or meningeal involvement. The patient's history of residence, travel, and occupation may also be used as a guide for applying these tests. The CF test is very sensitive; however, with currently available antigens, the test is not entirely specific. Cross-reactions may occur with sera from patients with blastomycosis, coccidioidomycosis, and other fungal infections. Sera from patients with leishmaniasis may cross-react in the CF test when *H. capsulatum* yeast forms

are used as the antigen. In addition, positive reactions cannot be obtained with anticomplementary specimens. The histoplasmosis ID and CF tests, with histoplasmin as antigen, will react with about 85% of histoplasmosis sera. The CF test with yeast-form antigen has greater sensitivity (10). This test with the yeast-form antigen should be used in the diagnostic laboratory, and where possible, it should be supplemented with either the ID or CIE test with histoplasmin (10). There is a greater than 90% agreement between results obtained with the ID and CIE tests. The latter tests are very useful for examining anticomplementary sera. Because of their greater specificity, they provide a more accurate diagnosis with those sera that cross-react in CF tests.

The histoplasmin LA test is satisfactory for detecting acute primary infections, but may be negative with sera from persons with chronic histoplasmosis (10). It is particularly valuable in detecting early disease. Because of the transitory nature of these agglutinins, the LA test cannot be considered a replacement for the CF test, especially with the intact yeast-form antigens.

Test 1. CF test

The standardized LBCF test with *H. capsulatum* yeast-form cells and histoplasmin antigens is recommended for titrating sera from persons with suspected cases of histoplasmosis. Details for performing the test have been previously published (19). In addition, see above under CF test procedure for blastomycosis. The microadaptation of the CF test for histoplasmosis gives results comparable to those of the macrotest (10).

Reagents. Two antigens are used in the CDC LBCF test. One antigen is a suspension of Merthiolate-treated, intact, yeast-form cells of *H. capsulatum*, and the other is a soluble mycelial-form filtrate antigen, histoplasmin, harvested after growth of the fungus for approximately 6 months in Smith asparagine medium (10). The optimal dilution for each antigen is determined by a block titration with low- and high-titered positive human sera. These antigens may be purchased from American Scientific Products, Immuno-Mycologics, M. A. Bioproducts, and Meridian.

Interpretation. CF tests are valuable in the diagnosis of acute, chronic, disseminated, and meningeal histoplasmosis. Antibodies in primary pulmonary infections are generally demonstrable within 4 weeks after exposure to the fungus or frequently by the time symptoms appear. These antibodies are usually antibodies to the yeast form of *H. capsulatum*. Antibodies to histoplasmin usually develop later in primary pulmonary cases, but titers are considerably lower than those with the yeast-form antigen. Histoplasmin titers are usually higher in sera from chronic cases. CF test results can be difficult to interpret, because cross-reactions or nonspecific reactions with the yeast-form or histoplasmin antigens are often encountered. In such instances, titers usually range between 1:8 and 1:32 and occur mainly with the yeast-form antigen. Many serum samples from culturally proven cases of histoplasmosis, however, give titers in the same range. Consequently, titers of 1:8 and greater with either antigen are generally considered presumptive evidence of histoplasmosis. Titers above 1:32 or rising titers offer strong presumptive evidence of histoplasmosis. The probability of infection increases in proportion to the increase in CF titer.

Nonetheless, one cannot rely solely on CF titers above 1:32 as a means of diagnosis, since false-positive reactions of that magnitude may occur in patients with other diseases. Titer changes are often of great assistance in diagnosing histoplasmosis. Fourfold changes in titer in either direction are significant indicators of disease progression or regression. However, cultural, clinical, and other laboratory data should also be considered in determining the patients' prognosis or in deciding whether or not to treat. Occasionally, in some patients, positive titers that slowly decline are noted for a long time after the patient has been cured. Reactions with heterologous antigens may complicate the interpretation of a result when only serum sample has been tested. For example, in some situations, the first serologic response noted in a person suffering from histoplasmosis may be obtained only with the nonpurified *B. dermatitidis* antigen. Some patients with histoplasmosis responses may even show antibody to the antigens of *H. capsulatum*, *B. dermatitidis*, and *C. immitis*, to only some of them, or to none. Furthermore, a lack of immunologic response does not exclude histoplasmosis, particularly when only one specimen has been tested and when the clinical picture strongly suggests pulmonary mycotic disease. In disseminated or terminal histoplasmosis, humoral antibody responses may or may not be positive. The CF test is usually positive with CSF specimens from cases of chronic meningitis. CF titers may range from 1:8 to 1:128 (11).

Attempts to replace the CF test with a primary binding assay, such as an EIA, have been frustrated by the presence of a galactomannan present even in column-purified M antigen that cross-reacts with *B. dermatitidis*, *C. immitis*, and *Paracoccidioides brasiliensis*. Recently Brock et al. (2) showed how specificity could be increased in the EIA to detect antibodies against the M antigen of histoplasmin. Column-purified M antigen was subjected to periodate oxidation, which inactivated the contaminating polysaccharide. The EIA was further modified by using a competitive binding format with enzyme-labeled rabbit anti-M IgG as the indicator antibody.

As indicated above, the test antigens may cross-react in cases of blastomycosis, coccidioidomycosis, other fungal diseases, and leishmaniasis. If cross-reactions are observed or suspected, the laboratorian should base the interpretation of results on a study of serial specimens in CF and ID tests used in combination, the clinical picture, and other laboratory tests.

Test 2. ID and CIE tests

ID test. The micro-ID procedure is recommended for detecting *H. capsulatum* precipitins against the H and M protein antigens of histoplasmin. Diagnostic precipitins can frequently be detected in CSF specimens from patients with meningeal histoplasmosis before isolates of *H. capsulatum* are obtained and when culture attempts are negative. The ID procedure used is the same as that described for blastomycosis, except that antigen and unknown and control sera

with H and M precipitins are added immediately. The reactants are then allowed to diffuse while the gel is incubating in a moist chamber for 24 h at 25°C.

CIE test. The histoplasmosis CIE procedure (10) is performed as follows. A 10-ml volume of an equal mixture of 0.85% agarose and 0.85% Ionagar no. 2 dissolved in 0.01 M Veronal buffer (pH 7.2) is applied to a 3.25- by 4-in. (8.2- by 10.2-cm) projector slide cover glass, and 5-mm wells are cut into the agar. Each antigen well is 3 mm from each of two serum wells. Sera are placed in the anodic wells of each pair, and histoplasmin is placed in the cathodic wells. A control serum containing H and M antibodies is placed in the well adjacent to the serum to be tested. Electrophoresis is performed at room temperature with 0.05 M Veronal buffer, pH 7.2, in each chamber. A constant current of 25 mA is applied across the narrow dimension of the slide for 90 min. After electrophoresis, the slides are removed and read for lines of identity. ID and CIE test results are valid only when control reference sera showing H and M bands are positive.

Reagents. Histoplasmin is made as described for the CF test. The mycelial-form filtrate antigen is concentrated 5 to 10 times and titrated to determine the optimal dilution that demonstrates well-defined H and M bands when the antigen is allowed to react with serum from a case of proven human histoplasmosis. Control antisera containing H and M precipitins may be prepared in animals by using precipitin arcs as vaccines (10). Histoplasmosis ID reagents or kits may be purchased from American Scientific Products, Immuno-Mycologics, M. A. Bioproducts, Meridian, and Nolan-Scott.

Interpretation. The ID or CIE test is a useful screening procedure or adjunct in the serologic diagnosis of histoplasmosis. The results usually obtained are qualitative. The ID test was first applied to the diagnosis of histoplasmosis in 1958 by Heiner (10). He demonstrated six precipitin bands when concentrated histoplasmin antigen interacted with serum from patients with histoplasmosis. Two of these bands had diagnostic value. One band, designated H, was found in the serum of patients with active histoplasmosis. The second band, designated M, was found in acute and chronic histoplasmosis and also appeared after normal sensitized persons had been skin tested with histoplasmin. Although the H band is usually associated with the M band, the M band frequently is the first to appear and frequently occurs without the H band. The M band has been considered presumptive evidence of infection with *H. capsulatum*. Finding only M antibodies in sera may be attributed to active disease, inactive disease, or skin testing (10).

The sera of about 70% of patients with proven histoplasmosis contain M precipitins, whereas only 10% demonstrate both the H and M precipitins. Detection of the H precipitin is increased by CIE.

To interpret the ID and CIE reactions properly, laboratory workers must know whether the patient whose serum sample is being analyzed was recently given a skin test. If the patient has not had a recent histoplasmin skin test, detection of an M band may serve as an indicator of early disease, since antibody to M appears before the H precipitin and disappears more slowly. The demonstration of both the M and H bands is highly suggestive of active histoplasmosis, regardless of other serologic results. An additional precipitin, Y, has been reported to indicate acute histoplasmosis, particularly when the patient's serum sample is devoid of M and H precipitins (10). Detection of M and H precipitins in CSF specimens indicates meningeal histoplasmosis (11).

Test 3. LA test

The LA test is useful for the early detection of acute histoplasmosis. Commercially prepared antigen in the form of histoplasmin-sensitized latex particles is available from Spectrum Diagnostics, Inc., Glenwood, Ill. When the test is performed, serial twofold dilutions of serum samples ranging from 1:4 to 1:512 are prepared in tubes, and optimally diluted antigen is added. The centrifuged reactants are then examined for strong agglutination (10).

Interpretation. The LA test yields results in 24 h and may even be used with anticomplementary sera. Although the test may be negative with sera from persons with chronic histoplasmosis, it is an excellent aid in the diagnosis of acute histoplasmosis (10).

Some workers consider an LA titer of 1:16 or greater to be significant, whereas other workers consider titers of 1:32 or greater strong evidence for active or very recent disease. Although a positive LA test can be demonstrated as early as 2 to 3 weeks after exposure to infection by *H. capsulatum* (10), such a reaction should be confirmed by an ID test or other laboratory data. False-positives can occur with the LA test, and results should be interpreted with caution, particularly if only one specimen has been examined and the titer is low.

Caution. Levels of complement-fixing antibodies, precipitins, and agglutinins to *H. capsulatum* antigens may be significantly increased in histoplasmin-sensitized persons after one histoplasmin skin test (10). This fact makes subsequent changes in serologic titers uninterpretable. For this reason, patients with suspected active histoplasmosis should not be skin tested. In the CF test, these antibody responses were detected in sera drawn 15 days after skin testing. Blood should be drawn for serologic studies before skin testing, but, obviously, the specimen can be taken within 2 to 3 days after the skin test, since antibodies do not develop that soon. Furthermore, it is the serum reaction with the histoplasmin antigen that is affected, although effects on the yeast titer have also been reported (10). One histoplasmin skin test does not produce a serologic response in unsensitized persons.

Actinomycotic HP

The ID test is widely used for screening or confirming a diagnosis of hypersensitivity pneumonitis (HP) or extrinsic allergic alveolitis resulting from sensitization to a thermophilic actinomycete. The CIE test, although more rapid and sensitive than the ID test, is not as specific or reproducible (10).

This section will be devoted to farmer's lung, but when the appropriate antigens are used (10), the tests described can also be applied to the diagnosis of other hypersensitivity diseases, such as bagassosis, mushroom worker's lung, and bird breeder's lung. Since the eliciting antigen is usually not known at the time of initial testing, it is a common practice to screen patients' sera with a battery of antigens including those from *Aspergillus* spp., *Aureobasidium pullulans*, and avian proteins as well as antigens from thermophilic actinomycetes.

Clinical indications

The demonstration of precipitating antibodies to antigens derived from thermophilic actinomycetes or other offending antigens is an important aid in establishing the diagnosis of farmer's lung and related HPs. The ID tests should be performed on patients who show respiratory disease that appears to be environmentally related, i.e., to occupation (farmer's lung), hobby (pigeon breeder's disease), or home or office (forced-air-system disease). The typical symptoms of these diseases are chills, fever, cough, and dyspnea, usually occurring 4 to 6 h after exposure to the antigen. Patients usually demonstrate crepitant rales in the lower lung fields. Chest X rays may show infiltrates with a pattern indistinguishable from patterns of other interstitial pneumonias. The demonstration of precipitating antibodies in the sera of patients with suspected HP is frequently used to determine the etiologic agent of the disease and to confirm the tentative diagnosis (10). Immediate hypersensitivity associated with elevated levels of IgE does not appear to play a role in HP. Quantitative IgE tests carried out at the same time as the ID tests would be expected to yield normal values in patients with HP.

Test

The ID test with antigens from *Faenia rectivirgula (Micropolyspora faeni), Thermoactinomyces candidus,* and *Thermoactinomyces vulgaris* and reference homologous rabbit antiserum is used to detect precipitating antibodies in the sera of patients with clinical and radiological evidence of farmer's lung. Many types of ID tests can be used, but the test performed at CDC is the same as that used for aspergillosis.

Reagents

Suitable *T. candidus, Thermoactinomyces sacchari, Saccharomonospora viridis,* and *T. vulgaris* antigens may be prepared in Trypticase soy broth (10). *F. rectivirgula* antigen can be prepared in an AOAC (Difco) synthetic broth containing 1.0% lactose (14).

HP test reagents may be obtained from Greer Laboratories or from Hollister-Stier.

Interpretation

The demonstration of precipitins to a particular antigen in a patient's serum is highly suggestive of a diagnosis of HP. The presence of precipitins per se is not diagnostic, since some healthy persons have precipitins. A proper diagnosis of hypersensitivity lung disease in a precipitin-positive patient must also be based on proper clinical, radiologic, and preferably biopsy or inhalation data. Precipitins provide information about the lung disease and the type of sensitizing antigen. A negative result does not rule out a diagnosis of HP (10).

Paracoccidioidomycosis

CF, ID, and CIE tests are useful in the diagnosis of paracoccidioidomycosis and in monitoring treatment response (10).

Clinical indications

Serologic tests for paracoccidioidomycosis should be performed on patients displaying symptoms of chronic disease with lung involvement or ulcerative lesions of the mucosa (oral, nasal, and intestinal) and the skin. In addition, patients with paracoccidioidomycosis often have lymphadenopathy. A history of travel or residence in Latin America also suggests the possibility of paracoccidioidomycosis.

The CF test will detect antibodies in 80 to 96% of patients with paracoccidioidomycosis (10). Complement-fixing antibodies are diagnostic. However, the CF test results with pooled filtrate antigens of the yeast form of *P. brasiliensis* are not always specific, and cross-reactions may be obtained with sera from patients with other diseases. These cross-reactions, however, are infrequent and occur mainly at the 1:8 level. The ID test (10), with concentrated yeast-form filtrate antigens, has a sensitivity of 94% with sera from patients with paracoccidioidomycosis. A 79% correlation was reported between the ID test results and the CF test results. The ID test used with reference sera is entirely specific (10). An initial serodiagnosis of paracoccidioidomycosis can be obtained in over 98% of cases with the use of both the ID and CF tests (10). Specific *P. brasiliensis* antigen may also be prepared from the mycelial form of the fungus grown in Sabhi broth with inocula derived from potato-glucose agar slants. This antigen in ID tests detected 103 (90%) of 114 proven cases of paracoccidioidomycosis, but did not appear to be suitable for use in CF tests (1).

Test. CF test

The standardized LBCF test with *P. brasiliensis* yeast-form filtrate antigens is recommended for titrating sera from suspected cases of paracoccidioidomycosis. Details for performing the test have been previously published (19). In addition, see the CF test described above under blastomycosis.

Reagents. Paracoccidioidin antigens for CF and ID tests are produced from yeast-form shake cultures of three CDC stock cultures of *P. brasiliensis* (B339, B341, and B1183) grown singly at 35°C in a Trypticase soy broth dialysate medium supplemented with glucose, ammonium sulfate, and vitamins (10). The 4-week culture filtrates of each isolate are dialyzed, concentrated 10 times, and mixed in equal volumes. The optimal dilution for each antigen pool is determined by titration with low- and high-titered CF-positive sera from human paracoccidioidomycosis cases or, in ID tests, with precipitin-positive sera. These antigens are not commercially available, but reference antigen can be obtained from CDC.

Interpretation. CF titers of 1:8 or greater are considered presumptive evidence of paracoccidioidomycosis. Titers may range from 1:8 to 1:16,384 depending on the severity and extent of infection. Serum samples from 85 to 95% of patients with active disease demonstrate CF titers of 1:32 or greater (10). Low CF titers are usually associated with localized disease or patients having reticuloendothelial involvement, whereas high CF titers are found in patients with pulmonary lesions or disseminating disease. Young children with disseminated paracoccidioidomycosis are an exception and ordinarily show low or negative CF reactions. Serial CF determinations are of prognostic value. Declines in titer generally indicate effective therapy, whereas clinical relapses are accompanied by increases in humoral antibodies. High and fluctuating titers suggest a poor prognosis. Complement-fixing antibodies at low levels may persist long after the patient is cured.

When examined in ID tests with paracoccidioidin, the sera of patients with paracoccidioidomycosis may contain one to three precipitins to *P. brasiliensis*. The ID test is excellent for the diagnosis of progressive pulmonary and disseminated paracoccidioidomycosis (17). Band 1 is found close to the antigen well, and band 3 is found near the serum well. Precipitin to antigen 1, the antibody most frequently encountered, is found in 95 to 98% of the seroactive cases of paracoccidioidomycosis (10). ID and CF tests for paracoccidioidomycosis are available at CDC.

A diagnostic precipitin that reacts with a specific soluble antigen, designated E, which demonstrates cationic electrophoretic mobility, has been consistently found in the sera of patients with paracoccidioidomycosis. The E arc appears to be identical to band 1 (10). High-titer antigen, equivalent to E and 1, may be produced in commercially prepared media in 2 weeks or less (1). The highest number of precipitin bands is usually found with sera from patients with lung involvement or disseminated disease. Precipitating antibodies, like those that react in the CF test, are long lasting. At least one of the three precipitins that might occur in blood could, however, disappear after successful treatment (10).

Sporotrichosis

Serologic tests can be used in establishing a diagnosis of sporotrichosis. These tests are especially helpful in diagnosing the extracutaneous or systemic form of sporotrichosis when distinct clinical features are lacking. Two tests, the TA and LA tests, are reliable and sensitive. The antigen that is the basis for the agglutinin test is the peptido-L-rhamno-D-mannan that is the outer layer of the cell wall. Comparable sensitivity is not obtained with the CF and ID tests with *Sporothrix schenckii* antigens. The slide LA and TA test are preferred because they are both highly sensitive and specific. The LA tests provides results in minutes, but the TA test must be incubated overnight (9). Both tests are performed at CDC.

Clinical indications

Serologic tests for sporotrichosis may be applied to sera from patients with skin lesions, subcutaneous nodules, bone lesions, lymphadenopathy, or pulmonary disease and to CSF from patients with undiagnosed chronic meningitis. The disease should be suspected in patients who handle thorny plants, timber, or sphagnum moss.

Because of its sensitivity (94%), high specificity, and ability to provide results in 5 min, the LA test is highly recommended for routine use in the clinical laboratory. The TA test has a comparable sensitivity, but sera being tested for sporotrichosis may show false-positive reactions with 1:8 and 1:16 dilutions of sera from patients with leishmaniasis (10).

Test. LA test for *S. schenckii* antibody

Equipment and reagents
1. GBS (pH 8.4)–0.1% BSA
2. Spectrophotometrically standardized suspension of 0.81-μm-diameter polystyrene latex particles sensitized with an optimal dilution of *S. schenckii* (yeast-form) culture filtrate antigen
3. Sera
   a. Positive reference human anti-*S. schenckii* serum with known titer
   b. Negative control human serum
   c. Patients' sera
4. Water bath, 56°C
5. Rotary shaker
6. Test tubes, 12 by 75 mm
7. Glass slides, 50 by 75 mm
8. Serologic pipettes, 0.1, 0.5, and 1.0 ml

Procedure
1. Inactivate all sera at 56°C for 30 min.
2. Prepare enough 50- by 75-mm slides (12 circles per slide) to accommodate the specimens to be tested. Ten sera plus negative and positive control specimens can be screened on each slide.
3. Place positive and negative control sera and patients' sera in a test tube rack in the order to be tested. These specimens should be diluted with GBS-BSA.
4. With a 0.1-ml pipette, add 0.02 ml of the optimally sensitized latex suspension to each of the circles on a slide.
5. With separate 0.1-ml pipettes, add 0.04 ml of each 1:4 dilution of the patients' sera and the positive and the negative controls to the circles on the slide. Mix the drops with applicator sticks.
6. Place the slide on a rotating shaker, and rotate at 150 rpm for 5 min.
7. Immediately read the test macroscopically over a dark background for agglutination. The positive control serum must show 2+ agglutination (small but definite clumps with a slightly cloudy background); the negative control must show no agglutination. Check the reactions of patients' sera, and record as positive all specimens showing agglutination equal to or greater than the 2+ positive reference serum.
8. All specimens positive in the screening test should be diluted serially with GBS-BSA to make 1:8, 1:16, 1:32, and 1:64 dilutions of each serum for titration.
9. The test is performed as described in steps 2 to 7. One slide will accommodate the four dilutions of each of two serum samples plus the positive and negative control serum samples.

10. Record as positive all dilutions that show agglutination equal to or greater than the 2+ positive reference serum.

If the reaction of a 1:64 dilution is greater than 2+, the specimen must be diluted through four more serial dilutions (1:128 to 1:1,024), and the testing procedure must be repeated until an endpoint is reached. The titer of each specimen is the highest serum dilution that gives a 2+ agglutination.

Controls. Positive and negative control sera must be included each time the test is performed.

Reagents. A properly standardized suspension of latex particles with an absorbance of 0.30 ± 0.02 when diluted 1:100 is sensitized with an equal volume of an optimal dilution of yeast-form *S. schenckii* culture filtrate antigens. The optimal quantity of filtrate is the highest dilution that produces a clear 2+ agglutination with the highest reactive dilution of rabbit *S. schenckii* reference antiserum or serum from a human sporotrichosis case (19). *S. schenckii* antibody test reagents are not commercially available.

Interpretation. Slide LA titers of 1:4 or greater are considered presumptive evidence of sporotrichosis. False-positive reactions have, however, been noted in the 1:4 to 1:8 range with sera from patients with nonfungal infections. Sera from patients with localized cutaneous, subcutaneous, disseminated subcutaneous, or systemic sporotrichosis may show titers ranging from 1:4 to 1:128. An increasing titer or sustained high titer is helpful in the diagnosis of pulmonary sporotrichosis. The test has limited prognostic value, since antibody levels may show little change during and after convalescence. Slide LA titers of 1:32 or greater with CSF are considered evidence of meningeal sporotrichosis (11).

Zygomycosis

An ID test in which homogenate antigens of *Absidia corymbifera*, *Rhizomucor pusillus*, *Rhizopus arrhizus*, and *R. oryzae* are used has been developed for the diagnosis of human and animal zygomycosis caused by the cited etiologic agents. Preliminary studies indicate that the test demonstrates a sensitivity of about 70%. The present state of research suggests that peptido-L-fuco-D-mannans are antigens that are common to zygomycetes and that differentiate them from other fungi. Cross-reactions occur among the zygomycete genera. The specificity of the test, however, appears good when reference precipitates are used (10). Studies, however, are needed to develop more sensitive and reliable methods for the immunologic diagnosis of zygomycosis.

Sera from patients with diabetic ketoacidosis who present evidence of rhinocerebral disease, from other compromised persons with renal disease or acute leukemia, and from debilitated patients who have signs of pulmonary or systemic infection should be tested for zygomycosis.

IN VITRO IDENTIFICATION OF MYCELIAL-FORM PATHOGENIC FUNGAL CULTURES BY EXOANTIGEN TECHNIQUES

Isolates of *B. dermatitidis*, *C. immitis*, *H. capsulatum*, and *P. brasiliensis* often vary in their gross and microscopic features and are frequently difficult or impossible to convert to their tissue forms in vitro or in vivo. A simple diagnostic procedure, the exoantigen technique, can be used to rapidly identify these four pathogens regardless of whether they are sporulating or nonsporulating (13). Studies have revealed that *B. dermatitidis*, *C. immitis*, *H. capsulatum*, and *P. brasiliensis* mycelial-form cultures readily produce cell-free antigens (exoantigens) that are homologous to the diagnostic precipitins discussed in the appropriate sections of this chapter.

Detection of specific exoantigens homologous to *B. dermatitidis* precipitin A, *C. immitis* precipitins HS, HL, or F, *H. capsulatum* precipitins H or M, or *P. brasiliensis* precipitins reactive with antigen 1 (E) or 2 in ID tests permits the early and accurate identification of these pathogens. A 10-day or older Sabouraud glucose agar slant culture with at least 15 by 30 mm of growth is extracted with 8 to 10 ml of 1:5,000 aqueous Merthiolate solution for 24 to 48 h at 25°C. Fungi that form arthroconidia are tested for *C. immitis* antigens. Those that form tuberculate or smooth, thick-walled macroconidia are tested for *H. capsulatum* antigens, and those devoid of characteristic conidia are tested for antigens to all four of the pathogens. The cellular extract is concentrated by ultrafiltration and tested in the ID test for diagnostic exoantigen(s). Technical details and information on the value of the method for identifying other hyaline species (*Aspergillus* spp., *H. capsulatum* var. *duboisii*, *H. farciminosum*, *Penicillium marneffei*, *Pseudallescheria boydii*, and *S. schenckii*) and dematiaceous fungi (*Cladosporium bantianum*, *Cladosporium carrionii*, *Exophiala jeanselmei*, and *Wangiella dermatitidis*) have been previously published (12, 13).

Reagents

Fungal reagents for use in ID tests for serodiagnosis are available from numerous commercial sources. These reagents are designed to detect antibodies and are not always reliable for use in exoantigen tests. They may, however, with proper concentration or dilution and after verifying the presence of specific antibodies and antigens, be used in exoantigen tests. At present, two companies sell kits specifically designed for the immunoidentification of *B. dermatitidis*, *C. immitis*, and *H. capsulatum* cultures. These companies are Immuno-Mycologics and Nolan-Scott.

IN VITRO AND IN VIVO IDENTIFICATION OF PATHOGENIC FUNGI BY FA TECHNIQUES

Fluorescent-antibody (FA) procedures provide mycologists with a valuable adjunct to conventional diagnostic tests. They permit the rapid acquisition of presumptive diagnostic data and the rapid screening of clinical material for pathogenic fungi. Above all, with fungus cultures, these procedures permit rapid identification, whereas conventional procedures might take 2 weeks or longer. They can be applied to viable as well as nonviable fungi in culture and in clinical materials or tissue sections. At the present time, these tests are available at CDC and at certain other reference laboratories in the United States.

With transmitted-light fluorescence microscopes, a combination of a 5113 Corning glass primary filter (3 mm thick) and a Wratten 2A secondary filter (2 mm thick) is satisfactory for use with the fungi. Some researchers use a BG-12 primary filter (3 mm thick) with a Schott GG-9 secondary filter. Recent studies indicate that an American Optical interference exciter filter used with a Schott GG-9 ocular filter gives excellent results with FA-stained fungi (10). Incident-light fluorescence microscopes are excellent for FA studies with fungi. These microscopes provide greater fluorescent intensity and offer the possibility of working with a completely dry system. The following information pertains to those FA procedures that have been developed to a practical level.

Actinomyces spp. and related organisms

Immunofluorescence procedures readily permit the detection and identification of the principal etiologic agents of actinomycosis. FA reagents have been produced for the specific staining of the serotypes of *Actinomyces israelii*, *A. naeslundii*, *A. viscosus*, and *Arachnia (Actinomyces) propionica* either in smears of tissues and exudates or in culture (9, 10).

B. dermatitidis

Specific FA preparations for *B. dermatitidis* have been developed (10) by adsorbing rabbit anti-yeast-form *B. dermatitidis*-labeled antiglobulins with yeast-form cells of *H. capsulatum* and *Geotrichum candidum*. These yeast-form-specific conjugates make possible the rapid and accurate detection of *B. dermatitidis* in culture and in clinical materials. FA techniques cannot identify the mycelial form of this fungus.

Candida spp.

Numerous investigators have studied the application of the FA technique to the detection and identification of *C. albicans* and other *Candida* species. All the investigators found that the *Candida* species are closely related antigenically. Attempts to isolate species-specific FA preparations useful for definitively identifying *C. albicans* in clinical materials and cultures have failed. As a result, single specific reagents are not available for use in the clinical laboratory. Some researchers have reported the successful use of a combination of reagents to identify *Candida* spp. isolates (10). Despite the lack of species-specific FA reagents, some reagents, that demonstrate broad intrageneric cross-staining properties, can be used for screening clinical specimens for the presence of *Candida* spp. (9).

Coccidioides immitis

FA reagents specific for the tissue form of *C. immitis* have been developed (9). These reagents have been produced from the antisera of rabbits infected with viable *C. immitis* cultures. The reagents generally stain the walls of endospores and the contents of spherules. Cross-staining of heterologous fungal antigens by the conjugates is eliminated by dilution or adsorption with yeast-form cells of *H. capsulatum*.

Alternatively, specific conjugates can be prepared from the antisera of rabbits immunized with suspensions of arthroconidia of *C. immitis* killed with Formalin. Cross-staining is eliminated by adsorption with yeast-form cells of *H. capsulatum*.

The specific conjugates are used to detect *C. immitis* in a variety of specimens from humans and animals with coccidioidomycosis. The conjugates can also be used in the diagnostic laboratory for the rapid and specific demonstration of the tissue form of *C. immitis* in clinical materials from laboratory animals injected with suspected *C. immitis* cultures.

Cryptococcus neoformans

Unadsorbed *C. neoformans* conjugates have successfully been used to study the distribution of *C. neoformans* and its polysaccharide products in Formalin-fixed tissue. One group of researchers (10) stained histopathological sections from patients with cryptococcosis with Mayer mucicarmine stain and FA preparations. They found that the conjugate, although nonspecific for *C. neoformans*, stained the yeast cells more intensely and rapidly than did mucicarmine. An effective and practical diagnostic FA reagent of higher specificity is produced by the adsorption of *C. neoformans* conjugates with cells of *C. diffluens* and *Candida krusei* (10).

H. capsulatum

A specific FA reagent for *H. capsulatum* is produced by adsorbing conjugated homologous antiglobulins with the yeast cells of *B. dermatitidis* (9). This conjugate is used to identify yeast-form cells of *H. capsulatum* in culture and in tissue impression smears from humans with histoplasmosis and from experimentally infected mice. Several workers have investigated the applicability of FA reagents to the rapid detection of *H. capsulatum* in human clinical specimens (10). The direct FA procedure has been recommended as a rapid screening procedure for *H. capsulatum* and for the staining of sputum smears as an adjunct to conventional cultural methods.

Serologic studies demonstrated the existence of five *H. capsulatum* serotypes (9). Of these, only one, the 1,4 type, consistently failed to react with the then available FA reagents. Recent studies indicate that antibodies to this serotype react with *H. capsulatum* var. *duboisii* and *B. dermatitidis* isolates.

A diagnostically useful polyvalent reagent has been developed (10) for detecting and identifying *H. capsulatum* var. *capsulatum*, regardless of serotype. Adsorption of labeled antibodies produced against the most complete *H. capsulatum* serotype, i.e., serotype 1,2,3,4, with cells of *C. albicans* yielded a reagent that intensely stained only *H. capsulatum* var. *capsulatum*, *H. capsulatum* var. *duboisii*, and *B. dermatitidis*. Despite this cross-staining, the *C. albicans*-adsorbed reagent can be used diagnostically by using the *B. dermatitidis*-specific FA reagent along with the polyvalent conjugate. Both of these FA reagents stain isolates of *B. dermatitidis*, whereas only the polyvalent conjugate stains *H. capsulatum*. The two varieties of *H. capsulatum* cannot be differentiated from each other with available FA reagents.

P. brasiliensis

FA reagents for the diagnosis of paracoccidioidomycosis have been developed (9). Tissue-form-specific reagents are produced from the antisera of rabbits immunized with suspensions of yeast-form cells of *P. brasiliensis* killed with Formalin. Cross-reactions are eliminated by multiple adsorptions with selected heterologous fungi. These reagents are used in the direct FA procedure to demonstrate *P. brasiliensis* cells in smears of clinical materials. The reagents are especially useful in clinical materials containing few *P. brasiliensis* cells or no morphologically typical cells.

Pseudallescheria boydii

Histopathology is not sufficiently definitive to permit a precise diagnosis of pseudallescheriasis. An FA reagent for detecting and identifying *Pseudallescheria boydii* in tissue has been developed (8). Labeled rabbit antiserum to mycelial and conidial antigens of *P. boydii* brightly stains all *P. boydii* isolates but cross-reacts with *A. flavus*, *A. fumigatus*, *A. nidulans*, *A. niger*, *A. terreus*, *Fusarium oxysporum*, *F. solani*, and a *Scopulariopsis* sp. Cross-staining antibodies can be removed by adsorption with *A. fumigatus* and *F. oxysporum* cellular elements. The adsorbed conjugate specifically stains *P. boydii* in Formalin-fixed tissues from humans and animals with pseudallescheriasis.

S. schenckii

Good quality reagents for detecting the tissue form of *S. schenckii*, both in clinical materials and in culture, have been developed (9). Such reagents are produced from antiserum obtained by immunizing rabbits with suspensions of whole yeast cells of *S. schenckii* killed with Formalin.

Cross-reactions are readily eliminated by dilution, which does not compromise staining qualities. Although, as a rule, few *S. schenckii* cells are found in exudates of lesions, they are readily detected with the FA tests. In a few cases, particularly if the patient is already under therapy, a number of fields may have to be searched before the fungal cells are found.

Comments on the application of FA reagents to clinical materials

The FA technique is most effective for detecting fungal antigens in cultures, pus, exudates, blood, tissue impression smears, and CSF specimens. It is, however, more difficult to use with sputum and tissue sections. Not only does one have to cope with tissue elements that autofluoresce, but for unknown reasons, the staining capacity of the conjugate is impaired in sputa and tissue sections. This impairment may result from a lack of surface interaction between antigen and antibody, because either enzymatic or chemical digestion of sputum specimens results in more effective staining of fungus elements (9). Such treatment may also be applied to tissue sections. FA work with tissue sections has shown that fungus elements are stained more intensely in thin sections (4 μm) than in thicker sections. Glass slides 1 mm or less in thickness are recommended.

Direct FA staining permits the rapid detection of fungi in paraffin sections of Formalin-fixed tissue. In addition, fungi in tissue sections previously stained with hematoxylin and eosin, Brown and Brenn, and Giemsa stains can also be identified. The conjugates, however, will not stain fungi in tissues stained previously by the Gomori methenamine-silver nitrate, the periodic acid-Schiff, or the Gridley procedures.

Prolonged storage of Formalin-fixed tissues, either wet or in paraffin blocks, does not appear to have adverse effects on fungal antigens. Therefore, the FA procedure can well be used to make retrospective immunohistologic diagnoses. Although fluorescein-labeled *H. capsulatum* antiglobulins regularly stain *H. capsulatum* in sections of fixed tissue from patients with active histoplasmosis, these antiglobulins do not regularly stain *H. capsulatum* in healed calcified lesions (9).

LITERATURE CITED

1. **Blumer, S. O., M. Jalbert, and L. Kaufman.** 1984. Rapid and reliable method for production of a specific *Paracoccidioides brasiliensis* immunodiffusion test antigen. J. Clin. Microbiol. **19**:404–407.
2. **Brock, E. G., E. Reiss, L. Pine, and L. Kaufman.** 1984. Effect of periodate oxidation on the detection of antibodies against the M-antigen of histoplasmin by enzyme immunoassay (EIA) inhibition. Curr. Microbiol. **10**:177–180.
3. **Cox, R. A., M. Huppert, P. Starr, and L. A. Britt.** 1984. Reactivity of alkali-soluble, water-soluble cell wall antigen of *Coccidioides immitis* with anti-*Coccidioides* immunoglobulin M precipitin antibody. Infect. Immun. **43**:502–507.
4. **de Repentigny, L., R. J. Kuykendall, F. W. Chandler, J. R. Broderson, and E. Reiss.** 1984. Comparison of serum mannan, arabinitol, and mannose in experimental disseminated candidiasis. J. Clin. Microbiol. **19**:804–812.
5. **de Repentigny, L., L. D. Marr, J. W. Keller, A. W. Carter, R. J. Kuykendall, L. Kaufman, and E. Reiss.** 1985. Comparison of enzyme immunoassay and gas-liquid chromatography for the rapid diagnosis of invasive candidiasis in cancer patients. J. Clin. Microbiol. **21**:972–979.
6. **de Repentigny, L., and E. Reiss.** 1984. Current trends in immunodiagnosis of candidiasis and aspergillosis. Rev. Infect. Dis. **6**:301–312.
7. **Green, J. H., W. K. Harrell, J. E. Johnson, and R. Benson.** 1980. Isolation of an antigen from *Blastomyces dermatitidis* that is specific for the diagnosis of blastomycosis. Curr. Microbiol. **4**:293–296.
8. **Jackson, J. A., W. Kaplan, L. Kaufman, and P. Standard.** 1983. Development of fluorescent-antibody reagents for demonstration of *Pseudallescheria boydii* in tissues. J. Clin. Microbiol. **18**:668–673.
9. **Kaplan, W.** 1975. Practical application of fluorescent antibody procedures in medical mycology, p. 178–186. *In* Mycoses, Proceedings of the Third International Symposium on Mycoses. Pan American Health Organization Scientific Publication no. 304. Pan American Health Organization, Washington, D.C.
10. **Kaufman, L.** 1980. Serodiagnosis of fungal diseases, p. 553–572. *In* N. R. Rose and H. Friedman (ed.), Manual of clinical immunology, 2nd ed. American Society for Microbiology, Washington, D.C.
11. **Kaufman, L.** 1983. Mycoserology: its vital role in diagnosing systemic mycotic infections. Jpn. J. Med. Mycol. **24**:1–8.
12. **Kaufman, L.** 1984. Antigen detection: its role in the diagnosis of mycotic disease and the identification of fungi, p. 203–212. *In* A. Sanna and G. Morace (ed.), New horizons in microbiology. Elsevier Science Publishers, Amsterdam.
13. **Kaufman, L., P. Standard, and A. A. Padhye.** 1983. Exoantigen tests for the immunoidentification of fungal cultures. Mycopathologia **82**:3–12.
14. **Kurup, V. P., and J. N. Fink.** 1977. Extracellular antigens of *Micropolyspora faeni* grown in synthetic medium. Infect. Immun. **15**:608–613.
15. **Lehmann, P. F., and E. Reiss.** 1980. Detection of *Candida albicans* mannan by immunodiffusion, counterimmunoelectrophoresis, and enzyme-linked immunoassay. Mycopathologia **70**:83–88.
16. **Lloyd, K. O.** 1970. Isolation, characterization, and partial structure of peptido-galactomannans from the yeast form of *Cladosporium werneckii*. Biochemistry **9**:3446–3470.
17. **Londero, A. T., J. O. S. Lopes, C. D. Ramos, and L. C. Severo.** 1981. A prova da dupla difusao em gel de agar no diagnostico da paracoccidioidomicose. Rev. Assoc. Med. Rio Grande do Sul **25**:272–275.
18. **Meckstroth, K. L., E. Reiss, J. W. Keller, and L. Kaufman.** 1981. ELISA detection of antibodies and antigenemia in leukemia patients with candidiasis. J. Infect Dis. **144**:24–32.
19. **Palmer, D. F., L. Kaufman, W. Kaplan, and J. J. Cavallaro.** 1977. Serodiagnosis of mycotic diseases. Charles C Thomas, Publisher, Springfield, Ill.
20. **Pappagianis, D.** 1980. Serology and serodiagnosis of coccidioidomycosis, p. 97–112. *In* D. A. Stevens (ed.), Coccidioidomycosis. Plenum Publishing Corp., New York.
21. **Reiss, E., R. Cherniak, R. Eby, and L. Kaufman.** 1984. Enzyme immunoassay detection of IgM to galactoxylomannan of *Cryptococcus neoformans*. Diagn. Immunol. **2**:109–115.
22. **Reiss, E., L. Stockman, R. J. Kuykendall, and S. J. Smith.** 1982. Dissociation of mannan-serum complexes and detection of *Candida albicans* mannan by enzyme immunoassay variations. Clin. Chem. **28**:306–310.
23. **Reiss, E., S. H. Stone, and H. F. Hasenclever.** 1974. Serological and cellular immune activity of peptidoglucomannan fractions of *Candida albicans* cell walls. Infect. Immun. **9**:881–890.
24. **Smith, C. E., M. T. Saito, R. R. Beard, R. M. Keep, R. W. Clark, and B. U. Eddie.** 1950. Serological tests in the diagnosis and prognosis of coccidioidomycosis. Am. J. Hyg. **52**:1–21.
25. **Stockman, L., and G. D. Roberts.** 1983. Specificity of the latex test for cryptococcal antigen: a rapid, simple method for eliminating interference factors. J. Clin. Microbiol. **17**:945–947. (Corrected version.)
26. **Weiner, M. H., and M. Coats-Stephen.** 1970. Immunodiagnosis of systemic aspergillosis. Antigenemia detected by radioimmunoassay in experimental infection. J. Lab. Clin. Med. **93**:111–119.
27. **Weiner, M. H., G. H. Talbot, S. L. Gerson, G. Filice, and P. A. Cassileth.** 1983. Antigen detection in the diagnosis of invasive aspergillosis. Utility in controlled, blinded trials. Ann. Intern. Med. **99**:777–782.
28. **Wieden, M. A., J. N. Galgiani, and D. Pappagianis.** 1983. Comparison of immunodiffusion techniques with standard complement fixation assay for quantitation of coccidioidal antibodies. J. Clin. Microbiol. **18**:529–534.

Chapter 72

Serodiagnosis of Parasitic Diseases

IRVING G. KAGAN

Many serological tests are currently in use for the diagnosis of parasitic diseases (120). Serological tests are especially useful for the diagnosis of echinococcosis (hydatid disease), trichinosis, amebiasis (25), and toxoplasmosis. Although demonstration of the parasite is not readily accomplished, antibody levels during active infections are often high, offering the physician a clue for further diagnostic studies. Serological tests are an aid in the diagnosis of other occult infections such as visceral larva migrans (62), cysticercosis, and filariasis (64). For schistosomiasis, toxoplasmosis, amebiasis, malaria, and Chagas' disease, serological tests have been effectively used as epidemiological tools to evaluate prevalence.

To date, immunodiagnostic tests have been developed for at least 24 infections with protozoan, trematode, cestode, and nematode species. Figure 1 shows the present status of tests for 20 parasitic diseases. I have classified each test according to whether it is extensively evaluated and used, partially evaluated, or still a research tool. The tests include complement fixation (CF); the particle agglutination tests, i.e., bentonite flocculation (BF), indirect hemagglutination (IHA), and latex agglutination (LA); special tests; indirect immunofluorescence (IF); the gel diffusion tests, i.e., double diffusion (DD), immunoelectrophoresis (IE), and countercurrent electrophoresis (CEP); and the enzyme-linked immunosorbent assay (ELISA). Radioimmunoassay and the detection of circulating antigen have been added to this figure since the last edition of this manual. Table 1 lists some of the parasitic antigens that can be purchased commercially.

Amebiasis

The CF test for amebiasis, although the oldest serological test, has generally been superseded by other techniques, such as IHA (68), DD, IF, CEP (73), and IE (25). All of these tests are very sensitive and specific with sera from patients with invasive amebiasis. The sensitivity of the tests decreases with sera from patients with intestinal amebiasis who have minimal tissue invasion. Serological techniques are less sensitive in detecting cyst carriers. Table 2 is a compilation of data on the reactivity of IHA, DD, and IF tests. Investigators using the IHA test have reported from 87 to 100% (61) positive results in cases of liver abscess and from 85 to 98% positive results in acute amebic dysentery. The diagnosis of asymptomatic carriers of *Entamoeba histolytica* cysts is very variable and appears to be dependent on the population from which the sample is drawn. The test was positive for 2 to 6% of the sera from noninfected controls and hospitalized patients sick with bacillary dysentery and other diseases. The percentage of serological reactors was as high as 44 in some areas in which the disease was endemic. IHA titers of 128 and above are reported as positive in my diagnostic laboratory.

Capron et al. (25) reported the sensitivity of the IF and IE tests to be 92 and 99%, respectively. With the advent of axenic cultivation of *E. histolytica* (70), improved soluble antigens have been made, and more reproducible and standardized tests have resulted. Such antigens have been used in the CF, IHA, LA, CEP, and IE tests. Commercial kits for CEP and LA tests are available; the former are more specific than the latter.

A new test that may prove of value in the routine diagnosis of amebiasis is the FIAX test, a new fluorescence technique in which fluorescence is measured by a fluorometer.

Bos et al. (18) and Voller et al. (145) found ELISA titers higher in patients with hepatic compared with intestinal amebiasis. Felgner (44) introduced a stick ELISA test, with polystyrene sticks as the solid phase. Variations of the ELISA test employing drops of antigen or antibody on nitrocellulose paper (spot ELISA) may play an important role in diagnostic laboratories in the future. In a continuing study, Krupp (74) reported on the IE antigen patterns of amebic sera as a method for differentiating various types of clinical amebiasis. The patterns obtained are complicated, and their clinical significance is not understood.

Four companies produce commercial reagents for these tests (Table 1).

Chagas' disease

Chagas' disease can be serologically diagnosed with a high degree of sensitivity and specificity. The serological tests used for diagnosis are the CF (79), IHA (56), IF (29), and a direct agglutination test (DAT). Sensitivity and specificity of the IHA test are shown in Table 3. The LA test has been found somewhat less sensitive and specific (92), but it is considered practical for surveys. The IHA test can also be readily adapted for epidemiological work. Eluates from blood samples collected on filter paper in population surveys can be tested (51). In the CF and IHA tests, titers of 8 and 128, respectively, are positive.

The DAT evaluated by Allain and Kagan (3) is very sensitive with sera from patients with acute infections. This method employs trypsinized, Formalin-fixed epimastigotes obtained from culture. Evaluations indicate high reactivity with sera from patients with acute Chagas' disease and relatively good specificity with regard to cross-reactions with leishmaniasis. The antibody involved in the DAT is sensitive to 2-mercaptoethanol and may be an immunoglobulin M (IgM; 93). Titers of 512 and above appear to be specific for Chagas' disease.

ELISA technique was evaluated by Voller et al. (146), who reported a sensitivity of 98%. An alkaline phosphatase enzyme, with *p*-nitrophenyl phosphate

PARASITIC DISEASES	Complement Fixation	Agglutination Tests				Indirect Immunofluorescence	Immunodiffusion	Immunoelectrophoresis	Countercurrent Electrophoresis	Enzyme Linked Immunoassay-Elisa-	Radio Immunoassay	Detection of Circulating Antigen
		Bentonite Flocculation	Indirect Hemagglutination	Latex	Special Tests							
African Trypanosomiasis	▲		▲							■		
Amebiasis	■	■	■	■	○▲ᶜ	■	■	■	■	▲		○
Ancylostomiasis	○		■	▲		○		○				
Ascariasis	■	■	■			▲	▲	○		■	○	
Chagas	■		■	■	■ᴬ	■	○	▲	■	▲		○
Clonorchiasis	■					○	○	○				○
Cysticercosis	▲	▲	■	▲		▲	▲	○	○	○		
Echinococcosis	■	■	■	■		■	■	■	■	■	○	
Fascioliasis	■	○	▲			■	■	■	■			
Filariasis	▲	▲	■	○		■			▲	▲	○	▲
Giardiasis						▲	○					
Leishmaniasis	■		■	■	■ᴬ	○	○	○	○	■		
Malaria	▲		■	▲		■	■	○	▲	○		▲
Paragonimiasis	■	○	○			▲	▲	○	○			○
Pneumocystosis	■			○		○						▲
Schistosomiasis	■	■	■	○	■ᴮᶜ	■	▲	■	▲	■	○	■
Strongyloidiasis			■			▲				○		
Toxocariasis	○	■	■			▲	■	○		○		○
Toxoplasmosis	■	■	■		■ᶜ	■	○		■	▲		○
Trichinellosis	■	■	■	■		■	■	▲	■	■	○	○

FIG. 1. Serodiagnostic tests for parasitic diseases. Symbols: ○, reported in the literature; ▲, experimental test; ■, evaluated test; A, DAT; B, COPT; C, FIAX automated fluoroimmunoassay.

as a substrate, was used. Sera from Brazil were tested, and a high level of correlation with the IF technique was obtained. Cross-reactions with sera from patients with African sleeping sickness were not observed. In the ELISA, eluates of blood samples collected on filter paper can be used.

The CEP test was evaluated by Knight et al. (71) with sera from 932 patients and 60 blood donors in Brazil. All were tested by CF, and a 92% agreement between the two techniques was obtained, but the sensitivity of the CEP test was less than that of the CF test. Aguilar-Torres et al. (2) evaluated sera from 180 people living in an area of Bolivia with endemic disease. They compared the CEP with the LA and IHA tests and found that the IHA test was more sensitive than the CEP test.

Cossio et al. (34) reported that the serum of 24 of 25 patients with Chagas' heart disease and the serum of 19 of 47 asymptomatic individuals with a positive CF test for Chagas' disease contained immunoglobulins which bind to cryostat sections of heart muscle obtained from a number of animals, including the mouse. The antibody binds to the endothelial lining of the blood vessels, the vascular musculature around the arteries, and the interstitium of striated muscles and is demonstrated by IF. The fluorescence of the triad of tissues constitutes a positive test. The test was negative with sera from 119 normal individuals and 286 patients with selected cardiovascular diseases. A high level of reactivity of the endocardial-vascular-interstitial factor in patients with Chagas' cardiomyopathies suggests that this technique may be prognostic for cardiac involvement in this disease. The endocardial-vascular-interstitial factor was found by Szarfman et al. (131) in sera from a few patients with malaria and leishmaniasis. Relatively high levels of cross-reactivity with sera from patients with leishmaniasis were reported by Hubsch et al. (59).

African trypanosomiasis

The serological detection of antibody against the African trypanosomes relied mainly on the detection by the Mancini test (78) of high levels of nonspecific IgM antibody in serum. The detection of specific antibody by the IF test (77) is more specific with homologous antigen than with heterologous antigen, and maximum sensitivity can be achieved when the serum is tested with trypanosomes of the homologous human species (76). Soltys and Woo (120) employed an indirect charcoal agglutination test for the diagnosis of West African sleeping sickness. Voller et al. (142) evaluated the ELISA for *Trypanosoma rhodesiense*, and Vervoort et al. (140) evaluated the ELISA for *T. gambiense* trypanosomiasis. Vervoort et al. (140), employing variable purified glycoprotein antigens of *T. brucei*, reported high sensitivity and specificity.

Leishmaniasis

Visceral leishmaniasis can be serologically diagnosed by IHA, IF, and CF tests and by DAT. The diagnosis of cutaneous leishmaniasis, especially in the Americas, is more difficult. For diagnosis, the IF test is being used routinely. Walton et al. (149) reported excellent results in cutaneous leishmaniasis from an IF test with amastigote antigen.

The application of the DAT with trypsinized culture forms of leishmania has increased the sensitivity of the serological diagnosis of American leishmaniasis (4). A simple card agglutination test for trypanosomiasis has been used (81), and an IHA test has been used in epidemiological studies. The CF test is still being used and is probably the test of choice for diagnosis (12, 82). Al-Qadhi and Haroun (5) evaluated an IHA test for kala azar. Desowitz et al. (37), using human kala azar sera or serum from a monkey infected with *Trypanosoma cruzi* with a promastigote antigen, evaluated a CEP test for serodiagnosis. Rezai et al. (102) reported that the CEP correlated with the IF test for the diagnosis of kala azar, and they favored the former test, since it is "rapid and sophisticated," for epidemiological surveys. Abdalla (1) also diagnosed Sudanese mucosal leishmaniasis by CEP, but found no correlation between the number and strength of precipitin lines and IF titer levels.

Antibodies to leishmaniasis cross-react with antigens to Chagas' disease. Amato Neto et al. (6) reported that leishmaniasis sera tested with Chagas' antigens cross-reacted in the IF, IF-IgM, and IHA tests, but were negative in the CF test. Edrissian and Darabian (41) found that the IF test was more specific than the ELISA for the diagnosis of cutaneous leishmaniasis, but neither test was as satisfactory as microscopic examinations. Both serological methods were adequate for the diagnosis of visceral leishmaniasis when promastigote forms of *Leishmania donovani* were used as antigen.

Two reviews of the serology of leishmaniasis for the period 1969 through 1973 (160) and to 1980 (21) are available. Hommel (55) reviewed the biology and clinical aspects of leishmaniasis.

Malaria

The test of choice for the serological diagnosis of malaria is the IF test. The use of a thick-smear antigen prepared from washed, parasitized blood cells showed

TABLE 1. Commercial sources for parasitic reagents by disease

Disease and company name	Country[a]	Test[b]	Reagent
African trypanosomiasis			
Behringwerke AG	FRG	IHA	Cellognost (antigen)
Calbiochem-Behring Corp.	USA	IHA	Cellognost (antigen)
Amebiasis			
Ames Co.	USA	LA	Serameba (kit)
ICN Medical Diagnostic Products	USA	IE, IHA, DD, CEP, CF	Antigen
Cordis	USA	ELISA, CEP	CORDIS-A
Behringwerke AG	FRG	CEP, IHA	Kit
Calbiochem-Behring Corp.	USA	CEP, IHA	Kit
Ascariasis			
G. S. Tulloch and Associates	USA	ELISA	Antigen
Chagas' Disease			
Behringwerke AG	FRG	LA, CF, IHA	Kit
Calbiochem-Behring Corp.	USA	LA, CF, IHA	Kit
Institute Adolpho Luz	Brazil	CF	Kit
Basco	Brazil	CF	Kit
Leo Serum	Brazil	DAT, CF	Kit
Trilab	Brazil	CF	Kit
Immuno-Serum	Brazil	DAT, IF	Kit
Polychaco	Argentina	DAT	Kit
Roche Diagnostics	Switzerland	DAT	Kit
Merieux	France	LA	Kit
Cysticercosis			
G. S. Tulloch and Associates	USA	IHA	Antigen
Echinococcosis			
Behringwerke AG	FGR	ID, CF, IHA	Antigen kit
Calbiochem-Behring Corp.	USA	ID, CF, IHA	Antigen kit
G. S. Tulloch and Associates	USA	IHA	Antigen
Laboratoires Fumouze	France	IHA	Kit
Ismunit	Italy	LA	Kit
Pasteur Institute	France	IE, CF	Kit
Commonwealth Serum Lab	Australia	ID	Antigen
Toxoplasmosis			
Menarini	Italy	IHA	Kit
Bouty	Italy	IHA	Kit
Ismunit (Telcolab)	Italy (USA)	LA, CF	Kit
Immunitalia	Italy	DAT	Kit
Behringwerke AG	FRG	CF, IHA, IF	Kit
Calbiochem-Behring Corp.	USA	CF, IHA, IF	Kit
Fisher Diagnostics	USA	ELISA	NIDAS (kit)
Clinical Science, Inc.	USA	IF	Kit
Electro-Nucleonics, Inc.	USA	IF	Kit
Microbiological Research Co.	USA	IF	Kit
International Diagnostic Technology	USA	FIAX	Kit
Cordis	USA	IF, ELISA	Kit
Wampole Laboratories	USA	IHA	Kit
M. A. Bioproducts (Microbiological Associates)	USA	ELISA	Kit, antigen antiserum
Syn-Kit, Inc.	USA	LA	Kit
Zeus Scientific, Inc.	USA	IF	Kit
Litton Bionetics	USA	ELISA	Bio-Bead (kit)
Laboratoires Fumouze	France	IF	Kit
Biotrol	France	IF, ELISA	Kit
Eurobio	France	IF	Kit
Merieux	France	DAT, IHA, IF	Antigen
Pasteur Institute	France	CF, IF	Antigen
National Veterinary Assay Laboratory	Japan	IHA	Antigen
Eiken Chemical	Japan	IHA, LA	Antigen
Kyowa Yakuhin	Japan	LA, IHA, IF	Kit
Kaketsuken	Japan	IHA	Kit
Tanabe	Japan	IHA	Kit
Kitazato	Japan	IF	Kit
Polychaco	Argentina	DAT	Kit
Immuno-Serum	Brazil	DAT	Kit
Leo Serum	Brazil	IF	Kit
Roche Diagnostics	Switzerland	IF	Kit
Toxocariasis			
G. S. Tulloch and Associates	USA	IHA, ELISA	Antigen

TABLE 1—*Continued*

Disease and company name	Country[a]	Test[b]	Reagent
Trichinosis			
Cordis Laboratories, Inc.	USA	CEP, DD	Kit
G. S. Tulloch and Associates	USA		Antigen
Difco Laboratories	USA	BF	Antigen
Fascioliasis			
Pasteur Institute	France	IE, CF	Kit
Merieux	France	CF	Kit
Laboratoires Fumouze	France	IHA	Kit
Fresenius	FRG	CF	Kit
Filariasis			
G. S. Tulloch and Associates	USA	ELISA	Antigen
Leishmaniasis			
Behringwerke AG	FRG	IHA	Cellognost (kit)
Calbiochem-Behring Corp.	USA	IHA	Cellognost (kit)
Malaria			
Merieux	France	IF	Kit
Schistosomiasis			
Behringwerke AG	FRG	ID, IHA	Antigen
Calbiochem-Behring Corp.	USA	IHA	Antigen kit
G. S. Tulloch and Associates	USA		Antigen
Ismunit	Italy	IHA	Kit
Pasteur	France	IE, CF	Kit
S.A.I.M.R	South Africa	IF	Kit

[a] FRG, Federal Republic of Germany.
[b] ID, Intradermal.

a false-positive rate of 1% at a titer of 16. Sensitivity of the test is 95% (128, 129). For high sensitivity and specificity, human homologous malaria antigen should be used. *Plasmodium falciparum* and *P. vivax* can be maintained in *Aotus trivirgatus*, the South American owl monkey; *P. malariae* can be maintained in *Ateles* sp., the spider monkey; and *P. ovale* can be maintained in the chimpanzee. In the IF test, a titer of 16 or greater is positive.

Stein and Desowitz (124) used an IHA test in which Formalin- and tannic acid-treated sheep erythrocytes sensitized with antigen from *P. cynomolgi* and *P. coatneyi* were used. Glutaraldehyde-sensitized cells (43), which enhance the usefulness and adaptability of the IHA test for malaria, have been evaluated by Meuwissen and Leeuwenberg (85). In my laboratory the IHA test was performed with sensitized double-aldehyde-fixed cells (43) and human malarial antigen for seroepidemiological studies.

The ELISA for malaria was evaluated by Voller et al. (141, 145). In a brief note, Bidwell and Voller (16) reported the use of CEP to detect antibodies to *P. falciparum* and *P. malariae* in owl monkeys. They also reported that preliminary tests with sera from human malaria infections gave similar results. Seitz (117) used the CEP test to detect malaria antigens or antibodies in the sera of rats and mice by using cellulose acetate membranes, but the reactions took at least 4 h to develop.

The in vitro cultivation of the malaria parasites (136) has been a significant achievement. Malaria parasites can be maintained in cell cultures over cell layers and will undergo maturation (123).

The literature on diagnosis for the period 1969 through 1974 was reviewed by Zuckerman (161) shortly before her untimely death and more recently by Voller and Houba (147).

Pneumocystosis

The tests of choice for pneumocystosis are the CF and IF tests. Depending on the disease status of the patient, serological procedures detect infection in approximately 85% of patients with *Pneumocystis carinii*. Antigens prepared from infected human or rat lung can be used in both tests. A direct fluorescent-antibody test has been developed for the detection of parasites in smears of mucus and sputum and in tissue from biopsies. The diagnosis and treatment of pneumocystosis was recently reviewed by Hughes

TABLE 2. Sensitivity and specificity of three serological tests in amebiasis as compiled from reports in the literature

Human serum	IHA		DD		Indirect IF	
	No. tested	% Positive	No. tested	% Positive	No. tested	% Positive
Amebic abscesses	314	91	622	92	484	98
Amebic dysentery	514	84	595	72	257	58
Asymptomatic cyst carriers	191	9	19	55	74	23
Patients with other diseases[a] and healthy people	658	2	198	10	1,667	1

[a] Including inflammatory bowel disease.

TABLE 3. Sensitivity and specificity of the IHA test with six parasitic antigens[a]

Human antiserum	No. positive/no. tested with antigen					
	Ascaris	Toxocara	Echinococcus	Filaria	T. cruzi[a]	Cysticercus[b]
Ascaris-toxocara	14/21	8/21	1/20	6/22	0/21	0/23
Bacteria-virus	3/39	2/39	0/49	7/84	1/24	0/33
Echinococcus	3/19	0/19	20/20	3/35	0/25	15/21
Filaria	2/23	14/23	2/32	27/37	0/22	4/23
Protozoa	3/18	1/8	1/21	3/38	3/14	1/18
Schistosoma	2/28	1/28	0/24	9/41	1/24	8/29
Trichina	4/33	7/33	1/29	15/43	2/30	1/31
Normal controls	1/24	1/24	0/25	4/84	0/23	1/24

[a] Sera from Chagas' disease, 11/11.
[b] Sera from cysticercus infections, 10/14.

(60). The serological diagnosis of pneumocystosis is very nonspecific. Antibodies are detected in "normal individuals" at about the same level of sensitivity as in infected individuals. Until more specific methods for diagnosis are developed, the serological test will be of little use.

Toxoplasmosis

The methylene blue dye test has established a firm basis for the serological diagnosis of toxoplasmosis. Most laboratories, however, use IHA and IF tests, since both tests employ a killed antigen, are technically simpler, pose no threat of infection to the laboratory worker, and are more economical to perform.

Jacobs and Lunde (61) introduced the IHA test for toxoplasmosis, and it has become accepted as a test for routine diagnosis in many laboratories. IHA has also been used in epidemiological studies. Recent evaluation, however, suggests that the IHA test with soluble cytosol antigens is very insensitive in the detection of recent acute infections. The use of a mixture of cytosol and membrane antigens yields test results that are more satisfactory.

The IF test is as sensitive and specific as the IHA and methylene blue dye tests. The IF test is also carried out with class-specific conjugates of the IgM type. An IgM titer is strongly suggestive of a recent exposure to the parasite. The test is especially important in detecting infection in the newborn. IHA titers of 64, 128, and 256 are considered of questionable clinical importance. These titers probably represent the low, persistent antibody levels detectable in a large percentage of the population. Titers higher than 256 may represent recent experience with the parasite and may be of clinical significance. Titers obtained with the IF test are slightly lower than those obtained with the IHA test, and an IF titer above 64 may be clinically significant.

In the detection of toxoplasma uveitis, Shimada and O'Connor (118) evaluated an immune adherence test and reported a relatively high sensitivity with this procedure. Hubner and Uhlikova (58) evaluated a gel diffusion technique and found it to be a more sensitive indicator of cure of toxoplasmosis after treatment than was the methylene blue dye or CF test. The ELISA (144) and FIAX (148) techniques are equivalent in sensitivity to the IF test, and both can measure IgM antibody.

HELMINTH DISEASES

Ancylostomiasis

LA, DD, and IF tests have been employed in the serology of ancylostomiasis. Ball and Bartlett (13) published a report on the IF, CF, and IHA tests for an experimentally induced infection in a volunteer. With serum from this person, the CF and IF tests become positive after infection. During the third year after the person had had three exposure to 100 larvae, the IF test indicated relatively high antibody levels, but the CF and IHA tests gave no reaction. The Prausnitz-Kustner tests were positive 4 weeks after infection, indicated the highest titers at 3 months, and became negative after 1 year. There was no observed correlation between concentration of ova in the stool and serological titer. Sood et al. (121) found the IHA and DD tests and the circumoval precipitin reaction test (COPT) of little value in the detection of antibody in infected individuals.

Ascariasis

One does not normally discuss the serology of ascariasis except as it relates to toxocariasis in humans. Soprunova et al. (122) reported the detection of four- to eight-branched carbon chain volatile fatty acids which correlated with the intensity of infection. This finding is important because, although it does not deal with serological diagnosis, it does open the door to the biochemical detection of infection. Little work has been done in this area, and the extension of this type of research to the detection of metabolites or antigens in the serum and body fluids is a most intriguing problem for future investigation.

For routine diagnosis, the IHA test, with perienteric fluid of Ascaris suum as antigen, has been employed (90). The same antigen can be used in the ELISA, but an extract of embryonated egg is more sensitive (35).

Clonorchiasis

Komiya (72) and Platzer (97) received the serology of clonorchiasis. The early serology of this disease was based mainly on the precipitin test. The urine precipitin reaction proved to be the most specific of the tests evaluated. Both CF and intradermal tests have also been used for diagnosis (110, 114). The percentage of positive intradermal reactions increased with the age of the population. With the DD test, high levels of cross-reactivity were found with sera from paragonimiasis patients (110). Melcher-type acid-soluble antigens of adult worms were found to be most sensitive in the intradermal reaction, whereas in the CF test the Melcher insoluble fraction was more satisfactory than the acid-soluble fraction (110). Sawada et al. (112) purified an intradermal antigen that proved to be a carbohydrate polyglucose antigen. The IHA test proved to be slightly more sensitive than CF or intradermal tests (91). A gel diffusion test with a metabolic antigen was found to be more sensitive in humans with liver disease (130). Kagan (63) reviewed more recent contributions.

Cysticercosis

The serology of cysticercosis is of interest from both the medical and veterinary points of view. CF, IHA, and DD reactions have been used for diagnosis, but recent workers are replacing these tests with CEP, IE, and IF. Results obtained with the CF test have been inconsistent. In South Africa, workers (100) have evaluated an IHA test and a DD test with sera from both human and hog cysticercosis. The IHA test yielded 85% positive results with sera from proven cases of cysticercosis in humans, 5% positive results with sera from African hospital patients, and 2% positive results with blood donor sera. The test was more sensitive with serum than with spinal fluid. Of sera from patients with intestinal tapeworm (Taenia saginata), 17% were serologically reactive. The IHA test on hog serum was 100% positive with sera from animals condemned because of heavy infection with cysticerci; only 26% of the sera from animals showing light infections were positive. Beltran and Gomez-Priego (14) reported the use of CEP in both human and experimental cysticercosis. Employing four antigens, these workers found an excellent correlation between the clinical condition of the cyst in the host and the number of precipitate bands formed. Flisser et al. (46) employed IE and DD tests in the diagnosis of human cysticercosis in Mexico. Rydzewski et al. (109) evaluated an antigen of T. saginata in the IHA, IF, and DD tests. The IF test was the most specific. Cross-reactions with sera from patients infected with echinococcosis, T. saginata, and coenuriasis have been reported.

An evaluation of the IHA test with cysticercal antigen is shown in Table 3. Strong cross-reactions are present with sera from patients with echinococcosis. Many nonspecific reactions were observed with sera from individuals with other parasitic infections. These nonspecific reactions can be eliminated if the serum is treated with 2-mercaptoethanol to remove nonspecific IgM antibody. A titer of 64 or higher is positive with human sera. In an unpublished study of 12 patients with seizures due to cerebral cysticercosis, titers were positive in 50% of the sera, but no positive titers were found in the spinal fluid specimens; of 12 patients with increased intracranial pressure, 100% had positive sera, and 93% had positive spinal fluid. In a group of 11 patients with chronic meningitis, 72% were positive by serum tests, and 87% were positive by spinal fluid tests. The literature on cysticercosis from 1930 to 1974 is available (33), and recent advances in the field have been published by Flisser et al. (47).

TABLE 4. Sensitivity and specificity of IHA and BF tests for the diagnosis of hydatid disease

Human antiserum	IHA		BF	
	No. positive/ no. tested	% Positive	No. positive/ no. tested	% Positive
Hydatid disease				
Liver	52/59	88	50/58	86
Lung	6/18	33	9/18	50
Controls				
Cysticercus cellulosae	9/9	100	4/8	50
T. saginata	0/16	0	2/16	12
Cancer	0/16	0	2/15	13
Other parasitic diseases	5/126	4	8/113	7
Miscellaneous diseases	0/61	0	0/52	0
Normal	0/47	0	0/52	0

Echinococcosis

Many serological tests are used successfully for the serological diagnosis of hydatid disease. The IHA, IF, and IE tests are extensively used. Sera with high IHA titers are usually indicative of an active infection; low IHA titers, however, may be equivocal. Low titers in the range of 64 to 128 have been observed with sera from patients with collagen diseases and liver cirrhosis (66), schistosomiasis (19), and other parasitic infections (Table 4). There is a strong cross-reaction between echinococcosis and cysticercosis sera. Hydatid cysts in the lung and dead or calcified cysts are less frequently detected by serological tests than are those in the liver. Antibodies can be detected by IHA, CF, and LA tests for many years after surgery (75), but CF and IF tests (7) may become negative within 1 year after surgery. The IF test performed with protoscolices from viable cysts of human or animal organs showed a sensitivity of 93% with 300 proven infections (7).

A combination of IHA with a BF, LA, CF, or DD test can lead to more accurate diagnosis. The IHA test is routinely performed on all diagnostic sera in my laboratory. The specificity is high only when titers of 256 and above are considered positive. The LA tests of Fischman (45) and Szyfres and Kagan (132) are somewhat simpler to perform. Their specificity is comparable to that of IHA, but their sensitivity is lower. LA particles sensitized with lyophilized hydatid fluid (as used in the IE test) are recommended for screening purposes.

IE analysis has identified a specific "band 5" among echinococcus antigens. The IE test has been evaluated in a number of countries, and the specificity of band 5 has been confirmed. In recent studies, band 5 was found in patients with Echinococcus vogeli (138). Since very large amounts of concentrated reagents are required for IE and the test is time-consuming, it does not lend itself to epidemiological studies. A DD band 5 test has been reported (31) to be more sensitive than the IE test and as specific. The ELISA has also been evaluated (42) with purified "antigen 5."

Fascioliasis

Fascioliasis in humans is a worldwide problem. Platzer (97) reviewed the serology of fascioliasis in his chapter on the trematodes of the liver and lung. Stork et al. (127) studied the prevalence of fascioliasis in 1,011 individuals in Peru and found that 9% of these people were passing eggs of *Fasciola hepatica* in their feces. Intradermal, CF, IF, and IE tests were performed on a group of 137 children with eggs in their stools. The results indicate that no one test gives conclusive diagnostic evidence of infection; i.e., 61% of the tests showed ova in the stools of these children, and 60% of the intradermal tests were positive, as were 14% of the CF tests, 49% of the IF tests, and 48% of the IE tests. Yuthsastr-Kosol et al. (159) prepared an antigen for *F. buski* and showed that antibody could be detected by CF. Cross-reaction with *Opisthorchis viverrini* was high. Fraga de Azevedo and Rombert (48) evaluated the IF test and reviewed serological work up to 1960. These workers employed miracidia as antigen and obtained good reactivity with animal (74%) and human (80%) sera. Hillyer (52) evaluated the CEP test and found that it could detect chemotherapeutic cure (54) and was also useful for routine diagnosis. Fascioliasis in Puerto Rico was also reviewed (53).

Filariasis

Because of the difficulty of obtaining human filarial antigens in an area in which filariasis is nonendemic, IHA tests with antigen prepared from *Dirofilaria immitis* adults are used routinely in my laboratory for the diagnosis of filariasis. The sensitivity of the tests varies with the clinical history of the patients. Specificity is not satisfactory. In *Loa loa* and *Onchocerca volvulus* infections, titers can be very high. On the other hand, very low titers are the rule with *Acanthocheilonema perstans* infections. Sera from patients with eosinophilic lung may be positive. Because of the many reactions with low titers in sera from people ill with other diseases, interpretation is difficult. The filariasis test cross-reacts with a wide variety of helminth infections and must be interpreted with caution.

In our evaluation, 27 (73%) of 37 filariasis sera were positive by the IHA test (Table 3). Of 152 sera from missionaries with microfilaria in the blood, 64% were positive. In addition, 14% of the approximately 2,877 sera from individuals without microfilaria in the blood (but who lived where the disease was endemic) were positive.

Filarial infections in humans perhaps epitomize the problems encountered in the nematode group, since broad cross-reactivities are evident. Niel et al. (87) found that antigen of *Ascaris suum* reacted in the DD test for filariasis. Petithory et al. (94) reported that *A. suum, Parascaris equorum,* and *Neoascaris vitulorum* gave 83 to 89% positive reactions in onchocerciasis. Capron et al. (24) reviewed their work on the use of IE with the sera of 172 patients with filariasis. The antigen used was *Dipetalonema viteae,* a filarial species found in rodents. With this antigen, they detected specific precipitin bands in sera of patients with *O. volvulus, L. loa,* and *Wuchereria bancrofti.* The sensitivity of the test was 80%.

The IF test has been extensively evaluated (8, 134, 135). Using frozen sections of *D. viteae,* Ambroise-Thomas and Kien-Truong (8) found a 90% sensitivity and a group reaction with all species of filaria. Homologous antigen reacted at a higher titer than heterologous antigen. Ten Eyck (134) employed frozen sections of *O. volvulus* and found the IF test to be comparable in sensitivity to skin biopsy for the diagnosis of onchocerciasis. Using both *O. volvulus* and *W. bancrofti* antigens, Ten Eyck (135) found that in bancroftian filariasis, the homologous antigen was superior, but for onchocerciasis, the antigens were of equal sensitivity. Specimens from patients with microfilaria but no local or systemic symptoms were nonreactive.

Cellular immune techniques have been used by Pinon and Gentilini (96). They applied the rosette and migration inhibition tests with peripheral leukocytes and compared these techniques of determining cellular hypersensitivity with IF and IHA tests on the sera of 15 patients with filariasis. Sera that were negative by IF and IHA tests were positive by the other methods. Bloch-Michel and Waltzing (17) have also worked with the rosette technique in the detection of filariasis, but they caution that until more purified antigens are available, results of the test are open to question.

Paragonimiasis

In his reviews of paragonimiasis, Yokogawa (157, 158) covered intradermal tests as applied to epidemiological studies; the purification of antigens; the evaluation of metabolic product antigen; the evaluation of extracts of adult worms, miracidia, and cercariae; and studies on precipitin, flocculation, urine precipitin, and CF tests. Yogore et al. (155) employed DD and IE tests and reported specific bands for paragonimiasis in the serum of infected rabbits and humans. Sawada et al. (113), using a variety of gel filtration and ion-exchange chromatographic methods, isolated a highly purified antigen that did not cross-react with serum from *Schistosoma japonicum,* ascaris, entamoeba, and trichuris infections. Capron et al. (26), employing IE, reported on the antigenic structure and host-parasite relationships for three species of *Paragonimus.* IF (30), CEP (11), and IHA (89) tests have been successfully used for diagnosis. In our laboratory we use the CF test routinely. A titer of 8 is diagnostic.

Schistosomiasis

A large number of serological tests have been evaluated for the diagnosis of schistosomiasis (57, 67). These tests include intradermal, CF, BF, IHA, cholesterol-lecithin (9), IF, and DD tests, plus special tests such as the "Cercarien Hüllen Reaktion" and COPT. Most tests are sensitive, and many detect antibody in people with chronic and acute infections. Specificity is not absolute. Positive trichina sera are usually positive in schistosomiasis tests. In my laboratory, IF tests are performed for routine diagnosis. The cholesterol-lecithin and BF tests were dropped for routine diagnosis because too many equivocal results were obtained. Cryostat sections of adult worms are used in the IF test. Cercariae were used as antigens in the

102. **Rezai, H. R., N. Behforouz, G. H. Amirhakimi, and J. Kohanter, Jr.** 1977. Immunofluorescence and counter immunoelectrophoresis in the diagnosis of kala-azar. Trans. R. Soc. Trop. Med. Hyg. **71**:149–151.

103. **Rombert, P. C., and J. M. Palmeiro.** 1973. Estudo da triquinose experimental do rato pela tecnica de imunofluorescencia, em cortes de congelacao. Medico **66**:88–97.

104. **Ruitenberg, E. J., A. Capron, D. Bout, and F. van Knapen.** 1977. Enzyme immunoassay for the serodiagnosis of parasitic infections. Biomedicine **26**:311–314.

105. **Ruitenberg, E. J., P. A. Steerenberg, and B. J. M. Brosi.** 1975. Micro-system for the application of ELISA (enzyme-linked immunosorbent assay) in the serodiagnosis of *Trichinella spiralis* infections. Med. Ned. **4**:30–31.

106. **Ruitenberg, E. J., P. A. Steerenberg, B. J. M. Brosi, and J. Buys.** 1974. Serodiagnosis of *Trichinella spiralis* infections in pigs by enzyme-linked immunosorbent assays. Bull. W.H.O. **51**:108–109.

107. **Ruitenberg, E. J., and F. Van Knapen.** 1977. Enzyme-linked immunosorbent assay (ELISA) as a diagnostic method for *Trichinella spiralis* infections in pigs. Vet. Parasitol. **3**:317–326.

108. **Ruiz-Tiben, E., G. V. Hillyer, W. B. Knight, J. Gomez de Rios, and J. P. Woodall.** 1979. Intensity of infection with *Schistosoma mansoni*: its relationship to the sensitivity and specificity of serologic tests. Am. J. Trop. Med. Hyg. **28**:230–236.

109. **Rydzewski, A. K., E. S. Chisholm, and I. G. Kagan.** 1975. Comparison of serologic tests for human cysticercosis by indirect hemagglutination, indirect immunofluorescent antibody and agar gel precipitin test. J. Parasitol. **61**:154–155.

110. **Sadun, E. H., B. C. Walton, A. A. Buck, and B. K. Lee.** 1959. The use of purified antigens in the diagnosis of *Clonorchiasis sinensis* by means of intradermal and complement fixation tests. J. Parasitol. **45**:129–134.

111. **Saunders, G. C., E. H. Clinard, M. L. Bartlett, and W. M. Saunders.** 1977. Application of the indirect enzyme-labeled antibody microtest to the detection and surveillance of animal diseases. J. Infect. Dis. **136**:258–266.

112. **Sawada, T., Y. Nagata, and K. Takei.** 1964. Studies on the substance responsible for the skin tests on clonorchiasis. Jpn. J. Exp. Med. **36**:315–322.

113. **Sawada, T., K. Takei, S. Sato, and G. Matsuyama.** 1968. Studies on the immunodiagnosis of paragonimiasis. III. Intradermal skin tests with fractionated antigens. J. Infect. Dis. **118**:235–239.

114. **Sawada, T., K. Takei, J. E. Wiliams, and J. W. Moose.** 1965. Isolation and purification of antigen from adult *Clonorchis sinensis* for complement fixation and precipitin tests. Exp. Parasitol. **17**:340–349.

115. **Schantz, P. M., D. Meyer, and L. T. Glickman.** 1979. Clinical, serologic and epidemiologic characteristics of ocular toxocariasis. Am. J. Trop. Med. Hyg. **28**:24–28.

116. **Schinski, V. D., W. C. Clutter, and K. D. Murrell.** 1976. Enzyme- and ^{125}I-labeled anti-immunoglobulin assays in the immunodiagnosis of schistosomiasis. Am. J. Trop. Med. Hyg. **26**:824–831.

117. **Seitz, H. M.** 1975. Counter-current immunoelectrophoresis for the demonstration of malarial antigens and antibodies in the sera of rats and mice. Trans. R. Soc. Trop. Med. Hyg. **69**:88–90.

118. **Shimada, K., and G. R. O'Connor.** 1973. An immune adherence hemagglutination test for toxoplasmosis. Arch. Ophthalmol. **90**:372–375.

119. **Singer, J. M., and C. M. Plotz.** 1958. Slide latex fixation test. J. Am. Med. Assoc. **168**:180–181.

120. **Soltys, M. A., and P. T. K. Woo.** 1972. Immunological methods in diagnosis of protozoan diseases in man and domestic animals. Z. Tropenmed. Parasitol. **23**:172–187.

121. **Sood, P., P. Prakash, and R. A. Bhujwala.** 1972. A trail of hemagglutination, circumoval precipitin and gel diffusion tests in hookworm infection. Indian J. Med. Res. **60**:1132–1133.

122. **Soprunova, N. J., F. F. Soprunov, and A. A. Lurie.** 1973. Nachweis von Helminthen-Metaboliten in Darm des Wirtes als ein neuer diagnostischer Test für Helminthiasen. Angew. Parasitol. **14**:11–17.

123. **Speer, C. A., P. H. Silverman, and S. G. Schiewe.** 1976. Cultivation of the erythrocytic stages of *Plasmodium berghei* in Leydig cell tumor cultures. Z. Parasitenkd. **50**:237–244.

124. **Stein, B., and R. S. Desowitz.** 1964. The measurement of antibody in human malaria by a formalized sheep cell hemagglutination test. Bull. W.H.O. **30**:45–49.

125. **Stek, M., Jr.** 1978. Micro-technique enzyme-linked immuno-sorbent assay (MELISA) for antibody and antigen detection in schistosomiasis. 4th Int. Congr. Parasitol., Short Commun. **E**:93–94.

126. **Stephanski, W., and A. Malczewski.** 1972. Specificity of migration inhibition test in parasitic invasion. II. Studies on *Trichinella spiralis*. Bull. Acad. Pol. Sci. Ser. Sci. Biol. **201**:26–28.

127. **Stork, M. G., G. S. Venables, S. M. F. Jennings, J. R. Beesley, P. Bendez, and A. Capron.** 1973. An investigation of endemic fascioliasis in Peruvian village children. J. Trop. Med. Hyg. **76**:231–235.

128. **Sulzer, A. J., and M. Wilson.** 1967. The use of thick-smear antigen slides in the malaria indirect fluorescent antibody test. J. Parasitol. **53**:1110–1111.

129. **Sulzer, S. J., M. Wilson, and E. C. Hall.** 1969. Indirect fluorescent antibody tests for parasitic diseases. V. An evaluation of a thick-smear antigen in the IFA test for malaria antibodies. Am. J. Trop. Med. Hyg. **18**:199–205.

130. **Sun, T., and J. B. Gibson.** 1969. Antigens of *Clonorchis sinensis* in experimental and human infections. Am. J. Trop. Med. Hyg. **18**:241–252.

131. **Szarfman, A., E. L. Khoury, P. M. Cossio, R. M. Arana, and I. G. Kagan.** 1975. Investigation of the EVI antibody in parasitic diseases other than American trypanosomiasis. An anti-skeletal muscle antibody in leishmaniasis. Am. J. Trop. Med. Hyg. **24**:19–24.

132. **Szyfres, B., and I. G. Kagan.** 1963. A modified slide latex screening test for hydatid disease. J. Parasitol. **49**:69–72.

133. **Tanaka, H., D. T. Dennis, B. H. Kean, H. Matsuda, and M. Sasa.** 1972. Evaluation of a modified complement fixation test for schistosomiasis. Jpn. J. Exp. Med. **42**:537–542.

134. **Ten Eyck, D. R.** 1973. Comparison of biopsy and fluorescent antibody staining techniques in the detection and study of onchocerciasis in an Ethiopian population. Am. J Epidemiol. **98**:283–288.

135. **Ten Eyck, D. R.** 1973. *Onchocerca volvulus* and *Wuchereria bancrofti*: fluorescent antibody staining of frozen homologous sections for diagnosis. Exp. Parasitol. **34**:154–161.

136. **Trager, W., and J. B. Jensen.** 1976. Human malaria parasites in continuous culture. Science **193**:673–675.

137. **Van Knapen, F., K. Framstad, and E. J. Ruitenberg.** 1976. Reliability of ELISA (enzyme-linked immunosorbent assay) as control method for the detection of *Trichinella spiralis* infections in naturally infected slaughter pigs. J. Parasitol. **62**:332–333.

138. **Varela-Diaz, V. M., E. A. Coltorti, and A. D'Alessandro.** 1978. Immunoelectrophoresis tests showing *Echinococcus granulosus* arc 5 in human cases of *Echinococcus vogeli* and cysticercosis-multiple myeloma. Am. J. Trop. Med. Hyg. **27**:554–557.

139. **Vattuone, N. H., and J. F. Yanovsky.** 1971. *Trypanosoma cruzi*: agglutination activity of enzyme-treated epimastigotes. Exp. Parasitol. **30**:349–355.

140. **Vervoort, T., E. Magnus, and N. Van Meirvenne.** 1978. Enzyme-linked immunosorbent assay (ELISA) with

variable antigen for serodiagnosis of *T.b. gambiense* trypanosomiasis. Ann. Soc. Belge Med. Trop. **58**:177–183.

141. **Voller, A., D. Bidwell, G. Huldt, and E. Engvall.** 1974. Microplate method of enzyme-linked immunosorbent assay and its application to malaria. Bull. W.H.O. **51**:209–211.

142. **Voller, A., D. E. Bidwell, and A. Bartlett.** 1975. A serologic study on human *T. rhodiense* infections using a microscale ELISA. Tropenmed. Parasitol. **26**:247–251.

143. **Voller, A., D. E. Bidwell, and A. Bartlett.** 1979. The enzyme linked immunosorbent assay (ELISA). Nuffield Laboratory of Comparative Medicine. The Zoological Society of London, London.

144. **Voller, A., D. E. Bidwell, A. Bartlett, D. G. Fleck, M. Perkins, and B. Oladehin.** 1976. A microplate enzyme-immunoassay for toxoplasma antibody. J. Clin. Pathol. **29**:150–153.

145. **Voller, A., D. E. Bidwell, and T. Edwards.** 1977. A comparison of isotopic and enzyme-immunoassays for tropical parasitic diseases. Trans. R. Soc. Trop. Med. Hyg. **71**:431–437.

146. **Voller, A., C. Draper, D. E. Bidwell, and A. Bartlett.** 1975. Microplate enzyme-linked immunosorbent assay for Chagas' disease. Lancet **i**:426–428.

147. **Voller, A., and V. Houba.** 1981. Malaria, p. 6–31. *In* V. Houba (ed.), Practical methods of clinical immunology, vol. 2. Immunologic investigations of tropical parasitic diseases. Churchill Livingstone, Ltd., Edinburgh.

148. **Walls, K. W., and E. R. Barnhart.** 1978. Titration of human serum antibodies to *Toxoplasma gondii* with a simple fluorometric assay. J. Clin. Microbiol. **7**:234–235.

149. **Walton, B. C., W. H. Brooks, and I. Arjona.** 1972. Serodiagnosis of Amerian leishmaniasis by indirect fluorescent antibody test. Am. J. Trop. Hyg. **21**:296–299.

150. **Wegesa, P., A. J. Sulzer, and A. Van Orden.** 1971. A slide antigen in the indirect fluorescent antibody test for *Trichinella spiralis*. Immunology **21**:805–808.

151. **Williams, J. P., R. W. Gore, and E. H. Sadun.** 1972. *Trichinella spiralis:* antigen-antibody interaction assayed by radioactive iodinatae antigen. Exp. Parasitol. **31**:299–306.

152. **Williams, J. S., E. H. Sadun, and R. W. Gore.** 1971. A radioactive antigen microprecipitin (RAMP) assay for schistosomiasis. J. Parasitol. **57**:220–232.

153. **Wilson, M., A. J. Sulzer, and K. W. Walls.** 1974. Modified antigens in the indirect immunofluorescence test for schistosomiasis. Am. J. Trop. Med. Hyg. **23**:1072–1076.

154. **Witebsky, F., P. Wels, and A. Heide.** 1984. Serodiagnosis of trichinosis by means of complement fixation. N.Y. State J. Med. **42**:431–435.

155. **Yogore, M. G., R. M. Lewert, and E. D. Madraso.** 1965. Immunodiffusion studies on paragonimiasis. Am. J. Trop. Med. Hyg. **14**:586–591.

156. **Yogore, M. G., M. A. Ozcel, and R. M. Lewert.** 1976. Study of the circumoval precipitate in schistosomiasis japonica by immunofluorescent technic. Am. J. Trop. Med. Hyg. **25**:353–354.

157. **Yokogawa, M.** 1966. Paragonimus and paragonimiasis. Adv. Parasitol. **3**:99–158.

158. **Yokogawa, M.** 1969. Paragonimus and paragonimiasis. Adv. Parasitol. **7**:375–387.

159. **Yuthsastr-Kosol, V., G. Manning, and C. Diggs.** 1973. *Fasciolopsis buski:* serum complement-fixing activity in human infection. Exp. Parasitol. **33**:100–104.

160. **Zuckerman, A.** 1975. Current status of the immunology of blood and tissue protozoa. I. Leishmania. Exp. Parasitol. **28**:370–400.

161. **Zuckerman, A.** 1977. Current status of the immunology of blood and tissue protozoa. II. Plasmodium. A review. Exp. Parasitol. **42**:374–446.

Chapter 73

Section H. Viral, Rickettsial, and Chlamydial Immunology

Introduction

JOHN L. SEVER

Immunological tests are used extensively to diagnose viral, rickettsial, and chlamydial infections. Some of the most frequently used tests are those for hepatitis B virus and the acquired immunodeficiency syndrome retrovirus. These are part of the routine screening performed on all donated blood and blood products in the United States, about 20 million tests annually. More than 7 million rubella antibody tests are also run each year, primarily for documenting immunity in children and women.

The importance of accurate diagnoses for the proper care of infected patients and for public health disease surveillance has resulted in the development of a variety of new rapid tests for detecting viruses. These tests are designed to detect viral antigens or nucleic acid without cultivation of the organisms. Also, immunoglobulin M-specific antibody tests are used increasingly to diagnose recent infections serologically on the basis of a single convalescent-phase blood sample. New monoclonal antibodies are now used by most laboratories for detecting and typing certain infectious agents. These highly uniform antibodies can be of great assistance when very specific tests are needed.

Simplified kits and automation have entered the field and are already a vital part of most diagnostic laboratories. Many of the kits use fluorescent or en-zyme-linked immunosorbent assay methods for detection of the agent. Antibody detection kits are also available involving these assays. New latex agglutination methods are becoming available for detecting specific immunoglobulin G antibody. These methods are very simple and can be completed in any laboratory in less than 10 min. Automation in the form of diluters, multiple pipetters, washers, and readers has simplified the performance of large volumes of tests. The first laboratory robot system has become available for enzyme-linked immunosorbent assay and other tests, and more robots are on the way. The robots can be "taught" most of the standard laboratory procedures. The most rapid increase in testing relating to infectious agents has been in blood banking (hepatitis B and acquired immunodeficiency syndrome) and for sexually transmitted diseases (herpesvirus, cytomegalovirus, and chlamydia). New methods for rapid diagnosis, monoclonal antibodies, commercial kits, and automation are all assisting the laboratory in the performance of these determinations.

The present chapters have all been rewritten and updated. Two new chapters have been added, the first on rapid viral diagnosis and the second on retroviruses. These areas represent very active and important new areas for the clinical laboratory.

Chapter 74

Rapid Viral Diagnosis

DAVID A. FUCCILLO, ISABEL C. SHEKARCHI, AND JOHN L. SEVER

The clinical microbiology laboratory, usually part of the hospital clinical laboratory, is responsible for the isolation and identification of microorganisms, i.e., bacteria, viruses, fungi, and protozoa, in specimens obtained from patients suspected of or diagnosed as suffering from infectious disease. Ideally, the microbiology laboratory should make a tentative identification of infecting organisms rapidly enough so that attending physicians can institute therapy or offer advice to eliminate potential spread of the disease. Unfortunately, until recently, isolation and identification of the causative agent, particularly when it is a virus, have been slow, and information obtained is retrospective, serving only to confirm the clinical diagnosis of the physician. The process used for virus isolation is not only slow but expensive. Cultivation requires inoculation of virus-containing materials into living cell cultures, which require costly reagents and, most important, handling by highly trained and skilled personnel. For these reasons only about 4% of the approximately 12,000 clinical microbiology laboratories in the United States perform diagnostic virology tests.

Immunological techniques offer an alternative to cell culture in the diagnosis of viral disease, and recent developments in precision instrumentation and hybridoma technology are making possible rapid, reliable, and less expensive methods for the clinical laboratory. Improved methods, many of which are described elsewhere in this manual, have decreased virus detection time from days or weeks to a few hours, and they show promise of being able to specifically detect a lower concentration of microorganisms than ever before. The improved immunologically based techniques involve assays for the detection of viral antigens and specific antiviral immunoglobulin M (IgM).

DIRECT DETECTION OF VIRAL ANTIGENS

In the past few years most efforts in rapid viral diagnosis have been placed on the development of methods permitting direct detection of viral antigen in a clinical specimen, thus avoiding the delay of waiting for cultivation of the virus in a cell culture system (9). This approach also allows the detection of viruses which are no longer viable or cannot be cultivated, such as hepatitis virus and human rotavirus. Success with these viruses has been possible because they are present in vivo in high concentrations. This is not true for most other viruses, and detection has been hampered by the lack of assays sensitive and specific enough to detect antigen in low concentrations, as immune complexes, and in the presence of interfering or nonspecific materials. Some progress is now being made in the production of specific immunological reagents, methodology, and equipment which will allow simple, sensitive, specific assays for detection of other viruses within minutes or a few hours. The status of some methods presently being used and changes that could produce better assays will be considered.

Immune electron microscopy

One of the most direct approaches for the detection of antigen has been the immune electron microscopy assay. The unknown specimen is classified, reacted with a specific viral antibody before it is negatively stained, and then examined by electron microscopy. The antibody clumps the virus and concentrates it, which aids in its detection and identification. This procedure has been used for noncultivatable agents such as hepatitis virus, rotavirus, and Norwalk gastroenteritis virus. A newer approach with a double-antibody method has increased the rapidity and sensitivity of the method. Unfortunately, small laboratories do not have an electron microscope available for their general use. Furthermore, the number of specimens that can be tested at any one time is rather limited.

Immunoassays

Various types of immunoassays which employ conjugated indicators to detect and measure antibody or antigen in a patient's specimen have been designed. These assays are diagrammed in Table 1. On the basis of the type of indicator used, these assays are designated radioimmunoassay (RIA), immunofluorescence assay (IFA), and enzyme immunoassay (EIA).

RIA. The RIA uses an isotope-labeled conjugate. Most of the early RIAs were basically isotope dilution methods and depended upon the competition between an antibody in a clinical sample and the same antibody labeled with an isotope (Table 1f).

The RIAs now used for detecting viral antigens or antibodies are noncompetitive solid-phase assays (Table 1b, c, g, and h), which require only a few hours to perform. RIA, while quite sensitive, is not widely used by small laboratories, however, because of expense and safety constraints; a fully automated gamma counter can cost over $100,000, fully trained personnel are required, and radiolabeled reagents present a health hazard and a waste disposal problem.

IFA. Immunofluorescence staining has long been used in rapid viral diagnosis (6). The method is based on tagging an antibody with fluorescein isothiocyanate and demonstrating the antibody-virus complex or viral antigens within or on the surface of the cells by examining the preparation microscopically with UV illumination. A number of procedures have been described, including the direct and indirect or anti-complementary IFAs (Table 1b, c, g, and h). Immunofluorescence staining has been a very useful technique in the past for detection of viral antigens and will continue to be important as a comparison technique for the new immunoassays being developed.

TABLE 1. Diagrams of various immunoassays with labeled antigen or antibody[a]

Assay type/method	Reaction
Homogeneous	
	(No solid phase)
a. CI/D	$Ab + \overline{Ag} + Ag^* \rightarrow \boxed{Ab\ Ag^{\circledR}}$
	$\rightarrow \boxed{Ab\ \overline{Ag}} + Ag^*$
Heterogeneous	
	Immobilized Ag
b. NC/D	$\underline{Ag} + Ab^* \rightarrow \boxed{\underline{Ag}\ Ab^*}$
c. NC/ID	$\underline{Ag} + \overline{Ab} \rightarrow \boxed{\underline{Ag}\ \overline{Ab}} + Ab^* \rightarrow \boxed{\underline{Ag}\ \overline{Ab}\ Ab^*}$
d. CI/D	$\underline{Ag} + Ab^* + \overline{Ag} \rightarrow \underline{Ag} + \boxed{Ab^*\ \overline{Ag}}\ \downarrow$
e. CI/ID	$\underline{Ag} + Ab + \overline{Ag} \rightarrow \boxed{\underline{Ag}\ Ab} + Ab^*\ \downarrow$
	$\rightarrow \underline{Ag} + \boxed{\overline{Ag}\ Ab}\ \downarrow + Ab^* \rightarrow \boxed{\underline{Ag}\ \ Ab^*}$
f. C/D	$\underline{Ag} + \overline{Ab} + Ab^* \rightarrow \boxed{\underline{Ag}\ \overline{Ab}} + Ab^*\ \downarrow$
	$\rightarrow \boxed{\underline{Ag}\ Ab^*}$
	Immobilized Ab
g. NC/D	$\underline{Ab} + \overline{Ag} \rightarrow \boxed{\underline{Ab}\ \overline{Ag}} + Ab^* \rightarrow \boxed{\underline{Ab}\ \overline{Ag}\ Ab^*}$
h. NC/ID	$\underline{Ab} + \overline{Ag} \rightarrow \boxed{\underline{Ab}\ \overline{Ag}} + Ab \rightarrow \boxed{\underline{Ab}\ \overline{Ag}\ Ab} + Ab^* \rightarrow \boxed{\underline{Ab}\ \overline{Ag}\ Ab\ Ab^*}$
i. CI/D	$\underline{Ab} + Ag^* + \overline{Ab} \rightarrow \boxed{\underline{Ab}\ Ag^*}$
	$\rightarrow \underline{Ab} + \boxed{\overline{Ab}\ Ag^*}\ \downarrow$
j. C/D	$\underline{Ab} + Ag^* + \overline{Ag} \rightarrow \boxed{\underline{Ab}\ Ag^*}$
	$\rightarrow \boxed{\underline{Ab}\ Ag} + Ag^*\ \downarrow$
k. IgM capture	$\underline{Ab} + Ab \rightarrow \boxed{\underline{Ab}\ \overline{Ab}} + Ag \rightarrow \boxed{\underline{Ab}\ \overline{Ab}\ Ag} + Ab^* \rightarrow \boxed{\underline{Ab}\ \overline{Ab}\ Ag\ Ab^*}$

[a] Symbols: D, direct; ID, indirect; *, labeled; NC, noncompetitive; C, competitive; CI, competitive inhibition; ↓, removed by washing; +, added reactant; □, bound reactants; Ag$^{\circledR}$, label inhibited; Ag, antigen; Ab, antibody; $\underline{Ag}$, immobilized antigen; $\underline{Ab}$, immobilized antibody; $\overline{Ab}$, sample antibody; $\overline{Ag}$, sample antigen; $\underline{\overline{Ag}}$, immobilized antigen from sample.

The IFA test, since it is performed microscopically, requires approximately 10^5 infectious units to be visualized. This limitation also applies to the immunoperoxidase assay in which the antibody is labeled with an enzyme and the production of an insoluble colored product from enzyme substrate is visualized. The specificity of visual detection by the IFA and immunoperoxidase methodologies is an advantage over all other assays based on colorimetric, fluorometric, or isotopic readings. The staining pattern and morphological location, which add specificity to a positive reading, are lost with other types of immunoassays. An important advantage of immunofluorescence staining compared with viral isolation has been its ability to detect the presence of viruses which cannot be cultured. This ability has been demonstrated quite effectively with respiratory viruses and varicella-zoster virus.

IFAs have been limited by the fluorescent probes used. Fluorescein, rhodamine, and umbelliferone all have small Stokes' shifts, which means that their absorption and emission maxima are very close together, and light scattering causes major interference while decreasing the capability of detection. Also, the absorption and emission bands of these labels occupy spectral regions similar to those of bilirubin, which can cause high background counts when determinations are made with sera. Many fluorescence-labeled materials combine nonspecifically to albumin, which will quench their fluorescence and block detection. The nonspecific absorption increases the background count and therefore decreases the sensitivity of the assay. Problems with deterioration of the fluorescence signal with time have been reported.

Recently workers have isolated from certain red and blue-green algae (cyanobacteria) a series of compounds called phycobiliproteins which, when purified, exhibit some spectral properties which make them extremely suitable for fluorescence labeling (7). They have high fluorescence quantum yields over a broad pH range, their absorption bands start at 440 nm, and their intense emission bands begin at 550 nm. They have fluorescence which is not quenched by most biomolecules, and they are highly soluble in aqueous solution. These materials have been successfully conjugated to immune sera and monoclonal antibodies and appear to remain stable reagents for long periods of time.

The production of antisera to be used in the detection of viral antigens by immunofluorescence has been another source of problems. Most of these antisera have been made with inocula containing residual materials from cell culture and therefore contain specific antibodies against extraneous proteins. Although these unwanted antibodies generally can be absorbed from reagent preparations, they still can interfere with a very sensitive assay. Furthermore, hyperimmune serum from animals used for immunization can have naturally occurring antibodies to the various viral agents under study. Because different animals respond differently to immunization, it is difficult to obtain consistent reagents over a period of time. The new techniques for producing monoclonal antibodies have dramatically overcome many of these problems. Monoclonal antibody technology offers the potential for virtually infinite supplies of antibodies of exceptionally well-defined specificity. These techniques provide reagents which markedly reduce the cause of false-positive reactions, thus increasing both the sensitivity and specificity of many different types of immunoassays. The full potential of immunofluorescence staining will be evident when monoclonal antibody becomes available for viruses of interest in the clinical laboratory.

EIA. In 1971 Engvall and Perlmann developed the enzyme-linked immunosorbent assay (2). This assay has been used extensively to detect either antigen or antibody and has been described as specific, sensitive, simple, inexpensive, and reproducible. The indicator in this technique is an enzyme which catalyzes a chemical reaction in a substrate. Various enzyme-substrate combinations have been used. The end product of the enzyme reaction can be quantitatively measured spectrophotometrically, fluorometrically, or by other means. EIA has proven to be a significant alternative to the traditional methods in viral immunology in terms not only of sensitivity and specificity but also of safety. It has proven to be as sensitive as RIA in detecting small quantities of antigen. The lower cost of equipment, longevity of test reagents, and decreased health hazards have made the use of EIA very attractive to a large number of microbiology laboratories. A number of modifications to the technique have expanded sensitivity and speed.

EIAs may be homogeneous or heterogeneous. With the homogeneous assay, no solid-phase matrix is used, and the enzyme-linked immunoreactant is dispersed in a solution. The homogeneous assay has received increasing attention in the past few years because it can be methodologically simpler to perform than the heterogeneous assay, since no separation of reagents is required. Its primary reagent is an antigen conjugated to an enzyme in such a way that the antigen is located at or near the enzyme catalytic site. In the presence of antibody to that particular antigen, the substrate will be excluded from enzyme activity, thus precluding color development. In the presence of free antigen in a clinical specimen, the antibody will bind to this free antigen and allow the substrate to react with the unbound enzyme-labeled antigen and produce color (Table 1a). Homogeneous methods have not been widely used because of difficulty in the preparation of the labeled antigen. The major problem is in retaining antigenicity while attaching an enzyme to the catalytic site of the antigen to interfere with enzymatic reaction. The assay is limited primarily to low-molecular-weight materials, such as drugs or hormones, and is not currently usable for the high-molecular-weight materials, such as viral antigens.

Recently, a homogeneous, colorimetric immunoassay system with one incubation step has been described which is capable of measuring macromolecular antigens. The system is called an enzyme membrane immunoassay (10). With this system the enzyme marker is encapsulated within liposomes and, when released, serves as a signal generator. The enzyme membrane immunoassay is based on the ability of guinea pig complement to damage antigen-tagged liposomes when antigen-antibody complexes are formed on the surfaces of the vesicles. Damage to the liposome membrane is monitored by measuring the released enzyme activity on a colorless substrate which is converted to a colored product. The amount of product reflects the extent of complement-mediated liposome damage. A test sample containing free antigen competes with the antigen on the liposome surface for antibody molecules in the mixture, and as a result, the number of antigen-antibody complexes that form on the liposome surface is reduced. Consequently, the amount of substrate converted to a colored product is also reduced. The amount of colored product formed is inversely correlated with the amount of free antigen present in the test sample. A number of immunoassay methods employing the liposomes and complement have been developed, and their potential for viral antigen detection remains to be evaluated.

The heterogeneous assay employs an enzyme-linked immunoreactant to either antibody or antigen which may be bound to a solid-phase matrix. In heterogeneous EIAs, an antigen can be quantitated by competitive or noncompetitive procedures (Table 1, b through k). Competitive assays are based on the blocking of labeled antigen or antibody from the solid phase by the antigen or antibody in a test specimen. These assays can be designed with either labeled antigen or labeled antibody. The advantage of competitive assays is that fewer incubation steps are required, and therefore the assays can be performed in less time. One major disadvantage, however, is that labeled antigen for these assays must be highly purified in sufficient quantity to be labeled with an enzyme. This is not a problem with materials that are synthesized, such as drugs, but can be quite a problem with infectious viral agents. The competitive method with labeled antibody is more practical for the detection of viral antigens, since large quantities of antibody can be made either by animal inoculation or by the production of monoclonal antibodies. A disadvantage with the labeled-antibody system is that endogenous antibody in a specimen will compete with the labeled antibody, thus yielding a false-positive reaction. This situation is especially true with viral infections where antigens for detection will be present in serum, in body fluids such as sputum and urine, and in fecal specimens. Therefore, to detect these antigens, endogenous antibodies must be denatured before the performance of the antigen-antibody reaction.

Because of the problems with competitive methods, the basic systems generally used for detection of virus have been noncompetitive. The simplest method involves the use of enzyme-labeled antibody specific for the particular antigen to be measured. In this assay, usually called direct, noncompetitive, capture, or sandwich (Table 1g), an unlabeled antibody is first bound to the solid phase. The unknown specimen is then added, and if antigen is present in the specimen, it will bind to the antibody, whereas unreactive material will be removed by washing. Specific enzyme-labeled antibody is then added. This antibody will bind to the antigen bound in the previous steps, whereas unreactive antibody will be removed by washing. The amount of bound antibody is measured by adding a substrate solution and measuring the formation of substrate products, whether they are colored, fluorescent, or luminescent.

The advantage of the direct procedure is that fewer reagents have to be used in the assay, which is therefore quicker. Also, since fewer reagents are used, the potential for nonspecific reactions is decreased, and, therefore, greater specificity may be possible than with the indirect assay.

The other noncompetitive method is called the indirect assay system (Table 1h). In this method the second antibody, or so-called detector antibody, is unlabeled and must be from an animal species different from that of the primary antibody on the solid phase. After the reaction of the second antibody, unreactive antibody is removed by washing, and an enzyme-labeled antibody against the species in which the second antibody was produced is added. This antibody will bind to the solid phase and then convert the substrates as described above. In this system, as with indirect immunofluorescence, only one labeled antiglobulin is required for the measurement of any antigen, provided that the second antibody is of the same animal species for all viral assays. Also, greater sensitivity than with the direct procedures is possible since increased surface areas of reactants are produced, which causes a corresponding increase in labeled antibody. One disadvantage is that the viral antisera must be prepared in two different species.

In noncompetitive assays an inherent problem involves the nonspecific binding of the materials in the specimens with the immunoreactants. A major nonspecific reacting substance can be rheumatoid-like factors present in body fluids. These can be removed (see the section below on rheumatoid factor [RF]). Controls for nonspecific binding should consist of testing the specimen with a solid phase coated with nonimmune serum from the same species and at the same concentration as the immune serum. An antiglobulin, if present, will result in equal binding to both the immune and nonimmune solid phases. A significant difference in activity between the two readings will demonstrate a positive reaction. A blocking or inhibition test can be performed in which the specimen is treated in parallel with viral antiserum and preimmunization serum before it is added to the test system. It should be remembered that the blocking antiserum must be from a different animal than the viral antisera used in the test proper. Blocking antiserum should inhibit reactivity of the specimen by more than 50%.

Increasing sensitivity for antigen detection

As mentioned above, the greatest success in the detection of virus by EIAs has been with agents that are present in high concentrations, such as hepatitis A and B viruses (surface antigens) and rotavirus. In viral infections with a lower virus concentration, such as adenovirus, cytomegalovirus, and respiratory syncytial, herpes simplex, influenza, and Epstein-Barr viruses, success of detection ranges anywhere from 60 to 90% in comparison to culture techniques. Therefore, to make a rapid diagnostic test reliable and practical, an increase in sensitivity is needed without a loss of specificity. In noncompetitive EIA systems, the sensitivity is determined by the interactions of the antigen and the antibody, the kinetics of the enzyme-substrate reaction, and the detectability of the substrate product. The antibodies used for the capture and detection of antigen must first have high specificity and contain minimal amounts of nonspecific reactivity. As previously mentioned, polyclonal antibody production can be controlled if pure preparations of antigens are made before inoculation of the animals. Antibodies can also be affinity purified after production. Monoclonal antibody production offers the greatest potential for specific antibody development and should help make possible the future production of highly specific and sensitive assays.

Antibody used for capture assays (Table 1k) must have a high affinity constant. It has been shown that the amount of antigen which can be detected is proportional both to the affinity constant of the antibody and to the affinity constant of the nonspecific reactions. Unfortunately, a large number of the monoclonal antibodies that have been produced have low affinity, and therefore their use in these antigen detection systems is limited. Selection for high-affinity-type monoclonal antibodies should eliminate this problem.

The limit of the detection of the enzyme-substrate reaction is determined both by the specific activity of the enzyme bound to the immunoreactant and the detectability of the substrate reaction products. Two enzymes that are quite popular for use in EIAs are alkaline phosphatase and horseradish peroxidase. Peroxidase has over twice the specific activity (900 U/mg) of alkaline phosphatase (400 U/mg). The molecular weight of peroxidase is less than half that of alkaline phosphatase, so theoretically, the potential of conjugating more enzyme activity per antibody molecule is present with peroxidase. The selection of enzyme, however, cannot be based solely on the specific activity or the molecular weight. For instance, although catalyase enzyme has a specific activity of 40,000 U/mg, the use of this enzyme is limited because it is difficult to maintain activity during conjugation to an antibody and, even more important, the availability of substrates is limited to hydrogen peroxide.

The substrate utilized is critically important to the eventual detection. As an example, the substrate for alkaline phosphatase, nitrophenyl phosphate, produces a colored end product which can be read by spectrophotometric instrumentation. It can be detected to 10^{-8} M. It has been determined that if alkaline phosphatase has a turnover rate of 10^5 molecules of enzyme per min, the amount that can be detected in a 10-min period is 10^{-14} M. If another substrate for alkaline phosphatase, such as 4:methylumbelliferone, which produces a fluorescent end product, is used, the level of detection is 10^{-11} M. Therefore, in a 10-min period, 10^{-17} mol of alkaline phosphatase per liter can be detected. It is evident that when a longer incubation period is used, theoretically it should be possible to detect even smaller amounts of enzyme. This is not the case, however, because to achieve extreme degrees of sensitivity, all nonspecific interactions must be controlled.

A number of different systems can be utilized for detection of the antigen-antibody reaction on a solid phase. One recent technique that has shown a great deal of sensitivity is the avidin-biotin technique (1). Avidin is a basic glycoprotein with a molecular weight of 68,000. Biotin is a vitamin with a molecular weight of about 244. There is a strong interaction between avidin and biotin, and this reaction has been used to link antibody to an enzyme which has been found to serve as an aid in amplifying the sensitivity of immunoassays. Each molecule of avidin has four binding sites for biotin. The affinity constant for avidin-biotin binding is 10^{-15}, or about 1 million times greater than for most antigen-antibody complexes. This bond is essentially irreversible and can be utilized quite effectively in amplifying the sensitivity and specificity of a particular assay system. Biotin molecules can be attached to an antibody or enzyme with very mild conjugation techniques. Avidin can also be bound to protein by a one- or two-step glutaraldehyde conjugation procedure. Assays employing avidin-biotin can therefore be quite flexible in design because both avidin and biotin can be bound to either antibody or enzyme. Methods have been described in which avidin serves as a linking molecule between biotinylated antibody and enzyme, forming an avidin-biotin complex. Avidin used in this manner causes an amplification effect due to several enzyme moieties being introduced at each antigen site. The sensitivities of these assays is limited only by the affinity of the antibody used and the stability of the enzyme, since the binding affinity of avidin-biotin is so great that it does not limit the final reaction. This new technique offers an enormous potential for detecting small quantities of antigen directly. A captured or localized antigen could be treated successively with biotinylated antibody, fluorescent avidin, biotinylated antiavidin, and finally, more fluorescent avidin. Amplification produced by the attraction between these molecules would greatly increase sensitivity. A direct reading could then be made for the presence of antigen. This would eliminate the problems of endogenous enzymes, with the specimen producing false-positives or inhibitors inactivating an enzyme label used for a detection assay. Also, the time required for performing the assay should be reduced, since the time necessary to turn over a substrate would not be required.

Handling time should be reduced with very little loss of sensitivity.

DNA PROBES

In the past few years, basic research in microbiology has developed the technology to produce small pieces of DNA called DNA probes (5). Simple, reproducible methods have been devised for synthesizing the probes by the use of purified biological enzymes, by cloned DNA procedures, and by chemical synthesis through the use of automated DNA synthesizers. These DNA probes make it possible to identify and isolate the genetic information of any organism. They should be particularly useful in the diagnosis of latent or slow virus infections because the DNA probe can detect the presence, rather than the expression, of genetic information.

DNA probe assays are based on the biochemical principle of the DNA double helix, in which complementary strands of nucleotides form stable double-stranded molecules. The methodology for performing the assay after the labeled probe is made is quite simple. The sample to be tested is dissolved with detergent and enzymes to remove non-DNA components. The mixture is then treated at a low pH, with the denatured DNA separating into two strands from the double helix. These strands are bound to a solid matrix such as a filter, and the single-stranded DNA is exposed to an excess of probe DNA. The probe seeks out the complementary sequences in the immobilized DNA and hybridizes to them. The filter is then washed to remove the unbound probe from the bound probe, which is detected by the presence of its label. In the past, the label was radioactive ^{32}P. However, as previously pointed out, other labels are replacing isotopes. Probes have now been made by a nick translation reaction which is catalyzed by an *Escherichia coli* DNA polymerase. A biotin-containing analog can then be incorporated into the DNA probe without altering its activity. Biotin can then be detected through the use of the avidin-biotin complex. Immunological reagents, however, have to be used with this assay to increase the sensitivity for detection. Usually goat antibiotin is used, and then a biotin-labeled rabbit anti-goat reagent, and finally the avidin-biotin complex reagent. It is claimed that 10^{-14} g of DNA can be detected with this methodology. Commercial kits are available which include the essential ingredients for constructing and labeling probes. These assays in combination with immunological reagents have the potential for many rapid viral diagnostic applications.

DETECTION OF VIRUS-SPECIFIC IgM ANTIBODIES

IgM antibodies characteristically appear 7 to 10 days after primary infection, reach maximum titers within 2 to 3 weeks, and then tend to decline to undetectable levels after about 3 months. The presence of IgM specific antibody therefore implies a current or recent infection and offers the potential of making a rapid diagnosis with a single serum specimen. In pregnancy, maternal IgM antibody does not cross the placenta; therefore, any detection of virus-specific IgM

TABLE 2. Comparison of various methods for IgM assay

Method	Advantages	Disadvantages
Solid-phase indirect immunoassay		
IFA	Speed; simplicity; can detect typical distribution of viral antigen (IFA)	Competition of IgG antibody for antigen binding sites can cause false-negatives and false-positives; low sensitivity (IFA) for detecting IgM antibody in congenital infections without absorption
EIA and RIA	Can test whole serum; high sensitivity	False-negatives with competing IgG if IgG is not removed; false-positive reactions due to RF without absorption
Solid-phase sandwich or capture immunoassay		
Solid-phase EIA with anti-human IgM as capture antibody	Can test whole serum; eliminates involvement of competing IgG antibody	Competition among IgM of various specificities for solid-phase binding sites, including RF; potential for false-positive reactions caused by RF without absorption
Solid-phase EIA with anti-human IgM F(ab')$_2$ fragment as capture antibody	No absorption of RF	Competition among IgM present; very expensive

in the cord blood or serum of a neonate can be assumed to be the result of a congenital infection.

Methods for separation and quantitation

In the past, a number of procedures have been developed for detecting specific viral antibodies of the IgM class (Table 2). Unfortunately, further research and sophistication of equipment and methods have revealed that the procedures were not sufficiently specific. Much of the information on IgM determined by older methods must be reviewed critically before it is accepted. Methods for quantitation of IgM and the problems involved with the various assays will be presented.

Sucrose density gradient centrifugation

One of the earlier techniques still often used to separate IgM from IgG and other serum proteins is sucrose gradient fractionation. This physical separation of IgM from other immunoglobulins based on its higher sedimentation coefficient (19S) compared with that of other immunoglobulins (7S to 11S) requires an ultracentrifuge. This requirement limits use of the technique by the average clinical laboratory lacking this equipment. When tested for purity by recently developed sensitive assays, IgM fractions prepared in this way have shown that they are not always pure IgM. Trailing of IgG into the IgM samples occurs, particularly if IgG is present in high concentrations or if the serum has been heat inactivated.

RF. RF is an IgM anti-IgG and in the presence of specific IgG antibodies can produce false-positive results in all of the various assays developed for specific IgM. In the indirect IgM immunoassays, the mechanism of interference is the attachment of RF to specific IgG antibodies in the serum of a patient which, when placed on solid phase with antigen, will result in the labeled anti-human IgM antibodies subsequently

binding to the RF, causing a false-positive IgM antibody result. RF is mainly associated with rheumatoid arthritis, but may also be present in subacute bacterial endocarditis, chronic liver disease, tropical infections, tuberculosis, and sarcoidosis and can be found in apparently healthy individuals. RF activation has been reported in connection with the acute phase of several viral infections, especially cytomegalovirus. Reimer, in 1975, was the first to show that RF was present in the serum of newborns and that it greatly complicated the diagnosis of congenital infections (8). The presence of high IgG antibody titers passively transmitted from the mother to the baby could interfere with the detection of the specific IgM response. As a consequence, much of the initial work reported on specific IgM assays with fluorescent-antibody tests has resulted in conflicting and confusing reports.

RF interference can be eliminated either by direct removal of RF or by removal of specific IgG antibodies. Methods proposed to remove RF include absorption with heat-aggregated IgG or with glutaraldehyde-polymerized IgG. There are differing opinions concerning the efficacy of these absorption procedures. Some investigators prefer to remove the IgG antibodies by absorption with staphylococcal protein A (staph A). Thus, by removing IgG, any problems caused by the presence of RF should also be removed. The advantages and disadvantages of serum pretreatments for IgM assays are presented in Table 3.

Investigators thought that by using a solid-phase anti-IgM assay or capture technique many of the problems caused by RF could be reduced. Recently, however, results have indicated that IgM-RF has the potential to reduce the sensitivity of a capture assay by competing with virus-specific IgM for binding sites on the solid phase (3). The RF bound in this manner can also produce false-positive results for the viral IgM antibodies, since RF complexes with the virus-specific IgG antibodies to which viral antigen attaches and subsequently binds the labeled antiviral antibod-

TABLE 3. Advantages and disadvantages of various pretreatments of sera for IgM assay

Method	Advantages	Disadvantages
Sucrose density gradient centrifugation	Good physical separation of IgG from IgM; separation of IgM from possible inhibitors	Time and expense of concentration and dialysis; requires ultracentrifuge; contamination by drifting IgG
Absorption with staph A	Fast and easy; removes IgG	Residual IgG$_3$ and IgA; loss of IgM
Absorption with staph A and streptococci (Staffinoc)	Same as for absorption with staph A but also removes IgG$_3$ and IgA	Possible loss of some IgM
Absorption with aggregated IgG capture M assay	Removes RF	Efficiency of aggregated IgG varies for removal of RF

ies. False-positive reactions can also result from IgM-RF binding directly to the labeled IgG antiviral antibody reagent used in the assay. Since RF binds the Fc part of the IgG molecule, this problem can be overcome by using F(ab')$_2$-labeled fragments as the indicative antibody. This solution, however, increases the expense of producing reagents. Detection of RF by latex agglutination is not a satisfactory method for evaluating specificity of results or for determining which sera contain RF. According to recent studies, many sera that show high levels of false-positivity in a specific assay give only weak-positive or no reactions by latex agglutination. Therefore, with the capture technique, as with the indirect solid-phase assay, absorption of test sera with aggregated human IgG for the former and staph A for the latter before testing is necessary to eliminate false-positive reactions.

ANA. Antinuclear antibodies (ANA) can be present simultaneously with IgM-RF. ANA activity has been observed both as RF cross-reactive with DNA histone complexes and as antibody molecules with no affinity for IgG. IgM-RF containing ANA activity has been found in patients with rheumatoid arthritis and systemic lupus erythematosus. In addition to consideration or RF and ANA, it is important, no matter which type of assay is used, to test each serum against noninfected tissue control antigen so that nonspecific reactivity of the test sera can be recognized and false-positive readings can be avoided.

It is quite apparent from various studies that in solid-phase immunoassay systems for specific IgM detection, whether indirect or capture assays, the problems of IgG competition and RF interference have to be eliminated by appropriate pretreatment or absorption before the results of the immunoassay system can be acceptable. In our laboratory we have found that an indirect EIA for IgM is quite useful for detecting antiviral IgM antibodies. Sera are preabsorbed with Staffinoc (M. A. Bioproducts), a commercial preparation containing staph A and streptococci, which effectively eliminates all nonspecific IgM reactions by removing all IgG, including IgG3, and IgA (4). This pretreatment of serum significantly increases the sensitivity of the specific IgM assay by removing most competing IgG. All positive IgM-containing sera should be checked after absorption with an EIA of equivalent sensitivity for detecting IgG antibodies. The elimination of most of the IgG activity against any specific antigen indicates that

pretreatment was appropriate and that the indication of the presence of specific IgM is accurate.

Significance of IgM in viral diagnosis

The value of determining specific IgM antibodies to viruses is variable, depending on the particular virus under study. Transient IgM responses seem to be a characteristic of infections caused by viruses which have antigenic uniformity and elicit a long-lasting immunity, such as the viruses that cause rubella, measles, and mumps (Table 4). With other viruses belonging to closely related strains or serotypes such as enteroviruses, adenoviruses, and parainfluenza viruses, IgM response can be weak or absent, and its use for diagnosis may be limited. Cross-reactions to related viruses or prolonged IgM responses in reactivation of the latent viruses such as herpesvirus may occur. These variable results and the technical pitfalls previously mentioned complicate the interpretation of IgM antibody results. The more sensitive methods now being developed for the detection of specific IgM may extend the time after infection during which IgM can be detected. Future studies may determine that it is necessary to artificially decrease the assay sensitivity so that the optimal persistence time of IgM antibody response is diagnostically useful.

FUTURE DEVELOPMENT

The development of new fluorescent compounds such as the phycobiliproteins, the modification of immunoassay techniques such as with liposomes and the avidin-biotin system, and the production of monoclonal antibodies should dramatically increase progress in the development of a rapid viral diagnostic capability. The current EIA techniques available for antibody determinations should prove quite adequate. Spectrophotometric readings of color endpoints should be sensitive enough for any future development of antibody assays. For detection of very low levels of antigen, however, detection of the color change is not sensitive enough. In spectrophotometric readings, the amount of light absorbed by a sample is independent of the intensity of the light source, whereas with fluorometry the intensity of fluorescence emission is directly proportional to the intensity of the incident beam. Therefore, the system more suitable for antigen detection should be fluorometry,

TABLE 4. Reported duration of virus-specific IgM response[a]

Virus	Usual duration (mo) or response	Unusual duration (yr) or response
Rubella	Adult: 1–3 Child: at birth 6–12	Adult: 1 year or more Child: 1–2 years
Cytomegalovirus	Adult: 2–9 Child: at birth with viruria 50% positive by IFA 90% positive by RIA	Adult and child: rare positive with reactivation
Herpes	Adult: 1–6 Child: positive	Adult and child: rare positive with reactivation
Epstein-Barr	1–3	
Varicella-zoster	1–2	
Hepatitis A	6–12	
Hepatitis B	12–18	
Measles	1–3	
Mumps	1–2	

[a] Many of these figures are based on older, less sensitive tests and should be reevaluated.

because this system allows for the development of more sensitive instrumentation. Detection capability by fluorescence, even at the present time, is similar to that obtained with gamma-emitting isotopes, which can extend into the range of picomoles per liter. The use of fluorescent materials also shares the advantage of isotopes in that immediate endpoint measurement is possible after completion of the immunological reaction. This measurement can be made by clearing bound from free fluorescence or by removing bound reactants from the path of the excitation light source.

The future use of hybridization techniques with nonisotopic labels should offer highly sensitive methods for the detection of the presence rather than the expression of genetic information. These methods have the potential to extend our capability to detect oncogenes and slow viral infections.

LITERATURE CITED

1. Bayer, E. A., and M. Wilcher. 1980. The use of avidin-biotin complex as a tool in molecular biology. Methods Biochem. Anal. 26:1–43.
2. Engvall, E., and P. Perlmann. 1971. Enzyme-linked immunosorbent assay (ELISA). Quantitative assay of immunoglobulin G. Immunochemistry 8:871–874.
3. Forghani, B., C. K. Myoraku, and N. J. Schmidt. 1983. Use of monoclonal antibodies to human immunoglobulin M in "capture" assays for measles and rubella immunoglobulin M. J. Clin. Microbiol. 18:652–657.
4. Kronvall, G., A. Simmons, E. B. Myhre, and S. Jonsson. 1979. Specific absorption of human serum albumin, immunoglobulin A, and immunoglobulin G with selected strains of group A and G streptococci. Infect. Immun. 25:1–10.
5. Leary, J. J., D. J. Brigati, and D. C. Ward. 1983. Rapid and sensitive colorimetric method for visualizing biotin-labeled DNA probes hybridized to DNA or RNA immobilized on nitrocellulose: Bio-blots. Proc. Natl. Acad. Sci. U.S.A. 80:4045–4049.
6. McIntosh, K., and L. Pierik. 1983. Immunofluorescence in viral diagnosis, p. 57–81. In J. D. Coonrod, L. J. Kune, and M. J. Ferraro (ed.), The direct detection of microorganisms in clinical samples. Academic Press, Inc., New York.
7. Oi, V. T., A. N. Glazer, and L. Stryer. 1982. Fluorescent phycobiliprotein conjugates for analyses of cells and molecules. J. Cell. Biol. 93:981–986.
8. Reimer, C. B., C. M. Black, D. J. Phillips, L. C. Logan, E. F. Hunter, B. J. Pender, and B. E. McGrew. 1975. The specificity of fetal IgM: antibody or anti-antibody? Ann. N.Y. Acad. Sci. 254:77–93.
9. Schmidt, N. J. 1983. Rapid viral diagnosis. Med. Clin. North Am. 67:953–972.
10. Tan, C. T., S. W. Chan, and J. C. Hsia. 1981. Membrane immunoassay: a spin membrane immunoassay for thyroxine. Methods Enzymol. 74:152–161.

Chapter 75

Herpes Simplex Virus

JOHN A. STEWART AND KENNETH L. HERRMANN

Human infections with herpes simplex virus (HSV) are ubiquitous throughout the world. The clinical course of HSV infections is extremely variable, and primary infection is subclinical or mild enough to be unrecognized in a majority of cases. Clinically apparent infection may range from mild pharyngitis to a severe generalized disease that causes death. The major clinical conditions associated with HSV infections are gingivostomatitis, keratitis and conjunctivitis, vesicular eruptions of the skin, aseptic meningitis, encephalitis, genital tract infections, and neonatal herpes. Infection in the newborn may be localized to the skin or generalized, seriously involving the central nervous system, eyes, and skin, as well as other organs. Other persons at increased risk for serious or prolonged HSV infections are those with eczema, severe burns, or a defect in their cell-mediated immunity.

Latent infection (8) with both type 1 (HSV-1) and type 2 (HSV-2) characteristically is established in most persons after primary infection. Recurrent infection in the form of fever blisters occurs in 10 to 15% of the seropositive group. Genital eruptions may recur commonly, but the exact frequency has not been as accurately described as that for fever blisters. It is important to appreciate that the initial clinically recognizable oral or genital HSV infection in a person is not synonymous with primary infection. The term primary infection should be reserved for an infection in which the person has not previously had either HSV-1 or HSV-2. There is little question that a previous oral HSV-1 infection does not protect a person against acquiring a genital HSV-2 infection; however, those persons with prior HSV-1 infection, when subsequently infected with HSV-2, may have a less severe clinical course.

A majority of persons in most population groups have been infected with HSV by the age of 20 years (8). Consequently, evidence of serum antibody against HSV by any serologic test provides no information regarding the time of infection with the exception of an immunoglobulin M (IgM)-specific antibody assay. Diagnosis of current infection by either virus type depends on demonstrating a significant increase in antibody titer. A serum collected as close as possible to the onset of illness and a convalescent-phase serum collected 10 days to 3 weeks later should be tested simultaneously. The two types of virus share many cross-reacting antigens, and a majority of the antibody produced in response to an initial infection is to the shared antigens. Type-specific antibody tests must be performed to differentiate the virus type involved.

When primary infection occurs with either HSV type, it is easily documented by testing paired sera in any of the common serologic tests. The immune response to recurrent infection or reinfection with either HSV type is much more complicated and may depend on the number and type of previous infections and the severity of the subsequent infection. After primary HSV infection, antibody levels may fall to low or undetectable levels and then be boosted by later clinical infections with the same type or a heterologous type. Patients who experience severe recurrences, particularly those associated with systemic or neurologic symptoms, may have a significant rise in antibody. On the other hand, most adults, after multiple recurrences of localized HSV-1 or -2 lesions, have stable titers by complement fixation (CF) and neutralization (NT) tests. Initial infection with HSV-2 in persons with prior experience with HSV-1 is likely to cause a significant antibody rise to both the common herpes antigens and HSV-2-specific antigens.

The only virus that shows some degree of cross-reactivity with HSV is varicella-zoster virus (VZV) (7). Paired acute- and convalescent-phase sera from patients infected with VZV who have preexisting HSV antibody may sometimes have a rise in antibody titer to HSV-1 and HSV-2. A similar rise in titer to VZV may occur in patients infected with HSV who have had prior infection and antibody to VZV. This heterotypic response has been observed using CF, NT, and immunofluorescence assay (IFA). Paired sera from patients with atypical-appearing skin vesicles should be tested against antigens of both viruses.

SERODIAGNOSTIC TESTS

The tests that have the widest application for serodiagnosis and serosurveys are CF, indirect IFA, NT, radioimmunoassay (RIA), enzyme immunoassay (EIA), indirect hemagglutination (IHA), and IHA inhibition tests.

CF tests

The CF test is most useful for those laboratories that normally perform this test with multiple antigens for serodiagnosis of other viral diseases. The exact titration required of its multiple components precludes its occasional use for the serodiagnosis of HSV alone. CF detects antibody directed to the intact virion and the soluble antigens produced by infected cells. The immune response in humans produces antibody to each of the structural components of the virus, the envelope, capsid, and internal proteins, as well as soluble nonvirion antigens specified by the virus.

The appearance of HSV CF antibodies after primary infection is readily detected when properly spaced acute- and convalescent-phase sera are obtained. CF-detected antibodies are stable and long lasting in the adult, and testing a single serum gives a reliable indication of prior infection with either HSV type. CF tests in which standard crude antigens obtained from HSV-infected cell extracts are used are usually incapable of distinguishing type-specific antibody because of the strong cross-reaction between the two HSV types. Better differentiation is obtained using enve-

The average acute *(X)* and convalescent *(Y)* log HI titers to influenza B/Maryland/1/59 were 1.20069 and 1.60206, respectively. The sample variances of the two log titer samples are given by $S_X^2 = 0.11327$ and $S_Y^2 = 0.20389$. To compare the acute and convalescent geometric mean titers, the usual *t* statistic is computed, where

$$t = \frac{\overline{X} - \overline{Y}}{S_p \sqrt{\dfrac{1}{n_X} + \dfrac{1}{n_Y}}}$$

S_p is the pooled standard deviation and is the square root of the weighted average of S_X^2 and S_Y^2, that is,

$$S_p = \frac{\sqrt{(n_X - 1)S_X^2 + (n_Y - 1)S_Y^2}}{n_X + n_Y - 2}$$

$$= \sqrt{\frac{(9 - 1)(0.11327) + (9 - 1)(0.20389)}{9 + 0 - 2}}$$

$$= 0.39822$$

where n_X and n_Y are the number of acute and convalescent titers, respectively. For these data,

$$t = \frac{1.20069 - 1.60206}{(0.39822) \sqrt{\dfrac{1}{9} + \dfrac{1}{9}}} = \frac{-0.40137}{0.18772} = 2.14$$

and there are $n_X + n_Y - 2 = 16$ degrees of freedom.

The tabulated value of the *t* statistic for 16 degrees of freedom is 2.120 at the $P = 0.05$ level and 2.583 at the $P = 0.02$ level. Since the absolute value of *t* for these data (2.14) is greater than 2.12, the null hypothesis, that the true geometric mean acute- and convalescent-phase HI titers are the same, can be rejected at the $P = 0.05$ level. This is strong presumptive evidence of an influenza B outbreak in the example.

LITERATURE CITED

1. **Frank, A. L., J. Puck, B. J. Hughes, and T. R. Cate.** 1980. Microneutralization test for influenza A and B and parainfluenza 1 and 2 viruses that uses continuous cell lines and fresh serum enhancement. J. Clin. Microbiol. **12**:426–432.
2. **Hammond, G. W., S. J. Smith, and G. R. Noble.** 1980. Sensitivity and specificity of enzyme immunoassay for serodiagnosis of influenza A virus infections. J. Infect. Dis. **141**:644–651.
3. **Kendal, A. P.** 1982. Newer techniques in antigenic analysis with influenza viruses, p. 51–78. *In* A. S. Beare (ed.), Basic and applied influenza research. CRC Press, Boca Raton, Fla.
4. **Kendal, A. P., and T. R. Cate.** 1983. Increased sensitivity and reduced specificity of hemagglutination inhibition tests with ether-treated influenza B/Singapore/222/79. J. Clin. Microbiol. **18**:930–934.
5. **Kendal, A. P., W. R. Dowdle, and G. R. Noble.** 1985. Influenza viruses, p. 755–762. *In* E. H. Lennette, A. Balows, W. J. Hausler, Jr., and H. J. Shadomy (ed.), Manual of clinical microbiology, 4th ed. American Society for Microbiology, Washington, D.C.
6. **Madore, H. P., R. C. Reichman, and R. Dolin.** 1983. Serum antibody responses in naturally occurring influenza A virus infections determined by enzyme-linked immunosorbent assay, hemagglutination inhibition, and complement fixation. J. Clin. Microbiol. **18**:1345–1350.
7. **Noble, G. R., H. S. Kay, A. P. Kendal, and W. R. Dowdle.** 1977. Age-related heterologous antibody responses to influenza virus vaccination. J. Infect. Dis. **136**(Suppl.): S686–S692.
8. **Stuart-Harris, C. G., and G. C. Schild.** 1976. Influenza. The viruses and the disease. Publishing Sciences Group, Inc., Littleton, Mass.

Chapter 80

Respiratory Syncytial Virus and the Parainfluenza Viruses

MAURICE A. MUFSON AND ROBERT B. BELSHE

The most common etiologic agents of bronchiolitis, croup, and pneumonia in infants and children are respiratory syncytial virus and the parainfluenza viruses, types 1, 2, 3, and 4 (1, 10). These viruses also cause upper respiratory tract illness in adults and occasionally severe respiratory infections in aged adults confined to nursing homes. Serological evidence of infection with respiratory syncytial virus and the parainfluenza viruses can be obtained by several methods, including complement fixation, neutralization procedures, enzyme-linked immunosorbent assay (ELISA), and, additionally, for the parainfluenza viruses, hemagglutination inhibition. Respiratory syncytial virus antigen can be detected in exfoliated nasal secretory cells by immunofluorescent procedures using either monoclonal antibodies or immune serum antibody directed against the whole virus.

As routine diagnostic antibody tests, complement fixation procedures for respiratory syncytial and parainfluenza viruses and hemagglutination inhibition tests for the parainfluenza viruses are easy methods for determining circulating antibody responses during infection except in children less than 6 months old (8). Infants and young children less than 6 months of age may not respond with a brisk and high-titered antibody response because they possess maternal antibody to these viruses and because of their immature immunological systems. For the survey among groups of individuals of the status of antibody to respiratory syncytial and the parainfluenza viruses, the ELISA procedure and virus neutralization test detect serum immunoglobulin G (IgG) antibody and reflect the level of immunity in individuals in the group. Neutralization tests can be conducted in roller tube cultures, petri dishes, or microtiter plates (3). Since antibody measured by hemagglutination inhibition correlates well with the level of antibody assayed by neutralization, such tests for the parainfluenza viruses provide a reliable and more rapid method for the survey of type-specific antibody than the neutralization procedures.

CLINICAL INDICATIONS

The choice of test to assay antibody to the parainfluenza and respiratory syncytial viruses depends on the information needed concerning the immunological status of the individual, the age of the patient, and the rapidity and ease of performance of the test. Both complement fixation and hemagglutination inhibition procedures provide specific and reliable assays for measurement of antibody in acute- and convalescent-phase paired sera and can be performed in hospital laboratories as routine tests. Since infants and young children less than 6 months old frequently do not develop sufficient antibody to be detected by these methods, the ELISA procedure can

provide a useful method for detecting antibody to respiratory syncytial virus in individuals in this age group. These tests are usually done by use of microtiter procedures (8, 9). By contrast, virus neutralization procedures seem too laborious for the measurement of antibody responses during the course of an individual patient's illness. The neutralization test is generally reserved for special surveys and research purposes rather than the routine measurement of parainfluenza or respiratory syncytial virus antibody responses that would usually be undertaken by hospital laboratories. As ELISA technology becomes refined, this test can be expected to supplant the more laborious neutralization assays for the measurement of protective antibody as well as for determining diagnostic rises.

Serological tests for the measurement of antibody responses during acute viral infections necessarily require paired sera for simultaneous testing to detect rising levels of antibody. The test cannot be performed until a convalescent-phase serum has been obtained late in the course of illness. Usually, the patient has recovered by this time. The measurement of antibody responses of individual patients can provide retrospective evidence of infection with respiratory syncytial and the parainfluenza viruses, especially in the absence of virus isolation, and signal the presence of an outbreak of these viruses in the community. Rapid diagnosis of respiratory syncytial virus infection is best accomplished by the demonstration of viral antigens in exfoliated respiratory tract mucosal cells in nasal secretions by use of indirect immunofluorescence procedures.

TEST PROCEDURES

Complement fixation

The measurement of antibody by complement fixation is performed with microtiter procedures because they conserve antigen, provide ease of operation, and allow the simultaneous testing of many sera quickly and accurately. The characteristics of this system have been described in detail (see chapter 10).

For the measurement of antibody to the parainfluenza viruses and respiratory syncytial virus in sera from infants and children, it is important that 8 U of the viral antigen be used; 4 U of antigen suffices for testing of sera from adults. Cell culture-grown antigens can be purchased from commercial sources. Respiratory syncytial virus antigen can be produced by a low-multiplicity infection of HEp-2 cells (supplemented with inactivated chicken serum), and parainfluenza virus antigen can be produced by infection of rhesus monkey kidney cells.

The guinea pig complement should be tested to ensure that it lacks antibody to the parainfluenza viruses and other paramyxoviruses, because guinea pigs can readily acquire these infections. Test each lot of guinea pig complement for parainfluenza, respiratory syncytial, and mumps virus antibodies before use; purchase additional complement from a negative lot.

Initially, test each serum for anticomplementary activity. Any serum found to be anticomplementary can be treated with mouse liver powder and then retested to determine whether or not the anticomplementary activity has been eliminated. Briefly, the procedure is as follows.

1. Mix 200 mg of mouse liver powder with 1.0 ml of serum and shake continuously for 1 h at room temperature.

2. Centrifuge the mixture at 2,000 to 2,500 rpm (700 to 1,000 × g) for 20 min.

3. Remove the serum with a fine-pointed pipette and inactivate at 56°C for 30 min.

The use of four dilutions, 1:8, 1:16, 1:32, and 1:64, for testing acute- and convalescent-phase sera provides an efficient scheme for the detection of antibody responses and at the same time conserves antigen. Occasionally, however, no endpoint is reached with this dilution series, and the test must be repeated with higher dilutions of sera, e.g., 1:8, 1:16, 1:32, 1:64, 1:128, 1:256, and 1:512. Low-level rises in paired sera from infants and children may be detected only with serum dilutions starting at 1:2. Acute- and convalescent-phase sera from a single patient must be tested in the same test.

Briefly, the procedure for the complement fixation test is as follows.

1. Dispense 0.025 ml of 0.85% saline containing magnesium and calcium (diluent) in appropriate wells of a disposable "U"-well plastic microtiter plate. Prepare diluent by adding 1 ml of magnesium-calcium solution ($MgCl_2 \cdot 6H_2O$, 10 g, and $CaCl_2 \cdot 2H_2O$, 4 g, in 100 ml of distilled water) to 1,000 ml of 0.85% saline. Use this diluent throughout the test.

2. Inactivate serum at 56°C for 30 min. Make twofold dilutions of serum with a 0.025-ml microdiluter (or "loop").

3. Add by pipette dropper 0.025 ml of antigen to each dilution of serum.

4. Prepare serial twofold dilutions of a positive serum control from 1:2 to 1:64 with a 0.025-ml microdiluter.

5. To the positive serum control, add with a pipette dropper 0.025 ml of diluent to each well; for an antigen control, add 0.025 ml of diluent to each of six wells; for the erythrocyte control, add 0.075 ml of diluent to each of four wells; and for the complement control, add 0.05 ml of diluent to each of eight wells.

6. Add 0.025 ml of antigen diluted to contain 4 or 8 U (as required) to each well containing dilutions of the positive serum control.

7. Make successive twofold dilutions, usually 1:2 to 1:64, of antigen, using 0.025 ml, and add 0.025 ml of diluent to each antigen control well.

8. Dilute complement in cold diluent to contain 2 U exactly. Further twofold dilutions of complement are made to contain 1, 0.5, and 0.25 U of complement.

9. Add 0.025 ml of each dilution of complement to the appropriate control wells.

10. Add 0.025 ml of the initial complement dilution containing 2 U to the remainder of the test, except for the erythrocyte control wells.

11. Tap the plates gently on all four sides to mix, cover with transparent adhesive cellophane tape, and incubate overnight at 4°C.

12. The next morning, warm the plates to room temperature for approximately 20 min, and add 0.05 ml of sensitized sheep erythrocytes to each well (prepared by mixing equal volumes of the erythrocyte suspension and hemolysin diluted to contain 2 U).

13. Tap the plate gently on all four sides to mix the erythrocytes, and incubate at 37°C for 30 to 45 min or until the complement controls show cell lysis. When the complement controls show the appropriate degree of hemolysis, transfer the plates from the 37°C incubator to a refrigerator at 4°C. The complement control wells containing 2 U should show complete hemolysis, and the 1-U wells should show nearly complete or complete hemolysis; the erythrocytes in the 0.5- and 0.25-U wells should not be hemolyzed. Remove the plates from 4°C after 1 h, warm to room temperature for 20 min, and read the test. Dilutions of test serum showing hemolysis of 75% or more of the erythrocytes are considered antibody positive.

Hemagglutination inhibition for parainfluenza virus antibody

Hemagglutination inhibition procedures easily provide data on serological responses in parainfluenza virus infection, especially when microtiter techniques are used. Antigen consisting of cell culture harvests of untreated virus can be prepared by low-multiplicity infection of rhesus monkey kidney cells and harvest of virus at maximal hemagglutination activity. Test a sample of culture media daily and harvest on the day of high-titer antigen, usually after day 5 of incubation. Freeze the untreated harvest in small portions at −70°C, incorporating bovine serum albumin at a final concentration of 0.5% for antigen stabilization. Add 0.1 ml of a 10% suspension of sterile bovine serum albumin to each 1.9 ml of virus antigen, and adjust to pH 7 with 1 or 2 drops of 1 N sodium hydroxide.

Treatment of cell culture harvests with Tween 80 and ether increases the hemagglutinin titer (5). Briefly, add Tween 80 to the cell culture harvest at a final concentration of 0.1%. Mix and add ether to increase the total volume by one-third. Mix vigorously for 5 to 15 min at 4°C. Centrifuge and pipette the lower aqueous phase into a flask gently. Bubble nitrogen through the antigen to remove residual ether. Hemagglutination antigens can also be purchased from commercial sources.

For the microtiter procedure, U-well plastic disposable plates are preferred. The hemagglutination patterns in U wells are easily interpreted. Initially, antigen lots must be titrated, and a dilution of antigen containing 1 hemagglutinin unit per unit of volume must be determined. Use 4 U of antigen per unit of volume in the hemagglutination inhibition test.

The procedure for determining the hemagglutinin content of the antigen preparation is as follows.

1. Dispense 0.05 ml of 0.85% phosphate-buffered saline (PBS) into duplicate columns of 10 wells each and into 5 additional wells for erythrocyte controls.

2. Make twofold dilutions of antigen with a 0.05-ml microdiluter in duplicate, starting in the 1st well and proceeding to the 10th well.

3. Dispense 0.05 ml of a 1% solution of guinea pig erythrocytes in PBS into each virus-containing well and into the erythrocyte control wells. Prepare erythrocyte dilutions fresh daily; the stock erythrocytes should be between 1 and 4 days old.

4. Tap gently on all four sides of the plate to mix.

5. Incubate at room temperature for 1 h and read the test.

6. The endpoint is the last dilution showing hemagglutination of about 50% of the cells. This represents 1 hemagglutinin unit per 0.05 ml. In the hemagglutination inhibition test, use 4 hemagglutinin units in a 0.025-ml volume (or eight times the concentration of the dilution containing 1 hemagglutinin unit as measured in the hemagglutination test in which 0.05-ml volumes are employed).

The procedure for the hemagglutination inhibition test is as follows.

1. Treat serum to remove nonspecific inhibitors of hemagglutination by using receptor-destroying enzyme, which can be purchased from commercial sources. Add 0.1 ml of receptor-destroying enzyme to 0.1 ml of serum and incubate the mixture overnight at 37°C. The next morning, add 0.3 ml of PBS to the mixture and inactivate at 56°C for 30 min. This is a 1:5 dilution of serum, which can be used immediately or stored at −20°C for testing later.

2. Test each serum in duplicate, and test acute- and convalescent-phase sera in the same test.

3. Serum should be tested starting at a dilution of 1:10; twofold dilutions are carried out to 1:1,280 or 1:2,560.

4. Dispense 0.025 ml of PBS in the appropriate number of wells.

5. Dip a 0.025-ml microdiluter into the 1:5 dilution of treated serum and loop it into the first well of PBS; mix and continue the dilution process. The initial serum dilution of the first well is now 1:10.

6. Add 0.025 ml of antigen, containing 4 U, to each serum dilution.

7. Tap gently on all four sides of the plate to mix, and incubate at room temperature for 1 h.

8. For the serum control, mix 0.025 ml of the 1:5 dilution of treated serum in a well with 0.025 ml of the PBS.

9. For the virus control titration (virus "back titration"), drop 0.05 ml of PBS in five wells, and in the first well, loop 0.05 ml of the dilution of virus antigen used in the test; continue the dilution process through the five wells. For interpretation, the first well (or highest concentration) is designated 4 U, and the succeeding dilutions are designated 2, 1, 0.5, and 0 U.

10. After 1 h of incubation at room temperature, add 0.05 ml of 1% guinea pig erythrocytes in PBS to each well, tap the plate gently on all four sides to mix, incubate at room temperature for 1 h, and read. Note that the erythrocytes in wells with serum will settle more quickly and may be read at 15 to 45 min, but the cell control and virus titration usually require the full 60 min of incubation.

11. The pattern of the virus control titration should show complete hemagglutination in the wells estimated to contain 4, 2, and 1 U of hemagglutination and no hemagglutination in the remaining two wells. Slight variations from this pattern are acceptable.

12. The serum hemagglutination inhibition endpoint is the last dilution showing complete inhibition of hemagglutination.

Neutralization test for determining antibody to respiratory syncytial virus

The measurement of neutralizing antibody to respiratory syncytial virus can be performed by plaque reduction, by tube neutralization procedures, or in microtiter plates (1–3). The plaque reduction assay provides an especially sensitive measure of neutralizing antibody. Its use and interpretation are facilitated by techniques which produce large clear plaques (1 to 2 mm in diameter) in susceptible cell monolayers (usually HEp-2 cells). The sensitivity of HEp-2 cells for replication of respiratory syncytial virus varies with the source of the cells, and several lines may have to be tested to find a sensitive one. Several plaque reduction procedures for respiratory syncytial virus antibody measurement have been described, each with slight but not major variations in the conduct of the test (3). The plaque reduction procedure used in our laboratory provides endpoints in 5 to 6 days.

Plaque reduction test. The plaque reduction tests for respiratory syncytial virus antibody is performed as follows.

1. HEp-2 or Vero cells grown in plastic (or glass), flat-sided bottles are treated with 0.25% trypsin for 15 to 20 min, and the dispersed cells are washed and suspended in growth media consisting of Eagle minimal essential medium supplemented with 10% calf serum and appropriate antibiotics.

2. Seed the cell suspension into plastic 16 mm wells of tissue culture trays and incubate in a 5% carbon dioxide atmosphere at 37°C.

3. Wash the confluent cell sheets twice with Hanks balanced salt solution.

4. Inactivate test sera at 56°C for 30 min and make dilutions of sera in growth media. Use 1:10, 1:40, 1:160, and 1:320 dilutions of sera in the initial test, but if no endpoint is reached, adjust dilutions in the repeat test. For sera obtained from older children and adults, the initial dilution is 1:50 and subsequent dilutions are carried to 1:2,000 or greater.

5. Mix 0.2 ml of respiratory syncytial virus (Long strain) suspension, diluted to contain approximately 20 to 30 PFU and containing 10% guinea pig complement, with an equal volume of each serum dilution, and incubate at room temperature for 1 h.

6. Inoculate duplicate dishes with 0.2 ml of virus-serum mixture.

7. Add 0.2 ml of Hanks balanced salt solution to each dish to prevent drying during virus adsorption.

8. Gently agitate the plates every 15 min during the 2-h adsorption period to allow equal distribution of the inoculum.

9. After adsorption, rinse the plates with Hanks balanced salt solution and overlay the cells with 10 ml of a fresh 1% methyl cellulose solution in Eagle minimal essential medium.

10. Incubate the plates for 5 to 6 days in a 5% carbon dioxide atmosphere at 37°C.

11. At the end of the incubation period, decant the overlay and add 5 ml of 10% Formalin to each dish to preserve the cells.

12. The next day, rinse the cells in tap water and air dry.

13. Plaques appear as 1- to 2-mm-diameter defects in the confluent cell monolayer. Microscopically, the defects of respiratory syncytial virus are syncytia, some of which become detached in part from the dish. Optionally, the cells can be stained with Giemsa stain.

14. Control plates include virus alone and diluent alone.

15. Express the plaque reduction neutralizing antibody titer as a reciprocal of the serum dilution producing a 50% reduction in plaque count from the virus control.

Tube neutralization procedure. Alternatively, a tube neutralization procedure can be used for the measurement of neutralizing antibody to respiratory syncytial virus. This test is more sensitive than the ELISA at detecting low levels of respiratory syncytial virus antibody.

1. Inactivate serum specimens at 56°C for 30 min and dilute in Eagle minimal essential medium supplemented with 5% inactivated chicken serum and appropriate antibiotics.

2. Serum dilutions used are 1:4, 1:8, 1:16, 1:32, 1:64, and 1:128.

3. Mix each serum dilution with an equal volume of virus diluted to contain approximately 10 to 30 50% tissue culture infective doses per ml. Add 10% guinea pig complement to the diluted virus before adding the virus to the serum dilutions (1).

4. Inoculate 0.2 ml of each serum-virus mixture into duplicate roller tube cultures containing a light growth of HEp-2 cells.

5. At daily intervals after day 3, examine the virus control tubes for cytopathic effects.

6. Read the test when the virus control tubes exhibit cytopathic effects involving all or nearly all of the cell sheet (75 to 100% cytopathic effects).

7. Add neutral red at a final concentration of 1:80,000 to each tube and incubate the tubes for 1 h at 37°C. Neutral red stains the syncytia of respiratory syncytial viruses red and facilitates their visual identification with a scanning objective. After neutral red has been added to the roller-tube cultures, they must be protected from light, usually by wrapping the entire rack of tubes in aluminum foil; once ready for reading, the tubes should be examined quickly and protected as much as possible from stray light.

8. The endpoint is the dilution of serum which inhibits the formation of cytopathic effects so that no more than one-fourth of the cell sheet shows involvement by respiratory syncytial virus.

Measurement of neutralization antibody for the parainfluenza viruses

For the measurement of antibody to the four parainfluenza viruses, individual tests must be carried out with the specific virus type as the challenge virus in the neutralization test. Since the parainfluenza viruses do not usually produce cytopathic effects in cell culture, but do exhibit hemadsorption, the endpoint of the neutralization procedure is the demonstration of hemadsorption inhibition.

1. Inactivate serum specimens at 56°C for 30 min and prepare serial twofold dilutions in Eagle minimal essential medium without serum but containing the appropriate antibiotics. Usually, the dilutions tested include 1:4, 1:8, 1:16, 1:32, 1:64, and 1:128.

2. Mix equal volumes of each serum dilution and virus containing approximately 100 50% tissue culture infective doses per 0.1 ml, and incubate the mixture at room temperature for 1 h.

3. Inoculate duplicate roller-tube cultures of rhesus monkey kidney cells or equivalent with 0.2 ml of each virus-serum mixture.

4. Include virus (back titration) and serum controls.

5. Incubate cell cultures on a stationary rack at 37°C.

6. After day 3, test all virus control tubes for hemadsorption by adding 0.25 ml of a 0.4% solution of sterile guinea pig erythrocytes in saline. Once the erythrocytes have been added to the roller-tube cultures, refrigerate the tubes for 20 min and then examine them for hemadsorption. On the day the virus titration shows a titer between 32 and 100 50% tissue culture infective doses of virus, add erythrocytes to all tubes, refrigerate for 20 min, and read the test.

7. The endpoint is the dilution of serum showing complete inhibition of hemadsorption.

ELISA for measurement of antibodies to respiratory syncytial virus

The antibody response among children aged 1 to 3 months with respiratory syncytial virus infection usually is not detected by the complement fixation or the plaque reduction test (1, 8). All children in this age range are seropositive as a result of the presence of maternal antibody, and this can prevent the detection of increasing antibody levels by techniques less sensitive than the ELISA procedure. The ELISA procedure can detect fourfold or greater antibody rises to respiratory syncytial virus in 50% of infected children in this age group. The plaque reduction and ELISA tests are equally efficient in detecting antibody response after infection with respiratory syncytial virus in children older than 6 months.

Materials. (i) Respiratory syncytial virus antigen. Antigen is prepared by infecting cell cultures and harvesting both cells and supernatant after a single cycle of freezing and thawing; the antigen can be used without further purification. Harvests of HEp-2 cells produce sufficiently high-titered viral antigen so that it can be diluted 10-fold for use. Since some human sera cross-react with HEp-2 cells, harvests of infected African green monkey kidney cells and supernatant can be used as antigen, but antigen prepared in these monkey kidney cells generally must be used undiluted.

(ii) Plates. Soft polyvinyl microtiter plates (Dynatech Corp., Alexandria, Va.) bind the viral antigen efficiently.

(iii) Enzyme conjugate. A satisfactory goat anti-human IgG conjugated with alkaline phosphatase is available from Miles Laboratories, Inc., Elkhart, Ind.

Performance

1. Dilute respiratory syncytial virus, grown in HEp-2 cells, in carbonate buffer (pH 9.8) and add 75 µl to each well of round-bottom polyvinyl microtiter plates.

2. Add to control wells uninfected HEp-2 cells harvested and treated in the same manner.

3. Store plates coated with antigen for at least 14 h at 4°C in a moist chamber. Additional storage for at least 3 months does not result in loss of activity.

4. At the time of testing, wash the plates three times with a solution of PBS containing polysorbate (Tween 20) at a concentration of 0.5 ml/liter (PBS-Tween).

5. Prepare fourfold dilutions of serum in the antigen-coated plates, using PBS-Tween supplemented with 1% fetal calf serum and 10% uninfected cell suspension. Calf serum and control cell suspension may be added to the diluent to reduce the nonspecific binding of test serum (8). The final volume of diluted serum in each well is 75 μl. The initial well contains a final dilution of 1:100, and subsequent dilutions carry the serum to a final dilution of 1:25,600.

6. After overnight incubation at 4°C, wash the plates three times with PBS-Tween and add a 75-μl sample of a 1:100 dilution of the enzyme-linked globulin fraction of goat anti-human IgG serum (Miles Laboratories, Inc.). Allow the mixture to react for 2 h at 37°C. Wash the plates again three times with PBS-Tween and add 75 μl of p-nitrophenyl phosphate disodium substrate (Sigma 104; Sigma Chemical Co., St. Louis, Mo.) diluted to contain 1 mg in 1 ml of diethanolamine buffer (pH 9.8). After 15 min of incubation at 37°C, measure the amount of yellow color (produced by the action of the enzyme on the substrate) in a colorimeter at an absorbance of 400 nm, or estimate the endpoint by visual reading.

7. The endpoint is considered the highest dilution which gives an absorbance value of 0.35 or greater.

Identification of respiratory syncytial virus antigens in epithelial cells shed in nasal secretions

Rapid diagnosis of respiratory syncytial virus infection has gained widespread acceptance with the development of commercially available reagents for the detection of respiratory syncytial viral antigens in epithelial cells. With this procedure, a diagnosis of respiratory syncytial virus infection can be confirmed in 4 h (7). The immunofluorescence procedure is as follows.

1. An adequate number of cells must be collected from infected infants for this assay. This is best accomplished by obtaining a nasal wash with normal saline. Alternatively, rhinorrhea fluid can be swabbed from the nose, and the swab is then agitated in normal saline to form a suspension.

2. Cells are washed repeatedly in PBS (pH 7.4). Cells are then dropped onto microscope slides, allowed to dry, and then fixed in cold acetone (4°C or colder) for 10 min. Slides of fixed cells can then be stained immediately or stored at −70°C for future evaluation.

3. Bovine antibody to respiratory syncytial virus is overlaid onto the fixed cells and allowed to incubate at 37°C for 30 to 45 min. The dilution of antisera must be in accordance with the strength of the reagent. Control nasal washes must be run to avoid both false-positive and false-negative results. A positive control can be nasal mucosal cells from a known infected individual or infected WI-38 cells or another infected cell line with which the test serum does not cross-react.

4. The slides are then washed three times in PBS and overlaid with fluorescein-conjugated anti-bovine serum.

5. After 45 min at room temperature, these slides are again washed in PBS three times; they should be given a final wash in distilled water before they are dried and mounted in buffered glycerol (pH 8 to 9) for observation with an immunofluorescence microscope.

Measurement of secretory antibodies

The class-specific antibody response in nasal secretions to respiratory syncytial virus infection has been studied by immunofluorescence and ELISA techniques (4, 6). However, these tests are as yet unstandardized for quantiative measurements of virus-specific secretory antibody. Large variations in the quantity of IgA antibodies appearing in nasal secretions complicate the interpretation of measured antibody responses. The data obtained by ELISA or immunofluorescence assay can be handled in two ways: (i) the measured antibody level can be adjusted to the total IgA per 100 ml of sample secretion (usually 10 or 20 mg of IgA per 100 ml of sample), or (ii) the measured antibody level may be interpreted as either the presence or absence of IgA antibody. The adjustment of titers based on milligrams of IgA per sample as a basis for quantitating antibody level has been questioned because of (i) the difficulty in measuring immunoglobulin concentrations in secretions, (ii) the possible production of antibodies directed against several antigens of the IgA class simultaneously with the production of the anti-respiratory syncytial virus antibodies, and (iii) variations in specimen collection procedure and anatomical location of the specimen collection.

REAGENTS

Small amounts of certified antigens for complement fixation and hemagglutination inhibition tests can be obtained from the Centers for Disease Control, Atlanta, Ga. These antigens should be used to evaluate and standardize commercial reagents. Seed virus for complement fixation and hemagglutination inhibition or virus neutralization tests is available from the American Type Culture Collection, Rockville, Md., and the Infectious Diseases Branch, National Institute of Allergy and Infectious Diseases, Bethesda, Md.

COMMERCIAL SOURCES

Complement fixation and hemagglutination inhibition antigens: M. A. Bioproducts, Walkersville, Md., and Flow Laboratories, Inc., McLean, Va.

Complement: Biological Laboratories, Inc., Fort Worth, Tex.

Cell culture media: M. A. Bioproducts; Flow Laboratories; GIBCO Laboratories, Grand Island, N.Y.

Methyl cellulose: Dow Chemical Co., Midland, Mich.

Immunofluorescence reagents for respiratory syncytial virus: Burroughs Wellcome, Research Triangle Park, N.C.

These reagents are also available from other sources. It behooves each user to evaluate the quality of purchased reagents.

Chapter 83

Rubella Virus

MAX A. CHERNESKY AND JAMES B. MAHONY

Reliable laboratory technology has been developed for (i) determination of immune status to rubella, (ii) diagnosis of postnatal rubella, and (iii) diagnosis of congenital rubella. Because antibody responses are rapid and specific and virus isolation procedures are slow and expensive, serological procedures are usually performed in disease diagnosis (the exception would be virus isolation in a congenitally infected newborn).

Immunity screening and infection diagnosis may be performed separately or together through the application of one or more of the following tests: passive hemagglutination (passive HA), latex agglutination, radial hemolysis, hemagglutination inhibition (HI), solid-phase immunoassay (SPIA), complement fixation (CF), neutralization, mixed hemadsorption, or time-resolved fluoroimmunoassay. Some of the newer techniques are quite sensitive and lend themselves to automation.

Although different methods are used in different laboratories to screen for immune status and to investigate sera for the diagnosis of rubella, we employ a passive HA test (Rubacell II; Abbott Laboratories, North Chicago, Ill.) on a routine basis with satisfactory results. All negative tests are confirmed at the end of each week by employing SPIA. Because Rubacell antibodies rise slowly after infection, this combination of tests may serve as a sentinel to rubella activity in the community.

Special cases with plateau HI titers are assayed by CF. If a change in titer is not achieved by CF, the sera may be fractionated by sucrose density gradient centrifugation and the immunoglobulin M (IgM) fraction may be tested by HI. Alternatively, whole sera may be tested by SPIA for rubella-specific IgM.

CLINICAL INDICATIONS

Rubella is a benign, self-limiting disease, usually of childhood, which is characterized by mild upper respiratory symptoms, suboccipital lymphadenopathy, and an erythematous rash. Mild complications of arthralgias and arthritis may occur after the disappearance of rash in young adults. The prime indication for laboratory diagnosis of rubella resides in the potential risk of this disease to the fetuses of women in the early stages of pregnancy. Susceptibility to rubella virus can be altered by administering live virus vaccine. Women of childbearing age should be assessed by antibody analysis for susceptibility to rubella; those found susceptible should be vaccinated with due regard taken for the potential dangers of vaccination during pregnancy. Some physicians determine the rubella antibody status of pregnant women at the patient's first prenatal visit. Those without antibodies are monitored through early pregnancy for seroconversion, and if negative, they are immunized postpartum.

Investigation of the pregnant patient who has been in contact with another person with rubella presents a challenge for a rapid and accurate serological diagnosis. If the patient develops clinical signs, a serum specimen should be collected at that time and paired with a second serum within 5 days. Both are investigated in parallel (same test, same day). A fourfold or greater rise in HI, CF, or neutralization antibodies, together with clinical symptoms, is diagnostic for recent infection. Alternatively, a significant change in optical densities or binding ratios of the sera would be diagnostic in SPIA. A seroconversion in any patient is conclusive for recent rubella infection. If SPIA is available for rubella IgM testing, a single serum collected more than 4 days after onset of rash can usually yield a positive diagnosis (2). Patients without clinical symptoms but with rising titers to rubella (the first serum containing antibodies) pose a special problem. They may have a primary infection or reinfection with a secondary antibody boost. To confirm these cases, a rubella IgM determination may be performed. The absence of late-rising passive HA or CF antibodies in the first serum of this type of patient would provide evidence that the infection was primary. The third type of case involves the patient whose sera are collected several days after the infection, when all serological tests are in plateau (Fig. 1). Testing for IgM may be helpful. If time is available, a third serum collected several weeks later and run in parallel with the others may demonstrate a fourfold decline in titer, which would be diagnostic. Serological examination of the suspected contacts may also be helpful in this situation.

The newborn infant who is of low birth weight for gestational age and who might have any one of a variety of symptoms (i.e., microcephaly, hepatosplenomegaly, thrombocytopenia, etc.) is a prime candidate to be investigated for congenital rubella. Specimens such as throat washings, urine, etc., should be submitted for virus isolation, and sera from the mother and infant can be examined. If the mother does not have rubella antibodies or has a very low titer, it is unlikely that the baby has congenital rubella. Serological investigation could involve two approaches. One approach is to make serial determinations of rubella HI or SPIA antibodies during the first 6 months of life; a persistence of titer in the infant during this time (Fig. 2) is highly suggestive of congenital rubella. As a second approach, the demonstration of rubella-specific IgM antibody in the infant's serum would be diagnostic of congenital rubella.

TEST PROCEDURES

Two popular passive HA tests are available from commercial sources (Rubacell II, Abbott; PHAST, Calbiochem-Behring, La Jolla, Calif.). Rubacell antibodies parallel CF and neutralization responses after

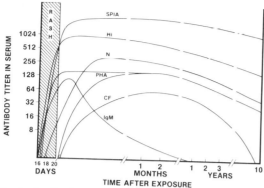

FIG. 1. Antibody responses to rubella virus infection. N, Neutralization; PHA, passive HA (PHAST, early rise; Rubacell, late rise).

infection, whereas PHAST responses are more closely aligned with HI and SPIA. Both antibodies remain measurable for years after infection or immunization as an index of immunity. Rubacell employs human erythrocytes, stabilized with formaldehyde-pyruvic aldehyde, which have been sensitized with a soluble rubella virus antigen (J. W. Safford, Jr., and R. Whittington, Fed. Proc. **35**:813, 1976). The erythroyctes agglutinate in the presence of specific rubella antibody. To perform the test, 25 μl of phosphate buffer is added to V-bottom microwells. Specimens, as well as positive and negative controls, are added (10 μl) and then mixed before the addition of 25 μl of the sensitized cells. We routinely set up alongside the test sera a row of erythrocytes without soluble rubella antigen as a control, which allows more objective scoring of results. The plates are incubated for 2 h at room temperature. A button of erythrocytes signifies the absence of antibody (susceptibility to rubella), whereas a disperse settling of erythrocytes indicates a positive reaction (immunity to rubella).

Radial hemolysis, which is popular in Europe, can be used to screen large numbers of sera by preparing plates in advance and storing them at 4°C. We have successfully used the method of Russell et al. (7). Freshly drawn sheep erythrocytes are washed with dextrose-gelatin-Veronal buffer, treated with 2.5 mg of trypsin (Difco, Detroit, Mich.) per ml in dextrose-gelatin-Veronal for 1 h at room temperature, and sensitized with rubella HA antigen (Flow Laboratories, McLean, Va.; 240 hemagglutination units [HAU] per ml) in HEPES (N-2-hydroxyethylpiperazine-N'-2-ethanesulfonic acid)-saline-albumin-gelatin buffer (HSAG) (pH 6.2) for 1 h at 4°C. Sensitized erythrocytes (0.15 ml of a 50% suspension) are mixed with 0.4 ml of guinea pig complement (Behringwerke, Marburg, West Germany) and then added to 10 ml of 0.8% agarose preheated to 43°C and poured into a square petri dish (100 by 15 mm). Plates can be stored at 4°C and used for up to 14 days. Prepoured radial hemolysis plates are available from Orion Diagnostics, Helsinki, Finland. Sera are inactivated at 56°C for 30 min, pipetted into 3-mm-diameter wells punched in the agarose, and allowed to diffuse overnight at 4°C in a humidified atmosphere. Plates are then incubated for 2 h at 37°C. Plates with incomplete hemolysis are flooded with 4 ml of guinea pig complement (diluted

1:3) and reincubated. All sera are tested in control plates containing unsensitized erythrocytes to monitor nonspecific hemolysis. Zones of hemolysis in control plates range from 3.5 to 5 mm in diameter. Zone diameters of >5 mm are taken to indicate immunity.

Two very rapid agglutination tests are commercially available and are predominantly used for immunity screening. Rubascan (Hynson, Westcott and Dunning, Baltimore, Md.) employs antigen-coated latex particles, and the test is performed on a card. Rubaquick (Abbott) is an agglutination test using rubella antigen-coated erythrocytes which are stabilized. The test is performed in a tray. Both kits lend themselves to processing smaller numbers of specimens.

Although different laboratories use modifications of the standard rubella HI test, the following is a description of the test which we have found consistently to give good results. The test is conveniently performed in disposable plastic or vinyl V-bottom microtiter plates. The rubella hemagglutinating antigen is titrated each time the test is performed. Serial two-fold dilutions of the antigen are made in 0.025 ml of HSAG (pH 6.2) to which 0.05 ml of a 0.25% washed suspension of pigeon erythrocytes is added. Control cups containing no antigen are included. The plates are sealed and placed at 4°C for 1 h, after which time they are placed at room temperature for 15 min before being read. The highest dilution that produces a pattern of complete hemagglutination is considered 1 HAU; 4 HAU is used in the HI test.

Before the HI test is performed, nonspecific inhibitors of hemagglutination and nonspecific agglutinins must be removed from sera. Test serum (0.1 ml) is added to 0.1 ml of HSAG and 0.6 ml of a 25% suspension of kaolin. The suspension is mixed and allowed to sit at room temperature for 20 min with frequent agitation. The kaolin is pelleted in a clinical centrifuge, and the supernatant fluid is transferred to a clean tube containing 0.05 ml of a 50% suspension of pigeon erythrocytes. After 60 min of incubation at 4°C the erythrocytes are centrifuged, and the supernatant fluid is removed and heated at 56°C for 30 min. This final sample, which represents a dilution of 1:8, is now ready to be incorporated into the test. Alternatively, nonspecific inhibitors may be removed by precipitation with heparin and manganous chloride. The serum sample is diluted 1:4 with 0.15 M NaCl. To each 0.8 ml of diluted serum are added 0.03 ml of sodium

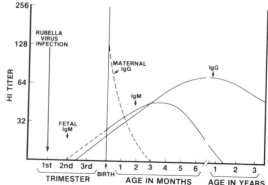

FIG. 2. Antibody responses in an infant congenitally infected with rubella virus.

applied in coating buffer to microtiter plates wells. After incubation and rinsing, Lassa virus antigen (Vero cell supernatant fluid inactivated by β-propriolactone or gamma radiation) is added, incubated, and rinsed. Test serum dilutions are added, incubated, and washed. Alkaline phosphatase-labeled anti-IgG is then added, incubated, and washed, followed by p-nitrophenylphosphate substrate in diethanolamine buffer. The reaction is read spectrophotometrically after 20 min at room temperature.

A μ-capture ELISA is used to measure IgM content. Goat anti-IgM is adsorbed to test wells and washed. Test serum dilutions are added, incubated, and washed, followed by Lassa virus antigen. After incubation and washing, guinea pig anti-Lassa virus IgG is added, incubated, and washed, followed by goat anti-guinea pig IgG. The plate is incubated and washed, p-nitrophenylphosphate substrate is added, and the reaction is read after 20 min as described above. For both IgG and IgM tests, samples are run on plates with Lassa virus antigen and on plates with uninfected Vero cell culture fluids substituted for antigen. A sample is considered positive if the difference in optical density between antigen-positive and control wells is more than the mean difference, testing 20 known negative sera + 3 standard deviations.

Although still being developed, ELISA for measurement of viral specific IgG and IgM antibodies may offer some advantages over the IFA test. The chief advantage is in testing sera with high background activity, which occur frequently in collections from seroepidemiology surveys in Africa. In the IFA test, these sticky sera produce bright green fluorescence in the uninfected control cells and sometimes preclude the detection of specific fluorescence in infected cells. Although these sera also produce high background activities in the antibody ELISA tests, this nonspecific binding can be quantitated in control antigen wells and subtracted from the optical density obtained in positive antigen wells, which in some cases allows interpretation of results. ELISA procedures have not yet been reported for Ebola, Marburg, Junin, Machupo, or LCM virus; for Lassa virus the procedures have yet to be field tested.

Neutralization tests

Neutralization tests for these viruses take many forms; depending on the virus, neutralization tests range from extremely sensitive and reliable (e.g., with Junin and Machupo viruses) to moderately insensitive but reliable (with Lassa and LCM viruses) to totally unreliable (with Marburg and Ebola viruses). The common denominator in all neutralization tests is measurement of an inhibition of viral replication by reaction with immune serum. Thus, the form of the test is determined in part by the availability of tools to measure infectious virus or viral antigens (e.g., direct fluorescent antibody, CF, or ELISA procedures, plaques, or animal infectivity) as well as the kinetics of the virus-antibody interactions. The unreliability of the Marburg and Ebola virus neutralization tests may be partially due to the primitive and cumbersome viral quantitation procedures available as well as to

low-avidity antibody. For the New World arenaviruses (Junin and Machupo), the most generally applied neutralization test is a plaque reduction test with Vero cells and the serum dilution-constant virus format. The serum dilution calculated (by probit analysis) to reduce the control number of plaques by 50% is usually taken as the endpoint, although in some laboratories, the highest serum dilution producing 80% reduction is used. The 80% plaque reduction test is commonly used to distinguish Junin from Machupo virus. For Lassa and LCM viruses, neutralizing antibody activity is rapidly lost on dilution; for this reason, the constant serum dilution-varying virus format is preferred. Neutralization of Old World arenaviruses is also markedly enhanced by the addition of complement; thus, 10% fresh guinea pig serum is routinely added to the diluent. Plaque reduction is further enhanced by the addition of either anti-immunoglobulin or protein A. Plaque reduction tests in various formats have largely replaced animal protection tests, which were notoriously imprecise for the measurement of arenavirus-neutralizing antibody.

LITERATURE CITED

1. **Casals, J.** 1977. Serologic reactions with arenaviruses. Medicina (Buenos Aires) **37**(Suppl. 3):59–68.
2. **Centers for Disease Control.** 1983. Viral hemorrhagic fever: initial management of suspected and confirmed cases. Morbid. Mortal. Weekly Rep. **32**(Suppl.):27S–40S.
3. **Centers for Disease Control and National Institutes of Health.** 1983. Biosafety in microbiological and biomedical laboratories. Centers for Disease Control, Atlanta.
4. **Goldwasser, R. A., L. H. Elliott, and K. M. Johnson.** 1980. Preparation and use of erythrocyte-globulin conjugates to Lassa virus in reversed passive hemagglutination and inhibition. J. Clin. Microbiol. **11**:593–599.
5. **International Committee on Taxonomy of Viruses.** 1982. Arenaviruses. Intervirology **17**:119–122.
6. **Jahrling, P. B.** 1985. Marburg virus, Ebola virus, and the arenaviruses, p. 796–804. In E. H. Lennette, A. Balows, W. J. Hausler, Jr., and H. J. Shadomy (ed.), Manual of clinical microbiology, 4th ed. American Society for Microbiology, Washington, D.C.
7. **Jahrling, P. B., B. S. Niklasson, and J. B. McCormick.** 1985. Early diagnosis of human Lassa fever by ELISA detection of antigen and antibody. Lancet **i**:250–252.
8. **Johnson, K. M., L. H. Elliott, and D. L. Heymann.** 1981. Preparation of polyvalent viral immunofluorescent intracellular antigens and use in human serosurveys. J. Clin. Microbiol. **14**:527–529.
9. **Kiley, M. P., E. T. W. Bowen, G. A. Eddy, M. Isaacson, K. M. Johnson, J. B. McCormick, F. A. Murphy, S. R. Pattyn, D. Peters, O. W. Prozesky, R. L. Regnery, D. I. H. Simpson, W. Slenczka, P. Sureau, G. Van der Groen, P. A. Webb, and H. Wulff.** 1982. Filoviridae: taxonomic home for Marburg and Ebola viruses? Intervirology **18**:24–32.
10. **Murphy, F. A., and S. G. Whitfield.** 1975. Morphology and morphogenesis of arenaviruses. Bull. W.H.O. **52**:409–419.
11. **Niklasson, B. S., P. B. Jahrling, and C. J. Peters.** 1984. Detection of Lassa virus antigens and virus-specific immunoglobulins G and M by enzyme-linked immunosorbent assay. J. Clin. Microbiol. **20**:239–244.
12. **Richman, D. D., P. H. Cleveland, J. B. McCormick, and K. M. Johnson.** 1983. Antigenic analysis of strains of Ebola virus: identification of two Ebola virus serotypes. J. Infect. Dis. **147**:268–271.

Chapter 86

Enteroviruses and Reoviruses

NATHALIE J. SCHMIDT

ENTEROVIRUSES

Introduction

The human enterovirus group, which is classified as a genus within the family *Picornaviridae*, consists of 67 distinct antigenic types. These include 3 polioviruses, 29 coxsackieviruses, 31 echoviruses, and 4 more recently recognized types which are classified as enterovirus types 68 through 71 without being assigned to any of the three subgroups. Hepatitis A virus has also been classified as a picornavirus which closely resembles enteroviruses, but different techniques are required for antibody assay because the virus replicates poorly in cell culture. Heterotypic, as well as homotypic, antibody responses commonly occur in human enterovirus infections, but unfortunately the heterotypic responses are not consistent enough or sufficiently well defined to permit the use of one or a few antigens for group-specific serologic diagnosis.

The neutralization test continues to be the most reliable serologic procedure for detection of type-specific enterovirus antibodies. Hemagglutination-inhibiting (HI) antibodies closely parallel neutralizing antibodies, but the HI test is severely limited by the fact that only about one-third of the enterovirus immunotypes contain strains which agglutinate erythrocytes (RBC). The complement fixation (CF) test is useful for serodiagnosis of poliovirus infections, but not for other enterovirus infections. In coxsackievirus infections, heterotypic CF antibody responses generally prevent type-specific diagnosis, and, further, high levels of CF antibody are often present in acute-phase sera, making it impossible to demonstrate diagnostically significant increases in antibody titer between acute- and convalescent-phase serum specimens. In echovirus infections heterotypic antibody responses are also a drawback to the CF test, and, in addition, some infected individuals fail to show a CF antibody response, even to the infecting virus type.

Various physical and chemical treatments of enterovirus antigens change the type-specific reactivity of the virion antigen to the heterotypic reactivity of procapsids, or H antigens; these treatments include heat inactivation at 56°C, acetone fixation for immunofluorescence staining, and fixation or adsorption onto microtiter plates. Therefore, indirect immunofluorescence staining (6) and enzyme immunoassays and radioimmunoassays which use antigen adsorbed to a solid phase (1, 4, 10) have not shown type specificity for assay of coxsackievirus and echovirus antibodies in human sera and thus have not been useful for serodiagnosis or for determination of past infections.

Immunoglobulin M (IgM) antibodies to enteroviruses can be assayed by neutralization tests on serum fractions separated by sucrose density gradient centrifugation (9) or, in the case of certain coxsackieviruses, by simpler immunodiffusion (9) or counterimmunoelectrophoresis (7) procedures. Enzyme immunoassays for coxsackievirus IgM antibodies which are based upon the "capture" of IgM antibodies by anti-IgM antibodies on a solid phase have also been described (8, 10), but their reliability requires further evaluation. The persistence and type specificity of enterovirus IgM antibody responses need to be better defined in human infections to establish the diagnostic value of IgM antibody assays.

Clinical indications

Although serologic methods are not generally used for laboratory diagnosis of enterovirus infections, neutralization tests may be employed in outbreak situations where the predominating enterovirus type(s) is known and tests can be limited to one or a few virus types. Tests against selected virus types may also be used in certain clinical syndromes in which only certain immunotypes have been implicated, e.g., hand-foot-and-mouth disease, acute hemorrhagic conjunctivitis, pleurodynia, or paralytic illness. Neutralizing antibody assays performed against the virus type isolated from a patient may strengthen the etiologic role of the isolate in the patient's illness; the demonstration of a significant rise in antibody titer establishes a temporal association of the enterovirus infection with the current illness. Neutralizing antibody assays for polioviruses are the only reliable means for determining immunity status, since CF antibodies persist for only a short time after infection and often are not produced in response to vaccination.

Although the neutralization test is the most reliable method for detection of enterovirus antibodies, its diagnostic value is limited to some extent by the rapid development of neutralizing antibodies in response to infection, which may preclude the demonstration of a diagnostically significant increase in antibody titer. Thus, early collection of the acute-phase serum specimen is particularly important.

Virus isolation is the most suitable method for laboratory diagnosis of enterovirus infections, but paired sera should also be submitted to the laboratory to be used in supporting the etiologic role of an enterovirus isolate, and also to rule out other viral infections which produce similar syndromes and for which satisfactory in vitro serologic tests are available, e.g. herpes simplex virus, mumps virus, and certain vector-borne viruses.

Test procedure

Enterovirus neutralization tests are based upon the ability of specific antibody to combine with virus and render it noninfectious for a susceptible host cell. Tests are performed in cell cultures in tubes or, more economically, in micro cell cultures grown in wells in plastic plates, and inhibition of the viral cytopathic effect (neutralization) is determined by microscopic reading. The cells most commonly employed are primary cynomolgus, grivet, or rhesus monkey kidney, human fetal diploid fibroblast lines, or continuous monkey kidney cell lines such as the BS-C-1 or Vero lines of grivet monkey kidney cells. Tube and bottle cultures or suspensions of these cell types are widely available from commercial sources. Detailed methods for initiating cultures and subpassaging various types of cells are given elsewhere (5). A satisfactory cell culture maintenance medium for enterovirus neutralization tests is Eagle minimal essential medium supplemented with 2% inactivated fetal bovine serum.

Seed enterovirus preparations produced under the auspices of the Research Resources Branch of the National Institutes of Health are available from the American Type Culture Collection, Rockville, Md., and these can be used to prepare working stocks. Before they are used in neutralization tests, the identity of stock virus preparations should be confirmed by testing against homotypic immune serum prepared in another, reliable laboratory. Well-characterized enterovirus reference antisera can be obtained from the American Type Culture Collection.

Certain enterovirus strains, or certain preparations of a virus type, may have a strong tendency to aggregate and thus to be insusceptible to neutralization by homologous antisera. If it is necessary to use such a preparation for neutralization tests, virus can be disaggregated by treatment with sodium deoxycholate or chloroform (3). Chloroform-treated virus preparations may be less toxic to cell cultures than are deoxycholate-treated preparations. Nine volumes of an undiluted virus suspension are shaken with 1 volume of chloroform for 15 min at room temperature, and after the mixture is centrifuged for 15 min at $1,500 \times g$, the supernatant fluid phase is removed for use in the test. For deoxycholate treatment, 1 volume of a 1% solution of sodium deoxycholate (prepared in distilled water) is mixed with 9 volumes of virus preparation; this is stirred on a Vortex mixer for 1 min and then incubated at 37°C for 15 min.

1. Infectivity titers of enterovirus preparations to be used as challenge virus are determined in the same cell type and culture vessels to be used for neutralization tests. Log_{10} dilutions of the virus are prepared in maintenance medium, and each dilution is inoculated into four tube cultures in a volume of 0.1 ml (0.05 ml for micro cell cultures). Tests are incubated at 36 to 37°C for 7 days and examined microscopically for viral cytopathic effect (CPE). The 50% tissue culture infective dose (TCD_{50}) endpoint is calculated by the method of Karber or Reed and Muench (5). The dilution of virus preparation containing a challenge dose of 100 TCD_{50} is determined by adding 2 to the negative log of the titer. Example: TCD_{50} titer = $10^{-6.0}$ per 0.1 ml; $-6.0 + 2.0 = -4.0$ = log of dilution of virus preparation containing 100 TCD_{50} in 0.1 ml.

2. Test sera are heated at 56°C for 30 min to inactivate heat-labile, nonspecific viral inhibitory substances, and twofold dilutions are prepared in maintenance medium.

3. Equal volumes of the serum dilutions and test virus diluted to contain 100 TCD_{50} per 0.1 ml are mixed and incubated at room temperature or 37°C for 1 h.

4. As a control on the test dose of virus, the working dilution and successive 10-fold dilutions prepared from this dilution are mixed with equal volumes of maintenance medium and incubated under the same conditions as the serum-virus mixtures. This control indicates the infectious dose of virus actually present in the test. A test dose below 32 TCD_{50} may give falsely high antibody titers, and one above 320 TCD_{50} may result in an insensitive test, as low levels of antibody may fail to neutralize the large challenge virus dose.

5. The serum-virus mixtures and virus-diluent mixtures are inoculated into tube cultures in a volume of 0.2 ml. Generally, two cell cultures are inoculated with each serum-virus mixture and four receive each virus dilution.

6. Known high- and low-titered positive sera and a negative serum should be included as controls in each run. The titers of the positive sera should vary by no more than twofold from their median titers, and the negative serum should show no neutralization.

7. Tests are incubated at 36 to 37°C and observed at 2- to 3-day intervals; final readings are made when the virus control shows that 100 TCD_{50} is present in the test. The antibody endpoint is the highest initial dilution of serum that inhibits CPE of the test virus dose.

Modifications for micro cell cultures

Cell cultures are prepared in microtiter plates with flat-bottom wells that have been processed for cell culture. BS-C-1 or human fetal diploid lung cells are suspended in growth medium (90% Eagle minimal essential medium and 10% fetal bovine serum) at a concentration of 100,000 to 150,000 cells per ml and planted in a volume of 0.2 ml per well. The plates are incubated in a CO_2 incubator for 2 to 3 days until the cells become confluent. Growth medium is then removed from each cup and replaced with 0.1 ml of maintenance medium (98% Eagle minimal essential medium and 2% fetal bovine serum).

Virus is diluted to contain 100 TCD_{50} in a volume of 0.05 ml, and serum-virus mixtures or virus-diluent mixtures are added in a volume of 0.1 ml per well.

Plates are incubated at 36 to 37°C in a 5% CO_2 atmosphere. A regular incubator can be used if 0.1 ml of sterile mineral oil (350 Seybold units viscosity) is added to each well and the plates are sealed with heavy Paklon tape. Alternatively, a HEPES (N-2-hydroxyethylpiperazine-N'-2-ethanesulfonic acid) buffer can be used in the medium and plates can be incubated in a humidified chamber in a regular incubator.

Tests are read using an inverted microscope.

Metabolic inhibition tests have been developed for large-scale enterovirus neutralizing antibody assays, e.g., for surveys to determine immunity status to polioviruses. The tests are based upon differences in the color of the phenol red indicator in cell cultures degenerated by virus (red) and in those protected by neutralizing antibody (yellow). The chief advantage of these tests is that they can be read visually without microscopic observation. The methods are described in detail elsewhere (5).

A few of the group A coxsackieviruses can be propagated only in suckling mice, and neutralization tests must be performed in this host system (5). However, these virus types appear to be of minor clinical importance, and serologic diagnosis is rarely attempted.

Interpretation

A fourfold or greater increase in neutralizing antibody titer to an enterovirus usually indicates a current infection with that virus type. Occasionally, however, there is recall of neutralizing antibody to closely related enteroviruses with which the patient has been previously infected, and this may confuse type-specific diagnosis, particularly in group B coxsackievirus infections. When neutralizing antibody titer rises occur to more than one enterovirus type, it is sometimes possible to identify the current infecting type by the fact that antibody is absent or at a low level in the acute-phase serum, while elevated titers of antibody to previous infecting virus types may be present.

REOVIRUSES

Introduction

Reoviruses of each of the three serotypes have been isolated from individuals with a wide variety of clinical syndromes, but their role in the etiology of human disease has not been well established. Most infections are inapparent and are acquired early in life. Antibody assays are rarely done for serodiagnosis of reovirus infections, but, as in the case of enteroviruses, they may be performed on individuals from whom virus is isolated in an effort to strengthen the association of the isolate with the patient's illness.

One important application of reovirus antibody assays is in monitoring infections in rodent colonies used for virus research and for preparation of viral immune reagents.

Methods available for assay of reovirus antibodies include HI, neutralization, and CF tests. Enzyme immunoassays and solid-phase immunofluorescence systems are now coming into use for serologic surveys in laboratory animals, and test components, or monitoring services employing these tests, are commercially available. The HI test has been the standard method for assay of reovirus antibodies because of its relative simplicity and its sensitivity, but it may be replaced in the future by newer immunoassays. Neutralization tests often lack sensitivity because low levels of antibody may fail to neutralize the large test doses of virus which are required to produce CPE in cell culture systems. Many infected individuals fail to produce detectable levels of reovirus CF antibody. On the other hand, most reovirus infections elicit the production of HI antibody. The HI test is based upon the fact that reoviruses have protein sites on their surfaces (hemagglutinins) which attach to human RBC (and bovine RBC in the case of reovirus type 3) and agglutinate them. This hemagglutination reaction is inhibited if specific antibody has reacted with the virus before the addition of the RBC.

HI test procedure

The following HI procedure is conducted by the microtiter method in "V" plates. The diluent used for erythrocytes, antigen, and serum is 0.01 M phosphate-buffered saline (pH 7.4) containing 0.2% bovine serum albumin.

Standardization of indicator (human group O) RBC suspension. RBC suspensions standardized by the cyanmethemoglobin (CMG) method (2) give the most accurate and reliable results, and the method is applicable for use with a wide variety of spectrophotometers. An alternative, but less satisfactory, method is to prepare an 0.5% suspension of RBC based upon packed cell volume. The CMG method is based upon lysing the RBC, converting the hemoglobin released to CMG with a reagent containing potassium cyanide and potassium ferricyanide (Cyanmethemoglobin Reagent; Boehringer Mannheim Diagnostics, Indianapolis, Ind.), and then reading the concentration of CMG against a standard on a spectrophotometer.

(i) Construction of a standard CMG curve. CMG is diluted in CMG reagent to contain 80, 60, 40, 20, and 0 (blank) mg of CMG per 100 ml. The optical density (OD) of each dilution is read on a spectrophotometer at 540-μm wavelength. These readings should fall on a straight line when plotted on regular graph paper against the milligrams of CMG per 100 ml.

(ii) Calculation of the factor to be used in determining the target OD. For each spectrophotometer the factor to be used in determining the target OD must be calculated from the OD readings obtained for the standards: Factor = sum of concentrations (milligrams of CMG per 100 ml) of standards (80 + 60 + 40 + 20 + 0) divided by the sum of the OD readings of the standards.

(iii) Calculation of the target OD for the 0.5% RBC suspension. Target OD = target milligrams of CMG per 100 ml, divided by the factor. In the case of an 0.5% suspension of mammalian erythrocytes, the target milligrams of CMG per 100 ml is 6.255.

The factor and target OD can be used for subsequent standardizations with the spectrophotometer if the instrument is not moved or unduly jarred. The reliability of the instrument should be checked before each use by reading the OD of the 40-mg/100 ml CMG standard; this standard will remain stable for several months if kept refrigerated and free of contamination.

(iv) Washing RBC. Human group O RBC collected in Alsever solution should be stored at 4°C for 18 to 24 h before use. The blood is then filtered through gauze, and the cells are washed three times in physiological saline by centrifugation at 700 × g for 7 min. The RBC are then packed in a graduated centrifuge tube at 700 × g for 10 min, and the volume of packed cells is noted. The supernatant fluid is removed, and a 4% suspension of RBC is prepared in dextrose-gelatin-Veronal solution in a volume sufficient to dilute for the day's test.

(v) Standardization of the 0.5% working dilution of human group O RBC.

1. One ml of the 4% suspension of RBC is transferred to a 25-ml volumetric flask, and 0.1 ml of a 5% aqueous saponin solution is added to enhance lysis of the cells. The flask is then filled to the mark with CMG reagent, and the contents are mixed well.

2. After standing at room temperature for 5 to 10 min, the OD of the solution is read at 540-μm wavelength against the reagent blank.

3. The dilution necessary to adjust the 4% RBC suspension to the desired OD for the 0.5% suspension is calculated:

$$\frac{\text{OD of 4\% suspension} \times \text{volume of 4\% suspension (1 ml)}}{\text{target OD}} = \text{dilution factor}$$

The 4% RBC suspension is diluted appropriately to prepare the working suspension, which is stored at 4°C until added to the test. A working suspension of RBC should be used only for a single day's tests.

Antigen titration. Reovirus hemagglutinating antigens are generally prepared from infected rhesus or cynomolgus monkey kidney cell cultures. The cells and fluids are harvested 72 h after the cultures show maximum viral CPE, frozen and thawed three times, and stored at −70°C. Reovirus type 3 antigen is commercially available. Before being used in the test, antigens are clarified by low-speed centrifugation (700 × g for 10 min).

1. Duplicate twofold dilutions of each antigen (starting with undiluted) are prepared in a volume of 0.025 ml using microdiluters.

2. To each antigen dilution is added 0.025 ml of diluent. Three wells in the plate receive only 0.05 ml of diluent. These are "cell controls" to indicate whether the RBC settle properly under the conditions of the test.

3. To each antigen and cell control well is added 0.025 ml of the standardized 0.5% human group O RBC suspension, and the reagents are mixed by shaking the plates or agitating them on a vibrating platform.

4. Tests are incubated at 37°C for 1 h, or until the RBC in the cell control wells settle into a tight button. Tests may also be incubated at room temperature, but settling of the RBC may require a longer time.

5. The endpoint of the antigen titration is the highest dilution producing complete agglutination of the RBC. This represents 1 hemagglutinating (HA) unit, and antigen is diluted to contain 4 HA units in a volume of 0.025 ml for the test proper. Example: final titer = 1:32; 1/32 × 4 = 1/8, or a 1:8 dilution of antigen contains 4 HA units.

6. The antigen concentration of the working dilution is checked before it is used in the test proper. Five dilutions are prepared in duplicate from the working dilution. To the first wells in each set is added 0.05 ml of antigen. Using microdiluters, four serial twofold dilutions are prepared from this in 0.025-ml volumes. The wells thus contain 4, 2, 1, 0.5, and 0.25 units of antigen. To each antigen well is added 0.025 ml of diluent, and wells containing 0.05 ml of diluent are prepared for cell controls. Each well then receives 0.025 ml of the 0.5% suspension of RBC, and the tests are mixed and incubated as described above. The first three antigen dilutions (containing 4, 2, and 1 HA units) should show complete agglutination, the fourth should show partial or no agglutination, and no agglutination should appear in the fifth. The antigen concentration of the working dilution is adjusted upward or downward as necessary.

HI test. For serodiagnosis of reovirus infection, acute- and convalescent-phase sera are tested in parallel in the same run against antigens to each of the reovirus types.

1. To remove nonspecific (nonantibody) inhibitors of reovirus hemagglutination, sera diluted 1:4 are absorbed with an equal volume of a 25% suspension of acid-washed kaolin (25 g of kaolin in 100 ml of phosphate-buffered saline, pH 7.4) for 20 min at room temperature with occasional shaking. After centrifugation at 700 × g for 15 min to sediment the kaolin, the supernatant fluid, representing approximately a 1:8 dilution of absorbed serum, is removed.

2. Human sera do not require absorption with human group O RBC, but animal sera must be absorbed to remove natural agglutinins. To each milliliter of kaolin-treated serum is added 0.1 ml of a 50% suspension of human group O RBC. After incubation at 4°C for 1 to 2 h, the RBC are sedimented by centrifugation at 700 × g for 15 min at 4°C, and the supernatant fluid (absorbed serum) is removed. Occasionally natural agglutinins encountered in animal sera may be absorbed more effectively at room temperature or 37°C than at 4°C. Sera are not heat inactivated for testing.

3. Twofold dilutions of serum (from 1:8 through 1:2,048) are prepared in 0.025-ml volumes for tests against each of the three reovirus antigen types, and dilutions of 1:8 through 1:32 are prepared in the same volumes for a "serum control." This set of dilutions receives diluent rather than antigen and indicates whether the test serum itself agglutinates the indicator erythrocytes.

4. The working dilution (continuing 4 HA units) of each reovirus antigen is added to the appropriate set of serum dilutions in a volume of 0.025 ml, and 0.025 ml of diluent is added to each of the serum control wells.

5. Again, controls on the working dilution of antigen are prepared as indicated in step 6 of antigen titration (above).

6. Cell control wells containing 0.025 ml of diluent are prepared.

7. Tests are incubated for 1 h at room temperature.

8. To each well is added 0.025 ml of the 0.5% human group O RBC suspension, and the contents of the wells are mixed.

9. Tests are incubated at 37°C for 1 h, or at room temperature until the RBC in the cell control wells show proper settling.

10. The HI antibody titer of a serum is the highest dilution which completely inhibits hemagglutination by the 4 units of test antigen.

The controls in the test should show the following results. Agglutination should not occur in the serum control dilutions; if it does, the test on that serum cannot be considered valid unless the inhibition titer of the serum is fourfold higher than the titer of natural agglutinins. The "back titration" of the working dilution of antigen should show the results indicated in step 6 of the antigen titration procedures (above); if fewer than 2 or more than 8 units of antigen were used in the test, it cannot be considered valid. Known positive and negative sera for each antigen should be included as controls in each run; these should be treated to remove inhibitors and agglutinins together with the test sera, rather than being pretreated. The titers of the positive control sera should vary by no more than twofold from their median titers, and the negative serum should show no inhibition. The RBC controls should show no agglutination.

Interpretation

A fourfold or greater increase in HI antibody titer to a reovirus antigen is considered evidence of a current reovirus infection, but it may not be possible to determine the infecting virus type. Infections with type 3 virus generally produce only a homotypic HI antibody response, but type 1 and type 2 infections usually elicit heterotypic HI antibody increases. The demonstration of reovirus HI antibody in a single serum specimen from a survey indicates a past reovirus infection, but again, the specific type(s) may be uncertain.

Literature Cited

1. **Hannington, G., J. C. Booth, C. N. Wiblin, and H. Stern.** 1983. Indirect enzyme-linked immunosorbent assay (ELISA) for detection of IgG antibodies against Coxsackie B viruses. J. Med. Microbiol. **16:**459–465.
2. **Hierholzer, J. C., and M. T. Suggs.** 1969. Standardized viral hemagglutination and hemagglutination-inhibition tests. I. Standardization of erythrocyte suspensions. Appl. Microbiol. **18:**816–823.
3. **Kapsenberg, J. G, A. Ras, and J. Korte.** 1979. Improvement of enterovirus neutralization by treatment with sodium deoxycholate or chloroform. Intervirology **12:**329–334.
4. **Katze, M. G., and R. L. Crowell.** 1980. Indirect enzyme-linked immunosorbent assay (ELISA) for the detection of coxsackievirus group B antibodies. J. Gen. Virol. **48:**225–229.
5. **Lennette, E. H., and N. J. Schmidt (ed.).** 1979. Diagnostic procedures for viral, rickettsial and chlamydial infections, 5th ed. American Public Health Association, Washington, D.C.
6. **McWilliam, K. M., and M. A. Cooper.** 1974. Antibody levels in human sera measured by the fluorescent antibody technique against the coxsackie B virus types 1-5 grown in HEp2 cells compared with results obtained by neutralization. J. Clin. Pathol. **27:**825–827.
7. **Minor, T. E., P. B. Helstrom, D. B. Nelson, and D. J. D'Alessio.** 1979. Counterimmunoelectrophoresis test for immunoglobulin M antibodies to group B coxsackievirus. J. Clin. Microbiol. **9:**503–506.
8. **Morgan-Capner, P., and C. McSorley.** 1983. Antibody capture radioimmunoassay (MACRIA) for coxsackievirus B4 and B5-specific IgM. J. Hyg. **90:**333–349.
9. **Schmidt, N. J., E. H. Lennette, and J. Dennis.** 1968. Characterization of antibodies produced in natural and experimental coxsackievirus infections. J. Immunol. **100:**99–106.
10. **Torfason, E. G., G. Frisk, and H. Diderholm.** 1984. Indirect and reverse radioimmunoassays and their apparent specificities in the detection of antibodies to enteroviruses in human sera. J. Med. Virol. **13:**13–31.

Chapter 87

Immunobiology of Hepatitis Viruses

F. BLAINE HOLLINGER AND GORDON R. DREESMAN

Viral hepatitis is one of 30 nationally reportable communicable diseases. Despite underreporting by physicians and laboratory directors—estimated to be 10 to 20% of actual cases—it currently ranks third behind the venereal diseases (gonorrhea and syphilis) and varicella. Because the agents of viral hepatitis produce characteristic but generally indistinguishable histopathological lesions in the liver and cannot be differentiated on clinical grounds alone, they are best grouped under a single heading. Diseases associated with these viruses include viral hepatitis type A (infectious hepatitis, epidemic catarrhal jaundice, short-incubation hepatitis) caused by hepatitis A virus (HAV); viral hepatitis type B (serum or transfusion hepatitis, homologous serum jaundice, long-incubation hepatitis) caused by hepatitis B virus (HBV); viral hepatitis type non-A, non-B caused by one or more non-A, non-B hepatitis viruses; and a new liver disease, viral hepatitis type D caused by a recently discovered agent provisionally designated hepatitis D virus (HDV). This is a defective virus which requires the presence of infectious HBV for its own replication. Other viruses that may occasionally be implicated in hepatitis include human cytomegalovirus, Epstein-Barr virus, rubella virus, yellow fever virus, herpes simplex virus, and some enteroviruses.

Acute viral hepatitis is associated with a broad spectrum of clinical manifestations, ranging from the absence of overt disease and minimal aberrations of liver function tests to acute fulminant disease that can be abruptly fatal. Clinical manifestations include a prodromal or preicteric phase characterized by low-grade fever (usually <39.5°C), easy fatigability, malaise, myalgia, blunting of taste and smell, anorexia, nausea, and vomiting. This is often followed by right upper quadrant discomfort or pain, hepatomegaly, and the appearance of jaundice. Extrahepatic manifestations of hepatitis (transient serum sickness-like syndrome that includes a rash, arthralgia or polyarthritis; polyarteritis nodosa; acrodermatitis; glomerulonephritis), death, and a severe and protracted clinical course are more likely to be associated with types B and non-A, non-B hepatitis, whereas asymptomatic infection is more common with type A hepatitis. Persons infected with HBV or the non-A, non-B hepatitis agent(s) (but not HAV) may become chronic carriers as a result of viral persistence in the liver. However, in most situations complete recovery is the rule (Table 1). The mortality rate is probably less than 2% for hospitalized patients with icteric hepatitis B whereas the frequency is less than 0.5% for hepatitis A. Infection with HDV in the presence of acute or chronic HBV can result in symptoms that are more severe and often more progressive than those observed with HBV alone.

In individual cases, it is not always possible to make a reliable clinical differentiation between the various agents of viral hepatitis. Because of this difficulty, the physician frequently faces a diagnostic dilemma when confronted with an icteric patient. However, recent characterization of the agents of type A and type B hepatitis according to various biochemical, biophysical, and immunoreactive properties has established the uniqueness of these etiological agents. This information, combined with the development of sensitive assays and a practical understanding of the complex serological and epidemiological profiles associated with these viruses, has provided the necessary tools to establish an accurate diagnosis in most cases.

ETIOLOGICAL AGENTS AND BIOLOGICAL FEATURES OF VIRAL HEPATITIS

Hepatitis A

Extensive investigations have demonstrated a close relationship between the nonenveloped HAV and the enteroviruses within the family *Picornaviridae*, and it has recently been classified as enterovirus type 72 (20, 23, 60). Similarities include its small size (27 to 32 nm); a buoyant density in CsCl of 1.33 to 1.34 g/cm^3, although both heavier and lighter particles exist; structural similarity (cubic capsid symmetry with a naked nucleocapsid); the presence of four major structural polypeptides with molecular weights of 30,000, 24,000, 21,000, and 7,000; the presence of RNA with a linear, single-stranded genome of approximately 2.3 × 10^6 daltons; and exclusive intracytoplasmic localization of viral particles in hepatocytes. A partial sequence from the 3' end of the RNA genome has recently been cloned (75). HAV is stable to ether and chloroform; thus, lipid is not an essential component of the virion. Virus can be preserved for years at −20°C and for at least 1 month in the dried state at 25°C. Formalin, autoclaving, boiling, and chlorine will destroy infectivity. Only one antigen, designated the HAV antigen, has been detected on the virus by polyclonal antibody or, more recently, with monoclonal antibody (9, 50). Antibody to HAV is abbreviated anti-HAV.

Immunological and biological events associated with HAV infection are illustrated in Fig. 1. The incubation period for type A hepatitis ranges from 14 to 49 days, with most symptoms developing 21 to 35 days after infection (Table 2). Infectivity studies performed in human volunteers have demonstrated fecal shedding of virus from 2 to 3 weeks before onset to 1 to 2 weeks after onset of jaundice. Subsequent to these studies, Feinstone et al. (18), using the technique of immune electron microscopy (IEM), reported the visualization of small 27-nm viruslike particles in acute-phase stool filtrates of hepatitis A patients. This technique, successfully employed by Kapikian et al. (44) to identify the viruslike "Norwalk agent" responsible for some cases of nonbacterial gastroenteritis, involves complexing virus particles with specific antibody to

TABLE 1. Predicted outcome following an infection with HAV or HBV[a]

Outcome	Patients affected (%) following infection with:	
	HAV	HBV
Subclinical (anicteric) or no disease	Children <5 yr: 90–95 Adults: 25–50	60–70
Icteric disease	Children <5 yr: 5–10 Adults: 50–75	20–35
Complete recovery	99	90
Chronic disease (% of total no. infected)	None	5–10
Mortality rate		
Based on infection	0.1	0.2–0.5
Based on icteric cases	0.5	0.5–1.5

[a] Hollinger (27).

form immune aggregates which are more easily detectable than monodispersed virions. In the hands of an experienced electron microscopist, as few as 10^5 to 10^6 particles per ml may be visualized, a level which is only slightly less sensitive than radioimmunoassay (RIA) but approximately 100 to 1,000 times more sensitive than that described for routine electron microscopy. Both "full" and "empty" viral capsids have been visualized by IEM similar to that observed with other enteroviruses. Care must be taken in differentiating between HAV particles and other virus-like particles that are occasionally present in fecal specimens.

Commercial RIA or enzyme-linked immunosorbent assay (ELISA) kits (HAVAB or HAVAB-EIA; Abbott Laboratories, North Chicago, Ill.) are available for measuring total anti-HAV antibody (immunoglobulin G [IgG] and IgM). They are competitive-binding assays in which anti-HAV in the test serum or plasma competes with ^{125}I-labeled or horseradish peroxidase-conjugated human anti-HAV for binding to HAV antigen that has been adsorbed onto a polystyrene bead. Because these assays measure total antibody to HAV, their primary function is to determine the immune status of an individual after exposure and to assess susceptibility to HAV in persons working in high-risk environments or traveling to endemic areas of the world. Recommendations regarding prophylaxis with conventional immune globulin can be made based on these results.

The advantages of RIA over other assays include excellent precision, ease of performance, and unexcelled specificity and sensitivity. ELISA is preferred where restrictive laws govern the handling of radioisotopes and the disposal of radioactive wastes. In addition, a shelf life of months to years versus 3 to 5 weeks for radionuclide-labeled antibody is also desirable, especially in laboratories where a limited number of specimens are to be examined.

An RIA method used in our laboratory to detect HAV in fecal specimens is based on modifications of the solid-phase immunoradiometric assay in which unlabeled anti-HAV is adsorbed to the polyvinyl matrix of a microtiter plate or to polystyrene beads (30, 31, 37, 78). These coated plastic surfaces can then extract immunologically reactive HAV antigen from stool filtrates. The bound HAV antigen is measured after interaction with a ^{125}I-labeled IgG preparation containing high-titer anti-HAV. Appropriate controls should include HAV-positive reference material, buffer, and an HAV-negative fecal specimen (or gradient material such as CsCl if the preparation was partially purified in that solution). Specificity can usually be ascertained by a blocking or inhibition test in which the reaction between HAV and labeled anti-HAV is

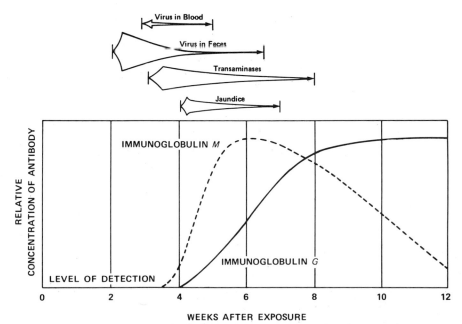

FIG. 1. Immunological and biological events associated with HAV infection.

TABLE 2. Epidemiological and clinical features of viral hepatitis types A, B, and non-A, non-B[a]

Feature	Type A	Type B	Non-A, non-B
Incubation period	2–7 weeks (avg, 4 ± 1)	4–20 weeks (avg, 11 ± 4)[b]	2–20 weeks (avg, 7 ± 2)
Principal age distribution	Children,[c] young adults	Adults[d]	?
Seasonal incidence	Throughout the year but tends to peak in autumn	Throughout the year	Throughout the year
Route of infection	Predominantly fecal-oral	Parenteral, sexual contact	Predominantly parenteral
Occurrence of virus			
Blood	2 weeks before to <1 week after jaundice	Months to years	Months to years
Stool	2 weeks before to 2 weeks after jaundice	Absent	Probably absent
Urine	Rare	Absent	Probably absent
Saliva, semen	Rare (saliva)	Frequently present	Unknown
Clinical and laboratory features			
Onset	Usually abrupt	Usually insidious	Insidious
Fever > 38°C	Common early	Less common	Less common
Duration of transaminase elevation	2–6 weeks	2–6+ months	2–6+ months
Immunoglobulins (IgM levels)	Elevated	Normal to slightly elevated	Normal to slightly elevated
Complications	Uncommon, no chronicity	Chronicity in 5 to 10%	Chronicity in 30 to 50%
Mortality rate (icteric cases)	<0.5%	<1–2%	0.5–1%
HBsAg	Absent	Present	Absent
Immunity			
Homologous	Yes	Yes	?
Heterologous	No	No	No
Duration	Probably lifetime	Probably lifetime	?
Gamma globulin (immune globulin USP) prophylaxis	Regularly prevents jaundice	Prevents jaundice only if gamma globulin is of sufficient potency against HBV	?

[a] Hollinger and Dienstag (32).

[b] Longer incubation periods, up to 9 months, have been observed, but the delay has usually been due to the administration of specific antibody (anti-HBs) after infection with HBV.

[c] Nonicteric hepatitis A is common in children.

[d] Among the 15- to 29-year age group, hepatitis B is often associated with drug abuse or promiscuous sexual behavior. Patients with transfusion-associated hepatitis B are generally over age 29.

blocked by convalescent-phase sera, but not by preimmune sera, obtained from patients or chimpanzees experimentally infected with HAV. Specificity is improved if sera from different species are used for coating the plastic matrix and for labeling. To modify the commercial HAVAB kit for the detection of HAV, specific anti-HAV can be immunologically bound to the HAV-coated beads. Extraction of HAV antigen from the test specimen and its subsequent detection with labeled anti-HAV can proceed as described above.

Although RIA is undoubtedly the most sensitive and specific assay available for detecting HAV antigen, the presence of viral particles can only be inferred from the results, a point in favor of IEM if this becomes a critical requirement.

Other assays used to detect HAV antigen include immunofluorescence (51), ELISA (17, 52), and the radioimmunofocus assay (48). All of these techniques have proved to be invaluable for the purification of HAV from stool or liver homogenates, for monitoring HAV in cell cultures as a measure of viral replication, and for pursuing the immunochemical analysis of purified HAV. However, their potential for assisting in the diagnosis of type A hepatitis by detecting virus or viral products in stools of acutely ill patients is limited because maximum shedding of viral particles occurs before the development of liver abnormalities in most HAV infections (13, 62; Fig. 1). This pattern of viral excretion, or virucopria, is well established and correlates with early experimental studies in chimpanzees (37) (Fig. 2). Less than one-third of the patients continue to excrete HAV at detectable levels by the time they see their physicians. However, this should not be construed to mean that virus is absent from these specimens, since over 10,000 particles per ml must be present to be detected by the most sensitive assays now available. Nevertheless, human volunteer studies indicate that communicability is markedly curtailed and virus shedding is essentially complete 2 to 3 weeks after the onset of symptoms (46). Viremia has been documented experimentally in volunteers (46) and serologically in chimpanzees (31) during the acute phase of the disease. However, the period of infectivity is both brief and minimal, precluding routine diagnosis by this route. Nevertheless, clinicians should recognize that posttransfusion hepatitis may, on rare occasions, be caused by HAV (36).

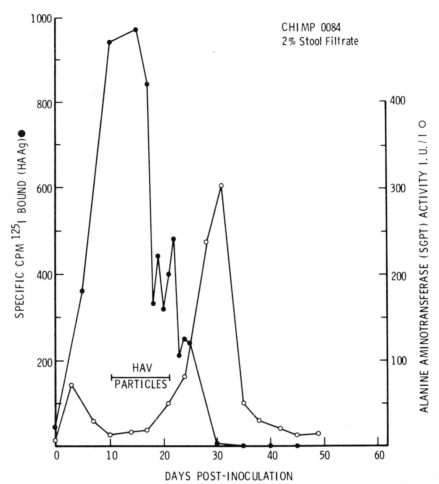

FIG. 2. Detection of HAV (by IEM) and HAV antigen (HA Ag; by RIA) in fecal specimens collected from a chimpanzee inoculated intravenously with a stool filtrate from another HAV-infected chimpanzee. Adapted from Hollinger and Maynard (37).

A more reliable method for the rapid diagnosis of type A hepatitis is to search for IgM-specific antibodies to HAV during the acute phase of the disease by RIA or ELISA (HAVAB-M or IIAVAB-M EIA; Abbott Laboratories) (10, 68). Conceptually, anti-HAV of the IgM class is extracted from the test specimen during interaction with polystyrene beads coated with anti-human IgM (μ-chain specific). A finite concentration of HAV is added which immunologically binds to any IgM-specific anti-HAV that is attached to the beads. The addition of radionuclide- or enzyme-conjugated anti-HAV to the beads completes the "sandwich" and documents the presence of IgM-specific anti-HAV in the sample being examined.

As shown in Fig. 1, IgM-specific anti-HAV is invariably present shortly after symptoms of hepatitis develop, and its detection provides presumptive evidence of a recent hepatitis A infection. Depending on the separation method employed, specific IgM anti-HAV antibodies can be detected for 6 to 16 weeks after onset of the illness before they are replaced by antibodies in the IgG class, which apparently persist for a lifetime (71).

Primary infection with HAV can also be documented by the immune adherence hemagglutination assay by demonstrating a fourfold or greater increase in anti-HAV titer using paired sera collected 4 weeks apart (12, 37, 55). In the United States, this test has been supplanted by RIA and ELISA, which are more sensitive and practical assays.

HAV isolated from human fecal material and blood has been used to successfully infect chimpanzees and several species of marmosets from the genus *Saguinus* (54, 60). Virus detected in the infected primate liver cells and excreted in the feces is morphologically identical to that of the original human HAV inoculum. In 1979, Provost and Hilleman (59) reported that a marmoset-adapted HAV strain, designated CR326, had been propagated in vitro in explant cultures of *Saguinus labiatus* marmoset livers and in fetal rhesus monkey kidney cell cultures. Since then, a number of investigators have successfully isolated and serially passaged HAV in a large variety of cell lines (2, 8, 21). However, recovery of virus from clinical specimens is hampered by a long eclipse period and limited sensitivity, making routine diagnosis by this method impractical. This noncytopathogenic agent can be detected by immunofluorescence microscopy, radioimmunofocus assay, or immunoassay of cellular extracts.

Hepatitis B

HBV is the prototype agent for a new virus family called *Hepadnaviridae*. Members of this group include woodchuck hepatitis virus, ground squirrel hepatitis virus, and duck hepatitis virus. These viruses have small circular DNA molecules that are partly single stranded and an endogenous DNA polymerase that repairs the DNA to make it fully double stranded. A strong tropism for hepatocytes and the development of persistent infection further characterizes this group.

The complete virion of hepatitis B consists of a complex double-layered structure with an overall diameter of 42 nm. An electron-dense core of 27 nm contains a circular double-stranded DNA with a molecular weight of 1.6×10^6 (67). Single-stranded gaps varying in length from 15 to 60% of the circle length are observed in isolated DNA, which serves as a primer template for the reactivity of the endogenous DNA polymerase enzyme incorporated within the virion. Core particles (containing hepatitis B core antigen [HBcAg]), isolated in CsCl from purified virus, have buoyant densities of 1.38 g/cm^3 (full particle containing DNA and DNA polymerase activity) and 1.28 to 1.33 g/cm^3 (empty cores). The latter particles have little or no DNA and do not contain DNA polymerase (45, 67). The 7-nm-thick outer envelope surrounding the core constitutes a biochemically heterogeneous complex, and this surface material, antigenically distinct from HBcAg, is designated HBsAg. HBsAg is produced in excess by the infected hepatocytes and is released into the blood as spherical particles with a size range of 17 to 25 nm (average diameter of 20 nm) and as tubular filaments with similar diameters but variable lengths, ranging from 100 to 700 nm. These 20-nm particles have a density of 1.20 g/cm^3 in CsCl and contain protein, lipids, and carbohydrates (16). Antibodies to the core antigen and to the surface antigen are designated anti-HBc and anti-HBs, respectively. Circulating titers of anti-HBs afford protection against reinfection with HBV. A third antigen-antibody system has also been observed in type B hepatitis infection and is designated HBeAg/anti-HBe. Current data would suggest that HBeAg is an integral part of the capsid of the hepatitis B virion. A 19,000-dalton polypeptide obtained following disruption of core particles by detergent appears to contain epitopes for both HBeAg and HBcAg. Larger polypeptides have also been observed (56, 74). The HBeAg may circulate either freely in the blood or in association with IgG. Because of its close relationship with the nucleocapsid of HBV, it is a reliable marker of virion concentration and thus for infectivity of the serum. In contrast, anti-HBe is associated with a much lower concentration of HBV.

There are four principal antigenic determinants (subtypes) of HBsAg, termed *adw*, *adr*, *ayw*, and *ayr*. The *adw* and *ayw* subtypes predominate in most parts of the world except in Southeast Asia and the Far East, where *adr* also is common. The *ayr* subtype is rarely observed. The group-reactive determinant *a* is cross-reactive among all four subtypes, and antibody to this determinant protects against reinfection by a second subtype. Antigenic heterogeneity of the *w* determinant results in 10 serotypes of HBV.

The prevalence of HBsAg in various United States populations ranges from 0.1 to 0.5%. Carriers are more likely to be found among populations that are nonwhite, male, and foreign born (73). Other predictive factors include socioeconomic status (crowded conditions, low income, and poor education), a history of hepatitis or tattooing, and sexual promiscuity. Older populations are less likely to be HBsAg positive.

The clinical course and serological changes that occur after exposure to HBV represent a complex interaction of the host, the virus, and specific antigens and antibodies. HBsAg typically appears 2 to 4 weeks before the development of liver abnormalities or 3 to 5 weeks before the onset of clinical symptoms. Peak concentrations of HBsAg are frequently present at the onset of clinical disease; the HBsAg level gradually declines within 4 to 6 months to levels undetectable by current methods (Fig. 3). As the aminotransferase (serum glutamic pyruvic transaminase or alanine aminotransferase [ALT]) levels rise, various HBV markers can be detected in the sera of many, but not all, patients. These serological markers include HBeAg, the 42-nm HBV (Dane) particles, specific endogenous DNA polymerase activity, and HBV-associated HBcAg. Free HBcAg, not associated with intact HBV particles, has occasionally been detected in icteric hepatitis patients before the development of anti-HBc when ALT levels were increasing (33).

As the ALT level increases, signifying necrosis of hepatocytes, HBcAg is released from the injured cells, resulting eventually in the appearance of anti-HBc of the IgM class. The presence of this IgM-specific antibody in high titer is evidence for acute infection and serves to distinguish this clinical entity from an acute exacerbation of chronic hepatitis B. Ultimately, these elevated levels of IgM-specific anti-HBc decline to nondetectable levels regardless of whether the disease resolves completely or becomes chronic. However, during early convalescence, when serum levels of HBsAg may be undetectable, IgM-specific anti-HBc may be the only serologic indicator of HBV activity (Fig. 3). A similar serologic pattern may be observed in patients with fulminant disease whose necrotic liver can no longer support the replication of HBV. If the IgM-specific anti-HBc assay is unavailable, the presence of both anti-HBe and anti-HBc (immunoglobulin type unspecified) in the absence of HBsAg and anti-HBs gives credence to a diagnosis of acute hepatitis B (41). This assumption is based on the rather transient nature of anti-HBe following acute infection.

Both anti-HBs and anti-HBc persist for many years. Anti-HBs may not be detected, or may rapidly disappear, in a small proportion of individuals with self-limited infections. Correspondingly, anti-HBc may ultimately disappear. When detectable, anti-HBe develops after anti-HBc and before anti-HBs.

SCHEMA FOR EVALUATING PATIENTS WITH HEPATITIS

Based on the preceding observations, a flow diagram can be constructed to assist the laboratory in arriving at a correct diagnosis of acute hepatitis A or B, chronic hepatitis B infection, past infection with HAV or HBV, the relative infectivity of the hepatitis B patient, and hepatitis B vaccine status (Fig. 4). IgM-

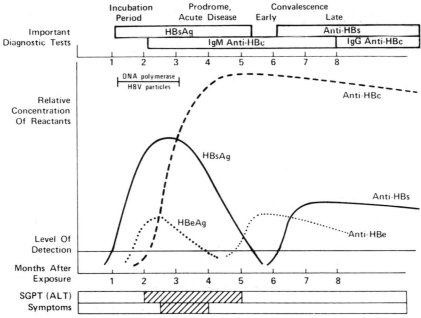

FIG. 3. Serological and clinical patterns observed during acute HBV infection.

specific anti-HAV, HBsAg, and total anti-HBc (immunoglobulin type unspecified) remain the procedures of choice for screening blood specimens for viral hepatitis. The presence of IgM-specific anti-HAV, regardless of the HBsAg status of the patient, is indicative of a recent HAV infection. Clinicians should be aware that

acute hepatitis A can occur simultaneously with hepatitis B in a chronic carrier. The presence of HBsAg is indicative of an active HBV infection, either acute or chronic. Anti-HBc is invariably positive when HBsAg is present in a clinically ill patient; an exception occurs only during the early stages of hepatitis B

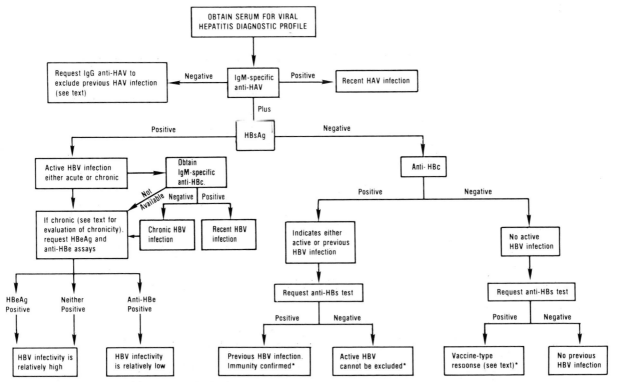

*Exclude recent transfusions, immune globulin, maternal antibody

FIG. 4. Algorithm for the serological diagnosis of HAV and HBV. Adapted from Hollinger et al. (35).

infection before the onset of symptoms (Fig. 3). High-titer IgM-specific anti-HBc differentiates acute from chronic hepatitis B. The potential for chronicity following acute disease can be determined by quantitative RIA testing of HBsAg in paired sera collected 2 to 3 weeks apart. Appropriate dilutions, which place the HBsAg test value on the descending slope of the RIA dose-response curve, permit comparisons to be made. A decline in HBsAg concentration during the sampling period predicts eventual recovery, whereas no change indicates that persistent hepatitis B infection is likely to develop. In a small percentage of acute type B hepatitis cases, perhaps less than 5%, HBsAg may be undetectable and only anti-HBc, with or without anti-HBs, may be present. This is particularly relevant in those situations where fulminant hepatitis has developed. Evaluation of these sera for IgM-specific anti-HBc may help to establish the correct diagnosis. In the absence of HBsAg or anti-HBc, active hepatitis B can be excluded.

If the specimen contains HBsAg, certain situations may warrant further testing of the serum for HBeAg or anti-HBe. These include assessing the risk of transmission of HBV after exposure to contaminated blood and advising health care professionals and others who are chronically infected concerning their potential for transmitting the disease to others. In general, there is little indication for determining the HBeAg/anti-HBe status of patients with acute hepatitis B. A strong correlation exists between HBsAg concentration and the presence of HBeAg. For example, we found that over 85% of blood donor units that were positive by RIA for HBsAg at a dilution of 1:10,000 were also HBeAg positive. Specimens positive for HBeAg are considered to be relatively infectious; i.e., they contain high concentrations of HBV and therefore have the potential for enhanced transmissibility. Infectivity is reduced, but probably not eliminated, in specimens containing anti-HBe (or low titers of HBsAg, i.e., ≤1:1,000).

A positive anti-HBc result (not IgM specific) in the absence of HBsAg requires further differentiation by examining the same serum specimen for anti-HBs. Simultaneous detection of anti-HBs is evidence of a previous infection with HBV and presumably lifelong immunity to the disease. However, the possibility of passively acquired antibody always should be entertained, and titers should be obtained on appropriately spaced samples when evaluating newborn infants or persons who have received immune serum globulin or blood transfusions. A decreasing level of anti-HBs would favor a diagnosis of passively acquired antibody. When anti-HBs alone is encountered during serologic evaluation, a number of possibilities should be considered. Such a response is expected following the administration of HBsAg vaccine. However, in the absence of such a history, anti-HBs RIA levels below a sample-to-negative counts per minute (cpm) ratio (S/N) of 10 (or even higher levels) should be viewed with caution since there is mounting evidence that many of these responses may be nonspecific. For this reason, clinicians should require the presence of anti-HBc in the same sample when determining susceptibility or immunity to HBV or deciding who should be vaccinated.

Delta hepatitis

The delta hepatitis virus (HDV), reviewed in reference 63, is a 35- to 37-nm virus that is encapsidated by HBsAg. It circulates in the blood of an HBV-infected host and requires the helper function of HBV for its own replication. Thus, HDV can infect only persons simultaneously or already infected with HBV. Within the virion is a delta antigen (HDAg)-expressing core that lacks structural definition and a small RNA genome (5.5×10^5 daltons) that shares no homology with the DNA of HBV. The virus particle has a buoyant density of 1.25 g/cm^3 in CsCl and a sedimentation coefficient intermediate between those of HBsAg and intact HBV particles. HDV is inactivated by Formalin (64). After infection, HDAg can be detected primarily in the nuclei of hepatocytes by immunocytochemical staining techniques. The antigen, a 68,000-dalton protein, is stable to Formalin fixation, thus permitting examination of paraffin-embedded tissue after digestion of the section with trypsin or pronase (7).

RIA and ELISA have been used to identify anti-HD in test specimens (6, 65). To accomplish this, a source of HDAg is required. Current commercial assays, such as the Abbott Anti-Delta RIA, use HDAg obtained from the liver of woodchucks that are experimentally infected with woodchuck hepatitis virus and HDV. This is a competitive-binding assay in which anti-HD in sera compete with ^{125}I-labeled human anti-HD for woodchuck liver-derived HDAg attached to polystyrene beads. Although the appearance of HDAg in the sera of HDV-infected patients is an infrequent and transient event, its presence can be detected by solid-phase RIA (65). Detection requires disruption of the HBsAg envelope with detergent to expose the sequestered antigen.

HDV occurs only in the presence of acute or chronic HBV infection. The duration of the latter disease determines the duration of HDV infection. Simultaneous infection with HBV leads to an illness whose clinical and biochemical features often are indistinguishable from acute HBV. Diagnosis is made by detecting HDAg in the liver or, more practically, by demonstrating IgM-specific anti-HD or anti-HD seroconversion or fourfold rise in titer in paired specimens. Prevalence studies to document previous acute, self-limited, simultaneous HBV and HDV infection are thwarted by the transient nature of the IgG response once HBsAg disappears.

Superinfection of a chronically infected HBV patient with HDV usually results in clinical exacerbation that frequently resembles acute viral hepatitis. In contrast to observations during acute HBV, patients with chronic HBV infection can support HDV replication indefinitely. In a patient with HBsAg and anti-HD, IgM-specific anti-HBc can help establish whether a coinfection or a superinfection has occurred. Its presence is a reliable indicator for a simultaneous acute infection, whereas its absence is evidence for acute delta hepatitis superimposed upon chronic HBV infection. The recent availability of cloned cDNA probes (72) provides a noninvasive approach for detecting HDV-associated RNA in sera, thus establishing the presence of ongoing HDV replication.

Non-A, non-B hepatitis

Non-A, non-B hepatitis accounts for 80 to 90% of the cases of transfusion-associated hepatitis seen in the United States today. In addition, up to 20% of sporadic hepatitis may be caused by the agent or agents responsible for this disease entity. The disease is clinically and epidemiologically similar to hepatitis B, except that chronic liver disease appears to occur more frequently with non-A, non-B hepatitis. The incubation period ranges from 5 to 10 weeks, although both shorter (2 weeks) and longer (4 months) intervals have been observed. Transmission to nonhuman primates has been accomplished (29, 34) and current studies indicate that more than one virus is responsible for this entity. Ultrastructural alterations have been detected by electron microscopy in the cytoplasm of hepatocytes obtained from chimpanzees infected with non-A, non-B hepatitis agents (70). Tubules, cylindrical complexes, undulating membranes, and protein matrices are characteristically observed. In the absence of a specific assay, these cytoplasmic inclusions have been adopted as the hallmark of non-A, non-B hepatitis even though the changes may represent only a cellular reaction to viral infection rather than specific viral components (43).

Viruslike particles have been recovered from the serum of infected patients, from liver homogenates, and from clotting factor concentrates. Most of these morphological forms appear to be approximately 27 nm in diameter, are often devoid of nucleic acid, and band at a density of 1.29 to 1.32 g/cm^3 (3, 53, 80, 81). Larger and smaller viruslike particles also have been described (reviewed in reference 11). At least one of the infectious agents, responsible for tubule formation, appears to be chloroform sensitive (4, 19).

Serological markers for active viral hepatitis A and B or other viral agents occasionally associated with hepatitis are absent. Thus, the diagnosis is one of exclusion in a patient with biochemical evidence of hepatitis. In the absence of specific markers for these agents, attention has turned to other risk factors associated with this disease. Currently, the most meaningful predictor of the disease in a blood donor appears to be the ALT (or serum glutamic pyruvic transaminase) value (26, 38). Transfusion of a donor unit with an elevated ALT value (≥45 IU/liter) significantly increases the recipient's risk of contracting non-A, non-B hepatitis

Several investigators recently have reported potentially significant findings that could lead to the identification of the agents of non-A, non-B hepatitis if the results can be confirmed. In one study, a biotin-avidin-amplified immunoperoxidase staining technique was used to localize a unique antigen in the cytoplasm of chimpanzees experimentally infected with non-A, non-B hepatitis (5). A related antigen also was detected in acute-phase chimpanzee plasma. This antigen could block the binding of human convalescent-phase antibody to tissue antigen in the staining reaction. In another study, particle-associated reverse transcriptase was detected in plasma-derived products and human sera which previously had been shown to transmit non-A, non-B hepatitis to humans and chimpanzees (69). Finally, chloroform-sensitive, membrane-coated virus particles, 85 to 90 nm in diameter with a core of 40 to 45 nm, were detected in chimpanzee liver cell cultures inoculated with sera previously shown to transmit non-A, non-B hepatitis (58). Cell homogenates from these cultures apparently caused hepatitis in chimpanzees. These findings await independent confirmation by other investigators.

TEST PROCEDURES FOR HEPATITIS A

IEM

The following procedure is recommended for detecting HAV particles in stool filtrates (13, 18). Appropriate biocontainment facilities should be available for those steps in which stool filtrates are prepared and utilized. One-tenth milliliter of a 1:10 dilution of convalescent serum (titer of 1:10,000 or more) is added to a 12- by 75-mm tube. Inactivation or clarification of the serum usually is not necessary. As a control for this procedure, 0.1 ml of phosphate-buffered saline (PBS) is added to another tube. To each of these tubes is added 0.9 ml of a 2% stool filtrate. The 2% filtrate is prepared as follows. An appropriate quantity of fecal material is mixed with veal infusion broth containing 0.5% bovine serum albumin. The mixture is agitated in the presence of 3-mm glass beads (8 to 10 beads per 1-ml volume) for 10 min to homogenize the stool and is then clarified in a refrigerated centrifuge for 1 h at 1,000 × g to remove debris. The supernatant fluid is collected and subsequently filtered through 1.2- and 0.45-μm Swinnex 47-nm filters (Millipore Corp., Bedford, Mass.) premoistened with 0.5% bovine serum albumin. The resulting filtrate represents the material to be examined. The serum-stool filtrate and the control (PBS)-stool filtrate mixtures are covered and mixed by inverting 15 to 20 times. The samples are incubated at room temperature for 1 h or overnight at 4°C. Immune aggregates are concentrated by pelleting in a refrigerated centrifuge at 47,000 × g for 90 min, using a fixed-angle rotor. The supernatant fluids are carefully discarded, and the tubes are inverted in a beaker to allow the remaining fluid to drain. The pellets or sedimented materials are resuspended with two drops (0.1 ml) of distilled water, negatively stained with an equal volume of 2% phosphotungstic acid (pH 7.2), and placed on a 400-mesh Formvar carbon-coated grid; the excess fluid is removed with the edge of a filter paper disk. The grid is examined at a magnification of about 40,000 with an electron microscope.

If aggregated particles are seen with an anti-HAV reference serum, the significance of these particles must be determined. This is done by performing the same test with a preillness serum and with a convalescent-phase serum from an HAV-infected patient in an attempt to show that a serological response occurred to that antigen. The paired serum preparations and the PBS control should be examined, as outlined above, under code to eliminate the possibility of biased interpretation.

The procedure for antibody quantification (12) is similar to that described above except that a known positive HAV stool filtrate is used to detect the presence of anti-HAV in the test serum. To quantitate the amount of antibody in each sample, five squares of each grid are routinely examined, and the relative concentration of antibody in each serum specimen is estimated by judging the amount of antibody causing aggregation of single particles on a 1 to 4+ scale (44). Three or more particles in a group are considered to constitute an aggregate. A rating of 0, i.e., no antibody, is assigned when single particles or doublets or groups of particles are observed without antibody. A 4+ rating indicates that particles are so heavily coated with antibody that they are almost obscured. A 1+ change in antibody between paired sera is considered significant.

In the IEM system, an interval of 4 to 6 weeks between paired acute and convalescent sera is considered ideal for establishing a diagnosis of hepatitis A. The IEM test is quite reproducible. Titrations of sera by IEM would be desirable, but are time-consuming.

RIA

The most specific and sensitive method for detecting HAV antigen is the solid-phase RIA (30, 31, 78). Samples to be tested are incubated with a solid-phase matrix (in this case, the wells of a microtiter plate or polystyrene beads) coated with human or chimpanzee anti-HAV. Adsorption of IgG to the plastic matrix is accomplished by diluting a high-titered reference plasma or serum containing anti-HAV (RIA titer ≥1:100,000) in 0.05 M glycine buffer, pH 7.2, and adding a predetermined optimal dilution of this material to the solid support system. A dilution between 1:500 and 1:5,000 is appropriate for most sera. Adsorption is carried out overnight at room temperature. The antibody is removed by aspiration, and the plastic matrix is washed three times with PBS. Subsequently, PBS containing 2% fetal bovine serum is added, and incubation is continued for an additional 30 min, at which time the buffer is removed and the specimen is added. Plates can be stored at 4°C for at least 6 months. After a 2-h incubation period at 45°C (or overnight at 4°C), the plates are washed and ^{125}I-labeled human IgG containing anti-HAV is added. Incubation is continued for 1 h at 45°C. After an additional wash step, the solid phase is evaluated for residual radioactivity in a gamma counter. Samples with residual count rates 2.1 times or greater than counts remaining in negative control samples are considered positive for HAV antigen.

Anti-HAV also can be measured by a solid-phase RIA. One modification that is commercially available (HAVAB; Abbott Laboratories) employs the principle of competitive protein binding. This measures the capacity of anti-HAV in serum or plasma to effectively compete with ^{125}I-labeled anti-HAV for binding sites on an HAV-coated polystyrene bead. After a bead has been incubated with the reactants, it is washed and counted in a gamma counter. In the presence of anti-HAV, less ^{125}I-anti-HAV will be bound to the bead. Within limits, the proportion of radioactive anti-HAV bound to the bead is inversely proportional to the concentration of anti-HAV present in the test specimen. Complete details of the procedure are provided in the brochure accompanying each kit or can be found in reference 32.

In our experience, a blocking or inhibition RIA is more sensitive than the competitive-binding assay for the detection of anti-HAV. In this method, a 1:10 dilution of serum is incubated for 30 min at room temperature with a finite quantity of HAV sufficient to provide 3,000 to 5,000 cpm in the absence of anti-HAV. The reactants are placed in a microtiter well previously coated with anti-HAV and incubated for 2 h at 45°C. The wells are rinsed, ^{125}I-labeled anti-HAV is added, and the incubation is continued at 45°C for 60 to 90 min. After an additional wash, the wells are cut out and counted. Specimens containing anti-HAV form complexes with the HAV antigen, reducing the amount of free antigen available for binding to the antibody-coated microtiter wells. Compared with the mean radioactivity observed with five anti-HAV–negative sera, a reduction in counts of 40% or more is consistent with the presence of anti-HAV in the test specimen.

A number of techniques are available for detecting specific IgM anti-HAV antibodies. These include physical separation of IgM from IgG by sucrose gradient ultracentrifugation; preferential adsorption of IgG from serum using staphylococcal protein A, leaving IgM remaining in the supernatant; and selective removal of IgM from serum by plant lectins that bind glycoproteins. The last technique is based on the observation that approximately 12% of the IgM molecule is composed of carbohydrates, whereas IgG molecules contain less than 3% carbohydrates. Concanavalin A (ConA), a plant lectin, avidly binds glycoproteins, and when linked to Sepharose 4B (ConA-Sepharose; Pharmacia Fine Chemicals, Inc., Piscataway, N.J.), it provides a solid support matrix for the removal of a large proportion of the IgM. To perform the test, ConA-Sepharose is washed three times in 0.05 M glycine buffer, pH 7.2, and then diluted to a final concentration of 25%; a 25% gel suspension of Sepharose 4B, without ConA, is used as a control. To 1 ml of each gel suspension is added 25 μl of the sample to be tested. Each sample is continuously shaken for 1 h at 45°C and then centrifuged at 2,500 × g for 15 min. Two hundred microliters of each supernatant is added to a H$\overline{A}$VAB bead (Abbott Laboratories) and incubated at 45°C for 2 h. After the beads are washed, 200 μl of ^{125}I-labeled anti-HAV is added and incubation is continued overnight at 25°C (or 2 h at 45°C). After a final wash cycle, the beads are counted. An N/D value is computed by dividing the negative control mean count rate (NCx̄) by the difference (D) between the ConA-Sepharose sample count rate and the Sepharose 4B sample count rate: $N/D = NC\bar{x}/(\text{ConA-Sepharose} - \text{Sepharose 4B})$. The presence of specific anti-HAV in the IgM fraction is indicated if the N/D value is ≤6.0.

Perhaps the most convenient RIA method for detecting IgM antibody to HAV is to use anti-human IgM (μ-chain specific), bound to a polystyrene bead, to preferentially remove IgM from serum (H$\overline{A}$VAB-M; Abbott Laboratories) (10, 68). The test is both sensitive and specific. The presence of IgM anti-HAV on the bead is recognized by the addition of HAV reagent followed, after an appropriate incubation period and wash stage, by a radiolabeled anti-HAV probe. A cutoff value is determined based on the IgM positive and negative control samples and on the potency of the HAV reagent and the labeled antibody. In our experience, false-positive reactions due to rheumatoid factor are unusual but can occur.

ELISA

ELISA is a third-generation assay that rivals RIA for the detection of anti-HAV, although nonspecific reactions may be somewhat more frequent. Simplified, standardized commercial ELISA test kits are now available to measure anti-HAV and IgM-specific anti-HAV (HAVAB EIA and HAVAB-M EIA; Abbott Laboratories). These tests are analogous in principle to the RIA procedures from the same manufacturer. The major differences are that horseradish peroxidase-conjugated human anti-HAV is substituted for the ^{125}I-labeled anti-HAV and a substrate (o-phenylenediamine solution containing hydrogen peroxide) is added, resulting in a color reaction after an additional period of incubation. Absorbance is determined in a spectrophotometer. Details of the procedures accompany each kit and have been reviewed elsewhere (32).

Radioimmunofocus assay

Propagation of HAV in cell cultures (2, 8, 21) has provided a method for the direct isolation of virus from clinical specimens. Recently, this approach was refined by a method known as the radioimmunofocus assay (48). The assay is performed by inoculating confluent cultures of continuous African green monkey kidney cells (BS-C-1) in 60-mm petri dishes with serial dilutions of HAV. Virus is adsorbed for 90 to 120 min and subsequently overlaid with maintenance medium containing 0.5% agarose MF (Seakem, FMC Corp., Marine Colloids Div., Rockland, Maine) at 45°C. The cultures are then incubated for 14 days at 35°C under 5% CO_2. If longer incubation periods are required, a second agarose overlay is added on day 14. Viral antigen is assayed by removal of the agarose, washing the monolayer with Hanks balanced salt solution, and then air drying. The cells are fixed for 2 min at room temperature with acetone. At that point, ^{125}I-labeled anti-HAV (5×10^5 cpm) is added to each plate and subsequently incubated at 35°C for 4 h. The radiolabeled antibody is then removed, and the monolayers are washed five times with PBS. Autoradiography is carried out by placing the cut-out bottom of each plate onto Kodak X AR5 film in a Kodak X-Omatic cassette with a regular intensification screen for 4 to 6 days at -70°C. The film is then processed through a Kodak RP automatic processor, and the autoradiograms of individual petri dishes are examined for foci of developed grains. From the number of such foci, the amount of virus in the inoculum can be estimated in terms of radioimmunofocus-forming units per milliliter.

TEST PROCEDURES FOR HEPATITIS B

Detection of HBV-specified antigens and their corresponding antibodies

Serum or plasma, stored either refrigerated or frozen, is suitable for essentially all diagnostic procedures. Because the third-generation methods are the most sensitive (Table 3), they are the preferred methods in most clinical situations, but there are valuable special applications of the other methods which merit their inclusion in this chapter. All commercially available reagents for HBsAg and anti-HBs detection are

TABLE 3. Relative sensitivity of methods used to detect HBV antigens and antibodies[a]

Relative sensitivity (HBsAg)	Assay method	Time to complete test (h)
Least (≥ 10 μg/ml)	Agarose gel diffusion	24–72
Intermediate (1–5 μg/ml)	Counterimmunoelectrophoresis	1–2
	Rheophoresis	24–72
	Complement fixation	18
Most (0.1–40 ng/ml)	Latex agglutination (third generation)	1
	Hemagglutination	3–6
	Immune adherence	4–24
	ELISA	4–24
	RIA	3–24

[a] Hollinger and Dienstag (32).

subject to federal licensure and control and are accompanied by detailed directions for use. A complete list of licensed manufacturers can be obtained by writing to the Director, Bureau of Biologics, Food and Drug Administration, Bethesda, MD 20209. Reference reagents may be obtained from the Reference Resources Branch, National Institute of Allergy and Infectious Diseases, Bethesda, MD 20892.

Agar gel diffusion

Historically, the presence of HBsAg in the blood of persons infected with HBV was observed by agar gel diffusion utilizing the method described by Ouchterlony. Although considerably less sensitive than other methods, agar gel diffusion has the advantages of demonstrating specificity by the formation of lines of identity between HBsAg in test samples and in positive control sera and of distinguishing among subtypes of HBsAg by lines of partial identity or spur formation. The method is relatively slow, requiring 24 to 72 h for optimal results (Table 3), but it is the simplest available method for HBsAg and anti-HBs detection, as no special equipment is required. Since agar gel diffusion is a relatively insensitive method for detecting anti-HBs as well as HBsAg, it provides a convenient method for identifying potent antisera. Based on its level of sensitivity, it was referred to historically as a first-generation test.

Counterelectrophoresis

Counterelectrophoresis is 5 to 10 times as sensitive as agar gel diffusion for HBsAg detection and provides results in 1 to 2 h (22). It is considered to be a second-generation test, along with the complement fixation test. Many variations of this technique have been described in the literature (15, 77; see also the previous editions of this manual for appropriate directions). Careful selection of the anti-HBs reagent is essential to obtain optimal sensitivity with counterelectrophoresis. By creating a discontinuous gradient between the electrophoresis cell buffer and the agarose buffer, endosmosis of IgG is facilitated and the sensitivity is enhanced (77).

Hemagglutination

Agglutination of erythrocytes coated with HBsAg (passive hemagglutination) or with anti-HBs (reversed passive hemagglutination) is the basis of very sensitive, rapid, and simple methods for detecting anti-HBs and HBsAg, respectively (40, 76). The tests are performed in microtiter plates in which dilutions of the test samples are mixed with the coated cells. Since both of these methods give nonspecific false-positive results with some sera, confirmation by specific inhibition of the agglutination reactions with HBsAg or anti-HBs or by testing the samples with another method of at least equivalent sensitivity is necessary before interpreting the results as positive or negative.

RIA

The most sensitive and specific methods for detecting HBsAg, anti-HBs, and anti-HBc are the RIAs (39, 47, 49, 61). RIA is at least 10-fold more sensitive than hemagglutination assays and 100 or more times more sensitive than second-generation tests. Assays with this level of relative sensitivity are generally referred to as third-generation tests. A solid-phase RIA system (78), the most widely used method for HBsAg testing, employs the "sandwich" principle, in which test samples are added to plastic tubes or beads coated with anti-HBs. After an initial incubation step, the sample is removed and the tubes or beads are washed before the addition of ^{125}I-labeled anti-HBs IgG. After a second incubation and a second washing step, the tubes or beads are counted in a gamma counter. Average cpm from at least five negative control sera are used to establish a cutoff point above which the samples are considered to contain HBsAg. Detailed procedures are included in each commercial kit and should be followed explicitly for best results.

Confirmation of positive results by showing that they are repeatable and are specifically inhibited by unlabeled human anti-HBs is essential because of the occurrence of an occasional nonspecific false-positive result. However, the occurrence of repeatedly positive test results which cannot be confirmed as positive by the blocking test is highly unusual (<0.1%). Additional verification of an HBsAg reaction is generated when antibody to HBcAg (anti-HBc) is also detected. The most common sources of error encountered in the solid-phase RIA are inadequate washing of the coated matrix or inadvertent contamination of the counting tubes or beads with radioactivity. Blood that contains anticoagulants or is obtained from a patient with clotting abnormalities may, on occasion, give rise to a false-positive HBsAg reaction. The absence of a corroborating positive anti-HBc test should alert the clinician to this possibility. In all RIA tests, the negative control sample should be similar to the unknown. For example, tests for HBsAg in urine should use "normal" urine as the negative control, not human serum. In general, protein-deficient samples and recalcified plasma result in higher levels of background counts.

For comparative purposes, semiquantitation of HBsAg can be accomplished as follows. Paired sera are diluted 1:10,000 in PBS containing 0.5% bovine serum albumin. Precision in preparing the dilutions is essential. The 1:10,000 dilution is selected because the capacity of the commercial antibody-coated beads for HBsAg molecules often is exceeded at lower serum dilutions, especially if the HBsAg concentration is greater than 1 μg/ml, as it generally is for most carriers or patients with acute hepatitis. In these situations, maximum binding occurs over a wide range, prohibiting quantitative comparisons until the descending slope of the RIA dose-response curve is reached. Occasionally, a lower dilution (1:1,000) is required for making comparisons of paired serum samples.

Commercial solid-phase RIA tests for detecting anti-HBs consist of incubating an unknown sample with plastic beads coated with HBsAg. During incubation, antibody, if present, combines with the solid-phase HBsAg. After the beads are washed, ^{125}I-labeled HBsAg is added and incubation is continued, creating an antigen–antibody–^{125}I-antigen sandwich. Increased counts signify increased levels of antibody present in the specimen. To avoid inter- and intralot variations in assays and to permit comparisons between laboratories, the anti-HBs can be expressed in milli-International Units per milliliter (mIU/ml) as reported by Hollinger et al. (28). Using a World Health Organization (WHO) anti-HBs reference preparation (lot 26.1.77) or a laboratory standard equivalent to this reagent, a sample-to-reference (S/R) cpm ratio is computed (after subtracting the negative control mean cpm from each). This value is incorporated into a formula that was derived by regression of the S/R ratio on various concentrations of the WHO reference standard using the computer nonlinear regression program, BMDP3R (14):

$$\text{mIU/ml} = 130.75(e^{0.66765(S/R)} - 1)(\text{reciprocal of dilution}).$$

In obtaining this regression, the R variable was the positive control cpm value for the anti-HBs kit (AUSAB; Abbott Laboratories) and the S variable corresponded to the cpm values of the diluted WHO standard. Over a 1-year interval, the AUSAB positive control remained constant at a concentration of 125 mIU/ml. However, to ensure against possible changes in the concentration of anti-HBs in future positive control lots, frozen samples of the WHO reference standard, diluted to contain 125 mIU/ml, were substituted for the positive reference (R) control. To conserve the WHO reference reagent, a laboratory standard can be prepared and compared with the WHO standard. The exponential value in the formula (0.66765) is adjusted proportionally to agree with the new laboratory standard when it is substituted for the WHO reference reagent as R in the S/R ratio. For further details, see reference 29. Anti-HBs concentrations of 0.7 mIU/ml or greater are considered positive. Dilutions are usually required when anti-HBs levels exceed 200 mIU/ml.

A commercially available RIA test for anti-HBc is based on the principle of competitive binding, in which nonradioactive anti-HBc from serum or plasma competes with ^{125}I-labeled human anti-HBc for binding sites on beads coated with HBcAg. After an incubation period and a wash step, the radioactive anti-HBc fixed to the bead is counted in a gamma counter.

The proportion of radioactive anti-HBc bound to the bead is inversely proportional to the concentration of anti-HBc in the sample being tested.

Another commercial RIA (Abbott HBe) can be used to detect either HBeAg or anti-HBe. The HBeAg test is a standard sandwich assay in which HBeAg in the sample binds to anti-HBe on a polystyrene bead; the captured antigen is subsequently disclosed by adding ^{125}I-labeled anti-HBe to the washed bead. For anti-HBe detection, the test sample and adsorbed anti-HBe on the bead compete for a standardized amount of HBeAg added to the reaction well before the addition of labeled anti-HBe. As with other competitive-binding assays, the proportion of radioactive antibody bound to the bead is inversely proportional to the concentration of homologous, unlabeled antibody present in the sample being tested (within limits).

ELISA

ELISA has recently become popular for diagnostic laboratories because it circumvents the problems of radioactive disposal and the relatively short half-life of isotopes inherent in RIA systems (24, 79). ELISAs are available for the detection of HBsAg, anti-HBc, IgM-specific anti-HBc, HBeAg, and anti-HBe. The principles of the ELISA are identical to those of the RIA described above. The only difference is that the antibody probe is conjugated to a purified enzyme instead of being labeled with ^{125}I. The two enzymes most often employed are horseradish peroxidase and alkaline phosphatase. After the addition of the enzyme-linked antibody, an additional step is required in that a specific substrate must be added. The reaction can be read visually as a color change or can be quantitated with a spectrophotometer. The IgM-specific anti-HBc ELISA, which is now available in a kit, is identical in principle to that described for the IgM-specific anti-HAV assay.

Subtype determinations

Subtype-specific antisera are prepared by hyperimmunization of guinea pigs or rabbits with purified HBsAg of a known subtype, followed by cross-adsorption with the heterologous subtype. More recently, subtype-specific monoclonal antibodies have been produced. These antisera may then be used in any of several methods, particularly agar gel diffusion, counterelectrophoresis, rheophoresis, passive hemagglutination, and RIA, for determining HBsAg subtypes (25, 40, 42). The subtype specificities of anti-HBs may be determined with the passive hemagglutination or RIA techniques by studying inhibition of the antibody reactions with different known HBsAg subtypes. Determination of HBsAg subtypes by any of a number of methods is of value as an epidemiological tool and also for answering basic questions regarding the importance of subtypes in protection against reinfection with HBV and in vaccine effectiveness.

Test for endogenous DNA polymerase

Endogenous DNA polymerase activity (66) is measured by incubating pelleted HBV particles with a reaction mixture consisting of dATP, dTTP, [^{3}H]dCTP, and [^{3}H]dGTP in Tris buffer (pH 8.0) with MgCl$_2$, NH$_4$Cl, 2-mercaptoethanol, and Nonidet P-40. After incubation of the reaction mixture at 37°C for 3 h, the reacted radioactive substrate is separated from the unreacted reagent on Whatman 3-mm paper and assayed for acid-precipitable ^{3}H in a beta particle spectrophotometer. The specificity of DNA polymerase activity is confirmed by demonstrating specific immune precipitation of polymerase activity, and hence of Dane particles, by anti-HBs before treatment with 2-mercaptoethanol and Nonidet P-40 and with anti-HBc after adding Nonidet P-40. This confirmatory test is necessary because contamination of sera with bacteria can result in false-positive DNA polymerase results (57).

Virus isolation: animal models

Since HBV has not been successfully isolated in tissue culture, presence of the virus can be directly demonstrated only by inoculation of susceptible animals. Although chimpanzees and gibbons have been experimentally infected with HBV, only the chimpanzee has been fully evaluated and demonstrated to be a sensitive indicator of HBV infectivity (1). HBV infection in the chimpanzee resembles HBV infection in humans but is generally less severe. All of the serological markers of type B hepatitis, including HBsAg, anti-HBs, anti-HBc, HBeAg, anti-HBe, and serum DNA polymerase activity have been detected in association with HBV infection in chimpanzees.

APPLICATIONS OF TEST METHODS

Until recently, most HAV testing was performed by research laboratories interested in the epidemiology of viral hepatitis. With the advent of commercial IgM and IgG antibody tests, routine testing for anti-HAV has become standard practice among clinicians. Physicians are now able to establish a diagnosis in clinical cases of hepatitis A based on the presence of circulating IgM anti-HAV and thereby determine the need for prophylaxis among close personal contacts. It is hoped that a commercial test for the detection of HAV in human fecal material will soon be available. Whether such information will facilitate the diagnosis of HAV remains to be determined.

The availability of a wide variety of laboratory techniques for detecting HBV infection necessitates discrimination in selecting the optimal method for each specific clinical and research situation as outlined above. The major applications for the HBV tests include identification of blood donors who are infected with hepatitis B and establishment of the etiology of clinical cases of hepatitis. The demonstration of HBsAg in serum or plasma provides the most direct, unequivocal evidence of active HBV infection for both of these purposes. The third-generation methods (reversed passive hemagglutination, ELISA, and RIA) are the methods of choice for these applications because of their high sensitivity; blood banks in the United States are required to test each unit by one of these methods. For diagnosis of clinical hepatitis when HBsAg is not detectable, sensitive methods should be employed to document anti-HBs seroconversion or the presence of IgM-specific anti-HBc. The

Chapter 89

The Acquired Immunodeficiency Syndrome and Related Diseases

H. CLIFFORD LANE, THOMAS FOLKS, AND ANTHONY S. FAUCI

The acquired immunodeficiency syndrome (AIDS) is one of the most destructive infectious diseases of the human immune system ever described. This disease, with its unique epidemiologic, virologic, immunologic, and clinical manifestations, has become one of the great public health challenges of the 20th century (3). In the United States the majority of cases (73%) are transmitted via male homosexual contact, while 17% of cases occur through needle sharing among intravenous drug abusers. A minority of cases in the United States (1%) at this time are transmitted through heterosexual contact. The overall mortality rate for patients with this disease is close to 50%. This figure does not impart the full severity of the illness, however, in view of the fact that there are no individuals who are known to have recovered from AIDS. Thus, the current epidemiologic data support the notion that AIDS is a lethal, sexually transmitted disease which can also be contracted through the intravenous administration of infected blood or blood products.

Perhaps the greatest single advance in the attempt to better understand this disease and to limit its impact was the discovery of the causative agent and the development of tests designed to detect antibodies to the agent. A human T-cell-tropic retrovirus referred to as either human T-lymphotropic virus type III (HTLV-III) or lymphadenopathy-associated virus (LAV) was initially isolated from several patients with AIDS or related conditions and was later conclusively shown to be the causative agent of this group of diseases. The most firm data supporting this point were the series of observations linking evidence of infection with the AIDS agent to the blood donors for individuals who developed AIDS subsequent to blood transfusions (1, 4, 6, 10).

The immune deficiency resulting from infection with the AIDS virus appears to be due to a selective elimination of the helper-inducer subset of T lymphocytes, and in particular the subset of helper-inducer T cells which respond to soluble antigens (7, 9). What remains unclear at the present time is why some people who have evidence of infection with the AIDS virus seem to do well with no evidence of immunologic dysfunction while others develop a progressive immunodeficiency state. The nature of the protective immunologic responses to the AIDS virus, if such exist, have yet to be delineated.

A variety of immunologic and clinical manifestations after infection with HTLV-III have been described. Among these are asymptomatic infection, the AIDS-related complex (ARC), and AIDS. Current epidemiologic data suggest that only about 10% of those individuals who have been infected with the AIDS virus will go on to develop AIDS. For these purposes AIDS is described as the occurrence of a disease that is at least moderately predictive of a defect in cell-mediated immunity, occurring in a person with no known cause for diminished resistance to that disease. Such diseases include *Pneumocystis carinii* pneumonia, cytomegalovirus retinitis, and Kaposi's sarcoma. Recently the definition has been expanded to include several diseases not always associated with a preexisting immunodeficiency state (lymphoreticular malignancies, Kaposi's sarcoma in individuals over the age of 60, disseminated histoplasmosis, and interstitial pneumonitis in children), when they occur in the context of a positive serology for HTLV-III. In addition, the definition has been modified to exclude individuals who do not have serologic evidence of infection with HTLV-III and who do not have a reduced number of helper-inducer T cells.

About 25% of individuals infected with the AIDS virus will develop a less serious disease known as ARC. The definition of this entity is constantly evolving with the current clinical and laboratory criteria for diagnosis. Clinical manifestations include fever, weight loss, diarrhea, lymphadenopathy, fatigue, and night sweats. Laboratory abnormalities included in the diagnostic criteria are decreased helper T cells (>2 standard deviations below the mean); leukopenia, thrombocytopenia, lymphopenia, or anemia; elevated serum immunoglobulins; decreased blastogenesis; and abnormal delayed-type hypersensitivity. To be diagnosed as having ARC, a patient must have two of the above clinical abnormalities for more than 3 months and two of the laboratory abnormalities in the absence of an obvious infectious etiology.

About 10% of ARC patients may go on to develop AIDS. Thus, the majority of patients who have evidence of infection with the AIDS virus do not develop clinical disease as best we know at this time. Due to the fact that many of these patients are viremic with the AIDS virus, however, it is felt that anyone with evidence of infection could potentially spread the disease. This latter group is the most difficult to counsel, for the length of follow-up of such cohorts is much too short to make any long-term prognosis.

The evaluation of individuals suspected of having an infection with the AIDS virus is currently a rapidly evolving area of science. As the testing procedures for detecting antibodies to the virus become more routine, the need to understand what impact the infection has had on the host's immune system will become more important. The enzyme-linked immunosorbent assay (ELISA) is currently the standard method for sensitive screening for antibodies to the AIDS virus. This test, however, lacks specificity, and in view of the impact of a positive antibody test, there is an absolute need for confirmation of the result with Western blot analysis or radioimmunoprecipitation assay when a positive ELISA test occurs in the absence of an appropriate clinical setting. In addition, viral isolation may be helpful in individuals who are seronegative for the virus but who clearly have the clinical disease. Thus, the diagnostic laboratory will be called upon not only to screen individuals for the presence of antibodies to the AIDS virus but also to provide confirmatory serologic testing, virologic isolation, and immunologic evaluation.

SEROLOGIC TESTING

The ELISA is the most commonly used test for screening sera for the presence of antibodies to HTLV-III/LAV. Among the companies which currently manufacture such kits are Abbott Laboratories, Travenol Laboratories, Biotech, and Litton. These kits all take advantage of the fact that certain cell lines have been developed which allow for the growth of the virus without killing the cell. Supernatants or purified virus from these infected cells are then used as the material adhered to the solid phase for the ELISA. Thus, in addition to placing viral proteins and nucleic acids on the plate, one is also adhering cell antigens. The sensitivity of such tests is quite good, ranging from 92 to 95%, whereas, depending upon the test population, the specificity may be as low as 30%.

A great deal of discussion surrounds the most appropriate way to present data generated from such ELISA tests and where to make the cut-off between negative and positive. One common formula used is to develop a ratio between the sample and the negative control and use that ratio to score samples as negative (≤ 2), borderline (2 to 5), or positive (>5). This type of system, while useful for declaring samples negative, especially for purposes such as screening in blood banks, is generally not helpful in declaring a person seropositive. If one desires to make a diagnosis of seropositivity to HTLV-III, then a more specific test must be done. The one most commonly used is the Western blot.

The specificity of the Western blot technique stems from the fact that it takes the whole virus, reduces it to a variety of protein fragments, separates those fragments electrophoretically, and then looks for antibodies directed toward any or all of the fragments.

To perform a Western blot one first needs a source of virus. Virus can be obtained either from zonal centrifugation of concentrated virus-containing supernatants of infected cells or via direct lysis of an infected cell line. The former source of virus is purer, while the latter has a higher content of high-molecular-weight protein. Regardless of the source of virus, the basic procedure of blotting is the same. A 300-µl sample of virus containing 10 to 100 µg of protein is placed in 300 µl of sodium dodecyl sulfate sample buffer (25 mM Tris, 10% glycerol, 2.3% sodium dodecyl sulfate) containing 7.0×10^{-6} M 2-mercaptoethanol (5%). The solution is boiled for 2 min and then placed onto a 3 to 27% gradient polyacrylamide gel (15 by 15 by 0.15 cm). The sample is then electrophoresed for approximately 16 h at 50 V. The electrophoresed proteins are then transferred to a nitrocellulose filter, and the filter is incubated with TN buffer (10 mM Tris, 155 mM NaCl, pH 7.4) containing 5% milk protein for 30 min at room temperature to saturate all protein-binding sites on the nitrocellulose. The nitrocellulose is next washed with TN-TN buffer (TN buffer, 0.3% Tween-

20, 0.05% Nonidet P-40) for 5 min to remove excess milk proteins. The nitrocellulose is then cut into approximately 1-cm strips, and each strip is identified using indelible ink. Care should be taken to keep the nitrocellulose moist throughout the entire procedure. The strips are then placed into a slot incubation tray or screw-top test tube with a 1:1,000 dilution of the test serum and allowed to incubate at room temperature for 2 to 16 h. The strips are then washed twice for 5 min with TN-TN buffer and then once for 5 min with TN-T buffer (TN, 0.3% Tween-20). The strips may be combined at this point. They are next incubated for 1 to 3 h at room temperature with 200,000 dpm of ^{125}I-protein A per ml in TN-T buffer containing 3% bovine serum albumin. The strips are then washed three times for 5 min each with TN-TN buffer containing 10 mM EDTA and then once for 5 min with TN buffer. The strips are then allowed to air dry, and autoradiography is performed at $-70°C$ with an intensifying screen.

A variety of protein bands may be seen on a positive Western blot (Fig. 1). Among these are high-molecular-weight bands (120,000 and 160,000) which correspond to viral envelope, mid-molecular-weight bands (65,000, 51,000, and 41,000) which correspond to core precursor proteins, and a component of the viral envelope and a low-molecular-weight band (24,000) which is felt to be the product of the *gag* gene of the virus. The 41,000-molecular-weight band, a transmembrane envelope protein, is generally the strongest band, and in fact reactivity with the next most prom-

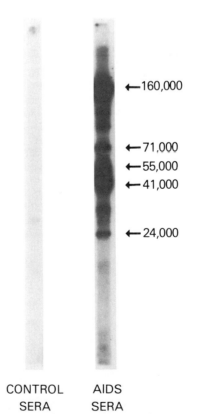

CONTROL   AIDS
SERA   SERA

FIG. 1. Positive and negative Western blots for antibodies to HTLV-III. The most characteristic antiviral bands are those at 24,000, 41,000, and 160,000.

inent band, p24,000, may disappear as the disease progresses (F. M. Barin, F. McLane, J. S. Allan, T. H. Lee, J. E. Groopman, and M. Essex, Science, in press). It should be stressed that the presence of a single positive band (especially 24,000) alone does not necessarily mean that an individual has antibodies to the AIDS virus. Western blots must be interpreted with caution and by someone with experience in the area. When many viral bands are positive, the sample is clearly positive. However, normal control sera will occasionally give patterns of single band reactivity which may or may not indicate true antiviral reactivity.

VIRAL ISOLATION

The AIDS retrovirus can be isolated most easily from the peripheral blood mononuclear cells of infected individuals. Although virus isolation has also been reported from bone marrow, saliva, semen, and tears, peripheral blood is the most reliable source. A variety of $T4^+$ cell lines have been described which will support the growth of the AIDS virus in vitro. Among these are the HT derivative H9 (6) and the CEM derivative 3.01 (5). In addition, the virus is perhaps most easily expressed by coculture of infected cells with normal peripheral blood phytohemagglutinin-activated blasts. It should be pointed out that, due to the biologic properties of this virus, anyone wishing to culture it should perform these cultures under Biosafety Level 3 precautions.

The AIDS retrovirus can be identified in culture by its cytopathic effect or by the production of the viral enzyme reverse transcriptase. The AIDS virus has the property of causing the formation of giant syncytia which appear to be due to the fusion of cells. These syncytia, which appear as fragile spheres containing multiple nuclei, are quite characteristic of the presence of the AIDS retrovirus (Fig. 2). The AIDS virus is an RNA virus which carries with it a virus-coded, RNA-dependent DNA polymerase known as reverse transcriptase. This reverse transcriptase catalyzes the transcription of a DNA copy of the RNA virus shortly after the virus infects the T4 cell. This DNA copy most likely then becomes incorporated into the host genome and serves as a template for the production of RNA virus. The presence of the enzymatic activity of this reverse transcriptase can thus be used as a marker for the presence of the AIDS virus.

The first step in attempting to isolate the virus is to obtain peripheral blood mononuclear cells, via standard Hypaque-Ficoll separation, from the patient suspected of being infected with the virus (2). Cells should be harvested as quickly after venipuncture as possible, and the blood and cells should be kept off ice. The mononuclear cells are suspended at 10^6/ml in RPMI 1640 culture medium containing glutamine, HEPES (N-2-hydroxyethylpiperazine-N'-2- ethanesulfonic acid), and 10% fetal calf serum. A sample (3 to 10 ml) of cells is placed in a 50-ml sterile flask, containing phytohemagglutinin phosphate at a final concentration of 2 μg/ml and 5 to 10 neutralizing units of anti-alpha interferon antibody per ml, and incubated at 37°C for 3 days. The flasks are observed daily for syncytium formation, which is a characteristic cytopathic effect of the AIDS retrovirus. Every 2 days after the initial 3-day activation period, approximately 95% of the medium is removed and fresh medium containing 10% interleukin 2-enriched, conditioned medium and 5 to 10 neutralizing units of anti-alpha interferon antibody per ml is added. The medium that was removed is spun at $500 \times g$ for 10 min and frozen at −70°C to be assayed later for reverse transcriptase activity. On day 3 of culture, fresh normal peripheral blood mononuclear cells which have been mitogen activated for 3 days with phytohemagglutinin are added to the cultures in a 1:1 ratio to enhance virus recovery by providing additional cell substrate for the virus. At the end of the culture (generally about 4 weeks), the frozen supernatants are all tested for Mg^{2+}-dependent reverse transcriptase activity. The peak of reverse transcriptase activity generally will correspond to the time when peak syncytium formation was noted.

IMMUNOLOGIC EVALUATION OF PATIENTS INFECTED WITH HTLV-III

A variety of immunologic abnormalities have been described in individuals with AIDS or related illnesses. Among them are a decrease in the number of helper-inducer T lymphocytes in the peripheral blood, a decrease in lymphocyte proliferative responses to mitogens and antigens, hypergammaglobulinemia, and a variety of serologic abnormalities including the presence of an unusual acid-labile form of alpha interferon, the presence of elevated levels of β_2-microglobulin, and the presence of suppressor substance(s) (8). Of these, the two defects which seem the most characteristic of the immunologic defect in AIDS are the decrease in the absolute number of helper-inducer T lymphocytes (9) and the absent reactivity to soluble antigen (7).

The evaluation of the patient suspected of having an immunodeficiency syndrome due to infection with the AIDS retrovirus is similar to that which would be appropriate for any patient with a suspected defect in cell-mediated immunity. The role of the clinician is to elicit facts from the history or physical which would suggest a defect. Among the things looked for are unexplained fever or weight loss, lymphadenopathy, oral Candida sp., evidence of other opportunistic infections, or evidence of Kaposi's sarcoma. The initial laboratory screen and clinical testing should include a complete blood count and differential, an erythrocyte sedimentation rate, serum immunoglobulin levels, and a battery of delayed-type hypersensitivity skin

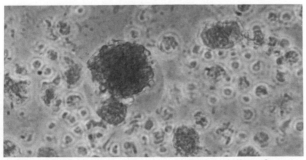

FIG. 2. Appearance of typical syncytia under phase-contrast microscopy. Note the spherical shape and thin outer membrane.

tests. If any of these clinical or laboratory parameters is abnormal, then there is a need for additional testing.

A test which is still considered only a research tool but which may provide valuable information is the determination of lymphocyte subset numbers. The immune systems of patients with AIDS are characterized by a profound defect in the number of cells bearing the helper-inducer phenotype (T4 or Leu 3). This determination is most easily made by utilizing monoclonal antibodies and a fluorescence-activated cell sorter-analyzer or a fluorescence microscope. In this procedure, peripheral blood mononuclear cells are obtained from Hypaque-Ficoll density gradient centrifugation in the standard fashion. A sample of 10^6 cells is then spun into a pellet and suspended in 5 μl of monoclonal antibody. The mixture is allowed to incubate for 45 min on ice, washed three times with 3 ml of FACS buffer (phosphate-buffered saline with 0.05% bovine serum albumin and 0.02% azide), and incubated with 3 μl of a goat anti-mouse immunoglobulin conjugated to fluorescein. The mixture is allowed to incubate for an additional 45 min on ice, and the cells are again washed three times, each time with 3 ml of FACS buffer. The resulting cell button is suspended in 1% paraformaldehyde for 30 min to fix the cells and inactivate the AIDS virus if present. The cells are then washed once in FACS buffer, resuspended in 1 ml of FACS buffer, and examined on the sorter-analyzer of the fluorescence microscope. Many variants of this technique exist, including some which utilize whole blood. We have chosen to describe this indirect immunofluorescence technique in detail due to its general applicability.

The patient with an immune system damaged by the AIDS virus will have a decrease in the total number of helper-inducer T lymphocytes. This is often seen in the context of an increased number of suppressor-cytotoxic T cells which can be identified by either the T8 or Leu 2 monoclonal antibodies. This latter finding is also seen in individuals who have experienced recent (within 1 year) infections with a variety of viruses, including cytomegalovirus and Epstein-Barr virus. Thus, an elevation in T8 number (which may cause a lowering of the T4/T8 ratio) by itself cannot be taken as an indicator of AIDS retrovirus-induced immunodeficiency unless it occurs in the context of a reduction in the number of T4 cells.

Virtually all measurable in vitro immunologic parameters have been reported to be abnormal in patients with AIDS. Among these are blast transformation to mitogens and antigens, autologous and allogeneic reactivity, specific and nonspecific cytotoxicity, monocyte-macrophage chemotaxis and cytotoxicity, specific and nonspecific immunoglobulin production, and lymphokine production. Most of these result from an alteration in the quantitative makeup of the peripheral blood mononuclear cell repertoire, while some result from chronic cellular activation. The one immunologic abnormality which appears to be directly due to the immunosuppressive activity of the AIDS virus is the inability of either peripheral blood mononuclear cells or purified T4 cells to recognize and proliferate in response to soluble protein antigens. For purposes of studying the standard 20- to 40-year-old American population, the easiest antigen

to use for this purpose is tetanus toxoid. Patients who have been infected with HTLV-III, as identified by a positive Western blot with the viral antigens, generally fall into two groups with respect to proliferative responses to tetanus toxoid: those who do respond and those who do not. Although formal proof is still lacking, the suspicion is that those individuals who retain their ability to respond to tetanus toxoid are in much better immunologic and clinical shape than those who do not. For these reasons, measurements of lymphocyte blast transformation to tetanus toxoid may be of value in attempting to determine whether or not a given immune system has been damaged by HTLV-III. This response, which is generally all or nothing, has been of much greater value than any of the standard mitogens in the evaluation of the immune systems of HTLV-III-positive individuals.

The measurement of lymphocyte blast transformation to tetanus toxoid utilizes a 5- or 6-day [³H]thymidine incorporation assay. Peripheral blood mononuclear cells are harvested, and 10^5 cells are cultured per well in 96-well microtiter dishes containing 15% human A serum, RPMI 1640 with glutamine, and 5 μg of tetanus toxoid per ml. The plates are incubated in a 37°C incubator containing 5% CO_2 for 5 to 6 days and then pulsed with 2 μCi of [³H]thymidine per well. Cells are allowed to incorporate the [³H]thymidine for 4 h, and the cells are then harvested with a MASH harvester or equivalent. Data are expressed as counts per minute of [³H]thymidine – background counts per minute (culture without tetanus toxoid). Normal values range from 5,000 to 50,000 cpm. As in all immunologic testing, this type of assay should be run in parallel with peripheral blood mononuclear cells from a healthy control individual.

CONCLUSION

The AIDS epidemic has become one of the most pressing medical problems of modern time. Although we are only in the early stages of our understanding of this complex illness, the discovery of the etiologic agent has greatly enhanced our ability to diagnose individuals who have been exposed to the virus and are thus potential carriers of the disease. Techniques exist not only for isolating the virus from infected individuals but also for testing sera for antibody responses to the virus. Our understanding of the way in which the virus affects the immune system is rapidly expanding and will, we hope, soon lead to effective therapeutic strategies designed to combat the etiologic retroviral agent and the immunodeficiency state it produces.

LITERATURE CITED

1. **Barré-Sinoussi, F., J.-C. Chermann, F. Rey, M. T. Nugeyre, S. Chamaret, J. Gruest, C. Dauguet, C. Axler-Blin, F. Brun-Vezinet, C. Rouzioux, W. Rozenbaum, and L. Montagnier.** 1983. Isolation of a T-lymphotropic retrovirus from a patient at risk for acquired immune deficiency syndrome (AIDS). Science **220:**868–871.
2. **Boyum, A.** 1968. Isolation of mononuclear cells and granulocytes from human blood. Scand. J. Clin. Lab. Invest. **21:**77–89.
3. **Fauci, A. S., A. M. Macher, D. L. Longo, H. C. Lane, A. H. Rook, H. Masur, and E. P. Gelmann.** 1984. Acquired immunodeficiency syndrome: epidemiologic,

clinical, immunologic, and therapeutic considerations. Ann. Intern. Med. **100**:92–106.

4. **Feorino, P. M., V. S. Kalyanaraman, H. W. Haverkos, C. D. Carbradilla, D. T. Warfield, H. W. Jaffe, A. K. Harrison, M. S. Gottlieb, D. Goldfinger, J.-C. Chermann, F. Barré-Sinoussi, T. J. Spira, J. S. McDougal, J. W. Curran, L. Montagnier, F. A. Murphy, and D. P. Francis.** 1984. Lymphadenopathy associated virus infection of a blood donor-recipient pair with acquired immunodeficiency syndrome. Science **225**:69–72.

5. **Folks, T., S. Benn, A. Rabson, T. Theodore, M. D. Hoggan, M. Martin, M. Lightfoote, and K. Sell.** 1985. Characterization of a continuous T-cell line susceptible to the cytopathic effects of the acquired immunodeficiency syndrome (AIDS)-associated retrovirus. Proc. Natl. Acad. Sci. USA **82**:4539–4543.

6. **Gallo, R. C., S. Z. Salahuddin, M. Popovic, G. M. Shearer, M. Kaplan, B. F. Haynes, T. J. Palker, R. Redfield, J. Oleske, B. Safai, G. White, P. Foster, and P. D. Markham.** 1984. Frequent detection and isolation of cytopathic retroviruses (HTLV-III) from patients with AIDS and at risk for AIDS. Science **224**:500–503.

7. **Lane, H. C., J. M. Depper, W. C. Green, G. Whalen, T. A. Waldmann, and A. S. Fauci.** 1985. Qualitative analysis of immune function in patients with the acquired immunodeficiency syndrome: evidence for a selective defect in soluble antigen recognition. New Engl. J. Med. **313**:79–84.

8. **Lane, H. C., and A. S. Fauci.** 1985. Immunologic abnormalities in the acquired immunodeficiency syndrome. Annu. Rev. Immunol. **3**:477–500.

9. **Lane, H. C., H. Masur, E. P. Gelmann, D. L. Longo, R. G. Steis, T. Chused, G. Whalen, L. C. Edgar, and A. S. Fauci.** 1985. Correlation between immunologic function and clinical subpopulations of patients with the acquired immune deficiency syndrome. Am. J. Med. **78**:417–422.

10. **Sarngadharan, M. G., M. Popovic, L. Bruch, J. Schupbach, and R. C. Gallo.** 1984. Antibodies reactive with human T-lymphotrophic retroviruses (HTLV-III) in the serum of patients with AIDS. Science **224**:506–508.

Chapter 90

Chlamydiae

JULIUS SCHACHTER

Chlamydia trachomatis is one of the most common human pathogens (15). Of the 15 recognized serotypes, 4 (A, B, Ba, and C) have been shown to cause hyperendemic blinding trachoma, a disease which afflicts hundreds of millions of people in developing countries (7). Three serotypes (L1, L2, and L3) are the causes of lymphogranuloma venereum (LGV), a sexually transmitted systemic disease. The other serotypes (D through K) have been associated with genital tract infections and sporadic cases of conjunctivitis in industrialized societies. These agents are the major recognized cause of nongonococcal urethritis in men, in whom they may also cause epididymitis. In women, *C. trachomatis* causes cervicitis and acute salpingitis. Infants born through an infected birth canal may contract the infection and then develop inclusion conjunctivitis of the newborn, the characteristic chlamydial pneumonia syndrome, or both (1). The only other species within this genus, *C. psittaci*, is a common pathogen of avian and lower mammalian species but is relatively uncommon in humans, in whom it may cause the disease psittacosis.

There are no wholly satisfactory serological methods for diagnosing the human chlamydial infections. The tests that are useful for diagnosing one of the diseases may be virtually useless in attempting to diagnose some of the other human infections. At best, the current status of chlamydial diagnostic serology leaves much to be desired. Problems stem from inadequate antibody response for certain tests, inability to obtain appropriately paired sera because of long incubation periods or inapparent infections, and a high background of antibody prevalence in high-risk populations.

For practical purposes, only two serologic methods can be recommended: the complement fixation (CF) test and the Wang microimmunofluorescence (Micro-IF) technique (25). The CF test (reviewed by Meyer and Eddie [9]) is most useful in the diagnosis of psittacosis and LGV (systemic infections), considerably less helpful in diagnosing oculogenital infections, and virtually useless in the diagnosis of trachoma (superficial infections). The Micro-IF test is most useful in the diagnosis of chlamydial oculogenital infections and trachoma, although it may be used in the routine diagnosis of psittacosis. Both tests are useful in serological surveys, perhaps more so than for diagnosing individual infections.

A variety of other serological tests have been used, largely in research projects (17). Among these are agglutination tests, immunodiffusion tests, radioisotope immune precipitation tests, enzyme-linked immunosorbent assays, and direct and indirect hemagglutination assays. Most recently, a series of enzyme immunoassay procedures have been described which use different types of chlamydial antigen preparations. An enzyme immunoassay using the major outer membrane protein as antigen is promising (12). Some of the tests are untried in the routine diagnosis of human infections; others have been tried and found wanting. Some of these tests may yet be refined and find some practical application, but currently none can be recommended for serodiagnosis of human chlamydial infections.

The CF test is a genus-specific test. It measures antibodies to an antigenic determinant common to all chlamydiae (the active moiety is apparently a 2-keto-3-deoxyoctanoic acid) (6). These antichlamydial antibodies react extensively with the lipopolysaccharide from *Acinetobacter calcoaceticus* (10). This organism may ultimately be a convenient source of genus-reactive antigen.

In contrast, the Micro-IF test measures specific antibodies that are not detected by the CF test. Wang and Grayston introduced the Micro-IF in 1970, initially for the serotyping of *C. trachomatis*, but further studies from the same and other laboratories showed it to be a highly sensitive and specific indicator of antichlamydial antibodies (8, 11, 13, 22, 25).

The CF and Micro-IF tests, when applied to individual sera, are generally carried through an appropriate dilution range to allow determination of endpoints against the antigen. In survey work, to determine prevalence of antichlamydial antibodies, it may be possible to simplify testing by screening sera at the specific dilutions which are considered to be indicative of significant titers. The Micro-IF test may involve many antigens (up to 15 serotypes may be used), but many studies could focus on antigenic types prevalent in the specific geographical area and associated with the disease condition under consideration. This is particularly applicable in studies on childhood trachoma. Even in other studies it may be possible to use only one or two serovars in the Micro-IF test. For instance, studies on genital tract infections in San Francisco, Calif., revealed that at least 75% of reactive sera had detectable antibodies to either serotype E or serotype L2. Similar results have been obtained in Washington (11). However, Wang and Grayston found type-specific patterns in 79% of their sera from isolate-positive patients (25). Even in that study, approximately 75% of patients' sera reacted with type E or LGV-2, although much higher titers were observed with homologous serotypes.

Attempts have been made to develop a more broadly reactive antigen for the Micro-IF test. One such test uses chlamydial inclusions in cultured cell monolayers as antigen (1, 14). Such intact inclusions tend to have less type-specific reactivity than the elementary-body suspensions used in the Micro-IF test. The inclusions show more broadly reactive responses and seem to have both genus- and species-specific reactivity. In some instances this could be an advantage since single inclusion types such as L2 are very broadly reactive and can be used to diagnose a variety of chlamydial infections, including psittacosis and chlamydial pneu-

TABLE 1. Antichlamydial antibodies in selected populations

Group	% with:		
	CF ≥1:16	Micro-IF ≥1:8	IgM ≥1:8
Screening studies			
Normal adults, all ages	2–3	25–45	2–3
Pediatric sera	<1	10	<1
Trachoma endemic population	5–15	>80	ND[a]
Venereal disease studies			
Males, young adults	5–10	20–25	<5
Females, young adults	15–20	50–70	<5
Prostitutes	30–60	≥85	ND
Proven chlamydial infections (isolation)			
LGV	100	100	80
Psittacosis	100	ND	ND
Adult inclusion conjunctivitis	50	100	70
Males, urethritis	15	90	30–50
Females, cervical infection	45	99	20–30
Infant pneumonia	ND	100	100
Newborn inclusion conjunctivitis	ND	100	30

[a] ND, Not determined.

monia in infants. Reticulate body suspensions have also been used as antigen. The reticulate body is more cross-reactive than the elementary body but it is not as sensitive for immunoglobulin M (IgM) and type-specific antibodies (26). Unfortunately, there is a price to be paid for simplifying the test procedures. Type-specific responses are not detected by single-antigen tests using inclusions or elementary-body suspensions. In addition, any single-antigen test will fail to diagnose some infections. This is most marked with infants, who tend to produce highly type-specific antibodies.

CLINICAL INDICATIONS

The CF test should be used routinely whenever LGV is considered in the differential diagnosis, usually in the case of young men being examined for inguinal lymphadenopathy, with or without systemic complications. In untreated cases, if a suitable laboratory is available, efforts should be made to isolate chlamydiae from aspirates of fluctuant nodes. The bubonic form of LGV is less often seen in women. Women usually present with what are considered to be the later sequelae of LGV (proctitis, rectal stricture, or rectovaginal fistula). Serological tests have taken greater importance in supporting the diagnosis of LGV now that the shortcomings of the Frei test (delayed hypersensitivity skin test) have been recognized and this skin test antigen is no longer commercially available (21).

The disadvantages of the CF test are not its lack of specificity (for there are no known cross-reactions), but rather the ubiquitous nature of some of the chlamydial parasites and the group specificity of the test. Thus, positive serology may support a diagnosis of LGV but cannot prove it. Serological proof of the diagnosis would be based on demonstration of rising titers (a greater than fourfold difference in paired acute- and convalescent-phase sera), but in most cases

the patient has had the chlamydial infection for too long a period of time before the test is performed. Even in acute lymphadenopathy in the male, there is usually a 3- to 4-week period from infection to presentation. Since there may have to be a reliance on a static titer, with LGV one will feel much more comfortable in accepting a serological diagnosis when the CF titers are high (1:64 or greater), although any titer above the 1:8 or 1:16 range is considered significant. The titers in men take on greater meaning than those in women because the common chlamydial infections causing nongonococcal urethritis in the male tend not to produce either as high a prevalence or as high a titer as do the genital tract infections in women (Table 1).

It is uncommon to find a man with chlamydial urethritis who has a CF titer above the 1:16 level (Table 2). Any patient tested for LGV should also have a serological test for syphilis. Some patients will have both diseases, and sera reactive in the Venereal Disease Research Laboratory test may also react with both LGV and normal yolk sac antigens.

The CF test should be performed whenever a diagnosis of psittacosis is considered. A pneumonitis or persistent influenza or any acute or chronic febrile disease following exposure to birds would be a clinical indication for considering psittacosis in the differential diagnosis. Here, the CF test is much more satisfactory for diagnosis since acute- and convalescent-phase sera can be obtained and often demonstrate rising titers. In fact, in our experience, the great majority of psittacosis cases can be diagnosed in this manner. The diagnosis may have to be based upon a single high titer if the patient has a persistent or relapsing disease, but such a titer would clearly support the clinical impression. The problems of cross-reactions and previous exposure to other chlamydiae are clearly the same. In general, psittacosis infections produce high CF antibody levels. If a patient has had early and persistent treatment with tetracyclines, the antibody levels may be suppressed. There have been a number of human infections (proven by agent isolation) in which no serologic response was obtained because of early therapy.

The CF test is useless in the diagnosis of trachoma and not particularly useful in the diagnosis of oculogenital infections (18, 20). At best, only 50% of individuals with eye and genital tract infections will have significant (>1:16) CF titers (18). In uncomplicated genital tract infections such as urethritis or cervicitis, the CF reactor rates are even lower. The CF

TABLE 2. Distribution of chlamydial CF titers in patients with proven infections

Disease	No. tested	No. with CF titer of:				
		<1:16	1:16	1:32	1:64	≥1:128
LGV	15	0	1	2	0	12
Psittacosis	30	0	2	5	5	18
Adult inclusion conjunctivitis	93	46	28	11	6	2
Cervicitis, females	55	30	9	6	4	6
Urethritis, males	60	51	8	1	0	0

test is almost useless in the diagnosis of urethritis, as only 15% of men with proven chlamydial urethritis have significant CF levels (Table 1). However, ca. 40% of women with chlamydial cervicitis have significant CF levels. CF titers in the background population, i.e., sexually active men or sexually active women, will show a similar distribution of reactor rates. Women will have a higher background rate of CF reactors than men.

C. trachomatis infection should also be considered in infants with pneumonia (1). Characteristically, chlamydial pneumonia occurs in infants less than 6 months of age, follows a chronic afebrile course, and is accompanied by a staccato cough and tachypnea. Many of the infants have conjunctivitis by history or by examination. The CF test is not useful, and such infants should be tested by the Micro-IF procedure. IgG antibody levels may be of maternal origin, and it is more important to test the sera for IgM antibodies, which reflect recent chlamydial infection. IgM titers of >1:32 are highly supportive of the diagnosis (19).

The Micro-IF test measures specific antibodies to antigenic determinants present in the cell walls of the elementary-body particles. It is much more sensitive than the CF test (11). For example, in one series of 55 isolate-positive patients, 29 were found to have significant CF reactions, while all 55 were positive in the Micro-IF test. The respective geometric mean titers were 1:12 and 1:164. The Micro-IF test can be applied to patients with LGV or with ocular or oculogenital infections caused by the trachoma-inclusion conjunctivitis agents. The presence of a reaction in a single serum specimen may reflect previous exposure. Changing titers may be seen in patients who are examined relatively early in the course of an infection, but this is usually not the case. One advantage of the Micro-IF test is that information on the specific serotype responsible for the infection may be obtained. The Micro-IF test offers the added advantage of determining the immunoglobulin class of the reactive antibodies since the presence of IgM antibodies may lend further support to diagnosis of active infection. Unfortunately, many chlamydial infections tend to be chronic, and the best assessment is that the IgM antibody response may last for ca. 1 month after infection (25). In one study only 33% of patients with active infections had IgM antibodies (11). The major disadvantage of the Micro-IF test is that its results reflect the high prevalence of chlamydial infection in certain groups (15). In other words, in appropriate populations there may be very high antibody prevalence rates from previous exposure to the chlamydiae, and these antibody levels may persist for life, although in some patients they disappear spontaneously (possibly reflecting brief antigenic exposure). The significant level in the Micro-IF test has been chosen as 1:8.

In sexually active women the high prevalence of antichlamydial antibodies is found not only in serum but also in cervical secretions. A number of workers have advocated testing cervical secretions for antichlamydial antibodies as a diagnostic test (5, 22). Although the great majority of *Chlamydia*-infected women will have antichlamydial antibodies in their cervical secretions, most women with such antibodies will not have current chlamydial infections (16). Thus,

the sensitivity of the test is very high but the specificity is very low, and the predictive value will be relatively poor (although somewhat better results are obtained in assaying IgA antibody in cervical secretions [4]). In fact, I have not found any of these serological tests applied to either serum or secretions to yield predictive values in excess of 40% for genital tract chlamydial infections in either men or women.

TEST PROCEDURES

CF

The CF test may be performed in either the tube system or the microtiter system. I strongly prefer the standardization of reagents in the tube system, regardless of which system is being used for the test. The microtiter systems are more useful in screening large numbers of sera, but it is preferable to retest all positive sera in the tube system. Occasionally, sera giving titers in the 1:4 and 1:8 range in the microtiter system are positive at 1:16 (the significant level) in the tube system. The microtiter system uses standard plates and volumes 1/10 of those used in the tube test. The CF test is performed on serum specimens heated at 56°C for 30 min (preferably acute- and convalescent-phase paired sera tested together). In each test a positive control serum of high titer is included together with a known negative serum. The reagents for the CF test are standardized by the Kolmer technique and include special buffered saline, group antigen, antigen (normal yolk sac) control, the positive serum, the negative serum, guinea pig complement, rabbit anti-sheep hemolysin, and sheep erythrocytes. The hemolytic system is titrated, and the complement unitage is determined. The standard units used in the test are 4 U of antigen and 2 exact U of complement. The test may be performed by either the water-bath technique or the overnight (icebox) technique; the former is preferable. Doubling dilutions of the serum (from 1:2) are made in a 0.25-ml volume of saline. The antigen is added at 4 U (0.25 ml), and 2 exact U of complement (0.5 ml) is added. Standard reagent controls are always included. The normal yolk sac control is used at the same dilution as the group antigen. The tubes are shaken well and incubated in a water bath at 37°C for 2 h. Then 0.5 ml of sensitized sheep erythrocytes is added, and the tubes are placed in the water bath for 1 h more. The tubes are read for hemolysis on a 1+ to 4+ scale roughly equivalent to 25 to 100% inhibition of erythrocyte lysis. The endpoint of the serum is considered the highest dilution producing at least 50% (2+) hemolysis after a complete inhibition of hemolysis has been observed. It is general practice in my laboratory to shake the tubes to resuspend the settled cells, refrigerate them overnight, and recheck the results the next morning.

Micro-IF

The Micro-IF test is performed against chlamydial organisms grown in yolk sac or cell culture. The individual yolk sacs are selected for elementary-body richness and pretitrated to give an even distribution of particles. It is generally found that a 1 to 3% yolk sac suspension (phosphate-buffered saline, pH 7.0) is satisfactory. The antigens may be stored as frozen aliquots, and after thawing they are well mixed on a Vortex mixer before use. Antigen dots are placed on a slide in a specific pattern, with separate pen points used for each antigen. Each cluster of dots includes all the antigenic types to be tested. The antigen dots are air dried and fixed on slides with acetone (15 min at room temperature). Slides may be stored frozen. When thawed for use, they may sweat, but they can be conveniently dried (as can the original antigen dots) with the cool air flow of a hair dryer. The slides have serial dilutions of serum (or tears or exudate) placed on the different antigen clusters. The clusters of dots are placed sufficiently separated to avoid the running of the serum from cluster to cluster. After addition of the serum dilutions, the slides are incubated for 0.5 to 1 h in a moist chamber at 37°C. They are then placed in a buffered saline wash for 5 min, followed by a second 5-min wash. The slides are then dried and stained with fluorescein-conjugated anti-human globulin. Conjugates are pretitrated in a known positive system to determine appropriate working dilutions. This reagent may be prepared against any class of globulin being considered (IgA or secretory piece for secretions, IgG, or IgM). Counterstains such as bovine serum albumin conjugated with rhodamine may be included. The slides are then washed twice again, dried, and examined by standard fluorescence microscopy. Use of a monocular tube is recommended to allow greater precision in determining fluorescence for individual elementary body particles. The endpoints are read as the dilution giving bright fluorescence clearly associated with the well-distributed elementary bodies throughout the antigen dot. Identification of the type-specific response is based upon dilution differences reflected in the endpoints for different prototype antigens (7). Monotypic reactions to serotype A may be spurious and should be interpreted with caution.

For each run of either CF or Micro-IF, known positive and negative sera should always be included. These sera should always duplicate their titers as previously observed within the experimental (±1 dilution) error of the system.

REAGENTS

The commercially available antigens have occasionally presented major problems. In the CF test an antigen with the highest possible titer should be used to allow greatest dilution of the crude preparations being used and for reasons of economy. Several commercial preparations are available, but none can be recommended. I have often seen commercial preparations with titers in the 1:8 or 1:16 range; the working dilution would be 1:2 to 1:4, which is unsatisfactory. A major problem in the CF test has been obtaining complement free from antibodies to chlamydiae. Guinea pig inclusion conjunctivitis is a very common chlamydial infection in guinea pig colonies. The CF antigens may appear to be anticomplementary, whereas they are simply reacting with the antibody present in guinea pig complement. This often is evident when the complement does not react with the normal yolk sac control. One should always attempt to purchase complement certified to be nonreactive

with chlamydial antigens. Unfortunately, the certification is not always accurate, and testing for antichlamydial antibodies before use is essential.

In the Micro-IF test the major reagent problem has been the reliability of immunoglobulin preparations against human IgM.

The CF hemolytic system reagents may be readily obtained commercially. M. A. Bioproducts (Los Angeles, Calif.) has proven to be a relatively reliable source of complement, although the previous warning on chlamydial antibodies in the complement still applies. Sheep erythrocytes can usually be obtained locally, and they must be checked for fragility. There is, however, no commercially available source of antigen which is highly potent; therefore, the antigens must be prepared in the laboratory. There are several methods that produce suitable antigens. The deoxycholate-extracted group antigen or the ether-extracted (and acetone-precipitated, if preferred) group antigens are perfectly satisfactory (24). Theoretically, any chlamydial strain can be used to prepare a group antigen, as it appears to be the major antigenic component for all strains. However, comparative tests have shown that some strains are to be preferred over others; for instance, the psittacosis antigens have been superior to the LGV antigens, even with LGV serum. The 6BC strain which has been used for many years is available from the American Type Culture Collection.

The technique of antigen preparation involves inoculation of 7-day-old embryonated hen eggs via the yolk sac route with a standardized inoculum (0.25 ml containing approximately 10^5 egg 50% lethal doses) which kills most of the embryos in approximately 96 h. Embryos dying before 72 h are discarded. When approximately 50% of the embryos are dead, all the eggs are refrigerated for 3 to 24 h. The yolk sacs are harvested and examined microscopically (Gimenez or Macchiavello strain) for elementary bodies. If rich in particles, they are pooled and weighed. Yolk sacs are then ground thoroughly with sterile sand, and a 20% suspension in nutrient broth (pH 7.0) is prepared. Bacterial sterility tests are performed, and the material is held in a refrigerator for 6 weeks. During this period, the antigen preparation is occasionally shaken. The suspension is then centrifuged lightly ($220 \times g$ for 30 min) to remove coarse tissue debris and steamed at 100°C for 30 min. After it has cooled, phenol is added to a final concentration of 0.5%. This antigen is divided into small portions and stored in a refrigerator. It should have a titer of at least 1:256 and, if stored properly and protected from contamination by using aseptic techniques, will be stable for years. The normal yolk sac control is prepared in a similar manner from uninfected embryos.

The routine immunofluorescence reagents used in the Micro-IF test are available from Kallestad Labs (Austin, Tex.) and Hyland Laboratories, Inc. (Costa Mesa, Calif.), among others. The yolk sac antigens, however, are not available commercially and must be prepared in the laboratory. For a complete battery of test antigens, types A, B, Ba, C, D, E, F, G, H, I, J, and K and LGV antigens L1, L2, and L3 must be included. For routine screening of human sera, a simplified antigen pattern involving fewer antigen dots is useful (27). Closely related antigens may be pooled, for example, D and E, L1 and L2, K and L3, G and F, and C and J. For diagnosis of psittacosis infections, a *C. psittaci* strain must be added. It is difficult to choose the appropriate strain in the absence of adequate information on serotype specificity, but in my laboratory the 6BC strain (isolated from a parakeet), which appears to be very broadly reactive, is used. The antigens are generally prepared from infected yolk sac suspensions. Cell culture preparations may be used although they tend not to be as rich in particles. The yolk sacs are inoculated with suspensions of chlamydiae titrated to kill the embryos in ca. 7 days. In some instances a greater time period may be required. When 50% of the eggs are dead, the rest are chilled, the yolk sacs are harvested, and individual yolk sacs are examined microscopically; those rich in elementary bodies are selected for use. They are homogenized to approximately 5% with sterile phosphate-buffered saline, and final antigen dilution is selected on the basis of morphological screening in a fluorescence system. The working dilution (usually 1 to 3%) may be frozen in aliquots at −60°C and stored until needed for making slides. The antigen suspensions and the slides when frozen are stable, but thawed suspensions should be used within 1 to 2 weeks.

Alternatively, the antigens may be prepared from cell culture monolayers. Heavily infected monolayers are incubated for 72 to 96 h and disrupted by either sonication or vigorous shaking with glass beads. To provide adequate contrast in microscopic examination and to enhance the attachment of the antigen to the slides, a 1% normal yolk sac suspension should be added to the cell culture antigen.

INTERPRETATION

The background prevalence of chlamydial antibodies (which reflect diseases prevalent in the community) will vary depending upon the geographical area where the assays are performed and the specific population group to be tested. Table 1 presents the results obtained in my laboratory, using these two tests in parallel in different population studies. For example, the prevalence of CF antibody at a 1:16 level in the general population in the San Francisco area is 2 to 3%. However, if one were testing veterinarians, one could find between 10 and 20% with significant CF levels. Further, if one were testing sexually active individuals, one would find the background to be approximately 5 to 10% for men and 15 to 20% for women. In patients with Reiter's syndrome there is approximately a 25% seropositivity rate, and approximately 10% of the patients with Reiter's syndrome have very high antibody levels such as those often seen in psittacosis or LGV. CF titers of 1:64 or higher are rarely seen in the normal population or in sexually active males, although they do occur in sexually active females. This is the level which would be highly supportive of a diagnosis of psittacosis or LGV.

There has not been similar broad experience with the Micro-IF test, but the published results together with unpublished data from the Hooper Foundation indicate little problem with group-specific cross-reactions. For example, psittacosis convalescent-phase sera with CF titers of 1:512 have been tested and found to be completely nonreactive in the Micro-IF test with *C. trachomatis* antigens. There is, however, a problem

of background antibody prevalence. For example, asymptomatic sexually active women have been found to have a background reactor rate of 60 to 70%. Thus, a single positive titer could be used only to determine previous exposure. In epidemiological studies, type-specific reactions could be of considerable interest in detecting predominant serotypes, transmission chains, patterns of clustering, etc. IgM antibodies in the Micro-IF test may give greater support for active infection, but experience indicates that only 28 to 33% of patients with active infections have these antibodies, and some patients who have IgM antibodies do not have demonstrable chlamydial infection (11, 25). Higher rates of IgM reactors are observed in selected patients having first attacks of chlamydial infection (3). There is an increasing antibody prevalence with age, with a background of ca. 10% in the pediatric population (2). The stimulus for this antibody is not known; this rate is higher than the rate of perinatal chlamydial infection.

Infants with proven *C. trachomatis* pneumonia invariably have high IgM antibody levels (19). A great majority are ≥1:256, and only the atypical young infant appears to have lower, but still appreciable, levels (≥1:64). On the other hand, infants with uncomplicated inclusion conjunctivitis have much lower titers (1). Patients with LGV tend to have high (≥1:128) CF titers and very high (≥1:2,000) and broadly reactive Micro-IF antibody responses. Specific antichlamydial IgA or IgG in tears may indicate active chlamydial infection of the conjunctiva, but it is likely that most antibodies in tears (8, 16) or cervical secretions reflect circulating antibody. As such, they may not be useful in diagnosing current infection. The prevalence of tear antibody in a trachomatous population may reflect the severity of trachoma in the community (23).

Most psittacosis cases can be diagnosed by CF, with which fourfold or greater rises, often to very high titers, can be shown. Paired sera from human psittacosis cases often show rising IgG levels by Micro-IF as well as the presence of IgM antibody in both acute- and convalescent-phase sera. IgM levels may rise but are often static or falling while the IgG levels tend to be rising.

In either CF or Micro-IF it is clear that a fourfold or greater rise in titer will support the diagnosis of chlamydial infection in the clinical syndrome being considered. Unfortunately, this is usually not observed with *C. trachomatis* infections, and often the clinician must simply use the titer of a late serum specimen in relation to background patterns to determine whether it supports the clinical diagnosis.

LITERATURE CITED

1. **Beem, M. O., and E. M. Saxon.** 1977. Respiratory-tract colonization and a distinctive pneumonia syndrome in infants infected with *Chlamydia trachomatis*. N. Engl J. Med. **296**:306–310.
2. **Black, S. B., M. Grossman, L. Cles, and J. Schachter.** 1981. Serologic evidence of chlamydial infection in children. J. Pediatr. **98**:65–67.
3. **Bowie, W. R., S.-P. Wang, E. R. Alexander, J. Floyd, P. Forsyth, H. Pollock, J.-S. Tin, T. Buchanan, and K. K. Holmes.** 1977. Etiology of nongonococcal urethritis: evidence for *Chlamydia trachomatis* and *Ureaplasma*

urealyticulum. J. Clin. Invest. **59**:735–742.

4. **Brunham, R. C., C.-C. Kuo, L. Cles, and K. K. Holmes.** 1983. Correlation of host immune response with quantitative recovery of *Chlamydia trachomatis* from the human endocervix. Infect. Immun. **39**:1491–1494.

5. **Carr, M. C., L. Hanna, and E. Jawetz.** 1979. Chlamydiae, cervicitis and abnormal Papanicolaou smears. Obstet. Gynecol. **53**:27–30.

6. **Dhir, S. P., G. E. Kenney, and J. T. Grayston.** 1971. Characterization of the group antigen of *Chlamydia trachomatis*. Infect. Immun. **4**:725–730.

7. **Grayston, J. T., and S.-P. Wang.** 1975. New knowledge of chlamydiae and the diseases they cause. J. Infect. Dis. **132**:87–105.

8. **Hanna, L., E. Jawetz, B. Nabli, I. Hoshiwara, B. Ostler, and C. Dawson.** 1972. Titration and typing of serum antibodies in TRIC infections by immunofluorescence. J. Immunol. **108**:102–107.

9. **Meyer, K. F., and B. Eddie.** 1956. Psittacosis, p. 399–430. *In* E. H. Lennette and N. J. Schmidt (ed.), Diagnostic procedures for viral and rickettsial diseases, 2nd ed. American Public Health Association, Inc., New York.

10. **Nurminen, M., M. Leinonen, P. Saikku, and P. H. Makela.** 1983. The genus-specific antigen of *Chlamydia*: resemblance to the lipopolysaccharide of enteric bacteria. Science **220**:1279–1281.

11. **Philip, R. N., E. A. Casper, F. B. Gordon, and A. L. Quan.** 1974. Fluorescent antibody responses to chlamydial infection in patients with lymphogranuloma venereum and urethritis. J. Immunol. **112**:2126–2134.

12. **Puolakkainen, M., P. Saikku, M. Leinonen, M. Nurminen, P. Vaananen, and P. H. Makela.** 1984. Chlamydial pneumonitis and its serodiagnosis in infants. J. Infect. Dis. **149**:598–604.

13. **Reeve, P., R. K. Gerloff, E. Casper, R. N. Philip, J. D. Oriel, and P. A. Powis.** 1974. Serological studies on the role of *Chlamydia* in the aetiology of nonspecific urethritis. Br. J. Vener. Dis. **50**:136–139.

14. **Richmond, S. J., and S. O. Caul.** 1977. Single-antigen indirect immunofluorescence test for screening venereal disease clinic populations for chlamydial antibodies, p. 259–265. *In* K. K. Holmes and D. Hobson (ed.), Nongonococcal urethritis and related infections. American Society for Microbiology, Washington, D.C.

15. **Schachter, J.** 1978. Chlamydial infections. N. Engl. J. Med. **298**:428–435, 490–495, 540–549.

16. **Schachter, J., L. Cles, R. Ray, and P. Hines.** 1979. Failure of serology in diagnosing chlamydial infections of the female genital tract. J. Clin. Microbiol. **10**:647–649.

17. **Schachter, J., and C. R. Dawson.** 1978. Human chlamydial infections, p. 273. Publishing Sciences Group, Littleton, Mass.

18. **Schachter, J., C. R. Dawson, S. Balas, and P. Jones.** 1970. Evaluation of laboratory methods for detecting acute TRIC agent infection. Am. J. Ophthalmol. **70**:375–380.

19. **Schachter, J., M. Grossman, and P. H. Azimi.** 1982. Serology of *Chlamydia trachomatis* in infants. J. Infect. Dis. **146**:530–535.

20. **Schachter, J., C. H. Mordhorst, B. W. Moore, and M. L. Tarizzo.** 1973. Laboratory diagnosis of trachoma: a collaborative study. Bull. W.H.O. **48**:509–515.

21. **Schachter, J., D. E. Smith, C. R. Dawson, W. R. Anderson, J. J. Deller, Jr., A. W. Hoke, W. H. Smartt, and K. F. Meyer.** 1969. Lymphogranuloma venereum. I. Comparison of the Frei test, complement fixation test, and isolation of the agent. J. Infect. Dis. **120**:372–375.

22. **Treharne, J. D., S. Darougar, P. D. Simmons, and R. Thin.** 1978. Rapid diagnosis of chlamydial infection of the cervix. Br. J. Vener. Dis. **54**:403–408.

23. **Treharne, J. D., and T. Forsey.** 1983. Chlamydial serology. Br. Med. Bull. **39**:194–299.

24. **Volkert, M., and P. M. Christensen.** 1955. Two orinthosis complement fixing antigens from infected yolk sacs. Acta Pathol. Microbiol. Scand. **37**:211–218.

25. **Wang. S.-P., and J. T. Grayston.** 1974. Human serology in *Chlamydia trachomatis* infection with microimmunofluorescence. J. Infect. Dis. **130**:388–397.

26. **Wang, S.-P., and J. T. Grayston.** 1982. Microimmunofluorescence antibody responses in *Chlamydia trachomatis* infection, a review, p. 301–316. *In* K. K. Holmes, J. D. Oriel, P. Piot, and J. Schachter (ed.), Chlamydial infections. Elsevier Biomedical Press, Amsterdam.

27. **Wang, S-P., J. T. Grayston, E. R. Alexander, and K. K. Holmes.** 1975. Simplified microimmunofluorescence test with trachoma-lymphogranuloma venereum (*Chlamydia trachomatis*) antigens for use as a screening test for antibody. J. Clin. Microbiol. **1**:250–255.

Chapter 91

Rickettsiae

CHRISTINE S. EISEMANN AND JOSEPH V. OSTERMAN

Rickettsial diseases affecting humans occur throughout the world. Table 1 gives the antigenic classification of rickettsiae, the diseases caused by various rickettsial species, the mode of transmission, and the geographic distribution of the etiologic agents. In the United States, only three rickettsial diseases occur with significant frequency: Rocky Mountain spotted fever (RMSF), murine typhus, and Q fever. RMSF continues to be the most severe of these diseases and the one most commonly reported to the Centers for Disease Control (CDC). The incidence of RMSF sharply increased during the 1970s, reaching a plateau from 1979 to 1983 of 0.48 cases per 100,000 population (12). Despite the increased efficiency of modern serological tests and an improved case report form introduced by the CDC in 1981, it is likely that the incidence of RMSF infection is still underreported, due to misdiagnoses and subclinical infections which have recently been shown to exist (36). The overall case fatality ratio for RMSF remains at approximately 4%, with the highest mortality rate (10%) in the adult population (≥30 years), despite the fact that the disease is diagnosed predominantly in children (<19 years; 52% of all cases in 1983) (5, 12). The name of this disease, derived from the initial studies of *Rickettsia rickettsii* conducted in the Rocky Mountains of the western United States, is misleading epidemiologically; RMSF has been reported in all 50 states, with the majority of cases reported in the South Atlantic (53% of the total number of cases in 1982) and South Central states (5, 9). The major incidence of RMSF occurs between early April and early September (5), when environmental conditions are optimal for tick activity. It is important to note, however, that RMSF has been diagnosed during the winter months and cannot be considered a strictly seasonal disease (22). Cases of murine typhus confirmed by the CDC have ranged from 20 to 70 per year and have occurred predominantly in Southern Texas, in both children and adults. These cases were not associated occupationally with grain handlers or dock workers (4) as has been traditional in the past. Q fever disease is reported mainly in the Mountain and Pacific states at a rate of approximately 30 to 60 cases each year. Since state health laboratories are not required to report Q fever to the CDC, however, the infection rate of Q fever may be higher than the reported incidence, especially in persons having contact with sheep and other livestock. California has the highest reported incidence of disease (8), but this may be a result of routine testing (since 1977) for Q fever in patients with respiratory infection. Rickettsialpox is seldom reported in the United States. Five serologically confirmed cases were reported in 1979, all occurring in New York City (4). It is likely that more cases of rickettsialpox occur in other major U.S. cities but that these go unrecognized due to diminished awareness by clinicians and diagnostic laboratories. Louse-borne epidemic typhus has been considered nonexistent in the United States since the last importation of this disease in 1950 (4). However, an agent indistinguishable from *R. prowazekii* was isolated from the eastern flying squirrel in 1975 (2, 25), and in the years between 1976 and 1979, 11 cases of epidemic typhus-like disease were serologically confirmed (4). These infections did not seem to be related to the louse contact usually associated with epidemic typhus, and the relationship of the flying squirrel agent with classical *R. prowazekii* is currently under investigation. However, the potential for this disease, especially in persons having contact with flying squirrels, should be recognized to help avoid misdiagnosis of the disease as RMSF or murine typhus. Brill-Zinsser disease, or recrudescent epidemic typhus, is rarely reported in the United States, usually in older individuals who previously contracted primarily epidemic typhus years earlier in Europe or Asia. Boutonneuse fever, other exotic spotted fever group diseases, and scrub typhus do not exist in the United States, but these diseases may be seen in persons exposed to infection during travel in endemic areas. In 1979, all of the four cases of boutonneuse fever confirmed by the CDC involved overseas travel (4), and it is notable that the incidence and severity of boutonneuse fever has increased drastically during the last decade in Sicily and other areas of Italy (24) and in Israel, South Africa, and France (40).

DIAGNOSIS

Early definitive diagnosis of rickettsial disease requires either the isolation of rickettsiae from the blood or the demonstration of rickettsiae in rash biopsies by fluorescent-antibody methods (20). Serological tests are of value in the confirmation of rickettsial infection; however, since treatment must be initiated before antibody usually is detectable, the diagnosis of rickettsial disease must be based on the patient's clinical symptoms, history of exposure to arthropod vectors, dogs, or livestock, or recent travel to endemic areas. The clinical features of RMSF include myalgia, fever, headache, maculopapular rash, palmar rash, muscle tenderness, photophobia, and stupor. Splenomegaly and thrombocytopenia frequently are associated with the disease. None of these clinical features is specific for RMSF, and the disease can be readily misdiagnosed as measles, meningococcemia, or an enteroviral or other type of viral infection. These features are not always present in every case of RMSF; in very severe cases, the maculopapular rash is often indistinct or absent. RMSF should be considered in the differential diagnosis of any illness involving fever and rash, even if the locale is not endemic for the disease (4). A history of travel, tick bite, or close contact with tick-infested dogs may be useful in diagnosis; recent studies have shown that as high as 85% of RMSF patients had been exposed to

TABLE 1. Rickettsial diseases of humans

Antigenic group and etiologic agent	Disease	Mode of transmission to humans	Geographic distribution
Spotted fever			
Rickettsia rickettsii	Rocky Mountain spotted fever	Tick bite	Western Hemisphere
R. conorii	Boutonneuse fever	Tick bite	Mediterranean littoral, India, Africa
R. sibirica	Siberian tick typhus	Tick bite	Siberia, Mongolia, central Asia
R. australis	Queensland tick typhus	Tick bite	Australia
R. akari	Rickettsialpox	Mite bite	North America, USSR, Korea
Typhus			
R. prowazekii	Epidemic typhus	Infected louse feces	Worldwide
R. prowazekii	Brill-Zinsser disease	Recrudescence of latent infection	Worldwide
R. typhi	Murine typhus	Infected flea feces	Worldwide
Scrub typhus			
R. tsutsugamushi	Scrub typhus	Mite bite	India, Asia, Australia, Pacific Islands
Q fever			
Coxiella burnetii	Q fever	Infectious aerosol, tick bite (?)	Worldwide
Trench fever			
Rochalimaea quintana	Trench fever	Infected louse feces	Mexico, Europe, Africa

tick-infested dogs that were serologically positive for *R. rickettsii* (13). Murine typhus is usually a relatively mild febrile illness also characterized by headache, chills, aches, and macular rash. During early stages of the infection, murine typhus is difficult to distinguish from the much more severe epidemic typhus, but it may be discriminated from RMSF by the evolution of the rash. In typhus, the rash appears on the body first, then spreads to the extremities, whereas in spotted fever infections, the rash ordinarily appears first on the exposed extremities and then extends to the trunk. Q fever takes the form of an acute systemic disease which varies in severity, and inapparent infections may occur in endemic areas. Clinical symptoms include general malaise, respiratory distress, fever, and severe headache. An interstitial pneumonia may develop, but unlike other rickettsial diseases, Q fever infection is not accompanied by a cutaneous rash.

ANTIGENS AND ANTIBODIES

The antigenic classification of typhus group and spotted fever group organisms shown in Table 1 is based upon the presence of group-specific, soluble complement-fixing antigens which are released from the rickettsiae after treatment with diethyl ether. All species shown within these two groups possess a group-specific antigen. The soluble complement-fixing antigen, after treatment with hot alkali, yields an erythrocyte-sensitizing substance (ESS) which spontaneously adsorbs to sheep or human group O erythrocytes or to latex beads (16, 18, 28, 35). ESS is the reactive antigen in both the indirect hemagglutination (IHA) test and latex agglutination (LA) test and exhibits group-specific reactivity when tested against the sera of patients convalescent from typhus or spotted fever infections. Scrub typhus rickettsiae do not release similar antigens after extraction with ether, and there are no scrub typhus antigens available for

use in the agglutination assays. Scrub typhus organisms exhibit a marked antigenic heterogeneity. The organisms undoubtedly share antigens since cross-reactivity is observed in serological procedures, but complement-fixing antigens are principally strain specific in reactivity. The scrub typhus group is defined on the basis of mouse cross-immunity tests. Animals surviving infection with any member of the group are resistant to subsequent challenge with heterologous scrub typhus strains. Q fever organisms also do not release a group-specific antigen after ether extraction and only minor differences in total antigenic composition have been detected in isolates recovered from widely separated geographical areas. These rickettsiae are known to undergo "phase variation," which is a host-dependent change in antigenic structure. Newly isolated strains from animals and ticks are characteristically in phase I, but after a variable number of passages in embryonated chicken eggs, the phase I strains are converted to phase II. This unexplained phenomenon is important in the preparation of diagnostic antigens, because the sera of individuals convalescent from Q fever generally are reactive in the complement fixation (CF) test only with phase II organisms. The presence of a significant level of antibody against phase I rickettsiae is suggestive of a chronic Q fever infection, such as subacute Q fever endocarditis.

Members of the typhus, spotted fever, and scrub typhus groups of rickettsiae share some minor antigens with *Proteus* bacteria. This antigenic relationship has provided the basis for the Weil-Felix (WF) test, a diagnostic agglutination procedure using several strains of the genus. The general pattern of reactivity is shown in Table 2. *Proteus vulgaris* strain OX-19 is agglutinated by the sera of individuals convalescent from epidemic or murine typhus but rarely by sera from those recovered from Brill-Zinsser disease. *Proteus* strains OX-2 and OX-19 are agglutinated by

TABLE 2. WF reactions in rickettsioses

Disease	WF reaction with *Proteus* strain:		
	OX-19	OX-2	OX-K
Epidemic typhus	+ + + +	+	0
Murine typhus	+ + + +	+	0
Brill-Zinsser disease	Variable[a]	Variable[a]	0
Spotted fever[b]	+ + + +	+	0
	+	+ + +	0
Rickettsialpox	0	0	0
Scrub typhus	0	0	+ + +
Q fever	0	0	0
Trench fever	0	0	0

[a] Usually negative.
[b] Spotted fever immune sera can agglutinate either strain OX-19 or strain OX-2, or both.

the immune sera of individuals following infection with most members of the spotted fever group. *Proteus* agglutinins are not observed following rickettsialpox infection, even though *R. akari* shares the group-specific CF antigen common to all spotted fever group organisms. Infection with scrub typhus rickettsiae may elicit the formation of agglutinating antibodies against *P. mirabilis* strain OX-K, but the human response is variable, and it is not unusual for only 50% of these patients to exhibit a meaningful rise in serum titer against this strain of bacteria.

Rickettsial antibodies can reach detectable levels within 1 week after the onset of symptoms and usually rise to maximum titer within a few months. In RMSF, immunoglobulin M (IgM) antibodies appear early (3 to 8 days) and are first detectable in acute sera by the IHA test or the indirect fluorescent-antibody (IFA) test (21). IgG antibodies are usually detectable within 3 weeks after onset, reach a maximum titer within 1 to 3 months, and can persist for a year or longer. The IgM antibody titer begins to decrease at about 4 weeks after onset and can become undetectable by 3 to 4 months.

The production of rickettsial antibodies may be influenced by the administration of antibiotics. Early treatment with tetracycline has been shown to reduce the antibodies measurable by the sensitive IFA test, with the greater decrease being in the IgG rather than the IgM class of antibody (15); thus, when antibiotic treatment has been initiated, the use of an IgM-specific conjugate in this test may be beneficial. Sera from patients treated with tetracyclines or chloramphenicol before the third day of infection may be only minimally reactive in the CF and microagglutination (MA) tests compared to the sera of patients treated later in the disease (29).

SEROLOGICAL TECHNIQUES

Procedures for rickettsial serology include the IFA test (30, 33), the IHA test (35), the LA test (16, 18), the enzyme-linked immunosorbent assay (ELISA; 7, 10, 14), the MA procedure (11), the CF test (34), and the WF reaction (31). Fluorescent-antibody staining of frozen (39, 41) or paraffin-embedded (38) tissue sections from biopsies of rickettsial skin lesions is an important technique for the early diagnosis of RMSF (37), since RMSF rickettsiae have been demonstrated

in biopsy specimens as early as 4 to 8 days after the onset of disease (41). This test, however, can be performed optimally only by experienced personnel and requires adequate containment facilities since the tissue may contain living and fully infectious rickettsiae. Specific fluorescence may also be used to demonstrate *R. rickettsii* organisms in the hemocytes of ticks isolated from suspected cases of RMSF (3).

Sensitivity

The IFA test is one of the most sensitive assays of antibodies resulting from RMSF, murine typhus, and epidemic typhus infections (26, 27, 29, 35). This test has been shown to be superior to most other tests both in the magnitude of observed titers and in the frequency of positive reactions. It is also the method of choice in scrub typhus serology because antigen preparation is simple and micromodifications of the procedure allow simultaneous testing of a single serum against multiple antigenic strains of scrub typhus organisms (33). In acute sera, the IHA and LA tests are the next most sensitive for the detection of rickettsial antibodies (21), but these tests are not sensitive for the detection of older infections and thus are not useful for epidemiological studies (7, 17). An ELISA has now been developed for each of the antigenic groups of rickettsiae. The sensitivity of this test compares favorably to that of the IFA procedure when used to examine the sera of patients with RMSF, murine typhus, and epidemic typhus (7, 10, 14). There is controversy over the sensitivity of the MA test, with some investigators reporting sensitivity similar to that of the IFA and IHA tests (27, 29) and others finding it less sensitive than the CF test (26). The MA test is not widely used, regardless of its sensitivity, because the antigen requirement of this test makes it too expensive to perform routinely. The CF test is widely used for the serological diagnosis of rickettsial infections, including Q fever, but it is much less sensitive than procedures based on immunofluorescence or IHA tests (21, 27, 29). The WF reaction is generally reported as the least sensitive procedure of all (19, 27, 35), and several rickettsial diseases, including Q fever, trench fever, and rickettsialpox, do not elicit WF agglutinins. Sera from individuals with recrudescent epidemic typhus (Brill-Zinsser disease) show a variable response in the WF test, and the results are often negative. Immunofluorescent staining of skin biopsies for *R. rickettsii* and *R. conorii* rickettsiae is a sensitive assay for the determination of an acute infection; however, performance and interpretation of this test demand a measure of experience, without which the sensitivity of the test is greatly diminished.

Specificity

The serological methods with intact rickettsiae (IFA, MA, ELISA, skin biopsy) or extracted rickettsial antigens (IHA, LA, CF) are specific for rickettsial infection and are accepted as confirmatory methods when fourfold rises in titers in paired sera are demonstrated. The infecting rickettsial species can generally be identified despite the existence of inter- and intragroup cross-reactivity (26, 34); homologous and heterologous titers are usually sufficiently different in magnitude to allow the reliable interpretation of results. The IFA and IHA tests exhibit the least cross-reactivity, and CF results can be made more specific for RMSF by using antigen derived from *R. rickettsii* rather than *R. akari* and by using 2 U of antigen rather than 8 U (34). Differentiation of infecting species among typhus and spotted fever group members may also be made by using extensively washed rickettsial organisms as corpuscular CF antigens or by a modification of the IFA test, in which group-specific antibodies are absorbed from serum before the IFA reaction. Identification of the etiologic agent from among scrub typhus strains is most clearly documented using specific CF antigens, although the IFA test usually shows a greater serum titer against the infecting strain than against heterologous strains. Antibodies against the Q fever agent are highly specific regardless of the diagnostic technique employed. No cross-reactions with other microorganisms or viruses are known to occur, and a positive serological finding is more important in establishing the identity of this etiologic agent than is the case for some other rickettsial diseases. The WF reaction, a test which utilizes a nonrickettsial antigen, is not specific for rickettsial diseases. The *Proteus* organisms used in this test are agglutinated not only by antibodies elicited by certain rickettsial organisms but also by antibodies occurring as a result of *Proteus* urinary tract infections. In one study, only 4 to 18% of WF-positive sera could be confirmed by the IFA test using spotted fever group rickettsial antigens (19). In another study, a majority of patients with positive WF reactions were shown by other criteria not to have RMSF, and this high false-positive rate was paralleled by a significant false-negative rate (37). The lack of specificity of the WF reaction has compelled the CDC to accept WF results as only provisional but not confirmatory for rickettsial infection.

IFA test

The rickettsial IFA test is conveniently performed by microimmunofluorescence methods which conserve time and reagents, particularly when a serum must be tested against several rickettsial antigens. IFA antigens and conjugates may be obtained by state health laboratories from the CDC, but antigens may also be obtained from infected chicken yolk sacs or from infected in vitro cell cultures. If purified organisms are used, they should be mixed with an equal volume of 5% normal yolk sac in phosphate-buffered saline (PBS) to improve antigen adherence and to diminish nonspecific fluorescence. Antigen slides are prepared by applying concentrated suspensions of rickettsiae to a microscope slide with a pen point. A premarked template serves as a guide (33), and nine different antigens can be delivered within a very small area. Each slide is prepared with several of the multiantigen arrays to facilitate the serum titration. Slides are air dried for 30 min and then fixed in acetone for 10 min at 26°C. After drying, they may be used immediately or stored dessicated at −70°C. Sera are initially diluted 1/16 with either PBS or PBS containing 5% normal yolk sac. If PBS is used, further dilutions of patient and control sera may be made in a microtiter plate. However, it has been our experience

that PBS containing 5% normal yolk sac is not transferred accurately by microtiter diluters and that dilutions should be made in test tubes. Patient and control sera undergo serial twofold dilutions, and a 5-μl portion from each dilution is placed on a multiantigen array on the antigen slide. The slides are then incubated at 37°C for 30 min in a humidified atmosphere, washed for 10 min in PBS, and air dried. Fluorescein-conjugated anti-human globulin, fluorescein-conjugated anti-human IgM (μ-chain specific) or fluorescein-conjugated anti-human IgG (γ-chain specific) are then added to the serum-treated antigen slides to determine the total serum antibody titer or the class-specific antibody response. Slides are incubated for 30 min at 37°C in a humidified chamber, washed for 10 min with PBS, and air dried. A cover slip is applied with glycerol mounting medium, and the fluorescence is observed with a microscope equipped with UV optics. The IFA titer is the reciprocal of the greatest dilution of serum which demonstrates fluorescence of morphologically recognizable rickettsiae. A fourfold rise in the titer of paired sera, a single serum titer of ≥64, or an IgM titer at any level (suggestive of recent infection) is diagnostically significant.

IHA test

The antigen used in the IHA test (ESS) can be prepared either from purified typhus group or spotted fever group rickettsiae (1) or from an ether extract of these organisms (6, 28) by adding sodium hydroxide to a final concentration of 0.2 N and boiling for 30 min. The resulting ESS is dialyzed for 24 h at 4°C against three changes of PBS. After dialysis, the ESS is adjusted to contain 0.1% sodium azide and stored at 4°C. Sheep erythrocytes used in the IHA test are treated with glutaraldehyde to preserve them and to eliminate the need for a constant supply of fresh cells. Erythrocytes that have been aged approximately 5 days are washed extensively with saline and suspended to 20% in phosphate-buffered glucose, pH 7.2 (76 ml of 0.15 M Na_2HPO_4, 24 ml of 0.15 M KH_2PO_4, 100 ml of 5.4% glucose solution). The erythrocytes are then mixed with an equal volume of 0.2% glutaraldehyde and incubated in a 37°C water bath for 15 min. After five washes in saline, the erythrocytes are suspended to 10% in saline containing 0.1% sodium azide and stored for 2 weeks at 4°C before use. For sensitization of erythrocytes with ESS, 1.25 ml of the glutaraldehyde-treated cells are pelleted, washed once with PBS, and resuspended in 2.4 ml of ESS. The erythrocyte-ESS mixture is incubated at 37°C for 1 h, with mixing every 10 min. The sensitized cells are washed twice with PBS and resuspended to 0.5% in PBS containing 0.4% bovine serum albumin (PBS-BSA). ESS-sensitized, glutaraldehyde-treated sheep cells may be used over a period of 10 months, but it is advisable to include a titration of a known positive control serum in each test to ensure that there has been no loss in reactivity of antigen-sensitized cells. Sera should be absorbed with unsensitized erythrocytes before testing to eliminate nonspecific agglutination. This is accomplished by adding 1 ml of serum to 0.25 ml of packed, stabilized erythrocytes and incubating for 10 min at 26°C. The erythrocytes are pelleted by centrifugation, and the absorbed serum is removed with a pipette. The IHA test is performed in U-bottom microtiter plates. All sera are initially diluted 1/40 with PBS-BSA, and subsequent twofold dilutions in PBS-BSA are made in the microtiter wells with conventional diluters. Two controls are usually included: unsensitized cells incubated with a 1/40 dilution of each serum and ESS-sensitized cells with a 1/40 dilution of normal serum. After the addition of sensitized erythrocytes, the plate is sealed, shaken, and incubated overnight at 26°C. The IHA titer is the reciprocal of the greatest serum dilution that shows agglutination of the erythrocytes. Agglutination is visualized as a layer of evenly dispersed erythrocytes covering the bottom of the well. Negative reactions appear as rings or buttons of erythrocytes. A fourfold rise in the titer of paired sera is diagnostically significant, and a titer of ≥128 in a single convalescent serum indicates a probable infection.

LA test

The rickettsial antigen used in the LA test is the same ESS antigen described for the IHA procedure. Latex beads (0.81 μm, 3.7×10^{10} beads per ml in 0.01 M glycine-buffered saline [GBS], pH 8.1) are mixed for 2 min with a volume of ESS previously determined to be optimal by box titration with human antirickettsial serum. GBS and then GBS plus 0.1% fatty-acid-free BSA are added with a 2-min agitation between each addition. Reagents are added in the proportion of 1 volume of latex beads, 0.6 volume of ESS-GBS, and 0.4 volume of GBS-albumin (16, 18). For the LA test, sera are initially screened at a 1/16 dilution in GBS-albumin, and the titers of positive specimens are subsequently determined by twofold serial dilutions. The test is performed by mixing the diluted sera (40 μl) and the latex-ESS suspension (20 μl) on a glass slide which is tilted by hand for 6 min and then incubated at 26°C in a humidified chamber. After 5 min, the agglutination titer is read macroscopically as the reciprocal of the highest dilution of serum which resulted in definite agglutination. Serum reactivities required for confirmed or probable cases are as for the IHA test.

ELISA

The rickettsial ELISA can be performed using a number of different antigen preparations, including sonic or ether extracts of density gradient-purified organisms or intact rickettsiae (7, 10, 14). Optimal concentrations of antigen, control sera, and the alkaline-phosphatase conjugate should be determined by box titration before use in a clinical assay. In the ELISA, 100 μl of rickettsial antigen diluted in 0.1 M sodium carbonate buffer, pH 9.6, is added to the wells of U-bottom polystyrene microtiter plates. A parallel set of wells is coated with buffer alone to serve as controls. Plates are incubated for 1 h at 37°C and then are washed three times for 3 min each with PBS containing 0.05% Tween 20 (PBS-T; pH 7.2). To minimize any further nonspecific binding to the plates, 100 μl of 0.5% gelatin in PBS is then added to the wells, and the plates are incubated and washed as described above. Dilutions of sera are prepared in PBS-T, and 100 μl is added to both test (antigen-containing) and control (buffer only) wells. The plates

are incubated for 1 h at 37°C and then washed three times. Diluted alkaline phosphatase-conjugated anti-human IgG or IgM (100 μl) is then added to each well, the plates are incubated and washed, and the substrate, p-nitrophenylphosphate (100 μl, 1 mg/ml in 10% diethanolamine buffer, pH 9.8), is added. The reactions are allowed to continue at 37°C for 45 min, and then they are stopped by the addition of 25 μl of 3 M NaOH. The optical density (OD) of each well is read at 400 nm using an ELISA microtiter colorimeter, and the net OD value for each serum dilution is calculated by subtracting the OD in the control well from the OD in the test well. The lowest OD at which an ELISA reaction is considered positive will depend on the particular ELISA utilized and the judgment of experienced personnel; however, the ELISA titer has been described as the dilution of serum which, by interpolation of the titration curve, yields an OD value approximately seven times greater than the OD of the negative serum control (14).

CF test

The CF test for rickettsial antibodies is performed by standard methods which have been described elsewhere in detail (23). Although the tube method may be used, the test is usually performed with microtiter equipment to conserve reagents. Rickettsial CF antigens can be prepared from either infected yolk sacs or infected cell cultures. These antigens are semipurified by differential centrifugation and then treated with diethyl ether to remove the soluble group-specific CF antigens from the residual intact rickettsiae (28). Extensive washing of the extracted rickettsial organisms results in a type-specific antigen which is also reactive in the CF test. Antigens are standardized for use in diagnostic tests by performing a box titration. Serial twofold dilutions of antigen are reacted against serial twofold dilutions of human convalescent serum. The greatest dilution of antigen which gives a positive result is considered to contain 1 U of antigen. The CF test is performed with either 2 or 8 U of antigen. Detection of early (IgM) antibodies to RMSF is enhanced by the use of 8 U of antigen, but cross-reactivity with typhus serum is minimized by the use of 2 U of antigen. Rickettsial CF antigens are stable when stored at −20°C, but a control antigen titration should be included with each clinical test to ensure that the correct concentration of antigen was used. The relative content of IgM and IgG antibodies in a serum may be assessed by treating a sample of serum with heat and ethanethiol and then comparing the resulting CF titer with that of an untreated control. Specifically, one sample of the serum is adjusted to contain 0.03 M ethanethiol, and another sample is similarly diluted with buffer. The samples are allowed to stand at 26°C for 3 h and then heated at 56°C for 30 min. Since ethanethiol acts principally against IgM antibodies, a decrease in the CF titer of the treated sample (compared to the control sample) reflects the IgM content of the serum. Residual IgG antibodies are responsible for the observed CF activity in a treated serum. Q fever CF antigens are available to state health laboratories from the CDC; however, the CDC no longer provides CF antigens for the other rickettsial groups. A fourfold rise in titer between paired sera, or a single serum titer of ≥16 is considered diagnostically significant.

WF test

Antigens for the WF test are suspensions of whole, unflagellated *P. vulgaris*, strains OX-19 and OX-2, and *P. mirabilis* strain OX-K. They may be purchased commercially or prepared in the laboratory according to the procedures described by Plotz (31). *Proteus* organisms may be obtained from the American Type Culture Collection, Rockville, Md., and are propagated by streaking on a veal infusion agar plate followed by incubation at 37°C. To prepare stock cultures, smooth, nonspreading colonies are transferred to dry agar slants and to nutrient broth cultures and incubated at 37°C for 18 to 24 h. The motility of the organisms is determined by examining a drop of the broth culture by the hanging drop method. It is imperative that only nonmotile organisms are used, since the flagellar H antigens prevent agglutination of the somatic O antigens by rickettsial antibodies. Pure cultures of nonmotile *Proteus* strains may be maintained on dry agar slants or lyophilized and should be checked routinely for purity. Antigens for the WF reaction are prepared by inoculating Roux bottles containing nutrient agar with 5 ml of broth culture and incubating them for 18 to 24 h at 37°C. The organisms are washed from the agar with normal saline containing 0.5% Formalin, washed three times by centrifugation, and resuspended to a concentration with turbidity equal to tube 3 of the McFarland nephelometer scale. Antigens are stored at 4°C. WF antigens should be tested with human antirickettsial sera of known titer and with a normal human serum. It is important that the positive control sera result from a rickettsial infection because animal antisera prepared by immunization with *Proteus* strains are agglutinated by WF antigens regardless of whether the bacteria are agglutinated by rickettsial antibodies. The WF test is most accurately performed by the tube agglutination method. Patient and positive control sera are initially diluted 1/10 in saline and then further diluted in twofold increments. Equal volumes (0.5 ml) of antigen and serum dilutions are mixed in Wasserman tubes, incubated at 37°C for 2 h, and then held at 4°C overnight. Agglutination is determined by holding the tubes at an angle against shielded light. Complete agglutination is visualized as large white masses of clumped organisms in the bottom of the tube, with a clear supernatant fluid. Gentle mixing will produce a granular suspension distinct from the fine, uniform turbidity of negative controls. Partial agglutination shows smaller masses at the bottom of the tube, with a partially clear supernatant fluid. The WF titer is the reciprocal of the greatest dilution of serum to show agglutination. A fourfold rise in the titer of paired sera or a single serum titer of ≥320 is considered suggestive of rickettsial infection.

Skin biopsy

A full-thickness section of skin is taken at the site of the rickettsial lesion, using a scalpel or a punch biopsy tool. It is important to obtain the macule itself, and marking the lesion with ink before excision may improve the success of the procedure. The specimen is placed in sterile saline and kept at 4°C. If further processing is not possible within 4 to 8 h, the tissue should be frozen and maintained at −70°C. For sectioning, the specimen is placed in embedding medium, frozen at −70°C for 30 min, and then cut into 4-μm sections using a cold microtome at −22°C. Since the vasculitis in both RMSF and boutonneuse fever is focal, it is important to cut and examine serial sections throughout the entire lesion before negative results can be accepted (32). Sections are mounted on alcohol-cleaned slides, fixed in acetone at −70°C for 10 min, and analyzed using either the direct or indirect fluorescent-antibody method. Regardless of the method selected, slides must be washed in 0.01 M PBS, pH 7.2 to 7.4, for 10 min to remove excess embedding medium. In the direct fluorescent-antibody method, the tissue section from a patient with suspected RMSF is flooded with fluorescein-conjugated anti-*R. rickettsii* serum, incubated for 30 min in a humidified atmosphere at 26°C, and rinsed with PBS for 10 min. After the slides have been air dried, cover slips are mounted using glycerol mounting medium (90 ml glycerol and 10 ml of PBS, adjusted to pH 8.0). For the IFA method, the skin section is flooded with anti-*R. rickettsii* serum, incubated in a humidified atmosphere at 26°C for 30 min, rinsed with PBS for 10 min, and dried. Fluorescein-conjugated antiglobulin is then added to the section. The slide is incubated as before for 30 min, washed with PBS, and air dried; a coverslip is then attached. Skin sections are examined with a fluorescence microscope equipped with a 40× or 100× objective. A positive skin biopsy will show morphologically distinct, brightly fluorescing rickettsiae lying predominantly around the small dermal capillaries. Fluorescein-conjugated rabbit anti-*R. rickettsii* serum for the direct fluorescent-antibody test is available to state health laboratories from the CDC.

LITERATURE CITED

1. **Anacker, R. L., R. K. Gerloff, L. A. Thomas, R. E. Mann, and W. D. Bickel.** 1975. Immunological properties of *Rickettsia rickettsii* purified by zonal centrifugation. Infect. Immun. **11**:1203–1209.
2. **Bozeman, F. M., S. A. Masiello, M. S. Williams, and B. L. Elisberg.** 1975. Epidemic typhus rickettsiae isolated from flying squirrels. Nature (London) **255**:545–547.
3. **Burgdorfer, W.** 1970. Hemolymph test: a technique for detection of rickettsiae in ticks. Am. J. Trop. Med. Hyg. **19**:1010–1014.
4. **Centers for Disease Control.** 1981. Rickettsial disease surveillance report no. 2, summary: 1979. Centers for Disease Control, Atlanta.
5. **Centers for Disease Control.** 1983. Rocky Mountain spotted fever: United States, 1982. Morbid. Mortal. Weekly Rep. **32**:229–232.
6. **Chang, R. S., E. S. Murray, and J. C. Snyder.** 1954. Erythrocyte-sensitizing substances from rickettsiae of the Rocky Mountain spotted fever group. J. Immunol. **73**:8–15.
7. **Clements, M. L., J. S. Dumler, P. Fiset, C. L. Wisseman, Jr., M. J. Snyder, and M. M. Levine.** 1983. Serodiagnosis of Rocky Mountain spotted fever: comparison of IgM and IgG enzyme-linked immunosorbent assays and indirect fluorescent antibody test. J. Infect. Dis. **148**:876–880.
8. **D'Angelo, L. J., E. F. Baker, and W. Schlosser.** 1979. Q fever in the United States, 1948–1977. J. Infect. Dis. **139**:613–615.

9. **D'Angelo, L. J., W. G. Winkler, and D. J. Bregman.** 1978. Rocky Mountain spotted fever in the United States, 1975–1977. J. Infect. Dis. **138:**273–276.

10. **Dasch, G. A., S. Halle, and A. L. Bourgeois.** 1979. Sensitive microplate enzyme-linked immunosorbent assay for detection of antibodies against the scrub typhus rickettsia, *Rickettsia tsutsugamushi.* J. Clin. Microbiol. **9:**38–48.

11. **Fiset, P., R. A. Ormsbee, R. Silberman, M. Peacock, and S. H. Spielman.** 1969. A microagglutination technique for detection and measurement of rickettsial antibodies. Acta Virol. **13:**60–66.

12. **Fishbein, D. B., J. E. Kaplan, K. W. Bernard, and W. G. Winkler.** 1984. Surveillance of Rocky Mountain spotted fever in the United States, 1981–1983. J. Infect. Dis. **150:**609–611.

13. **Gordon, J. C., S. W. Gordon, E. Peterson, and R. N. Philip.** 1984. Epidemiology of Rocky Mountain spotted fever in Ohio, 1981: serologic evaluation of canines and rickettsial isolation from ticks associated with human case exposure sites. Am. J. Trop. Med. Hyg. **33:**1026–1031.

14. **Halle, S., G. A. Dasch, and E. Weiss.** 1977. Sensitive enzyme-linked immunosorbent assay for detection of antibodies against typhus rickettsiae, *Rickettsia prowazekii* and *Rickettsia typhi.* J. Clin. Microbiol. **6:**101–110.

15. **Hays, P. L.** 1985. Rocky Mountain spotted fever in children in Kansas: the diagnostic value of an IgM-specific immunofluorescence assay. J. Infect. Dis. **151:**369–370.

16. **Hechemy, K. E., R. L. Anacker, R. N. Philip, K. T. Kleeman, J. N. MacCormack, S. J. Sasowski, and E. E. Michaelson.** 1980. Detection of Rocky Mountain spotted fever antibodies by a latex agglutination test. J. Clin. Microbiol. **12:**144–150.

17. **Hechemy, K. E., E. E. Michaelson, R. L. Anacker, M. Zdeb, S. J. Sasowski, K. T. Kleeman, J. M. Joseph, J. Patel, J. Kudlac, L. B. Elliott, J. Rawlings, C. E. Crump, J. D. Folds, H. Dowda, Jr., J. H. Barrick, J. R. Hindman, G. E. Killgore, D. Young, and R. H. Altieri.** 1983. Evaluation of latex-*Rickettsia rickettsii* test for Rocky Mountain spotted fever in 11 laboratories. J. Clin. Microbiol. **18:**938–946.

18. **Hechemy, K. E., J. V. Osterman, C. S. Eisemann, L. B. Elliot, and S. J. Sasowski.** 1981. Detection of typhus antibodies by latex agglutination. J. Clin. Microbiol. **13:**214–216.

19. **Hechemy, K. E., R. W. Stevens, S. Sasowski, E. E. Michaelson, E. A. Casper, and R. N. Philip.** 1979. Discrepancies in Weil Felix and microimmunofluorescence test results for Rocky Mountain spotted fever. J. Clin. Microbiol. **9:**292–293.

20. **Kaplowitz, L. G., J. V. Lange, J. J. Fisher, and D. H. Walker.** 1983. Correlation of rickettsial titers, circulating endotoxin, and clinical features in Rocky Mountain spotted fever. Arch. Intern. Med. **143:**1149–1151.

21. **Kleeman, K. T., J. L. Hicks, R. L. Anacker, R. N. Philip, E. A. Casper, K. E. Hechemy, C. M. Wilfert, and J. N. MacCormack.** 1981. Early detection of antibody to *Rickettsia rickettsii:* a comparison of four serological methods: indirect hemagglutination, indirect fluorescent antibody, latex agglutination, and complement fixation, p. 171–178. *In* W. Burgdorfer and R. L. Anacker (ed.), Rickettsiae and rickettsial diseases. Academic Press, Inc., New York.

22. **Lange, J. V., D. H. Walker, and T. B. Wester.** 1982. Documented Rocky Mountain spotted fever in wintertime. J. Am. Med. Assoc. **247:**2403–2404.

23. **Lennette, E. H., J. L. Melnick, and R. L. Magoffin.** 1974. Clinical virology: introduction to methods, p. 667–677. *In* E. H. Lennette, E. H. Spaulding, and J. P. Truant (ed.), Manual of clinical microbiology, 2nd ed. American Society for Microbiology, Washington, D.C.

24. **Mansueto, S., G. Vitale, M. Bentivegna, G. Tringali, and R. DiLeo.** 1985. Persistence of antibodies to *Rickettsia conorii* after an acute attack of boutonneuse fever. J. Infect. Dis. **151:**377.

25. **McDade, J. E., C. C. Shephard, M. A. Redus, V. F. Newhouse, and J. D. Smith.** 1980. Evidence of *Rickettsia prowazekii* infections in the United States. Am. J. Trop. Med. Hyg. **29:**277–284.

26. **Newhouse, V. F., C. C. Shepard, M. A. Redus, T. Tzianabos, and J. E. McDade.** 1979. A comparison of the complement fixation, indirect fluorescent antibody, and microagglutination tests for the serological diagnosis of rickettsial diseases. Am. J. Trop. Med. Hyg. **28:**387–395.

27. **Ormsbee, R., M. Peacock, R. Philip, E. Casper, J. Plorde, T. Gabre-kidan, and L. Wright.** 1977. Serologic diagnosis of epidemic typhus fever. Am. J. Epidemiol. **105:**261–271.

28. **Osterman, J. V., and C. S. Eisemann.** 1978. Rickettsial indirect hemagglutination test: isolation of erythrocyte-sensitizing substance. J. Clin. Microbiol. **8:**189–196.

29. **Philip, R. N., E. A. Casper, J. N. MacCormack, D. J. Sexton, L. A. Thomas, R. L. Anacker, W. Burgdorfer, and S. Vick.** 1977. A comparison of serologic methods for diagnosis of Rocky Mountain spotted fever. Am. J. Epidemiol. 105:56–67.

30. **Philip, R. N., E. A. Casper, R. A. Ormsbee, M. G. Peacock, and W. Burgdorfer.** 1976. Microimmunofluorescence test for the serological study of Rocky Mountain spotted fever and typhus. J. Clin. Microbiol. **3:**51–61.

31. **Plotz, H.** 1944. The rickettsiae, p. 559–578. *In* J. S. Simmons and C. J. Gentzkow (ed.), Laboratory methods of the United States Army, 5th ed. Lea & Febiger, Philadelphia.

32. **Raoult, D., C. deMicco, H. Gallais, and M. Toga.** 1984. Laboratory diagnosis of Mediterranean spotted fever by immunofluorescent demonstration of *Rickettsia conorii* in cutaneous lesions. J. Infect. Dis. **150:**145–148.

33. **Robinson, D. M., G. Brown, E. Gan, and D. L. Huxsoll.** 1976. Adaptation of a microimmunofluorescence test to the study of human *Rickettsia tsutsugamushi* antibody. Am. J. Trop. Med. Hyg. **25:**900–905.

34. **Shepard, C. C., M. A. Redus, T. Tzianabos, and D. T. Warfield.** 1976. Recent experience with the complement fixation test in the laboratory diagnosis of rickettsial diseases in the United States. J. Clin. Microbiol. **4:**277–283.

35. **Shirai, A., J. W. Dietel, and J. V. Osterman.** 1975. Indirect hemagglutination test for human antibody to typhus and spotted fever group rickettsiae. J. Clin. Microbiol. **2:**430–437.

36. **Taylor, J. P., W. B. Tanner, J. A. Rawlings, J. Buck, L. B. Elliott, H. J. Dewlett, B. Taylor, and T. C. Betz.** 1985. Serological evidence of subclinical Rocky Mountain spotted fever infections in Texas. J. Infect. Dis. **151:**367–369.

37. **Walker, D. H., M. S. Burday, and J. D. Folds.** 1980. Laboratory diagnosis of Rocky Mountain spotted fever. South. Med. J. **73:**1443–1446.

38. **Walker, D. H., and B. G. Cain.** 1978. A method for specific diagnosis of Rocky Mountain spotted fever on fixed, paraffin-embedded tissue by immunofluorescence. J. Infect. Dis. **137:**206–209.

39. **Walker, D. H., B. G. Cain, and P. M. Olmstead.** 1978. Laboratory diagnosis of Rocky Mountain spotted fever by immunofluorescent demonstration of *Rickettsia rickettsii* in cutaneous lesions. Am. J. Clin. Pathol. **69:**619–623.

40. **Walker, D. H., and J. H. S. Gear.** 1985. Correlation of the distribution of *Rickettsia conorii*, microscopic lesions, and clinical features in South African tick bite fever. Am. J. Trop. Med. Hyg. **34:**361–370.

41. **Woodward, T. E., C. E. Pedersen, Jr., C. N. Oster, L. R. Bagley, J. Romberger, and M. J. Snyder.** 1976. Prompt confirmation of Rocky Mountain spotted fever: identification of rickettsiae in skin tissues. J. Infect. Dis. **134:**297–301.

Chapter 92

Section I. Immunohematology

Introduction

BRUCE C. GILLILAND

The development of sensitive and reproducible immunologic techniques has greatly enhanced the field of immunohematology. Blood typing and cross-matching, the mainstay of this field, are excellently described by Crookston in chapter 93. Blood typing in clinical medicine is important for accurate matching of donors and recipients of blood transfusion or tissue transplantation, protection against alloimmunization of women exposed to the D antigen of the Rh system during pregnancy or delivery, diagnosis and treatment of hemolytic disease of the newborn due to alloantibodies, and investigation of erythrocyte destruction caused by autoantibodies or alloantibodies. The incidence of hemolytic disease of the newborn has been dramatically reduced by the administration of immunoglobulin G anti-D to the mother before or soon after delivery of an Rh-positive infant.

In chapter 94, an excellent description is given by Papayannopoulou and Nakamoto of the detection of fetal hemoglobin in erythrocytes of adults by immunofluorescence. The immunofluorescence technique is more sensitive and reproducible than the acid elution method. While detection of hemoglobin F (Hb F) is largely investigative, semiquantitation of fetal erythrocytes in maternal circulation has been utilized in the design of treatment protocols for preventing Rh immunization of Rh-negative women during pregnancy. Studies of cellular distribution of Hb F in the adult are of value in defining conditions associated with increased levels of Hb F. These conditions include acute erythropoietic stress after severe bleeding and hereditary persistence of Hb F.

The methods for diagnosing autoimmune and drug-induced immune hemolytic anemia are detailed in an outstanding fashion by Petz in chapter 95. He points out that approximately 26% of patients with acquired immune hemolytic anemia will have a negative direct Coombs test unless an antiserum with specificity for C3d is used. C3d is the fragment from C3b left on the cell membrane after cleavage by C3b inactivator. Petz's studies also demonstrate the enhanced sensitivity of antiglobulin tests with the use of enzyme-treated erythrocytes, especially in the detection of erythrocyte antibodies in serum.

Autoimmune hemolytic anemia may occur in a small number of patients (2 to 10%) who have negative antiglobulin tests. The amount of antibody on these patients' erythrocytes is below the level of detection by conventional direct antiglobulin tests. A concentration of at least 100 to 500 molecules of immunoglobulin G antibody per cell is required for a positive direct antiglobulin test. Antibody can be detected on the erythrocytes of these Coombs-negative patients by several techniques. In chapter 95, a practical method that uses the polyvalent cation hexadimethrine bromide (Polybrene) is detailed. Polybrene acts by reducing the electrostatic repulsive charges of erythrocytes, allowing antibodies on one cell to cross-link with another cell to produce agglutination. The test is delicate and requires experience in interpretation.

A distinct disorder, combined cold and warm autoimmune hemolytic anemia, is also described by Petz. This form of hemolytic anemia was found in 8% of patients in a recent study. Patients responded initially to steroids, but some patients had relapses and a chronic clinical course.

Techniques for detecting antibodies to neutrophils and platelets are elegantly presented in chapter 96 by Lalezari. Antibodies to either of these cell types have been demonstrated in the serum of mothers who have newborns with alloimmune neonatal neutropenia or thrombocytopenia. Autoantibodies to either or both cell types may occur in patients with systemic lupus erythematosus or other connective-tissue disorders as well as in otherwise normal persons. Detection of cell-bound antibody by antiglobulin serum has been greatly facilitated by the use of paraformaldehyde, which removes nonspecific immunoglobulin G from the surface of the neutrophils or platelets.

Godwin and Roberts in chapter 97 give an excellent description of tests for recognizing and characterizing inhibitors to clotting proteins. The majority of acquired inhibitors to clotting proteins are antibodies. Persons with genetic coagulation factor deficiencies may develop alloantibodies to their missing component, especially after replacement therapy. Autoantibodies to clotting factors are found in some patients with systemic lupus erythematosus or other disorders, after drug administration, and, rarely, in normal persons. The lupus anticoagulant has attracted attention because of its association with thrombotic events or fetal loss in patients with systemic lupus erythematosus or in normal women. Recent studies suggest that antibodies to cardiolipin rather than the lupus anticoagulant are associated with fetal distress or death in women with systemic lupus erythematosus. Lupus anticoagulants are antibodies that interact with phospholipids and inhibit prothrombin activation in phospholipid-dependent coagulation tests. Their anticoagulant effect is usually not observed when platelets are substituted for phospholipid in coagulation tests. The lupus anticoagulant, therefore, is not an anticoagulant in vivo and may even induce thrombosis by interacting with phospholipids. Antibodies to clotting proteins represent an important clinical problem and are useful tools in the structural mapping and sensitive measurement of clotting factors.

Chapter 93

Blood Typing and Cross-Matching Procedures for Blood Transfusion

MARIE C. CROOKSTON

The term blood type or blood group could be applied to all the genetic markers in the blood, including the serum proteins and erythrocyte (red cell) enzymes (1). However, by convention, the term is reserved for inherited antigens detected on the red cell surface by specific antibodies. Excluding the rare private antigens (which are often restricted to one or two families), there are about 200 red cell antigens detectable, directly or indirectly, by agglutination tests (2, 7). The majority of these antigens belong to 1 of 15 systems listed in Table 1; most were recognized as the result of investigation of antibodies stimulated by pregnancy or blood transfusion. Almost all red cell antigens vary in frequency in different populations (5).

The antigens are assigned to a blood group system when genetic studies show that they are the products of alleles (i.e., alternative forms of a gene at a single locus). Almost all blood group genes are inherited as codominant characters (i.e., in the heterozygote, both genes are expressed). With the exception of Xg, all the blood group loci are on autosomes (e.g., the ABO locus is on chromosome 9; the Rh locus is on chromosome 1). It is customary to denote genes and loci by italic letters.

The notation for blood group antigens and antibodies is inconsistent (Table 1). There may be a sequence of uppercase (e.g., A and B, M and N), a sequence of upper and lowercase letters (e.g., S and s, K and k), a symbol with a superscript (e.g., Lu^a and Lu^b), or a symbol with numbers (e.g., Sc1 and Sc2). In most cases the name of the system is derived from the name of the patient in whom the antibody was first detected.

Clinical importance

Blood typing and antibody detection procedures are important in clinical medicine for (i) matching donors and recipients of blood transfusions or organ grafts; (ii) identification and protection against alloimmunization of women exposed to D, an antigen of the Rh system, during pregnancy or delivery; (iii) prediction, diagnosis, and treatment of hemolytic disease of the newborn due to alloantibodies; and (iv) diagnosis and investigation of red cell destruction caused by autoantibodies or alloantibodies.

Blood typing also plays an important role in forensic medicine, anthropology, and genetics (7). Some blood types are associated with disease (4, p. 203). For example, a malarial parasite (*Plasmodium vivax*) invades red cells that carry a Duffy antigen (Fy^a or Fy^b) but does not invade Fy(a−b−) cells; the red cells of some patients with chronic granulomatous disease have greatly weakened Kell antigens. Among the many blood group systems, two are of outstanding clinical importance, i.e., the ABO system in which anti-A and anti-B, active at 37°C, occur regularly and the Rh system in which the antigen D is a potent immunogen.

ABO blood types (groups)

In the ABO system, the three major alleles are A, B, and O. Based on the reactions of red cells with anti-A and anti-B, four phenotypes (O, A, B, and AB) are recognized. When the cells lack A, the plasma (serum) contains anti-A; when the cells lack B, the plasma (serum) contains anti-B (Table 2). The O gene does not produce a red cell antigen. Its presence can be recognized only in the homozygote (O/O) whose red cells are not agglutinated by anti-A or anti-B; routine agglutination tests cannot distinguish between the cells of A/A and A/O individuals or the cells of B/B and B/O individuals. With few exceptions, type A individuals can be classed as A_1 or A_2, depending on the reactions of their red cells with anti-A_1 (Table 3). About 20% of type A (and AB) individuals are A_2 (and A_2B). Although the number of A antigen sites is significantly greater on A_1 than on A_2 cells (1×10^6 and 2.5×10^5, respectively), these subtypes cannot ordinarily be distinguished in tests with anti-A. There is no specific anti-A_2. The serum of some A_2 and A_2B individuals contains anti-A_1; the serum of some B, A_1, and A_1B individuals contains anti-H. (The H antigen, a precursor in the synthesis of A and B, is the product of the H gene at a different locus from ABO.) Based on the strength of the red cell reactions with anti-H, the common ABO types can be ranked in descending order as follows: O, A_2, A_2B, B, A_1, A_1B. Individuals of the very rare phenotype O_h (genotype h/h) lack H; their serum contains anti-H, as well as anti-A and anti-B.

In individuals who have H, A, and B genes, the corresponding antigens are present on almost all body cells. In about 80% of individuals, these antigens are also present in secretions such as milk, saliva, and seminal fluid. The ability to secrete H, A, and B is controlled by a secretor gene (Se); its allele (se) has no known function. The presence or absence of the Se gene does not affect the number of H, A, and B antigen sites on the red cell. In a secretor (genotype Se/Se or Se/se), the ABO blood type can be determined by testing the secretions: type O secretors secrete H; type A secretors secrete H and A; type B secretors secrete H and B. This phenomenon has been exploited in forensic medicine and in the typing of patients massively transfused with blood of an ABO type different from their own.

Naturally occurring anti-A and anti-B may be present at a low titer and mainly as immunoglobulin M (IgM); they are weak or absent at birth. After a person is exposed to the A or B antigen in blood (by transfusion of incompatible cells or plasma) or in other

TABLE 1. Main human blood group systems

Yr of discovery	System (abbreviation)	Main antigens on red cells	Naturally occurring antibodies[a]
1901	ABO	H, A, B	Always
1926	MNSs	M, N, S, s	
1926	P	P_1, P	Sometimes
1940	Rh	D, C, E, c, e	
1945	Lutheran (Lu)	Lu^a, Lu^b	
1946	Kell	K, k, Kp^a, Kp^b, Kp^c Js^a, Js^b	
1946	Lewis (Le)	Le^a, Le^b	Sometimes
1950	Duffy (Fy)	Fy^a, Fy^b	
1951	Kidd (Jk)	Jk^a, Jk^b	
1955	Diego (Di)	Di^a, Di^b	
1956	Cartwright (Yt)	Yt^a, Yt^b	
1962	Xg	Xg^a	
1965	Dombrock (Do)	Do^a, Do^b	
1967	Colton (Co)	Co^a, Co^b	
1974	Scianna (Sc)	Sc1, Sc2	

[a] In normal subjects who lack the corresponding antigen and who have not been transfused or pregnant.

biological products (e.g., certain vaccines), a rapid secondary response almost always occurs, and the antibody titer rises to high levels. The antibody is then mainly IgG (especially in type O individuals). Transfusion of ABO-incompatible blood is likely to produce an acute and severe reaction with intravascular hemolysis, shock, hemorrhage, and renal damage. IgG anti-A (or anti-B) is transferred to the fetus via the placenta and is a common cause of hemolytic disease of the newborn (HDN). However, HDN due to ABO incompatibility is almost always milder than HDN due to antibodies of the Rh system (4, p. 675–698).

The Rh blood group system

Discussion of the Rh system is complicated by the existence of competing terminologies (Table 4). The DCE terminology of Fisher and Race and the terminology of Wiener are based on different concepts of the genetic basis of the Rh antigens. A numerical terminology was devised by Rosenfield et al. (9) to be genetically neutral and uncommitted to any theory of the genetic representation.

In 1977, the World Health Organization Expert Committee on biological standardization recommended that the DCE nomenclature be universally adopted. The DCE theory assumes the existence of three pairs of closely linked genes, i.e., D and d, C and

TABLE 2. ABO blood typing of cells and plasma (serum)

Phenotype	Red cell reactions with antisera[a]		Plasma (serum) reactions with red cells of type:		
	Anti-A	Anti-B	A	B	O
O	−	−	+	+	−
A	+	−	−	+	−
B	−	+	+	−	−
AB	+	+	−	−	−

[a] Agglutination absent (−) or present (+) in tests at room temperature.

TABLE 3. ABO blood group phenotypes and genotypes

Phenotype	Genotype
O	O/O
A_1	A^1/A^1 A^1/O A^1/A^2
A_2	A^2/A^2 A^2/O
B	B/B B/O
A_1B	A^1/B
A_2B	A^2/B

c, and E and e. Although there is no d antigen, it is convenient to denote the absence of D by using the symbol d in genotypes. The set of Rh antigens determined by the genetic material on one chromosome may be designated the Rh haplotype, by analogy with the term applied to the histocompatibility antigens.

At present, the most commonly used notation is a combination of short symbols and DCE. The short symbol R^1 is used to describe the haplotype that gives rise to the antigens D, C, and e (Rh1, Rh2, and Rh5, respectively). The numerical notation is indispensable for Rh antigens other than D, C, E, c, and e (10, p. 125).

It should be noted that individuals who are D negative are termed Rh negative; those who are D positive are termed Rh positive. Thus, in this context, the terms anti-D and anti-Rh are synonyms.

The D antigen is clinically the most important antigen of the Rh system because it is the most immunogenic. For this reason, D-negative patients who require transfusion are given D-negative blood; D-negative women who have not formed anti-D are given an injection of IgG anti-D (Rh immune globulin) soon after the delivery of a D-positive infant or fetus. This prophylactic measure can reduce the incidence of alloimmunization after pregnancy to less than 1% of D-negative women at risk and has helped to reduce the incidence of HDN in several countries by about

TABLE 4. Various nomenclatures[a] used to describe Rh alleles and antigens

Allele (haplotype)[b]		Antigenic determinants	
Short symbol	DCE	DCE	Numerical
R^1	(DCe)	D, C, e	Rh1, Rh2, Rh5
r	(dce)	c, e	Rh4, Rh5
R^2	(DcE)	D, c, E	Rh1, Rh3, Rh4
R^0	(Dce)	D, c, e	Rh1, Rh4, Rh5
r'	(dCe)	C, e	Rh2, Rh5
r''	(dcE)	c, E	Rh3, Rh4
R^z	(DCE)	D, C, E	Rh1, Rh2, Rh3
r^y	(dCE)	C, E	Rh2, Rh3

[a] Cells that are D positive (Rh:1) are Rh positive, and cells that are D negative (Rh:−1) are Rh negative.
[b] In descending order of frequency.

two-thirds in the past decade. The incidence is lower in centers where women receive antenatal as well as postnatal injections of Rh immune globulin (4, p. 382–401).

Antibodies to other Rh antigens (such as c or E) and to antigens of other systems (such as those of Kell, Kidd, and Duffy) can cause HDN and can shorten the survival of transfused cells. However, these antibodies are relatively uncommon. It is therefore not practical to type the cells of patients or donors for antigens other than A, B, and D, unless an unexpected antibody is found in the patient's serum during screening and cross-matching tests.

TEST PROCEDURES

Choice of procedure

Red cell antigens and antibodies are commonly detected, directly or indirectly, by agglutination techniques. The speed of the antigen-antibody reaction and the strength of agglutination observed are affected by many variables. Unlike IgM antibodies, IgG antibodies do not cause direct agglutination unless (i) the antigen site number is relatively great (e.g., A and B), (ii) the cell surface properties are altered by using enzymes or colloid media, (iii) the antibody-coated cells are brought into contact by centrifugation, or (iv) the span of the IgG molecule is increased by cleaving disulfide bonds in the hinge region, thus allowing the two antigen-binding sites to move further apart (8; 10, p. 140–141).

IgG antibodies of most specificities are readily detected by the indirect antiglobulin test, a two-stage procedure in which red cells are exposed to the antibody-containing serum and then washed free of unbound globulin before being tested with an antiglobulin reagent. Some antibody will elute from the cells during the washing process; the washed cells must each carry at least 100 to 150 IgG molecules to be agglutinated by anti-IgG (4, p. 511). When appropriate reagents are used, the indirect antiglobulin test also detects complement components (C3 and C4) remaining on the cell after complement activation by IgG or IgM antibodies.

Choice of controls

In all methods for phenotyping (typing) red cells, controls must be included to show that the standard cells and antisera are giving the reactions expected of them and that the test cells and test sera are not giving false reactions. For example, in testing cells for antigen c, at least the following three controls are needed: (i) c-positive cells versus anti-c, (ii) c-negative cells versus anti-c, and (iii) test cells in their own serum (or compatible serum or medium recommended by a supplier of anti-c).

For all cell-typing tests, the positive control cells should contain only a single dose of the relevant antigen (e.g., for tests with anti-c, the positive control cells are *DCe/dce* rather than *dce/dce*). Conversely, for antibody detection, cells containing a double dose of the relevant antigen are used (e.g., to detect anti-c, the screening cells are *dce/dce* or *DcE/DcE*, rather than *DCe/dce*).

When the indirect antiglobulin test is used, the control cells and test cells must first be shown not to give a positive direct antiglobulin test.

Reagents and equipment

Antisera. Antisera of most specificities are obtainable commercially from many sources such as Biological Corp. of America, Div. of Cooper Biomedical, Inc., Malvern, Pa.; American Dade, Div. of American Hospital Supply Corp., Miami, Fla.; Gamma Biologicals, Inc., Houston, Tex.; Ortho Diagnostic Systems, Inc., Raritan, N.J.; and Immucor, Inc., Norcross, Ga. Each antiserum must be used as recommended by the supplier; other techniques might reveal an unexpected antibody.

Anti-A is obtained from type B human volunteers who have responded to injections of porcine A substance to boost the level of their naturally occurring antibody. Commercially available anti-A is usually colored with a blue dye. Some blood transfusion centers in Europe use anti-A prepared from the albumin gland and eggs of a snail (*Helix pomatia*); the addition of one *H. pomatia* egg to 100 ml of saline produces a potent anti-A typing reagent.

Anti-B is obtained from type A human volunteers who have responded to injections of equine B substance. Commercially available anti-B is usually colored with a yellow dye.

Potent monoclonal anti-A and anti-B is produced by Service des Hybridomes, Centre National de Transfusion Sanguine, 75739 Paris Cedex 15, France.

Anti-A_1 lectin is prepared from the seeds of *Dolichos biflorus*. When suitably diluted, the extract agglutinates A_1 cells, but not A, B, or O cells.

Anti-H lectin (Ulex I) is prepared from the seeds of *Ulex europaeus* (common European gorse). This lectin is used in hemagglutination inhibition tests to detect the H antigen in saliva.

The peanut lectin, prepared from the seeds of *Arachis hypogaea*, detects T, Tk, and Th activation of red cells by bacterial enzymes (4, p. 468–476).

Anti-D is obtained from D-negative individuals immunized by transfusion or pregnancy or from male volunteers who respond to injections of a small volume of D-positive cells. Antibodies to other antigens (C, c, E, e, K, Fy^a, Jk^a, etc.) are obtained from individuals immunized by transfusion or pregnancy. Synthetic A and B antigens (e.g., Synsorbs, Chembiomed, Edmonton, Alberta, Canada) can be used to remove anti-A and anti-B from the serum so that the serum is suitable for testing cells of all ABO types.

Antiglobulin reagents are prepared from the serum of animals (usually rabbits) immunized with human IgG or with complement components (e.g., C3). The reagent must be free of heteroagglutinins against normal human red cells. Antiglobulin serum supplied for use in other techniques (e.g., immunoelectrophoresis) usually contains potent hemagglutinins and must be either absorbed with normal human red cells or diluted to a point where it no longer reacts with normal cells. Monospecific antiglobulin reagents (e.g., anti-IgG and anti-C3) are available, but for most tests (e.g., cross-matching), a polyspecific reagent containing anti-IgG and anti-complement components (anti-C3b, -C3d, and -C4) is used.

Bovine serum albumin (BSA) and a low-ionic-strengthsolution (LISS) are available commercially (e.g., from Ortho).

Reagents used for specific inhibition of agglutination. Saliva containing secreted blood group antigens (A, B, H, Le^a, Le^b) is obtained from donors of appropriate ABO, Lewis, and secretor types (4, p. 302 and 493–494). The saliva (2 to 5 ml) is centrifuged, and the supernatant is poured into a hard glass test tube to be heated in a boiling-water bath for 10 min; the supernatant can be used immediately after centrifugation and cooling. To obtain a clear fluid, freeze the saliva for several days and then thaw it and remove the debris by centrifugation. The fluid can be stored for many years at −20°C. It is hypotonic; to avoid lysis of indicator red cells, the saliva must be diluted 1:10 in saline before being added to the test serum. A preparation containing H, Le^a, and Le^b is available commercially (e.g., from Ortho).

Hydatid cysts (larval forms of small tapeworms of the genus *Echinococcus*) contain a fluid that inhibits anti-P$_1$; it does not inhibit anti-P. A preferable preparation (from the tissues or egg albumin of the domestic pigeon) that inhibits anti-P$_1$ is available commercially (e.g., from Ortho).

Human serum samples containing complement C4 of known Chido and Rodgers type are stored at −20°C until required for the identification of anti-Chido and anti-Rodgers; these antibodies react with red cells when C4d is attached to the cell membrane after activation of complement.

Standard cells. Standard cells (red cells typed for many antigens) are used for controls in typing tests and for the detection of antibodies. From each selected donor of standard cells, a venous sample is taken into an anticoagulant containing glucose (e.g., acid-citrate-glucose or Alsever solution). Evacuated tubes containing acid-citrate-glucose are available commercially (e.g., Vacutainer tubes, Becton-Dickinson and Co., Rutherford, N.J.). The blood samples are stored at 4°C for 1 to 21 days. Standard screening cells (from 2 type O donors) and panel cells (usually from 10 to 16 type O donors) are available commercially (e.g., from companies that supply antisera). The screening cells are selected for their sensitivity in detecting clinically important antibodies (i.e., the donors are homozygous for genes such as *E*, *c*, *Fy^a*, and *Jk^a*).

For most tests, the cells are washed free of their own plasma; otherwise clots form when fibrinogen (in the plasma) is mixed with thrombin (in the antiserum). Macroscopically, it is sometimes difficult to distinguish cells that are agglutinated from cells that are enmeshed in fibrin. (Commercially available cell samples contain preservatives but do not usually contain plasma and therefore can be used without washing.) Each cell suspension must be adequately labeled; the work sheet must include appropriate information about the blood type, storage age, and source of the cells.

Enzyme-treated cells. The enzymes most commonly used for the treatment of cells are proteases, i.e., papain (from papaya, *Carica papaya*), bromelin (from the pineapple, *Ananas sativus*), ficin (from the fig, *Ficus carica*), and trypsin (from pig stomach). Some preparations are available commercially.

By removing sialopeptides, protease treatment of red cells enhances the reaction of the cells with certain antibodies (e.g., Rh, Lewis, and Kidd systems) but may impair their reaction with others (e.g., Duffy system). Enzymes can be used in two ways, i.e., a simple one-stage technique in which the enzyme is mixed directly with the serum and test cells or a two-stage technique in which the test cells are enzyme treated and washed before being mixed with serum. Enzyme-treated cells are used in antibody screening tests and for large-scale cell phenotyping (e.g., in centers that process blood donations). However, for cross-matching blood, the technique is too sensitive, unless the cells and serum are kept strictly at 37°C. In tests at lower temperatures, clinically insignificant IgM antibodies are detected; their investigation may cause needless postponement of a transfusion.

Equipment. Recommended equipment is as follows: racks (usually with 5 rows of 10 holes each) to fit small tubes (10 or 12 by 75 mm); disposable Pasteur pipettes; indelible marking pens (several colors); small centrifuge (e.g., Serofuge, Clay Adams, Parsippany, N.J., or Immufuge, American Dade); microscope and microscope slides; inverted microscope (Olympics Corp. of America, New Hyde Park, N.Y. 11042); illuminated viewing box with opal glass surface; 37°C water bath; and a refrigerator with a −20°C freezer.

CROSS-MATCHING BLOOD FOR TRANSFUSION

When transfusion is ordered for a patient, 10 to 15 ml of the patient's blood (preferably clotted) is sent to the laboratory with appropriate information (patient's full name, history number, sex, date of birth, diagnosis, pregnancies, previous transfusions, adverse reactions to transfusion, and antibodies previously identified). The patient's identification on the blood sample must be the same as that on the requisition form.

Before proceeding to the final step of matching the patient's serum with the donor's cells, the following four tests are performed on the patient's blood: (i) ABO typing, (ii) D typing, (iii) direct antiglobulin test, and (iv) detection and identification of unexpected antibodies in the serum.

Although in practice these four tests are performed simultaneously, each test is described below as a separate procedure. To avoid errors that could endanger the health of the transfused patient, each laboratory must define (in writing) its own procedures and the sequence in which the tests are done (10, p. 206–220). The methods described below are often modified, particularly in laboratories that process many samples.

ABO typing

The ABO type of a blood sample is determined by testing the cells and serum separately.

Cell testing (forward typing). The cells of the patient are tested in tubes with anti-A and anti-B. Standard cells (types A$_2$, B, and O) are tested once a day as controls.

1. Add 1 drop of cell suspension (2 to 5% in saline) to 1 drop of antiserum.

2. Centrifuge the tubes at 3,400 rpm (1,000 × *g*) for 15 to 30 s or at 1,000 rpm (100 to 125 × *g*) for 1 min. (Unless otherwise specified, this centrifugation technique is used in all methods described below.)

3. Gently dislodge the cell button; resuspend the cells, and examine them for agglutination (use an optical aid if necessary).

4. Grade and record the results (e.g., as 0, +, ++, or +++).

Serum testing (reverse typing). The serum is tested in tubes with A_1, B, and O cells. It is important to use A_1 rather than A_2 cells to detect weak anti-A. Type O screening cells are used here to detect unusual properties of the serum that might affect the interpretation of ABO typing and other tests.

1. Add 1 drop of cell suspension (2 to 5% washed cells in saline) to 1 drop of serum or plasma.

2. Centrifuge the tubes.

3. Examine for free hemoglobin (evidence of hemolysis).

4. Gently dislodge the cell button; resuspend the cells, and examine them for agglutination (use an optical aid if necessary).

5. Record the results (agglutination and hemolysis).

Interpretation and pitfalls. The ABO type deduced from the cell testing should be the same as the ABO type deduced from testing the serum (or plasma) of that sample (Table 2). When the cell and serum typing are in accord, the deduced ABO type is correct unless the patient has recently been transfused with whole blood of an ABO type different from his or her own. Discrepancies may be caused by unsuitable techniques or by some unusual property of the patient's cells or serum. If tubes are overcentrifuged, vigorous shaking necessary to dislodge the cell button may disperse weak agglutinates and cause a false-negative result. If the majority of the cells are lysed by antibodies in the patient's serum, agglutinates will be sparse; it is therefore important to record lysis in reverse typing. Commercially available type A and B standard cells, if used unwashed, are not lysed by antibodies because the suspending medium contains EDTA.

The first step in investigating a discrepancy is to check that the cells and serum are from the same blood sample; then repeat the tests (use washed red cells). Clinical information may be helpful in solving a problem. Some typing discrepancies due to causes other than technique are listed below.

(i) Forward-typing anomalies

1. The A or B antigen may be too weak to be detected by standard techniques. For example, the cells of some patients with leukemia or with weak subtypes (A_x, B_x, or A_3) may require special procedures.

2. A "mixed-field" or "partial" agglutination may be observed when the patient has a weak A or B subtype or has been recently transfused (e.g., type A cells in a type AB recipient are not agglutinated by anti-B). In patients who have a permanent dual population of cells, a mixed-field agglutination may be the first clue to the blood group chimerism.

3. The cells may be polyagglutinable due to exposure of the T-receptor by bacterial enzymes in vivo or in vitro. Such cells are agglutinated by anti-T in peanut lectin and by anti-T present in most normal adult sera. Polyagglutinability is usually first recognized when the ABO typing is discrepant (e.g., a patient appears to be type AB on cell testing, but type A, B, or O on serum testing).

4. Type A_1 cells may be agglutinated by anti-B when some of the A antigen has been changed to a B-like antigen by the action of a bacterial deacetylase. This antigen is termed "acquired B."

5. In very rare patients, the plasma contains an excessive amount of A or B antigen; it is then necessary to wash the patient's red cells several times in saline to prevent a false-negative cell typing due to the inhibition of anti-A or anti-B.

6. When an antibody such as anti-I is attached to the patient's cells, autoagglutination may occur. Anti-I can usually be removed by washing the cells repeatedly in warm (40 to 45°C) saline.

(ii) Reverse-typing anomalies

1. About 1% of random blood samples contain unexpected agglutinins; some (e.g., anti-A_1, -H, -HI, -P_1, -Le^a, and -M) cause ABO reverse-typing anomalies.

2. The patient's serum may contain a potent autoantibody such as anti-I reacting with the A, B, and O standard cells and with the patient's own cells. If the serum is tested at 37°C, interference by anti-I is diminished, but agglutination by anti-A and anti-B is also weakened.

3. The serum of some patients with dysproteinemias, such as myeloma, causes cells to form intense rouleaux which may be difficult to distinguish from agglutination. Rouleau formation can sometimes be diminished by washing the aggregated cells once in saline or by diluting the patient's serum in saline before it is tested. The patient's own cells should be included as a control.

4. In patients with hypogammaglobulinemia or in elderly individuals, anti-A and anti-B may be weak and undetectable in routine reverse typing.

5. In newborn infants, the ABO type cannot be correctly deduced from the results of reverse typing. The expected antibody may be missing (because the infant's own antibodies are weak or absent), or an unexpected antibody may be present (because maternal IgG antibodies are transferred via the placenta).

6. Anti-A or anti-B may be missing in a blood group chimera who is immunologically tolerant to A or B antigens acquired by a graft of hemopoietic tissue.

7. In patients who have been transfused with large volumes of blood, the forward and reverse typing may be discrepant; e.g., a type A patient transfused with type O packed cells may appear to be type O lacking the expected anti-A.

Rh typing (D typing)

The patient's cells are typed for the D antigen by using anti-D in direct agglutination tests. In some individuals, a very weak Rh antigen (D^u) is not detectable in direct agglutination tests. However, the detection of D^u is not important for prospective transfusion recipients, since D^u-positive patients who type as D negative by routine tests can be treated as D negative and given D-negative blood.

Two anti-D reagents are commercially available, i.e., anti-D in a high concentration of protein, "for slide and modified tube test," and anti-D in a low concentration of protein, "for saline tube test," which is often prepared by chemical modification (i.e., reduction and alkylation) of IgG anti-D.

Anti-D for slide and modified tube test. Provided that adequate controls are included, the D type of

fluorescence, an appearance that tends to further exaggerate their size difference (Fig. 2). However, prospective studies to evaluate the immunofluorescence approach for the detection of fetal cells in the maternal circulation have not been conducted. Clearly, for this purpose, conditions should favor the staining of fetal cells rather than maternal F cells. Such a flexibility in the application of the method, coupled with the absence of ambiguity in the evaluation of preparations, is a performance advantage which cannot easily be matched by the acid elution technique. Furthermore, the fluorescence approach, in contrast to the acid elution method, can be used in bone marrow smears (5) or in in vitro erythroid colonies for identification of Hb F containing erythroblasts (4). In the latter preparations, fluorescing eosinophils may be present (due to enhanced autofluorescence), but their granular appearance renders them easily discernible from the truly positive erythroid precursors. No labeling of other nonerythroid cells is observed when the procedure described above is followed and our antibody is used.

In our experience, the most important factors in obtaining optimal results by the fluorescence method are the high purity and affinity of the antibodies used. A drawback of the fluorescence approach is the fact that useful antibodies for the technique are not commercially available at present. Some experience with techniques with fluoresceinated probes is needed to evaluate differences in background fluorescence, to choose the optimal dilution of antibodies, and to select appropriate combinations of filters.

LITERATURE CITED

1. Boyer, S. H., T. K. Belding, L. Margolet, and A. N. Noyes. 1975. Fetal hemoglobin restriction to a few erythrocytes (F cells) in normal human adults. Science 188:361–363.
2. Kleihauer, E., H. Braun, and K. Betke. 1957. Demonstration von fetalem Hämoglobin in den Erythrocyten eines Blautausstrichs. Klin. Wochenschr. 35:637–638.
3. Ley, T. J., J. DeSimone, N. P. Anagnou, G. H. Keller, K. Humphries, P. H. Turner, N. S. Young, P. Heller, and A. W. Nienhuis. 1982. 5-Azacytidine selectively increases γ-globin synthesis in a patient with β+ thalassemia. N. Engl. J. Med. 307:1469–1475.
4. Papayannopoulou, T., M. Brice, and G. Stamatoyannopoulos. 1977. Hemoglobin F synthesis in vitro: evidence for control at the level of primitive erythroid stem cells. Proc. Natl. Acad. Sci. U.S.A. 74:2923–2927.
5. Papayannopoulou, T., T. C. McGuire, G. Lim, E. Garzel, P. E. Nute, and G. Stamatoyannopoulos. 1976. Identification of haemoglobin S in red cells and normoblasts, using fluorescent anti-Hb S antibodies. Br. J. Haematol. 34:25–31.
6. Papayannopoulou, T., and G. Stamatoyannopoulos. 1979. On the origin of F-cells in the adult: clues from studies in clonal hemopathies, p. 73–86. In G. Stamatoyannopoulos and A. W. Nienhuis (ed.), Cellular and molecular regulation of hemoglobin switching. Grune & Stratton, New York.
7. Reiss, A. M., and W. Pollack. 1980. Detection and semiquantitation of fetal cells (fetal hemoglobin) in the maternal circulation, p. 764–766. In N. R. Rose and H. Friedman (ed.), Manual of clinical immunology, 2nd ed. American Society for Microbiology, Washington, D.C.
8. Stamatoyannopoulos, G., M. Farquhar, D. Lindsley, M. Brice, T. Papayannopoulou, and P. E. Nute. 1983. Monoclonal antibodies specific for globin chains. Blood 61:530–539.
9. Tomoda, Y. 1964. Demonstration of foetal erythrocyte by immunofluorescent staining. Nature (London) 202:910–911.
10. Weatherall, D., and J. B. Clegg. 1981. The thalassemia syndromes, 3rd ed., p. 450–507. Blackwell Scientific Publications, Ltd., Oxford.
11. Wood, W. G., G. Stamatoyannopoulos, G. Lim, and P. E. Nute. 1975. F-cells in the adult: normal values and levels in individuals with hereditary and acquired elevations of Hb F. Blood 46:671–682.
12. Woodrow, J. C., and R. Finn. 1966. Transplacental hemorrhage. Br. J. Haematol. 12:297–309.

Chapter 95

Autoimmune and Drug-Induced Immune Hemolytic Anemia

LAWRENCE D. PETZ

This chapter describes the means of definitively diagnosing the autoimmune hemolytic anemias (AIHAs) and drug-induced immune hemolytic anemias on the basis of their distinctive serological characterics. A classification of immune hemolytic anemias follows.

I. AIHAs
   A. Warm-antibody AIHA
      1. Idiopathic
      2. Secondary (chronic lymphocytic leukemia, lymphomas, systemic lupus erythematosus, etc.)
   B. Cold-agglutinin syndrome
      1. Idiopathic
      2. Secondary
         a. *Mycoplasma pneumoniae* infection, infectious mononucleosis, virus infections
         b. Lymphoreticular malignancies
   C. Paroxysmal cold hemoglobinuria
      1. Idiopathic
      2. Secondary
         a. Viral syndromes
         b. Syphilis
   D. Atypical AIHA
      1. Antiglobulin test-negative AIHA
      2. Combined cold- and warm-antibody AIHA
II. Drug-induced immune hemolytic anemia
III. Alloantibody-induced immune hemolytic anemia
   A. Hemolytic transfusion reactions
   B. Hemolytic disease of the newborn

It is essential that a precise diagnosis be made in each case since prognosis and management differ strikingly among the various hemolytic anemias. Characteristic clinical features of the various kinds of AIHAs and drug-induced immune hemolytic anemias are as follows.

Warm-antibody AIHA

Clinical manifestations. Variable, usually symptoms of anemia, occasionally acute hemolytic syndrome
Prognosis. Fair, with significant mortality
Therapy. Steroids, splenectomy, immunosuppressive drugs

Cold-agglutinin syndrome

Clinical manifestations. Moderate chronic hemolytic anemia in middle-aged or elderly persons, often with signs and symptoms exacerbated by cold
Prognosis. Good, usually a chronic and quite stable anemia
Therapy. Avoidance of cold exposure, chlorambucil

Paroxysmal cold hemoglobinuria

Clinical manifestations. Acute hemolytic anemia often with hemoglobinuria, particularly in a child with history of recent viral or viruslike illness
Prognosis. Excellent after initial stormy course
Therapy. Not well defined, steroids empirically and transfusions if required

Combined cold plus warm AIHA

Clinical manifestations. Severe anemia (hemoglobin about 6 g/dl) usually
Prognosis. Initial good response to corticosteroids followed by variable course
Therapy. Corticosteroids initially, splenectomy and immunosuppressive drugs often required ultimately

Drug-induced immune hemolytic anemia

Clinical manifestations. Variable, most commonly subacute or chronic in onset but occasionally acute hemolytic syndrome
Prognosis. Excellent
Therapy. Stop drug, occasionally a short course of steroids empirically

INDICATIONS FOR A DETAILED SEROLOGICAL EVALUATION

The hematological studies required to determine the presence or absence of hemolytic anemia should precede any serological study. Generally, simple tests suffice, e.g., blood counts, reticulocyte counts, serum haptoglobin, total serum bilirubin with direct and indirect fractions, and serum lactate dehydrogenase. When the presence of hemolytic anemia is confirmed, further tests are indicated to determine if the hemolysis is caused by an immune mechanism. If the direct antiglobulin (Coombs) test (DAT) is positive in a patient with an acquired hemolytic anemia, detailed serological tests are necessary to diagnose a specific immune hemolytic anemia.

Occasionally, an unexpected positive DAT may be discovered during pretransfusion compatibility test procedures. If this result occurs, further serological studies may not be indicated, since clinically insignificant positive DATs occur in approximately 8% of hospitalized patients. Further testing is necessary if other laboratory tests confirm the presence of hemolytic anemia or, in the absence of hemolytic anemia, if a patient has been transfused in recent weeks. In the latter case, an erythrocyte eluate should be prepared and tested, since this eluate may contain antibody and be the first manifestation of a clinically significant alloantibody.

Finally, if a nonimmunological cause for an acquired hemolytic anemia cannot be established, serological studies are indicated as described below, even if the DAT is negative, since a small percentage of patients with AIHA do have a negative DAT.

LABORATORY DIAGNOSIS OF IMMUNE HEMOLYTIC ANEMIAS

The diagnosis of immune hemolytic anemias is based on the finding of characteristic serological abnormalities in a patient with clinical evidence of hemolysis (4, 6). To distinguish among the diagnostic possibilities listed above, a detailed laboratory evaluation is required. The serological tests to be performed determine whether the patient's erythrocytes are coated with immunoglobulin G (IgG), complement components, or both, and whether the erythrocytes are weakly or strongly sensitized. The results of the DAT and antiglobulin test titrations supply such information. Further tests must be performed to determine the characteristics of the antibodies in the patient's serum and in an eluate from his or her erythrocytes. Screening tests followed by steps required for a more detailed characterization of the antibodies are described below.

DAT

Collection of specimens

Blood for the DAT should be collected in EDTA anticoagulant (0.01 M) to inactivate complement and thus prevent in vitro sensitization of erythrocytes by clinically insignificant cold antibodies (e.g., normal incomplete cold antibody), which would result in a false-positive reaction. Vacutainer tubes (Becton Dickinson & Co., Parsippany, N.J.) containing EDTA are adequate for this purpose. If positive reactions are obtained with erythrocytes that have been separated from a clotted specimen or are in another anticoagulant and have been allowed to cool to room temperature or lower, the DAT should be repeated on a specimen anticoagulated with EDTA.

Method

The instructions of the manufacturer should be followed carefully, and the reactivity of the serum should be checked with the use of appropriate controls (see below). In general, the technique is as follows.

1. Place 2 drops of a 2 to 5% saline suspension of erythrocytes in a labeled tube (10 by 75 mm). Wash the erythrocytes three or four times with saline. After the last wash, centrifuge and decant the wash fluid completely, add 1 or 2 drops of anti-human globulin serum (AGS), and mix.

2. Centrifuge for approximately 15 s at 900 to 1,000 $\times g$ (equivalent to centrifugation in a Serofuge [Clay-Adams, Inc., Parsippany, N.J.] at 3,400 rpm). Examine the mixture for agglutination macroscopically and, if negative, microscopically. The manner in which the erythrocytes are dislodged from the bottom of the tube is critical. The tube should be held at an angle and shaken gently until all cells are dislodged. Then it should be tilted back and forth gently until an even suspension of cells or agglutinates is observed.

3. If results are negative with polyspecific or anti-C3 antiglobulin sera (see below), the tubes are allowed to incubate at room temperature for 5 to 10 min. They are then recentrifuged and read again for macroscopic or microscopic agglutination. This step is necessary because the sensitivity of the antiglobulin test for detection of C3 is significantly enhanced by a short incubation.

Agglutination is graded as follows: 4+, one solid aggregate, no free cells; 3+, several large aggregates, very few free cells; 2+, medium-sized aggregates, free cells in the background; 1+, small aggregates with turbid reddish background; $\frac{1}{2}$+, tiny aggregates with turbid reddish background or microscopic aggregates; 0, no agglutination.

Controls

1. Add 2 drops of 1% bovine serum albumin or manufacturer's AGS diluent to 1 drop of the patient's washed erythrocytes as a control test. The DAT is truly positive only if the AGS reacts and the diluent control remains negative.

2. IgG-coated erythrocytes (commercially available) should always be added to negative tests obtained with polyspecific or anti-IgG antisera; ideally, C3-coated erythrocytes should be added to negative tests with anti-C3, but these cells are not readily available. After recentrifugation, the tests should now be positive, ensuring that AGS has not been inhibited (e.g., by inadequate washing).

Polyspecific antiglobulin serum

It is convenient first to perform the DAT with a "polyspecific" antiglobulin serum which is defined as one which contains anti-IgG and anti-C3d and may contain antibodies of other specificities. A positive result in a patient with acquired hemolytic anemia almost always indicates that the patient's erythrocytes are coated with IgG, C3d, or both, even though it is theoretically true that other proteins coating the patient's erythrocytes may react with antibodies of other specificities to cause a positive reaction. Antibodies against the C3d fragment of C3 are essential, since this is the fragment of C3 that is readily detectable on erythrocytes that have been coated with C3 in vivo.

Monospecific antiglobulin sera

When it has been determined by use of a polyspecific reagent that the DAT is positive, it is then a simple matter to determine whether the erythrocytes are sensitized with IgG or C3d. Licensed monospecific antisera against IgG and C3 (containing anti-C3d) that have been standardized for use in the DAT are available from commercial manufacturers.

Other monospecific antiglobulin sera

Generally, it is not helpful to perform the DAT with monospecific antiglobulin reagents other than anti-IgG and anti-C3. Although some autoantibodies are of

TABLE 1. DAT results obtained with anti-IgG and anti-C3 in immune hemolytic anemias

Diagnosis	Presence of:	
	IgG	C3[a]
Warm-antibody AIHA (% of patients)		
67	+	+
20	+	−
13	−	+
Cold-agglutinin syndrome	−	+
Paroxysmal cold hemoglobinuria	−	+
Penicillin- or methyldopa-induced immune hemolytic anemia[b]	+	−
Other drug-induced immune hemolytic anemias[c]	−	+
Warm-antibody AIHA associated with systemic lupus erythematosis	+	+

[a] Such cells are primarily sensitized with the C3d component of C3 (see the text).

[b] Weakly positive reactions with anti-C3 may occur; invariably, reactions are strongly positive with anti-IgG.

[c] The most common pattern of erythrocyte sensitization is indicated, but occasionally IgG may be detected with or without C3.

the IgM immunoglobulin class, IgM sensitization of erythrocytes is difficult to detect with the antiglobulin test. Furthermore, IgM antibodies that cause immune hemolytic anemia characteristically, if not invariably, fix complement which is much more readily detected. IgA antibodies only infrequently play a role in erythrocyte sensitization, and in such cases, other immune globulins or complement components or both are almost always, although not invariably, found on the cell surface as well. Performance of the DAT with antisera against additional complement components is superfluous for diagnostic purposes, because if erythrocytes from patients with immune hemolytic anemia are sensitized with complement components other than C3, C3 can always be detected as well.

Interpretation

The DAT must be interpreted in conjunction with clinical and other laboratory data. The role of the DAT is to aid in the evaluation of the etiology of acquired hemolytic anemias. It cannot be used to determine the presence or absence of hemolysis; indeed, positive reactions occur in about 8% of hospitalized patients who do not have hemolytic anemia. The significance of a positive DAT with monospecific anti-IgG and anti-C3d antisera is outlined in Table 1 and may be described in more detail as follows.

In warm-antibody AIHA, there is no diagnostic pattern of antiglobulin test reactivity. Most commonly, positive reactions are obtained with both anti-IgG and anti-C3 antisera, but in a minority of cases, only IgG or C3 is found on the patient's erythrocytes. In contrast to the variable findings in warm-antibody AIHA, the DAT in cold-agglutinin syndrome is invariably positive when anti-C3 antiserum is used. Equally important is the fact that reactions are also invariably negative with anti-IgG antiserum; that is, a positive DAT with anti-IgG excludes cold-agglutinin syndrome as the sole diagnosis.

Paroxysmal cold hemoglobinuria is caused by an IgG complement-fixing antibody, but, nevertheless, the DAT is usually positive only with anti-C3 antiserum. The reactions may be only weakly positive even during episodes of acute hemolysis. Negative reactions with anti-IgG antisera are probably caused by the fact that the Donath-Landsteiner antibody readily elutes from the erythrocyte membrane during in vitro washing, whereas complement components remain fixed to the cell membrane.

Methyldopa and penicillin are the most common causes of drug-induced immune hemolytic anemia, and the DAT in both instances is characteristically strongly positive with anti-IgG and negative with anti-C3. Although this pattern of antiglobulin test reactivity remains the most common, there are a number of reports of the sensitization of erythrocytes with IgG and complement components in penicillin-induced immune hemolytic anemia.

The DAT in patients with hemolytic anemias caused by drugs other than methyldopa or penicillin is usually positive only with anti-C3, and the reactions are often very weakly positive. In some instances, the drug-related antibody is of the IgM class, and in other cases the antibody (which may be IgG or part of an immune complex) apparently elutes from the erythrocytes after fixing complement or is present on the erythrocytes in concentrations too low to be detectable by the antiglobulin test. In a minority of patients, the DAT is positive when anti-IgG antiglobulin serum is used.

Systemic lupus erythematosus deserves particular consideration since many patients with this disorder have C3 on their erythrocytes even at times when no evidence of hemolysis exists. When patients with systemic lupus erythematosus do develop AIHA, their erythrocytes are regularly coated with C3 and IgG.

One point that is evident from the above discussion, but which must be emphasized, is that performance of the DAT with an antiglobulin serum that does not contain anti-C3d antibodies will frequently result in misleadingly negative results in patients with immune hemolytic anemias. This result occurs in all patients with cold-agglutinin syndrome, 13% of patients with warm-antibody AIHA, essentially all patients with paroxysmal cold hemoglobinuria, and most patients with drug-induced immune hemolytic anemia caused by drugs other than methyldopa or penicillin. Altogether, this accounts for about 26% of patients with acquired immune hemolytic anemias.

ANTIGLOBULIN TEST TITRATIONS AND SCORES

It is useful to perform titrations of monospecific antiglobulin reagents against antiglobulin test-positive erythrocytes to assess more accurately the relative strength of the reactions. Commercially available anti-IgG and anti-C3 antiglobulin reagents are suitable for this purpose.

The strength of agglutination resulting with each dilution of the antiglobulin sera may then be used to develop an antiglobulin test titration score. Scores are of value in more accurately assessing the strength of the antiglobulin test than is possible by the use of only a single dilution of antiglobulin serum.

TABLE 2. DAT (Coombs test) titers[a]

Dilution	Agglutination grade for:	
	Anti-IgG	Anti-C3
Neat	4+	4+
1:2	4+	3+
1:4	4+	3+
1:8	3+	2+
1:16	2+	1+
1:32	1+	0
1:64	0	0
Control	0	0

[a] Anti-IgG titration score, 48; anti-C3 titration score, 36. Titration score is derived by assigning a value of 10 for complete agglutination (4+), 6 for a strong reaction with a number of large agglutinates (2+), etc. The score is the sum of the values obtained at each dilution of antiglobulin serum. The examples illustrate reactions obtained when potent monospecific antiglobulin sera were allowed to react against erythrocytes strongly sensitized with IgG and moderately strongly sensitized with C3. Such reactions are frequently found in patients with warm-antibody AIHA. See the text for an explanation of agglutination grades.

Since the titration score obtained is arbitrary and is dependent on the antiglobulin serum utilized, each laboratory will need to develop experience to be able to recognize the range of scores that occur with the antisera used and then arbitrarily divide them into categories such as weak, moderate, strong, and very strong.

Method

1. Prepare doubling dilutions of the antiglobulin serum in saline (neat [undiluted], 1:2, 1:4, 1:8, 1:16, 1:32, etc.). If DAT titrations are performed frequently, make up a large volume (e.g., 10 ml) of each dilution (to 1:1,024), and store it at 4°C.

2. One drop of a 2 to 5% suspension of the patient's cells is added to each of 10 tubes labeled neat through 1:512. Positive results are rarely obtained at dilutions beyond 1:512, but if further dilutions are required, they can be made, starting with the 1:1,024 dilution.

3. The labeled tubes are washed four times with isotonic saline. The last wash is decanted completely, leaving a dry button of erythrocytes in the bottom of the tube.

4. Two drops of each antiglobulin serum dilution are added to the correspondingly labeled tube.

5. The contents of the tubes are mixed, and the tubes are centrifuged at 1,000 × g for 15 to 20 s.

6. Inspect for agglutination as in the DAT.

7. A numerical score may be assigned to specific degrees of agglutination so that an antiglobulin test titration score can be developed for each antiglobulin test. One such method assigns a value of 10 for 4+ agglutination, 8 for 3+, 6 for 2+, 4 for 1+, 2 for $\frac{1}{2}$+, and 0 for negative reactions (Table 2).

Interpretation

Antiglobulin test titration scores are of significance in various ways in evaluating patients with AIHA, but, on the other hand, their significance must not be exaggerated. Although the amount of antibody on the erythrocyte membrane is generally proportional to the rate of erythrocyte destruction, exceptions to this correlation are frequent. The strength of the DAT titer or score is not used to determine the presence or absence of hemolysis. Nevertheless, clinical evidence of hemolysis is usually present when erythrocytes are strongly sensitized with IgG. Similarly, the strength of C3 sensitization of erythrocytes is an important additional determinant of hemolysis in human immune hemolytic anemias.

Patients with methyldopa-induced AIHA have DAT titers and scores which are quite characteristic. When anti-IgG is used, the titers and scores almost always indicate strong erythrocyte sensitization, whereas reactions with anti-C3 are negative or very weakly positive. Thus, the DAT titer and score may lead to a suspicion of methyldopa-induced hemolytic anemia (very strong sensitization with IgG, negative with anti-C3) or may essentially exclude the diagnosis (negative or weak sensitization with IgG or strong sensitization with C3 or both).

Antiglobulin test titers and scores are of some value in follow-up of an individual patient during response to therapy. Although it is not rare for the antiglobulin test to remain positive in AIHA even when the patient is in remission as assessed by other laboratory findings, the titer and score are generally markedly reduced.

CHARACTERIZATION OF ANTIBODIES IN SERUM AND ELUATE

Although the DAT provides useful information, the definitive diagnosis rests upon the characterization of the antibodies present in the patient's serum and erythrocyte eluate. It is wise to initiate such studies with screening tests to develop a preliminary diagnosis and then perform additional tests as necessary for confirmation of the diagnosis and exclusion of alternative possibilities.

The patient's serum is examined to determine whether it contains antibodies. If so, one must determine the characteristics of the antibodies, particularly their thermal range and specificity. Also of significance are whether they are agglutinins or "incomplete" antibodies and whether they have hemolytic activity. In addition, an erythrocyte eluate is tested for reactivity by the indirect antiglobulin test (IAT) and by agglutination of enzyme-treated erythrocytes; if it is reactive, the specificity of the antibody should be determined.

Screening tests should first be performed by several different techniques and at various temperatures. Information derived from such screening tests with the patient's fresh serum and with an erythrocyte eluate is useful in planning the best procedures for definitive evaluation.

Before describing an approach to the diagnosis of various kinds of AIHA, I shall describe methods for the preparation of enzyme-treated erythrocytes, low-ionic-strength saline (LISS) solution, and erythrocyte eluates.

Enzyme-treated erythrocytes

Enzymes enhance the reactivity of erythrocytes with certain alloantibodies such as those of the Kidd, Lewis, Rh, and P systems. In warm-antibody AIHA, autoantibody is detectable in the patient's serum in about 90% of cases by use of enzyme-treated erythrocytes, whereas the IAT will detect antibody in only about 60%.

It must be stressed that enzymes considerably enhance the reactivity of cold autoagglutinins. Therefore, the great majority of normal sera will react with enzyme-pretreated cells at room temperature and in some instances demonstrate "carry-over reactivity" at 37°C. Thus, it is important to warm the enzyme-pretreated cells and serum under test separately to 37°C before mixing. This technique prevents the cold autoagglutinins from reacting with their antigen at temperatures below 37°C.

It should also be noted that, if enzyme-pretreated cells are used with antiglobulin serum, the reagent must be shown to be free from unwanted antibody activity (i.e., anti-A, anti-B, anti-H, and antispecies) that might demonstrate increased reactivity with enzyme-pretreated cells.

Enzymes commonly used are bromelin, trypsin, papain, ficin, and multienzyme preparations. Enzymes may be employed in a simple one-stage (direct) technique, in which the enzyme is mixed directly with the test cells and serum to be tested, or in a two-stage (indirect) technique, in which the test cells are pretreated before use. I recommend the two-stage technique utilizing papain or ficin since it is more sensitive than the one-stage technique.

One-stage papain technique

1. Place in a tube 2 volumes of the patient's serum, 1 volume of a 5% suspension of erythrocytes, and 1 volume of cysteine-activated papain solution (pH 5.4; see below).
2. Incubate at 37°C for 15 to 30 min.
3. Centrifuge; examine for hemolysis and agglutination.
4. Record the results.

Two-stage papain technique

1. Place in a small tube 2 volumes of the patient's serum and 1 volume of premodified cells (see below).
2. Incubate at 37°C for 15 to 60 min.
3. Centrifuge; examine for hemolysis and agglutination.
4. Record the results.

Preparation of 1% cysteine-activated papain

1. With a mortar and pestle, grind 2 g of powdered papain (Difco Laboratories, Detroit, Mich.) into a small amount of 0.01 M phosphate-buffered saline (PBS; pH 5.4).
2. Make up to 100 ml with 0.01 M PBS (pH 5.4).
3. Allow papain-buffered saline solution to stand at 4°C overnight.
4. Centrifuge for 15 min at 1,000 × g to remove debris, and transfer the supernatant to a 200-ml flask.
5. Add 10 ml of 0.5 M L-cysteine hydrochloride (Eastman Organic Chemicals, Rochester, N.Y.).
6. Make up to 200 ml with PBS (pH 5.4).
7. Incubate at 37°C for 1 h.
8. Dispense in 1-ml quantities, and keep frozen (−20°C) until use.

Procedure for treating erythrocytes with papain. Dilute 0.5 ml of 1% papain with 4.5 ml of PBS (pH 7.3) to give a 0.1% papain solution.

1. One volume of well-washed packed erythrocytes is incubated with 2 volumes of 0.1% papain for the predetermined length of incubation for optimal proteolytic effect (usually 15 to 30 min; see below, Standardization of papain).
2. After incubation, the erythrocytes are washed four times with large volumes of isotonic saline and then suspended to 2 to 5% in saline or LISS for testing.
3. If the enzyme-premodified erythrocytes are to be stored for more than 8 h, they should be suspended in a modified Alsever solution (Gamma Biologicals, Houston, Tex.). Enzyme-treated cells are stable for approximately 5 days if stored at 4°C in modified Alsever solution.

Standardization of papain. Standardization of the papain should be performed by incubating Fy^a and c-positive erythrocytes with the papain solution over a range of incubation times (e.g., 10 min, 15 min) up to 45 min. The incubation time at which the Fy^a antigen is denatured when tested with a potent anti-Fy^a while the c antigen is enhanced when tested with a very weak (diluted) anti-c is considered optimal.

Procedure for treating erythrocytes with ficin. The procedure for treatment of erythrocytes with ficin is modified slightly from that given in the instructions of the manufacturer.

1. To 1 volume of washed packed erythrocytes, add 2 volumes of ficin solution (Accugenics, Costa Mesa, Calif.).
2. The mixture is incubated at 37°C for 10 min.
3. The erythrocytes are washed four times with isotonic saline and then suspended to 2 to 5% in saline or LISS for testing.

Preparation of LISS solution

1. It is convenient to use an empty carboy saline container (greater than 10-liter capacity).
2. Weigh and put into the carboy 180 g of glycine (Eastman Kodak Co., Rochester, N.Y.).
3. Add 17.55 g of NaCl.
4. Add 10 liters of sterile water (McGaw Laboratories, Irvine, Calif.), and mix the solution by agitation.
5. Add 3 g of NaN$_3$ (Sigma Chemical Co., St. Louis, Mo.).
6. Add 120 ml of 0.15 KH$_2$PO$_4$ and 80 ml of 0.15 M Na$_2$HPO$_4$.
7. Leave the solution at room temperature, and agitate it intermittently for about 30 min.
8. Adjust the pH to 6.7 with 1 N NaOH (approximately 5.3 ml).
9. The Na$^+$ ion content, pH, and osmolality should be measured and recorded. The values for these should fall within the following ranges: Na$^+$, 30 to 36 meq/liter; pH, 6.65 to 6.75; and osmolality, 280 to 300 mosmol/kg of H$_2$O.

Periodically, these measurements should be checked. Ideally, measurement of the specific conductivity of the LISS solution should be made and should fall within the range of 3.4 to 3.9 mS/m. LISS solution is stable for up to 1 year when stored at room temperature.

LISS solutions are also available through commercial suppliers as suspending medium or additive medium. Although LISS suspending medium is used for the procedures in this chapter, LISS additive medium used according to the manufacturers' instructions should also be satisfactory.

Preparation of eluate from patient's erythrocytes

The ether elution method described below is simple and generally produces potent eluates. However, it requires the use of a highly flammable reagent, and, because of this, the chloroform elution technique is recommended (1). Landsteiner and Miller's heat elution method requires no special reagents, but the eluates produced are often not as potent. A necessary control, regardless of the method used, is to test saline from the last wash in parallel with the eluate (see below).

Ether elution method
1. Allow the patient's whole-blood sample in EDTA to incubate at 37°C for 10 min to allow any cold autoantibodies present to dissociate.
2. Wash the erythrocytes to be eluted (preferably at least several milliliters of erythrocytes) four times in large volumes of saline; keep approximately 1 ml of the last saline wash for the control.
3. To the washed packed erythrocytes, add ether at twice the volume of the erythrocytes, and add saline at half the volume. Mix thoroughly for 1 min.
4. Incubate at 37°C for 15 to 30 min.
5. Centrifuge at 900 to 1,000 × g for 10 min.
6. Separate the eluate which is the red bottom layer into a labeled, unstoppered test tube, and incubate it at 37°C for 30 min to allow excess ether to evaporate.

Landsteiner and Miller method. One volume of isotonic saline, group AB serum, or 6% albumin is added to washed packed erythrocytes and mixed thoroughly. Approximately 1 ml of the last saline wash should be kept for the control. The mixture is placed in a water bath at 56°C for 5 to 10 min, with repeated shaking. At the end of this time, the mixture is centrifuged rapidly while still hot, and the cherry-red supernatant fluid is removed; this fluid is the eluate.

Since antibodies may deteriorate rapidly in saline, there is a possible advantage in using group AB serum or 6% albumin rather than saline in the elution process. The actual volume of the suspending medium that is added to the washed packed cells may be varied depending on the strength of the antiglobulin test; if this test is very strong, a volume of medium twice that of the erythrocytes should be used; if the test is moderately strong, use a volume equal to that of the erythrocytes; and, if the test is weak, use a volume half that of the erythrocytes.

Chloroform elution method. For more information, see reference 1.
1. Wash the erythrocytes four times; keep about 1 ml of the last saline wash for the control.
2. To the packed washed erythrocytes, add an equal volume of diluent (saline, LISS, or 6% bovine serum albumin).
3. Add a volume of chloroform (Matheson, Coleman, and Bell, Norwood, Ohio) equal to the combined volumes of packed cells and diluent.
4. Stopper the tube and shake it vigorously for approximately 10 s, and then mix the contents by repeated inversion for a total of 1 min.
5. Place the tube, uncorked, into a 56°C water bath for 5 min. Stir the contents vigorously with a wooden applicator stick periodically throughout the 5-min period. Do not allow the incubation time to exceed 5 min.

6. Remove the tube, and centrifuge it at 1,000 × g for 5 min.
7. Three layers will be apparent. The eluate is the top layer.
8. With a Pasteur pipette, transfer the eluate to another tube to be used for testing.

Control: check of last saline wash fluid. The last saline wash should always be tested in parallel with the eluate. This step ensures that the erythrocytes have been washed free from serum and thus the eluate has only erythrocyte-sensitizing antibody and is not contaminated with diluted serum antibody.
1. Wash the erythrocytes four to six times with large volumes of isotonic saline.
2. Withdraw 2 drops of saline from the last wash, and add them to a tube (10 by 75 mm).
3. Add 2 drops of polyspecific or anti-IgG antiglobulin serum. Mix the contents, and let them incubate for 30 s to 1 min.
4. Add 1 drop of IgG-coated antiglobulin test control cells.
5. Centrifuge at 1,000 × g for 15 to 20 s, and observe for agglutination.
6. If 3+ to 4+ agglutination is seen, the erythrocytes have been washed sufficiently and can be processed for elution. If negative or weak agglutination is seen, the erythrocytes need additional washing.

This technique relies on the fact that anti-IgG contained in the antiglobulin reagent can be completely inhibited when as little as 2 μg of IgG per ml remains in the supernatant.

Screening tests for serum antibodies

The patient's serum is tested against erythrocytes suitable for antibody detection (i.e., either a single sample of group O cells or, preferably, a pool of equal volumes of commercially available screening cells I and II). The screening cells are suspended in isotonic saline or LISS (see below) and are used both untreated and enzyme premodified (e.g., papain treated) at 20 and 37°C as indicated in Table 3.

Screening tests for serum antibodies at 20°C
1. Untreated pooled antibody detection cells are suspended to 5% in isotonic saline or to 2% in LISS.
2. Four volumes of serum are added to 1 volume of the 5% saline suspended cells, or 2 volumes of serum are added to 2 volumes of the 2% LISS-suspended cells.

TABLE 3. Antibody screening in immune hemolytic anemia

Temp (°C)[a]	Test with pooled I and II[b]	
	Untreated	Enzyme premodified
20	Lysis, agglutination	
37[c]	Lysis, agglutination, IAT[d]	Lysis, agglutination, IAT[e]

[a] Incubation for 30 min.
[b] Pooled I and II is a mixture of commercially available erythrocytes selected for the purpose of screening "unexpected" erythrocyte antibodies.
[c] Prewarmed serum and erythrocytes.
[d] With polyspecific reagent.
[e] With anti-IgG reagent.

3. The cells and serum are mixed and incubated at 20°C (or room temperature, if <25°C) for 30 min.

4. The tube is centrifuged at 1,000 × g for 15 to 20 s and read first for lysis and then for agglutination (macroscopic only).

Screening tests for serum antibodies at 37°C

1. Untreated and enzyme-premodified pooled antibody detection cells are suspended to 5% in isotonic saline or to 2% in LISS. If saline-suspended erythrocytes are used, 2 drops of 22 or 30% bovine serum albumin should be added to the untreated cells only.

2. The antibody detection cells and patient's serum must be prewarmed separately at 37°C for 5 to 10 min before mixing.

3. Four volumes of prewarmed patient's serum are added to 1 volume of the prewarmed 5% saline-suspended cells, or 2 volumes of prewarmed patient's serum are added to an equal volume of prewarmed LISS-suspended cells.

4. The cells and serum are mixed and incubated at 37°C for 30 min.

5. After incubation, the tubes are centrifuged in a centrifuge that is maintained at 37°C. (This can be accomplished by having a centrifuge placed in an incubator or by using centrifuge "cups" prewarmed to 45°C before centrifugation). After centrifugation at 37°C, the samples are first read for lysis and then for macro- and microscopic agglutination (the enzyme test is read only for macroscopic agglutination).

6. The samples are then washed four times with saline prewarmed to 37 to 40°C.

7. Polyspecific antiglobulin serum is added to the tubes containing the dry button of untreated test cells; anti-IgG antiglobulin serum is added to the tubes containing the dry button of enzyme-premodified test cells.

8. The tubes are centrifuged at 1,000 × g for 15 to 20 s. The untreated erythrocytes are read for macro- and microscopic agglutination; the enzyme-premodified cells are read only for macroscopic agglutination.

Testing of eluate for autoantibody

1. The eluate is first screened against pooled antibody detection cells (I and II), both untreated and enzyme premodified.

2. If the eluate is nonreactive against untreated test cells and positive against enzyme-premodified cells, it will be further characterized with enzyme-premodified cells.

3. If the eluate is nonreactive against both untreated and enzyme-premodified test cells, it can be concentrated at least twofold with a Minicon concentrator (B125; Amicon Corp., Lexington, Mass.) and retested for activity. Also, if the patient is receiving a drug that has been documented as causing immune hemolysis (i.e., high-dose penicillin), the eluate should be tested for possible antibody to the drug (see below, Drug-Induced Immune Hemolytic Anemias).

4. Positive eluates are serially diluted, with doubling dilutions in saline from neat to 1:512 (0.5-ml volumes).

5. Transfer 2 drops of each dilution to three tubes labeled R_1, R_2, and r.

6. Add 1 drop of a 2 to 5% saline or LISS suspension of group O R_1R_1 (CDe/CDe), R_2R_2 (cDE/cDE), and rr

TABLE 4. Typical results of serum screening tests in warm-antibody AIHA[a]

Temp (°C) and test	Test with pooled I and II[b]	
	Untreated	Enzyme premodified
20		
Lysis	0	
Agglutination	0	
37		
Lysis	0	$\frac{1}{2}$+
Agglutination	0	2+
IAT	2+	3+

[a] Reprinted with permission from reference 4.
[b] See Table 3, footnote b.

(cde/cde) erythrocytes to each appropriate row of tubes.

7. Incubate at 37°C for 15 to 30 min.

8. Wash four times in isotonic saline.

9. Add antiglobulin serum to the dry button of washed cells.

10. Examine for agglutination and record results.

Results of serological tests in warm-antibody AIHA

The results of screening tests in a typical patient with warm-antibody AIHA are listed in Table 4, and a summary of screening test results in a series of 244 patients (6) is given in Table 5.

If the screening test results are suggestive of warm-antibody AIHA, further testing is indicated to confirm the diagnosis. In particular, the specificity of the warm antibody must be determined. This determination is made by testing against a panel of erythrocytes, usually from about 10 carefully selected persons. The donors are chosen so that the various erythrocyte antigens are represented on some erythrocyte samples but not others. (Such erythrocyte panels are commercially available and are standard blood bank reagents.) In addition, to gain additional information about possible Rh "relative specificity" (see below), one may determine the titer of the patient's serum against cells of various Rh phenotypes, i.e., R_1R_1 (CDe/CDe), R_2R_2 (cDE/cDE), and rr (cde/cde).

The antibody may demonstrate clear-cut specificity by reacting only with erythrocytes containing a particular Rh antigen (e.g., e or hr"). If that erythrocyte antigen is absent from the patient's own erythrocytes, the antibody is an alloantibody which has developed as a result of exposure to foreign antigens by blood transfusion or pregnancy. Such antibody may cause

TABLE 5. Results of serum screening in 244 patients with warm-antibody AIHA

Kind of erythrocytes	Temp (°C)	Test	% Positive sera
Untreated	20	Lysis	0.4
		Agglutination	34.8
	37	Lysis	0.4
		Agglutination	4.9
		IAT	57.4
Enzyme treated	37	Lysis	8.6
		Agglutination	88.9

hemolytic transfusion reactions if the patient is transfused with erythrocytes containing the antigen, but since the antibody cannot react with the patient's own erythrocytes, it is not an autoantibody and is irrelevant in a diagnosis of AIHA. However, if the antigen is present on the patient's own erythrocytes, one has a clear demonstration of an erythrocyte autoantibody. The finding of such clear-cut specificity of a warm autoantibody does occur, but is rare. More commonly, the antibody, while reacting with all cells on the panel, will consistently react more strongly with erythrocytes containing a certain Rh antigen than with cells lacking this antigen. If the patient's own erythrocytes contain this antigen, it is customary to consider that the antibody is an autoantibody with specificity, even though it reacts with all cells tested. I refer to autoantibodies that react with all erythrocytes of common Rh phenotypes but which react with a higher titer against erythrocytes having a certain Rh antigen than with erythrocytes lacking that antigen as demonstrating Rh "relative specificity."

The most common result obtained when testing for specificity of the antibody in warm-antibody AIHA is that the antibody in the patient's serum and eluate will react about equally strongly with all erythrocytes on the panel. It may not be possible to test the antibody for reactivity against the patient's own erythrocytes because they are already coated with antibody. However, it is inferred from its reactivity with all normal erythrocytes that the antigen with which the antibody is reacting is on the patient's own erythrocytes as well; this inference may be further supported by finding that the antibody eluted from the patient's own erythrocytes demonstrates a similar broad reactivity. Such an inference has been confirmed by freezing some of the serum and eluate and retesting them against the patient's own erythrocytes after a remission has been induced.

Although the testing described thus far may not have identified the specificity of the antibody found in the screening test, further studies utilizing rare donor cells and additional serological tests such as absorption and elution will very frequently demonstrate specificity of the autoantibody. However, such detailed tests are generally not considered essential for the diagnosis of warm-antibody AIHA.

A diagnosis can usually be reached on the basis of the serological tests described thus far. Despite the seemingly complicated nature of the foregoing, the usual or "typical" essential diagnostic tests that lead to a reasonably confident diagnosis of warm-antibody AIHA may be very simply summarized as follows: (i) the presence of an acquired hemolytic anemia, (ii) a positive DAT, and (iii) an incomplete antibody in the serum and eluate which reacts optimally at 37°C. The antibody usually reacts with all normal erythrocytes, but in some cases can readily be shown to react preferentially with antigens on the patient's own erythrocytes.

Several points concerning the above laboratory tests merit emphasis. Enzyme-treated erythrocytes are not routinely utilized in most blood transfusion laboratories for compatibility test procedures but must be used for adequate detection and characterization of autoantibodies in warm-antibody AIHA. These erythrocytes are used because only 57% of patients with warm-antibody AIHA have antibody detectable in their serum when tests at 37°C are performed utilizing only "normal" erythrocytes (i.e., non-enzyme treated). In contrast, autoantibodies are detectable in 89% of patients when enzyme-treated cells are utilized (Table 5).

Enzyme-treated erythrocytes are also essential since warm autoantibodies only rarely are capable of lysing untreated erythrocytes. Warm hemolysins may occur in association with incomplete IgG autoantibodies. However, in approximately 10% of patients with warm-antibody AIHA, the serum antibody will cause lysis of enzyme-treated erythrocytes but, when reacted against normal erythrocytes, will not cause lysis, agglutination, or a positive IAT. The DAT in these patients is positive with anti-C3 and negative with anti-IgG antisera. Almost all of these warm hemolysins are IgM antibodies, but, rarely, IgG antibodies have also been described. In contrast to autoantibodies reactive by the IAT, specificity tests do not reveal specificity within the Rh system; they are maximally reactive at a pH of 6.5.

A summary of results found in patients with warm-antibody AIHA is given in Table 6.

COLD-AGGLUTININ SYNDROME

The results of screening tests in a typical case of cold-agglutinin syndrome are given in Table 7, and a summary of results of screening tests for a series of 57 patients is given in Table 8.

Cold-agglutinin syndrome must be considered for all patients with acquired hemolytic anemia who have a positive DAT when anti-C3 is used and a negative DAT when anti-IgG is used. The most distinctive screening test is the agglutination of normal erythrocytes at 20°C, which occurs in essentially all patients with cold-agglutinin syndrome (Table 8). With these findings, further studies are necessary to determine the titer and thermal amplitude of the cold agglutinin. The titer at 4°C in saline is usually greater than 500, and antibodies that do not cause agglutination of erythrocytes suspended in albumin to a temperature of at least 30°C seem to be incapable of causing chronic cold-agglutinin syndrome (2) (although they may be of clinical significance in association with unusual exposure to cold). The cold-agglutinin titer and thermal amplitude may be determined as follows and, if desired, one can simultaneously determine the specificity of the cold agglutinin within the Ii blood group systems.

Cold-agglutinin titration, thermal amplitude, and specificity

A master series of doubling dilutions of serum is made in 0.9% NaCl, starting with undiluted serum and ending at a dilution of 1:2,000 or 1:4,000. One drop of each serum dilution is then pipetted into separate tubes (10 by 75 mm) in each of three rows so that three replicate titrations are made. The tubes are placed in a 37°C water bath until the contents reach 37°C (i.e., 10 min), and 1 drop of a 2% suspension of saline-washed erythrocytes that have been warmed to 37°C is added to each tube as follows: normal pooled group O adult erythrocytes are added to the first row,

TABLE 6. Characteristic serological findings in acquired immune hemolytic anemias[a]

Type of anemia	Result of DAT	Eluate	Tests for serum antibody	Antibody specificity
Autoimmune				
Warm-antibody AIHA (most common type)	IgG or complement (C3) or both	IgG antibody	IAT positive (57%), agglutinating enzyme-premodified cells (89%), hemolyzing enzyme-premodified cells (9%)	Usually within Rh system; other specificities include LW, U, I^T, K, Kp^b, K13, Ge, Jk^a, En^a, and Wr^b
Cold-agglutinin syndrome	Complement (C3) alone	Negative	Agglutinating activity up to 30°C in albumin; high titer at 4°C (usually >500)	Usually anti-I; other specificities include i, Pr, Gd, and Sd^x
Paroxysmal cold hemoglobinuria	Complement (C3) alone	Negative	Biphasic hemolysin[b]	Anti-P[c]
Drug induced				
Alpha-methyldopa (Aldomet)	IgG alone	IgG autoantibody	Similar to warm-antibody AIHA	Usually within Rh system
Penicillins	Usually IgG alone, but complement (C3) may also be detected	Negative unless penicillin-coated erythrocytes are tested	Negative unless penicillin-coated erythrocytes are tested	Reacts with penicillin-coated erythrocytes
Other drugs[d]	Usually complement (C3) alone, but IgG may also be detected	Usually negative	Negative unless drug, normal erythrocytes, and patient's serum are incubated together	Positive reaction occurs in presence of appropriate drug

[a] Reprinted with permission from reference 4.
[b] Sensitizes erythrocytes in the cold and hemolyzes them when they are moved to 37°C in the presence of complement.
[c] Reacts with all normal erythrocytes except p or P^k cells.
[d] For example, quinidine and phenacetin (usually reactive due to immune complex formation).

normal pooled group O cord erythrocytes are added to the second row, and, if available, the rare adult i cells are added to the third row. The contents of the tubes are mixed, and the tubes are incubated for 1 to 2 h. Agglutination is read macroscopically, with each tube being read directly from the water bath to prevent cooling. The tubes are then incubated at 30°C for 60 min, and agglutination is again read macroscopically. The procedure is repeated at 20 and 4°C. If centrifugation is employed, it must be carried out strictly at the required temperature (e.g., 4°C).

The cold-agglutination titrations may also be performed in albumin by adding 2 drops of 30% albumin to each tube before the erythrocytes are added.

By utilizing clinical information, the results of the DAT, and the above screening tests, a reasonably confident assessment of the presence or absence of cold-agglutinin syndrome can be made. Cold-agglutinin syndrome may be diagnosed if the following criteria are met (2): (i) clinical evidence of acquired hemolytic

anemia, (ii) a positive DAT caused by sensitization with C3, (iii) a negative DAT when anti-IgG antiglobulin serum is used, and (iv) the presence of a cold agglutinin with reactivity up to at least 30°C in albumin.

An alternative diagnosis must be sought for patients who do not satisfy all these criteria.

A few final comments are necessary concerning the diagnostic tests described above. Determining the cold-agglutinin titer at 4°C and the thermal amplitude is crucial in avoiding diagnostic errors, because cold agglutinins are frequently reactive at room temperature, are noticed because they cause difficulty in compatibility testing, and may cause agglutination visible to the naked eye in an anticoagulated blood sample. Commonly, it is assumed that such cold agglutinins must be potent enough to cause in vivo shortening of erythrocyte survival, and if the patient has a hemolytic anemia, an erroneous diagnosis of cold-agglutinin syndrome is made without further characterization of the antibody.

Although the titer of the cold agglutinin at 4°C is not a direct measurement of its in vivo significance, nev-

TABLE 7. Typical results in serum screening tests for cold-agglutinin syndrome[a]

Temp (°C) and test	Test with pooled I and II[b]	
	Untreated	Enzyme premodified
20		
Lysis	1+	
Agglutination	4+	
37		
Lysis	0	0
Agglutination	0	0
IAT	0	0

[a] Reprinted with permission from reference 4.
[b] See Table 3, footnote b.

TABLE 8. Results of serum screening for 57 patients with cold-agglutinin syndrome

Type of erythrocytes	Temp (°C)	Test	% Positive sera
Untreated	20	Lysis	2.0
		Agglutination	98
	37	Lysis	0
		Agglutination	10.7
		IAT	5.4
Enzyme treated	37	Lysis	12.2
		Agglutination	28.6

ertheless such information is usually of distinct value. When the titer is greater than 1,000 at 4°C in saline, patients usually have hemolytic anemia, and I have not observed a patient with a titer greater than 2,000 without hemolytic anemia. Thus, for patients with very high titers at 4°C (2,000 in saline, assuming proper technique, with separate pipettes used for each dilution to avoid carry-over) who otherwise satisfy the criteria for the diagnosis of cold agglutinin syndrome, diagnostic error is very unlikely to result from failure to determine the thermal amplitude. However, many cold agglutinins in patients with cold-agglutinin syndrome have titers at 4°C of 1,000 or less in saline, and it is in these patients that determination of thermal amplitude (especially in albumin) is extremely important.

Although results of specificity of the cold agglutinin are of interest, they are not essential either for diagnosis or for selection of blood for transfusion. The specificity, whether in the idiopathic disease or secondary to *M. pneumoniae* infection or lymphoma, is usually anti-I. Other antibodies, including those from some of the patients with infectious mononucleosis, have anti-i specificity. Rarely, the antibody is anti-Pr (anti-Sp$_1$).

The ability of cold antibodies to cause lysis of enzyme-treated erythrocytes is a rather common characteristic of antibodies from patients with cold-agglutinin syndrome, but is also a characteristic of antibodies from some patients with no evidence of hemolysis. Thus, positive in vitro tests for lysis are not diagnostic of cold-agglutinin syndrome. What is more important is that cold antibodies will cause a decreasing amount of lysis at progressively higher temperatures. If results for lysis are more strongly positive at 37 than at 20 or 30°C, a warm hemolysin, which may be a separate antibody, must be suspected.

The serological findings for cold-agglutinin syndrome are summarized and compared with findings for other types of acquired immune hemolytic anemias in Table 6.

PAROXYSMAL COLD HEMOGLOBINURIA

The diagnosis of paroxysmal cold hemoglobinuria or the exclusion of that diagnosis in the laboratory is usually considerably easier than the diagnosis or exclusion of either warm-antibody AIHA or cold-agglutinin syndrome. The results of screening tests in paroxysmal cold hemoglobinuria are usually negative, since the Donath-Landsteiner test (see below) is necessary to demonstrate the responsible antibody. The essential laboratory test is the biphasic hemolysis test originally described by Donath and Landsteiner in 1904.

Donath-Landsteiner test

For the Donath-Landsteiner test, serum from the patient is obtained from blood allowed to clot undisturbed at 37°C. One volume of a 50% suspension of washed, normal group O, P-positive erythrocytes is added to 9 volumes of the patient's serum. The suspension is chilled in crushed ice at 0°C for 1 h and then placed in a water bath at 37°C. The tube is centrifuged after 30 min at 37°C.

Lysis visible to the naked eye indicates a positive test. In some cases, this lysis occurs within 1 min or so of warming. An additional tube containing the patient's serum diluted with an equal volume of normal serum should be subjected to the same procedure to allow the possibility that the patient's serum is deficient in complement, as it may be soon after a hemolytic attack. A further control tube, kept strictly at 37°C throughout, should show no hemolysis.

Interpretation

Since paroxysmal cold hemoglobinuria is quite rare, one may justifiably question the advisability of routinely performing a Donath-Landsteiner test in patients with acquired hemolytic anemia. My attitude is to be liberal with the indications for performance of the test, since the test is very simple and specific. A negative test excludes the diagnosis of paroxysmal cold hemoglobinuria, and a positive test is essentially diagnostic of the disorder. Ordinarily, only a one-tube test need be performed initially, and, if positive, this test can be repeated with appropriate controls. Performance of the test is indicated in any child, any patient with hemoglobinuria, patients with a history of hemolysis exacerbated by cold, and in all cases of AIHA with atypical serological findings. If, however, tests for warm-antibody AIHA or cold-agglutinin syndrome quickly lead to perfectly characteristic findings for these disorders, the Donath-Landsteiner test may be omitted as superfluous. If positive results are obtained in the Donath-Landsteiner test, determination of the specificity of the autoantibody is indicated. In almost all reported cases, the autoantibody reacts with clear-cut anti-P specificity. This result is of some diagnostic significance since autoantibodies of this specificity have only very rarely been reported in any other type of AIHA. Erythrocytes necessary for determining anti-P specificity are rare, but with the assistance of reference laboratories, specificity testing can be carried out. Table 6 compares serological findings for paroxysmal cold hemoglobinuria with findings for other acquired immune hemolytic anemias.

AIHA ASSOCIATED WITH A NEGATIVE DAT

Patients with acquired hemolytic anemia whose erythrocytes are not agglutinated by antiglobulin serum have been reported by numerous investigators. In same instances, the hemolysis is clearly not antibody induced, as in cases of hemolytic anemia caused by oxidant drugs in patients with glucose-6-phosphate dehydrogenase deficiency, mechanical hemolytic anemias, and paroxysmal nocturnal hemoglobinuria (PNH). However, in other patients, extensive evaluation fails to reveal a nonimmunological etiology, and clinical findings are suggestive of AIHA; that is, these patients destroy transfused normal compatible erythrocytes at a rate approximating destruction of their own erythrocytes, thus indicating an extrinsic mechanism for erythrocyte destruction. In addition, these patients usually respond to steroid therapy, splenectomy, or both, as do those patients with more typical serological findings of AIHA. In many such patients, evidence supporting the hypothesis that these cases are AIHAs can be obtained through techniques more sensitive than standard serological procedures.

The frequency of patients with AIHA with a negative DAT has varied from 2 to 10% in various reported series.

The inability to demonstrate autoantibodies on erythrocytes of patients with DAT-negative immune hemolytic anemia is often due to the fact that the concentration of antibody on the cell is too low for detection by the usual antiglobulin test. However, the antiglobulin test result depends not only on the concentration of IgG on the erythrocyte surface, but also on characteristics of the erythrocyte antibody and on the antiglobulin serum. With manually performed antiglobulin tests and potent antiglobulin serum, erythrocytes coated with either IgG anti-A or anti-Rh_o(D) are generally weakly agglutinated when they are coated with 100 to 500 antibody molecules per cell.

Measurement of small amounts of erythrocyte antibodies

Several groups have reported new laboratory procedures for identifying small concentrations of IgG on erythrocytes. Such techniques are needed since the complement fixation antibody consumption test, used for this purpose by earlier investigators, is hopelessly cumbersome even for most research laboratories. Yam et al. (9) described a method with radiolabeled purified staphylococcal protein A, which has an affinity for the Fc receptor of human IgG. The assay detects as few as 70 molecules of IgG per erythrocyte and is therefore as sensitive as the complement fixation antibody consumption test. The assay is easier to perform and uses a commercially available protein which requires no further purification.

A similar assay with radioactive anti-IgG was reported by Schmitz et al. (7). IgG was detected by this method in all cases (33 of 33) with a positive direct IgG antiglobulin test, in 13 of 20 patients in whom the DAT was negative with anti-IgG but positive with anticomplement reagents, and in four of six patients with DAT-negative acquired hemolytic anemia Although the sensitivity of the direct radioactive test with ^{125}I-labeled anti-IgG far exceeded that of the DAT, the indirect test with radiolabeled anti-IgG was no more sensitive than the IAT.

One other test, which may prove to be the most practical, is the manual Polybrene test. This technique uses the polyvalent cation hexadimethrine bromide (Polybrene) to overcome the erythrocyte electrostatic repulsive charges and force the erythrocytes together. If the erythrocytes are sensitized with IgG and forced together with Polybrene, they become juxtaposed in a way that allows for antigen crosslinking by antibody molecules. This juxtaposition results in agglutination, which persists after the Polybrene is neutralized with a citrate resuspending medium.

Manual Polybrene test. (i) Reagents required

1. 10% normal human serum (single donor, untransfused male; group AB preferable) diluted in isotonic saline

2. Low-ionic medium (LIM). 5% glucose (Mallinckrodt, Inc., Paris, Ky.) in distilled water containing 2 g of disodium EDTA (J. T. Baker Chemical Co., Phillipsburg, N.J.) per liter

3. 0.1% Polybrene (Aldrich Chemical Co., Milwaukee, Wis.) distilled in isotonic saline; store in plastic container

4. Resuspending solution. 60 ml of 0.2 M trisodium citrate (J. T. Baker) in distilled water with 40 ml of 5% glucose (Mallinckrodt)

All reagents are stable indefinitely if stored at 4°C. Care must be taken to ensure that the reagents do not become contaminated with low levels of immunoglobulin; therefore it is best to divide into aliquots sufficient reagents for each assay and discard any reagents not used.

(ii) Polybrene procedure. The direct Polybrene test detects small concentrations of IgG on erythrocytes.

1. Allow all reagents and erythrocytes to reach room temperature before use.

2. Add 0.1 ml of 10% normal human serum to a glass culture tube (12 by 75 mm).

3. Add 0.1 ml of a 3% saline suspension of erythrocytes.

4. Add 0.1 ml of LIM; invert the tube gently to mix, and incubate for 1 min at room temperature.

5. Add 0.1 ml of 0.1% Polybrene; shake gently, using a back-and-forth motion to mix; allow to stand for 15 min.

6. Centrifuge the sample for 10 s at 1,000 × g.

7. Completely decant the supernatant.

8. Dislodge the cell aggregate by tapping the base of the tube on the counter top, being careful to keep the cells from adhering to the wall of the tube.

9. Add 0.1 ml of resuspending solution.

10. Shake very gently, using a back-and-forth motion three or four times.

11. Apply a large drop onto a clean glass slide directly from the tube by inverting the tube over the slide, at a slight angle, being careful not to touch the tube to the glass. Pour back into the tube any excess, and read with a microscope for agglutination along the thin edge of the droplet.

In an indirect Polybrene test for the detection of low levels of antibodies in serum samples, substitute 0.1 ml of patient's serum for the 10% normal human serum in step 2 above.

(iii) Controls. A commercial slide and rapid tube anti-D reagent is serially diluted in 10% normal human serum from 1:5,000 to 1:80,000. The dilutions are tested with R_2R_2 (cDE/cDE) and rr (cde/cde) erythrocytes by the indirect Polybrene technique. The highest dilution that gives a clear-cut positive result with the R_2R_2 erythrocytes and a negative result with the rr erythrocytes is selected as the dilution to be used with a positive (R_2R_2) and negative (rr) control cell with each direct or indirect Polybrene assay. Usually this dilution is 1:20,000 or 1:40,000, but it will vary depending on the potency of the anti-D. It is helpful to read the negative control test before reading the positive control; this control becomes the cutoff activity for the interpretation of a weak-positive result.

The following recommendations must be followed to achieve reliable results by the Polybrene technique.

1. All reagents and erythrocytes must be at room temperature before they are tested.

2. Normal human serum (10%; or patient's serum if an indirect Polybrene test is being performed) must be

added to the test tube before the addition of erythrocytes.

3. LIM is added in the direct test simply to maintain a standardized technique for both direct and indirect Polybrene testing. In the indirect Polybrene technique, LIM causes increased uptake of IgG antibody onto test erythrocytes and is extremely important.

4. After the addition of 0.1% Polybrene followed by centrifugation, the tubes need not be processed further immediately. Therefore, multiple tubes can be taken to this point before the test is continued.

5. Add resuspending solution to only two tests at a time.

6. It is important to read tubes individually and immediately after resuspending medium is added and to use a gentle, rocking back-and-forth motion to suspend the erythrocytes.

7. The drop onto the glass slide helps to disperse any residual Polybrene aggregates and must be done on all tests before they are read (along the thin edges of the droplet under a low-power light microscope).

Evaluation of a patient with acquired hemolytic anemia and a negative DAT

From my experience with acquired hemolytic anemias with a negative DAT, I suggest that one first consider nonimmune causes for the hemolysis; however, if such a diagnosis cannot be made, emphasis should be placed on practical serological methods that are more sensitive than routine methods. Often erythrocyte antibodies can be detected in the serum or erythrocyte eluate simply by using enzyme-premodified erythrocytes. In particular, tests with an erythrocyte eluate from just 3 to 5 ml of erythrocytes may be positive, especially if the eluate is concentrated two to five times before testing. Eluates are easily prepared by standard methods and can be readily concentrated using Minicon filters (Amicon). Methods with ^{125}I-staphylococcal protein A or ^{125}I-labeled anti-IgG for detection of IgG on the patient's erythrocytes are more sensitive than the DAT but are not practical for most routine laboratories. For this purpose, the manual Polybrene test is likely to prove the most valuable of available procedures. It needs no expensive reagents or equipment and is extremely rapid, requiring less than 3 min. However, the test is rather delicate, requiring some experience in interpretation, and positive and negative controls must be performed with each test.

With these tests, convincing evidence of erythrocyte autoantibodies can be found in many patients with acquired hemolytic anemia with a negative DAT in whom a nonimmune etiology cannot be determined. Such patients should be diagnosed as having warm-antibody AIHA and treated accordingly. However, there are some cases in which even the most sensitive techniques fail to demonstrate the presence of erythrocyte antibodies on the patient's erythrocytes or in the serum. I suspect that increasing the sensitivity of methods to detect IgG antibodies will not resolve this problem. Hemolysis may be caused by other mechanisms such as by IgM antibodies that are not readily detected by present methods or by abnormalities in the effector arm of the immune system (e.g., monocyte macrophages). Indeed, whether or not the hemolysis is immunologically mediated is conjectural and should be investigated further.

If it is impractical to perform one of the sensitive tests for erythrocyte-bound IgG or if results of the test are negative, clinical judgment must prevail. If the acquired hemolytic anemia is severe enough to require treatment and if nonimmunological causes have been carefully excluded, a trial of therapy appropriate for warm-antibody AIHA is warranted.

COMBINED COLD AND WARM AIHA

Patients who have AIHA with a positive DAT and who simultaneously satisfy diagnostic criteria for warm-antibody AIHA and cold-agglutinin syndrome appear to represent a distinct category of AIHA. Although previously thought to occur rarely, such patients may be a significant proportion of those patients with AIHA. In a recent study of 144 patients having AIHA with a positive DAT, 12 (8.3%) satisfied diagnostic criteria for both warm-antibody AIHA and cold-agglutinin syndrome. All 12 patients had IgG and C3d sensitizing their erythrocytes, and their sera contained an IgM cold autohemagglutinin optimally reactive at 4°C, but with a thermal amplitude to 37°C, and an IgG warm autoantibody. All erythrocyte eluates contained IgG warm autoantibody. Except for one patient who had a cold autoanti-i, no apparent blood group specificity was found for either the cold or warm autoantibodies. All 12 patients presented with severe hemolytic anemia which responded dramatically to steroid therapy, the mean hemoglobin level increasing from 6.3 to 12.9 g/dl. Five patients (42%) had systemic lupus erythematosus, one patient (8%) had a non-Hodgkin's lymphoma, and six patients (50%) had idiopathic AIHA; four patients (33%) had concomitant thrombocytopenia (Evans' syndrome). Nine patients (75%) were female. Four patients had unexpected alloantibodies potentially capable of causing in vivo hemolysis of transfused blood.

Thus, combined cold- and warm-antibody AIHA represents a unique catgory of AIHA and appears to affect a significant proportion of those patients having AIHA. The disorder responds well to initial therapy with corticosteroids but may be followed by relapse and a chronic clinical course. Because of the dramatic clinical response to steroid therapy, these patients should be started on steroids as soon as possible.

DRUG-INDUCED IMMUNE HEMOLYTIC ANEMIAS

Approximately 15% of acquired immune hemolytic anemias are related to drug administration (3, 6; L. D. Petz and D. R Branch, in H. Chaplin, ed., Methods in Hematology: Acquired Immune Hemolytic Anemias, in press), and by far the most common causes are methyldopa and penicillin. Methyldopa is the prototype of drugs which cause the development of AIHA, whereas penicillin is the prototype of drugs which cause immue hemolysis by the "drug absorption" mechanism. Still other drugs cause hemolysis as a result of development of immune complexes consisting of drug (or drug metabolite) and anti-drug antibody.

Methyldopa-induced AIHA

Immune hemolytic anemia caused by methyldopa is different than that caused by most other drugs because patients receiving methyldopa produce antibodies which react directly with normal erythrocytes, even in the absence of the drug (8). Indeed, the antibody seems to be directed mainly against the rhesus blood group antigens. In contrast, most other drug-induced antibodies are generally directed against the drug itself and not the erythrocyte.

The other drugs that have been described as acting in a fashion similar to methyldopa are levodopa and mefenamic acid. Levodopa causes positive DATs in about 6% of patients and also causes hemolytic anemia. Mefenamic acid is chemically unrelated to methyldopa but has been described as causing positive DATs and AIHA. Rarely, procainamide, phenacetin, chlorpromazine, and ibuprofen have also been implicated.

Characteristics of methyldopa-induced abnormalities

1. The serological findings caused by methyldopa-induced abnormalities are indistinguishable in the laboratory from idiopathic warm-antibody AIHA.

2. A positive DAT is found in ~15% of patients receiving methyldopa (reported values vary from 10 to 36%).

3. The positive DAT is due to sensitization with IgG. One of the most distinctive aspects of the serological results in patients with methyldopa-induced hemolytic anemia is the fact that the DAT titration score (see above, Antiglobulin Test Titrations and Scores) is extraordinarily high with anti-IgG antiglobulin serum and negative with anticomplement serum. This combination of results occurs uncommonly in AIHA not associated with methyldopa administration.

4. The DAT usually becomes positive after 3 to 6 months of treatment. (It is interesting to note that this delay is not shortened when a patient who previously exhibited a positive test is restarted on the drug.)

5. The development of the positive DAT appears to be dose dependent. One report indicated that 36% of patients taking more than 2 g of the drug daily have a positive DAT. In contrast, only 11% of patients taking less than 1 g daily have a positive test; 19% become positive on 1 to 2 g daily.

6. Various reports indicate that from 0 to 5% of patients receiving methyldopa have hemolytic anemia. The cumulative incidence is 0.8%.

7. The positive direct antiglobulin reaction gradually becomes negative once methyldopa is stopped. This change may take from 1 month to 2 years. Fortunately, the clinical and hematological values improve much more rapidly, i.e., usually within 1 to 3 weeks.

In conclusion, methyldopa is one of the most common causes of a positive DAT due to drugs. The total of methyldopa-induced AIHAs exceeds the total of all other drug-induced immune hemolytic anemias so far described. The laboratory evaluation of methyldopa-induced hemolytic anemia is identical to that for warm-antibody AIHA described above. Final proof that methyldopa is responsible for causing hemolytic anemia can be obtained clinically only by stopping methyldopa administration and observing resolution of the hemolysis.

Penicillin-induced immune hemolytic anemia

Penicillin is one of the few drugs which binds firmly to normal erythrocyte membranes both in vivo and in vitro. The drug cannot be removed even by multiple washes in saline. This fact means that one very easily can "sensitize" cells with penicillin in the laboratory and then use these treated cells for the detection of penicillin antibodies. This situation is in contrast to that with most other drugs, with which it is not possible to prepare drug-coated cells for antibody detection.

Considerable experimental work has demonstrated that the immunogenicity of penicillin is due to its ability to react chemically with tissue proteins to form several different haptenic groups. The major haptenic determinant is the benzylpenicilloyl group. It is not yet clear whether the benzylpenicilloyl group is formed by the direct reaction of penicillin with amino groups of protein or through the intermediate formation of benzylpenicillinic acid.

Penicillin can be detected on the erythrocyte membranes of all patients receiving large doses of intravenous penicillin.

Approximately 3% of patients receiving large doses of intravenous penicillin will develop a positive DAT. A small percentage of these patients will develop hemolytic anemia. The mechanism of the positive DAT and hemolytic anemia seems clear. The drug is absorbed onto the erythrocytes, and an immune antibody, i.e., antipenicillin, is produced by the patient and will react with the penicillin on the erythrocytes. The end product, therefore, is an erythrocyte sensitized by IgG. This mechanism of erythrocyte sensitization by penicillin and anti-penicillin antibody has been referred to as the drug absorption mechanism. Other drugs that bind tightly to the erythrocyte membrane and cause hemolysis by the drug absorption mechanism are some cephalosporins (see below), tolbutamide, erythromycin, cisplatin, and tetracycline (Table 9).

Complement is not usually involved in this reaction, and generally no intravascular hemolysis occurs. The erythrocytes are destroyed extravascularly by the reticuloendothelial system, probably in the same way as erythrocytes sensitized with Rh antibodies (i.e., non-complement-fixing IgG antibodies).

The essentials for penicillin-induced immune hemolytic anemia are as follows (3–6).

1. Administration of large doses of penicillin (on the order of more than 20×10^6 U/day)

2. High-titer IgG penicillin antibody present in serum

3. Strongly positive DAT, due to sensitization with IgG

4. Antibody eluted from the patient's erythrocytes, reactive against penicillin-treated erythrocytes but not against nontreated erythrocytes

Exceptions to the above typical findings occur. Complement activation may contribute to immune hemolysis in some cases. In these patients, the erythrocytes are sensitized with both IgG and complement, and intravascular hemolysis may ensue.

TABLE 9. Drugs that have been reported to cause hemolytic anemia by the immune complex mechanism

Drug	Intravascular hemolysis[a]	Renal failure[a]
Acetaminophen	×	
Aminopyrine	×	
p-Aminosalicylic acid	×	×
Antazoline	×	×
Chlorpromazine	×	×
Chlorpropamide	×	
Dipyrone[b]	×	×
Hydralazine		
Hydrochlorothiazide[c]	×	×
9-Hydroxymethyl ellipticinium	×	×
Insulin[b]		
Isoniazid[b]	×	
Melphalan		
Methotrexate		
Nomifensine[d]	×	×
Phenacetin[e]	×	×
Probenecid		
Quinidine[b]		
Quinine	×	
Rifampin	×	×
Stibophen	×	×
Streptomycin[b,d]		
Sulfonamides	×	×
Teniposide (VM-26)[d]	×	×
Triamterene[b]	×	×

[a] ×, Intravascular hemolysis or renal failure reported on at least one occasion.

[b] May also bind to erythrocytes, and hemolysis may be caused in part by drug adsorption mechanism.

[c] Intravascular hemolysis and renal failure occurred only with an overdose of the drug.

[d] Also caused development of erythrocyte autoantibody.

[e] May also cause hemolysis by drug adsorption mechanism and has been associated with the development of AIHA.

One should also appreciate that a positive DAT occurring during penicillin administration is not, in itself, an indication for cessation of the drug. Approximately 3% of patients receiving high doses of intravenous penicillin will develop a positive DAT. Hemolysis may not ensue, even with continued administration of the drug.

Hemolytic anemia caused by cephalosporin antibiotics

Immune hemolytic anemia probably as a result of the drug absorption mechanism has also been caused by several cephalosporin drugs including cephalothin, cephaloridine, cephalexin, cefazolin, and cefamandole. Such cases are, however, rare.

Detection of antibodies to penicillin and cephalosporins

Standard saline agglutination and IATs are employed in which the drug-coated erythrocytes and the patient's serum and eluate are used as follows.

1. The eluate and the patient's serum should be tested against both normal group O cells and the same cells treated with the appropriate drug. Usually, serial dilutions of the patient's serum are tested.

2. Two volumes of eluate or serum dilutions should be incubated in saline with 1 volume of a 2% suspension of drug-treated and untreated group O cells.

3. Incubate at room temperature for 15 min; centrifuge and inspect for agglutination.

4. Move the tubes to 37°C for 30 min; centrifuge and inspect for agglutination.

5. Wash the cells four times in saline.

6. Add antiglobulin serum to the button of washed cells, centrifuge, and inspect for agglutination.

IgM penicillin antibodies will agglutinate saline-suspended penicillin-treated cells but not the same cells untreated. IgG penicillin antibodies will react by the IAT against penicillin-treated cells but not against the same cells untreated.

If IATs are used to detect cephalothin or cephaloridine antibodies, it must be remembered that erythrocytes treated with these drugs can absorb proteins nonimmunologically. Therefore, normal sera may give a positive IAT with drug-treated erythrocytes. The reaction does not usually occur once the normal serum is diluted to more than 1:20. The amount of protein present in erythrocyte eluates does not seem to be enough to give nonspecific results, so a positive result usually indicates the presence of antibody to the cephalosporin or a cross-reacting penicillin antibody. The coupling of cephalothin to erythrocytes at acid pH (described below) virtually eliminates nonimmunological protein absorption.

Also, some β-lactam antibiotics may not be effectively coupled to erythrocytes by a pH coupling technique, and the use of the cross-linking technique for coupling these drugs to erythrocytes may be more efficacious.

Preparation of penicillin-sensitized cells. (i) pH coupling technique

1. Wash group O cells (preferably fresh) three times in saline.

2. Prepare sodium barbital buffer (0.1 M [20.5 g/liter]); adjust to pH 9.6 with 0.1 N HCl.

3. Add 10^6 U (approximately 600 mg) of potassium benzylpenicillin G dissolved in 15 ml of barbital buffer (pH 9.6) to 1 ml of packed washed cells.

4. Incubate for 1 h at room temperature with gentle mixing.

5. Wash the cells three times in saline.

Slight lysis may occur during incubation, and a small "clot" may form in the erythrocytes, which can be removed with applicator sticks before washing the cells. Once prepared, the cells may be kept in acid-citrate-glucose at 4°C for up to 1 week, but they do deteriorate slowly during this time.

Although penicillin-coated erythrocytes may be prepared by using isotonic saline, maximum coupling of the penicillin to the erythrocyte membrane can only be achieved with an alkaline solution at about pH 9.6. If the particular penicillin under study has a phenylacetamide side chain (e.g., ampicillin), the pH coupling method may not be effective.

(ii) Cross-linking technique

1. Dissolve 700 mg of the appropriate penicillin in 30 ml of 0.01 M PBS (pH 7.3). Adjust the pH to around 7.0.

2. Add 1 ml of a 50% saline suspension of human erythrocytes, and place the mixture at 0 to 4°C (wet ice).

3. 1-Ethyl-3-(3-dimethylaminopropyl)carbodiimide (ECDI) is obtained from commercial sources and must be stored desiccated at −20°C. Add 5 ml of a 50-

mg/ml solution of ECDI in PBS (pH 7.3; must be freshly made).

4. Incubate in the cold for 50 min.

5. Pour the erythrocytes into cold PBS (pH 7.3) containing 2% dipotassium EDTA, and then wash the erythrocytes three times with PBS (pH 7.3)–2% dipotassium EDTA.

6. Suspend the erythrocytes in isotonic saline for testing.

If gross lysis occurs, the concentration of the penicillin being used should be reduced until there is minimal lysis. If the particular penicillin under study has an additional carboxyl group as part of the side chain (e.g., carbenicillin) or an amino group alpha to the phenyl on the side chain (e.g., amoxicillin), the ECDI may also cross-link these groups to the erythrocyte membrane. This cross-linking may result in a conformational change in the penicillin which might position the side chain in a way that interferes with antibody binding.

Preparation of cephalosporin-coated erythrocytes. (i) pH coupling technique

1. Dissolve 400 mg of the appropriate cephalosporin preparation in 10 ml of 0.01 M sodium barbital-buffered saline. Adjust the pH to 8.5.

2. Wash group O erythrocytes (preferably fresh) three times in saline.

3. Add 1 ml of washed packed erythrocytes to the cephalosporin solution and mix.

4. Incubate for 2 h at 37°C with frequent mixing.

5. Wash the erythrocytes three to four times in isotonic saline. If gross lysis occurs, the concentration of the cephalosporin being used should be reduced until there is minimal lysis. Once prepared, the cells may be kept in Alsever solution at 4°C for up to 2 weeks. When moxalactam is used, 200 mg of the cephalosporin should be used in step 1 above. If the particular cephalosporin under study has a phenylacetamide side chain (e.g., cephalexin), the pH coupling method may not be effective.

(ii) Cross-linking technique

1. Dissolve 200 mg of the appropriate cephalosporin in 30 ml of 0.01 M PBS (pH 7.3). Adjust the pH to around 7.0.

2. Add 1 ml of a 50% saline suspension of human erythrocytes, and place the mixture at 0 to 4°C (wet ice).

3. ECDI is obtained from commercial sources and must be stored desiccated at −20°C. Add 5 ml of a 50-mg/ml solution of ECDI in PBS (pH 7.3; must be freshly made).

4. Incubate in the cold for 50 min.

5. Pour the erythrocytes into cold PBS (pH 7.3) containing 2% dipotassium EDTA, and then wash the erythrocytes three times with this buffer.

6. Suspend the erythrocytes in isotonic saline for testing.

If the particular cephalosporin under study has an additional carboxyl group as part of the side chain structure (e.g., moxalactam) or a free amino group on the side chain (e.g., cephradine, cephaloglycin, cefotaxime), the ECDI may also cross-link these groups to the erythrocyte membrane. This cross-linking may result in a conformational change in the cephalosporin which might position the molecule in a way that interferes with antibody binding.

(iii) Coupling of cephalothin to erythrocytes at acid pH

1. Dissolve 300 mg of cephalothin in 10 ml of 0.01 M PBS (pH 6.0). Check the pH and adjust it to 6.0 if necessary.

2. Wash group O erythrocytes (preferably fresh) three times in saline.

3. Add 1 ml of washed packed erythrocytes to the cephalothin solution, and mix.

4. Incubate for 1 h at 37°C with frequent mixing.

5. Wash erythrocytes three to four times in isotonic saline.

If gross lysis occurs, recheck the pH; it may be below 6.0. Once prepared, the cells may be kept in Alsever solution at 4°C for up to 1 week. By this method, cephalothin can be bound to erythrocytes, but nonimmunological protein binding by these cephalothin-coated cells is virtually eliminated.

Drugs causing hemolysis by an immune complex mechanism

A number of drugs have been reported to cause immune hemolytic anemia by an immune complex mechanism (Table 9). This mechanism, which is accepted by most investigators as the most probable explanation for the reactions seen with the drugs listed in Table 9, is related to the fact that drugs such as quinine, quinidine, and stibophen have a far stronger affinity for their respective antibodies than for cell membranes. Such drugs, when present with antibody in the patient's plasma, will combine to form an immune complex which may be absorbed to the cell membrane, often activating complement in the process. It is not known why this immune complex, once formed, sometimes causes erythrocyte destruction only and at other times causes platelet destruction only.

The patient usually presents with acute intravascular hemolysis, with hemoglobinemia and hemoglobinuria. Renal failure is frequent. A sensitized patient need take only a small quantity of the drug to precipitate these reactions.

The serum antidrug antibody is often IgM and is capable of activating complement. The DAT is positive often as a result of the presence of complement components on the erythrocyte surface, usually without detectable immunoglobulins. This situation may be explained by the fact that the immune complex does not bind very firmly to the erythrocytes and may dissociate from the cells and be free to react with other cells. This dissociation in turn may explain why such a small amount of drug complex can cause so much erythrocyte destruction. Furthermore, erythrocyte sensitization by IgM antibodies is not readily detectable by the antiglobulin test. Some reports of negative DATs, particularly in the earlier literature, may be due to inadequate anticomplement properties of the antiglobulin serum. In vitro reactions (agglutination, lysis, and sensitization to antiglobulin sera) are usually observed only when the patient's serum, drug, and erythrocytes are all incubated together.

Detection of drug antibodies reacting by an immune complex mechanism. (i) General methods

1. Prepare a saturated solution of the suspect drug in 0.01 M PBS (pH 7.0 to 7.4). Crush the tablets with a mortar and pestle. Incubate the solution at 37°C until

the drug seems adequately dissolved. Vigorous shaking may help dissolve the drug. *Caution*: Check the solubility of the drug before proceeding. Some drugs (e.g., chlorpropamide) are insoluble at pH 7.3; others (e.g., prednisone) are not soluble in aqueous media, and this procedure cannot be used. Other methods, obtained from the manufacturer or from specific publications, may be needed to dissolve adequate quantities of drug.

2. Centrifuge the solution, and save the clear supernatant. Many drugs, especially pharmaceutical preparations containing certain inert "filler" materials, will not dissolve completely, but even if the drug preparation appears to be only slightly soluble in aqueous media, the supernatant may contain enough drug for testing.

3. Check the pH of the drug solution, and adjust it to approximately 7.0 if necessary. Again, the final pH may depend upon the solubility of the drug.

4. Using serial doubling dilutions of the drug solution, test for nonspecific hemolysis against a 5% saline suspension of group O erythrocytes by incubating each dilution at 37°C for 1 h. If hemolysis is evident, select the lowest dilution at which no visible hemolysis is seen; this dilution is used in further testing.

5. Set up two tests with the following combinations:

   a. Patient's serum plus drug solution
   b. Patient's serum plus PBS
   c. Patient's serum plus normal serum (source of complement) plus drug solution
   d. Patient's serum plus normal serum plus PBS
   e. Drug solution plus normal serum

Usually, these tubes contain 2 to 4 volumes of each mixture.

6. To one set of tubes, add 1 volume of a 5% saline suspension of normal group O erythrocytes. To the other set, add 1 volume of a 5% saline suspension of enzyme-premodified group O erythrocytes.

7. Incubate both sets of tubes at 37°C for 1 to 2 h with periodic gentle mixing.

8. Centrifuge the tubes and examine the mixture for hemolysis and agglutination.

9. Wash the erythrocytes four times, and add antiglobulin serum to the button of washed erythrocytes. Centrifuge, observe for agglutination, and record the results.

(ii) Interpretation. Hemolysis, agglutination, and a positive IAT may occur together or separately. A positive result in any of the tubes to which the drug was added and a negative result in the corresponding control tubes (those with PBS added instead of drug and those with no patient's serum) suggest the presence of an antidrug antibody.

Technique for dissolving drugs which are only slightly soluble or are insoluble in aqueous media

1. Mix 30 mg of the drug with 1 ml of acetone.

2. Incubate the mixture at room temperature for 30 min with frequent agitation.

3. Add 5 ml of 0.15 N NaOH to the acetone-treated drug, and dissolve with low heating and stirring.

4. Neutralize the drug mixture with 5 ml of 0.15 N HCl (check the pH and adjust it to neutrality if necessary).

5. Incubate the mixture at room temperature for 60 min.

6. Centrifuge at $1,700 \times g$ for 20 min, and remove the supernatant solution.

7. If the supernatant solution alone causes lysis of test cells, dilute the supernatant 1:2 with isotonic saline before testing with erythrocytes.

Detection of antibodies to drugs with PNH or "PNH-like" erythrocytes

1. Add 0.2 ml of the drug solution (2 to 3 mg/ml) to 0.2 ml of patient's acidified serum. Acidified serum can be prepared by making a 1:10 dilution of 0.15 N HCl in patient's serum or fresh normal human serum and adjusting the pH to 6.5.

2. Add 0.2 ml of fresh, acidified, ABO-compatible serum as a source of complement.

3. Add 0.2 ml of a 10% suspension of PNH cells (or chemically modified PNH-like cells).

4. Bring the mixture to a final volume of 2 ml with PBS (pH 7.3) containing 0.005 M $NaCl_2$ and 0.0015 M $MgCl_2$.

5. Incubate the mixture at 37°C for 60 min.

6. Centrifuge at $1,000 \times g$ for 5 min, and observe for lysis.

7. A control consisting of patient's serum, normal human serum, and PNH cells, but no drug, should be run in parallel.

Preparation of PNH-like erythrocytes

1. Prepare an 8% solution of 2-aminoethylisothiouronium bromide (AET) in distilled water. Adjust the pH to 8.0 with 10 N NaOH. Make the solution immediately before use. (AET is obtained from commercial sources and is stored at $-20°C$.)

2. Add 4 volumes of AET solution to 1 volume of normal group O packed erythrocytes that have been washed three times.

3. Incubate the mixture at 37°C with gentle agitation for exactly 19 min.

4. Wash the erythrocytes four times with large volumes of saline or until the supernatant is free from hemoglobin.

Interpretation and comments. Methods described for the detection of drug-induced immune hemolytic anemia due to the immune complex mechanism vary widely, and, in addition to the methods described in this chapter, it may be of value to refer to a review for methods used for the detection of antibodies to individual drugs (3, 6; Petz and Branch, in press). In principle, the patient's serum and erythrocyte eluate should be tested against normal untreated and enzyme-treated erythrocytes in the presence of the suspected drug.

Several important points deserve emphasis. (i) The suspect drug must be soluble under the conditions used. If it is not soluble, the method described above for dissolving drugs which are insoluble in aqueous media can be substituted. (ii) It is preferable to test the pure-drug preparation and the pharmaceutical preparation in parallel. If only the pharmaceutical preparation is tested, positive results may be due to any number of excipient compounds contained in the pharmaceutical product, and the results may be misinterpreted.

The sensitivity of in vitro detection of drug antibodies may be increased by erythrocytes which have been premodified with proteolytic enzymes (e.g., papain or ficin).

The use of LISS for suspending drug-coated erythrocytes may be helpful in the detection of drug antibodies which are of low titer or have low avidity. This result may be because LISS significantly increases the sensitivity of tests for detecting antibodies to certain erythrocyte antigens.

The use of erythrocytes from patients having PNH or of normal erythrocytes which have been chemically modified to resemble PNH erythrocytes can be informative in the investigation of drug-induced immune hemolytic anemia caused by drug antibodies reacting by the immune complex mechanism. Such erythrocytes demonstrate exquisite sensitivity to complement lysis by drug-antibody complexes.

Previously, it has been shown that normal erythrocytes which have been chemically treated with AET become modified in such a way that their in vitro behavior closely resembles that of PNH erythrocytes. Thus, artificially prepared PNH-like erythrocytes may be as useful in the evaluation of drug-induced immune hemolytic anemias as true PNH erythrocytes.

A summary of characteristic serological findings for drug-induced immune hemolytic anemias and a comparison with findings for AIHAs are listed in Table 6.

LITERATURE CITED

1. **Branch, D. R., A. L. Sy Siok Hian, and L. D. Petz.** 1982. A new elution procedure using chloroform, a nonflammable organic solvent. Vox Sang. **42**:46–53.
2. **Garratty, G., L. D. Petz, and J. K. Hoops.** 1977. The correlation of cold agglutinin titrations in saline and albumin with haemolytic anaemia. Br. J. Haematol. **35**:587–595.
3. **Petz, L. D.** 1980. Drug-induced immune haemolytic anaemia. Clin. Haematol. **9**:455–482.
4. **Petz, L. D., and D. R. Branch.** 1983. Serological tests for the diagnosis of immune hemolytic anemias, p. 9–48. *In* R. McMillan (ed.), Methods in hematology: immune cytopenias. Churchill Livingstone, New York.
5. **Petz, L. D., and H. H. Fudenberg.** 1966. Coombs-positive hemolytic anemias caused by penicillin administration. N. Engl. J. Med. **274**:171–178.
6. **Petz, L. D., and G. Garratty.** 1980. Acquired immune hemolytic anemias. Churchill Livingstone, New York.
7. **Schmitz, N., I. Djibey, V. Kretschmer, I. Mahn, and C. Mueller-Eckhardt.** 1981. Assessment of red cell autoantibodies in autoimmune hemolytic anemia of warm type by a radioactive anti-IgG test. Vox Sang. **41**:224–230.
8. **Worlledge, S. M.** 1973. Immune drug-induced hemolytic anemias. Semin. Hematol. **10**:327–344.
9. **Yam, P., L. D. Petz, and P. Spath.** 1982. Detection of IgG sensitization of red cells with ^{125}I-staphylococcal protein A. Am. J. Hematol. **12**:337–346.

Chapter 96

Neutrophil and Platelet Antibodies in Immune Neutropenia and Thrombocytopenia

PARVIZ LALEZARI

Antibodies specific for blood neutrophils can be readily demonstrated in sera of mothers who have children afflicted with alloimmune neonatal neutropenia (10, 11), a disorder analogous to erythroblastosis fetalis. Similar antibodies have been found in sera of patients who develop autoimmune neutropenia (13, 25). Multitransfused patients also develop neutrophil antibodies which often have multiple specificities and are produced in combination with anti-HLA antibodies. We have classified the neutrophil antigens into those which are shared with other tissue cells (i.e., I, i, HLA, and 5) and those which have been detected only on the cells derived from the myeloid lineage (12). The latter group includes antigens such as NA (NA1, NA2), NB (NB1, NB2), Vaz (NC), ND (25), and NE (4) which appear to be expressed only on mature polymorphonuclear neutrophils. Neutrophil antibodies primarily reacting in the cold also have been described (14) and have been implicated in the pathogenesis of autoimmune neutropenia (10, 14). Platelet antibodies have been demonstrated in neonatal thrombocytopenia due to fetal-maternal incompatibility, in association with posttransfusion purpura syndrome and in autoimmune thrombocytopenic purpura. Platelet antigens, like neutrophil antigens, can be divided into those shared with cells of other tissues and those which are detected only on platelets. The latter group includes Zw (Zw^a, Zw^b), Ko (Ko^a, Ko^b), Duzo (21, 23), and Bak^a (27). Pl^{A1} and Pl^{A2} antigens, described by Shulman et al. (21), are identical to Zw^a and Zw^b. Shulman described another platelet system designated Pl^E (Pl^{E1}, P1^{E2}). Suggestive evidence exists that in some cases of autoimmune thrombocytopenic purpura, as in autoimmune neutropenia, the antibodies may be directed against platelet-specific antigens (7). Van Leeuwen et al. (24) have demonstrated that 80% of platelet autoantibodies fail to react with thrombocytes of patients who have Glanzmann's disease, a finding suggestive of specificity for epitopes on GpII^b or GpIII^a, the platelet membrane glycoproteins that are missing in this disorder. A wide variety of techniques have been described for the detection of neutrophil and platelet antibodies. The agglutination and immunofluorescence (IF) tests for neutrophils and the IF test for platelets are described in detail in this chapter, but only references are provided for other procedures.

For the study of neutrophil antibodies, a combination of the agglutination and IF tests should be used because some antibodies are selectively detected with only one of the two methods. For platelet antibodies, the indirect IF test is most useful for the detection of transfusion-induced alloantibodies and the antibodies involved in neonatal thrombocytopenia. In autoimmune thrombocytopenia, however, the IF test often produces weak reactions, so other procedures for measuring platelet-associated immunoglobulins should be used as well. Erythrocyte antibodies, mainly demonstrated by the use of automated techniques (9), were found to coexist with platelet and neutrophil antibodies in an appreciable number of patients studied in this laboratory. Indeed, the autoimmune nature of the leukopenia or thrombocytopenia, or both, has been frequently established by demonstrating coexisting erythrocyte antibodies even in the absence of manifest anemia.

AGGLUTINATION ASSAY FOR DETECTION OF NEUTROPHIL ANTIBODIES

Principle

Understanding the mechanism of antibody-mediated leukoagglutination and the causes of nonspecific leukocyte aggregation is a prerequisite for the proper performance of this test. Neutrophil agglutination by warm-reactive antibodies depends upon cell viability, mobility, and ability to form pseudopods. In cold agglutination, by contrast, the leukocytes appear to aggregate passively. Neutrophils lack ABH antigens (12) and, unlike erythrocytes, cannot be agglutinated by the ABH antibodies. However, when hemolytic erythrocyte antibodies and complement are added to a mixture of erythrocytes and neutrophils, mixed agglutination occurs which may be mistaken for true leukoagglutination (10). Another potential cause of artifact is the tendency of the isolated neutrophils to aggregate spontaneously. EDTA in critical concentrations prevents both of these nonspecific reactions without affecting test sensitivity.

Reagents

22% Bovine serum albumin (BSA) (Ortho Diagnostics, Inc., Raritan, N.J.)

Dextran-T500 (Pharmacia Fine Chemicals, Inc., Piscataway, N.J.)

Lymphocyte separation medium, density 1.077 (Bionetics Laboratory Products, Litton Bionetics, Kensington, Md.)

Citrate-phosphate-glucose anticoagulant solution

Citric acid (hydrous) . . . . 3.27 g
Trisodium citrate (hydrous) . . . . 25.40 g
Sodium biphosphate . . . . 2.22 g
Glucose (hydrous) . . . . 25.56 g
Distilled water to . . . . 1,000 ml
Solution A
  10% EDTA . . . . 0.5 ml
  Phosphate-buffered saline
  (PBS), pH 7.2 . . . . 99.5 ml

Solution B
    22% BSA . . . . 1.50 ml
    10% EDTA . . . . 0.44 ml
    PBS, pH 7.2 . . . . 9.06 ml
Solution C
    22% BSA . . . . 0.25 ml
    10% EDTA . . . . 0.50 ml
    PBS, pH 7.2 . . . . 10.00 ml
Ammonium chloride solution
    NH_4Cl . . . . 0.83 g
    $KHCO_3$ . . . . 0.10 g
    10% EDTA . . . . 0.05 ml
    Distilled water to 100   ml

The last three solutions must be prepared biweekly and kept at 4°C.

Neutrophil-specific typing reagents (anti-NA1, -NA2, -NB1, -NB2, and -Vaz) are available from the National Institute of Allergy and Infectious Diseases serum bank.

Method for isolation of neutrophils

1. Freshly drawn blood samples are anticoagulated by adding 0.15 ml of 10% EDTA/10 ml of blood. If blood samples are to be stored or mailed, 10-ml portions may be collected in tubes containing 1.3 ml of citrate-phosphate-glucose solution and 0.15 ml of 10% EDTA. Glucose, present in citrate-phosphate-glucose solution, enables leukocytes to remain viable for about 24 h at room temperature (22 to 24°C), and EDTA prevents spontaneous cell aggregation and disintegration. Blood samples should not be refrigerated.

2. Centrifuge the blood samples at 1,300 × g for 5 min. Remove the cell-free supernatants and save for use in the test as the source of antibody or as control. Replace the plasma with solution A.

3. Add 0.2 ml of 6% dextran in PBS (pH 7.2) per ml of original volume, and mix well. (Wipe adherent erythrocytes from the top of the tubes with a cotton applicator.)

4. Allow the erythrocytes to sediment at room temperature for 15 min.

5. Transfer the leukocyte-rich supernatant to a glass tube, and add 0.03 ml of 10% EDTA/ml.

6. Place 0.15 ml of lymphocyte separation medium in each of several Fisher centrifuge tubes (model 59; Fisher Scientific Co., Pittsburgh, Pa.), and then gently layer 0.9 ml of the cell suspensions on top.

7. Centrifuge at 2,500 × g for 2 min.

8. Discard the supernatant. Resuspend the pellets in ammonium chloride solution, and keep suspensions at room temperature for 3 min to lyse the contaminating erythrocytes.

9. Centrifuge the tubes and wash the pellets twice in solution A, performing all centrifugation at 2,500 × g for 15 s.

10. Wash the cells once in solution B. The cells must be kept in this solution if they are not used immediately.

11. Before the cells are plated, centrifuge the tubes, resuspend the pellet in solution C, and adjust the cell count to 4,000/µl.

Preparation of trays for neutrophil typing and antibody screening

The stored typing sera often contain debris and denatured proteins that must be removed by centrifugation. Serial twofold dilutions of these monospecific typing sera in solution C are prepared and dispensed in 5-µl volumes into Terasaki trays under oil with 1 µl of NaN_3 added as a preservative. The same procedure is used for antibody screening and for normal control sera obtained from nontransfused males. The trays can be kept at 4°C for 2 months or at −80°C indefinitely.

Agglutination test

Dilutions of the leukocyte donor's own plasma are first prepared and dispensed into Terasaki trays as an additional control. Then 1 µl of the cell suspension is added to each well. The trays are incubated at 30°C, and the results are read after 5 h and again after 18 h using an inverted phase microscope. The strength of the reaction is arbitrarily graded from 1+ to 4+ according to the percentage of cells agglutinated and the size of the aggregates.

Interpretation

The results read after 4 to 5 h are particularly important because on many occasions cell lysis occurs after prolonged incubation in wells containing undiluted sera. The second reading allows endpoints for antibody titers to be determined. "Prozone" is not infrequent, particularly when anti-NB1 reagent is used. Thus, serum must always be tested at various dilutions. It has already been indicated that ABO incompatibility does not interfere with this test.

DETECTION OF COLD-REACTIVE LEUKOAGGLUTININS

Normal neutrophil suspensions, washed free of plasma, are prepared and mixed with antisera dispensed into Terasaki trays as described above. The trays are kept at 4°C for 2 h and then examined by phase-contrast microscopy. More than 25% of normal individuals have "naturally occurring" cold-reactive leukoagglutinins, with titers not exceeding 8. Pathologic cold-reactive leukoagglutinins usually produce massive aggregates with titers greater than 16. Aggregates produced by cold-reactive agglutinins have a tendency to dissociate upon warming. The results of the test must therefore be evaluated rapidly.

IF TEST FOR DETECTION OF NEUTROPHIL ANTIBODIES

Principle

This test is used for the detection of both circulating and cell-bound antibodies, the latter indicating in vivo cell sensitization. Verheugt et al. (25) demonstrated that the treatment of neutrophils with paraformaldehyde facilitates removal of nonspecific immunoglobulins which exist in large quantities on normal neutrophil membranes. This treatment, however, leaves intact the membrane antigens and the specific antibodies coating these antigens. Membrane-bound antibodies can thus be detected by the use of fluorescein-labeled anti-human immunoglobulins (25).

Reagents

In addition to the reagents used for the isolation of neutrophils (see above) and PBS-BSA (0.22% BSA in PBS, pH 7.2), the following two reagents are needed.

(i) A 4% stock solution of purified paraformaldehyde (Fisher) is prepared by dissolving 4 g of paraformaldehyde in 90 ml of 0.85% NaCl. Solubilization is facilitated by warming at 70°C and the dropwise addition of 1 M NaOH. The pH is readjusted to 7.2 by dropwise addition of 1 M HCl. A 1% working solution is prepared by diluting the stock solution with 3 volumes of PBS (pH 7.2). The working solution must be prepared every week, and both solutions must be stored in the dark at 4°C.

(ii) Fluorescein isothiocyanate (FITC)-labeled anti-human immunoglobulin G (IgG) and anti-human IgM are prepared as follows. The key to success in the test is the availability of suitable FITC-labeled reagents. Antiglobulin reagents prepared in the goat are preferred to those prepared in the rabbit. Commercially available reagents may be conveniently used once their suitability and the optimal dilutions have been determined experimentally. Some investigators have recommended the use of FITC-labeled F(ab')$_2$ antiglobulin reagents to avoid a nonspecific fluorescence caused by a possible reaction between the antiglobulin molecules and the Fc fragment receptors on neutrophils. We found this step unnecessary for the procedure described here.

Method for isolation and paraformaldehyde treatment of neutrophils

1. Isolate neutrophils as described for the agglutination test, following steps 1 through 9.
2. Concentrate the neutrophils in Fisher tubes, and fill the tubes with 1% paraformaldehyde. Keep them at room temperature for 5 min.
3. Centrifuge the tubes, and wash the cells twice with PBS-BSA. The cells are then resuspended in PBS, and the concentration is adjusted to 10,000/μl. The paraformaldehyde-treated neutrophils lose their tendency to aggregate and so can be suspended in PBS without EDTA.

Direct IF test on neutrophils

1. Dilute FITC-antiglobulin reagents to optimal dilution. In our laboratory, the commercially available goat anti-human IgG and reagents (lot numbers 77724 and 88337; Meloy Laboratories, Inc., Springfield, Va.), diluted from 1:30 to 1:60 in PBS, have given optimal results.
2. Place 50-μl samples of the patient's cells in Fisher tubes.

3. Add 100 μl of diluted FITC-labeled anti-IgG and anti-IgM antibodies to separate tubes containing the patient's cells. A negative control, consisting of neutrophils obtained from a normal donor, must be tested in parallel. The tubes are then incubated in the dark at room temperature for 30 min.
4. Wash the cells twice with PBS.
5. Resuspend the cells in 0.1 ml of PBS, and keep cells at 4°C in the dark until examined.
6. The cells may be treated with paraformaldehyde again if the results are not to be read immediately. Such cells can be preserved for 4 days at 4°C in the dark.

Indirect IF test for neutrophil antibodies

1. Isolate neutrophils from the blood of normal donors, treat with paraformaldehyde, and wash as described above.
2. The test sera are used undiluted, the optimal dilutions for the typing sera being determined experimentally.
3. Dispense 50-μl portions of the cell suspensions in the required number of Fisher tubes.
4. Add 50 μl of the test sera (or typing reagents) to each tube, and incubate at 37°C for 30 min with gentle, continuous mixing.
5. Wash the cells four times with PBS-BSA.
6. Follow instructions as for the direct IF test described above. The indirect IF test for the detection of cold-reactive anti-neutrophil antibodies is performed as described for the warm-reactive antibodies except that incubation with the test sera should be at 4°C and the cells should be washed with precooled PBS-BSA at 4°C. FITC-anti-IgM and -anti-IgG should then be incubated with the sensitized cells for 30 min at 4°C and for 30 min at room temperature, not exceeding 18°C.

Interpretation of the results

The treated leukocytes are examined by using a phase-contrast fluorescence microscope, a mercury lamp, and filters suitable for FITC testing (25). Positive reactions are recognized by the appearance of sharp fluorescent rings around neutrophils, which indicate membrane localization of the antigens. In negative tests, a faint and homogeneous fluorescence may appear but membrane distinction cannot be made. The positive reactions may be graded 1+ to 4+ according to the intensity of the membrane-associated fluorescence. ABO incompatibility does not interfere with the test. The results can be more precisely quantitated by flow cytometry (25), in which a minimum of 10^5 sensitized cells are required for each test. The flow cytometer measures and analyzes the fluorescence of individual cells and gives the results in graphs in which the x axis represents the scale (channel) of fluorescence intensity and the y axis represents the number of cells in each channel. The final results are thus presented as fluorescence distribution curves. The shape of these curves and the channel in which the highest number of cells fluoresce (the peak) characterize the results.

IF TEST FOR DETECTION OF PLATELET-BOUND AND CIRCULATING PLATELET ANTIBODIES

Principle

As described for neutrophils, the immunoglobulins normally present on platelet membrane can be removed by paraformaldehyde treatment without affecting antigen-antibody reactions. This property of paraformaldehyde has made the difficult task of platelet antibody detection by an antiglobulin reaction possible (28). Paraformaldehyde-treated platelets also lose their normal reactivity to thrombin. Consequently, for detection of antibodies, platelets treated with paraformaldehyde may be incubated with serum. In the test described here, modifications have been introduced to prevent nonspecific platelet clumping which can be a major cause of false reactions.

Reagents

FITC-labeled antiglobulins (as described above for neutrophils).
PBS-BSA-EDTA (pH 6.8):

0.1 M Na$_2$HPO$_4$	7	ml
0.1 M KH$_2$PO$_4$	1	ml
10% Disodium EDTA	1	ml
22% BSA	1.5	ml
0.85% NaCl	89.5	ml

Paraformaldehyde solution (as described above for neutrophils except that the pH must be 6.8 to 7.0).

Method for isolation and paraformaldehyde treatment of platelets

1. Blood is anticoagulated using 0.15 ml of 10% EDTA/10 ml of whole blood.
2. The tubes are centrifuged at 500 × g for 10 min. The centrifuge is decelerated slowly (with the aid of an auxiliary rheostat) to minimize leukocyte and erythrocyte contamination.
3. Samples (1.5 ml) of platelet-rich plasma are dispensed into glass tubes (12 by 75 mm), diluted with an equal volume of PBS-BSA-EDTA, and then centrifuged at 1,300 × g for 4 min at room temperature.
4. The supernatants are discarded, and the pellet in each tube is resuspended using a Vortex mixer, mixed with 1 ml of paraformaldehyde solution, and incubated for 5 min at room temperature.
5. PBS-BSA-EDTA (1 ml) is added and mixed with paraformaldehyde-treated platelets, and the tubes are centrifuged at 1,300 × g for 3 min.
6. The pellets are washed twice in 2 ml of PBS-BSA-EDTA, with centrifugation at 1,300 × g for 3 min.
7. The washed platelets are pooled and resuspended in PBS-BSA-EDTA, and the concentration is adjusted to 2 × 10^8/ml.

Direct IF test on platelets

1. Appropriate dilutions of FITC-labeled antiglobulin reagents are prepared using PBS (pH 7) as the diluent. The optimal dilution must be determined experimentally.
2. Portions (100 μl) of platelet suspensions are dispensed into separate glass tubes and incubated with 100 μl of the labeled antiglobulin reagents (anti-IgG and anti-IgM) for 30 min at room temperature. Controls consist of platelet suspensions prepared from normal donors.
3. The platelets are washed twice, each with 2 ml of PBS-BSA-EDTA (all washes must be carried out at 4°C, with centrifugation for 5 min at 1,000 × g).
4. The pellets are resuspended in 0.1 ml of PBS (pH 7) and kept in the dark at 4°C until examined.

Indirect IF test for platelet antibodies

1. Isolate platelets from normal donors, treat with paraformaldehyde, and wash as described above.
2. Dispense into the required number of tubes 100 μl each of platelet suspensions and test sera. Sera obtained from ABO-compatible, nontransfused normal male donors and from the platelet donors are used as controls.
3. Incubate the tubes at 37°C for 60 min, with periodic mixing.
4. Wash the cells four times with PBS-BSA-EDTA at 4°C, each time using 2 ml of wash solution and centrifugation for 5 min at 1,000 × g.
5. Follow instructions for the direct IF test.

The indirect IF test for the detection of cold-reactive platelet antibodies is performed as described above except that incubation with the test sera is done at 4°C and FITC-labeled anti-IgM is incubated with the sensitized cells for 30 min at 4°C and then for 30 min at a temperature not exceeding 18°C.

Interpretation of results

Platelet IF tests are evaluated by fluorescence microscopy and flow cytometry as described for neutrophils (28). Attention must be paid to nonspecific platelet aggregation which may occur during the test procedure if BSA is omitted from the wash solutions, if the centrifugation step in the cold is neglected, or if the centrifugal force is excessively high. The nonspecific aggregates entrap trace amounts of serum proteins which can react with FITC-labeled antiglobulins and produce nonspecific fluorescence. Such platelet aggregation could also render a true positive reaction negative if the entrapped serum proteins are released during incubation with the antiglobulin reagents.

OTHER TECHNIQUES

Most of the techniques used for detection of neutrophil antibodies have been reviewed elsewhere (17). The details of capillary agglutination are given in reference 23a, and other methods include quantitation of cell-bound immunoglobulins (15, 22), assay of opsonic activity against neutrophils (2), and tests based on the ability of antineutrophil antibodies to interfere with neutrophil functions (20). In addition, antibodies identified by cytotoxic assays have been implicated in autoimmune neutropenia (1, 5). Techniques (other than IF tests) used to detect platelet antibodies have been reviewed by Shulman et al. (21), scribed because they must be distinguished from immune inhibitors. Inhibitory activity was resistant to boiling, proteolytic digestion with pronase, and precipitation with trichloroacetic acid. One inhibitor was separated on a platelet factor 4-Sepharose 4B affinity column (23), and the other inhibitor was separated by DEAE ion exchange and a protamine affinity column (32). Both inhibitors had heparin-like anticoagulant properties and the biochemical characteristics of heparan sulfate. The release or altered metabolism of endogenous proteoglycans from the vasculature of these patients was postulated as the cause of the appearance of the anticoagulants.

Laboratory diagnosis

Procedure. The TCT and immediate mix tests are used to detect heparin-like inhibitors.

Interpretation. The heparin-like anticoagulants can be confused with some of the immune inhibitors or with dysfibrinogenemia and exogenous heparin. In all of these cases, the TCT is prolonged and will not be corrected by mixing with normal plasma. The APTT may be prolonged, though generally much less than the TCT. A simple test to exclude these inhibitors is the Reptilase test. The Reptilase clotting time is normal in the presence of heparin-like or heparin inhibitors, but will be abnormal in the presence of inhibitors of fibrinogen or in the presence of dysfibrinogenemia. Immune inhibition of fibrinogen can be distinguished from dysfibrinogenemia by procedures described above in the fibrinogen section. Isolation and biochemical characterization of the anticoagulants can be performed by published methods (23, 32).

CONCLUSION

The human antibodies to coagulation factors are an important clinical problem, even though these antibodies occur infrequently. Patients who develop inhibitors to clotting factors may be very difficult to treat. Patients with factor VIII or factor IX alloantibodies offer a particular challenge to the physician because of the frequency of occurrence of the alloantibodies.

Antibodies to coagulation factors, nonetheless, are useful clinical and research tools. Their limited specificity allows structural mapping of the antigen as well as detection of clotting factors in assays not dependent upon clotting activity. The recent factor VIII coagulant radioimmunoassays attest to the usefulness of factor VIII:C antibodies for very sensitive immunologic measurements. In general, immunologic methods have allowed significant contributions to our knowledge of the clotting mechanism, the nature of some coagulation defects, and the characteristics of the immune response to these proteins.

We express our heartfelt appreciation for the excellent assistance of Dianne Partin in the preparation of the manuscript. We also appreciate the assistance of our coagulation laboratory personnel in reviewing the text and providing test examples.

This work was supported in part by Public Health Service grant HLO7149 from the National Institutes of Health.

LITERATURE CITED

1. **Aalberse, R. C., R. van der Gaag, and J. van Leeuwen.** 1983. Serologic aspects of IgG$_4$ antibodies. I. Prolonged immunization results in an IgG$_4$-restricted response. J. Immunol. **130**:722–726.
2. **Bajaj, S. P., S. I. Rapaport, D. S. Fierer, K. D. Herbst, and D. B. Schwartz.** 1983. A mechanism for the hypoprothrombinemia of the acquired hypoprothrombinemia lupus anticoagulant syndrome. Blood **61**:684–692.
3. **Bidwell, E., K. W. E. Denson, G. W. R. Dike, R. Augustin, and G. M. Lloyd.** 1966. Antibody nature of the inhibition to antihaemophilic globulin (factor VIII). Nature (London) **210**:746–747.
4. **Biggs, R., D. E. G. Austen, K. W. E. Denson, C. R. Rizza, and R. Borrett.** 1972. The mode of action of antibodies which destroy factor VIII. I. Antibodies which give second-order concentration graphs. Br. J. Haematol. **23**:125–135.
5. **Briët, E., H. M. Reisner, and H. R. Roberts.** 1984. Inhibitors in Christmas disease, p. 123–139. In L. W. Hoyer (ed.), Factor VIII inhibitors. Alan R. Liss, Inc., New York.
6. **Castro, O., I. R. Farber, and L. P. Clyne.** 1972. Circulating anticoagulants against factors IX and XI in systemic lupus erythematosus. Ann. Intern. Med. **77**:543–548.
7. **Coleman, M., E. M. Vigliano, M. E. Weksler, and R. L. Nachman.** 1972. Inhibition of fibrin monomer polymerization by lambda myeloma globulins. Blood **39**:210–223.
8. **Dahlback, B., I. M. Nilson, and B. Frohm.** 1983. Inhibition of platelet prothrombinase activity by a lupus anticoagulant. Blood **62**:218–225.
9. **Ewing, N. P., and C. K. Kasper.** 1982. In vitro detection of mild inhibitors to factor VIII in hemophilia. Am. J. Clin. Pathol. **77**:749–752.
10. **Feinstein, D. I.** 1982. Acquired inhibitors against factor VIII and other clotting proteins, p. 563–576. In R. W. Colman, J. Hirsh, V. J. Marder, and E. W. Salzman (ed.), Hemostasis and thrombosis: basic principles and clinical practice. J. B. Lippincott Co., Philadelphia.
11. **Feinstein, D. I., S. I. Rapaport, and M. N. Y. Chong.** 1969. Immunologic characterization of 12 factor VIII inhibitors. Blood **34**:85–90.
12. **Fiore, P. A., L. D. Ellis, H. L. Dameshek, and J. H. Lewis.** 1971. Factor XIII inhibitor and antituberculosis therapy. Clin. Res. **19**:418.
13. **Furie, B.** 1982. Acquired coagulation disorders and dysproteinemias, p. 577–581. In R. W. Colman, J. Hirsh, V. J. Marder, and E. W. Salzman (ed.), Hemostasis and thrombosis: basic principles and clinical practice. J. B. Lippincott Co., Philadelphia.
14. **Furie, B., L. Voo, K. McAdam, and B. C. Furie.** 1981. Mechanism of factor X deficiency in systemic amyloidosis. N. Engl. J. Med. **304**:827–830.
15. **Gandolfo, G. M., A. Afeltra, A. Amoroso, F. Biancolella, and G. M. Ferri.** 1977. Circulating anticoagulant against factor XII and platelet antibodies in systemic lupus erythematosus. Acta Haematol. **57**:135–142.
16. **Gawryl, M. S., and L. W. Hoyer.** 1982. Inactivation of factor VIII coagulant activity by two different types of human antibodies. Blood **60**:1103–1109.
17. **Gill, F. M.** 1984. The natural history of factor VIII inhibitors in patients with hemophilia A, p. 19–29. In L. W. Hoyer (ed.), Factor VIII inhibitors. Alan R. Liss, Inc., New York.
18. **Graham, J. E., W. J. Yount, and H. R. Roberts.** 1973. Immunochemical characterization of a human antibody to factor XIII. Blood **41**:661–669.
19. **Hoyer, L. W., and R. T. Breckenridge.** 1968. Immunologic studies of antihemophilic factor (AHF, factor VIII): cross-reacting material in a genetic variant of hemophilia A. Blood **32**:962–971.
20. **Hoyer, L. W., M. S. Gawryl, and B. de la Fuente.** 1984.

Immunochemical characterization of factor VIII inhibitors, p. 73–85. *In* L. W. Hoyer (ed.), Factor VIII inhibitors. Alan R. Liss, Inc., New York.

21. **Iizuka, A., and T. Nagao.** 1983. Analysis of IgG heavy chain subclasses of alloantibodies to factor IX by crossed immunoelectrophoresis of factor IX using the intermediate gel technique. Br. J. Haematol. **53:**687–688.

22. **Kane, W. H., M. J. Lindhout, C. M. Jackson, and P. Majerus.** 1980. Factor V-dependent binding of factor X_a to human platelets. J. Biol. Chem. **225:**1170–1174.

23. **Khoory, M. S., M. E. Nesheim, E. J. W. Bowie, and K. G. Mann.** 1980. Circulating heparan sulfate proteoglycan anticoagulant from a patient with a plasma cell disorder. J. Clin. Invest. **65:**666–674.

24. **Lewis, R. M., H. M. Reisner, R. L. Lundblad, K. S. Chung, and H. R. Roberts.** 1979. Binding of allo- and heteroantibodies to human factor IX (F.IX). Thromb. Haemostasis **42:**364.

25. **Lorand, L., N. Maldonado, J. Fredera, A. C. Atencio, B. Robertson, and T. Urayana.** 1972. Haemorrhagic syndrome of autoimmune origin with a specific inhibitor against fibrin stabilizing factor (factor XIII). Br. J. Haematol. **23:**17–27.

26. **Lossing, T. S., C. K. Kasper, and D. I. Feinstein.** 1977. Detection of factor VIII inhibitors with the partial thromboplastin time. Blood **40:**793–797.

27. **Mannucci, P. M., and D. Mari.** 1984. Antibodies to factor VIII-von Willebrand factor in congenital and acquired von Willebrand's disease, p. 109–122. *In* L. W. Hoyer (ed.), Factor VIII inhibitors. Alan R. Liss, Inc., New York.

28. **Marchesi, D., A. Parbtani, G. Frampton, M. Livio, G. Remuzzi, and J. S. Cameron.** 1981. Thrombotic tendency in systemic lupus erythematosus. Lancet **i:**719.

29. **Marciniak, E., and M. F. Greenwood.** 1979. Acquired coagulation inhibitor delaying fibrinopeptide release. Blood **53:**81–92.

30. **Menache, D.** 1973. Abnormal fibrinogens: a review. Thromb. Diath. Haemorrh. **29:**525–535.

31. **Owen, W. G., and R. H. Wagner.** 1972. Antihemophilic factor: separation of an active fragment following dissociation by salts or detergents. Thromb. Diath. Haemorrh. **27:**502–515.

32. **Palmer, R. N., M. E. Rick, P. D. Rick, J. A. Feller, and H. R. Gralnick.** 1984. Circulating heparan sulfate anticoagulant in a patient with a fatal bleeding disorder. N. Engl. J. Med. **310:**1696–1699.

33. **Parekh, V. R., P. M. Mannucci, and Z. M. Ruggeri.** 1978. Immunological heterogeneity of haemophilia B: a multicentre study of 98 kindreds. Br. J. Haematol. **40:**643–655.

34. **Peake, I. R., A. L. Bloom, J. C. Giddings, and C. A. Ludlam.** 1979. An immunoradiometric assay for procoagulant factor VIII antigen. Results in haemophilia, von Willebrand's disease, and fetal plasma and serum. Br. J. Haematol. **42:**269–281.

35. **Poon, M.-C., H. Saito, and W. J. Koopman.** 1984. A unique precipitating autoantibody against plasma thromboplastin antecedent associated with multiple apparent plasma clotting factor deficiencies in a patient with systemic lupus erythematosus. Blood **63:**1309–1317.

36. **Robinson, A. J., P. M. Aggeler, G. P. McNicol, and A. S. Douglas.** 1967. An atypical genetic haemorrhagic disease with increased concentration of a natural inhibitor of prothrombin consumption. Br. J. Haematol. **13:**510–527.

37. **Rosenberg, R. D., R. W. Colman, and L. Lorand.** 1974. A new hemorrhagic disorder with defective fibrin stabilization and cryofibrinogenemia. Br. J. Haematol. **26:**269–284.

38. **Ruggeri, Z. M., N. Ciavarella, P. M. Mannucci, A. Molinair, F. Dammacco, J. M. Lavergue, and D. Meyer.** 1979. Familial incidence of precipitating antibodies in von Willebrand's disease: a study of four cases. J. Lab. Clin. Med. **94:**60–75.

39. **Sarji, K. E., R. D. Stratton, R. H. Wagner, and K. M. Brinkhous.** 1974. Nature of von Willebrand factor: a new assay and a specific inhibitor. Proc. Natl. Acad. Sci. U.S.A. **71:**2937–2941.

40. **Schiffman, S., R. Marglit, M. Rosoue, and D. Feinstein.** 1981. Pseudo-factor-XI deficiency: effect of an inhibitor of factor XI adsorption to surface. Blood **57:**437–443.

41. **Schmaier, A. H., M. Schapira, and R. W. Colman.** 1983. Methods to study the proteins of the contact phase of coagulation, p. 24–47. *In* R. W. Colman (ed.), Disorders of thrombin formation. Churchill Livingstone, New York.

42. **Shapiro, S. S., and M. Hultin.** 1975. Acquired inhibitors to the blood coagulation factors. Semin. Thromb. Hemostasis **1:**336–385.

43. **Stern, M. D., H. L. Nossel, and J. Owen.** 1982. Acquired antibody to factor XI in a patient with congenital factor XI deficiency. J. Clin. Invest. **69:**1270–1276.

44. **Stratton, R. D., R. H. Wagner, W. P. Webster, and K. M. Brinkhous.** 1975. Antibody nature of circulating inhibitor of plasma von Willebrand factor. Proc. Natl. Acad. Sci. U.S.A. **72:**4167–4171.

45. **Suomela, H., M. Blomback, and B. Blomback.** 1977. The activation of factor X evaluated by using synthetic substrates. Thromb. Res. **10:**267–281.

46. **Thiagarajan, P., and S. S. Shapiro.** 1983. Lupus anticoagulants, p. 101–108. *In* R. W. Colman (ed.), Disorders of thrombin formation. Churchill Livingstone, New York.

47. **Thiagarajan, P., S. S. Shapiro, and L. DeMarco.** 1980. Monoclonal immunoglobulin M coagulation inhibitor with phospholipid specificity. J. Clin. Invest. **66:**397–405.

48. **Triplett, D. A., J. T. Brandt, D. Kaczor, and J. Schaeffer.** 1983. Laboratory diagnosis of lupus inhibitors: a comparison of the tissue thromboplastin inhibition procedure with a new platelet neutralization procedure. Am. J. Clin. Pathol. **79:**678–682.

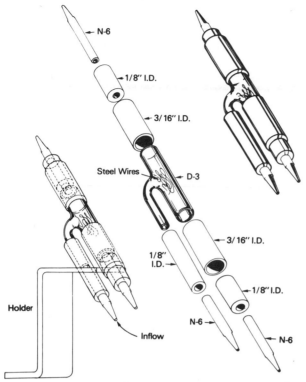

FIG. 2. Extractor used to separate organic-aqueous phases. The ends of the N-6 should be directly in contact with the glass of the D-3 connector.

1 N NaOH, and sample uptake. All of the manifold pump tubes are changed after 160 h of operation. These tube replacements are important when analyzing samples at high-sensitivity settings.

Operational suggestions. The fluorometer requires about 45 min for warm-up; it is suggested that the system be tested with histamine standards (10 ng/ml) before any experimental samples are analyzed. The aperture setting on the fluorometer is usually at 5 with the damping set at 2. If the sensitivity of the system is not adequate, the 5-57 secondary filter can be removed. Similarly, if the fluorometer cannot be "blanked" at aperture setting 5, an extra secondary

TABLE 1. Changes in automated system for analyzing samples with and without dialysis

Analysis	Sample pump tube flow rate (ml/min)	Sample vol required (ml)[a]	Histamine concn for full-scale deflection (ng/ml)[b]
Without dialysis[c]	0.16	0.3	15
	0.23	0.4	6
With dialysis	0.16	0.3	30
	0.23	0.6	20
	0.32	0.6	15

[a] Total volume in the sample cup; actual volume analyzed is about 25% less.

[b] The readability of the graph is 0.5 to 1% of the full-scale value; therefore, the amount of histamine that can be quantitated is 25 to 100 pg.

[c] Protein less than 3 mg/ml.

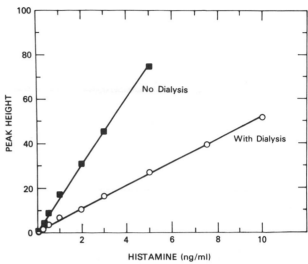

FIG. 3. Histamine standard curves. Histamine-containing samples were analyzed by the automated system with (○) or without (■) dialysis. Sample uptake pump tube is 0.23 ml/min; total volume of sample analyzed is ~0.35 ml.

filter should be used to decrease the light (e.g., neutral density filter). Samples on the machine are analyzed at the rate of 30/h; after every 25 to 50 samples a histamine-containing standard and a tube containing saline should be run to check for machine drift and also to serve as a marker on the recorder chart. It is advisable to run a sample containing only saline after analyzing samples with high histamine concentrations (e.g., completes or standards) to allow the machine to return to base line.

If after several months of use there is a decrease in the sensitivity of the system, it is usually due to a decrease in the output of the UV excitation lamp in the fluorometer and the lamp should be replaced. If used daily the system does not ordinarily require rinsing after use if the tubes are left clamped. However, for prolonged storage the system should be rinsed with 0.1 N HCl followed by distilled water.

Manual histamine assay

Usually 48 samples are extracted at one time; this requires about 3 to 4 h. See references 3 and 4. The supernatant fluids after centrifugation of the histamine release reaction are poured into a plastic tube (12 by 75 mm); a 1.0-ml sample of the supernatant fluid is then transferred into a 15-ml screw-cap glass culture tube (13 by 100 mm with Teflon-lined caps) containing 300 mg of NaCl (a heaping of no. 1 Coor spatula; Thomas Scientific, Swedesboro, N.J.) and 1.25 ml of n-butanol (added with an automatic pipette). After all of the 1.0-ml samples are added to the butanol-NaCl tubes, 0.10 ml of 3 N NaOH is added quickly and accurately with an automatic pipette. After the NaOH is added to three to five tubes, the tubes are capped and shaken for a few seconds. After all of the samples are transferred, the rack is shaken for 1 min. The tubes are centrifuged at 600 × g at 4°C for 5 min. A 1.0-ml sample of the butanol (top) layer is removed with a pipette filler and transferred to a screw-cap glass tube (12 by 100 mm, 15 ml) containing 0.6 ml of 0.12 N HCl and 1.9 ml of n-heptane (add both with automatic pipettes). The tubes are capped and shaken for 1 min by rapid inversion by hand. They are allowed to stand upright for 5 min for the clear separation of the two phases. Then 0.5 ml of the 0.12 N HCl (bottom layer) is transferred into a glass cuvette (10 by 75 mm), making sure that none of the top organic solvent layer is present and wiping the outside of the pipette. The rack of tubes is transferred to an ice bath; extra tubes are added which receive either 0.12 N HCl or histamine standards of 25 to 100 ng/ml. To each tube, 0.1 ml of 1 N NaOH is added with an automatic pipette, the contents of the tube are mixed by vortexing, and immediately 0.025 ml of 0.2% o-phthalaldehyde solution is added and the contents are mixed again. The reaction is allowed to proceed for 40 min in an ice bath, 0.05 ml of 2 M H_3PO_4 is added to each tube, and the tubes are mixed and allowed to equilibrate to room temperature (about 15 min). The samples are then read in either a spectrofluorometer or a simple fluorometer with an activation wavelength of 350 nm and a fluorescent wavelength of ~450 nm.

A 4-min histamine standard is run before analyzing the experimental samples to check the activity of the fluorophore reagents: 0.5 ml of histamine (100 ng/ml) in 0.12 N HCl is reacted with NaOH and o-phthalaldehyde at room temperature for 4 min. The sample is read immediately after the addition of the 2 M H_3PO_4. The fluorometer readings should be 60 to 80% of the levels of the 40-min 4°C reaction system.

Histamine is stable at an acid pH; therefore, during the extraction, tubes can be left for several hours after the transfer of the butanol samples into heptane-HCl tubes. The extraction procedure requires modification if the samples contain appreciable amounts of protein (e.g., 10% serum); the protein should be removed by perchloric acid precipitation before proceeding with the extraction steps (e.g., 0.2 ml of 8% $HClO_4$ is added to 1.0 ml of the supernatant fluid). The tubes are mixed, incubated at 37°C for 30 min, and then centrifuged (4°C, 15 min, 500 × g). The supernatant fluids are poured off, and portions are transferred into the next step. With acid-precipitated samples, care should be taken that excess NaOH is added at the first extraction step to alkalinize the aqueous phase so that histamine will be extracted into the butanol.

Calculations

The experimental results are expressed as the percentage of histamine release relative to the total cellular histamine content: histamine release (%) = $[(E - B)/(C - B)] \times 100$, where E is the fluorometric reading of the experimental sample, B is the fluorometric reading of samples with cells and buffer (and serum), and C is the fluorometric reading of completes (cells with $HClO_4$).

Cell sensitivity (HR_{50}) is the antigen concentration, expressed in micrograms, required to release 50% of the cellular histamine. This concentration can be determined by plotting the histamine release (as a percentage) versus the antigen concentration on semilogarithmic paper. The antigen concentration on the ascending part of the curve is read from this

graph. Similarly, if the histamine release is less than 50%, an HR_{30} can be determined.

Cell reactivity is the maximal amount of histamine release obtained with any amount of inducing agent (e.g., allergen or anti-IgE).

Reaginic antibody titer (PLS_{50}) is defined as the reciprocal of the dilution of allergic serum required for passive sensitization of normal leukocytes to release 50% of their histamine is response to the addition of antigen. A known standard reaginic serum is used to normalize the values.

The blocking-antibody concentration can be determined in several ways. When antigen dose-response curves are determined in 10% normal or allergic human serum, the results are usually expressed as the allergen-neutralizing capacity (ANC): ANC = $G_{50}AHS/G_{50}NHS$, where $G_{50}AHS$ is the antigen concentration for 50% histamine release in allergic human serum and $G_{50}NHS$ is the antigen concentration for 50% histamine release in normal human serum. Similarly, the $G_{30}NHS$ can be calculated utilizing the antigen concentration for 30% histamine release. In contrast, where different dilutions of the allergic serum are tested, the blocking-antibody titer is the reciprocal of the dilution at which the tested serum inhibits antigen-induced leukocyte histamine release by 50%.

REAGENTS

All solutions are made with distilled water and all chemicals are of reagent-grade purity unless otherwise specified.

Solutions for histamine release studies

A 10× concentrated stock PIPES buffered medium is prepared by dissolving 75.60 g of PIPES (Sigma Chemical Co.), 69.28 g of NaCl, 3.72 g of KCl, and 43 ml of 10 N NaOH in 1 liter. The pH of this stock should be 7.48. The pH of a 1:10 dilution should be 7.40 at 37°C. It is stored at 4°C. The human serum albumin is obtained as a 25% sterile solution (normal human serum albumin; American Red Cross, Blood Services, Washington, D.C.) and stored at 4°C.

A 0.1 M EDTA solution is prepared by dissolving 37.23 g of disodium EDTA in about 600 ml of water and slowly adding 50% NaOH (~5 ml) to bring the pH to between 7.18 and 7.20. The EDTA goes into solution at that pH; the volume is then adjusted to 1 liter. This solution is stored at 4°C. Perchloric acid solutions of 12, 6, and 2% are prepared by diluting a 60% solution of $HClO_4$.

The Ca^{2+} and Mg^{2+} solutions are prepared from the respective salts ($CaCl_2 \cdot 2H_2O$ and $MgCl_2 \cdot 6H_2O$). The stock solutions are 0.1 M each and are kept at 4°C.

The following solutions are prepared fresh daily: the dextrose-dextran solution, PIPES A, PIPES A-EDTA, and PIPES ACM. The dextrose-dextran solution is prepared by adding 600 mg of dextrose to 20 ml of sterile 6% clinical dextran (dextran-75 with NaCl, 0.9%; Abbott Laboratories, North Chicago, Ill.); 2.5 ml of this solution is added per 10 ml of blood. The PIPES A medium is prepared by diluting 10 ml of 10× stock PIPES to 100 ml and adding 0.125 ml of the 25% human serum albumin solution. The PIPES A-EDTA (4 mM EDTA) is prepared by diluting 10 ml of 10×

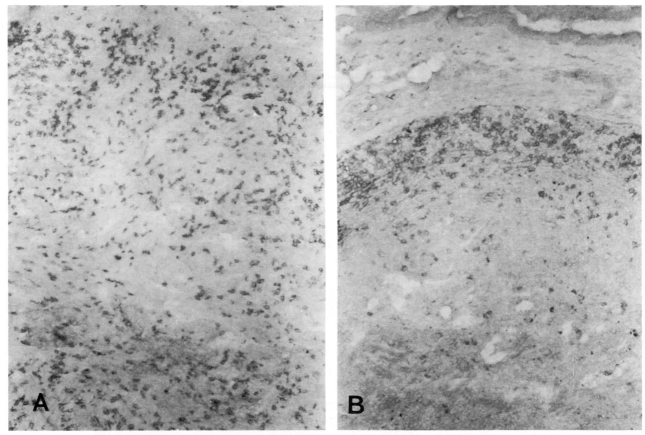

FIG. 4. Technique as for Fig. 3. Node from common variable immunodeficiency with predominant B-cell and some T-cell deficiency. (A) T cells are scattered without normal organization and are sparse in number. (B) B cells are few, not arranged in follicles, and scattered thinly at the periphery of the node.

not diagnostic of AIDS. The presence of risk factors, lymphopenia, elevated immunoglobulins, and characteristic infections in addition to the reversed ratio is necessary to make a justified diagnosis.

Any combination of surface marker abnormalities can be seen in immunodeficiency. An absolute decrease in the total number of all or some of the subsets requires further investigation. It is not uncommon for lymphocytes to show inappropriate surface phenotypes such as $T6^+$ (a cortical thymocyte marker not ordinarily found on peripheral cells), or be $T11^+$ but T4 or T8 negative.

Patients with significant T-cell deficiency can demonstrate normal responses to mitogenic and allogeneic cell stimulation and even have normal numbers of total T cells. Usually, responses to all of the above stimulatory agents are decreased and the diagnosis is clear; however, certain notable exceptions exist. In Wiskott-Aldrich syndrome and ataxia telangiectasia there may be variable loss of T-lymphocyte function depending upon the duration of the disease. To demonstrate abnormalities of some in vitro lymphocyte responses, multiple doses of stimulating agents may have to be employed. In some cases of CID and in Ommen's disease, normal responses to phytohemagglutinin and allogeneic cells have been observed. In my experience, however, the constant in vitro abnormality in all T-cell-deficient states is an

inability to respond to antigens. Unfortunately, thymic deficiency is not the only cause of nonreactivity to antigens, for failure to respond may be due to inadequate sensitization or to a macrophage defect. Also, any in vitro tests of T-lymphocyte function may be temporarily depressed if the patient is suffering from a virus infection or has had a recent rubeola vaccination. Therefore, repeated testing must be done for confirmation of any abnormal finding.

It can be seen that assessment of the thymic system can be a complicated procedure requiring great experience and sound clinical judgment.

ASSESSMENT OF B CELLS

The key presented at the start of this chapter shows the clinical manifestations of B-cell deficiency diseases. Assessment is in general more straightforward than for T cells. Determination of quantitative immunoglobulin levels by the single radial diffusion method is a reliable screening technique (see section A of this volume). Immunoelectrophoretic analysis and simple protein electrophoresis are unreliable for screening and should not be employed for that purpose. There is virtually no overlap of the maximal values of truly deficient patients having primary immunodeficiency with the minimal values of normal subjects. Patients with true B-cell immunodeficiency usually show def-

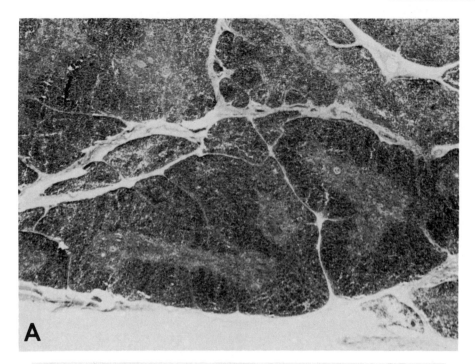

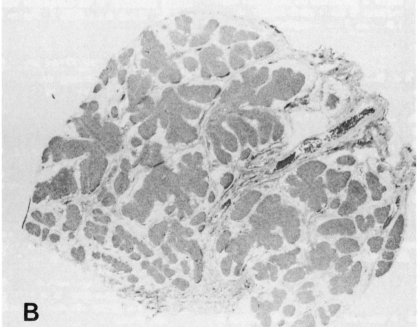

FIG. 5. (A) Normal thymus. Note the dense thymocyte composition, giving rise to well-demarcated corticomedullary differentiation. In the medulla, Hassall's corpuscles, remnants of epithelial-thymocyte interactions, are prominent (original magnification, ×25). (B) Dysplastic thymus of SCID. The lobules are very small, and no lymphocytes or Hassall's corpuscles are seen (original magnification, ×25).

icits of all major classes of immunoglobulins. Thus, a pattern of an abnormally low IgG (less than 2 standard deviations below mean for age) but normal IgA and IgM levels in a 4-month-old infant is still probably within normal limits. Such a deficiency can be termed transient hypogammaglobulinemia of infancy. These patients form normal amounts of IgG antibody, however, and do not require exogenous IgG

injections. When some but not all values are low, immunodeficiency should be suspected with the finding of immunoglobulin patterns or characteristics shown in Table 2.

Uncertainty is most clearly resolved by functional assessment. Antibodies to previously administered antigens (diphtheria, tetanus, polio) can be measured, often by state or local health agencies. Isohemag-

TABLE 1. Interpretation of proliferation assays

Stimulus	Significance of response
Mitogens	
Phytohemag-glutinin, concanav-alin A	Nonspecific stimulators of both helper and suppressor subsets. Indicates that some of the normal populations are present.
Pokeweed mitogen	Particularly helpful in stimulating T cells for B-cell help to yield immunoglobulin synthesis and secretion.
Staphylococcus cowan protein A	Stimulates B-cell secretion in presence of additional factors (T-helper, antigen, anti-mu, etc.).
Allogeneic lymphocytes	Proliferative stimulus to T-helper cells; results in generation of specific cytotoxic cells against the stimulating histocompatibility antigens. May be normal even in the face of severe T-cell deficiency.
Antigens	Requires genetically restricted antigen-presenting cell. Most stringent test of immunological competence; correlates better with state of health than other tests. The cytotoxic T cell which is generated by allogeneic cell stimulus is also a good marker of functional T-cell competence.

glutinins can be determined. Patients with normal immunoglobulin levels but deficient functional capability are being seen more and more.

When normal immunoglobulin levels are observed in the face of persistent severe bacterial infections (not recurrent colds), an IgG subgroup deficiency may be present. IgG subgroup deficiency may coexist with IgA deficiency. Quantitation of these variants is performed by Peter Schur, Clinical Immunology Laboratory, Brigham and Women's Hospital, 75 Francis St., Boston, MA 02115.

Enzyme-Linked Immunosorbent Assay for Isotype Determinations

Materials

Antigens
Escherichia coli: A mixture of desired serotypes is grown on nutrient agar and suspended to a concentration of approximately 1.2×10^9 organisms per ml. Boil the suspension for 2 h and centrifuge for 30 min at $5,000 \times g$. Store in aliquots at $-20°C$.
Tetanus toxoid and diphtheria toxoid from Massachusetts State Department of Health
PBS
PBS with 0.05% Tween-20 (PBS-T)
PBS–0.05% Tween–2% bovine serum albumin (PBS-TBSA)
Sodium bicarbonate buffer

Na_2CO_3 .... 1.59 g
$NaHCO_3$ .... 2.93 g
NaN_3 .... 0.20 g

Bring to approximately 1,000 ml with water. Adjust pH to 9.6. Bring to final volume of 1,000 ml.
Bovine serum albumin, 2% (wt/vol) in bicarbonate buffer
Diethanolamine buffer

Diethanolamine (Sigma) 48   ml
$MgCl_2$ .... 0.245 g

Add approximately 400 ml of water. Adjust pH to 9.8 with concentrated HCl. Make to final volume of 500 ml.
Dynatech Immulon micro-ELISA plates (Dynatech Laboratories, Alexandria, Va.)
Antisera: anti-human IgG, IgA, and IgM, alkaline phosphatase labeled (TAGO, Inc., or Sigma)

Coating plates

Dilute *E. coli* antigen 1:1,000 in PBS. Add 0.2 ml to wells of a 96-well Immulon plate. Erratic results are sometimes obtained if the outer row is used. If this occurs, use only the innermost 60 wells. Incubate overnight at 4°C. Wash with PBS-T. (A Water-Pik is convenient for this purpose.) Add 0.2 ml of 2% bovine serum albumin in bicarbonate buffer. Incubate for 2 h at 37°C. Wash with PBS-T. Plates can be stored for up

TABLE 2. Immunoglobulin patterns in deficiency states

Deficiency of all immunoglobulins
Usual type of hypogammaglobulinemia; occasionally normal IgE levels

Selective deficiencies
1. IgA[a]: Most common primary deficiency, occurs in 70% of ataxia telangiectasia, may be associated with mild or severe T-cell deficiency
2. IgM: Most common secondary deficiency
3. IgE: Deficiency of unknown significance, may occur in association with IgA deficiency, especially in ataxia telangiectasia
4. IgG: Never well documented as an isolated deficiency; IgG subgroup deficiencies are known
5. IgG and IgA[b]: associated with elevated IgM (dysgammaglobulinemia I), elevation in part artifactual and due to 7S IgM
6. IgA and IgM[b]: IgG normal or elevated in amounts and usually monoclonal (K or λ), single or multiple electrophoretic peaks common; associated T-cell defect usually present

Unique patterns
1. Markedly elevated IgA and diminished IgM common in Wiskott-Aldrich syndrome (nonresponsivity to carbohydrate antigens is the most characteristic functional abnormality)
2. In multiple myeloma or Waldenstrom's macroglobulinemia, noninvolved immunoglobulins are usually nondetectable[b]

[a] Serum IgA determinations usually screen for secretory IgA deficiency. Normal levels of secretory IgA with absent serum IgA have been observed but usually not the reverse.

[b] There is usually no formation of antibody in response to administered antigens despite normal or elevated levels of one or more classes of immunoglobulin in these diseases. In type 5, however, some agglutinin response has been observed.

to 6 months. For storage, add at least 0.2 ml of PBS-T to each well and store in a container with a tight lid or in plastic bags at 4°C.

Dilute toxoid antigens 1:1,000 in bicarbonate buffer. Fill wells as for *E. coli* antigen, and follow with 2% bovine serum albumin solution.

Assay

Do not allow wells to dry.

Add samples diluted in PBS-TBSA. Usual dilutions are 1:10 and 1:50. Add 0.2 ml of sample.

Incubate overnight at 4°C.

Wash with PBS-T three times.

Fill wells with diluted alkaline phosphatase-conjugated anti-immunoglobulin directed against the relevant isotype. We usually use a 1:1,000 dilution. Incubate for 4 h.

Wash with PBS-T three times.

Add 0.2 ml of substrate (*p*-nitrophenyl phosphate). Vary substrate concentration to produce optimal rate of color development. The positive control should yield an optical density at 405 nm (OD_{405}) of ca. 1.0 in 30 to 45 min.

A serum pool can be used as a daily positive reference control. A dilution which will produce an OD_{405} of approximately 1.0 in 30 to 60 min is used. This internal standard is diluted 20-fold, and the OD_{405} generated by this dilution is taken as the background or zero value.

The sample value is calculated as a normalized percentage of the reference values:

Normalized value =

$$\frac{\text{sample } OD_{405} \times \text{dilution} - \text{zero value } OD_{405}}{\text{reference } OD_{405} \times \text{dilution} - \text{zero value } OD_{405}}$$

This treatment of the OD is taken because the OD values vary from day to day and it is difficult to compare results between analyses performed on different days. Therefore, each result is expressed in terms of a daily reference standard.

Antibody response to φX174 offers a very helpful assessment of antibody response and can define many patterns of response. The study can be performed in collaboration with Ralph Wedgwood, Department of Pediatrics, University of Washington Medical School, Seattle (8).

Lymphoid Morphology

See above.

Surface Immunoglobulins

See chapter 31.

In Vitro Production of Immunoglobulins

See chapter 45.

In common variable immunodeficiency (B- and T-cell systems involved to variable degrees and deficiency state tending to be less severe than in SCID), overactivity of T-suppressor cells is found in 50 to 70% of cases (7).

Materials

(All available from GIBCO Laboratories, Grand Island, N.Y.)
Pokeweed mitogen
RPMI 1640 with L-glutamine and bicarbonate
Fetal calf serum
Penicillin-streptomycin solution, 10^4 U of each per ml

Method

Lymphocytes (2×10^6/ml) from a normal subject are cocultured with 2×10^6 T cells per ml, obtained from a patient with common variable hypogammaglobulinemia. T cells are prepared by rosetting with neuraminidase-treated sheep erythrocytes. The culture is carried out in RPMI 1640 medium supplemented with glutamine, penicillin, streptomycin, and 10% fetal calf serum. Cultures are stimulated with 50 µg of pokeweed mitogen per tube. Nonstimulated cultures produce a mean of 212 ng of IgG, 303 ng of IgA, and 537 ng of IgM per 2×10^6 lymphocytes after 7 days of culture. Stimulated cultures produce, per 2×10^6 lymphocytes, means of 1,641, 1,691, and 3,715 ng of IgG, IgA, and IgM, respectively. When cocultured with T-lymphocyte populations with excess suppressor activity, the amount of synthesis is depressed (for all immunoglobulins) by from 40 to 100%. Recently, class-specific suppressors for IgA have been described.

Antibodies to IgA

Antibodies to IgA should be sought for in patients with selective IgA deficiency.

Reagents

Draw human O-negative erythrocytes into EDTA tubes. Ordinarily, these cells can be used immediately; however, when erythrocytes are difficult to coat, let cells stand in tube, with stopper loosened or removed, for 24 to 48 h at 4°C before coating. Wash cells three times in 0.9% sodium chloride before coating.

Chromic chloride, granular ($CrCl_3 \cdot 6H_2O$; Mallinckrodt Chemical Works, St. Louis, Mo.), 10 mg in 10 ml of distilled water. Prepare fresh.

IgA (1 mg/ml) in 0.9% sodium chloride (protein available from Cappel Laboratories, Malvern, Pa.)

PBS (pH 7.2).

PBS-BSA: 100 ml of PBS plus 1.6 ml of 30% bovine serum albumin (Dade Division, American Hospital Supply Corp., Miami, Fla.)

PBS-Tween: 100 ml of PBS, 50 µl of Tween 80 (Fisher Scientific Co., Chicago, Ill.), 2.5 mg of polyvinyl pyrrolidone, 1.6 ml of 30% bovine serum albumin

Method

1. Dilute stock $CrCl_3$ 1:6 in 0.9% sodium chloride just before use.

2. Mix in test tube in the following order:

IgA solution . . . . 0.05 ml
Washed packed erythrocytes . . . . 0.05 ml
$CrCl_3$ solution . . . . 0.1 ml

TABLE 3. Classification of immune response to bacteriophage φX174

Classification	Antigen clearance	Primary response		Secondary response		Memory amplification
		Antibody amt	Immunoglobulin class	Antibody amt	Immunoglobulin class	
Normal	Yes	Normal	IgM	Normal	IgG	Yes
Type 0	None	None		None		None
Type I	Yes	None		None		None
Type II	Yes	Decreased	IgM	Decreased	IgM	None
Type III	Yes	Decreased	IgM	Decreased	IgM	Yes
Type IV	Yes	Decreased	IgM	Decreased	IgM > IgG	Yes
Type V	Yes	Decreased	IgM	Decreased	IgG > IgM	Yes

Agitate constantly at room temperature for 5 min. Stop reaction immediately by dilution if macroscopic agglutination is observed.

3. Add saline to stop reaction and immediately wash three times with saline.

4. Add 3.0 ml of PBS-BSA to erythrocyte button.

5. Perform hemagglutination in V-bottom microtiter trays; use polyvinyl pyrrolidone-Tween buffer for dilution of test sera.

Interpretation

The absence or marked diminution (less than 5th percentile) of all major classes virtually establishes the diagnosis of hypogammaglobulinemia. In protein-losing states, IgM levels are normal to only slightly decreased; the marked diminution of albumin and transferrin confirms the true cause of the deficiency state.

A special problem arises in selective IgA deficiency. Fifty percent of these patients have antibodies to ruminant proteins. If the antiserum used for quantitation is of goat origin, there will be a detectable ring in the radial diffusion analysis. This will produce an erroneous reading of IgA presence when, in fact, deficiency exists. If such a patient's serum is used as an antibody in immunoelectrophoretic analysis and normal goat serum is used as antigen, the IgG arc of the goat will be revealed.

Antibodies to IgA are common in patients with selective IgA deficiency and are not found in normal blood.

In interpreting immunoglobulin levels any uncertainty can be resolved by functional assessment. Measurement of diphtheria and tetanus antibodies is a simple technique. No matter what the immunization history, one must restimulate the patient if low antibody values are initially detected, before a deficiency state can be defined with certainty. For this reason, we rely extensively on *E. coli* antibody responses, as all individuals can be assumed to have a high degree of constant exposure to this antigen.

Immune responses to bacteriophage φX174 are shown in Table 3. One advantage of testing the φX174 response is that a rapid presumptive diagnosis of B-cell deficiency can be made at birth, since normal subjects can clear the virus immediately after birth whereas abnormal subjects show persistence of phage for more than 1 week. The antibody response will not be affected by placentally transmitted IgG since the mother would not ordinarily have antibodies to φX174. It has been suggested that those with type 0, I, II, or III responses will require IgG therapy. Patients

showing type IV responses may or may not benefit from IgG, whereas those who manifest a type V response, even though they are immunodeficient, do not require IgG therapy (8).

BIOCHEMICAL TESTS

Deficiency of adenosine deaminase has been observed in numerous children with CID. The symptoms tend to occur later in infancy than other forms of SCID, and there is a suggestion that the deficiency is "acquired." Bony abnormalities are characteristic and common. Nucleoside phosphorylase, which catalyzes the metabolism of inosine, the next step in the adenosine pathway, has also been found to be absent in some patients with CID. A characteristic feature of nucleoside phosphorylase deficiency is primary red cell aplasia and normal B-cell activity (2).

Gel Method for Screening for Adenosine Deaminase or Nucleoside Phosphorylase Deficiency

Reagents

Gel for purine nucleoside phosphorlyase detection

MTT-tetrazolium	10 mg
Phenazine methosulfate	10 mg
Xanthine oxidase	0.16 U
Inosine	10 mg

Dissolve the above ingredients (available from Sigma) in 50 ml of 0.025 M sodium potassium phosphate buffer (pH 7.5), warmed to 55°C. Then add 50 ml of 2% Noble agar (Difco Laboratories, Detroit, Mich.) prepared in 0.025 M sodium potassium phosphate buffer (pH 7.5) and cooled to 55°C after dissolving.

Gel for adenosine deaminase detection

Replace inosine in the above mixture with 40 mg of adenosine and add 1.6 U of nucleoside phosphorlyase (Sigma). Fill plastic petri dishes with either gel. Use filter paper for collecting blood spots.

Method

Cut a piece of blood-impregnated filter paper approximately 9 mm in size and press onto the gel. Incubate in a 37°C incubator for 1 h.

Interpretation

In the presence of the appropriate enzyme, the substrate is finally converted to uric acid if purine nucleoside phosphorylase or adenosine deaminase is in the blood sample. The subsequent oxidation of hypoxanthine causes a reduction of the MTT-tetrazolium to a blue insoluble formazan, forming an easily detected ring around the filter paper.

Procedure for Electrophoretic Screening of Adenosine Deaminase

Materials

Adenosine
MTT-tetrazolium
Phenazine methosulfate
Nucleoside phosphorylase
(All from Sigma.)

Method

1. Draw blood into acid-citrate-glucose containing 20 U of heparin per ml. Volume of acid-citrate-glucose = 15% of blood drawn.
2. Centrifuge at 1,500 rpm for 15 min.
3. Remove plasma and wash erythrocytes three times in 0.9% sodium chloride. Remove as much buffy coat as possible each time. Erythrocyte sedimentation tubes half filled with cells are convenient for this purpose.
4. Sonically treat cells for 3 min, or freeze and thaw cells three times to produce a lysate. The lysate is introduced into the gel on a strip of Whatman no. 3 filter paper.
5. Samples are run in 12% starch gel using 0.01 M PO_4 (pH 6.5) for the gel and 0.1 M PO_4 (pH 6.5) for the bridge solution. Electrophoresis conditions: 16 h at 4°C; 3 to 3.5 V/cm. Slice gel parallel to the surface into two equal halves.
6. Make staining gel by dissolving 40 mg of adenosine, 10 mg of MTT-tetrazolium, 10 mg of phenazine methosulfate, 1.6 U of nucleoside phosphorylase, and 0.16 U of xanthine oxidase in 50 ml of 0.025 M PO_4 (pH 7.5). Warm to 55°C and add to 50 ml of 2% special Noble agar in 0.025 M PO_4 (pH 7.5) at 55°C. Overlay cut surface of starch with staining gel and let stand at 37°C for 1 h. Positive bands are intense blue.

Procedure for Quantitative Determination of Adenosine Deaminase in Erythrocytes

Materials

Phosphate buffer, 0.05 M, pH 7.5
Sodium chloride, 0.9%
Adenosine, 1 mg/ml in water (Sigma)
Xanthine oxidase (Sigma)
Nucleoside phosphorylase (Sigma)

Method

1. Dilute lysate from preparation for electrophoresis 1:5 with water and add 50 μl to tubes containing 3.0 of 0.05 M PO_4 (pH 7.5) each (a blank tube and a reaction tube).
2. Read and record absorbance at 541 nm against a buffer blank.
3. Add 0.04 U of xanthine oxidase and 0.4 U of nucleoside phosphorylase to each of the tubes.
4. Allow to equilibrate at 37°C for 15 min.

5. Add 75 μl of adenosine stock to the reaction tube only and mix well
6. Immediately read and record the absorbance at 293 nm and start the timer (zero time).
7. Incubate the tubes at 37°C in a water bath for 10 min.
8. Read the absorbance at 293 nm again and stop the timer. Record the absorbance and time elapsed.

Notes

1. When assaying more than one sample in a group, allow the same amount of time to elapse between each sample reading in the group at the beginning of the assay and at the end as well.
2. If a calibrated recording spectrophotometer is used, the assay may be done in cuvettes with continuous recording. The instrument must have a jacketed cuvette chamber held at 37°C. The change in absorbance and time may also be calculated from the graph as well as from the recorded absorbance and time done manually.

Calculations. The needed data for caculations are the initial and final absorbance at 293 nm (A_{293}), the elapsed time, and the absorbance at 541 nm:

micromoles of adenosine deaminated per minute =

$$\left(\frac{\Delta A_{293}}{min}\right)\left(\frac{\text{total volume}}{11.6}\right)$$

Activity is expressed as micromoles of adenosine deaminated per minute per unit of optical density at 541 nm.

Addendum: stability of adenosine deaminase activity. Erythrocytes may be kept frozen at −70°C with preservation of adenosine deaminase activity. Lysates are stable for up to 1 month at −70°C. Serum appears to be stable indefinitely at −70°C. Lymphocyte lysates are unstable; activity of adenosine deaminase falls off rapidly after the cells are separated.

Procedure for Electrophorectic Screening of Nucleoside Phosphorylase

Materials

Inosine
Phenazine methosulfate
Xanthine oxidase
(All from Sigma.)

Method

1. Prepare erythrocyte lysate as in steps 1 through 4 for electrophoretic screening of adenosine deaminase.
2. Use 11% starch gel in the following buffer system:
Gel (pH 7.2): 12.4 mM Tris, 3.3 mM citric acid, 3.6 mM boric acid, and 0.33 mM lithium hydroxide
Bridge (pH 7.2): 0.44 mM boric acid and 0.04 M Tris
Electrophoretic conditions: 4 h at room temperature; 10 V/cm for 45 min, 6 V/cm for the remainder of the time.
3. For staining, dissolve 5 mg of inosine, 5 mg of MTT-tetrazolium, 5 mg of phenazine methosulfate, and 0.04 U of xanthine oxidase in 25 ml of 0.05 M phosphate buffer (pH 7.5). Warm to 55°C and mix with 25 ml of 2% aqueous special Noble agar at 55°C. Stain at 37°C for a few minutes. Positive bands are intense blue.

Procedure for Quantitative Determination of Erythrocyte Nucleoside

Materials

Inosine (Sigma), 1 mg/ml in distilled water
NaCl, 0.9%
PO_4, 0.05 M (pH 7.5)

Method

1. Dilute erythrocyte lysate prepared for electrophoresis 1:50 with water and add 50 μl of this to two tubes, each containing 3.0 ml of 0.05 M PO_4 (pH 7.5) (blank tube and reaction tube).

Steps 2, 3, and 4 are the same as for quantitative adenosine deaminase determination.

5. Add 0.16 ml of inosine stock to the reaction tube, mix well, and immediately proceed to steps 6, 7, and 8, which are the same as for quantitative adenosine deaminase determination.

Interpretation

Each laboratory should determine its own set of normal values from a large group of normal subjects. Deficiency of adenosine deaminase has been observed only in immunodeficiency disease (with one exception) and is probably causally related. The gel method for screening is adequate for detecting adenosine deaminase deficiency but provides less information than the electrophoretic method. Quantitative tests should be done to confirm the deficiency and to detect the heterozygous carrier state. Patients studied to date have had undetectable levels of enzyme. Most heterozygous carriers for adenosine deaminase deficiency show values less than 2 standard deviations of the normal mean. In the single case of nucleoside phosphorylase deficiency described, both parents had values less than 50% of the mean control value. At present, the complete spectrum of symptomatology associated with biochemical defects is unknown. Determinations of adenosine deaminase and nucleoside phosphorylase are indicated in all cases of SCID and, if facilities permit, would be of interest in all forms of immunodeficiency.

POLYMORPHONUCLEAR LEUKOCYTE ABNORMALITIES

Polymorphonuclear leukocyte (PMN) abnormalities can result in significant increased susceptibility to infection. For the PMNs to exert their full biological capability, they must perform three major functions: (i) mobilize to the area of need, (ii) phagocytize, and (iii) kill the infectious agent. The tests of neutrophil function fall into categories which measure these three basic functions. The subject has been recently reviewed (4).

Assessment of Mobility

Epinephrine stimulation

Inject 0.4 ml of 1:1,000 epinephrine per m² subcutaneously. Capillary blood samples are taken before and at 5, 15, 30, 45, and 60 min after the injection of epinephrine. Normal subjects increase the total PMN count >45% over the base-line values.

Cortisone stimulation

Hydrocortisone hemisuccinate (100 mg) is given intravenously. Samples are drawn before and at hourly intervals after the administration of hydrocortisone. The normal response is to increase the total PMN by 2,000 over the base-line value.

Rebuck skin window

A superficial abrasion is made on the volar surface of the forearm. Fine punctate capillary oozing should be seen, but frank bleeding should not be present. A sterile cover slip is covered by a small piece of cardboard cut slightly larger and held in place by adhesive tape. Cover slips are removed and new ones are placed at 2, 4, 6, 8, 12, 16, and 20 h. PMN assessment is based upon the cover slips removed at 2, 4, and 6 h, and mononuclear cell assessment is based upon the studies at 12, 16, and 20 h. Scoring is performed by counting the total number of cells on the cover slip and assigning scores as follows: 0 cells = 0; 1–10 = 1; 11–100 = 2; 101–1,000 = 3; greater than 1,000 = 4. If the total score of three slides is 6 or less, deficient migration is present.

Random mobility

Materials
Earle balanced salt solution (GIBCO Laboratories) plus 0.01 mg of rabbit serum albumin per 100 ml (ERA solution)
Heparin (The Upjohn Co., Kalamazoo, Mich.)
Dextran, 6% in saline (Abbott Laboratories, North Chicago, Ill.)

Preparation of leukocytes
1. Blood is drawn into heparin-containing syringes (100 U/ml of blood).
2. Add 4 ml of dextran to each 20 ml of blood. Allow to settle for 30 to 60 min at 37°C.
3. Transfer plasma to Falcon plastic disposable tubes (17 by 100 mm), and centrifuge for 5 min at 450 × g (room temperature).
4. Wash cells in ERA solution. Resuspend cells in ERA at a concentration of 5 × 10⁶ neutrophils per ml.

Method
1. Fill heparinized glass capillary tubes (Scientific Products, Evanston, Ill.) to approximately 70% of the total volume with the neutrophil solution.
2. Centrifuge for 20 min at 200 × g or in a microhematocrit centrifuge.
3. Incubate vertically for 4 h at 37°C.
4. Measure migration from the leading edge of the packed neutrophil suspension. This can be conveniently done with a hand-held magnifier (Bausch & Lomb, catalog no. 81-34-35).

Chemotaxis (see also chapter 40)

Materials
Neuroprobe blind well chambers (catalog no. FH013BW31201; Nuclepore Corp., Pleasanton, Calif.)

Nuclepore chemotactic membranes, 13 mm (catalog no. N 300 CPC 013 00; Nuclepore)
Manual for use of chemotactic chambers (Nuclepore)
Yeast zymosan (Schwarz-Mann, Orangeburg, N.Y.).
Gey balanced salt solution (GIBCO Laboratories)

Method. The studies of chemotaxis are detailed in the Nuclepore manual described above. A convenient attractant can be made from activated serum. For each 1 ml of fresh serum, 0.025 g of zymosan is needed. Weigh out appropriate amount of zymosan and wash with PBS. Remove PBS and add serum to zymosan precipitate. Mix well and incubate at 37°C for 30 min. Spin at 500 × g for 10 min; remove supernatant fluid and save. A mixture of 200 μl of activated serum per ml of Gey balanced salt solution is a good attractant solution. Various amounts of patient serum can be added to the activated serum mixture to detect inhibitors of chemotaxis. It is probably important to have the total concentration of serum in the attractant at least 10% but no more than 20%. The effect of normal serum or plasma at various concentrations must be studied by the individual investigator. An alternative method for chemotaxis under agarose has been described.

Interpretation. For a complete assessment, all of the tests of mobility must be performed. Epinephrine stimulation measures the ability to derive leukocytes from the marginal pool. Cortisone stimulation measures the marrow reserves. The Rebuck skin window simulates the actual neutrophil response at a local inflammatory site. Chemotactic experiments measure the ability of the PMNs to respond to a chemotactic stimulus and, furthermore, can be used to test for the presence of inhibitors of chemotaxis in the serum. Inhibitors to chemotaxis have been observed in Hodgkin's disease, Chediak-Higashi syndrome, diabetes mellitus, rheumatoid arthritis, elevated IgE syndromes, chronic granulomatous disease, and mucocutaneous candidiasis and as an isolated defect. Defective chemotaxis due to intrinsic cellular abnormality of the leukocyte has been observed in Chediak-Higashi syndrome, diabetes mellitus, "lazy leukocyte syndrome," postrenal dialysis, active infection, and other diseases.

Screening Test for Granulomatous Disease, Formazan Test

Materials

Nitro Blue Tetrazolium dye (Sigma), 0.28 g in 100 ml of 0.9% NaCl; filter through ultrafine sintered-glass filter and freeze in small portions
Safranin O (Fisher), 1 g of dye plus 100 ml of distilled water and 40 ml of glycerol
Incubation medium: 0.5 ml of normal serum plus 0.3 ml of sterile saline plus 0.6 ml of Nitro Blue Tetrazolium dye

Method

1. Collect 1 drop of patient's blood on a cover slip.
2. Incubate the cover slip in a humid chamber for 20 min at 37°C.
3. Carefully wash the clot off with sterile saline.

4. Invert the cover slip on a slide which contains 1 drop of medium.
5. Incubate for 30 min in a humid chamber at 37°C.
6. Remove cover slip from slide and air dry rapidly.
7. Fix with absolute methanol for 60 s and wash with distilled water.
8. Stain with 0.77% safranin for 5 min; wash off with water and mount on a slide.

Interpretation

Formazan-positive cells are large and blastlike and bear no resemblance to normal PMNs. They are filled with blue precipitate. Thirty percent or more of the granulocytes are converted to the formazan type normally. Patients with chronic granulomatous disease form no formazan cells, and this test is useful as a screen. Heterozygous carriers of the disease show less than normal conversion; however, this is not a reliable test of the carrier state.

Bactericidal Killing Assay, Method 1

Materials

Penicillin and streptomycin (5,000 U of each per ml)
Hanks balanced salt solution (HBSS)
(From GIBCO Laboratories, Lawrence, Mass.)

Method

(From the laboratory of B. Holmes, University of Minnesota, Minneapolis)
1. Prepare leukocytes.
   a. Draw blood into heparin-containing syringes (100 U/ml of blood).
   b. Add 4 ml of dextran to each 20 ml of blood. Allow to settle for 30 to 60 min at 37°C.
   c. Transfer plasma to Falcon plastic disposable tubes (17 by 100 mm), and centrifuge for 5 min at 450 × g (room temperature).
   d. Wash cells in HBSS and resuspend at 10^7 cells per ml.
2. Bacterial suspension.
   a. Inoculate overnight culture of *Staphylococcus aureus* 502A.
   b. Spin culture at 1,800 × g for 10 min.
   c. Wash pellet in 10 ml of 0.9% NaCl.
   d. Resuspend in ca. 7 ml of 0.9% NaCl.
   e. Take a Klett reading (should be about 80) or an OD reading (should be about 0.16 at 540 nm).
   f. Make a 1:50 dilution in HBSS; 0.1 ml contains approximately 10^6 bacteria.
3. Reaction mixture.
   a. Combine in a sterile, disposable Falcon plastic tube (12 by 75 mm) (prepare in duplicate if doing with and without antibiotics added): 0.3 ml of HBSS, 0.1 ml of pooled normal human serum (from five donors; stored in small portions at −70°C; DO NOT REFREEZE), 0.5 ml of leukocyte suspension, and 0.1 ml of bacterial suspension. Run bacterial control without leukocytes; substitute 0.5 ml of HBSS.
   b. Incubate all tubes in a Lab-Tek Aliquot Mixer which is in a 37°C incubator.

cluding neoantigens such as keyhole limpet hemocyanin or plague vaccine or recall antigens such as tetanus toxoid. This approach, while inherently more appealing, has also led to conflicting results. There are several possible explanations for the discrepancies found between the results of different studies. One is that different antigens were used in different studies. Another problem is that the B-cell system for antibody production simply does not appear to be as severely affected by neoplasia as the T-cell system is.

Thus, the quantitation of immunoglobulin production in cancer patients has essentially no clinical value. However, several laboratories have shown a correlation between the level of circulating immune complexes (CIC) and the degree of tumor burden or the prognosis of cancer patients. A discussion of the techniques for the measurement of CIC and their evaluation is beyond the scope of this chapter, but a recent review by Gupta and Morton (R. K. Gupta and D. L. Morton, Contemp. Top. Immunobiol., in press) has addressed this issue. While detection of CIC suffers from the same conceptual problem as does measurement of immunoglobulin, i.e., only a portion of the CIC will represent tumor-associated complexes, the correlations between CIC and clinical parameters have been encouraging. Furthermore, improved technology may soon lead to the capacity to measure CIC that contain tumor-associated antigens or antibodies, and this refinement may prove of significant value.

LYMPHOCYTE PROLIFERATIVE FUNCTIONS

Lymphocyte transformation is an extremely popular in vitro technique used to measure cellular immunocompetence. Small resting lymphocytes are exposed to a mitogen and are transformed into large lymphoblastic cells. Lymphocyte transformation measures the capacity of lymphocytes to proliferate and is thus restricted to one necessary, but not sufficient, component of the immune response. The most popular mitogens are phytohemagglutinin (PHA) and concanavalin A, both primarily T-cell mitogens, and pokeweed mitogen, which activates both B and T cells. There are many reports of correlations between PHA response and stage of disease and of correlations between the response to mitogens and recurrence of disease. However, there are also conflicting reports which do not show these relationships.

The mixed lymphocyte culture is another type of lymphocyte activation assay in which lymphocytes respond to foreign histocompatibility antigens on unrelated lymphocytes. The proliferative response is activated by the antigens of the human major histocompatibility complex (HLA antigens). The mixed lymphocyte culture measures both the afferent and efferent lines of the immune response in vitro and thus closely parallels the in vivo DNCB test. Many studies report a correlation of the proliferative response induced in mixed lymphocyte culture and the stage or prognosis of disease. However, the proliferative assays do not always correlate to each other or to other readily assessed parameters such as skin test responses. Presumably, each assay involves sufficiently different cellular mechanisms that none is clearly redundant.

Variability in results from different sources may be due to differences in the patient populations studied or to the lack of standardization of assay systems. Roux et al. (8), in an analysis of the PHA assay, pointed out the importance of a dose-response curve, of established quantitative criteria for the maximal response of each patient, and of determining the optimal time course for the assay, which appears to vary among individuals. Dean (3) examined variation in lymphoproliferative assays and noted problems related both to the assay itself and to the study design. Assay problems include inherent variation and nonstandardization of methods and measurement parameters, while study design problems include the choice of appropriate normal controls, differences in patients' disease groupings, and the influences of chemotherapy and immunotherapy on the lymphoproliferative response. Thus, the most common and readily available assays such as PHA response have proven more difficult to use and interpret than expected.

There is also no consensus on how to express proliferation data. The simplest method for assaying lymphoproliferation is tritiated thymidine ($[^3H]$thymidine) incorporation. This measures the counts per minute (cpm) or disintegrations per minute of tritiated thymidine incorporated into DNA for a standard number of cells. Simply reporting the cpm incorporated does not include the background, or unstimulated, response in the formulation. To attempt to compensate for this, one may use the net cpm (stimulated cpm − unstimulated cpm) or the "stimulation index" (net cpm/unstimulated cpm). Although the stimulation index is a very popular way to report such data, it is fraught with problems. These include statistical problems, namely, the fact that the unstimulated cpm is always a smaller number and therefore statistically less reliable, so that the index converts good data (stimulated cpm) into less reliable data. There are also biological problems with the index, as the assumption is made in this formula that there is a direct relationship between unstimulated activity and mitogen-stimulated activity while there is no evidence for this. We have felt that it is safest to deal with the stimulated responses without modification by the unstimulated results, and simply calculate the unstimulated response as a separate parameter of responsiveness.

The final way to analyze data is by some mathematical transformation of the cpm results. Golub et al. (4) examined a number of such transformations and found that $\log_{10}$ provided the most reliable transformation. Repeated samplings from the same individual showed the greatest reproducibility when data were expressed as $\log_{10}$ units. This transformation is particularly appealing because lymphocyte proliferation is a geometric function and probably should be expressed in log units.

QUANTITATION OF LYMPHOCYTE SUBSETS

It has now become very clear that lymphocytes represent a very heterogeneous group of cells and that surface markers can be used to identify many of the functional subgroups of lymphocytes. It remains to be determined whether the quantitation of lymphocytic subpopulations can be of general clinical significance. There are several obvious situations in which measurement of lymphocyte populations is quite important, e.g., acquired immune deficiency syndrome (AIDS) and the identification of T and B leukemias, but the general applicability of these procedures in oncology remains to be determined.

T cells are frequently identified by rosette formation with sheep erythrocytes (SRBC), with those lymphocytes which bind at least three SRBC considered to be T lymphocytes. The most common technique to measure rosette-forming cells involves the formation of E-rosettes by mixing SRBC and peripheral blood lymphocytes at 100:1, briefly incubating at 37°C, pelleting the cells, and then incubating at 4°C for 1 to 24 h. Results are usually reported as the percentage of lymphocytes forming E-rosettes or as the absolute number of E-rosettes, obtained by multiplying the percent E-rosettes by the total lymphocyte count.

A modification of the E-rosette test is the "active" E-rosette test. This measures the rosettes formed after 5 min of incubation between low ratios of SRBC and lymphocytes. Some workers distinguish between two rosette-forming populations on the basis of relative rosette-forming affinity. "High-affinity" rosettes are those formed at high temperature (29°C) and at low SRBC/lymphocyte ratios. "Low-affinity" E-rosette-forming cells are those that require optimal conditions (4°C and SRBC excess). The level of low-affinity rosettes in normal individuals correlates with the proportion of Fc receptor-bearing cells and reactivity in antibody-dependent cellular cytotoxicity (ADCC) assays (9).

Several studies have shown a relationship between the level of E-rosettes and other tests of immunocompetence. However, the overall number of rosette-forming cells may not be an accurate indicator of the total T cells, as it has been found that even with a normal level of T cells there may be a defect in the ability to form rosettes or respond to PHA (2). Jerrells et al. (5) concluded that some cancer patients have a decreased lymphoproliferative response in association with low levels of T lymphocytes, and some have decreased functional activity with completely normal E-rosette levels.

The rosette technique is now being superseded by other markers for lymphocyte subpopulations, including Fc receptors for immunoglobulin and markers identified by monoclonal antibodies (usually using flow cytometry). Some T cells have receptors for immunoglobulin G (IgG) (Tg), others for IgM (Tm). Tm has been associated with helper activity, and Tg is associated with suppressor activity. Some studies show a decrease in Tm/Tg ratios with malignancy. However, when monoclonal antibodies against T-helper (OKT4) and T-suppressor (OKT8) cells were used in a study of malignant melanoma patients, no correlation was found between OKT4 or OKT8 and stage or outcome (6). The markers for T-suppressor cells and T-helper cells have proven to be important in AIDS, but there is little evidence at present that such determinations are of significance in malignant disease.

There are probably several factors responsible for the failure of lymphocyte markers to identify patient populations clearly according to clinical parameters. (i) Technical variables can cause difficulty; a slight change in the temperature of incubation, the ratio of SRBC to lymphocytes, the freshness of the SRBC, or the choice of serum as a stabilizing agent can considerably alter rosette results. There is a lack of standardization so that virtually every study employs a somewhat different technique. (ii) The assumption is made that measurement of a cell type by the presence of a receptor is a direct indication of function, and this may not be true. Furthermore, the available markers appear to identify broad groups of cells, and the truly relevant subpopulations may have to be analyzed with several markers simultaneously. (iii) Peripheral blood lymphocytes may not be the most appropriate choice for the study of T-cell subset variations. Study of lymph node lymphocytes or tumor-infiltrating lymphocytes may be more revealing, as these compartments may be more directly influenced by the tumor.

LYMPHOCYTE CYTOTOXIC FUNCTIONS

Many laboratories have measured the function of K ("killer") cells and NK ("natural killer") cells, which do not require previous exposure to an antigen to express cytotoxicity and therefore qualify as measures of general immune function. Excluded from this discussion are tumor-specific cytotoxic T lymphocytes. These may actually be among the most important factors in determining host-tumor relationships, but their measurement is not a function of "immunocompetence," and no currently available methods allow standardized testing of cytotoxic T lymphocytes against single known tumor antigens. K cells are nonadherent, nonphagocytic lymphoid cells which do not possess T- or B-cell markers although they may sometimes have low-affinity SRBC receptors or other T markers. They have an Fc receptor for IgG that interacts with the specific IgG bound to the surface of the target cell.

ADCC can be mediated by various populations of cells in the peripheral blood. The ADCC assay is more technically complex than other measures of general immune function, and there have been fewer clinical studies using this assay. The reports that are available on ADCC mediated by K cells in cancer patients are conflicting. The discrepancies may be due to variables imposed on the system by use of several different target cells and undefined or unpurified effector cells.

NK cells are cells of lymphoid appearance whose cytotoxic capabilities are not dependent on prior sensitization. They are nonphagocytic, nonadherent, and heterogeneous with regard to other markers. NK activity in the peripheral blood is mediated by cells with an Fc receptor for IgG, although some activity is associated with cells bearing an Fc receptor for IgM. The myeloid leukemia cell line K562 is the most popular target cell to test NK activity. This is usually done using a chromium release assay, in which cells that are to be tested for NK activity are incubated with chromated K562 cells; after 3 to 4 h, the supernatant from each test well is collected, and the amount of chromium released into it is measured. The amount of chromium released is taken as an indication of the number of target cells that have been lysed by the NK cells.

Some studies that have attempted to correlate NK activity with the clinical situation show a decrease in NK cytotoxicity with malignancy and a correlation of diminished NK activity with stage of disease. Howev-

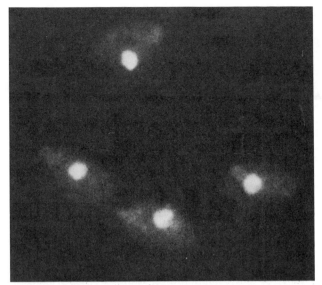

FIG. 3. Indirect immunofluorescence preparation of *C. luciliae* demonstrating fluorescence of the kinetoplast (×1,000).

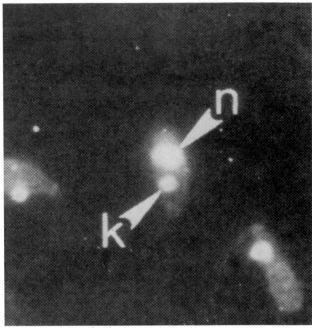

FIG. 4. Indirect immunofluorescence preparation of *C. luciliae* demonstrating kinetoplast (k) fluorescence alone in some organisms and kinetoplast and nuclear (n) fluorescence in others (×1,000).

for 10 min. Excess buffer is then removed by tapping the slide against a paper towel.

3. The substrate is layered over with 20 μl of an appropriate dilution (normally 1:10) of FITC-conjugated anti-human immunoglobulin, and the slide is incubated in a humid chamber for 30 min.

4. The slide is again washed, as described in step 2, in PBS in a Coplin jar for 10 min.

5. Excess buffer is removed, and cover slips are mounted with a drop of PBS-glycerol.

6. The slides are examined at ×1,000 with a fluorescence microscope, and kinetoplast fluorescence is scored on a scale of 0 to 4+.

Positive and negative controls are tested concurrently with each group of slides. If a serum proves positive at 1:10, serial dilutions are carried out.

For the detection of anti-DNA of individual immunoglobulin classes, specific FITC-conjugated antisera against human IgG, IgM, or IgA are used in step 3 above. For the detection of complement-fixing antibodies to DNA, the test serum is initially heated at 56°C for 30 min, after which the above procedure is followed through step 2. Fresh normal human serum is then layered on the substrate and the slide is incubated in a humid chamber for 30 min. After being washed in PBS as described in step 2 above, the substrate is then overlaid with FITC-conjugated anti-human C3 or C4 and again incubated in a humid chamber for 30 min. The slides are then washed, mounted, and evaluated as described in step 6 above.

INTERPRETATION

A positive test for anti-DNA is observed as a brightly stained kinetoplast. This structure is somewhat smaller than the nucleus and is often located near the periphery of the organism (Fig. 3). Nuclear staining may be observed in some instances also, since sera may contain antibodies directed against other nuclear

antigens in addition to DNA (Fig. 4). Kinetoplast staining can be differentiated from nuclear staining on the basis of the smaller size, brighter staining, and peripheral location of the kinetoplast. Two additional staining patterns (Fig. 5) which are occasionally observed are as follows. (i) The organism is stained near

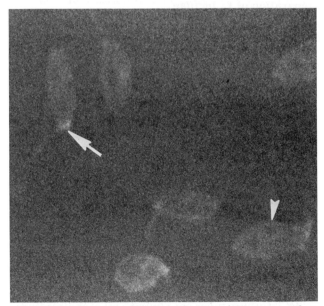

FIG. 5. Indirect immunofluorescence preparation of *C. luciliae* showing a negative test for anti-DNA. Faint immunofluorescent staining near the insertion of the flagellum (arrow) and an absence of background immunofluorescence in the area of the kinetoplast (arrowhead) are of no significance (×1,000).

the insertion of the flagellum or at the region of the basal body. This staining is of uncertain significance. (ii) There is perikinetoplast staining with a total absence of staining of the kinetoplast itself, which appears as a "hole." This pattern is also of uncertain significance and should be considered negative for antibodies to DNA.

Detection of antibodies to DNA by this technique in a serum dilution of 1:10 or greater is considered a positive test. The finding of a positive test only with undiluted serum has less diagnostic specificity for SLE and is associated with unreliable reproducibility. If the serum is positive at a dilution of 1:10, further dilutions should be carried out to determine the maximum titer of positivity. Titers of 1:160 or greater strongly suggest active lupus and are often present in patients with active lupus nephritis (2, 5). A positive test with a titer of 1:10 or in undiluted serum only is more characteristic of patients with inactive lupus.

The disadvantages of the *C. luciliae* immunofluorescence test are relatively minor compared with those of other tests for the detection of anti-DNA. It is necessary to repeatedly standardize the test against known positive and negative controls when one of the commercial kits is being used, since there may be some variability in the preparation of the *Crithidia* substrate. Another disadvantage is that results are expressed in semiquantitative, rather than quantitative, terms. Finally, a theoretical disadvantage is related to whether antibodies directed against DNA of parasitic origin are adequately reflective of the range of antibodies to DNA in human SLE. This concern, however, has not detracted from the substantial practical clinical utility of the test.

CONCLUSIONS

The quantitation of antibodies to DNA has become an established medical practice for patients with SLE and for those in whom SLE is suspected. The relatively high degree of specificity of these antibodies for the clinical disease and the unique association of antibody levels with disease activity have been repeatedly confirmed and have probably contributed to the improved management of patients with SLE. The *C. luciliae* immunofluorescence test described here has proven to be among the most satisfactory of tests for anti-DNA because of its relative immunochemical specificity for antibodies against double-stranded DNA, its ease of performance, and its low cost. It is readily adaptable to and can be carried out in any laboratory which has immunofluorescence capabilities. These factors contribute to its widespread clinical use in the diagnosis and management of lupus and related rheumatic diseases.

SUPPLIERS

The following is a partial list of suppliers of *C. luciliae* immunofluorescence anti-DNA kits.

Antibodies, Inc., Davis, Calif.
Calbiochem-Behring, San Diego, Calif.
California Immuno Diagnostics, San Marcos, Calif.
Electro-Nucleonics, Inc., Columbia, Md.
International Diagnostic Technology, Inc., Santa Clara, Calif.
Kallestad Laboratories, Inc., Austin, Tex.
Meloy Laboratories, Inc., Springfield, Va.
M. A. Bioproducts, Walkersville, Md.
Zeus Scientific, Inc., Raritan, N.J.

LITERATURE CITED

1. **Aarden, L. A., E. R. deGroot, and T. E. W. Feltkamp.** 1975. Immunology of DNA. III. *Crithidia luciliae*, a simple substrate for the determination of anti-dsDNA with the immunofluorescence technique. Ann. N.Y. Acad. Sci. **254**:505–515.
2. **Ballou, S. P., and I. Kushner.** 1979. Anti-native DNA detection by the *Crithidia luciliae* method. An improved guide to the diagnosis and clinical management of systemic lupus erythematosus. Arthritis Rheum. **22**:321–327.
3. **Ballou, S. P., and I. Kushner.** 1979. Immunochemical characteristics of antibodies to DNA in patients with active systemic lupus erythematosus. Clin. Exp. Immunol. **37**:58–67.
4. **Beaulieu, A., F. P. Quismorio, Jr., R. C. Kitridou, and G. J. Friou.** 1979. Complement fixing antibodies to DS-DNA in systemic lupus erythematosus: a study using the immunofluorescent *Crithidia luciliae* method. J. Rheumatol. **6**:389–396.
5. **Chubick, A., R. D. Sontheimer, and J. N. Gilliam.** 1978. An appraisal of tests for native DNA antibodies in connective tissue diseases. Clinical usefulness of *Crithidia luciliae* assay. Ann. Intern. Med. **89**:186–192.
6. **Crowe, W., and I. Kushner.** 1977. An immunofluorescent method using *Crithidia luciliae* to detect antibodies to double-stranded DNA. Arthritis Rheum. **20**:811–814.
7. **Laurent, M., S. Van Assel, and M. Steinert.** 1971. Kinetoplast DNA. A unique macromolecular structure of considerable size and mechanical resistance. Biochem. Biophys. Res. Commun. **43**:278–284.
8. **Samaha, R. J., and W. S. Irvin.** 1975. Deoxyribonucleic acid strandedness. Partial characterization of the antigenic regions binding antibodies in lupus erythematosus serum. J. Clin. Invest. **56**:446–457.
9. **Sontheimer, R. D., and J. N. Gilliam.** 1978. DNA antibody class, subclass, and complement fixation in systemic lupus erythematosus with and without nephritis. Clin. Immunol. Immunopathol. **10**:459–467.
10. **Tan, E. M., A. S. Cohen, J. F. Fries, A. T. Masi, D. J. McShane, N. F. Rothfield, J. G. Schaller, N. Talal, and R. J. Winchester.** 1982. The 1982 revised criteria for the classification of systemic lupus erythematosus. Arthritis Rheum. **25**:1271–1277.

Chapter 113

Enzyme-Linked Immunosorbent Assay for Anti-DNA and Antihistone Antibodies†

ROBERT L. RUBIN

Antibodies to native DNA (anti-nDNA) are of considerable interest in the diagnosis and management of patients with systemic lupus erythematosus (SLE). These autoantibodies are rarely found in patients with other rheumatic diseases, and their levels, especially of those with complement-fixing ability, often correlate with disease activity (4). Antihistone antibodies are also very common in SLE and probably account for the lupus erythematosus cell phenomenon. Antibodies to histones are also found in lower frequencies in other diseases and are the predominant autoantibody in patients with drug-induced lupus.

Numerous assays for anti-nDNA have been devised. The first quantitative assay, which still remains the standard reference method, is the Farr assay (10). The original procedure, in which ammonium sulfate is used to precipitate immunoglobulin along with bound, radiolabeled DNA, and variants, in which free DNA is separated from antibody-bound DNA by cellulose ester membranes, anti-immunoglobulin, or polyethylene glycol, all require radiolabeled DNA of reproducible high quality. The difficulties in obtaining such DNA, the associated hazards and disposal problems of radioisotopes, and the expensive equipment required to perform these assays have led to the development of alternative methods.

Anti-nDNA can also be detected in a semiquantitative fashion by an immunofluorescence (IF) assay utilizing *Crithidia luciliae* as the substrate (1), as detailed elsewhere in this section. This assay, which requires no special equipment other than a fluorescence microscope, has the advantage of high reproducibility and is readily modifiable for measuring immunoglobulin class-specific or complement-fixing anti-nDNA. It is particularly suitable for a limited number of determinations but becomes cumbersome with large numbers of samples and is not quantitative unless the titer is determined by assaying serial dilutions of the sample.

Reliable, sensitive assays for quantitating antihistone antibodies have only recently become available. Previous assays were hampered by the tendency of histones to aggregate and to bind nonimmune immunoglobulin or other serum proteins such as alpha-2 macroglobulin and complement components. Another approach utilized an IF assay modified to render it specific for histone-reactive antibodies (8). This histone reconstitution IF assay shows good specificity for antihistone antibodies and requires only a fluorescence microscope. However, it is insensitive to antihistone antibodies reactive with histones H3 and H4 and cannot be used with sera in which anti-nDNA coexists (6).

†This paper is publication number 3698BCR from the Research Institute of Scripps Clinic, La Jolla, Calif.

Solid-phase assays have begun to replace conventional assays for anti-DNA and antihistone antibodies. Many macromolecules (although not nDNA) readily bind to polystyrene microtiter plates. nDNA can be made to bind to polystyrene either directly, through limited single-stranded regions, or through a basic protein-polypeptide precoating the vessel wall. If an enzyme-conjugated anti-immunoglobulin is used as the detecting reagent, many of the safety and disposal problems associated with radioisotopes are precluded. These enzyme-linked immunosorbent assays (ELISAs) are particularly conducive to semiautomation and are versatile in permitting a variety of immunoglobulin class-specific or complement-fixing antibodies to be used as detecting reagents. ELISAs are quantitative methods for a wide range of antibody activities and are easily scaled up for screening large numbers of samples. However, this method may not be cost-effective for laboratories with only a modest number of samples to be screened. In addition, careful control of the reagents and reaction conditions are required in any ELISA format.

CLINICAL INDICATIONS

An anti-nDNA test is often useful diagnostically for patients who have antinuclear antibodies or clinical findings suggestive of SLE. The presence of anti-nDNA is one of the American Rheumatism Association criteria for SLE, and the antibody is rarely found in patients with other rheumatic diseases (9).

Criteria for selecting a type of anti-nDNA assay should depend more on the quality of the laboratory operation and source of reagents than on the method itself. All anti-nDNA assays require a DNA preparation which is essentially free of single-stranded regions, since antibodies to single-stranded DNA are common in a variety of diseases and, therefore, are not specific for SLE (3). Liquid-phase methods such as the Farr assay (10) can give reliable results when a high-quality, radiolabeled DNA preparation is available, and generally this assay shows good agreement with solid-phase ELISA methods. The specificity of the *Crithidia* IF method for anti-nDNA is essentially unambiguous, but its sensitivity may be low with certain fluorescent anti-immunoglobulin-detecting reagents. ELISA should be considered the method of choice for a clinical or research laboratory engaged in screening substantial numbers of samples.

The presence of antihistone antibodies can be used to verify a diagnosis of lupus induced by such drugs as procainamide and hydralazine. Antihistone antibodies can be assayed by the modified IF method with histone-reconstituted mouse kidney sections (8) or by ELISA (7). The IF method is sensitive and specific for antihistone antibodies in patients with procainamide-

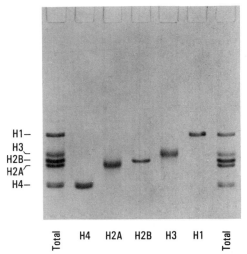

H1—
H3
H2B—
H2A
H4—

Total H4 H2A H2B H3 H1 Total

FIG. 1. Polyacrylamide gel electrophoretic profile of total histones from calf thymus and of purified preparations of each individual histone class. Purification was based on the procedure of Bohm et al. (2). Redrawn from R. L. Rubin, *in* R. G. Lahita, (ed.), *Systemic Lupus Erythematosis*, 1985, with permission from John Wiley & Sons, Inc.

induced lupus. However, sera from patients with hydralazine-induced lupus often are false-negative by this method (5), and the assay is cumbersome and expensive to perform because of the requirement of three substrate preparations. ELISA with total histones as the screening antigen detects antihistone antibodies of the wide specificities encountered in drug-induced and idiopathic SLE and, therefore, is preferable. In addition, antihistone antibodies reactive with individual histone classes can be readily detected when pure preparations are available (Fig. 1) (2), and these antibodies may have special diagnostic

significance. For example, immunoglobulin G antibodies to a complex of histones H2A and H2B are very common in patients with procainamide-induced lupus, whereas antihistone antibodies of other specificities are induced by procainamide in patients who remain asymptomatic.

INTERPRETATION

The extent of elevated reactivity in ELISA for anti-nDNA and antihistone antibodies is shown in Fig. 2 and 3, respectively, for a panel of sera from patients with a variety of diagnoses. The upper limit of the normal range for these assays is shown as a horizontal line two standard deviations above the mean of normal serum binding.

A polyvalent anti-immunoglobulin capable of reacting with all classes of antibody can be used to establish the anti-nDNA and antihistone activity of an unknown serum. A substantially elevated reaction to nDNA is virtually diagnostic of SLE. Anti-nDNA is not found in patients with drug-induced lupus (Fig. 2). Antihistone antibodies with total histones as the antigen (Fig. 1) are also usually elevated in SLE and are also found in patients with drug-induced lupus and in 10 to 15% of patients with other rheumatic diseases (Fig. 3). Therefore, a serum displaying positive antihistone and anti-nDNA is consistent with idiopathic lupus, whereas elevated antihistone without anti-nDNA is expected in patients with drug-induced lupus. Since drug-induced lupus sera also commonly have antibodies to denatured or single-stranded DNA, the lack of reactivity of drug-induced lupus sera in the anti-nDNA assay can be used to document the absence of denatured DNA in the anti-nDNA assay.

PRINCIPLE OF THE ASSAY

The reagents and procedure described below are generally applicable for measuring antibodies in se-

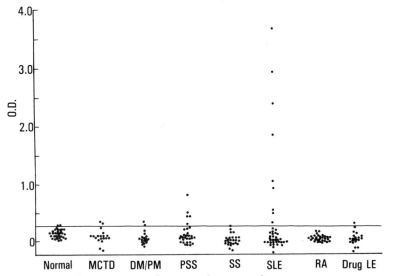

FIG. 2. ELISA for anti-nDNA. Sera from patients of various rheumatic disease groups were assayed for anti-nDNA with peroxidase-conjugated anti-human immunoglobulin as the detecting reagent. MCTD, Mixed connective tissue disease; DM/PM, dermatomyositis/polymyositis; PSS, progressive systemic sclerosis; SS, Sjögren's syndrome; RA, rheumatoid arthritis; Drug LE, drug-induced lupus. Reprinted from R. L. Rubin, F. G. Joslin, and E. M. Tan, J. Immunol. Methods **63:**359–366, 1983, with permission from Elsevier Biomedical Press B.V.

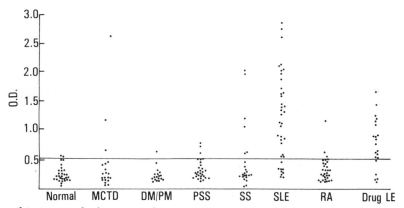

FIG. 3. ELISA for antihistone antibodies. Sera from patients of various rheumatic disease groups were assayed for antibodies to total histones with peroxidase-conjugated anti-human immunoglobulin as the detecting reagent. See the legend to Fig. 2 for abbreviations. Reprinted from R. L. Rubin, *in* R. G. Lahita (ed.), *Systemic Lupus Erythematosus*, 1985, with permission from John Wiley & Sons, Inc.

rum, plasma, and other fluids, such as spinal, pleural, or joint, as well as in cell culture media. The assay requires purified antigen that is immobilized in a polystyrene microtiter plate well. Proteins passively adsorb to plastics to various extents, depending on protein hydrophobicity and the characteristics of the plastic. Denatured DNA also binds to polystyrene, but nDNA does not unless it is partially denatured or contaminated with protein. nDNA is immobilized by binding to a basic protein such as methylated bovine serum albumin (BSA).

After immobilizing the antigen, unoccupied protein binding sites are blocked with the inert protein gelatin. Human test serum is diluted in a medium containing nonhuman immunoglobulins and a weak detergent to minimize nonspecific binding, and the serum is incubated in the antigen-coated wells. Nonbound or loosely bound immunoglobulin is removed by repeated rinsing. The wells are then incubated with peroxidase-conjugated anti-human immunoglobulin (polyvalent or class specific). After the wells are rinsed, hydrogen peroxide and a secondary substrate are added, and these substances form a chromogenic product upon enzymatic action of peroxidase. The optical density (OD) of the contents of each well is determined, and these values are used as measures of the amount of specific antibody bound to the wells.

MATERIALS

Reagents

Methylated BSA. Some preparations of methylated BSA (Calbiochem-Behring, La Jolla, Calif.) may be overmethylated, giving high background values, and should not be used. A stock solution at a concentration of 1 mg/ml in water can be stored frozen.

S1 nuclease. A stock solution of S1 nuclease (New England Nuclear Corp., Boston, Mass.) at a concentration of 300 U/ml in 50% glycerol can be stored at −20°C.

Peroxidase-conjugated anti-human immunoglobulin. Commercial sources of affinity-purified antibod-

ies are recommended (Tago, Inc., Burlingame, Calif., or Kirkegaard & Perry Laboratories, Gaithersburg, Md.). The reagents should be stored undiluted at 5°C and should contain thimerosal, not azide.

Histones. Total histones from calf thymus should consist of the five polypeptides shown in Fig. 1. Good preparations have been obtained from Calbiochem-Behring and United States Biochemical Corp., Cleveland, Ohio, but preparations from other sources are variable in quality. In addition, DNA must be considered a potential contaminant of any histone preparation. Digestion of histones with DNase in the presence of phenylmethylsulfonyl fluoride (Calbiochem-Behring) to inhibit possible endogenous proteases is currently the most exhaustive method for DNA removal. This procedure is performed as follows.

1. Dissolve histones at a concentration of approximately 1 mg/ml in H_2O. Dialyze at 5°C against phosphate-buffered saline (PBS) containing 1 mM $MgCl_2$ and 0.25 mM $CaCl_2$.

2. Add phenylmethylsulfonyl fluoride to a concentration of 0.5 mM. Add DNase 1 (Millipore Corp., Bedford, Mass.) to a concentration of 100 U/ml. Incubate at 37°C for 4 h.

3. Cool to 0°C. Gradually add 2 N H_2SO_4 at 0°C to a final concentration of 0.4 N H_2SO_4. Incubate at 0°C for 30 min.

4. Centrifuge at 10,000 rpm for 15 min. Save the supernatant.

5. Dialyze against two changes of 0.05 M acetic acid at 5°C and then against two changes of water.

DNA. The species of origin and the size of the DNA are unimportant, but the preparation should be free of contaminating protein, RNA, and single-stranded regions. Calf thymus DNA of the highest quality commercially available is usually used. The removal of single-stranded regions is described below.

Solutions

Stock phosphate buffer (0.5 M, pH 7.4). Dissolve 56.8 g of Na_2HPO_4 and 13.8 g of $NaH_2PO_4 \cdot H_2O$ in water to volume of 1 liter. Store frozen in 20-ml aliquots, and make up larger volume for PBS and PBS-Tween.

Gelatin stock solution (1%). Dissolve 0.1 g of gelatin (Baker Chemical Co., Phillipsburg, N.J.) in 1 liter of water by heating (not boiling). Store frozen in 100-ml aliquots.

Gelatin postcoating solution (0.1% gelatin in PBS). Mix 100 ml of gelatin stock solution (preheated to 50 to 60°C) with 880 ml of water and 20 ml of stock phosphate buffer, and dissolve 8.2 g of NaCl and 0.1 g of thimerosal in this solution.

PBS. For PBS (0.14 M NaCl, 0.01 M phosphate buffer [pH 7.2]), dissolve 65.4 g of NaCl and 0.1 g of thimerosal in water, and add 160 ml of stock phosphate buffer and water to a volume of 8 liters. Store at 5°C for less than 6 weeks.

PBS-Tween. For PBS-Tween (0.14 M NaCl, 0.01 M phosphate buffer, 0.05% Tween 20), dissolve 163.6 g of NaCl and 2.0 g of thimerosal in water, and add 400 ml of stock phosphate buffer, 10 ml of Tween 20 (polyoxyethylene sorbitan monolaurate; Sigma Chemical Co., St. Louis, Mo.), and water to a volume of 20 liters. Store at 5°C for less than 6 weeks.

Serum diluent A. Serum diluent A contains (per ml) 1 mg of gelatin, 5 mg of bovine gamma globulin (BGG), and 1 mg of BSA in PBS-Tween. Dissolve 8.2 g of NaCl, 0.1 g of thimerosal, 5 g of BGG (Cohn fraction II, Sigma), and 1 g of BSA (Cohn fraction V, Sigma) in 875 ml of water. Add 100 ml of gelatin stock solution (preheated to 50 to 60°C), 20 ml of stock phosphate buffer, and 0.5 ml of Tween 20. Store at 5°C for less than 2 weeks.

Serum diluent B. Serum diluent B contains (per ml) 1 mg of gelatin, 0.75 mg of BGG, and 1 mg of BSA in PBS-Tween. Dissolve 8.2 g of NaCl, 0.1 g of thimerosal, 0.75 g of BGG (Cohn fraction II, Sigma), and 1 g of BSA (Cohn fraction V, Sigma) in 875 ml of water. Add 100 ml of gelatin stock solution (preheated to 50 to 60°C), 20 ml of stock phosphate buffer, and 0.5 ml of Tween 20. Store at 5°C for less than 2 weeks.

Anti-immunoglobulin diluent. Anti-immunoglobulin diluent contains (per ml) 1 mg of BGG and 5 mg of BSA in PBS-Tween. Dissolve 8.2 g of NaCl, 0.1 g of thimerosal, 1 g of BGG, and 5 g of BSA in 975 ml of water, and add 20 ml of stock phosphate buffer and 0.5 ml of Tween 20. Store at 5°C for less than 2 weeks.

S1 nuclease buffer. S1 nuclease buffer contains 0.03 M sodium acetate, 0.1 M NaCl, 5 mM $ZnCl_2$, and 0.1 mg of BSA per ml, pH 4.4. Dissolve 4.1 g of $NaC_2H_3O_2 \cdot 3H_2O$, 5.9 g of NaCl, and 0.70 g of $ZnCl_2$ in approximately 900 ml of water. Adjust the pH to 4.4 with approximately 2 ml of glacial acetic acid. Adjust the volume to 1 liter, and add 0.1 g of BSA.

Peroxidase substrate solution

1. ABTS (2,2'-azino-di-(3-ethylbenzthiazoline-6-sulfonic acid) stock solution, 10 mg/ml (Sigma). Dissolve 0.5 g of ABTS in water to a volume of 50 ml. Store at 5°C for less than 1 month.

2. Hydrogen peroxide stock (1% H_2O_2). Dilute 30% H_2O_2 to 1%. Store at 5°C for less than 1 week.

3. McIlvaine buffer (0.2 M Na_2HPO_4, 0.1 M citric acid [pH 4.6]). Dissolve 35.61 g of $Na_2HPO_4 \cdot 2H_2O$ to a volume of 1 liter (0.2 M) and 21.01 g of monohydrated citric acid (0.1 M) to a volume of 1 liter. Mix 234 ml of 0.2 M Na_2HPO_4 with 266 ml of 0.1 M citric acid. Adjust the pH of the mixture to 4.6 by adding the appropriate component. Buffer and components can be stored at 5°C, but Na_2HPO_4 may need to be heated to be redissolved.

4. Working substrate solution (1 mg of ABTS per ml, 0.005% H_2O_2 in McIlvaine buffer [pH 4.6]). Mix 1 part ABTS stock with 9 parts McIlvaine buffer, and add 1/200 of a volume of H_2O_2 stock. Use within a few hours at room temperature.

nDNA stock solution. nDNA stock solution is S1 nuclease-treated DNA at a concentration of approximately 0.5 mg/ml. Dissolve calf thymus DNA at a concentration of approximately 0.5 mg/ml in 1 mM phosphate buffer, pH 7, at 0 to 5°C. Dialyze against 0.03 M sodium acetate–0.1 M NaCl–1 mM $ZnCl_2$, pH 4.4. Add S1 nuclease to 0.1 U of DNA per μg. Incubate at 37°C for 3 h. Dialyze against PBS, and store over chloroform at 5°C. Determine the DNA concentration based on A_{260} of 1.07 OD units for a 0.05-mg/ml solution.

Histone stock solution. Dissolve histones at a concentration of 0.5 to 1.0 mg/ml in distilled water. Determine the histone concentration based on A_{230} of 1.65 OD units for a 0.5-mg/ml solution. Store frozen.

Equipment

Flat-bottom 96-well microtiter plates with lids (Immulon 2 from Dynatech Laboratories, Inc., Alexandria, Va., are recommended)

Repetitive, mechanical pipetting devices

Aspiration manifolds (at least 8 well)

Plate-washing apparatus (at least 8 well)

Spectrophotometer, preferably an automatic machine capable of absorbance determinations directly through the wells (Dynatech or Flow Laboratories, McLean, Va.)

PROCEDURES

Preparation of nDNA-coated plates

1. Dilute methylated BSA stock to 10 μg/ml in PBS, and place 0.2 ml in each well of a microtiter plate. Incubate at 5°C for 6 to 18 h.

2. Decant the contents, and rinse with 0.3 ml of PBS.

3. To methylated BSA-coated wells, add 0.2 ml of nDNA solution which has been prediluted to 20 μg/ml in PBS. Incubate for 6 to 18 h at 5°C.

4. Decant the contents, and add 0.3 ml of gelatin postcoating solution. Store for at least 18 h.

5. For long-term storage, replace the standard gelatin postcoating solution with a solution of gelatin at 1 mg/ml in 1 mM phosphate buffer, pH 7, and store at 5°C in a sealed container. Plates stored in low-ionic-strength gelatin solution are stable for at least 2 months.

Redigestion of nDNA-coated plates with S1 nuclease

Redigestion with S1 nuclease may be unnecessary, depending on the quality of the DNA originally used to coat the plates and on the age of the DNA-coated plates. Redigestion is normally done just before plates are used.

Test tubes, 10 by 75 mm.

Pipettes, adjustable.

Centrifuge. Any serofuge is suitable.

Photometer capable of measuring light transmission at 650 nm.

Reagents

GBS (0.1 M, pH 8.2).

Stock solution of Cohn fraction II. To 0.25 g of lyophilized fraction II add 10-ml increments of GBS, mixing well until 50 ml has been added and the powder is completely dissolved. Dilute to 150 ml with GBS, and store the solution at 4°C (maximum storage time is 4 weeks). Before use, spin the solution at 1,000 × g for 10 min to remove the particulate debris.

Latex particles sensitized with stock solution of fraction II. Add 1.0 ml of latex particles to 100 ml of GBS. The concentration (volume/volume) of the latex particles is then checked by adding a sample of the latex to a square cuvette (13 by 13 by 100 mm) and measuring light transmission at 650 nm; an appropriate concentration should be in the range of 5 to 7%. Add 5.0 ml of fraction II solution and incubate the mixture at 37°C for 90 min. The sensitized latex particles should be prepared fresh daily.

Procedure

1. Heat inactivate serum for 30 min at 56°C and dilute it 1:20, using 0.1 ml of serum and 1.9 ml of GBS in a test tube (10 by 75 mm).

2. Place 1.0 ml of GBS in each of eight additional tubes and serially dilute the test sera with 1.0 ml from the first tube, discarding 1.0 ml from the ninth tube.

3. Add 1.0 ml of latex-human IgG reagent (prepared as described above) to each tube and to an additional control tube containing 1 ml of GBS alone. Incubate for 30 min at 4°C, for 90 min at 56°C, and for 5 min at room temperature.

4. Centrifuge in a serofuge (1,000 × g) for 5 min.

5. Read the flocculation reaction by gently tapping the tube to dislodge the pellet, and view in front of a microscope lamp having a light intensity of 60 W. If the precipitate breaks into small particles and the supernatant remains clear, the reaction is positive. If the precipitate breaks up into a smoky pattern, the test is negative. The highest tube dilution showing flocculation defines the titer of rheumatoid factor. The test is considered positive when flocculation occurs at a titer greater than 1:160.

6. Standardize the test with batches of reference sera of known titers.

ELISA for IgM rheumatoid factor

Materials

Microtiter plates, 96 well (round-bottomed plastic).

pH meter.

Pipettes.

Photometer capable of measuring light transmission at 405 nm (micro-ELISA ELISA reader, Dynatech Laboratories, Inc., Alexandria, Va.).

Reagents

Purified human IgG (Sigma Chemical Co., St. Louis, Mo.) diluted in phosphate-buffered saline (PBS) (0.1 M pH 7.4) to 5 μg/ml.

PBS–Tween 20: PBS (0.1 M pH 7.4) containing 0.05% Tween 20 (polyoxyethylene sorbitan monolaureate; Sigma).

Patient and control sera.

Alkaline phosphatase-conjugated anti-human IgM (μ-chain-specific antibody developed in goats; Sigma).

Distilled water.

Substrate: para-nitrophenyl phosphate (Sigma) at 1.0 mg/ml in glycine buffer (0.1 M pH 7.4) containing 0.001 M $MgCl_2$ and 0.001 M $ZnCl_2$.

3 M NaOH.

Procedure

1. Microtiter plate wells are coated with 100 μl of human IgG and left overnight at room temperature.

2. After one wash with PBS–Tween 20 (add 100 μl of PBS–Tween 20, and shake out by inverting the plates and shaking three times), 100 μl of test serum, diluted 1/100 in PBS–Tween 20, is added to the wells, which are again left at room temperature overnight.

3. The plates are then washed three times (twice with PBS and once with distilled water), and 100 μl of the substrate solution is added. The color reaction is stopped after 10 min by the addition of 100 μl of 3 M NaOH, and the absorbance values are read at 405 nm.

4. The test results are standardized with portions of reference sera of known titer run with each assay.

INTERPRETATION

Numerous commercial kits are available for testing rheumatoid factor; almost all employ either the slide or tube method. In a recent College of American Pathologists survey utilizing 18 serum specimens sent to participating laboratories (4), 11 different commercial tube and slide kits were compared. Slide tests on negative samples performed better than tube tests, while equally good performance was obtained on the positive high-titer samples. On the low-titer samples better performance was obtained with tube tests. It should be realized that all tests for rheumatoid factor are inhibited by serum IgG to some extent. In its extreme form, depletion of IgG from the serum may be required for detection of the rheumatoid factor (1).

An attempt to eliminate interlaboratory variability by the use of World Health Organization standard serum comparison (international units) has not, with the possible exception of nephelometry, narrowed titer variations (4). As the ELISA and radioimmunoassay tests become better standardized, objective measurements (in milligrams per milliliter) of rheumatoid factors of various immunoglobulin classes will become available, and their respective significance both in the joint cavity and in serum will be better appreciated.

With the latex fixation test, rheumatoid factors are found in 1 to 4% of the general population, whereas the incidence is about 1% when the sensitized sheep erythrocyte agglutination test is utilized. The highest incidence of rheumatoid factors occurs in persons over 65 years of age, reaching approximately 20% when the latex fixation is used.

The clinical correlation of an elevated rheumatoid factor should be interpreted cautiously. Increased titers may accompany a variety of acute immune responses, particularly viral infections (e.g., infectious mononucleosis), and, as noted, may also be observed in the normal elderly population. The clinician has little difficulty interpreting markedly elevated rheumatoid factors. Diagnostic difficulty may occur during the evaluation of titers ranging from 1:20 to 1:80. The significance of these values, which may be present during early rheumatoid arthritis or as a normal variant, should be deemphasized unless symptoms and physical signs are highly suggestive of rheumatoid arthritis.

Rheumatoid factors, although of diagnostic utility for rheumatoid arthritis, may be observed in a number of other diseases. For example, chronic infectious diseases (tuberculosis, leprosy, various parasitic diseases, subacute bacterial endocarditis), liver disease (chronic active hepatitis), sarcoidosis, and lymphoproliferative syndromes (Waldenstrom's macroglobulinemia) all may be associated with the presence of rheumatoid factors. A variety unlike the common rheumatoid factors, which demonstrate a restricted polyclonal pattern and do not react with IgG at 4°C, is termed cold-reactive rheumatoid factor. Such antigamma globulins may be monoclonal, forming a cryoprecipitate when cooled to 4°C. Although observed in systemic lupus erythematosus, Sjogren's syndrome, and viral infections, cold-reactive rheumatoid factors may be associated with cryoglobulinemic states complicated by lymphoreticular malignancy. This type of rheumatoid factor is detected by measurement of circulating cryoglobulins, followed by solubilization of the cryoprecipitate at 37°C and the subsequent determination of rheumatoid factor activity on separated products.

LITERATURE CITED

1. **Allen, J. C., and H. G. Kunkel.** 1966. Hidden rheumatoid factors with specificity for native γ-globulin. Arthritis Rheum. **9:**758–768.
2. **Faith, A., O. Pontesilli, A. Unger, G. S. Panayi, and P. Johns.** 1982. ELISA assays for IgM and IgG rheumatoid factors. J. Immunol. Methods **55:**169–177.
3. **Finley P. R., M. J. Hicks, R. J. Williams, J. Hinlicky, and D. A. Lichti.** 1979. Rate nephelometric measurement of rheumatoid factor in serum. Clin. Chem. **25:**1909–1914.
4. **Rippey, J. H., and J. L. Biesecker.** 1983. Results of tests for rheumatoid factor on CAP survey specimen. Am. J. Clin. Pathol. **80:**599–602.
5. **Rose, H. M., C. Ragan, E. Pearce, and M. O. Lipmann.** 1948. Differential agglutination of normal and sensitized sheep erythrocytes by sera of patients with rheumatoid arthritis. Proc. Soc. Exp. Biol. Med. **68:**1–11.
6. **Singer, J. M., and C. M. Plotz.** 1956. The latex fixation test. I. Application to the serologic diagnosis of rheumatoid arthritis. Am. J. Med. **21:**888–892.
7. **Waaler, E.** 1940. On the occurrence of a factor in human serum activating the specific agglutination of sheep blood corpuscles. Acta Pathol. Microbiol. Scand. **17:**172–178.
8. **Weinblatt, M. D., and P. C. Schur.** 1980. Rheumatoid factor detection by nephelometry. Arthritis Rheum. **23:**777–779.

time, although there are only sparse data on this question.

5. Control sera must be included in every test, using a positive control and a negative control for each semen sample. If the controls do not each give the expected result, the test results must be discarded. A saline solution should not be used as a negative control (although it may be an extra control); a negative serum is needed. A positive serum control for Kibrick tests may well be a different serum from that used as a positive control in other techniques.

6. The semen source may be completely unimportant. In a detailed study, it was found that in the vast majority of cases the same results were obtained for each serum, whether the semen was autologous (from the husband) or homologous (from a donor).

7. The ABO blood group status of the semen source has no influence on the results.

8. The mode of agglutination may be of interest. From other kinds of observations, it is known that clumping may occur head to head, tail to tail in the main part of the tail, tail tip to tail tip, and also in various tangled modes. The GAT is much more sensitive to tail-to-tail agglutination; a positive GAT result indicates the presence of tail antibody, but a negative GAT result does not prove the absence of head antibody (1).

9. Several studies have shown that the GAT type of agglutination is caused by immunoglobulin. This can be either IgG or IgM, although the former class is more common.

10. Application can be made to other fluids. The Kibrick test can be applied to seminal plasma and also to cervical mucus. Regarding seminal plasma, one may find lower or higher titers than in serum or no activity at all. It should be emphasized that a lack of activity does not necessarily mean that antibody is absent, since it may well be that the semen antibody has adhered to the sperm cells without showing any agglutination or immobilization. Sperm antibody in cervical mucus has been discussed elsewhere in some detail (8).

11. The tissue specificity has been explored. Positive sera have been tested against erythrocytes, leukocytes, and platelets; these were always negative. Various other clinical sera, containing antibodies to these three types of blood cells, were tested against spermatozoa; these were always negative also. Hence, it has been concluded that the Kibrick-positive sera are specific for spermatozoa (8).

PERFORMANCE OF THE TSAT

A method was introduced by Franklin and Dukes (reviewed in reference 8) for studying antibodies in women's sera. In this test, the final sperm concentration is quite low. It is diluted to 1:11 from the initial 50×10^6 cells per ml when mixed with the serum, thus giving 4.5×10^6 cells per ml. In our modification, introduced as the F-D test, we take readings only at 2 h.

Detailed test procedure (F-D method)

1. The serum samples are inactivated by heating at 56°C for 30 min. Each serum sample is diluted 1:4 with Baker buffer.

2. A fresh semen sample is diluted with Baker buffer to 50×10^6 cells per ml. The original semen sample should have a high degree of motility.

3. In a small test tube, 0.5 ml of each serum sample is mixed with 0.05 ml of the sperm suspension. The tubes are incubated at 37°C.

4. After 2 h of incubation, a drop is removed from each mixture and placed on a microscope slide under a cover slip for observation.

5. The total number of motile sperm cells is counted in each of 12 (or more) high-power fields, and the number of cells free or agglutinated is also noted, as well as the number of clumps and the nature of the agglutination (head to head, tail to tail, etc.).

6. The number of motile, clumped cells is divided by the total number of motile cells, to give a percentage. This should be at least 10% for the result to be considered positive.

Comments

1. Only a diluted serum should be studied; in our laboratory, we always use a 1:4-diluted serum, both in screening and in the repeat tests. Other investigators have used a dilution series and report a titer from the limiting dilution. Instead of a titer, we express TSAT results as a percentage index, as explained above. At any rate, sera that are concentrated at more than a 1:4 dilution should be used only with caution.

2. The total number of cells in clumps, of whatever size, is divided by the number of free and clumped cells, and this percentage is taken to be an index of the reaction. If this index is less than 10%, it is not significant; in other words, the serum is considered positive only if it gives a percentage of more than 10 (8). However, variations in values greater than 10% are of little significance with regard to the antibody titer.

3. In the method as modified by Boettcher and co-workers, the mixtures are made by using 10 drops of inactivated serum and 1 drop of the semen suspension. After incubation, the specimen, when observed on a slide, is quantitated and judged by criteria similar to those given above. In this system, one counts the number of clumps that are seen in a number of fields sufficient to permit one to count 100 motile, nonagglutinated sperm cells. The judgment is made by considering only those sample mixtures that give a result of 12/100 (6 agglutinates per 100 free cells) or greater to be positive.

PERFORMANCE OF THE TRAY AGGLUTINATION TEST

A microscopic method was developed by Friberg. This test is performed in disposable microchambers of a sort that are used in tissue-typing studies. The samples of semen and serum are measured in microliter quantities, using microsyringes to place the components of each reaction mixture in a circled area on the plate; as many as 18 tests can be performed in each microchamber. By using this technique, as many as 200 to 300 sera may be tested simultaneously with one sperm sample. The occurrence of a positive reaction and the intensity of such a reaction can be judged for each mixture by a single examination. However, an inverted microscope is needed, and the semen should have a preliminary processing to obtain better motility and clarity. The type of agglutination can be clearly revealed. Two main types of sperm agglutination have been distinguished, namely, tail to tail and head to head. The tail-to-tail sperm agglutination has been found more often in sera from men than in sera from women, whereas the head-to-head agglutination was more common in sera from women. Occasionally sera show a third variety, namely, tail tip-to-tail tip agglutination.

Detailed test procedure (Friberg method)

1. The serum to be tested is diluted with phosphate-buffered saline to give 1:4, 1:8, 1:16, and 1:32 dilutions.
2. A 5-µl quantity of each dilution is transferred by microsyringe to a sample site of a disposable microchamber, putting the sample under paraffin oil. The microsyringe is rinsed four times with saline between different serum samples.
3. Semen from a suitable donor is diluted with the saline to give a sperm concentration of 40×10^6 cells per ml.
4. A 1-µl quantity of the sperm suspension is added to 5 µl of each serum sample.
5. Each site is observed under the microscope, and agglutination is judged.

Comments

1. A large number of sera can be examined at one time, and many tests can be made with a small amount of semen.
2. It is easy to make titrations of each serum, since one can judge a positive result almost at a glance, rather than going through the labor of counting cells in a number of fields.
3. In contrast to the TSAT, there is no agitation of the sample mixture, as is done in the TSAT by transferring a drop from the tube to the slide.

PERFORMANCE OF THE CAPILLARY TUBE AGGLUTINATION TEST

One drop each of sperm suspension and antiserum are mixed, and the mixture is aspirated into a capillary tube of about 1-mm diameter. No addition of gelatin is necessary. Various dilutions of antiserum can be used, as well as normal serum for negative-control mixtures. Nonspecific agglutination is considerably inhibited (as compared with the situation in wider tubes), whereas the anticipated agglutination by antiserum proceeds well. Positive results are readily seen as a formation of clumps inside these capillaries, whereas the negative systems retain a uniform turbid appearance.

Detailed test procedure

1. Serum dilutions are prepared, using serological pipettes and tubes, with saline (0.15 M NaCl) or Baker buffer as the diluent.
2. A semen sample is diluted with Baker buffer to 40×10^6 cells per ml. The degree of motility of the

spermatozoa is not of critical importance, but the sperm cells should not be washed.
3. A small volume, generally 0.1 ml, of each serum dilution (beginning with the 1:4 dilution) is placed in a clean serological tube.
4. An equal volume of the sperm suspension is added to each tube, and the contents are gently mixed.
5. Each mixture is allowed to rise into and fill an unsealed capillary tube, 1.1 mm in diameter and 75 mm long. Blu-tip tubes are very satisfactory. One end of each tube is sealed with soft putty, and the tubes are stood upright (sealed end down) in a putty plate.
6. The tubes are incubated at room temperature (20 to 23°C), and results are recorded at 1 and 2 h.
7. Agglutination is seen as the appearance of white floccules, along with a clearing of the suspending medium.

Comments

1. The most important point to note is that immotile sperm cells can be used for this method; in fact, immotile spermatozoa may give a better titer with the antiserum than motile spermatozoa. It is not difficult, of course, to obtain immotile cells, since freshly available spermatozoa can be readily immobilized.
2. The technique as described above is for human spermatozoa. It was originally developed for guinea pig spermatozoa (8), using an initial sperm count of 10×10^6 cells per ml. Mixtures of this type are incubated at 4°C for 1 and 2 h, and observations of clumping can then be made. With rabbit spermatozoa, it was found that the best conditions for the test were a sperm concentration of 40×10^6 cells per ml, a temperature of about 20 to 25°C, and the use of washed rather than unwashed sperm cells. This is a most striking point; namely, much better activity is obtained by using well-washed spermatozoa. It was also found that the best incubation temperature was about 23 to 25°C. The preferred use of room temperature for incubation was in contrast to the preferred 4°C for guinea pig spermatozoa. Washing could be done with saline, phosphate-buffered saline, or Baker buffer. Motility was of no consequence to the results. In general, the titers were comparable to those obtained in Kibrick tests.
3. With human antisera, positive results could be obtained, but the titers were somewhat lower than in Kibrick tests. The optimum conditions were a sperm concentration of 40×10^6 cells per ml, a temperature of about 20 to 25°C, and the use of unwashed sperm cells. Unwashed spermatozoa gave much better results than washed spermatozoa.

SPERM IMMOBILIZATION PROCEDURES

The fact that some antibodies to spermatozoa can cause the immobilization of sperm cells, as long as the system contains complement, gave rise to the very first method developed for the detection of sperm antibody. However, the application of this method to the human clinical situation developed much later. The first extensive work with this method was that of Fjällbrant (reviewed in reference 8), who applied it to a number of clinical studies. His method, in essence, was to determine the time required for 90% or more of the motility to be lost in the test mixture, compared with the control mixture with negative serum. This control value was about 60 h. This method does not seem to have become widely used; its usefulness should be explored.

The second approach to an immobilization method for clinical purposes was that reported by Isojima and colleagues (4); they strongly recommended it as a good procedure for the exploration of human infertility problems. Their method was based on a different approach; it compared the ratio, after a standard time interval, of the surviving motility in the test mixture with that of the control mixture, and it selected those mixtures as positive in which the motility fell to one-half or less of that in the control mixture. The technique has become popular, and it has been used in a large number of studies; it is often referred to as the Isojima immobilization method.

PERFORMANCE OF THE SPERM IMMOBILIZATION TEST OF ISOJIMA

1. Human sperm cells of at least 70% motility and good forward progression are diluted to 60×10^6 cells per ml in Baker buffer.

2. As a source of complement, pooled fresh rabbit normal serum is used. Human and guinea pig sera may also be used.

3. As a positive-control serum, an appropriate dilution of rabbit anti-human sperm serum is used, such that it will immobilize about 90 to 95% of the sperm cells in 1 h in the presence of complement.

4. As a negative-control serum, a negative human serum (having no immobilizing activity) is used.

5. The control and test sera are inactivated at 56°C for 30 min.

6. To a small tube, 0.25 ml of inactivated test serum or control serum, 0.05 ml of complement solution, and 0.025 ml of fresh human semen dilution are added.

7. There should be a mixture for detecting any nonspecific sperm-immobilizing activity of the test serum; this mixture consists of 0.25 ml of the test serum plus the semen sample. There should be no immobilization in this mixture.

8. Incubate the mixtures at 37°C for 1 h.

9. Examine a drop of each mixture on a microscope slide at 100× to 250×, studying several fields for a reliable estimate. Measure the percentage of motility. Positive mixtures are those that have motilities one-half or less that of the negative-control mixture.

10. The initial study of each test serum is made at full concentration; those which are positive can then be titrated, for example, from 1:2 to 1:128 or more.

SOME NEWER METHODS FOR SPERM ANTIBODY

1. One method was proposed by Mathur and her colleagues (reviewed in reference 10); it is a rather complicated method, and I shall not discuss it in detail. It involves the preparation of erythrocytes that are coated with sperm extracts or seminal plasma for passive hemagglutination titrations with sera from patients. The method has not been fully evaluated; in particular, it was not standardized against a classical method.

2. The second new procedure was proposed by Haas et al. (reviewed in reference 10); it is quite simple in concept, although there are many technical maneuvers. This is a radiolabel-antiglobulin test; it is not a radioimmunoassay. Briefly, this method requires a rabbit anti-human IgG serum, from which the rabbit IgG is isolated and then radiolabeled with ^{125}I. A diluted donor sperm sample is incubated with undiluted plasma from the patient and then centrifuged and washed four times. The sample is then incubated with a measured amount of the radiolabeled anti-IgG and again centrifuged and washed four times. The remaining amount of sperm-associated radioactivity is determined in a gamma counter; above a certain numerical value, the result is called positive. The authors make great claims for the method, especially in calling it more specific and also more sensitive than other methods. However, it is not clear that these claims are fully justified; the authors do not have enough data for that. Instead, it can be said that this method is not worse than the GAT; on the other hand, it is more cumbersome.

3. A third new method is the application of the principles of the popular enzyme-linked immunosorbent assay. This has been attempted by several groups. The first, perhaps, was the effort by Ackerman et al. (reviewed in reference 10); they found this method to be quite satisfactory. Similar results were reported by Zanchetta et al., although they found it to be less sensitive than the Kibrick method. Again, similar results and conclusions were presented by Lenzi.

4. A fourth new method was proposed by Hancock (reviewed in reference 10). This method is a hemadsorption procedure.

5. Finally, a new method, which is a variation of complement-dependent cytotoxicity of spermatozoa, was proposed by Suominen et al. (reviewed in reference 10). It is based on measuring the release of ATP from the damaged cells.

INCIDENCE OF SPERM ANTIBODIES IN HUMAN POPULATIONS

Many worthy studies have been reported by various investigators (8, 10). Only a few main points can be considered here.

A large number of infertile couples have been analyzed in my own laboratory, using the classical methods described in this chapter. These couples were referred by a number of gynecologists; in the majority of cases, the couples had organic causes for infertility. Occasionally, a serum sample was not available from one of the partners, and so the summations are not equal.

Table 1 shows the antibody incidence for an accumulated total of about 400 infertile couples. For the GAT (Kibrick method), there were positive findings in 18% of the women and 9% of the men, and for the TSAT (F-D method) there were positive findings in 15% of the women and 5% of the men. Other studies, from a number of investigators, have given similar results.

Serum samples from about 100 fertile women, including pregnant women (antepartum patients) and immediate postpartum patients were also tested, us-

TABLE 1. *Incidence of positive results in serum samples from infertile couples*

Method	No. of patients tested		No. (%) positive	
	Female	Male	Female	Male
Kibrick (GAT)	409	381	72 (17.6)	33 (8.7)
F-D (TSAT)	389	347	58 (14.9)	17 (4.0)

ing the GAT and TSAT procedures. We found less than 3% to be positive in each of the tests (10).

The immobilization method should also be evaluated in terms of the incidence of positive results. According to Isojima et al. (4), positive findings were made in 18% of a group of 74 women from couples with unexplained infertility, whereas the incidence was zero in a group of 83 pregnant women. On the other hand, Vaidya and Glass have also used this method, and they found positive results in only 2.5% of a group of 40 women from infertile couples. It may be important to make further studies of the results of this method on several large groups of various types of populations (8).

LITERATURE CITED

1. **Boettcher, B., T. Hjort, P. Rümke, S. Shulman, and O. E. Vyazov.** 1977. Auto- and iso-antibodies to antigens of the human reproductive system. I. Results of an international comparative study. Clin. Exp. Immunol. **30:**173–180.

2. **Bronson, R. A., G. W. Cooper, and D. L. Rosenfeld.** 1982. Correlation between regional specificity of antisperm antibodies to the spermatozoan surface and complement-mediated sperm immobilization. Am. J. Reprod. Immunol. **2:**222–224.

3. **Clarke, G. N., and H. W. G. Baker.** 1982. Treatment of sperm antibodies in infertile men: sperm antibody coating and mucus penetration, p. 337–340. *In* K. Bratanov (ed.), Immunology of reproduction. Proceedings of the 5th International Symposium, Varna, 1982. Bulgarian Academy of Sciences, Sofia.

4. **Isojima, S., K. Tsuchiya, K. Koyama, C. Tanaka, O. Naka, and H. Adachi.** 1972. Further studies on sperm-immobilizing antibody found in sera of unexplained cases of sterility in women. Am. J. Obstet. Gynecol. **112:**199–207.

5. **Jager, S., J. Kremer, and T. van Slochteren-Draaisma.** 1978. A simple method of screening for antisperm antibodies in the human male. Detection of spermatozoal surface IgG with the direct mixed antiglobulin reaction carried out on untreated fresh semen. Int. J. Fertil. **23:**12–21.

6. **Rose, N. R., T. Hjort, P. Rümke, M. J. Harper, and O. Vyazov.** 1976. Workshop on techniques for detection of iso- and auto-antibodies to human spermatozoa. Clin. Exp. Immunol. **23:**175–199.

7. **Rümke, P.** 1954. The presence of sperm antibodies in the serum of two patients with oligospermia. Vox Sang. **4:**135–140.

8. **Shulman, S.** 1975. Reproduction and antibody response. CRC Press, Cleveland.

9. **Shulman, S.** 1978. Agglutinating and immobilizing antibodies, p. 81–99. *In* J. Cohen and W. F. Hendry (ed.), Spermatozoa, antibodies and infertility. Blackwell Scientific Publications, Ltd., Oxford.

10. **Shulman, S.** 1985. Autoimmune aspects of human reproduction, p. 189–227. *In* J. M. Cruse (ed.), Concepts in immunopathology. S. Karger, Basel.

Interpretation

See immune adherence assay above.

MIXED HEMADSORPTION ASSAY

Materials and reagents

Fresh sheep blood
Alsever solution
0.15 M NaCl
VBM
GGF-FCS
Sodium azide
PBS

Preparation of indicator cells

1. The mixed hemadsorption assay works best when sheep erythrocytes (SRBC) have been in Alsever solution at 4°C for 1 to 4 weeks.
2. Wash SRBC in a large volume of sterile 0.15 M NaCl three times by graduated centrifugation (see above).
3. Suspend the final pellet to make a 20% suspension of SRBC in a 5% solution of GGF-FCS in VBM (GGF-VBM). This suspension can be stored for 1 week at 4°C.
4. The optimal dilution of the amboceptor should be determined by hemagglutination tests. In these tests, 50 µl of serial double dilutions of human serum containing antibody to SRBC, or of nonhuman primate serum containing antibody to SRBC, in 5% GGF-VBM is incubated with 50 µl of 2% SRBC in microtiter plates for 1 h. Agglutination is determined macroscopically. The concentration of amboceptor used for the preparation of indicator cells is the highest concentration that does not produce agglutination.
5. Add 1 volume of the chosen dilution of the amboceptor to 1 volume of 2% SRBC and incubate, with gentle shaking, for 1 h at room temperature.
6. Wash twice with sterile 1% GGF-VBM by graduated centrifugation.
7. Suspend in 5% GGF-VBM to a final SRBC concentration of 2%. Add sodium azide to a final concentration of 1:1,000 (a 1:100 dilution of a 10% [wt/vol] stock solution in PBS).
8. The indicator cells can be stored for up to 2 weeks at 4°C. If hemolysis occurs, wash the cells twice with 1% GGF-FBM before they are used.

Test procedure and interpretation

See PA hemadsorption assay above.

ROSETTING ASSAYS WITH NONADHERENT CELLS

For further information, see reference 3.

Materials and reagents

FCS
Microtest plates
Dulbecco PBS (DPBS)
Concanavalin A
PBS

Preparation of target cell plates

1. Add 10 µl of 5% FCS in minimal essential culture medium to the wells of the Microtest plates.
2. Incubate the plates overnight at 37°C in a 5% CO_2 incubator.
3. Add 10 ml of DPBS to each plate, and wash three times.
4. Blot the plates with gauze.
5. Add 10 µl of a 0.1% concanavalin A solution in DPBS. Keep the concanavalin A solution at −20°C until it is used.
6. Incubate the plates at room temperature for 45 min.
7. Wash the plates twice with DPBS, and blot them with gauze.
8. Add 10 µl of a 0.5% (vol/vol) suspension of target cells in DPBS to the wells.
9. Keep the plates for 45 min at room temperature.
10. Wash the plates twice with 5% FCS-PBS; they are now ready for use in serological assays.

ABSORPTION TESTS

Materials and reagents

Cell culture flasks
FCS
PBS
Absorption tubes (6 by 50 mm)
Conical tubes (15 and 50 ml)

Test procedure

1. Grow the cells to be used for absorption in flasks with 150 cm^2 of bottom surface area.
2. When cultures are confluent, remove the culture medium and add 10 ml of 3% FCS in PBS (3% FCS-PBS).
3. Scrape off the cells with a rubber policeman.
4. Wash the cells twice with 50 ml of 3% FCS-PBS by centrifugation at $170 \times g$ for 10 min.
5. Transfer the cells to 15-ml conical tubes, fill the tubes with 3% FCS-PBS, and pellet the cells by graduated centrifugation (see above).
6. Estimate the cell pellet volume, drain the tubes, and dry the edges of the tubes carefully with gauze.
7. Suspend the cells at a 20% (vol/vol) concentration in 3% FCS-PBS. Transfer the cell suspension to absorption tubes (6 by 50 mm). For qualitative absorption tests, 150 µl of the 20% cell suspension is transferred. For quantitative absorption tests, the volume of cell suspension used ranges from 10 to 300 µl.
8. Centrifuge the absorption tubes by graduated centrifugation.
9. Remove the supernatant carefully with a Pasteur pipette. The cell pellet will be 30 µl for qualitative absorptions.
10. Add 30 µl of the appropriately diluted test serum to the absorption tubes. In quantitative absorption tests, the volume of serum is kept constant, and the volume of absorbing cells is titrated.

To determine the appropriate serum dilution to be used in an absorption test, a pretest should be done. For absorption, serum is used at a concentration four times higher than the concentration at which 50% of the target cells form rosettes with the indicator cells. It is critical to determine in this way the dilution at which the serum should be absorbed.

11. Incubate the cell suspension for 30 min at room temperature and for 30 min at 4°C, with frequent vortexing.

12. Recover the absorbed serum by graduated centrifugation.

13. Remove absorbed serum with a Pasteur pipette, and prepare serial double dilutions of the serum in medium appropriate for the assay. These dilutions will be used to determine remaining antibody reactivity.

14. Perform antibody assays as indicated above.

LITERATURE CITED

1. **Albino, A. P., K. O. Lloyd, A. N. Houghton, H. F. Oettgen, and L. J. Old.** 1981. Heterogeneity in surface antigen expression and glycoprotein expression of cell lines derived from different metastases of the same patient: implications for the study of tumor antigens. J. Exp. Med. **154**:1764–1778.

2. **Carey, T. E., T. Takahashi, L. A. Resnik, H. F. Oettgen, and L. J. Old.** 1976. Cell surface antigens of human malignant melanoma. I. Mixed hemadsorption assays for humoral immunity to cultured autologous melanoma cells. Proc. Natl. Acad. Sci. U.S.A. **73**:3278–3282.

3. **Mattes, M. J., M. Tanimoto, M. S. Pollack, and D. H. Maurer.** 1983. Preparing monolayers of non-adherent mammalian cells. J. Immunol. Methods **61**:145–150.

4. **Old, L. J.** 1981. Cancer immunology: the search for specificity. G. H. A. Clowes Memorial Lecture. Cancer Res. **41**:361–375.

5. **Pfreundschuh, M., H. Shiku, T. Takahashi, R. Ueda, J. Ransohoff, H. F. Oettgen, and L. J. Old.** 1976. Serological analysis of cell surface antigens of malignant human brain tumors. Proc. Natl. Acad. Sci. U.S.A. **74**:5122–5126.

6. **Real, F. X., M. I. Mattes, A. N. Houghton, H. F. Oettgen, K. O. Lloyd, and L. J. Old.** 1984. Class I (unique) antigens of human melanoma. Identification of a 90,000 dalton cell surface glycoprotein by autologous antibody. J. Exp. Med. **160**:1219–1233.

7. **Shiku, H., T. Takahashi, H. F. Oettgen, and L. J. Old.** 1976. Cell surface antigens of human malignant melanoma. II. Serological typing with immune adherence assays and definition of two new surface antigens. J. Exp. Med. **144**:873–881.

8. **Shiku, H., T. Takahashi, L. A. Resnik, H. F. Oettgen, and L. J. Old.** 1977. Cell surface antigens of human malignant melanoma. III. Recognition of autoantibodies with unusual characteristics. J. Exp. Med. **145**:784–789.

9. **Ueda, R., H. Shiku, M. Pfreundschuh, T. Takahashi, L. T. C. Li, W. F. Whitmore, Jr., H. F. Oettgen, and L. J. Old.** 1979. Cell surface antigens of human renal cancers defined by autologous typing. J. Exp. Med. **150**:564–579.

10. **Watanabe, T., C. S. Pukel, H. Takeyama, K. O. Lloyd, H. Shiku, L. T. C. Li, L. R. Travassos, H. F. Oettgen, and L. J. Old.** 1982. Human melanoma antigen AH is an autoantigenic ganglioside related to GD2. J. Exp. Med. **156**:1884–1890.

3. Surgical resection, though not curative, was associated with a decrease in CEA levels.

4. CEA levels progressively increase in patients with widespread metastatic pancreatic carcinoma.

Since extrahepatic obstruction, by cancer of the head of the pancreas or of the bile ducts, may raise the CEA level, the clinician may assume an even worse prognosis than is warranted. Thus, in the nonjaundiced patient, a CEA level above 20 ng/ml appeared to preclude resectability in Barkin's study; this indication was not correct when the CEA elevations were due in part to extrahepatic biliary obstruction. Transhepatic percutaneous catheter drainage of bile to release the obstruction allows one to distinguish the degree of elevation of CEA in plasma attributable to the obstruction alone from the residual elevation due to persistent tumor production (39). The presence of CEA in pancreatic juice may also provide a clue to the presence of cancer.

CEA IN BREAST CANCER

CEA measurement is of no use for the diagnostic screening for breast carcinoma (12), since it is not specific, and elevations observed in patients with "operable" breast carcinoma overlap the range of levels encountered in benign breast disease. CEA levels in plasma correlate with staging (from 14.8 ng/ml with stage I to 73 ng/ml with stage IV) and with the size of the local tumor.

Postoperative CEA measurements are useful for indicating the presence or absence of metastasis. Neville (see reference 12) showed that in 11% of patients monitored postmastectomy, rising CEA levels were observed before the clinical detection of metastasis, and in 45%, the elevation was synchronous with the clinical detection of metastasis. Elevations of CEA (>10 ng/ml) are reported to appear from 1 to 15 months (4 to 6, average) before the clinical detection of metastatic disease. Some reports define elevations as >10 ng/ml, and others define them as low as >2.5 ng/ml. Hence, reported figures given for the clinical usefulness of CEA vary.

Response to therapy

There is agreement that serial CEA levels correctly monitor clinical response to therapy for metastatic breast cancer.

Serial CEAs in 168 patients with metastases and elevated CEA levels monitored well the effect of therapy on disease status (14a). Lokich et al. found 100% correlation between serial changes in CEA level and response to therapy in patients with CEA levels above 35 ng/ml, but a poor correlation in those with CEA levels between 5 and 15 ng/ml (18).

Because CEA levels are infrequently elevated in patients with operable breast cancer and elevated in only about 50% of patients with overt metastases, there is an active search for other tumor markers to supplement or replace CEA measurements. At present, only CEA is in widespread clinical use.

SMALL-CELL CANCER OF THE LUNG

Eight-five cases of small-cell cancer of the lung (9, 11) were reviewed to evaluate the clinical usefulness of CEA levels in plasma. All patients with CEA > 10 ng/ml had extrathoracic metastases, and all patients with CEA > 50 ng/ml had liver metastases. Serial CEAs in 60 patients showed that all patients with elevated pretreatment CEAs had a fall in CEA with therapeutic response or a rise with progression.

Eighteen cases (nine with CEA < 5 ng/ml, nine with CEA > 5 ng/ml) were selected for histological review and CEA immunoperoxidase staining. In summary, (i) plasma CEA was useful in staging and monitoring response to chemotherapy, (ii) CEA tissue staining predicted the clinical usefulness of CEA in 15 of 18 patients studied, and (iii) no correlation was seen between histological subtype and immunoperoxidase staining of tumor.

CEA IN MTC

The distribution of CEA and its relationship to calcitonin in early, localized, and disseminated (virulent) medullary thyroid carcinoma (MTC; 23) was studied by immunoperoxidase methods. CEA was demonstrated within C cells though all stages of progression of MTC. In early disease (C-cell hyperplasia and microscopic carcinoma), CEA and calcitonin were present in virtually every cell. There was a similar, homogeneous distribution among cells in gross medullary carcinoma confined to the thyroid region. In patients with virulent, disseminated MTC, there was an inverse relationship between calcitonin and CEA distribution.

Rougier and associates (27a) also showed that CEA appeared to be capable of defining a subgroup of patients with MTC at high risk for aggressive behavior. Thus, the finding of persistently high or increasing circulating CEA levels in the face of falling or stable calcitonin levels may predict aggressive clinical behavior.

ROLE OF THE LIVER: MECHANISM OF CLEARANCE AND EXCRETION OF CEA

The liver plays a key role in regulating CEA levels (36). All varieties of liver disease, i.e., hepatitis, cirrhosis, and cholestasis (benign and malignant, intra- and extrahepatic), are associated with increased levels of CEA in plasma.

The failure to detect elevated CEA levels in the plasma of patients with early colonic cancer may be due in part to the ability of the normal liver to clear CEA and prevent such rises. There is a need to devise strategies for reversibly impeding this clearance so that the circulating level will more directly reflect the load of CEA produced by the tumor. See Thomas and Zamcheck (36) for a recent review. Inhibition of this mechanism or of the initial Kupffer cell uptake should be accompanied by a rise in CEA levels in plasma, reflecting true production by a tumor source. Kupffer cell function and thus CEA clearance may be impaired by obstructive jaundice. Approximately 50% of patients with benign extrahepatic obstructive jaundice have mildly elevated CEA levels which fall on decompression. The mechanism of this effect is not known, although damage to cell membranes by high concentrations of bile salts is a possibility. The measurement of lysosomal enzymes such as β-N-acetyl hexosaminidase that are normally cleared by the Kupffer cell may be useful in this regard (E. Scapa, P. Thomas, M. S. Loewenstein, and N. Zamcheck, Gastroenterology **84**:1394, 1983). Such measurements help to distinguish benign from malignant extrahepatic biliary obstructions. All of 16 patients with malignant obstruction had hexosaminidase levels above 30 U/liter, whereas only 1 of 12 patients with benign biliary tract obstruction had hexosaminidase levels that high.

Menard et al. (22) pointed out that many anticancer agents may damage the liver by interfering with liver cell metabolism, by impairing biliary excretion, or by direct hepatotoxicity. Savrin and Martin reported a patient whose CEA levels increased in the absence of tumor recurrence with the administration of 5-fluorouracil (29). Since drug therapy may influence clinical decision making based on CEA changes, these changes need much more study.

The major factor in the elevation of CEA levels in plasma in the patient with advanced cancer remains increased production of CEA and increased entry into the circulation caused by tumor invasion. Patients with hepatic metastases tend to have the highest levels.

Recent studies have shown that the carbohydrate heterogeneity of CEA may affect its clearance by the liver (R. A. Byrn, P. Thomas, P. L. Medreck, and N. Zamcheck, Clin. Res., **31**:694A, 1983). In a series of patients with very high CEA levels but with good-performance status, we found that their CEA (obtained from ascites) cleared much more slowly from the circulation of rats than did other CEAs. This slowly clearing CEA had an increased sialic acid and decreased fucose content compared with CEAs that cleared rapidly.

Saravis is developing a clinically useful test to distinguish between the low- and high-sialated CEAs by utilizing sophisticated isoelectric focusing separations (P. Thomas, C. A. Toth, R. A. Byrn, C. A. Saravis, M. S. Loewenstein, G. D. Steele, R. J. Meyer, and N. Zamcheck, Clin. Res. **31**:696A, 1983).

The use of substances to inhibit CEA clearance by the liver may allow the direct measurement of CEA input into the circulation and help in the detection of tumors now undetectable.

A FEW METHODOLOGICAL CONSIDERATIONS

Two commercially available reagent kits are approved by the Food and Drug Administration for clinical use. The Roche radioimmunoassay has been in clinical use for more than 10 years. It requires perchloric acid extraction and dialysis or gel chromatography of the plasma sample before the determination. Abbott Laboratories produced an enzyme immunoassay kit which utilizes a heat extraction procedure. Both procedures have been reported to be technically sound and to provide reproducible results. The two methods produced equivalent determinations in about 80% of the cases, with the remaining determinations discordant. In general, the serial assay findings tend to show the same trend as the clinical course of a given patient, i.e., they reflect the response or lack of response to treatment. The absolute levels obtained by the methods may differ. The Food and Drug Ad-

ministration requires that CEA assay reports identify the method used and urges that the same assay be used throughout the clinical course of a single patient. Clinical decisions (for surgery or for changing chemotherapy, for example) based on an unexpected change in CEA levels in blood may be misleading if the change is caused by a switch in assay method. The Consensus Conference Panel recommended that each laboratory performing CEA assays establish its own "normal" range.

In Europe, a number of other commercial assays are now available, and new methods for measuring CEA are emerging steadily. The degree to which variations in findings by different methods reflect the heterogeneity of cancer cells and of the amounts and nature of their products requires further study.

There is a considerable structural variability in the carbohydrate portions of the CEA molecule; also, several different antigenic determinants are known to be present on CEA, some shared with molecules biochemically different from CEA. Thus, in CEA analysis the method of sample preparation, the antibody utilized for CEA recognition, and the matrix utilized for the assay (solid or liquid phase) may all affect the amount of CEA measured. As new CEA assays are clinically tested, the methodology should be stated, and the findings should be compared with those of established assay procedures.

Need to standardize CEA assay and reagents

The Gastrointestinal Tumor Study Group conducted an experiment to address the issue of reproducibility of CEA assays performed at participating institutions and at a central laboratory (15). Samples were drawn in quadruplicate from 37 patients representing five participating institutions. Systematic biases were observed in four of the five institutions; i.e., two series were consistently higher and two series were consistently lower than those measured by the central laboratory. Significantly higher variations were found in three of the five series when the sample variances associated with the matching assay series were compared. Overall, the standard deviation associated with the central laboratory findings was one-third that of the participating institutions. These results point out a limitation in the pooling of multiinstitutional CEA data. The use of multivariate models with parameters for institution comparison was proposed as a solution to this problem.

This study was done at a time when there was only one assay method available, the radioimmunoassay of Roche, the single supplier of reagents. The problem is now more complex, and the need for standardization is even greater. In this regard, the use of monoclonal antibodies has the great potential advantage of providing a large supply of monospecific reagents.

New candidate markers and the remarkable durability of CEA

Studies performed on CEA, both basic and applied, have proved to be prototype studies (38). They have stimulated the development of many new candidate markers for cancers of many organs (including the digestive tract, pancreas, lung, ovary, breast, and prostate). Comparison of these markers with CEA is essential. The pancreatic cancer marker pancreatic oncofetal antigen and other markers are under study. The initial report that galactosyl transferase II was more specific than CEA for pancreatic cancer has not yet been confirmed. CA 125 from Centocor shows promise of being a useful monitor for ovarian adenocarcinoma, and large-scale studies of this antigen, as well as of CA 19-9 from Centocor, are under way (see chapters 126 and 127).

The use by Goldenberg, Order, and others of tagged antibodies for directly targeting therapy to the tumor has opened new therapeutic opportunities beyond the scope of this chapter.

The application of monoclonal antibody technology, first to CEA and then to its several epitopes, has yielded potentially useful candidate antibodies of different specificities. Shively (31) has summarized the burgeoning work on the new monoclonal antibodies to CEA. The widespread availability of these antibodies has sparked a renewal of both clinical and basic research on CEA and CEA-related antigens in normal and malignant tissues. Whether these antibodies will prove useful for the detection and monitoring of cancers of specific cell types and for the selection of specific therapy remains to be studied (14). Despite the greater specificity of the assays utilizing single monoclonal antibodies, these antibodies are unlikely to entirely replace polyclonal CEA antibodies. The "broad spectrum" reactivity of polyclonal antibodies used in immunoassays for measuring CEA may be advantageous in monitoring some patients. Combinations of monoclonal antibodies to several epitopes are now being recommended by some investigators in the effort to achieve more specificities useful for clinical purposes.

The durability of CEA as a useful clinical marker derives in part from the fact that one or more of the CEA-reactive epitopes produced by most of the common adenocarcinomas are "picked up" by the broad-spectrum polyclonal anti-CEA antibodies used initially in commercially available test kits. The very nonspecificity of the antibody may account for its usefulness.

Does the heterogeneity of the CEA molecule reflect the changing nature of tumor cells during a changing clinical course? Will the use of antibodies of different specificities prove advantageous when tumor cells produce glycoproteins of altered antigenic specificity, possibly caused by chemotherapy or by other means?

The investigation of the biology, pathology, physiology, and metabolism of CEA and its related glycoproteins continues to elucidate the nature of human cancer at the same time it helps us manage the cancer patients.

This work was supported by Public Health Service grant CA-04486 from the National Cancer Institute.

LITERATURE CITED

1. Barkin, J. S., M. H. Kalser, R. Kaplan, D. Redlhammer, and A. Heal. 1978. Initial levels of CEA and their rate of change in pancreatic carcinoma following surgery, chemotherapy and radiation therapy. Cancer 42:1472–1476.

2. Bronstein, B. R., G. D. Steele, Jr., W. Ensminger, W. D. Kaplan, M. S. Loewenstein, R. E. Wilson, J. Forman, and N. Zamcheck. 1980. The use and limitations of serial plasma carcinoembryonic antigen (CEA) levels as a monitor of changing metastatic liver tumor volume in patients receiving chemotherapy. Cancer 46:266–272.

3. Dhar, P., T. Moore, N. Zamcheck, and H. Z. Kupchik. 1972. Carcinoembryonic antigen (CEA) in colonic cancer. Use in preoperative and postoperative diagnosis and prognosis. J. Am. Med. Assoc. 221:31–52.

4. Gastrointestinal Tumor Study Group. 1984. Phase II study of methyl-CCNU, vincristine, 5-fluorouracil, and streptozotocin in advanced colorectal cancer. J. Clin. Oncol. 2:770–773.

5. Go, V. L. W., and N. Zamcheck. 1982. The role of tumor markers in the management of colorectal cancer. Cancer 50:2618–2623.

6. Goldenberg, D. M., E. E. Kim, S. J. Bennett, M. O. Nelson, and R. H. Deland. 1983. Carcinoembryonic antigen radioimmunodetection in the evaluation of colorectal cancer and in the detection of occult neoplasms. Gastroenterology 84:524–532.

7. Goldenberg, D. M., M. Neville, A. C. Carter, V. L. W. Go, E. D. Holyoke, K. J. Isselbacher, P. S. Schein, and M. Schwartz. 1981. Carcinoembryonic antigen: its role as a marker in the management of cancer. A National Institutes of Health Consensus Development Conference. Ann. Intern. Med. 94:407–409.

8. Goslin, R., M. J. O'Brien, G. Steele, R. Mayer, R. Wilson, J. M. Corson, and N. Zamcheck. 1981. Correlation of plasma CEA and CEA tissue staining in poorly differentiated colorectal cancer. Am. J. Med. 71:246–253.

9. Goslin, R., G. Steele, Jr., J. MacIntyre, R. Mayer, P. Sugarbaker, K. Cleghorn, R. Wilson, and N. Zamcheck. 1980. The use of preoperative plasma CEA levels for the stratification of patients after curative resection of colorectal cancer. Ann. Surg. 192:747–751.

10. Goslin, R. H., M. J. O'Brien, A. T. Skarin, and N. Zamcheck. 1983. Immunocytochemical staining for CEA in small cell carcinoma of lung predicts clinical usefulness of the plasma assay. Cancer 52:301–306.

11. Goslin, R. H., A. T. Skarin, and N. Zamcheck. 1981. Carcinoembryonic antigen: a useful monitor of therapy of small cell lung cancer. J. Am. Med. Assoc. 246:2173–2176.

12. Haagensen, D. E., Jr. 1982. Tumor markers for breast carcinoma, p. 543–565. In B. E. Statland and P. Winkel (ed.), Clinics in laboratory medicine, vol. 2, no. 3. Symposium on laboratory measurements in malignant disease. The W. B. Saunders Co., Philadelphia.

13. Herrera, M. A., T. M. Chu, and E. D. Holyoke. 1976. Carcinoembryonic antigen (CEA) as a prognostic and monitoring test in clinically complete resection of colorectal carcinoma. Ann. Surg. 183:5–17.

14. Kupchik, H. Z., V. R. Zurawski, Jr., J. G. R. Hurrell, N. Zamcheck, and P. H. Black. 1981. Monoclonal antibodies to carcinoembryonic antigen produced by somatic cell fusion. Cancer Res. 41:3306–3310.

14a. Lamerz, R., A. Leonhardt, H. Ehrhart, and H. von Lieven. 1980. Serial carcinoembryonic antigen (CEA) determinations in the management of metastatic breast cancer. Oncodev. Biol. Med. 1:123–135.

15. Lavin, P. T., N. Zamcheck, and E. D. Holyoke (for the Gastrointestinal Tumor Study Group). 1979. A CEA standardization experiment for the conduct of multi-institutional clinical trials. Cancer Treat. Rep. 63:2031–2033.

16. Lokich, J., S. Ellenberg, B. Gerson, W. E. Knox, and N. Zamcheck. 1984. Plasma clearance of carcinoembryonic antigen following hepatic metastatectomy. J. Clin. Oncol. 2:462–465.

17. Lokich, J. J., S. Ellenberg, and B. Gerson. 1984. Criteria for monitoring carcinoembryonic antigen: variability of sequential assays at elevated levels. J. Clin. Oncol. 2:181–186.

18. Lokich, J. J., N. Zamcheck, and M. Loewenstein. 1978. Sequential carcinoembryonic antigen levels in the therapy of metastatic breast cancer. Ann. Intern. Med. 89:902–906.

19. Mach, J. P., P. H. Jaeger, M.-M. Bertholet, C.-H. Ruegsegger, R. M. Loosli, and J. Pettavel. 1974. Detection of recurrence of large bowel carcinoma by a radioimmunoassay of circulating carcinoembryonic antigen (CEA). Lancet ii:535–540.

20. Martin, E. W., K. J. James, P. E. Hurtubise, P. Catalano, and J. P. Minto. 1977. The use of CEA as an early indicator for gastrointestinal tumor recurrence and second-look procedures. Cancer 39:440–446.

21. Mayer, R. J., M. B. Garnick, G. D. Steele, and N. Zamcheck. 1978. Carcinoembryonic antigen (CEA) as a monitor of chemotherapy in disseminated colorectal cancer. Cancer 42:1428–1433.

22. Menard, D. B., C. Gisselbrecht, M. Marty, F. Reyes, and D. Chumeaux. 1980. Antineoplastic agents and the liver. Gastroenterology 78:142–164.

23. Mendelsohn, G., S. A. Wells, Jr., and S. B. Baylin. 1984. Relationship of tissue carcinoembryonic antigen and calcitonin in tumor virulence in medullary thyroid carcinoma: an immunohistochemical study in early, localized, and virulent disseminated states of disease. Cancer 54:657–662.

24. Minton, J. P., and E. W. Martin, Jr. 1978. The use of serial CEA determinations to predict recurrence of colon cancer and when to do a second look operation. Cancer 42:1422–1430.

25. Moertel, C. G., A. J. Schutt, and V. L. W. Go. 1978. Carcinoembryonic antigen test for recurrent colorectal carcinoma. Inadequacy for early detection. J. Am. Med. Assoc. 239:1065–1100.

26. O'Brien, M. J., B. Bronstein, N. Zamcheck, C. Saravis, B. Burke, and L. S. Gottlieb. 1980. Cholestasis and hepatic metastases: a factor contributing to extreme elevations of carcinoembryonic antigen. J. Natl. Cancer Inst. 64:1291–1294.

26a.Ravry, M., V. L. W. Go, A. J. Schutt, and C. G. Moertel. 1973. Usefulness of serial serum carcinoembryonic antigen (CEA) during anti-cancer therapy or long term follow up of gastrointestinal cancer. Cancer Chemother. Rep. 57:493–495.

27. Riittgers, R. A., G. Steele, N. Zamcheck, M. S. Loewenstein, P. H. Sugarbaker, R. J. Mayer, J. J. Lokich, J. Maltz, and R. E. Wilson. 1978. Transient carcinoembryonic antigen (CEA) elevations following resection of colorectal cancer: a limitation in the use of serial CEA levels as an indicator for second-look surgery. J. Natl. Cancer Inst. 61:315–318.

27a.Rougier, P. H., C. Calmettes, A. Laplanche, J. P. Travagli, M. Lefevre, C. Parmentier, G. Milhaud, and M. Tubiana. 1983. The values of calcitonin and carcinoembryonic antigen in the treatment and management of nonfamilial medullary thyroid carcinoma. Cancer 51:855–862.

28. Rule, A. H. 1984. A decade of CEA testing. J. Clin. Immunoassay 7:101–132.

29. Savrin, R. A., and E. W. Martin. 1981. The relationship of the possible hepatic toxicity of chemotherapeutic drugs and carcinoembryonic antigen evaluation. Cancer 47:481–485.

30. Shani, A., M. J. O'Connell, C. G. Moertel, A. J. Schutt, A. Silvers, and V. L. W. Go. 1978. Serial plasma carcinoembryonic antigen measurements in the management of metastatic colorectal carcinoma. Ann. Intern. Med. 86:627–630.

31. Shively, J. E. 1984. Monoclonal antibodies to CEA. J. Clin. Immunoassay 7:112–119.

32. Staab, H. J., F. A. Anderer, E. Stumpf, and R. Fischer. 1978. Carcinoembryonic antigen follow-up and selection of patients for second look operation in management of gastrointestinal carcinoma. J. Surg. Oncol. 10:273–280.

33. Steele, G., Jr., S. Ellenberg, K. Ramming, M. O'Connell, C. Moertel, H. Lessner, H. Bruckner, J. Horton, P. Schein, N. Zamcheck, J. Novak, and E. D. Holyoke. 1982. CEA monitoring among patients in multiinstitutional adjuvant G.I. therapy protocols. Ann. Surg. 196:162–169.

34. Steele, G., Jr., R. T. Osteen, R. E. Wilson, D. C. Brooks, R. J. Mayer, N. Zamcheck, and T. S. Ravikumar. 1984. Patterns of failure after surgical cure of large liver tumors: a change in the proximate cause of death and a need for effective systemic adjuvant therapy. Am. J. Surg. 147:554–559.

35. Steele, G., Jr., N. Zamcheck, and R. E. Wilson. 1981. Serial CEA in the follow-up of patients after "curative" resection of colorectal cancer, p. 150–155. In T. O'Connel (ed.), Controversies in surgical oncology. G. K. Hall & Co., Boston.

36. Thomas, P., and N. Zamcheck. 1983. Role of the liver in clearance and excretion of circulating carcinoembryonic antigen (CEA). Dig. Dis. Sci. 28:216–224.

37. Wanebo, H. J., M. Stearns, and M. K. Schwartz. 1978. Use of CEA as an indicator of early recurrence and as a guide to a selected second-look procedure in patients with colorectal cancer. Ann. Surg. 188:481–493.

38. Zamcheck, N. 1981. The expanding field of colorectal cancer markers: CEA, the prototype. Cancer Bull. 33:141–151.

39. Zamcheck, N., and E. W. Martin. 1981. Factors controlling the circulating CEA levels in pancreatic cancer: some clinical correlations. Cancer 47:1620–1627.

Chapter 125

Monitoring of Patients with Testicular Cancer by Assays for Alpha-Fetoprotein and Human Chorionic Gonadotropin

ROBERT L. VESSELLA AND PAUL H. LANGE

BACKGROUND

AFP

Alpha-fetoprotein (AFP) is a single-chain glycoprotein with a molecular weight of approximately 70,000. It is produced by the fetal yolk sac and proximal structures of the liver and gastrointestinal tract. In the human fetus, AFP is a major serum protein which reaches a level of several milligrams per milliliter at week 12 of gestation and then drops to 50 μg/ml at birth. After 1 year of age, the concentration of AFP declines to less than 16 ng/ml and remains at this low level throughout life unless certain normal or pathological events occur. For example, elevations in AFP concentration always accompany pregnancy and sometimes accompany benign liver diseases, especially those that are acute and severe. Furthermore, tumors that are derived from the fetal structures that produce AFP may also begin producing this protein (thus, AFP is classified as an oncodevelopmental protein). The tumors which most commonly produce AFP are primary hepatocellular carcinoma and the germ cell tumors. In this chapter we will discuss AFP in the clinical context of germ cell tumors of the testes. The clinical situations which are associated with elevated circulating levels of AFP are listed in Table 1.

The clinical value of AFP as a tumor marker was not immediately appreciated because the assays used for quantitation were not sensitive enough to detect the nanogram amounts associated with early disease. As more sensitive radioimmune assays became available (see below) the utility of AFP as a tumor marker became increasingly apparent, and today it is an important serum marker for germ cell tumors and for primary hepatocellular carcinoma. But for germ cell tumors, AFP as a tumor marker cannot be studied alone; it must be measured along with human chorionic gonadotropin (hCG).

hCG

hCG is normally secreted by the syncytiotrophoblastic cells of the placenta, and its early appearance after conception made it the universally accepted pregnancy marker. hCG is a glycoprotein with a molecular weight of approximately 38,000. Like many ectopic hormones, hCG consists of two noncovalently linked polypeptide chains, designated alpha and beta. The alpha chain is nearly identical both immunologically and biochemically to the alpha subunits of the pituitary hormones lutenizing hormone (LH), follicle-stimulating hormone, and thyroid-stimulating hormone. The beta subunit of hCG shares considerable structural homology with the beta subunit of LH, although the hCG beta subunit does contain a unique carboxyl terminus consisting of approximately 30 amino acids which is not found in the other glycoprotein hormones. This distinction confers biological specificity and substantial, although not absolute, immunological specificity.

Zondek (10) is credited with making the first observation that hCG was present in the sera of some men with germ cell tumors. As with AFP, the value of this marker was not realized until more sensitive radioimmune assays revealed hCG in the serum of 40 to 60% of patients with nonseminomatous germ cell tumors (NSGCT). hCG elevations also have been associated with other malignancies (Table 1). Neoplasms associated with hCG production occasionally secrete abnormal forms of the molecule or its subunits. For example, some tumors have been shown to secrete alpha or beta chains exclusively, or mixtures of subunits and whole molecules. Free chains have relatively short serum half-lives, 20 min for the alpha chain and less than 45 min for the beta chain. Whole-molecule hCG has a metabolic half-life of between 24 and 48 h. As a result, some caution is necessary in interpreting the rate of decline of circulating hCG levels before treatment (see below).

Purification of the tumor markers and development of immunoassays

The purification of AFP is complicated by the fact that it must be separated from albumin, which is present in all source materials (reviewed in reference 7). Also, because AFP is microheterogeneous, the proportion of AFP molecules which bind to concanavalin A is dependent on the source of AFP; this proportion ranges from approximately 90% reactive if the AFP is primarily derived from liver components to 50% or less if the source of AFP is yolk sac or malignantly transformed yolk sac progeny (8). The most common sources of AFP include cord serum (15 μg of AFP per ml), second trimester amniotic fluid (15 μg/ml), amniotic fluid from an early pregnancy with an encephalic fetus (600 μg/ml), or ascitic fluid or serum from patients with primary hepatocellular carcinoma (200 μg/ml). All of these sources are rich in the concanavalin A-binding fraction.

Purified hCG can be obtained commercially or can be prepared, although the techniques are laborious. As previously described, a discriminating hCG assay requires antibodies that recognize the N terminus of the beta subunit so that high physiological concentrations of LH do not give false-positive indications of elevated hCG.

TABLE 1. Clinical situations associated with elevated AFP or hCG

Condition	AFP	hCG	Comments
Ataxia telangiectasia	+	−	
Hereditary tyrosinemia	+	−	
Nonmalignant liver disease	+	−	With severe disease AFP levels usually are <1,000 ng/ml
LH	−	+	Apparent hCG elevation (see text)
Marijuana use	−	+	
Hepatocellular carcinoma	+	+	
Pancreatic carcinoma	+	+	
Gastric carcinoma	+	+	
Lung carcinoma	+	+	
Breast carcinoma	−	+	
Renal carcinoma	−	+	Rare; levels usually low
Bladder carcinoma	−	+	Rare; levels usually low
Seminoma	−	+	
NSGCT	+	+	
Benign genitourinary disease	−	−	

Assay sensitivity requirements for AFP and hCG vary with the disease in question. Germ cell tumors have a very high requirement: for AFP at least 5 ng/ml and for hCG at least 5 mIU/ml. In fact for monitoring, assays with greater sensitivity are desirable so that the marker can be reproducibly quantitated at levels significantly below the upper limit of normal. For example, at our laboratory with an enzyme immunoassay, our upper limit of normal for AFP is 4 IU/ml (1 IU = 1.22 ng), and the sensitivity of this assay is approximately 0.4 IU/ml; the upper limit of normal for hCG is 6 mIU/ml, with an assay sensitivity of 0.8 mIU/ml.

For many years the most widely accepted assays for AFP and hCG were based on radioimmunoassays. Recently, enzymatic assays have gained popularity and in many laboratories have replaced these classical isotopic assays. These recent assays are based on the enzymatic conversion of a substrate to a colored end product which can be accurately quantitated spectrophotometrically. There are now very sensitive enzyme immunoassays for AFP and hCG. Most, but not all, of the β-hCG immunoassays commercially available measure both the amount of intact molecule and any free beta chains containing the antigenic determinant of the particular β-hCG antibody used. Since some tumors produce significant levels of free beta chain alone or in combination with intact molecule, it is not yet known whether assays which only measure the intact molecule are appropriate for monitoring patients with trophoblastic tumors.

Tumor marker terminology

Certain terms are used to indicate whether an immunoassay will be useful in clinical practice. Sensitivity is a term used in two contexts, one referring to clinical use and the other referring to assay performance. Clinically, sensitivity refers to the proportion of true-positive results obtained in a population of pa-

tients known to have the tumor in question. Several factors influence this percentage, including the smallest number of tumor cells required to produce a detectable level of the marker, the number of those cells actively producing the marker, and the somewhat subjective upper limit of normal for the marker in sera from individuals without cancer. Sensitivity may also refer to the lowest level of detectable marker that the assay can discriminate from a serum control without marker. Sensitivity in this context is influenced by variables of assay design and the antisera selected. High-affinity antisera provide for immunoassays with greater sensitivity.

Another important term is specificity, which is a measure of the uniqueness of the marker for the tumor and reflects the incidence of true-negative results in a subject population known to be free of the tumor in question. Obviously, specificity is influenced not only by the quality of the antibody used in the assay but by the prevalence of the marker in various clinical conditions. Thus, AFP or hCG can never be specific for germ cell tumors since elevated levels of these markers are found in other clinical conditions. Nonetheless, a marker may still have great value if these other conditions can be consistently and accurately separated from the illness of interest.

The third important term is the false-negative rate, or the proportion of patients with the tumor in whom the marker is not elevated. Of course, this relates to the established value or the upper limit of normal. The corollary term, the false-positive rate, is the proportion of donors without the tumor in whom the marker is elevated. With any given assay, even those that are commercially available, it is recommended that each laboratory determine its own upper limit of normal.

CLINICAL CONSIDERATIONS

Background about testicular tumors

To properly use AFP and hCG for monitoring of testicular tumors, one must understand the clinical spectrum of the disease. Briefly, more than 95% of testicular cancers arrive from the germ cells of the seminiferous tubules. These germ cell tumors are classified pathologically as seminomas or as NSGCT, with the latter being further divided into embryonal cell carcinoma, teratoma, and choriocarcinoma. Usually metastasis occurs to lymph nodes high in the retroperitoneum along the aorta and inferior vena cava. Subsequently, metastasis spreads to the lung and to other organs.

The treatment of testicular cancer begins with the removal of the testes, surrounding tissue, and spermatic cord (i.e., radical orchiectomy). Pathological classification often necessitates extensive tissue evaluation, for if seminoma is found, it is important to be certain that nonseminomatous elements are not present also. When they are, the patient is treated as if he had NSGCT. If the pathologist diagnoses pure seminoma, the retroperitoneal lymph nodes are irradiated, although seminomas normally grow slowly and only a minority of patients have metastasis at the time of orchiectomy. If there is evidence of metastasis beyond the retroperitoneum, the mediastinum and other sites may be irradiated or chemotherapy may be given. Since seminomas are very sensitive to radiation and chemotherapy, cure rates of 95% are common.

For nonseminomatous cancer with or without the presence of seminoma, most centers in the United States remove the retroperitoneal lymph nodes (lymphadenectomy), provided that preoperative tests determine that the disease in the retroperitoneum is minimal or absent and that no disease exists beyond the retroperitoneum. However, about 30% of patients believed to have only localized disease actually do have metastatic tumors, as shown by pathological evaluation of the retroperitoneal lymph nodes after surgery. In patients with known high-stage disease (bulky retroperitoneal disease or spread beyond it), chemotherapy replaces or proceeds the lymphadenectomy.

Specificity and sensitivity

AFP and hCG should be measured simultaneously to achieve the maximal clinical benefit, since elevated levels of one or both of these proteins will be found in 50 to 90% of patients with active NSGCT. In a series of 400 patients with metastatic NSGCT, 25% had increased levels of AFP only, and approximately 15% had hCG as the only marker (3). It is also known that nonparallelism (discordance) occurs with AFP and hCG; that is, as fluctuations in the levels occur due to treatment or progression of disease, one marker may remain stable while the other rises or decreases. Similarly, one marker may be at normal levels despite the presence of tumor, only to increase later during progression or recurrence. Also, up to 30% of patients with stage II NSGCT and 10% of those with untreated stage III disease have elevation of neither AFP nor hCG. In addition, among patients with pure seminoma, elevated levels of these markers are infrequent, as discussed below.

Neither AFP nor hCG is specific for germ cell tumors, since these markers may be significantly elevated in other malignant and nonmalignant conditions (Table 1). Nevertheless, experience has demonstrated that for practical purposes these markers, when used together, are quite specific and invaluable in monitoring the status of patients with testicular tumors. In studies of more than 300 patients, we have had only one case of an elevated marker (AFP) caused by another disease (in this instance, hepatitis). However, today patients with advanced disease are being rendered free of disease for years by use of chemotherapy. Thus, recently it has become apparent that occasionally patients with testicular tumor develop elevated AFP levels 5 years or more after becoming free of disease. While recurrent testicular tumor seems to be the cause of the elevated levels in most of these cases, the other AFP-related conditions, especially benign liver disease, become increasingly possible causes as these patients age.

False-positives and false-negatives

There are certain qualifications to the statement that false-positives rarely occur for AFP and hCG in testicular cancer. For example, if a serum sample is obtained too soon after orchiectomy for testicular tumor, elevated marker levels may be observed due to the residual marker in the serum. This is seen more frequently with AFP, due to its 5-day half-life, than with β-hCG (30-h half-life). Accordingly, it is good practice to obtain serial samples to establish trends; single determinations may be misleading. A second caveat is that small elevations of β-hCG can occur among patients who have high LH levels. This is particularly relevant in the patient with testicular cancer who may exhibit elevated LH levels because of hypogonadism induced by chemotherapy or orchiectomy. The best solution to this problem is to utilize only β-hCG assays which have negligible cross-reactivity with LH. Also, one can wait and watch: if recurrent tumor is the cause of β-hCG elevation, the levels will usually rise significantly. Alternatively, a short course of testosterone to suppress LH production may resolve the issue (2).

True false-negatives (i.e., normal marker levels in patients with known germ cell cancer) do occur in testicular tumor patients. The frequency of this event varies with the clinical stage and circumstances of the disease. We explain below why the markers are not very useful in screening or diagnosis, why they may be useful in staging, and why they are essential for monitoring.

Diagnosis

Patients with masses in the testicles and elevated marker levels almost certainly have NSGCT. However, normal levels do not rule out the diagnosis of testicular cancer. Surgical excision and pathological examination of the mass remains the only certain method of diagnosis. However, it is important to obtain marker levels before orchiectomy for later comparison during monitoring. Our current preorchiectomy marker data (5) can be summarized as follows. First, in patients whose scrotal masses are found to be benign or composed of non-germ cell tissues (i.e., lymphomas, Leydig cell tumors), marker levels are not elevated (n = 43). Second, if AFP is elevated, the patient has NSGCT; if hCG alone is elevated, the diagnosis may be pure seminoma, pure NSGCT, or a mixed germ cell testicular tumor. Third, marker levels are normal in the majority of men with pure seminoma and in about 60% of men with NSGCT localized to the testicle (i.e., stage A). Thus, marker levels help in the diagnosis only if they are elevated, in which case the diagnosis of testicular cancer is a virtual certainty. As will now be discussed, the frequency of elevated markers in preorchiectomy sera coincides with increasing stage of disease.

Staging

Analysis of AFP and hCG levels after diagnosis but before treatment can help in staging a patient, that is, in making a determination as to whether the extent of the disease is local, slight metastasis, or distant and extensive metastasis. However, to interpret accurately the meaning of these levels, one must understand the importance of marker metabolic decay. For example, it is not appropriate to conclude that an elevated marker after orchiectomy signifies remaining tumor. If one is attempting to detect retroperitoneal metastases after orchiectomy, one must be certain that any elevation is due to continued production of the marker by remaining tumor and not to residual marker in the serum from the resected tumor. Accordingly, after orchiectomy, at least two values obtained several days apart often are required to distinguish between the two possibilities. If the marker originated from the excised tumor, the rate of biological decay or clearance from the circulation would be in accordance with the physiological half-life of the marker. When two or more postsurgery values are available, one can calculate the expected marker level from the following equations:

$$\text{for AFP, } X_F = X_0 e^{-0.139(t_d)}$$
$$\text{for hCG, } X_F = X_0 e^{-0.023(t_h)}$$

where X_0 is the initial concentration and X_F is the concentration at time t in hours (h) or days (d) (6).

In patients with only retroperitoneal disease, the incidence of positive markers is about 40% for stage B1 (microscopic disease only), 60% for stage B2 (gross disease with tumors < 2 cm in diameter), and 80% for stage B3 (bulky disease). Only ca. 11% of patients with metastasis beyond the retroperitoneum are marker negative, but here also the percent positive is directly proportional to the extent of the disease.

Monitoring of disease

Without question, the most important role of AFP and hCG analysis in germ cell cancers is in the monitoring of disease during and after initial therapy. In fact, these markers have become indispensable for the follow-up of patients with testicular cancer because they often reflect or predict progression of disease several months before any other methods do so. Unequivocal persistent elevated blood levels of either marker in a patient who has completed a definitive course of treatment indicates that residual tumor is present, taking into account, of course, metabolic decay and possible LH cross-reactivity. In these and related circumstances, it is now common practice to begin or resume appropriate therapy (even toxic chemotherapy) without pathological proof of malignancy when to obtain such proof would require major surgery for tissue diagnosis.

There are several principles that should be remembered when these markers are used for monitoring therapy or recurrence.

(i) Marker levels often fall rapidly during chemotherapy and reach normal levels while the tumor masses are still evident. Planned therapy should be completed. Some physicians give at least two additional courses of chemotherapy after normalization of the markers.

(ii) Recurrent or persistent disease does occur with completely normal marker levels. This is most commonly observed after planned chemotherapy when a mass is still present. Most of the time these masses contain only fibrosis/necrosis or mature teratoma. However, sometimes elements of NSGCT are present in the mass. It has become apparent that it is usually not advisable to operate on patients who have positive markers and residual masses after chemotherapy because the cancers almost invariably recur quickly.

(iii) The decline of serum markers during chemotherapy is variable and can provide useful information. In many patients there is an initial rise which peaks at about 3 to 5 days after chemotherapy is started. We have called this the release phenomenon (9). Thereafter in some patients, the levels may fall as though no more markers are being released (that is, in a manner predicted by metabolic decay), while in others, the levels fall more slowly or not at all. The prognostic importance of this decline (or apparent half-life) varies with the type of chemotherapy given. With modern platin-based chemotherapy programs, the slow decline probably portends a less favorable outcome, although the more normal decline does not guarantee against relapse.

(iv) After therapy is completed, marker levels should be checked regularly. The frequency and duration of this surveillance is a matter of debate and ultimately should depend on the patient's disease type and severity. As a general guideline, we perform marker determinations monthly for 1 year and every 2 months for the second year. In patients who have had chemotherapy for disseminated disease, especially bulky disease, the markers should be measured at least yearly for many years. As previously mentioned, this is because we have seen some cases in which an elevated AFP level is detected 5 years or more after the patient was declared free of disease. In many cases these marker levels have plateaued at between 100 and 400 IU/ml for months to years before ascending to higher levels. So far, of the patients whose levels have risen further, all eventually had firm evidence of recurrent NSGCT and no evidence of liver pathology. Until more is known about the incidence and natural history of these later marker elevations, and because all of these patients have had extensive courses of chemotherapy already, it is reasonable to observe these patients closely and wait for unequivocal (visible) evidence of recurrence before beginning further chemotherapy. Presumably these patients had persistent foci of apparently mature teratoma which (as previously discussed) may exist after chemotherapy and which may convert into frank malignancy after years of dormancy.

It is probably important to develop a method to biochemically or immunologically distinguish AFP species based on their major sources: liver versus yolk sac and malignant liver cells versus benign hepatocytes. Currently there is no test which can make these distinctions. Concanavalin A lectin-binding studies can often distinguish the AFP of yolk sac from the liver type, but the distinction is not absolute (8).

Marker levels and prognosis

A controversial issue of tumor marker use in NSGCT has been the value of marker levels to determine prognosis. Production of high levels of β-hCG or AFP was thought to be an adverse prognostic indicator; however, these studies often did not take into account such important variables as histologic type, tumor stage, or both. Recently this issue has been studied with more sophisticated statistical methods, including multivariate analysis which can determine independent prognostic variables (1). However, in our opinion this issue is still unresolved.

Marker immunohistochemical analysis

AFP, hCG, and a variety of other markers have been successfully applied to immunohistochemical analysis of testicular tumor section (4). Generally AFP "stains" yolk sac elements, while hCG reacts with syncytiotrophoblastic cells. Some cells without the classic characteristics of these types also seem to contain the markers, although undoubtedly the cells are of the same lineage. Immunohistochemical analysis has generated a large body of work and some increase in our understanding about the characteristics of germ cell tumors, but the approach has not yet contributed a great deal to the clinical management of patients with such tumors.

CONCLUSION

The serum markers AFP and hCG, when used together in germ cell tumors of the testes, are some of the best tumor markers in clinical oncology. There are significant restrictions: these markers are of limited value for diagnosis, and they provide useful information for staging only if they are elevated. Their greatest value is for monitoring disease, in which they are indispensable, but here also there are limitations. To use AFP and hCG correctly, one must have a thorough understanding of the pathophysiology of the marker and also of the disease. These lessons have great application to other tumor markers for other human cancers.

LITERATURE CITED

1. **Bosl, G. J., N. L. Geller, C. Cirrincione, N. J. Vogelzang, B. J. Kennedy, W. F. Whitmore, Jr., D. Vugrin, H. Scher, J. Nisselbaum, and R. B. Golbey.** 1983. Multivariate analysis of prognostic variables in patients with metastatic testicular cancer. Cancer Res. **43:**3403–3407.
2. **Catalona, W. J., J. L. Vaitukaitis, and W. R. Fair.** 1979. Falsely positive specific human chorionic gonadotropin assays in patients with testicular tumors: conversion to negative with testosterone administration. J. Urol. **122:**126–128.
3. **Kohn, J., and D. Raghavan.** 1981. Tumour markers in malignant germ cell tumors, p. 50–69. *In* M. J. Peckham (ed.), The management of testicular tumors. Edward Arnold, London.
4. **Kurman, R. J., P. T. Scardino, K. R. McIntire, T. A. Waldmann, and N. Javadpour.** 1977. Cellular localization of alpha-fetoprotein and human chorionic gonadotropin in germ cell tumors of the testis using an indirect immunoperoxidase technique. Cancer **40:**2136–2151.
5. **Lange, P. H., and D. Raghavan.** 1983. Clinical applications of tumor markers in testicular cancer, p. 111–130. *In* J. P. Donohue (ed.), Testis tumors. The Williams & Wilkins Co., Baltimore.
6. **Lange, P. H., N. J. Vogelzang, A. Goldman, B. J. Kennedy, and E. E. Fraley.** 1982. Marker half-life analysis as a prognostic tool in testicular cancer. J. Urol. **128:**708–711.
7. **Norgaard-Pedersen, B.** 1976. Human alpha-fetoprotein. A review of recent methodological and clinical studies. Scand. J. Immunol. Suppl. **4:**7–45.
8. **Vessella, R. L., M. A. Santrach, D. Bronson, C. J. Smith, M. J. Klicka, and P. H. Lange.** 1984. Evaluation of AFP glycosylation heterogeneity in cancer patients with AFP producing tumors. Int. J. Cancer **34:**309–314.
9. **Vogelzang, N. J., P. H. Lange, A. Goldman, R. L. Vessella, E. E. Fraley, and B. J. Kennedy.** 1982. Acute changes of alpha-fetoprotein and human chorionic gonadotropin during induction chemotherapy of germ cell tumors. Cancer Res. **42:**4855–4861.
10. **Zondek, B.** 1930. Versuch einer biologischen (hormonalen) Diagnostik beim malignen Hodentumor. Chirug **2:**1072–1073.

Chapter 126

CA 19-9

R. E. RITTS, JR., AND DEBORAH A. JACOBSEN

CA 19-9 is a tumor-associated antigen reported by Koprowski et al. (5), who used the human colorectal carcinoma cell line SW 1116 to produce monoclonal antibodies. This monoclonal antibody (19-9) was found to be specific for an oligosaccharide antigenic determinant which shares structural features with Lewis blood group substance and has been identified as a sialylated lacto-N-fucopentaose II (7). Several reports (4, 6, 9) have suggested that CA 19-9, as measured by an inhibition radioimmunoassay, is elevated in patients with cancer of the pancreas, stomach, colon, or rectum, particularly in those with recurrence after surgical removal of colorectal cancer. An improved forward immunoradiometric assay (3) has confirmed the initial findings on CA 19-9. As is the case for other human tumor-associated antigens, CA 19-9 is not qualitatively unique with the development of cancer, but may be found in embryonal gut tissue as well as adult pancreatic and liver duct epithelium (1). However, CA 19-9 shows a significant quantitative rise in patients with cancer, and its relatively rare increases in patients with benign gut and pancreatic diseases make it potentially valuable for clinical application.

CLINICAL INDICATIONS

It is important to recognize that the application of the CA 19-9 assay is not routine at this time (1984) but is still an investigational matter. Because of the high sensitivity initially reported for the assay for pancreatic cancer (70% overall, 80% in untreated patients), gastric cancer (62%), hepatobiliary cancer (62%), and advanced colorectal cancer ($\sim$30%), coupled with low sensitivity, ranging from 16% in lung cancer to 3% for breast and prostatic cancer, and a high specificity of >90% (0 to 1.4% of normal persons and 1.3% of patients with benign diseases were positive) (8), it is obvious that this test may be a useful noninvasive adjunct in discriminating between benign and malignant diseases in the gut and pancreas and in monitoring treatment, particularly surgical removal of these cancers. It is this latter use toward which most of the current work is directed and for which its proponents are seeking approval from the Food and Drug Administration.

By blind use of CA 19-9 and other assays, we have studied a high-risk gastrointestinal clinic population (R. E. Ritts, Jr., D. A. Jacobsen, D. C. Ilstrup, and E. DiMagno, Cancer Detect. Prev. 7:525, 1984). In this group of 4,916 patients, 82% had benign disease and 96% were CA 19-9 negative (<40 U/ml), and the previously noted high sensitivities were confirmed, especially in those patients having pancreatic cancer. Indeed, three "false-positive" patients diagnosed as having benign diseases later died from cancer of the liver or pancreas. The overall sensitivity for gut cancer was not as impressive as the specificity, but was acceptable at 36%, which is better than for other tumor-associated antigens put to such an examination. Because of this high specificity and reasonable sensitivity, when CA 19-9 is used with one or two assays of less desirable sensitivity, such as the assay with CEA or CA 125 (an antigen expressed primarily in patients with ovarian carcinoma, as reported by Bast et al. [2], but also elevated in pancreatic cancer), the CA 19-9 assay yields a predictive value near 100% (R. E. Ritts, Jr., T. Klug, D. A. Jacobsen, E. DiMagno, and V. A. Zurawski, Jr., Cancer Detect. Prev. 7:459, 1984). It is appropriate to record that the greatest sensitivity of CA 19-9 is in pancreatic cancer, which is not usually diagnosed early enough for an effective cure to be possible and for which the disease-free interval is not generally long enough for monitoring. Consequently, the proposed current monitoring application is largely for colorectal cancer in which, in our experience, CA 19-9 is only $\sim$30% positive in metastatic or Dukes' D disease (8). However, Sears et al. (9) have shown that patients who were initially CA 19-9 negative (<37 U/ml) before surgery may express elevated levels of CA 19-9 months before CEA rises and clinical recurrence can be detected. It is premature to say whether a simple doubling of CA 19-9 levels, even below the reference value of 37 to 40 U/ml, or three successive rising CA 19-9 values should be the indicator for "second-look" surgery, because these findings are new, the cases studied are necessarily few, and there is a lack of substantive information on the frequency of documented recurrences in which CA 19-9 did not rise. In any event, the early studies on CA 19-9 in several institutions in this country and a number of institutions in Europe and Japan are promising and encourage further application.

LABORATORY ASSAY AND INTERPRETATION

The CA 19-9 assay is a forward sandwich solid-phase radioimmunometric assay utilizing a single polystyrene bead coated with capture murine monoclonal antibody to CA 19-9 and the same ^{125}I-labeled antibody as the indicator (3), the bound CA 19-9 being determined by gamma scintillation counting. The test is supplied as a kit with all components from Centocor, Inc., Malvern, Pa. To the best of our knowledge, individual components, including the anti-CA 19-9 antibody or its producer clone, are not otherwise available.

Neither a firm reference or cutoff value nor a formula for rising values can be stated with assurance at this time, but 37 U/ml (3) to 40 U/ml (8) would appear to be the correct range, with nearly all investigators finding a mean value of 7 to 9.4 U/ml in several thousand normal volunteers and patients with benign disease. Patients with severe benign hepatobiliary disease, but not pancreatitis, are most frequently the individuals with values > 40 U/ml, some values being even as high as 200 to 500 U/ml. These values are to be contrasted with mean values of >5,000 U/ml for hepatobiliary cancer and >6,400 U/ml for pancreatic cancer (8).

Currently, the cost effectiveness of the CA 19-9 assay is not known. It is reasonable at present to regard this assay as comparable to, if not potentially better than, CEA appropriately used in selected surgical cases for postsurgical monitoring. We believe that the best applications are to use CA 19-9 during and after therapy for recurrence to monitor patients with treated gastrointestinal cancer, and quite possibly to use CA 19-9 with other tests to screen high-risk patients or unresolved diagnostic problems. As a general principle, the more frequent application of the assay (e.g., every 3 to 4 weeks) provides the best opportunity to detect rises in the circulating antigen. It is doubtful that more definitive information can be had on these or other uses until 1986.

The detailed test procedure is provided with the kit, and since this kit is the only source of the reagent, it is inappropriate to reproduce the procedure here beyond noting that the test configuration is ingeniously packaged and easily performed by anyone familiar with a radioimmunoassay, and it includes positive controls and five human standards in doubling concentrations for the construction of a standard curve from which the test data can be read. The assay components appear to be well standardized over nearly 2 years by having purified antigen and excellent quality control. The interlaboratory coefficient of variation of coded aliquots has been 4 to 6%, and the interassay variation among three laboratories has been 10 to 12% in the linear range of results to 999 U/ml. The minimal detectable quantity of CA 19-9 is 1.5 U/ml, which corresponds to 0.89 ng/ml.

LITERATURE CITED

1. Atkinson, B. F., C. S. Ernst, M. Herlyn, Z. Steplewski, H. F. Sears, and H. Koprowski. 1982. Gastrointestinal cancer-associated antigen in immunoperoxidase assay. Cancer Res. 42:4820–4823.
2. Bast, R. C., M. Feeney, H. Lazarus, L. M. Nadler, R. B. Colvin, and R. C. Knapp. 1981. Reactivity of a monoclonal antibody with human ovarian carcinoma. J. Clin. Invest. 68:1331–1337.
3. Del Villano, B. C., S. Brennan, P. Brock, C. Bucher, V. Liu, M. McClure, B. Rake, S. Space, and V. R. Zurawski, Jr. 1983. Radioimmunometric assay for a monoclonal antibody-defined tumor marker, CA 19-9. Clin. Chem. 29:549–552.
4. Herlyn, M., H. F. Sears, Z. Steplewski, and H. Koprowski. 1982. Monoclonal antibody detection of a circulating tumor-associated antigen. I. Presence of antigen in sera of patients with colorectal, gastric, and pancreatic carcinoma. J. Clin. Immunol. 2:135–140.
5. Koprowski, H., H. F. Sears, M. Herlyn, and Z. Steplewski. 1981. Sera from patients with adenocarcinoma of the colon inhibit binding of a monoclonal antibody to colon carcinoma cells. Science 212:53–55.
6. Koprowski, H., Z. Steplewski, K. Mitchell, M. Herlyn, D. Herlyn, and P. Fulner. 1979. Colorectal carcinoma antigens detected by hybridoma antibodies. Somatic Cell Genet. 5:957–972.
7. Magnani, J. L., B. Nilsson, M. Brockhaus, D. Zopf, Z. Steplewski, H. Koprowski, and V. Ginsburg. 1982. A monoclonal antibody-defined antigen associated with gastrointestinal cancer in a ganglioside containing sialylated lacto-N-fucopentaose II. J. Biol. Chem. 257:14365–14369.
8. Ritts, R. E., Jr., B. C. Del Villano, V. L. W. Go, R. B. Herberman, T. L. Klug, and V. R. Zurawski, Jr. 1984. Initial clinical evaluation of an immunoradiometric assay for CA 19-9 using the NCI Serum Bank. Int. J. Cancer 33:339–345.
9. Sears, H. F., M. Herlyn, B. Del Villano, Z. Steplewski, and H. Koprowski. 1982. Monoclonal antibody detection of a circulating tumor-associated antigen. II. A longitudinal evaluation of patients with colorectal cancer. J. Clin. Immunol. 2:141–149.

Chapter 127

Antigenic Markers for Ovarian Carcinoma

ROBERT C. BAST, JR., AND ROBERT C. KNAPP

Carcinomas can arise from the ovarian surface epithelium, stroma, or germ cells. In adults, approximately 90% of ovarian cancers are derived from epithelium which covers the ovarian surface or which lines subcapsular cysts. Epithelial ovarian cancers can metastasize hematogenously or through lymphatics, but most frequently they spread over the peritoneum, studding serosal surfaces, blocking diaphragmatic lymphatics, and producing ascites. Once the primary ovarian mass has been resected, many small tumor nodules often remain on the peritoneal surface. Cytotoxic chemotherapy will produce regression of residual tumor in a majority of patients. Monitoring residual tumor burden has, however, proven difficult. In most cases, the tumor can be neither palpated nor detected by computerized axial tomography. In this setting, antigenic markers which reliably reflect the amount of residual tumor would be of great value in judging the efficacy of treatment.

ONCOFETAL MARKERS

A modest elevation of carcinoembryonic antigen (CEA) is found in sera from as many as 50% of ovarian cancer patients, but elevations of CEA sufficient to permit effective monitoring are observed in only an occasional individual. CEA is most likely to be elevated in patients with widespread, poorly differentiated mucinous ovarian cancer (22). Among the germ cell tumors, alpha-fetoprotein and human chorionic gonadotropin have provided useful markers. Human chorionic gonadotropin is elevated in nongestational choriocarcinomas and in some embryonal tumors, but not in endodermal sinus tumors. Alpha-fetoprotein is associated with endodermal sinus tumors and embryonal carcinomas, but not with choriocarcinomas. In contrast to the germ cell tumors, human chorionic gonadotropin and alpha-fetoprotein have not proven useful for monitoring epithelial ovarian malignancy.

MARKERS DEFINED BY HETEROANTISERA

In early studies, rabbit heteroantisera were used to define ovarian tumor-associated antigens. Radioimmunoassays were developed for two markers: ovarian cystadenocarcinoma-associated antigen and ovarian carcinoma antigen. Both markers can be detected in serous and in mucinous carcinoma. Levels of ovarian cystadenocarcinoma-associated antigen are elevated in approximately 70% of patients with epithelial ovarian carcinoma, as well as in a smaller fraction of patients with metastatic colon, breast, and cervical cancer (4). Increases or decreases in this antigen have correlated with disease activity in approximately 60% of cases. Ovarian carcinoma antigen is a high-molecular-weight glycoprotein which has partial cross-reactivity with CEA (14). A 70,000-dalton component (NB/70K) has been isolated which is antigenically distinct from CEA. NB/70K levels are elevated in sera from a majority of patients with epithelial ovarian cancer (15).

ANTIGENIC MARKERS DEFINED BY MONOCLONAL ANTIBODIES

CA125 determinants

Murine monoclonal reagents have been prepared against several ovarian tumor-associated antigens. The first monoclonal antibody reported to react with epithelial ovarian carcinoma (OC125) was raised against a serous cystadenocarcinoma cell line (1). OC125 is a murine immunoglobulin G (subclass 1) which recognizes multiple CA125 determinants on a mucinlike glycoprotein of greater than 200,000 daltons (17). CA125 is expressed by the coelomic epithelium and amnion during embryonic development (10). By using biotin-avidin immunoperoxidase, traces of CA125 can be found in adult pleura, pericardium, and peritoneum, as well as in the epithelial lining of the fallopian tube, endometrium, and endocervix. The antigen is not associated with the normal ovary either in the fetus or in the adult. CA125 is expressed by more than 80% of nonmucinous epithelial ovarian tumors (11). Benign, borderline, and malignant ovarian neoplasms express the antigen. CA125 is not a specific marker for tumors of ovarian origin and can be detected in a majority of carcinomas which arise from the fallopian tube, endometrium, endocervix, pancreas, and liver as well as in a smaller fraction of tumors derived from the colon, breast, and lung.

CA125 assay

A double-determinant simultaneous sandwich immunoradiometric assay has been developed to detect CA125 in serum (3, 13). Antigen in 100-μl portions of serum is trapped on a polystyrene bead (outer diameter, 0.64 cm) which has been coated with OC125. Since more than one CA125 determinant is associated with each antigen molecule, bound antigen can be detected by simultaneous incubation of the bead with 130,000 dpm of ^{125}I-labeled OC125 (9 to 12 μCi/μg) in 100 μl of trace buffer (pH 5.9; 100 mM sodium citrate, 50 mM EDTA, 150 mM sodium chloride, 2 g of bovine serum albumin per liter, 0.4 g of murine immunoglobulin G per liter). After incubation at ambient temperature for 20 h, serum and excess ^{125}I-labeled OC125 are washed from the system, and the activity associated with the immunoabsorbent is measured in a gamma counter. A kit has been prepared for clinical investigation by Centocor, Inc., Malvern, Pa.

Antigen units are arbitrarily defined relative to a standard specimen of CA125 from tissue culture supernatants of an epithelial ovarian cancer cell line. The assay can detect 1.4 U of CA125 per ml and is

TABLE 1. CA125 levels in ovarian cancer patients[a]

Investigators	Antigen level (U/ml)	No. positive/ no. studied	% Positive
Bast et al. (3)	35	84/101	83
Chatal et al.[b]	30	35/38	92
Sarmini et al.[b]	35	14/27	52
Canney et al. (7)	35	45/58	83
Crombach et al.[b]	35	71/91	78
Auvray et al.[b]	35	43/49	83
Kreienberg and Melchart[b]	65	36/57	63
Lien[b]	65	29/30	97
Kimura et al. (12)	35	19/23	83
Eerdekens et al. (8)	35	10/20	50
van Dalen et al. (25)	35	13/14	92

[a] Revised from Bast et al. (R. C. Bast, Jr., V. R. Zurawski, and R. C. Knapp, in *Roche-UCLA Symposium on Monoclonal Antibodies and Cancer Therapy*, in press).

[b] Cited in Bast et al., in *Roche-UCLA Symposium on Monoclonal Antiboldies and Cancer Therapy*, in press.

linear up to 500 U/ml. With dilution, more than 10,000 U of antigen activity can be detected in serum and ascites fluid. The day-to-day coefficient of variation is 12 to 15%. Consequently, a doubling or halving of antigen levels has been considered significant.

CA125 for monitoring tumor growth

Using the CA125 assay, 83 (82%) of 101 patients with epithelial ovarian cancer had greater than 35 U of antigen per ml (3). A similar antigen level was found in 1% of apparently healthy women, 6% with benign disease, and 28% of patients with nongynecologic neoplasms. Subsequent reports have confirmed that CA125 is elevated in 399 (78%) of 508 ovarian cancer patients (Table 1).

In a restrospective analysis (3), increases or decreases in CA125 paralleled growth or regression of tumor in 93% of the instances studied (Fig. 1). Tumor regression has sometimes been associated with a decrease in antigen level of as much as 1,000-fold. The half-life of CA125 in serum has been estimated at approximately 4.8 days (7). Failure of CA125 to fall below 35 U/ml by 3 months has been strongly correlated with the persistence of disease at "second-look" surveillance operations after 9 to 12 months of cytotoxic chemotherapy (P. T. Lavin et al., manuscript in preparation). CA125 may, however, return to an activity of less than 35 U/ml without complete regression of disease (3, 19). In 36 of 56 surveillance procedures, CA125 had returned to less than 35 U/ml before operation. In 14 (39%) of the 36, surgical exploration failed to reveal residual tumor. In 22 (61%) of the 36, tumor was detected macroscopically or on microscopic examination of biopsies and washings, but in no case was the largest tumor nodule greater than 1 cm in diameter. Persistently elevated CA125 has been consistently associated with residual tumor. A sufficient number of cases has now been studied to conclude that if CA125 is elevated preoperatively, there is a greater than 90% chance of finding residual disease by a surgical surveillance procedure.

Serum CA125 may be elevated in 1 to 11 months (median, 3 months) before clinical recurrence of ovar-

ian cancer. Persistently rising CA125 values have consistently been associated with recurrent tumor. Elevations of CA125 have been found in some benign conditions, including first-trimester pregnancy, chronic liver disease, acute pancreatitis, cholecystitis, peritonitis, acute pelvic inflammatory disease, and endometriosis (19b, 21; R. L. Barbieri, J. M. Niloff, R. C. Bast, Jr., E. Schaetzl, R. W. Kistner, and R. C. Knapp, submitted for publication). Most of these conditions are not likely to confuse the oncologist who is monitoring patients with previously diagnosed epithelial ovarian carcinoma. Whether or not CA125 will prove useful in monitoring patients with endometrial, fallopian tube, or pancreatic carcinoma remains to be determined (19a).

CA125 for detecting ovarian cancer

Clinically, more than two-thirds of ovarian cancers are diagnosed in an advanced stage where tumor has spread outside the pelvis. Earlier detection of the neoplasm might permit more effective treatment. At present, there is no useful screening test for ovarian cancer aside from pelvic examination.

In one fortuitous case monitored retrospectively, serum CA125 was greater than 35 U/ml at 12 months and greater than 65 U/ml at 10 months before diagnosis of a primary epithelial ovarian cancer (3a). CA125 has been elevated preoperatively in 8 of 11 patients with stage I or stage II ovarian cancer. Among 100 women with pelvic masses studied preoperatively in

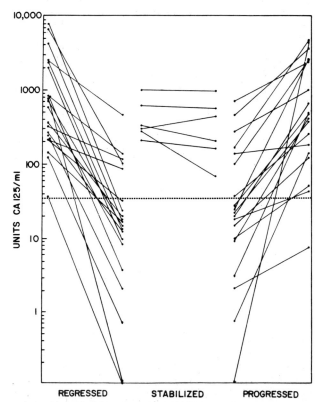

FIG. 1. CA125 levels before and after treatment in patients whose disease regressed, stabilized, or progressed. Reprinted with the permission of the *New England Journal of Medicine* (3).

TABLE 2. Monoclonal antibodies reactive with epithelial ovarian carcinomas[a]

Source of immunogen	Antibody	Investigators
Ovarian carcinoma	OC125	Bast et al. (1)
	ID3	Bhattacharya et al. (6)
	MOV-2	Tagliabue et al. (24)
	OC133	Berkowitz et al.[b]
	MD144	Mattes et al.[b]
	MF61	Mattes et al.[b]
	MF116	Mattes et al.[b]
	632	Fleuren et al.[c]
	OV-TL-3	Poels et al.[d]
	4F4, 7A1	Bhattacharya et al. (5)
Endometrial carcinoma	MH55	Mattes et al.[b]
	MH94	Mattes et al.[b]
Colorectal carcinoma	CA19-9	Koprowski et al. (16)
Pancreatic carcinoma	DUPAN-2	Metzgar et al. (18)
Breast carcinoma	F36/22	Croghan et al.[b]
	DF3	Sekine et al.[e]
	72.3	Johnston et al. (9)
Milk fat globule protein	HMFG2, AUA1	Epenetos et al.[b]
Laryngeal carcinoma	CA1	Woods et al.[b]
Osteogenic sarcoma	791-T/36	Embleton et al.[b]
Placental alkaline phosphatase	NDOG2	Sunderland et al. (23)
	E6	Nouwen et al. (20)

[a] As in Table 1, footnote a.
[b] As in Table 1, footnote b.
[c] Fleuren et al., Int. Meet. Monoclonal Antibodies Oncol.: Clin. Appl., 1984.
[d] Poels et al., in press.
[e] H. Sekine, D. F. Hayes, T. Ohno, K. A. Keefe, E. Schaetzl, R. C. Bast, R. Knapp, and D. W. Kufe, J. Clin. Oncol., in press.

the Stockholm area, only 1 of 68 patients with benign disease at exploratory laparotomy had greater than 65 U of CA125 per ml (N. Einhorn, R. C. Knapp, V. A. Zurawski, and R. C. Bast, Jr., Obstet. Gynecol., in press). A similar antigen elevation was found in 9 of 11 patients with frankly malignant nonmucinous epithelial ovarian cancer. Consistent with previous observations, the CA125 was not elevated in patients with mucinous or borderline tumors, but was increased in patients with endometrial and fallopian tube carcinomas. Overall, 13 of 14 women with a pelvic mass and an elevated CA125 had some form of gynecologic cancer. Similar results have been obtained in a prospective study of women seen at the Dana-Farber Cancer Institute, the Mayo Clinic, and the University of California, Los Angeles (G. Malkasian et al., manuscript in preparation). Taken together, these studies suggest that a preoperative CA125 of >65 U/ml is associated with a greater than 90% chance that a pelvic mass will be malignant. Although the test is not sufficiently sensitive to eliminate the need for exploratory operations which are otherwise indicated, patients who have CA125 values of >65 U/ml and an adnexal mass might be referred directly to surgeons who could perform definitive cytoreductive operations, if necessary, at the time of initial surgical exploration.

Whether or not CA125 will prove useful as a screening test remains to be determined. Use of 65 U/ml as a cutoff would exclude 99.5% of healthy individuals. Among 1,020 patients seen at a gynecology clinic, CA125 was elevated in 20 (2%) (19b). When pregnant individuals were excluded, the positive rate fell to 1%, and when two serial determinations were performed, the positive rate was 0.5%. In a group of 937 nuns with a median age of more than 50 years, CA125 was greater than 65 U/ml in 7 (0.75%) (V. R. Zurawski, P. Lavin, S. Broderick, P. Pickens, T. Klug, R. C. Knapp, and R. C. Bast, Jr., manuscript in preparation). Even with a relatively low rate of positivity in benign disease, given the low prevalence of ovarian cancer, effective screening will still require the development of confirmatory radioimmunoassays or the application of noninvasive staging techniques to eliminate false-positives.

Other monoclonal reagents

A number of other murine monoclonal antibodies have been reported which react with epithelial ovarian carcinoma (Table 2). Many reagents have been raised against ovarian tumors or their products, but several have been developed against human neoplasmas which have arisen from other sites. DUPAN-2 was raised against a pancreatic carcinoma (18), and CA19-9 was raised against a colorectal carcinoma cell line (16). The CA19-9 antibody reacts with a sialylated Lewis blood group determinant and binds to 40% of ovarian carcinomas in tissue section. CA19-9, however, was elevated in serum from only 18 (17%) of 105 ovarian cancer patients. Some reagents which react with breast, such as the DF3, 72.3, and anti-milk fat globule protein, cross-react with ovarian cancers. In addition to identifying potential markers for radioimmunoassays, some of these monoclonal reagents may prove useful for cytologic diagnosis or radionuclide imaging. Some of these antibodies react only with mucinous tumors, whereas others recognize both mucinous and nonmucinous histologies. ID3 reacts with mucinous ovarian tumors as well as colonic, rectal, and gastric cancers (6). Reactivity with normal tissues is limited to the colon. In general, antibodies have reacted with at least one normal tissue, although the 632 (G. Fleuren, E. Coerkamp, M. Nap, and S. Warnaar, Int. Meet. Monoclonal Antibodies Oncol.: Clin. Appl., Nantes, 1984) and OV-TL-3 (L. Poels, D. Peters, V. van Megen, G. P. Vooijs, R. Verheyen, A. Willemen, C. van Niekirk, P. Jap, G. Mungyer, and P. Kennemans, J. Natl. Cancer Inst., in press) reagents may be exceptions to this generalization.

Several antibodies recognize determinants which are expressed on high-molecular-weight mucinlike molecules, including CA125, CA19-9, MOV-2, DUPAN-2, and ID3. Preliminary studies indicate that CA125, CA19-9, MOV-2, and DUPAN-2 are antigenically distinct. CA125 and CA19-9 can, however, be coexpressed on the same molecule. As CA19-9, MOV-2, and DUPAN-2 are carbohydrate determinants, their expression probably reflects the aberrant glycosyl transferase and glycosidase profiles of ovarian tumor cells. Coexpression of different determinants on the same glycoprotein might be utilized as a more specific marker for ovarian cancer.

COMBINATIONS OF MARKERS

Use of markers in combination might provide more sensitive tests for detecting or monitoring ovarian cancer. In monitoring disease progression, CA125 proved superior to α-acid glycoprotein, C-reactive protein, phosphohexosisomerase, serum albumin, and CA50 ganglioside (T. Hogberg, S. Hammarstrom, A. Hedin, and L. Lindholm, Abstr. European Conf. Clin. Oncol., 3, p. 135, 1985; M. E. L. van der Burg, W. L. J. van Putten, and P. H. Cox, Proc. Am. Soc. Clin. Oncol., 4:116, 1985). A combination of CA125, CA19-9, and CEA was no more effective than CA125 alone for monitoring a group of 41 ovarian cancer patients (2). A combination of CA125 and tissue polypeptide antigen has, however, been more useful than CA125 alone in some studies (B. Tholander, L. Tamsen, U. Stendahl, O. Sjoberg, A. Kiviranta, and K. Hollman, Abstr. European Conf. Clin. Oncol., 3, p. 135, 1985). Additional information may also be obtained by monitoring both CA125 and lipid-associated sialic acid (P. E. Schwartz, S. K. Chambers, J. T. Chambers, J. Gutmann, R. S. Foemmel, and H. R. Behrman, Proc. Am. Soc. Clin. Oncol., 4:118, 1985). Recent reports suggest that NB/70K and CA125 recognize different moieties (S. Knauf, D. Anderson, R. C. Knapp, and R. C. Bast, Jr., submitted for publication) and that their use in combination may include most of the ovarian cancer population (A. J. Dembo, P.-L. Chang, A. Malkin, and G. Urbach, 16th Annu. Meet. Soc. Gynecol. Oncol., Miami, 1985, p. 30).

We thank Wenice G. Wells for outstanding secretarial assistance.

LITERATURE CITED

1. **Bast, R. C., Jr., M. Feeney, H. Lazarus, L. M. Nadler, R. B. Colvin, and R. C. Knapp.** 1981. Reactivity of a monoclonal antibody with human ovarian carcinoma. J. Clin. Invest. **68**:1331–1337.
2. **Bast, R. C., Jr., T. L. Klug, E. Schaetzl, P. Lavin, J. Niloff, T. F. Greber, V. R. Zurawski, Jr., and R. C. Knapp.** 1984. Monitoring human ovarian carcinoma with a combination of CA125, CA19-9, and carcinoembryonic antigen. Am. J. Obstet. Gynecol. **149**:553–559.
3. **Bast, R. C., Jr., T. L. Klug, E. St. John, E. Jenison, J. Niloff, H. Lazarus, R. S. Berkowitz, T. Leavitt, C. T. Griffiths, L. Parker, V. R. Zurawski, and R. C. Knapp.** 1983. A radioimmunoassay using a monoclonal antibody to monitor the course of epithelial ovarian cancer. N. Engl. J. Med. **309**:883–888.
3a. **Bast, R. C., Jr., F. P. Siegal, C. Runowicz, T. L. Klug, V. R. Zurawski, D. Schonholz, C. J. Cohen, and R. C. Knapp.** 1985. Elevation of serum CA125 prior to diagnosis of an epithelial ovarian carcinoma. Gynecol. Oncol. **22**:115–120.
4. **Bhattacharya, M., and J. J. Barlow.** 1979. Ovarian cystadenocarcinoma-associated antigen (OCAA), p. 527–531. *In* R. B. Herberman (ed.), Compendium of assays for immunodiagnosis of human cancer. Elsevier/North-Holland Biomedical Press, Amsterdam.
5. **Bhattacharya, M., S. K. Chatterjee, and J. J. Barlow.** 1984. Identification of a human cancer-associated antigen defined with monoclonal antibody. Cancer Res. **44**:4528–4534.
6. **Bhattacharya, M., S. K. Chatterjee, J. J. Barlow, and H. Fuji.** 1982. Monoclonal antibodies recognizing tumor-associated antigen of human ovarian mucinous cystadenocarcinomas. Cancer Res. **42**:1650.
7. **Canney, P., M. Moore, P. Wilkinson, and R. James.** 1984. Ovarian cancer antigen CA125: a prospective clinical assessment of the role as a tumor marker. Br. J. Cancer **50**:765–769.
8. **Eerdekens, M. W., E. J. Nouwen, D. E. Pollet, T. W. Briers, and M. E. De Broe.** 1985. Placental alkaline phosphatase and cancer antigen 125 in sera of patients with benign and malignant diseases. Clin. Chem. **31**:687–690.
9. **Johnston, W. W., C. A. Szpak, S. C. Lottich, A. Thor, and J. Schlom.** 1985. Use of a monoclonal antibody (B72.3) as an immunocytochemical adjunct to diagnosis of adenocarcinoma in human effusions. Cancer Res. **45**:1894–1900.
10. **Kabawat, S. E., R. C. Bast, Jr., A. K. Bhan, W. R. Welch, R. C. Knapp, and R. B. Colvin.** 1983. Tissue distribution of a coelomic epithelium related antigen recognized by the monoclonal antibody OC125. Int. J. Gynecol. Pathol. **2**:275–285.
11. **Kabawat, S. E., R. C. Bast, Jr., W. R. Welch, R. C. Knapp, and R. B. Colvin.** 1983. Immunopathologic characterization of a monoclonal antibody that recognizes common surface antigens of human ovarian tumors of serous, endometrioid and clear cell types. Am. J. Clin. Pathol. **79**:98–104.
12. **Kimura, E., M. Murae, R. Koga, Y. Odawara, Y. Nakabayashi, K. Yokoyama, H. Nakata, T. Totake, K. Ochiai, M. Yasuda, Y. Terashima, and S. Hachiya.** 1984. Clinical significance of new tumor marker CA125 in gynecological cancer. Acta Obstet. Gynaecol. Jpn. **36**:2121–2128.
13. **Klug, T. L., R. C. Bast, Jr., J. M. Niloff, R. C. Knapp, and V. R. Zurawski.** 1984. Monoclonal antibody immunoradiometric assay for an antigenic determinant (CA125) associated with human epithelial ovarian carcinomas. Cancer Res. **44**:1048–1053.
14. **Knauf, S., and G. I. Urbach.** 1980. A study of ovarian cancer patients using a radioimmunoassay for human ovarian tumor associated antigen OCA. Am. J. Obstet. Gynecol. **138**:1222–1223.
15. **Knauf, S., and G. I. Urbach.** 1981. Identification, purification and radioimmunoassay of NB/70K, a human ovarian tumor-associated antigen. Cancer Res. **41**:1351–1357.
16. **Koprowski, H., Z. Steplewski, K. Mitchell, M. Herlyn, D. Herlyn, and J. P. Fuhrer.** 1979. Colorectal carcinoma antigens detected by hybridoma antibodies. Somatic Cell Genet. **5**:957.
17. **Masuho, Y., M. Zalutsky, R. C. Knapp, and R. C. Bast,**

Jr. 1984. Interaction of monoclonal antibodies with cell surface antigens of human ovarian carcinomas. Cancer Res. **44**:2813–2819.

18. **Metzgar, R. S., M. T. Gaillard, S. J. Levine, F. L. Tuck, E. H. Bossen, and M. J. Borowitz.** 1982. Antigens of human pancreatic adenocarcinoma cells defined by murine monoclonal antibodies. Cancer Res. **42**:601.

19. **Niloff, J. M., R. C. Bast, Jr., E. M. Schaetzl, and R. C. Knapp.** 1985. Predictive value of CA125 antigen levels at second-look procedures in ovarian cancer. Am. J. Obstet. Gynecol. **151**:981–986.

19a.**Niloff, J. M., T. L. Klug, E. Schaetzl, V. R. Zurawski, R. C. Knapp, and R. C. Bast, Jr.** 1984. Elevation of serum CA125 in carcinomas of the fallopian tube, endometrium, and endocervix. Am. J. Obstet. Gynecol. **148**:1057–1058.

19b.**Niloff, J. M., R. C. Knapp, E. Schaetzl, C. Reynolds, and R. C. Bast, Jr.** 1984. CA125 antigen levels in obstetric and gynecologic patients. Obstet. Gynecol. **64**:703–707.

20. **Nouwen, E. J., D. E. Pollet, J. B. Schelstraete, M. W. Eerdekens, C. Hansch, A. Van de Voorde, and M. E. De Broe.** 1985. Human placental alkaline phosphatase in benign and malignant ovarian neoplasia. Cancer Res. **45**:892–902.

21. **Ruibal, A., G. Encabo, E. Martinez-Miralles, J. A. Murcia, J. A. Capderhal, L. A. Salgado, and J. M. Martinez-Vasquez.** 1984. CA125 seric levels in nonmalignant pathologies. Bull. Cancer **71**:145–148.

22. **Stall, K. E., and E. W. Martin.** 1981. Plasma carcinoembryonic antigen levels in ovarian cancer patients: a chart review and survey of published data. J. Reprod. Med. **26**:75–79.

23. **Sunderland, C. A., J. O. Davies, and G. M. Stirrat.** 1984. Immunohistology of normal and ovarian cancer tissue with a monoclonal antibody to placental alkaline phosphatase. Cancer Res. **44**:4496–4502.

24. **Tagliabue, E., S. Menard, G. Della Torre, P. Barbanti, R. Mariani-Costantini, G. Porro, and M. I. Colnaghi.** 1985. Generation of monocolonal antibodies reacting with human epithelial ovarian cancer. Cancer Res. **45:** 379–385.

25. **van Dalen, A., J. Favier, and W. N. Eastham.** 1984. Preliminary observations with a new monoclonal antibody in ovarian carcinoma. Tumor Diag. Ther. **5**:67–69.

Chapter 128

Section N. Immunogenetics and Transplantation Immunology

Introduction

DEVENDRA P. DUBEY AND EDMOND J. YUNIS

Investigations carried out in the past three decades have established the role of genes in the major histocompatibility complex region in controlling the outcome of tissue transplantation. The success of transplantation, an alternative in the treatment of several diseases involving loss in the function of organs, depends on the degree of histocompatibility between donor and recipient. An HLA typing laboratory is now an important component of any hospital conducting organ transplants and transfusions of blood components. The laboratory procedures described in this section were selected to meet the needs of clinical HLA laboratories to keep abreast with the rapid developments which are occurring in the theory and practice of use of the HLA systems.

The genes of major histocompatibility complex region H-2 in mice are located on chromosome 17, and those of HLA in humans are located on the short arm of chromosome 6. While the HLA region contains many different genes, two sets of genes coding for cell surface antigens are class I HLA-A, -B, and -C genes, which are expressed on all nucleated cells, and class II HLA-D-related genes (HLA-DP, -DQ, and -DR), which are expressed primarily on B lymphocytes and macrophages. In addition to the HLA class I and II genes, another class of genes identified within this complex is class III, which consists of the structural genes for serum complement C2, factor B (BF), serum complement C4, and the structural gene 21 hydroxylase (21-OH). Moreover, genes encoding for specific enzyme molecules (superoxide dismutase-2, phosphoglucomutase-2, and glyoxylase-1) are linked to the HLA complex.

It has been known for some time that the class I and II genes of the HLA complex are polymorphic to various degrees; this polymorphism is discussed by Sullivan and Amos (chapter 130). Recent research findings have indicated that the four HLA-linked structural genes for the serum components C2, BF, C4A, and C4B are also polymorphic. At least two alleles exist for C2, four for BF, and seven each for C4A and C4B. Furthermore, the nucleotide sequences of the genes for C2 and BF appear to indicate that these two genes belong to the same gene family. An extensive homology between C4A and C4B genes and 21-OHA and 21-OHB has been observed, suggesting tandem gene duplications in the class III region. Studies using molecular biology and recombinant families have shown the overall order of genes in the HLA region to be D, C2, BF, C4B, 21-OHA, C4A, 21-OHB, B, C, A.

Despite increasing application of biochemical and molecular biological techniques in HLA studies, the use of conventional serological techniques will continue in typing patients for organ transplantation, blood component transfusion, disease association studies, and paternity testing. One of the essential reagents required in such typing studies is a well-characterized HLA antibody. The demand for such reagents will undoubtedly continue in the future, and the screening for such sera will require careful planning and organization. Although the basic methodology of HLA typing has not changed since the publication of the 2nd edition of this manual, a tremendous amount of new information has been gathered during the past 5 years. Many new HLA antigens were identified and old antigens were established during the international workshops held in Los Angeles (1980) and Munich (1984). The chapters by Zachary et al. (chapter 129) and Sullivan and Amos (chapter 130) discuss technical aspects relevant to the planning and organization of serum screening and HLA typing. The chapter by Sanfillipo and Amos (chapter 134) discusses both the significance and the limitations of interpretation of the HLA data obtained by use of the various methodologies.

Cellular typing using homozygous typing cells in mixed lymphocyte culture has played a valuable role in the discovery of the HLA-D region. Cell-mediated lympholysis can also be used as a typing method to identify surface molecules that are recognized by cytotoxic T lymphocytes generated in mixed lymphocyte culture. In the majority of cases the molecules recognized by cytotoxic T cells correlate with serologically defined HLA (A, B, C, and D/DR) specificities. In addition, cell-mediated lympholysis can detect HLA determinants that are not identified by serology. The traditional methods utilized for cellular typing are described by Dubey et al. (chapter 131). A more recent cellular method used specifically to type the DP locus antigens of the HLA-D region is primed-lymphocyte testing. Recent developments in the techniques of cloning of cells of unique specificity used in conjunction with primed-lymphocyte testing have made it possible to type HLA-DP specificities easily and rapidly. This method is described by Hartzman and Sheehy (chapter 132). It is worth mentioning here that the earlier concept that antigens defined by cellular methods are distinctly different from those identified by serological methods no longer holds, since monoclonal antibodies can identify antigens that have been defined by using cellular methods. The use of monoclonal antibodies has made it possible, for example, to sort out the three sets of products DP, DQ, and DR as subregions of HLA-D.

Molecular biological techniques combined with serological and cellular techniques provide a very powerful method to study the HLA system. A spectacular development in our understanding of class I and II genetic systems became possible with the application of these techniques, and typing by gene probes may soon become a routine technique in clinical HLA laboratories. The chapter by Biro and Glass on restriction fragment length polymorphism (chapter 133) is indicative of this trend. Restriction fragment length polymorphism may prove to be an extremely valuable technique in the diagnosis of inherited diseases. This technique has already been applied in the study of hemoglobinopathies and diagnosis of Huntington's chorea. The important aspect of this technique is that it can be used even with those diseases where no genetic markers are presently known. Moreover, it can be successfully utilized in prenatal diagnosis of inherited diseases.

Studies on disease associations with the various HLA haplotypes have provided interesting information on disease heterogeneity and clinical subclassification. Svejgaard (chapter 139) has provided up-to-date information on disease association with various haplotypes and on methods employed in estimating sample size and in calculating relative risks and the level of significance indicated by χ^2. This chapter includes material that can be useful in experimental design for disease association studies and interpretation of HLA data.

Another important clinical application of HLA typing is in the areas of kidney and bone marrow transplantation. Despite continuous immune suppression treatment, most patients undergo clinical episodes of graft rejection. A complex network of cellular processes is responsible for the cellular and humoral responses of organ rejection. By employing sensitive techniques which are directed toward determining both cellular and humoral responses, a comprehensive picture of the rejection process can emerge. The methods used in monitoring the status of graft rejection are described by Garovoy and Carpenter in chapter 136. Donor selection and recipient-monitoring strategies in bone marrow transplantation are discussed by Hansen et al. in chapter 137.

The correlation between hyperacute renal allograft rejection and the presence of antibody against HLA-A, -B, and -C on donor tissue is well established. The probability of graft rejection can be reduced, however, by presensitization of the potential recipient to the donor's lymphocytes for HLA antigens. Approaches to detect cross-matching are described by Johnson (chapter 135).

HLA typing has reached the courtrooms as an important and acceptable method in paternity testing. Since an increasing number of HLA laboratories must deal with the question of paternity testing, a greater understanding of genetics and statistics is necessary for the interpretation of HLA typing data for use in this area. Bias and Zachary have presented a very lucid exposition of this difficult subject (chapter 138).

In summary, this section reviews the basic principles and present state of knowledge in the rapidly developing field of human immunogenetics and transplantation immunology. The practical applications of HLA to clinical settings are presently limited to clinical transplantation, blood transfusion therapy, and the study of certain HLA-linked and -associated diseases. Since the major goal of HLA studies is to understand the functional relationship, if any, between the HLA genetic system and transplantation and disease association, and since function is intimately related to structure, the application of monoclonal antibodies, protein chemistry, and molecular biology techniques should provide the tools necessary for further practical application of immunogenetics in clinical medicine.

Chapter 129

Screening Sera for HLA Antibodies

ANDREA A. ZACHARY, NANCY B. MURPHY, ALAN R. SMERGLIA, AND WILLIAM E. BRAUN

Because of the great variety in the types of laboratories interested in screening sera for HLA antibodies, the approach to serum screening will have to fit the needs of each laboratory. Included among the various objectives of a serum screening program are: the detection of HLA antibodies which have relevance to transplantation, the evaluation of HLA antibodies for use as routine typing reagents, and the characterization of antibodies useful in the biochemical analysis of HLA gene products. As the understanding of the function of the HLA system and the application of this knowledge to organ transplantation, transfusions, forensic medicine, and disease studies increase, the need for greater quantities of well-characterized HLA reagents will also increase.

A laboratory can establish a basic serum screening program with a moderate amount of equipment and concentrated effort. However, a program should be flexible enough to expand in both size and sophistication to meet additional or different objectives as the needs of the laboratory change.

In this chapter we discuss various aspects of serum screening, including specimen acquisition, cell panel construction, test methodologies, data analysis, record keeping, applications, and computerization. We have attempted to present concepts as well as specifics. The reader is urged to keep in mind that these examples are drawn from our own experience and may require modification to suit the needs of other programs.

SPECIMEN ACQUISITION

Sources of antibody

An effective approach to specimen acquisition will take into account when and how HLA antibodies occur as well as the logistics of sample collection. In this chapter we will be concerned with antibodies directed to the products of class I and class II HLA genes. Both classes of genes are highly polymorphic, encoding glycoprotein products which can be found distributed throughout the body (4). Class I products are found on the surface of nucleated cells, while class II products are located primarily on B lymphocytes, monocytes, endothelial cells, and sperm. These glycoproteins are expressed early in fetal development (9) and, as implied by the designation "histocompatibility antigens," differentiate self from non-self. Therefore, it is not surprising that such antibodies may arise after organ transplantation, transfusion, or pregnancy. In addition to HLA antibodies occurring in humans, monoclonal antibodies have been produced by immunization of animals with lymphocyte membranes or purified HLA antigen.

Patients awaiting transplantation may have been immunized by blood transfusions, previous organ transplant, pregnancy, or a combination of these.

Generally, these antibodies are duo- to polyspecific. Although there is often an increase in sensitization with increasing numbers of transfusions, some individuals may never make antibody or may experience a reduction of antibody. Hemodialysis patients awaiting kidney transplantation may have drastic fluctuations in both the specificity and the number of antibodies being produced. Identification of the different antibodies may be important. Therefore, to establish an accurate profile of antibody reactivity, it is necessary to collect samples on a monthly basis, as well as after sensitizing events like transfusion or allograft nephrectomy. Patients awaiting heart, liver, or pancreas transplantation present a different problem. Due to the severity of their illness, expediency in acquiring and testing a serum sample may be an urgent objective. The major goal in testing patients' sera is to detect and define presensitization. Generally, transplant patients, either because of the polyspecificity and transiency of their antibody response or because of their poor state of health, are not good sources of reagent-quality HLA antibodies. However, exceptions to this rule do occur, and when a useful reagent is detected, the patient's physician should be approached to determine if acquisition of additional serum is possible. All patients' sera, particularly that from dialysis patients, carry a risk of transmitting hepatitis, and appropriate precautions must be taken by those handling the specimens.

To date, parous females have been, as a group, the largest single source of reagent-quality HLA antisera. Antibodies are produced in response to the fetus's paternal HLA antigens in about 10 to 19% of primigravidae (1, 13) and 20 to 30% of women with two or more children (3, 13). In primigravidae, there is a single peak of antibody production at 6 months, whereas in multiparidae, two peaks occur in the 3rd and 6th months (13). The antibodies may develop as early as the 2nd month in multiparidae (13) and show a rising incidence and titer from 16 to 32 weeks, after which the antibodies either level off (3) or decrease (13). The range of antibody specificities may narrow at the time of delivery (12), and both the number and titers of the various antibodies will decline in a variable fashion after delivery (3, 10, 11). Clearly, the antibody activity observed in the laboratory will depend on the time(s) at which the samples are acquired as well as on the frequency of immunization, the immunogenicity of the paternal antigens, and the immune responsiveness of the mother.

The HLA antibody produced by the mother is absorbed onto the placenta (6), preventing its entrance into the fetal circulation. The placenta is then a potential source of antibody, and many laboratories, particularly those unable to obtain samples of peripheral blood from parous females, routinely perform antibody extraction procedures on placental material (2).

Other sources of HLA antibody that have been pursued for the purpose of procuring typing reagents, including polytransfused patients, immunized animals, and hybridomas, have been only moderately successful. However, it is likely that monoclonal antibodies will play a significant role in the biochemical analysis of the HLA gene products. A discussion of the production and analysis of monoclonal antibodies is beyond the scope of this chapter. Therefore, we will limit our consideration to programs for screening antibody from more conventional sources.

Specimen handling

Specimens should be labeled in a way which minimizes the possibility of misidentification without requiring an inordinate amount of time. For patients, the label should include, minimally, the patient's name, a unique subject identification number (e.g., social security or case history number), and the date the sample was drawn. Samples from parous females may be coded with a sequential number system for the sake of expediency.

Samples should be handled in a manner which does not alter the biologic properties pertinent to their use. That is, they should be protected from temperature extremes, collected aseptically if extended storage at 4°C or higher is anticipated, and subjected to a minimum of freeze-thaw cycles, aeration, and dehydration. Addition of sodium azide to a final concentration of 0.1% may be used to retard microbial growth in sera to be used in the lymphocytotoxicity test, but should be avoided for sera to be used in a functional assay such as lysostripping. Successful specimen collection, therefore, requires planning and coordination.

Although sample size has not been mentioned and although it seems obvious that the size should be adequate to perform all necessary tests, 5 ml of serum is generally sufficient.

Once the sample has been obtained, it should be subjected to all necessary treatments and dispensed into aliquots. All appropriate record keeping should be performed. Most small samples will arrive as clotted blood, and the serum requires only clarification by centrifugation to be ready for use in lymphocytotoxicity assays. On the other hand, large samples obtained by plasmapheresis are usually citrated plasma that requires easily performed recalcification (7). Samples obtained from patients on hemodialysis will contain heparin and must be treated with an agent such as protamine sulfate before they will clot. Other treatments may be necessary for use of the samples in different assays. In addition to treatments necessary to allow the use of a sample in a particular type of test, it may be desirable to remove certain antibodies. For example, in tests that use purified B lymphocytes to screen for class II-specific antibodies, it is desirable to remove antibodies to class I antigens which are also expressed in B cells, because reactions with class I antigens may mask class II antibodies and make analysis difficult. Removal of class I-specific antibodies can, in most cases, be achieved by absorption with pooled platelets (14), since platelets express class I but not class II antigens. If the antibody to be removed is specific for an uncommon antigen or for an antigen which is poorly expressed on platelets, such as HLA-B12, more extensive absorption may be necessary to assure complete removal of the antibody.

It is usually advisable to dispense a serum sample into several aliquots at the beginning. This reduces the chance of damaging antibodies by repeatedly freezing and thawing a single specimen. Furthermore, it is possible to sort samples according to the type of screening they are to receive, when a single specimen is to be tested in several different ways. In the labeling of aliquots, it is important to designate any treatment that has been performed on a specimen. Color-coded tubes can be used to differentiate these different preparations without requiring additional time for labeling.

Good record keeping throughout the screen program is essential, and various examples of different records will be provided throughout this chapter. Laboratories responsible for evaluating potential renal transplant patients usually receive serum specimens each day. Under these circumstances, and especially when different treatments are to be performed on the sera, it is practical to batch process the specimens. When batch processing is performed, a log sheet of specimens received can be used to designate what treatments and tests are to be performed on the specimens. An example of a log sheet is provided in Fig. 1.

LYMPHOCYTE PANEL

The lymphocyte panel should have adequate representation of all known antigens and verified "blanks" reflecting unknown antigens. The adequacy of the panel will be determined by the objectives of the screening program, but, in general, all antigens listed as easy or moderately difficult in Table 1 should be included. The antigens listed as rare and difficult are those with low population frequencies or for which good reagents are so scarce that some laboratories may have difficulty in detecting them. Genotyping of cell donors provides the best definition of an antigen and is necessary for establishing homozygotes and blanks, but clearly phenotyped donors are certainly useful. Periodic retyping of the cell panel with additional new reagents is important for refining and expanding the antigens of the panel. Each antigen should be represented on three or four different panel lymphocytes, because with fewer cells a technical problem with one cell could result in an antiserum specificity being missed or misinterpreted. Because of the large number of recognized specificities, panels which have multiple representations of each antigen are becoming unmanageably large; it is therefore important to keep in mind the objectives or information desired when establishing the cell panel. For example, the detection and identification of antibody in serum from a potential transplant patient is important, but the precise knowledge of the quality of this antibody as a reagent is not important to providing health care to the patient. Therefore, it may be possible to achieve this goal with fewer cell donors than are needed for reagent evaluation. By making certain assumptions about serum samples in advance, it is possible to reduce the size of the cell panel used in certain cases. For example, in a panel comprising 50

Name _____ Serum# _____

Address _____ Specif. _____

_____ Date _____

Phone _____ Sample# _____

No. Preg. _____ No. Child. _____ Yngst. _____ Blood Tx _____

ABO _____ Rh _____ RhoGam _____

1st screen _____ tray ____ Immzg. donor _____

BLEEDINGS

Date   Amount   Pd   Preg   Screen   Results

FIG. 8. Reagent donor card.

the antibody specificity. The exact results of the screening of a serum should include the number of concordant and discordant reactions, the strength of the reactions, and subjective comments about the serum that can be included on a card such as that shown in Fig. 9. Of course, this card can be filed by serum name, antibody specificity, or both. The usefulness of a reagent is affected by its accessibility, and therefore an accurate and current serum inventory is essential. This inventory is most useful when it is indexed by specificity and includes the precise volume and location of a serum and even, when there is a large volume of the serum, a record of the number of aliquots of different sizes.

It is evident that suitable record keeping involves time-consuming duplication. In the final section of this chapter, we discuss the application of computers to a serum screening program, not only for the more traditional data analysis, but also to perform clerical and managerial functions.

COMPUTERIZATION OF DATA MANAGEMENT AND ANALYSIS

The use of a computer in the tissue typing laboratory can increase the efficiency of personnel, reduce the number of tedious tasks, and facilitate data analysis. Therefore, computers can be used as aids in laboratory management as well as in the analysis of HLA data.

Among the managerial chores which can be computerized are (1) the generation of worklists, (2) the production of billing records, and (3) the production of test result reports. Any of these tasks is simple to perform manually, but with a computer these tasks can be integrated to eliminate duplication. For example, if a typing is requested for a particular day, the name of the subject to be tested is added to a worklist of typings for that day. At the initial entry, all information necessary for billing and generating a report is also entered so that when the test results are entered, all necessary paperwork can be generated automatically by the computer. This same procedure can be applied to serum screening. However, instead of a daily worklist, the computer can maintain a running log of sera to be screened. Characteristics assigned to a serum would include the type of screen (i.e., cell type and technique to be performed) as well as the dilutions at which the serum is to be tested. The computer would then assign a particular serum at a particular dilution to a single well of a specified tray, thus designing the screen trays. If the program is designed to keep track of the status of a serum sample, the patient's serum records can be updated automatically so that one would know what samples exist, if and when they have been tested, and what the test results were. Again, a billing record and eventually a report of the test results could be generated automatically.

It is possible to quickly amass a large number of patient and reagent samples so that an accurate in-

SERUM B

Tray	Dil	Freq	Specificity	Serum vs Group				Remarks
				++	+	-	--	
					False			
343	1:1	40%	B5	11	4	0	30	1 Bw35±
			Bw35	5		1	29	
..	1:2	32%	B5	11	0	0	34	2 Bw35±
			Bw35	5		1	33	
..	1:4	18%	B5	6	0	5	36	1 B5± , 3 Bw35
			Bw35	3		3	38	

FIG. 9. Reagent evaluation record.

	A					B			
	S1	S2	S3	S4		S1	S2	S3	S4
S2	.77				S2	+			
S3	.70	.76			S3	+	+		
S4	.77	.70	.60		S4	+	+	−	
S5	.86	.70	.62	.70	S5	*	+	−	+

FIG. 10. Examples of cluster analysis printouts. In A, the numerical value of the correlation coefficient for each serum comparison is given. In B, value ranges are represented by symbols as follows: −, $r = 0.60$ to 0.69; +, $r = 0.70$ to 0.79; *, $r = 0.80$ to 0.89.

ventory system is a necessity. For patients' samples, a single record by patient name may be adequate. However, for reagents, it is desirable to organize various types of information, such as screen data and sample volume and location, by both serum name (or donor name) and specificity. As noted earlier, manual data management would require multiple files to facilitate cross-indexing; however, only a single file would be needed for computerized data management. By using the appropriate inquiry one can call up information by the character of interest. For example, one could request a listing of all HLA-A1 antibodies. The request could be more specific, such as for all A1 antisera which have a certain minimum volume or all antisera which correlated with A1 with an r value of ≥ 0.9.

For the maintenance of records of the HLA antibody history for transplant patients, a computer is very helpful. With the aid of database management software, a graph of a patient's antibody activity versus time can be prepared. This is a relatively easy task to perform manually on 1 patient or even 10 patients, but it is prohibitive for 100 patients unless a computer is available.

Several types of computer programs are used for the analysis of serum screening data, including inclusion analysis, cluster analysis, pattern analysis, and serograph (8). The inclusion analysis is one of the most popular programs for the identification of antibody specificities in a system in which at least some of the antigens have been defined. As in the manual analysis, a serum pattern is compared with each antigen pattern to find the best match. The evaluation of the correlation between antigen and antibody is based on the value of the correlation coefficient discussed earlier. Thus, the antigen specificity which yields the highest r value for a serum reaction pattern is assigned to that serum. The process continues as concordantly positive cells are deleted, and for the remaining cells, the serum reaction pattern is compared with each antigen pattern to find the best fit. The process is carried out in an iterative fashion until no further significant associations are found. The remaining reactions are referred to as the "tail."

A typical printout from an inclusion analysis provides a listing of the assigned specificities, the numbers of concordant and discordant reactions for each assigned specificity, and the phenotypes of the cells in the tail. Some inclusion analysis programs are designed to differentiate the various reaction scores and print the phenotypes of the cells in each reaction score category.

On the assumption that a significant positive association between two (or more) sera is due to antibodies which react either with the same antigen or epitope or with different antigens which themselves are nonrandomly associated, the initial recognition of a new antigen is often based on the identification of positively associated sera. Cluster analysis programs are used to identify similarly reacting sera as measured by criteria such as the Pearson correlation coefficient or the Dice similarity index. That is, a minimum value for the association between sera is determined by the investigator, and the cluster is composed of sera which have an association equal to or greater than that value. The cluster may be constructed in several different ways. A cluster may consist of sera which have a positive association with a specified key serum, or it may consist of sera that all have a positive association of a specified minimum value with each of the other sera in the cluster. For systems with a large number of antigens already identified, such as the HLA system, cluster analysis is most useful in identifying new subgroups or "splits."

Printouts for cluster analysis display comparisons of all sera included within a cluster. The exact numerical value of the correlation can be provided, or symbols, designating different value ranges, may be used. Examples of these two cluster displays are given in Fig. 10.

Another approach to the recognition of antigen splits is the pattern analysis. In this analysis, sera known to react with a certain antigen are examined for the different patterns of reactivity displayed within the group. The number of times each pattern is observed is determined. The occurrence of different patterns according to racial group can also be tabulated. The pattern analysis can thus provide information on possible splits and racial variants of a known antigen. The occurrence of only one or two individuals for a particular pattern is not very informative since this could represent technical error or random serum variability. Therefore, the pattern analysis is best utilized when sera have been tested against a large number of individuals.

A serograph is a graph of the reactions of various sera, listed on one axis, with cells from a group of donors listed on the other. The rows or columns are usually rearranged until any patterns are clearly visible. The serograph and pattern analysis are complementary, the former providing a clearly discernible picture of significant patterns and trends and the latter providing a quantitative evaluation of those patterns. As with the other types of analyses discussed above, serographs can be prepared manually, but they are tedious and consume a great deal of time. A computer can perform these analyses quickly and without error, provided the data are entered correctly. A computer cannot, however, recognize errors in data entry or make inferences about the biologic significance of data. Therefore, computer-generated analyses should always be reviewed by experienced serologists to determine their validity and biologic significance.

Computers can provide a major enhancement to an HLA laboratory; however, finding computer software tailored to an HLA laboratory is difficult. There are very few computer programmers who have learned the jargon of HLA, and very few HLA people who have learned the computer jargon necessary to define their nccds to the computer programmer, thus creating a Tower of Babel. One must select help in this area with great care.

LITERATURE CITED

1. **Ahrons, S.** 1971. Leukocyte antibodies: occurrence in primigravidae. Tissue Antigens **1**:178–183.
2. **Doughty, R. W., and K. Gelsthorpe.** 1974. An initial investigation of lymphocyte antibody activity through pregnancy and in eluates prepared from placental material. Tissue Antigens **4**:291–298.
3. **Doughty, R. W., and K. Gelsthorpe.** 1976. Some parameters of lymphocyte antibody activity through pregnancy and further eluates of placental material. Tissue Antigens **8**:43–48.
4. **Hood, L., M. Steinmetz, and B. Malissen.** 1983. Genes of the major histocompatibility complex of the mouse. Annu. Rev. Immunol. **1**:529–568.
5. **Hopkins, K. A., and J. M. MacQueen.** 1981. Basic microlymphocytotoxicity technique, p. II-1-1–II-1-9. *In*

A. A. Zachary and W. E. Braun (ed.), AACHT laboratory manual. AACHT, New York.
6. **Oh, J. H., and L. D. Maclean.** 1975. Comparative immunogenicity of HLA antigens: a study in primiparas. Tissue Antigens. **5**:33–37.
7. **Perkins, H.** 1974. Conversion of plasma to serum, p. 147–148. *In* J. G. Ray, Jr., D. B. Hare, P. D. Pedersen, and D. E. Kayhoe (ed.), Manual of tissue typing techniques. Publication no. (NIH) 75-545. U.S. Department of Health, Education and Welfare, Washington, D.C.
8. **Pickbourne, P., S. Richards, J. G. Bodmer, and W. F. Bodmer.** 1978. Data organization and methods of analysis, p. 295–324. *In* W. F. Bodmer, J. R. Batchelor, J. G. Bodmer, H. Festenstein, and P. J. Morris (ed.), Histocompatibility testing 1977. Munksgaard, Copenhagen.
9. **Seigler, H. F., and R. S. Metzger.** 1970. Embryonic development of human transplantation antigens. Transplantation **2**:478–486.
10. **Stastny, P.** 1972. Tissue typing antisera from immunization by pregnancy. Tissue Antigens **2**:123–127.
11. **Tongio, M. M., A. Benebi, B. Pfeiffer, and S. Mayer.** 1971. Serological studies on lymphocytotoxic antibodies in primiparous women. Tissue Antigens **1**:243–257.
12. **Tongio, M. M., and S. Mayer.** 1977. Narrowing of fetomaternal immunization at time of delivery. Tissue Antigens **9**:174–176.
13. **Vives, J., A. Gelabret, and R. Castillo.** 1976. HLA antibodies and period of gestation: decline in frequency of positive sera during last trimester. Tissue Antigens **7**:209–212.
14. **Ward, F. E., J. F. Shaw, and A. A. Zachary.** 1981. Serum characterization and donor-recipient crossmatching, p. III-1-1–III-2-43. *In* A. A. Zachary and W. E. Braun (ed.), AACHT laboratory manual. AACHT, New York.
15. **Willoughby, P. B., F. E. Ward, and J. M. McQueen.** 1981. Modifications of the microcytotoxicity test, p. II-1-2–II-2-13. *In* A. A. Zachary and W. E. Braun (ed.), AACHT laboratory manual. AACHT, New York.

Chapter 130

The HLA System and Its Detection

KAREN A. SULLIVAN AND D. BERNARD AMOS

HLA, the major histocompatibility complex of humans, is an assembly of closely linked genes of chromosome 6 which regulate or control numerous immunological processes. Most of the genes are highly polymorphic, and many variants or alleles can be distinguished. One set of genes codes for the cell surface glycoprotein antigens of the HLA-A, HLA-B, and HLA-C series. These are called class I antigens and provide "fingerprints" that determine the distinction between self and nonself. A second set codes for the cell surface glycoproteins of the class II antigens, the HLA-DP, HLA-DQ, and HLA-DR series (formerly SB, DC/DS/MB, and DR). These are the antigens of immunoregulation which are expressed on B lymphocytes and other cells that have been activated. Because they were originally identified in sera which could specifically block the mixed-lymphocyte reaction (MLR) that measures HLA-D, they are also referred to as D-related or D-region antigens. HLA-D is a functional expression of HLA. Another set of genes, sometimes called class III, code for or regulate a variety of complement components of both the classic and alternate pathways. Other genes within or near the major histocompatibility complex are structural genes for various enzymes.

Genes which determine susceptibility or resistance to disease are also linked to the major histocompatibility complex. HLA-associated diseases include many autoimmune, allergic, and metabolic disorders. Transplant rejection, leukemogenesis, oncogenesis, and resistance to a variety of infections are other associated characteristics being studied.

Inheritance of HLA

HLA is inherited in Mendelian fashion. The set of class I, class II, and class III genes carried by each chromosome is called an HLA haplotype. The HLA haplotype includes a minimum of six genetic loci: HLA-A, B, and C (class I genes) and the HLA-D region loci, DP, DQ, and D/DR (class II genes). The haplotype also carries three genes for complement components (class III genes), two 21-hydroxylase genes plus at least one gene that regulates the expression of class I and class II antigens on T cells (7a, 12a) (Fig. 1). These loci have been shown to be distinct entities which can be separated by recombination, lost through deletion in certain mutant cell lines, or isolated through hybridization to complementary DNA probes. It is believed that some of the characteristics of the major histocompatibility complex result from interactions between its constituents (as well as from its components), e.g., HLA-D expression or the ability to stimulate primed cells in mixed culture, which is attributable to interactions involving DP alleles. Since HLA loci comprising the haplotype are closely linked, they are inherited as a genetic unit. Each individual, therefore, has two HLA haplotypes, one contributed by

each parent. As the HLA gene products are codominantly expressed, each person expresses two antigens per locus. The identification of antigens at each locus constitutes a phenotype, e.g., A3, A11, B8, Bw22, Cw3, Cw4, DR3, DR4. The assignment of each antigen to its locus on a parental chromosome is a genotype, e.g., *A3, B8, Cw4, DR3, A11, Bw22, Cw2, DR4*. By convention, paternal haplotypes are arbitrarily labeled a and b and maternal haplotypes are designated c and d. The haplotypes of offspring, therefore, become ac, ad, bc, and bd, resulting in a 25% chance of identity between siblings. Codominant expression of the antigens and the Mendelian mode of inheritance is the basis for many clinical tests such as matching for transplant or paternity testing.

Nomenclature

The current system of HLA terminology was adopted in 1975 by the World Health Organization Committee on HLA Nomenclature. Each HLA locus as it is defined is assigned a letter in alphabetical order, e.g., HLA-A, HLA-B, etc. Universally accepted specificities are designated by Arabic numerals, such as HLA-A1, HLA-B5, HLA-DR1, etc. Specificities that are less well defined (but not less in significance) are given provisional status and are indicated by the prefix "w" before the numeral; examples are HLA-Aw33, HLA-Bw22, and HLA-DRw6. HLA-C locus specificities will always retain the prefix "w" before the numeral to avoid confusion with the complement components. At all loci except HLA-A and HLA-B, specificities are numbered consecutively, preceded by their locus designation, i.e., HLA-Cw1, HLA-Cw2, HLA-DR1, HLA-DR2, etc. The antigens of the HLA-A and HLA-B series (previously the 1st or LA and 2nd or Four locus antigens, respectively), were defined before it was recognized that HLA is a multilocus system. Rather than change the names of well-known and accepted antigens, therefore, HLA-A and HLA-B antigens continue to be numbered jointly, e.g., B8, A9, A26, B27, etc. A rather different strategy may become necessary for the HLA-D region alleles. A complete list of specificities is given in Table 1. See also Antigenic Determinants of HLA, below.

Class I antigens, HLA-A, HLA-B, HLA-C

HLA-A, HLA-B, and HLA-C antigens are present on the membranes of most nucleated cells. Antigen concentrations are especially high on lymphocytes, but the antigens are also found on blood platelets, vascular endothelium, fibroblasts, macrophages, epidermal cells, and kidney parenchymal cells. All of these cell types have been used in antigen assays.

The genes and antigens of HLA-A and HLA-B have been extensively characterized (8). The genes, which have a typical intron-exon structure, belong to a large

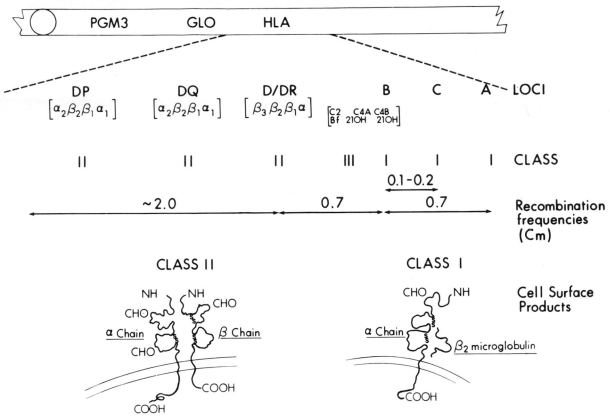

FIG. 1. HLA chromosome and products.

gene family of 30 or more members, many of which are regarded as pseudogenes as no products have been identified. The class I antigenic product, a glycoprotein (α chain) with a molecular weight of 45,000 has three extracellular domains each consisting of about 90 amino acid residues and designated α_1, α_2, and α_3. The α_1, amino (N)-terminal domain contains a glycosylation site at an asparagine residue (position 86). The α_2 and α_3 domains have internal disulfide bonds. The α-chain molecule is inserted through the membrane via a hybrophobic sequence (of 24 amino acids) which can be cleaved from the membrane by papain. Noncovalently bound to the α chain is a smaller (β) chain of 11 kilodaltons which corresponds to β_2-microglobulin found in serum and urine and encoded by chromosome 15.

HLA-B is the most highly polymorphic of all the HLA antigens (Table 1). HLA-A is less polymorphic, and fewer than a dozen alleles of HLA-C have been identified. HLA-C has been less well characterized serologically, functionally, or biochemically than either HLA-A or HLA-B. It appears to be less immunogenic; antibodies to HLA-C are not as common, and the product has been thought to be less stable.

Class II antigens, HLA-DP, HLA-DQ, HLA-DR

The HLA-D region antigens, DR, DQ, and DP, also glycoproteins, are less polymorphic and have a more restricted distribution than the class I antigens, but have a more complex genetic and structural composition. The class II antigens are characteristic of B lymphocytes. They are not expressed on platelets. The

HLA-DR antigens have the widest distribution, being present also on macrophages, Langerhans cells of the epidermis, activated T cells, and endothelial cells. HLA-DP antigens are also detected on macrophages (at 10% the expression of DR) and activated T cells; the distribution of HLA-DQ antigens on other than B cells has not yet been clarified. It is likely that the concentration of all class II antigens increases as cells are activated.

The HLA-DR, HLA-DQ, and HLA-DP serologically detectable antigens are composed of two noncovalently associated chains: in this instance, both chains are inserted through the cell membrane via hydrophobic regions and both are HLA-encoded products (6). The respective molecular weights are 33,000 (heavy or α chain) and 27,000 (light or β chain). Class II molecules have a membrane orientation similar to that of the class I α-chain molecules, with the N terminus extracellular and the carboxyl (C) terminus intracellular. The α and β chains of class II molecules have two extracellular domains: both β-chain domains (β_1, β_2) and the α-chain domain nearer the C terminus (α_2) contain an intrachain disulfide bridge. The C-terminal extracellular domains of class II molecules (α_2, β_2) have sequence homology to the corresponding domains of class I molecules (α_3, β_2-microglobulin) and to the CH_3 domain of immunoglobulins (see Fig. 1).

Molecular genetic studies using complementary DNA clones have shown that there are at least seven nonallelic β-chain genes and five nonallelic α-chain genes encoded within the HLA-D region (see Fig. 1). The HLA-DR locus encodes for one α- and three β-chain genes, while the HLA-DQ and HLA-DP loci

TABLE 1. Complete listing of recognized HLA specificities[a]

HLA-A	HLA-B		HLA-C	HLA-D	HLA-DR	HLA-DQ	HLA-DP
HLA-A1	HLA-B5	HLA-B49(21)	HLA-Cw1	HLA-Dw1	HLA-DR1	HLA-DQw1	HLA-DPw1
HLA-A2	HLA-B7	HLA-Bw50(21)	HLA-Cw2	HLA-Dw2	HLA-DR2	HLA-DQw2	HLA-DPw2
HLA-A3	HLA-B8	HLA-B51(5)	HLA-Cw3	HLA-Dw3	HLA-DR3	HLA-DQw3	HLA-DPw3
HLA-A9	HLA-B12	HLA-Bw52(5)	HLA-Cw4	HLA-Dw4	HLA-DR4		HLA-DPw4
HLA-A10	HLA-B13	HLA-Bw53	HLA-Cw5	HLA-Dw5	HLA-DR5		HLA-DPw5
HLA-A11	HLA-B14	HLA-Bw54(w22)	HLA-Cw6	HLA-Dw6	HLA-DRw6		HLA-DPw6
HLA-Aw19	HLA-B15	HLA-Bw55(w22)	HLA-Cw7	HLA-Dw7	HLA-DR7		
HLA-A23(9)	HLA-B16	HLA-Bw56(w22)	HLA-Cw8	HLA-Dw8	HLA-DRw8		
HLA-A24(9)	HLA-B17	HLA-Bw57(17)		HLA-Dw9	HLA-DRw9		
HLA-A25(10)	HLA-B18	HLA-Bw58(17)		HLA-Dw10	HLA-DRw10		
HLA-A26(10)	HLA-B21	HLA-Bw59		HLA-Dw11(w7)	HLA-DRw11(5)		
HLA-A28	HLA-Bw22	HLA-Bw60(40)		HLA-Dw12	HLA-DRw12(5)		
HLA-A29(w19)	HLA-B27	HLA-Bw61(40)		HLA-Dw13	HLA-DRw13(w6)		
HLA-A30(w19)	HLA-B35	HLA-Bw62(15)		HLA-Dw14	HLA-DRw14(w6)		
HLA-A31(w19)	HLA-B37	HLA-Bw63(15)		HLA-Dw15			
HLA-A32(w19)	HLA-B38(16)	HLA-Bw64(14)		HLA-Dw16	HLA-DRw52[c]		
HLA-Aw33(w19)	HLA-B39(16)	HLA-Bw65(14)		HLA-Dw17(w7)	HLA-DRw53[c]		
HLA-Aw34(10)	HLA-B40	HLA-Bw67		HLA-Dw18(w6)			
HLA-Aw36	HLA-Bw41	HLA-Bw70		HLA-Dw19(w6)			
HLA-A43	HLA-Bw42	HLA-Bw71(w70)					
HLA-Aw66(10)	HLA-B44(12)	HLA-Bw72(w70)					
HLA-Aw68(28)	HLA-B45(12)	HLA-Bw73					
HLA-Aw69(28)	HLA-Bw46						
	HLA-Bw47	HLA-Bw4[b]					
	HLA-Bw48	HLA-Bw6[b]					

[a] Bodmer et al. (3).

[b] The following are the generally agreed inclusions of HLA-B specificities into Bw4 and Bw6. Bw4: B5, B13, B17, B27, B37, B38(16), B44(12), Bw47, B49(21), B51(5), Bw52(5), Bw53, Bw57(17), Bw58(17), Bw59, Bw63(15). Bw6: B7, B8, B14, B18, Bw22, B35, B39(16), B40, Bw41, Bw42, B45(12), Bw46, Bw48, Bw50(21), Bw54(w22), Bw55(w22), Bw56(w22), Bw60(40), Bw61(40), Bw62(15), Bw64(14), Bw65(14), Bw67, Bw70, Bw71(w70), Bw72(w70), Bw73.

[c] The following specificities are generally agreed to be associated with DRw52 and DRw53. DRw52: DR3, DR5, DRw6, DRw8, DRw11(5), DRw12(5), DRw13(w6), DRw14(w6). DRw53: DR4, DR7, DRw9.

each encode for two α- and two β-chain genes, all of which, at each locus, may not be expressed. Immunochemical as well as serological studies have shown that the α- and β-chain gene products of HLA-DR are distinctly different from the α- and β-chain gene products of HLA-DQ and HLA-DP, which are, in turn, different from each other.

The HLA-D series is functionally defined. The alleles are not detectable by antisera and have not been characterized biochemically or by molecular genetics. HLA-D antigens were first identified in families by MLR and called MLR-S determinants (16). Investigation was slow and tedious in populations because of the length of time to perform MLR and the requirement for homozygous cells. A more convenient definition was provided by van Rood et al. (14), who showed that sera which blocked MLR would bind with the stimulating B cells. They thus thought MLR-S was the same as DR. Exceptions were soon reported and were most common when Asiatics or blacks were studied. Since no HLA-D gene has been isolated and no product has been found, it is thought that HLA-D is the functional expression of HLA-DR together with other class II antigens and may result from interactions involving various D-region α and β gene products. Procedures for assigning HLA-D alleles to the haplotype are described elsewhere in this manual, so they will not be further mentioned here. A similar situation seems to apply to the HLA-DP antigens (formerly SB). The serologic detection of DP was, like HLA-DR antigens, subsequent to the original definition of the SB locus by functional studies using

primed lymphocyte testing. Since very few alloantisera or polymorphic monoclonal antibodies to DP have been generally available, the relationship between DP molecules and SB as defined by primed lymphocyte testing is still uncertain.

Antigenic determinants of HLA

The antigens of HLA have been defined by a consensus of acclamation. The first antigen to be universally recognized was HLA-A2, which was described as "MAC" by Dausset, as 8a by van Rood, and as LA2 by Payne and was also independently identified in several other laboratories. Since A2 has a gene frequency approaching 0.3 in Caucasians, it was possible for Bodmer and Payne to deduce that HLA-A1, A3, and A9 (initially designated LA1, LA3, and LA4, respectively) were alleles of HLA-2. Once the A series of antigens had been separated, it was possible to recognize the alleles of HLA-B, e.g., HLA-B5, B7, B8, etc. The separate identity of the two series was confirmed by the identification of recombinant individuals within families who inherited the A allele from one haplotype with the B allele of the homologous chromosome of the same parent. The identification of HLA-C was more difficult because the sera were often weak and mixed with antibodies to HLA-B, recombinants between B and C are rare, and linkage disequilibrium is high. In this instance a comparison of different populations was helpful as linkage disequilibrium changes markedly between different ethnic groups. (Linkage disequilibrium is an attribute of genetic systems whereby alleles at two or more loci are found on the same haplotype more [or less] frequently than is expected on the basis of random assortment. For example, the HLA haplotype HLA-A1, B8, Cw7, DR3 is found in Caucasian populations roughly four times more often than is expected based on the individual gene frequency for each allele in the same population.)

The definition of antigens was refined through antiserum screening. Many thousands of antisera have been screened. Occasionally a serum is identified which reacts strongly with cells from some donors carrying a given specificity (e.g., B5) and not with others also identified as carrying B5. This suggests a "split." If a second serum is identified which reacts only with the other panel donors at first characterized as B5, the split is confirmed and the two components are now given special designations as "subtypic" antigens, e.g., B51 and B52, while B5 is regarded as "supertypic." This system of antigen identification cannot readily accommodate broader categories of antigen. An antibody reacting with panel members carrying (say) B7, B8, and Bw22 does not fit into the general scheme, and most such antisera are set aside or disposed of. Recently, through the studies of a few investigators and because of the bizarre patterns of reactivity of many monoclonal antibodies, a new concept is being accepted under which the HLA molecules would carry two or more polymorphic determinants. The concept itself is not new and was suggested by Dausset and others many years ago. The difference is that proof of the existence of several epitopes on one molecule can now be tested by competitive inhibition (or failure of inhibition) using monoclonal antibody binding. The concept has great relevance because, in other systems, different epitopes on the same molecule can have different effects (help versus suppression), and the same may be true of HLA.

The precise nature of the antigenic sites (epitopes) on either class I or class II molecules has not yet been fully defined. In general terms, antigenicity can be conferred by a linear sequence of amino acids, as in the case of sperm whale myoglobin, or by the juxtaposition of amino acids in close proximity on the cell surface, held as a structure by the short-range forces generated by the tertiary or quaternary structure of the molecule, as in the case of egg white lysozyme. Both classes of determinants may be present in HLA.

The HLA-B7 molecule and most of the HLA-A2 molecule have been sequenced, as have several molecules of the homologous H-2 system of the mouse, in which spontaneous mutants are frequent. Variability in amino acid substitution appears to be greatest in the α_1 and α_2 domains, whereas the α_3 domain, nearer the C-terminal end, is more constant. Since single amino acid substitutions can give alterations in antigenic specificity of immunoglobulin allotypes and of the K^b molecule of H-2, it is clear that the known substitutions in the HLA-A and HLA-B molecules thus far sequenced can more than account for the extraordinary polymorphism of the HLA alleles (Table 1).

Similar arguments apply to HLA-D region antigens, where the involvement of the α chain and the β chain in alloreactivity remains to be decided. At least one monoclonal antibody will react only with the intact DR molecule and will not react with dissociated α or β chains (12). Other monoclonal antibodies will react

with free β chains (12). The β chain of the DR molecule appears to carry the polymorphism, while the α gene product is constant. The supertypic DR antigens HLA-DRw52 (previously MT2 or BR3) and HLA-DRw53 (formerly MT3 and BR4) are antigenic sites that may be on the same β chain as the DR subtypic antigen (i.e., $\alpha\beta_1$), or on a second DR-encoded β chain (3, 10). The DQ molecules can be constituted of chains coded by either α-and-β-gene pair. Both components are polymorphic, and both are thought to contribute to specificity. The DP products, so far, seem to be the result of expression always of the same α-and-β-gene pair, both contributing to polymorphism. The second α-and-β-gene pair do not appear to be expressed. Note that although α chains exhibit polymorphism, in all these loci the β chains are the most polymorphic.

Cross-reactivity

A single HLA molecule is thus thought of as potentially carrying more than one "antigen." We must here consider the problem of cross-reactivity, the bane of tissue typing. Cross-reactions occur most frequently between specificities on the same locus. As stated earlier, sera defining a subtypic specificity are very rare. Most sera tend to be "broadly" or "cross"-reactive; that is to say, most anti-B7 sera will react with cells from individuals carrying HLA-B27 or HLA-Bw22 and occasionally even with individuals carrying HLA-B8 (Fig. 2). In the past, the terms "private" and "public" have been substituted for subtypic and supertypic, but their use is generally infrequent in HLA serology.

While almost all HLA sera exhibit some degree of cross-reactivity (and even monoclonal antibodies can be cross-reactive), the reaction of an antiserum is strongest with its homologous antigen; e.g., in a homologous cytotoxic reaction, more cells will be killed and at a greater dilution of serum than in a cross-reaction. To minimize cross-reactivity, many antisera are, therefore, diluted so that only the homologous reaction is detected. It is important to note that cross-reactivity and multispecificity are not equivalent terms. Multispecific sera frequently contain two or more distinct antibodies easily identified by absorption of one without affecting reactivity of the other(s). Cross-reactive sera, when absorbed for the homologous reactivity, also lose reactivity to the cross-reacting specificity. The distinction between cross-reactive specificities, such as HLA-A3 and HLA-A11, is often quite sharp, while the distinction between some other cross-reactive series can be extremely difficult. Even highly experienced workers may, on occasion, have difficulty in distinguishing between highly cross-reactive specificities such as HLA-A30 and HLA-A31 or HLA-B40 and HLA-Bw41. P. I. Terasaki distributes a series of blindly coded cells to a large number of laboratories for HLA typing. Almost all laboratories usually agree on the identification of well-defined specificities such as HLA-A2, but there are many discrepancies in the characterization of certain of the newer "w" specificities.

Leukocyte typing

There are many subtle difficulties in tissue typing, not all of which are recognized by inexperienced

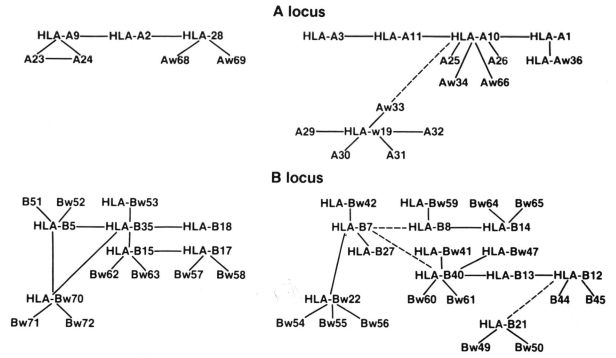

FIG. 2. Minimum representation of cross-reacting antigen groups.

laboratories. Some of the technical considerations are discussed by Ward et al. (15). Questions of antigenic specificity and definition of antigens occupy many volumes and are the subject of continuing international workshops.

The sera available for the detection of many HLA specificities (especially the provisional specificities) are frequently limited in number and in volume. Many are also highly technique dependent. Technique dependency is a phenomenon whereby minor differences in the dilution of antiserum, the activity of the complement used, the time and temperature of incubation, and the use or avoidance of a wash step can give wide variations in the results obtained. Because of these and other variables, numerous procedures for the detection of HLA specificities have been developed, and for each procedure there are multiple variations. Major centers frequently standardize a particular procedure which is then used by other laboratories in the same region or by those using the same antisera.

The first method to gain wide acceptance was leukoagglutination. Numerous variations were introduced to conserve reagents and to improve reproducibility. The procedures of van Rood and van Leeuwen (11), Dausset (11), or Amos and Peacocke (2) are still occasionally employed and are based on similar principles. In all procedures, one or more drops of buffy-coat lymphocytes, variously prepared, were mixed with serum in small test tubes, incubated at room temperature, and read microscopically for agglutination after mixing. The procedures gave about 95% reproducibility with cells from most subjects. Leukoagglutination is unsuitable for cells from severely ill donors, and the cells cannot be stored or shipped. Microagglutination methods were devel-

oped, but they never came into widespread use. Other procedures, such as complement consumption or platelet agglutination, have also been largely discontinued. Platelet complement fixation is a precise procedure giving excellent results in experienced hands (5). Its use is, however, restricted to a very few laboratories, largely because of difficulties in obtaining antisera. For routine use, microcytotoxicity has been the method of choice for nearly 20 years. Its advantages are the minute (1.0 μl or less) volumes of antiserum required and the concomitantly small requirement for target cells; the applicability to typing of cadaveric lymphocytes from blood, spleen, or lymph nodes; reproducibility; and speed in reading. The development of procedures for the shipment of live or frozen cells and for long-term preservation of cells (e.g., by controlled-rate freezing and storage in liquid nitrogen) (17) has also furthered the use and standardization of the microcytotoxicity test.

BASIC REQUIREMENTS

Donor panel

It is important to select reliable donors who will be available for repeat donations. Cells may be frozen at various concentrations and stored in the vapor state of liquid nitrogen, or, less desirably, they may be prepared on the day required. It is necessary to characterize the antigens of 60 or more individuals as a reference panel. The specificities typed for should be represented at least twice. It may be necessary to recruit additional subjects (Nordic, Mediterranean, Oriental, Hispanic, or black) to cover some of the rare specificities. From the full panel, a screening panel of 20 to 40 subjects representing all available specificities is frequently selected. This is adequate for the preliminary screening of new sera, especially if the antigens of the husband of a multiparous donor can also be characterized. Obviously, it is desirable to have each specificity represented more than once. For more detailed testing, an extended panel should be used.

Collection of antisera

About one in five multiparous women has detectable levels of HLA antibody. Some antibodies are lost soon after delivery, so antibodies (antisera) are often collected at the time of discharge from the hospital. Not infrequently, antibody persists for months or years, and female blood donors constitute a major source of antisera. Other sera are obtained from multiply transfused individuals, from patients who have rejected a transplant, or directly from placentas. Placentas (kept cold or frozen) are sliced with a scalpel, sealed in strong plastic storage bags, and weighted with bricks to press or squeeze out the serum. The serum is poured into sterile culture tubes and centrifuged until contaminating red cells and debris are removed. As much as 200 ml of sera can be obtained (and as little as 25 ml). In our experience, 91 of 920 placental sera that we have tested contain antibody to class I antigens. Amniotic fluid is an occasional antibody source. Since this material is frequently heavily bacterially contaminated, it is essential that the fluid be kept cold and be separated and filtered as soon as possible.

Monoclonal antibodies are a newer source of anti-HLA reagents but are at present used mostly in research laboratories. The specificity of monoclonal antibodies can be exquisite, and some of them are extremely high titered ($>1/1,000$). At the Ninth International Workshop (see reference 3), two monoclonal antibodies were identified which recognize a new specificity (Aw69) not previously identified with alloantisera. On the other hand, monoclonal antibodies often demonstrate cross-reactions between specifications of different loci (e.g., HLA-A2 and HLA-B17) or may be of an immunoglobulin class that does not fix complement and therefore is not useful in the microcytotoxicity assay. Enzyme-linked immunosorbent assay, radioimmunoassay, and direct binding assays are especially well suited for monoclonal antibodies.

Serum is screened for anti-HLA activity against separated B and T lymphocytes from the panel. It is useful to screen the serum at dilutions of 1:2 or 1:4, since sera that react only weakly are of less value. Of the sera that do react, many will be valueless for routine typing because of their multispecificity (or cross-reactivity). In general, only those sera giving strong and highly specific reactions are retained. However, if the serum reacts exclusively with T cells or B cells, or if it detects, e.g., only one HLA-A and one HLA-B locus specificity, especially where one or both are rare, the serum may be valuable. Selected antisera that are strongly reactive with both B and T cells and give discordant reactions with one subset may be chosen for platelet absorptions and further screening for possible DR or T-cell antibodies. Donors with useful antibodies are later bled for larger quantities, and, preferably, plasmaphoresed. Immediately after separation from the clot, serum is divided into smaller quantities and stored frozen at −20°C or colder. It is advisable to have the pattern of reactivity checked by a collaborating laboratory. Precious sera may be stored in liquid nitrogen. Several sizes of containers are useful, especially those holding about 8 to 10 ml, 1 ml, and 400 μl. Although sera slowly deteriorate at −20°C, they often retain activity for 15 or more years. Many laboratories prefer either to lyophilize sera in bulk and then to weigh out small quantities for reconstitution or to lyophilize them in 1-ml quantities. Reconstitution is done with distilled water, and the pH is adjusted to near neutrality.

Sera should not be kept in contact with CO_2 vapor for more than 24 h. Such sera (or cells) become very acidic and will deteriorate. This is most marked with small volumes, as in microtiter plates. Some sera are extremely sensitive, whereas others are more resistant. This adds to the danger, since a plate may seem to be intact, yet some of the sera may have become inactivated.

Additional sera may be obtained from commercial sources in the United States or abroad (including Pel-Freeze, Geometric Data, Hocht, and One-Lambda) and from other laboratories. The National Institutes of Health-American Red Cross serum bank maintains a collection of lyophilized sera for research purposes, proficiency testing, and upgrading of local lymphocyte donor panels. The American Society for Histocompatibility and Immunogenetics also maintains a reference bank of well-characterized sera for use in defining local reagents and cell panels.

Loading and storing microtiter plates

It is frequently convenient to load microtiter plates with sera and to keep them frozen at −80°C, or colder, in a mechanical freezer. Two methods are used to prevent evaporation. In one procedure, a small quantity of lightweight mineral oil, usually 1 or 2 μl (although the amount is not critical), is placed in the well with a multiple dispenser. The serum is then dispensed through the oil. The second method relies on saturation of the air inside the microtiter plate with water vapor. Collars of bibulous paper (as noted below) are prepared. Each collar is U shaped and approximately 7 mm wide. The collar fits on three sides of the moat surrounding the wells, leaving the fourth side free for ease in identifying rows. The paper is saturated with buffer or saline. The top of the microtiter plate is kept in place as much as possible during filling.

The microtubes of antisera should be microfuged for about 3 to 10 min before dispensing. The supernatant is then transferred to a clean tube. This is a beneficial pretreatment for all sera, but is essential for DR, DQ, and DP antisera which have been platelet absorbed to remove HLA-A, HLA-B, or HLA-C antibodies. Fat-laden serum can be centrifuged in a plastic tube and frozen, and the lipid layer is then cut off with a single-edge razor blade before the serum is transferred to microtubes. Alternatively, sera may be clarified by Freon extraction in which 2 volumes of serum is agitated with 1 volume of Freon II on a Vortex mixer for 1 min and then centrifuged. The lipids are discarded with the heavy Freon layer. A 1- or 2-μl volume of trypan red or neutral red, added to the serum before dispensing, provides easy visual confirmation that all the wells are indeed filled.

In the United States, microtiter plates usually have six columns of 10 or 12 wells. Before loading, the plates are labeled with the lot number and date by use of a marker (Markette Thin-Rite). For loading, a Hamilton dispenser, single- or six-place, or a Greiner (or other) multidispenser is used. It is necessary when loading a six-place dispenser to prepare a Lucite block with holes drilled to hold serum-filled microtubes so that the tubes have the same spacing as the wells in the row of the plate. Drilled blocks are also commercially available.

Sixty or 72 microtubes containing antisera are placed in the block. The syringes are filled with the sera of row 1 after a thorough mixing with the dye, and the Hamilton dispenser is clicked several times while in the microtubes to eliminate air in the needle. This helps ensure the delivery of a uniform quantity of antisera. Approximately 45 plates are filled by pressing the button once for each row in each plate. Batches of 45 plates may be filled sequentially. Before dispensing the next group of six antisera, the Hamilton syringes are washed 15 times with buffer and distilled water, and the plungers are wiped with moistened new gauze so as to avoid the slightest possibility of serum carry-over. The danger of carry-over cannot be overemphasized, especially if any of the sera are particularly strong. Alternatively, an entire plate of antisera can be loaded at one time with a multidispenser. When using the multidispenser, be certain that each delivery tube is clear of debris (a fine wire can be used to unclog any that are blocked) and check to see that all wells receive sera. Be certain to wash the dispenser repeatedly before loading a different set of antisera.

It is usual to include a negative control (normal human group AB serum) and a positive control for each plate. The positive control for HLA-A, HLA-B, and HLA-C typing trays is an antilymphocyte serum diluted to the point where it just gives 100% kill. For DR and DQ typing trays we use a heterologous rabbit antiserum raised against a pool of solubilized membranes from B-cell lines and absorbed with pooled T-cell lines. Anti-B-cell sera also can be obtained commercially. After all serum is dispensed and plates are inspected, the trays are placed in the bottom of an Ultra Low freezer (at least 70°C, and the colder the better). Plates are removed only 5 to 10 min before use. Note that after prolonged storage, serum in trays loaded without oil may become freeze-dried. This does not appear to affect their activity significantly.

TEST PROCEDURES

Two cytotoxicity procedures for HLA-A, HLA-B, and HLA-C typing will be described, the most widely used being that developed by Terasaki and standardized in agreement with the National Institute of Allergy and Infectious Diseases. This procedure is generally known as the NIH technique (13). The other procedure, that of Amos and his colleagues, is similar to the NIH technique but with the important difference of a wash step being introduced (Amos-modified technique) (1). This greatly increases the sensitivity of the test. The minor modifications made for the HLA-DR, HLA-DQ, and HLA-DP cytotoxicity assay on isolated B cells will also be described.

CELL PREPARATIONS

Isolation of unfractionated lymphocytes from whole peripheral blood

A variety of methods for the isolation of unfractionated lymphocytes from whole blood are in use (17). Most are modifications of a technique based on the gradient flotation method introduced by Boyum (4), and the variations relate to the methods of blood collection, volume of blood handled, and the removal of platelets, granulocytes, and monocyte/macrophages. Two of the most commonly used techniques for HLA-A, HLA-B, and HLA-C typing are detailed here.

Technique 1. Best results are obtained from defibrinated blood, as this will yield a platelet-free lymphocyte preparation. Six to eight glass beads are added to each 10 ml of blood immediately upon drawing, and the tube is continuously inverted for approximately 7 min. The blood is then diluted 1:2 with Hanks balanced salt solution (HBSS), layered over Ficoll-Hypaque solution (about 3 ml/10 ml of blood), and centrifuged at 600 or 800 × g for 40 or 20 min. The lymphocyte layer is removed with a Pasteur pipette, diluted 1:3 or greater, and spun for 10 min at 450 × g. Defibrinated cells for typing, if contaminated with erythrocytes, should be suspended in 1 to 3 ml of Tris-buffered NH_4Cl (see Materials) and incubated for 10 min in a 37°C water bath. After incubation, the cells are spun for 7 min at 800 × g, resuspended in HBSS, and adjusted to $2.0 × 10^6$ to $2.5 × 10^6$ cells per ml. Blood drawn into heparin (or other anticoagulants) can also be handled as described above, starting with the dilution of the blood 1:2 with HBSS and an additional step to remove platelets. The most commonly used methods of platelet removal are by differential sedimentation or use of ADP or thrombin (see Appendix). ADP and thrombin also remove granulocytes. Platelets (and granulocytes) also can be removed by incubation on nylon columns. However, there is the problem of selective depletion of B lymphocytes which are retained by the column.

Technique 2. In the alternative and equally good method, methylcellulose (2 ml of a 1% solution in phosphate buffered saline [PBS] per 10 ml of blood) and a small amount of carbonyl iron powder are added to whole blood. The amount of carbonyl iron powder clinging to an applicator stick is usually sufficient. The tubes are incubated on a rotator or rocker for 15 min at 37°C and then in a vertical position for an additional 15 min at 37°C. Use of carbonyl iron takes advantage of the adherent and phagocytic properties of platelets, macrophages, and granulocytes for iron particles. Methylcellulose increases the sedimentation differences of lymphocytes, erythrocytes, and iron ingesting/adhering cells, yielding a lymphocyte-rich plasma layer. The lymphocyte-rich plasma is carefully layered over 0.3 ml of Ficoll-Hypaque (or lymphocyte separation medium) solution in two to four microcentrifuge tubes (1-ml capacity). The tubes are placed in a microcentrifuge (e.g., Fisher model 59 centrifuge), and speed is adjusted slowly to 2,000 × g, then maintained for 3 min. With a Pasteur pipette, the top plasma layer is discarded and the mononuclear cells at the interface are transferred to new microtubes. The cells are washed twice by centrifugation to remove any remaining platelets, first at $3,000 \times g$ for 2 min and then at $1,000 \times g$ for 1 min; supernatant is discarded and cells are suspended in fresh medium between centrifugations. After the last spin, cells are resuspended, combined in a 5-ml culture tube, and adjusted to 2.0×10^6 to 2.5×10^6 cells per ml.

For the two-color fluorochromasia technique (17), crude lymphocyte suspensions, as described above, are used. This technique, although it gives good results in the research laboratory and is useful for screening serum samples that react exclusively with T cells and B cells, is used only in a few laboratories in the United States for routine clinical typing. The great majority of laboratories test for HLA-D region antigens on separated B cells.

B-cell separation procedures

Several techniques are used for the separation of B cells (17). All work best in the absence of contaminating platelets, granulocytes, and monocytes. In our experience, satisfactory B-cell preparations cannot be made from certain individuals. Such individuals are excluded from the cell panel.

The three most widely used methods, described in detail below, include the depletion of T cells by sheep erythrocyte (SRBC) rosetting (E-rosetting) (7), the adherence and subsequent elution of B cells from nylon-wool columns (9), and the adsorption and elution of B cells from goat anti-HuF(ab')$_2$-coated tissue culture flasks. The last technique is the technique of choice in one of our laboratories (D.B.A.) for various reasons, one being the positive selection of immunoglobulin-positive lymphocytes rather than negative selection dependent on depletion of other lymphocyte populations. The technique, although perhaps more elaborate to adapt, when once established offers reliable B-cell isolation in a technically expedient and facile procedure. Purity can be expected to exceed 90% consistently, while background is consistently less than 5%. This technique can also be amended to deplete cell contaminants (null cells, macrophages, myeloblasts, etc.), which are often present in high concentration in certain disease states, without affecting the reliable results of the final B-cell isolation. Frozen cells give excellent results.

The adherence and elution of B cells from nylon-wool columns is the technique of choice in the other of our laboratories (K.A.S.; a clinical laboratory) because of the simplicity of the technique and the short time necessary to recover T-enriched as well as B-enriched populations. This technique utilizes the property of B cells, but not T cells, to adhere to nylon wool (among other surfaces), from which they can subsequently be recovered. This method also yields excellent B and T preparations (>90% purity).

The third most commonly employed method for enrichment of B lymphocytes, the E-rosetting technique, utilizes the fact that T cells have receptors on their cell surface which are specific for SRBC while B cells do not. The yield of E-rosetted cells is generally 60 to 80% (optimal conditions, 85%). Therefore, some nonrosetting T cells and other nonrosetted cells will be present in the B-cell population to varying degrees.

Detailed procedures

Monocyte depletion treatment and anti-HuF(ab')$_2$ technique

1. Suspend the lymphocyte pellet in 2 ml of heat-inactivated fetal calf serum (FCS) and transfer it to a 15-ml conical plastic Corning centrifuge tube. Add 8 ml of carbonyl iron solution and incubate the tube with rocking for 30 min at 37°C. After incubation, pull down carbonyl iron by passing the tube over a strong magnet. Layer the supernatant onto 3 ml of lymphocyte separation medium and centrifuge at $700 \times g$ for 20 min. Harvest the lymphocyte layer, dilute with HBSS, and spin for 10 min at $250 \times g$. Resuspend the pellet, and adjust the cell concentration to 15×10^6 to 40×10^6 cells per 3 ml of HBSS with 10% FCS.

2. Prepare anti-HuF(ab')$_2$ flasks for B-cell separation as follows:
   a. Coat the bottom of a 25-cm^2 tissue culture flask with 2 to 3 ml of affinity-purified anti-HuF(ab')$_2$ (see Appendix).
   b. Incubate the flask for 30 min at 37°C, coated side down.
   c. Remove and reserve anti-HuF(ab')$_2$ for future use (see Appendix). Then wash the flask once with about 5 ml of HBSS, decant, and wash once with about 5 ml of HBSS with 10% FCS. Store until use with 3 ml of HBSS + FCS.

3. Decant the HBSS with FCS from precoated anti-HuF(ab')$_2$ tissue culture flasks, and add the cell suspension from step 1 to the flask, allowing the cells to rest on the coated surface. Incubate for 30 min at 37°C. During the final 10 min of this incubation, prepare 10 ml of elution medium per flask:
   4 ml of pooled human serum (heat inactivated)
   1 ml of 5% EDTA (see Materials)
   5 ml of HBSS

4. After incubation, remove the supernatant containing nonadherent, predominantly T cells. These cells, after being washed once with HBSS, are perfectly suited for routine HLA-A, HLA-B, and HLA-C typing, as well as for any other functional studies. Platelets may be removed with the supernatant at this stage by differential centrifugation.

5. Wash the flask twice with 7 to 10 ml of HBSS with 10% FCS. Washes should include fairly vigorous pipetting down the sides of the flask while avoiding any bubbles. All traces of media should be drained before the addition of the elution medium. Combine the washes with the initial supernatant to yield the immunoglobulin-negative T-cell population.

6. Add 10 ml of elution medium per flask and incubate for 30 min at 37°C. After incubation, vigorously rap the flask on the desk top, then remove the supernatant containing immunoglobulin-positive "B" cells to a 40-ml, siliconized glass, conical centrifuge tube. Vigorously wash the flask as before, combining washes with supernatant for total B-cell yield. Pellet the cells for 10 min at $250 \times g$. Extreme care should be taken to remove all supernatant because it includes EDTA, which is inhibitory in the cytotoxicity test. Add HBSS and adjust the cells to a final concentration of 2.0×10^6 per ml for anti-DR cytotoxicity testing. Transfer the cells to a 3-ml, siliconized glass, conical centrifuge tube to facilitate dispensing.

Adherence and elution of B cells from nylon-wool columns

1. Nylon-wool columns are prepared from plastic drinking straws (0.6 cm diameter), cut to ca. 12 to 14 cm in length. Heat seal one end at a 45° angle. Tease apart and soak in HBSS 0.1 g of "scrubbed nylon wool" (Leukopak). Pack the nylon wool gradually and evenly into the straw to a height of approximately 6 cm. Columns can be kept overnight at 4°C or stored frozen. If stored, seal both ends of the straw until ready for use. Snip off the tip of the straw (~2-mm opening) so the medium drips through. Wash the column with 5 ml of HBSS and then add 3 ml of McCoy's 5a medium supplemented with 5% FCS (medium). Turn horizontally when the medium just covers the nylon wool, and bring to 37°C.

2. Add the lymphocytes, which have been suspended in 0.5 ml of warm medium, to the top of the column. Hold vertically and allow the cells to move all the way into the nylon. Add 0.2 ml of warm medium to the column to prevent drying, and incubate horizontally at 37°C for 30 to 45 min.

3. Elute the nonadherent T cells by placing the column vertically over a 5-ml culture tube and allowing 5 ml of warm medium to drip through. This yields purified T cells. Repeat the wash, collecting the cells in a second culture tube. Discard cells from the second wash, as they tend to be a mixture of cell populations.

4. The adherent B lymphocytes are recovered in a third culture tube by adding 3 ml of room-temperature or cold medium to the column and gently squeezing the straw at the level of the nylon while the medium drips through. Repeat twice. Wash the purified T- and B-cell preparations in standard McCoy's 5a medium and adjust to 2×10^6 cells per ml.

Depletion of T cells by E-rosetting

1. A number of enzymes and chemical compounds are used to unmask or increase the accessibility of the receptor sites on SRBC and to increase the stability of the rosettes. Treatment with neuraminidase is the most widely used and is therefore given here. To a 5% suspension of well-washed SRBC add 0.2 ml of *Vibrio cholerae* neuraminidase (500 U/ml, specific activity), mix, and incubate at 37°C for 30 min. Wash three times in HBSS (or PBS) and adjust the neuraminidase-treated SRBC (SRBC-N) to a 1% suspension. SRBC-N must be prepared daily.

2. One milliliter of a lymphocyte suspension (3×10^6 to 7×10^6 cells per ml of HBSS) is mixed with 1 ml of the 1% SRBC-N suspension in round-bottom test tubes, the sides and bottom of which have been fully coated with 0.1 ml of heat-inactivated serum. The serum may be human AB serum, pooled serum from nontransfused males, or FCS pretested for cytotoxic activity. The serum should be preabsorbed with SRBC at a ratio of 1 volume of packed SRBC to 2 to 3 volumes of serum and used immediately (or stored frozen at −70°C). Centrifuge the lymphocyte-SRBC-N mix for 10 min at $200 \times g$ and incubate the pelleted cells at room temperature for 20 min.

3. The cell pellet is resuspended by gentle rocking until visible clumps have dispersed. Add a drop of toluidine blue to the cells and, using a light microscope (×45 objective), score the number and viability of rosette-forming cells. A rosette is formed by a lymphocyte with three or more SRBC-N attached.

Viable lymphocytes stain blue; dead lymphocytes appear purple.

4. Gently underlay the suspension with 1.5 ml of Ficoll-Hypaque. Centrifuge (slowly increasing the speed) at $400 \times g$ for 2 min at 4°C. Because of their density, E-rosettes settle to the bottom of the Ficoll-Hypaque; B-cells and other nonrosetted cells are found at the interface.

CYTOTOXICITY

NIH technique for HLA-A, HLA-B, and HLA-C testing

1. One microliter of cells which have been adjusted to a concentration of 2.5×10^6 cells per ml is dispensed into each well of a preloaded Falcon plastic microtiter plate (as described above in the loading and storing section) with a Hamilton dispenser. A single-place dispenser is most frequently used. Note that when oil is used it is essential to check each well microscopically to show that the droplets have fused. False-negative reactions are scored when serum and cells do not come in contact.

2. The cells and sera are mixed by placing the microtiter plate against a Yankee pipette shaker (or similar vibrator) and are left to incubate at room temperature for 30 min.

3. Five microliters of pretested and titered rabbit complement is then added to each well. (A few microliters of trypan blue, eosin, or neutral red may be added to the complement to serve as a marker.) Incubation is continued at room temperature for 60 min. (*Note:* Results are greatly influenced by the complement. It is usually convenient to buy a quantity of a single batch from a large supplier after requesting a small portion for testing. An effective complement will usually give 90% lysis when diluted 2:3, 1:2, or even 1:3 in HBSS and with most antisera. Some complement batches give more intensive cross-reactivities than others; these are to be avoided, as are those batches that give backgrounds in the absence of antibody. Complement must be stored at −70°C or below in small volumes. Enough for 1 day's use is thawed, diluted if necessary, and kept on ice. Any excess from a day's test is discarded.)

4. By use of a multiple dispenser, 3 μl of 5% aqueous eosin is added to each well. A 2-min period is allowed to elapse to let the dead cells stain (for B cells allow 10 min). The wells are then filled with Formalin (pH 7.2; a 10% solution is sufficient). A cover glass (50 by 75 mm) is placed over the wells to flatten the top of the droplet (or the plate is flooded with oil) before reading.

Wash step or flick procedure in HLA-A, HLA-B, and HLA-C typing

1 and 2. These steps are identical to the NIH technique, but trays must be set up with less than 2 μl of oil per well, or without oil and with buffer-soaked collars.

3. After 30 min of incubation, the wells are filled with HBSS with a thinly drawn Pasteur pipette, employing gentle, steady pressure to produce a swirling action which allows thorough mixing. The cells are left to settle for 10 min or are gently centrifuged ($200 \times g$, 1 to 2 min) in a plate holder (many different holders are available).

4. Excess fluid is removed by inverting the plate over a sink or waste container with a snapping motion of the wrist (flick). Although difficult to describe, the flick is rapidly learned. The motion resembles that used by erythrocyte serologists to remove supernatants from erythrocyte pellets. Early learning attempts may result in the loss of some cells; proficiency comes with practice. Alternatives are to blot or pipette off excess fluid, but these are time-consuming and may also cause loss of cells.

5. Five microliters of pretested and pretitered rabbit complement is then added to each well with a 250-µl Hamilton syringe. Incubation is for 60 min at room temperature.

6. The plates are then flicked as in step 4.

7. Wells are filled with filtered reagent made of trypan blue (3 ml of 1% trypan blue) plus EDTA (7 ml of 2% EDTA) by use of the finely drawn Pasteur pipette, and plates are allowed to stand for 10 min or are centrifuged as before.

8. The plates are flicked and filled, again using the drawn pipette with HBSS, to permit better visualization. Two drops of undiluted Formalin is applied to the collar or margin of the plate for preservation.

HLA-DR cytotoxicity

1. One microliter of cells adjusted to 2.0×10^6–2.5×10^6 cells per ml is added to each well as for HLA-A, HLA-B, and HLA-C typing: the tray contents are similarly mixed.

2. Incubation of cells and serum in DR testing is for 60 min at room temperature (some laboratories incubate at 37°C).

3. Five microliters of rabbit complement is added to each well with a Hamilton syringe, and incubation is continued for 60 to 120 min at room temperature. Particular attention should be devoted to the selection of complement to be used with B cells because of the increased sensitivity of these cells to xenoantibody in the complement. Young rabbits (type I), 8 to 10 weeks old, are used most often. Alternatives are baby rabbit serum (<5 weeks of age) or adult rabbit serum (usually from more than 50 rabbits) absorbed with spleen cells.

4. The rest of this procedure is identical to steps 6 through 8 of the wash step or flick procedure and step 4 of the NIH technique for HLA-A, HLA-B, and HLA-C testing. This method also is applied to detection of the more recently defined HLA-DQ locus and HLA-DP locus, class II antigens.

Reading

Determinations of the incidence of staining are made by placing the plate under a standard (wash step technique) or inverted (NIH technique) microscope at ×150 (×10 objectives, ×15 oculars). Scoring is based on the percent lysis (Table 2) as detected by stain uptake of dead cells. The degree of staining is usually by estimation, but stained and unstained cells may also be counted. Eosin may be substituted for trypan blue in the wash step procedure, but trypan blue is not always a reliable stain in the presence of serum in the NIH procedure.

The most frequent sources of error or difficulty in determining the percentage of lysed cells are as fol-

TABLE 2. Reading: two techniques for incidence of staining

Wash step scoring system		Interpretation	NIH scoring system	
% Lysis	Scoring		% Lysis	Scoring
0–14	1	Negative	0–10	1
15–19	2	Doubtful negative	10–19	2
20–29	3	Doubtful positive	20–39	4
30–59	4	Positive	40–79	6
60–92	5	Positive	80–100	8
93–100	6	Positive		

lows. (i) Uneven distribution of cells: in some wells cells may accumulate on the walls as a result of faulty technique. Further mixing may be required. (ii) Clots in the wells: this is often due to improperly clotted serum. (iii) Debris in solutions used or dust in the wells before the serum was introduced: it is recommended that all reagents be filtered or centrifuged before use. Dusty plates can be cleaned with an air jet before filling. (iv) No cells in some wells: this may have several causes, including a faulty dispenser (usually due to worn mechanical parts, or inadequate cleaning and maintenance), uneven flicking, or overlysis. Over-lysis may be corrected by checking the pH of all reagents, by diluting the serum, or by retitrating and diluting the complement. (v) Contamination of the lymphocyte suspension with platelets or granulocytes: granulocyte contamination is often a special problem with some cadaver donors, granulocytic leukemia patients, and patients with infections. The granulocytes often remain unstained, but may stain after exposure to some antisera. Platelets, while resembling debris or dust in the wells, can give false-negative reactions since they express HLA and are known to absorb the antibody. This problem can be alleviated by more efficient anticoagulation of whole blood, by differential centrifugation of a lymphocyte suspension, or by using defibrinated blood. (vi) "Small blues," sometimes a problem with trypan blue, can occur if the protein concentration in the wells is high, e.g., if the dye and final solutions are dropped onto the cells rather than swirled and completely mixed. (vii) Bubbles in the well: bubbles obscuring the cells can form if cover slips are placed carelessly (i.e., "dropped on"). Bubbles also occur over long storage of the plates. Cover slips can be carefully removed and replaced. If bubbles form in oil they can be pricked, or the oil can be poured off and fresh oil added. (viii) Old serum in the wells: this is only a problem in laboratories reusing old plates and can cause a variety of problems.

Background level of staining is determined from the well containing AB serum. The proportion of stained cells should rarely exceed 5%. High backgrounds are due to: (i) cells prepared too long before testing; (ii) cells improperly handled (centrifugation too vigorous, or incorrect pH or isotonicity of solutions); (iii) reactions of xenoantibodies in rabbit complement (this is especially a problem with lymphoblastoid cell lines or with cells from leukemic donors; preabsorption of complement with spleen cells or leukemic lymphocytes is advisable for use with leukemic cells). Also, occasionally and for no apparent reason, the control well may contain a high proportion of stained cells, while many wells containing antiserum give clear negative results. With due caution, the background may in such cases be based on the negative reactions. HBSS often is toxic with complement for B cells and should be avoided as a control.

MATERIALS

The materials listed have been found to give acceptable definition of specificities. Equivalents from local or other suppliers may give equally good results.

Barbital buffer. Consolidated Laboratories, Inc. (Chicago Heights, Ill.), Oxoid Barbitone, C.F.T. diluent, 100 tablets.

Bibulous paper. Fisher Scientific Co. (Fair Lawn, N.J.), no. 611, 8 by 10 in. (20 by 25 cm). Often a local printer will be willing to cut out the collars.

Carbonyl iron powder. G A G Corp. (140 West 51st St., New York, N.Y.), 1-163763, B#560.

Conical centrifuge tubes. Kimax, 40 ml, catalog no. 5-537; Pyrex, 3 ml, catalog no. C4101-3. American Scientific Products (McGaw Park, Ill.).

EDTA. Disodium EDTA no. S-300, Fisher Scientific Co. Make 2 or 5% EDTA by adding 20 or 50 g of EDTA to 1,000 ml of barbital buffer. Adjust to pH 7.0 to 7.4 with NaOH.

Eosin. Eastman Kodak Co. (Rochester, N.Y.). Dye content, 85%. Five grams per 100 ml of distilled water = 5% solution. Filter before use.

Fetal calf serum, heat inactivated. GIBCO Laboratories (Grand Island, N.Y.), catalog no. 230-6140. Order samples of several lot numbers, test in separation procedure, and order a large quantity of a good lot number.

Ficoll. Sigma Chemical Co. (St. Louis, Mo.), 500 g per bottle, F4375. For a 9% solution, use 9 g of Ficoll per 100 ml of distilled water.

Ficoll-Hypaque. Combine 24 ml of 9% Ficoll and 10 ml of 34% Hypaque (see below). Final specific gravity should be 1.078 to 1.080. Store at 4°C. Use at room temperature.

Formalin. Formaldehyde solution, 37% (wt/wt). American Scientific Products, catalog no. 5016-030. Can be used as is or diluted.

Hamilton dispenser syringes. Hamilton Co., Inc. (Whittier, Calif.), 50-μl capacity, 1-μl delivery, no. 705N. Repeating dispenser, PB-600-1 Terasaki dispenser with six 705SN syringes, 0.050 ml, no. 83726, or with six 7255N syringes, 0.25 ml, no. 83790.

HBSS. Hanks balanced salt solution without sodium bicarbonate no. K-12, GIBCO Laboratories. Make up with distilled water, add HEPES (see below) to make a 15 mM solution, and adjust the pH to 7.2 with NaOH. Filter for long-term storage.

HEPES. N-2-Hydroxyethylpiperazine-N'-2-ethanesulfonic acid, Sigma Chemical Co., catalog no. 3375, or GIBCO Laboratories.

Human serum, pooled. GIBCO Laboratories, catalog no. 200-6150. Order a sample, test in assay, and then order a large quantity of the lot number.

Hypaque. Hypaque sodium, 50% (wt/vol), 50-ml vials, Winthrop Laboratories (New York, N.Y.). Use 6.8 ml of Hypaque and 3.2 ml of distilled water to make a 34% solution, or a commercially prepared gradient as described below.

Lymphocyte separation medium. Bionetics Laboratory Productions, Litton Bionetics, Inc. (Kensington, Md.), catalog no. 8410-01, 500 ml per carton.

Microplates. Scientific Products, Inc. (Detroit, Mich.), Falcon Plastics (Oxnard, Calif.), microtest plates no. 3034, one case = 100 units.

Mineral oil. Atlas Mineral Oil or Squibb Light Weight Mineral Oil, E. R. Squibb & Sons (Princeton, N.J.).

Nylon wool. Fenwal Laboratories (Deerfield, Ill.), Fenwal scrubbed nylon fiber; 3 denier, 3.81 cm, type 200. In some countries nylon fiber is unavailable. Locally available fiber used for throat swabs, dressings, etc. should be tried.

Phosphate-buffered saline (Dulbecco). GIBCO Laboratories, no. 450-1300.

Rabbit complement. Pel-Freeze Biologicals, Inc. (Deerborn, Mich.), pooled complement. Order several sample lots and test for cytolysis and titer in an appropriate cytotoxicity assay, then order several months' supply, aliquot in small tubes, and store at −70°C.

Technicon Lymphocyte Separation Reagent (carbonyl iron solution). Technicon Corp., Inc. (Tarrytown, N.Y.), product no. T01-0507-62. Lot number variable.

Tissue culture flasks, 25 cm². Scientific Products, canted neck, no. 25100-25-Corning, 20 per sleeve.

Toluidine blue. Fisher Scientific Co. Color index no. 52040.

Tris buffer. Trizma base, Sigma Chemical Co., or Tris buffer, General Biochemicals (Chagrin Falls, Ohio), three times crystallized. Use 20.6 g of Tris per 1,000 ml of distilled water. Make up a flask to one-half to three-fourths of its volume and adjust the pH with concentrated HCl to 7.2 to 7.4 (starting pH will be about 11.0). Do this at room temperature. Transfer to a volumetric flask and add distilled water to the desired volume.

Tris-NH₄Cl. Mix 1 part Tris buffer (see above) in 9 parts of NH₄Cl (0.83 g of NH₄Cl per 100 ml of distilled water).

Trypan blue. K & K Laboratories, Inc. (Plainview, N.Y.) or Harleco (Hartman-Leddon Co., Philadelphia, Pa.). One gram per 100 ml of distilled water, filtered = 1% stock solution. For daily use in cytotoxicity testing, dilute 3 ml of 1% stock solution with 7 ml of 2% EDTA (see above) = 0.3% trypan blue in EDTA. Needs filtration before each use.

APPENDIX

Goat Anti-HuF(ab')₂ Reagent: Preparation and Standardization

Procurement of anti-F(ab')₂

Anti-F(ab')₂ may be obtained commercially from Miles Laboratories, Inc. (Elkhart, Ind.) or Atlantic Antibodies, Inc. (Scarborough, Maine), or the antibody can be made by standard immunization procedures.

Affinity purification of anti-HuF(ab')₂

1. Use a column of Sepharose 4B with CNBr-conjugated human immunoglobulin G (commercial Cohn fraction II).

2. Ten milliliters of serum is applied to a 50-ml bed-volume column with 2 mg of conjugated immunoglobulin G per ml of Sepharose at 4°C.

3. The column is washed overnight with about 500 ml of PBS. The optical density (280 nm) of the eluate should then be less than 0.03.

4. The column is eluted with 200 ml of 0.1 M sodium acetate buffer (pH 3.5); 5-ml fractions should be collected. The peak is determined by reading the optical density of the fractions at 280 nm.

5. The peak fractions are pooled, concentrated to about 20 ml (if necessary) by ultrafiltration, and then dialyzed overnight (or for 6 h minimum) against PBS.

Standardization of anti-F(ab′)$_2$

Each batch of affinity-purified anti-F(ab′)$_2$ must be ultracentrifuged at $100,000 \times g$ for 45 min and titrated before routine use. Dilutions of anti-F(ab′)$_2$ are made in PBS plus 0.025% sodium azide and tested against two or more reliable panel cells in the routine separation procedure. Criteria for selection of a working dilution should be based on both the quantity and quality of the B-cell population, the quality being determined by percent lysis in a cytotoxicity assay with a known heterologous anti-DR serum, or percent fluorescent cells in the immunofluorescence assay.

Standardization of the anti-F(ab′)$_2$ reagent should also include a determination of the number of separations per sample of the affinity-purified antibody. It is normal for the antibody to be used at least three times; it is then ultracentrifuged again to remove aggregates, and this allows two or three more uses before discarding, for a total of five or six uses. It is important to emphasize the necessity of standardization of each affinity-purification product due to the inevitable variabilities.

Platelet removal techniques

1. Differential sedimentation (low platelet contamination), based on the density differences between lymphocytes (1.077) and platelets (1.03). Centrifuge the cell suspension at 600 to 800 $\times$ g for 1 min. Discard the platelet-containing supernatant. Repeat as necessary.

2. ADP or thrombin (heavy platelet contamination). Resuspend the cell button in medium containing either 2 to 3 drops of 0.1% ADP in saline or 1 drop of autologous plasma and 1 drop of thrombin (100 U/ml of saline). Rotate the tube until small clumps form, and centrifuge for 3 s at 100 $\times$ g. Collect the lymphocyte-containing supernatant and wash once in medium.

LITERATURE CITED

1. **Amos, D. B., R. Corley, D. Kostyu, Y. Delmas-Marsalet, and M. Woodbury.** 1972. The serologic structure of HL-A as indicated by crossreactivities: the inclusion of HL-A loci into major histocompatibility complex H-1, p. 359–366. *In* J. Dausset and J. Colombani (ed.), Histocompatibility testing 1972. Munksgaard, Copenhagen.
2. **Amos, D. B., and N. Peacocke.** 1963. Leukoagglutination. A modified technique and preliminary results of absorption with tissues, p. 1132–1140. *In* H. Ludin (ed.), Proceedings of the 9th Congress of the European Society of Hematology. S. Karger, Basel.
3. **Bodmer, W. F., E. Albert, J. B. Bodmer, J. Dausset, F. Kissmeyer-Nielsen, W. Mayr, R. Payne, J. J. Van Rood, Z. Trinka, and R. L. Walford.** 1984. Nomenclature for factors of the HLA system 1984. *In* E. D. Albert, M. P. Baur, and W. R. Mayr (ed.), Histocompatibility testing 1984. Springer-Verlag, Heidelberg.
4. **Boyum, A.** 1968. Isolation of mononuclear cells by one centrifugation and of granulocytes by combining centrifugation and sedimentation at 1 g. Scand. J. Clin. Lab. Invest. **21**(Suppl. 97): 77–89.
5. **Colombani, J., M. Colombani, A. Benajam, and J. Dausset.** 1967. Leukocyte platelet antigens defined by platelet complement fixation test, p. 413–418. *In* E. S. Curtoni, P. L. Mattuiz, and R. M. Tosi (ed.), Histocompatibility testing 1967. Munksgaard, Copenhagen.
6. **Cresswell, P.** 1977. Human B cell alloantigens: separation from other membrane molecules by affinity chromatography. Eur. J. Immunol. **7**:636–641.
7. **Gilbertson, R. B., and R. S. Metzgar.** 1976. Human T and B lymphocyte rosette tests. Cell Immunol. **24**:97–100.
7a. **Howell, D. N., and P. Cresswell.** 1983. Expression of T-lymphoblast-encoded HLR-DR antigens on human T-B lymphoblast hybrids. Immunogenetics **17**:411–425.
8. **Johnson, A., R. J. Hartzman, and M. A. Robinson.** 1984. HLA: the major histocompatibility complex. Immunogenetics of HLA antigens, p. 790–821. *In* John B. Henry (ed.), Clinical diagnosis and management by laboratory methods. W. B. Saunders, Philadelphia.
9. **Lowry, R. P., A. E. Person, J. E. Goguen, C. B. Carpenter, and M. R. Garovoy.** 1978. T and B cell separation by nylon wool columns. Transplant. Proc. **10**:4–8.
10. **Markert, M. L., and P. Cresswell.** 1982. Human B cell alloantigens: expression of MB and MT determinants. J. Immunol. **128**:2004–2008.
11. **National Academy of Science Research Council (ed.).** 1965. Histocompatibility testing. Publication 1229. U.S. Government Printing Office, Washington, D.C.
12. **Radka, S. F., D. B. Amos, L. J. Quackenbush, and P. Cresswell.** 1984. HLA-DR7-specific monoclonal antibodies and a chimpanzee anti-DR7 serum detect different epitopes on the same molecule. Immunogenetics **19**:63–76.
12a. **Salter, R. D., D. N. Howell, and P. Cresswell.** 1983. Genes regulating HLA class I antigen expression in T-B lymphoblast hybrids. Immunogenetics **21**:235–246.
13. **Terasaki, P. I., J. D. McClelland, M. S. Park, and B. McCurdy.** 1973. Microdroplet lymphocyte cytotoxicity test, p. 54. *In* Manual of tissue typing techniques. DHEW Publ. (NIH) 74-545. U.S. Government Printing Office, Washington, D.C.
14. **van Rood, J. J., A. van Leuwen, J. J. Keuning, and B. van Oud Albas.** 1975. The serological recognition of the human MLC determinants using a modified cytotoxicity technique. Tissue Antigens **5**:73–80.
15. **Ward, F. E., D. B. Amos, W. B. Bias, J. C. Pierce, and R. D. Stulting, Jr.** 1971. Report of three histocompatibility testing workshops in the Southeast Regional Procurement program. Transplantation **12**:392–398.
16. **Yunis, E. J., and D. B. Amos.** 1971. Three closely linked genetic systems relevant to transplantation. Proc. Natl. Acad. Sci. U.S.A. **68**:3031–3035.
17. **Zachary, A., and W. Braun (ed.).** 1981. The American Association for Clinical Histocompatibility testing laboratory manual. American Society for Histocompatibility and Immunogenetics, New York.

Chapter 131

Cellular Typing: Mixed Lymphocyte Response and Cell-Mediated Lympholysis

DEVENDRA P. DUBEY, IVAN YUNIS, AND EDMOND J. YUNIS

Cell-mediated immunity plays an important role in allograft rejection and graft-versus-host diseases. In animal studies, it has been observed that after in vivo immunization with allogeneic cells, host lymphoid cells recognize and lyse immunizing cells without the aid of antibody or complement.

The cell-mediated immune response has two important phases: (i) recognition, when host cells recognize the donor cell as foreign in the context of the major histocompatibility complex (MHC), and (ii) destruction, when the host cells respond by attacking the foreign cells. A small number of responder cells acquire cytotoxicity and proliferate. Thus, cell-mediated immunity can be described in terms of two measurable functions, i.e., proliferative (2) and cytotoxic (3) activities. It has been further shown that the cytotoxic activity generated during the allostimulation is specific to MHC antigens.

Development of cell culture techniques has led to the establishment of in vitro methods which mimic the in vivo immunization process, thus providing measures for the assessment of cell-mediated immunity in vitro. These in vitro techniques are (i) the mixed lymphocyte culture (MLC) assay, which assesses host proliferative response, and (ii) the cell-mediated lympholysis (CML) assay, which tests the ability of responder cells to generate cytotoxic T cells (CTL) against the immunizing cell.

In the MLC assay, cells are generated which are cytotoxic to allogeneic cells. The scheme of reaction is shown in Table 1. Lymphocytes from individual A (responder) are mixed with X-irradiated lymphocytes from individual B (B_x) (stimulator). During the 6-day culture, a fraction of lymphocytes from A differentiates to become cytotoxic (effector) and proliferates with specificity directed against the HLA-A, B, and C antigens on immunizing cell B. The cytotoxic cell becomes able to recognize and kill the immunizing (stimulating) cell. This phenomenon is known as CML and is mediated by T cells generated in MLC. Lightbody et al. (7) were the first to demonstrate that normal human peripheral blood lymphocytes can be activated by phytohemagglutinin (PHA) to become sensitive targets for cytotoxic cells generated in MLC. Early studies of CML suggested that CTL recognized serologically defined gene products of HLA-A, B, C, and D/DR loci. However, several studies, including recent international collaborative studies reported by Schendel et al. (8), have shown that CTL can detect antigens not identified by serology techniques. Serologically defined HLA antigens have often been invoked as target antigens in CTL-mediated lysis, but although the expression of HLA antigens on the cell surface is necessary for lysis of the cell, other molecular structures may also be involved in recognition.

The mixed lymphocyte reaction in humans is controlled by the HLA-D region of the MHC of HLA in humans (1). That locus is separate from the HLA-A and HLA-B loci on chromosome 6. The human HLA-D region is identified as a region analogous to the immune response gene in mice (9). A disparity in the HLA-D loci between two cells causes a stimulatory response, whereas an identity may lead to a mutual lack of stimulation of lymphocytes. This concept forms the basis of HLA-D typing. The cellular typing techniques have been primarily exploited to explore the HLA-D region of the MHC. With homozygous typing cells as reagent, the HLA-D region has been studied. The HLA-D region is highly polymorphic. Thus far, 19 alleles have been identified (see chapter 130).

Clinical application of cell-mediated immune functions and cellular typing

The MLC assay is considered a predictor of host response to transplantation (4). Evidence suggests that MLC tests predict the acute rejection episodes and graft survival in living recipients when the transplant donors are either living related or cadaver donors. Thus the primary clinical use of the MLC assay is in the selection of a compatible donor for organ transplantation, especially among family members. This test is used in selection of an HLA-identical donor for kidney or bone marrow transplant. To prevent rejection of graft or graft-versus-host disease, the donor and recipient cells must be mutually nonstimulatory. HLA typing alone may not be satisfactory for donor selection, since not all alloantigens important for transplantation have been identified. It is possible for lymphocytes from two HLA-identical individuals to stimulate each other in MLC. Indeed, bone marrow transplantation between HLA-identical, MLC-negative siblings may occasionally result in graft-versus-host disease. The cause of this disease in such situations is not known.

The use of the CML assay as a predictor of transplant rejection or graft survival has not been extensively studied. Since the cells responsible for lytic activity in CML are not the same as those that proliferate in MLC and since the CML assay detects histocompatibility differences at loci other than HLA-D, it is possible that the CML assay may provide additional information concerning transplant outcome. When the results of CML and MLC assays are combined, the predictive accuracy appears to be greater than when either test is used alone (4).

MLC TEST PROCEDURES

Collection of blood specimens

Standard blood collection procedures used for clinical tests are followed. First, informed consent from the donors is obtained prior to drawing of the blood.

TABLE 1. MLC and CML assays

Operation	Culture time	Outcome
AB_x	5–6 days	Proliferation of cell A[a]
AB_x	5–6 days	CTL generation[b] (A anti-B)
A anti-B_x + A	4 h	A not destroyed[c]
A anti-B_x + B	4 h	B destroyed
A anti-B_x + C	4 h	C not destroyed or C destroyed if B and C share HLA-A,B,C antigens

[a] Proliferation is assayed by [^{3}H]TdR uptake.
[b] Cytotoxic activity is assayed in 4-h ^{51}Cr release assay.
[c] Lysis of cells A, B, and C is facilitated when these cells are previously activated with PHA (see text).

To avoid any possible bacterial and fungal infections, lymphocyte techniques and cell culture procedures are performed in a laminar-flow hood under sterile conditions. Care is taken in handling the blood, serum, or cells from patients or normal donors to avoid the possibility of hepatitis infection. All plastic ware and glassware are separately autoclaved and disposed of.

Blood is drawn with either a sterile heparinized syringe or a VACUTAINER tube containing 10 IU of heparin per ml of blood. It is important to label each tube clearly with the name of the donor. When a large volume of blood is being drawn, the use of a 19- or 21-gauge butterfly needle is convenient, since this kind of needle facilitates the interchange of syringes during the collection of multiple samples. Fresh blood is diluted 1:2 (vol/vol) with Hanks balanced salt solution (Microbiological Associates, Walkersville, Md.) before separation. The blood sample is transferred to a flask, diluted with an equal volume of sterile medium without any serum, and kept at room temperature (22°C). Generally, the blood sample is processed on the day of collection. A variable response is observed when blood samples are processed 24 h after being drawn. When blood is not drawn on the premises of the laboratory where the test is to be performed, the blood is diluted before transportation.

Lymphocytes are separated from whole blood by Ficoll-Hypaque density centrifugation. Ficoll-Hypaque can be purchased from commercial sources (e.g., Pharmacia Fine Chemicals, Piscataway, N.J.) or prepared as described below in the section on reagents. About 3 to 4 ml of Ficoll-Hypaque is transferred to a 15-ml tube, and 6 to 8 ml of the diluted blood is carefully layered over it. Dilution of the blood increases the recovery of lymphocytes. Care must be taken not to disturb the blood-Ficoll interface. If large volumes of blood must be separated, 10 ml of Ficoll-Hypaque is transferred to 50-ml tubes (Falcon no. 2070; Becton Dickinson Labware, Oxnard, Calif.) in which as much as 35 ml of diluted blood can be overlaid. In either case, tubes are centrifuged at 400 × g for 30 min at room temperature. A white ring-shaped layer will appear. This layer (the buffy layer) contains mononuclear cells, including lymphocytes, monocytes, and macrophages. Erythrocytes settle at the bottom of the tube.

With a sterile pipette, the buffy layer is carefully removed and transferred to another tube. The volume is brought to about 15 ml with the medium, and the combination is mixed gently by Vortex mixer (Vortex Genie; Scientific Industries, Inc., Bohemia, N.Y.). The tube is spun at 200 × g for 15 min, and the supernatant fluid is discarded. This washing procedure is repeated twice. Finally, the cells are suspended in 1 ml of culture medium. Cells are counted with a hemacytometer or Coulter Counter. If a hemacytometer is used, at least 200 cells should be counted to evaluate cell concentration. If the number of samples is large, a Coulter Counter is preferable. In our hands, the typical yield of mononuclear cells is about 1×10^6 to 2×10^6 cells per ml of whole blood. We generally obtain 95 to 100% viability of macrophages, as determined by the trypan blue uptake method. The cell population consists mainly of 75 to 85% lymphocytes and 15 to 25% monocytes. Cell concentration is adjusted by experimental design. The cells can either be used fresh or be frozen for future testing. Cell-freezing techniques are briefly described below.

Freezing procedures

Lymphoid cells separated from blood by the Ficoll-Hypaque procedure can be frozen for future use. The cells are suspended in culture medium at the desired concentration. The initial concentration should be twice the concentration needed to freeze the cells. The composition of freezing medium containing dimethyl sulfoxide (DMSO) (Sigma Chemical Co., St. Louis, Mo.) is described below in the section on reagents. The precooled (4°C) freezing medium is added, drop by drop, to the cell suspension and gently mixed with a Pasteur pipette. The cell mixture is always kept on ice. Then 1 ml of cell suspension is quickly transferred to screw-top polypropylene ampoules for freezing.

Sometimes it is necessary to freeze cultured cells or clones. It is important to remember that the procedure used in freezing one kind of cell may not work for other kinds of cells.

T cells generated in MLC are quite sensitive to freezing in the presence of DMSO. These cells can be frozen in the presence of 50% fetal calf serum or pooled human serum (PHS) and 10% DMSO. With this procedure, more than 90% cell recovery can be achieved.

The cells in ampoules can be frozen directly by cooling in liquid-nitrogen vapor. The advantage of this method is that it does not require controlled freezing equipment. It is also quick and yields cells with good viability and without significant change in functional properties. A major disadvantage, however, is variation in viability in different freezings. In this procedure, ampoules or tubes containing cells are precooled for 1 h in a vapor of liquid nitrogen. After 1 h of precooling, the cells are transferred to a liquid-nitrogen tank for storage. Cells can also be frozen by cooling at a controlled rate, i.e., first at 1°C/min to −40°C and then rapidly to −100°C. Although the required equipment is expensive, it provides consistent and reproducible results. The frozen cells can be stored for several years without a significant decrease in viability.

Several types of freezing equipment are commercially available. Operating instructions are provided by the manufacturers. In general, it is important to determine that thermocouple probes are working and that they are placed in the vial chamber. Also, before starting the machine, the liquid-nitrogen supply should be checked. Subsequently it should be confirmed that the temperature recorder is operative and the switch is in the "on" position. After the cells have been frozen, they should be transferred as soon as possible to a liquid-N$_2$ storage tank.

Thawing of cells

Vials containing frozen cells are removed from the liquid-nitrogen storage tank and kept on dry ice until used. Frozen vials are shaken manually in a 37°C water bath until few crystals are left in the vial. The thawed cell sample is immediately transferred to a sterile 15-ml tube and slowly diluted with 10 to 12 ml of ice-cold RPMI 1640 medium containing 10% fetal calf serum or PHS. Cells are spun at $150 \times g$ for 5 min, and the supernatant is removed. The washing procedure is then repeated. Two washes are sufficient to completely remove DMSO. After being washed, cells are suspended in 1 to 2 ml of culture medium for counting. Assessment of viability of the recovered cells is determined by the trypan blue exclusion method. If viability is less than 80%, dead cells should be removed by centrifugation on Ficoll-Hypaque. It is important to have some protein present in the medium at the time of thawing, since the protein protects cells from damage. Also, cells should never be left at room temperature in the presence of DMSO.

Functional studies show that frozen cells provide responses similar to those of fresh cells when used in MLC. The frozen-cell response may be somewhat lower; however, stimulation by cells does not appear to be affected by freezing, suggesting that there is no loss in functional capacity of cells during freezing and thawing.

MLC assay

An MLC setup requires lymphocytes from two individuals, i.e., recipient (responder) and possible organ donor (stimulator). After blood is obtained from these donors and lymphocytes are separated by the procedure outlined above, the next steps are to adjust both groups of cells to the desired concentrations by the addition of an appropriate amount of culture medium and to inactivate the stimulator cell. The culture medium contains 10 or 20% PHS (see below, Reagents).

Cell inactivation can be performed by X-radiation or by treatment with mitomycin C, an inhibitor of DNA synthesis. A ^{137}Cs or ^{60}Co source is commonly used. If a radiation source is not available, stimulators may be inactivated by treatment with mitomycin C. This treatment is performed in the following manner. To a 2.0-ml (5×10^6-cell) cell suspension, add 0.2 ml of mitomycin C (0.25 mg/ml). The mixture is then incubated for 20 min in a 5% CO$_2$–95% air atmosphere. After the incubation, the cells are washed three times in culture medium. It is important to note that up to 50% of the cells may be lost in this procedure.

Although both methods are widely used to inactivate stimulator cells, radiation is the method of choice. It is quick and simple, with 100% cell recovery. It is important to note that the effect of radiation dose on the mixed lymphocyte reaction is variable and dose dependent. The contribution of surviving stimulator cells to the uptake of tritiated thymidine ([^{3}H]TdR) by MLC cells is seen even on day 5 at 2,500 rads, though it is small (<1%) (Fig. 1). In contrast, a dose greater than 5,000 rads diminishes the stimulation capacity of responder cells. The reason for this discrepancy is not known. It is likely that, due to decreased survival of the stimulating population at high doses (Fig. 2), responder cells are not stimulated to the same extent as at lower doses, so the response is diminished. The effect is particularly noticeable in the first 24 to 48 h after radiation, which is the most critical time in MLC stimulation.

The contribution of [^{3}H]TdR uptake by irradiated cells surviving on day 6 is small. As low as 500 rads may be sufficient to completely inactivate stimulator cells (Fig. 3). In a two-way MLC, two cells were given equal and increasing amounts of radiation. [^{3}H]TdR uptake by surviving cells was measured on day 6. The results show that the counts drop off to very low levels even after each cell has received as little as 500 rads.

Culture setup

The MLC is set up in checkerboard fashion in sterile, 96-well, round-bottom plates (Fig. 4). It is particularly important to mix a precise amount of responding cells with inactivated stimulator cells. Each responder-stimulator combination is set up in triplicate. To each well, 100 μl each of the appropriate responder and stimulator cells is added. Pipetting is best done with an Eppendorf or Oxford pipette, with autoclavable and disposable sterile tips. Note that autologous as well as allogeneic combinations are set up for each responder.

The plate is then placed in a 5% CO$_2$ incubator at 37°C for 5 to 6 days, with humidity maintained at 100% (Fig. 5). After 5 or 6 days, the culture is pulsed with 25 μl of [^{3}H]TdR. The plates are then returned to the incubator and incubated for another 6 h. After incubation, the plates are either removed and harvested immediately or stored at 4°C until harvested. In the latter case, plates are covered with a pressure-sensitive film (Falcon Plastics). In our hands, cells thus stored for up to 30 days showed results similar to those from cells harvested immediately after removal from the incubator.

The labeling time of 6 h appears to be optimal (Fig. 6). The [^{3}H]TdR uptake by the autologous cells is also low at this time. For experiments in which it is desirable to estimate the number of cells synthesizing DNA, a labeling time in the linear portion of the uptake curve must be chosen. The [^{3}H]TdR uptake is then a linear function of the number of cells synthesizing DNA during the labeling period. Consequently, comparisons between two sets of MLC are valid. The dose of [^{3}H]TdR at 1.0 μCi per well is the optimum and is consistent with economical use of the radioactive substance. No statistical advantage is gained by increasing the dose (Fig. 7).

After incubation of cells with [^{3}H]TdR, the labeled cells are recovered by filtration on glass fiber filters or by trichloroacetic acid precipitation determination of radioactivity incorporated. The filtration method is convenient and allows rapid and effective cell removal, thus making possible large-scale harvesting in a short time. Basically, the cells and medium are removed by suction from the wells, the wells are thor-

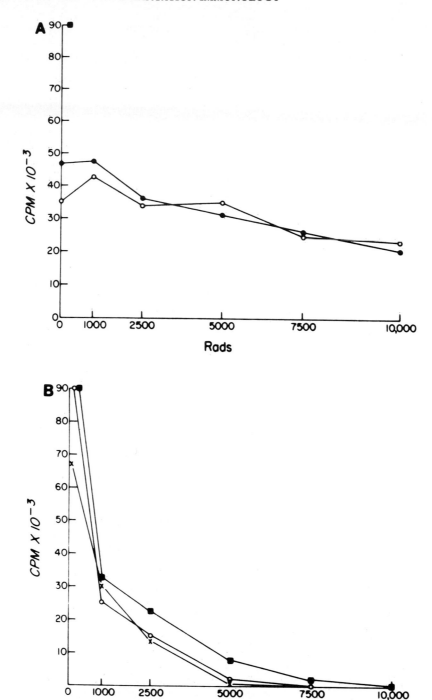

FIG. 1. (A) Results of unidirectional MLC, i.e., AB (○) and AC (●), after stimulator cells (B or C) were inactivated by various doses of X rays. Cells were cultured for 120 h and then given an 18-h pulse with 1.0 μCi of [³H]TdR. (B) Response of the same responding cells as in panel A to stimulation by concanavalin A (×), PHA (Difco) (○), and HA-17 (■) after the cells had been inactivated by various doses of X rays. Cells were cultured for 96 h and then given an 18-h pulse with 1.0 μCi of [³H]TdR.

oughly flushed, and any unbound [³H]TdR is washed off the filters. The cellular material is bound to the filter by ionic interaction and denatured. Whatman GF/C glass filters are suitable for collection of cells. A number of harvesting devices are commercially available. Regular maintenance of the harvestor is essential for accuracy in counting.

The filter is thoroughly air dried. A small amount of water can result in quenching of fluorescence of the scintillation fluid, thus introducing errors in counting. The individual circles from the filter are carefully removed and placed in scintillation vials. To each vial, 2 to 3 ml of scintillation cocktail is added, and vials are capped to avoid evaporation and spillage.

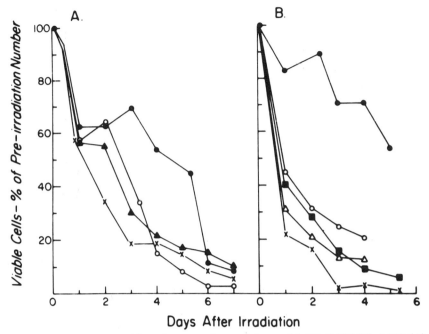

FIG. 2. (A) Percent survival of unseparated lymphocytes after rad doses of 0 (●), 2,500 (○), 5,000 (▲), and 7,500 (×), with survival determined by trypan blue dye exclusion. (B) Percent survival of B or T lymphocytes after various doses of X ray. T cells with rad doses of 0 (●), 2,500 (■), and 7,500 (×); B cells with rad doses of 2,500 (○) and 7,500 (△).

Counting is performed on a beta scintillation counter 6 to 8 h after the cocktail is added, with windows set for ^{3}H counting.

Presentation and treatment of MLC data

To identify suitable organ donors, the MLC test is usually performed between members of the family or close relatives of the patient. Ideally, family members should include the patient, both parents, and at least one sibling. In addition to family members, at least three unrelated healthy individuals are used as control stimulators as well as responders. All of the specific culture conditions should be indicated in the report as follows (for example): number of stimulator cells = responder cells = 10×10^3; 5,000 rads; [^{3}H]TdR, 1.0 µCi per well; labeling time, 6 h; culture time, 5 days.

The results of a family MLC assay are presented in Table 2. The data are given in counts per minute (cpm), taken over a 1-min period. It is convenient to present the data in tabular form, with the stimulator cells along the side and the responders across the top. Values of the triplicate counts are averaged, and for every combination, the mean cpm are given. The data can be expressed in a number of ways, as shown in Table 2. The methods of calculation and the usefulness of the various expressions are discussed below. Since none of these methods unambiguously distinguishes a negative from a positive result in all cases, an arbitrary decision is made about the value which is consistent with certain hypotheses.

One method for the expression of MLC data is simply to tabulate the average difference in cpm between test and control. The autologous counts are commonly used as a control. In this method, the autologous value (in cpm) of a given responder cell is subtracted from the test value of that responder, for example, $AB_x - AA_x$.

A second method for the expression of MLC data is in terms of the stimulation index (SI). The SI is the test value divided by the autologous cpm, with both values in cpm. There are two main drawbacks to the SI method, as follows: (i) the SI value depends strongly on autologous counts, which are generally low but show a great deal of variability; and (ii) use of the SI value implies some quantitative relationship between autologous responder cells which divide spontaneously (AA_x) (autologous cell proliferation) and response to allogenic stimulation (AB_x). In fact, there is no relation between these two types of responses. Since the control value is not precisely determined, the ratio is susceptible to significant variation, rendering comparisons between different sets of responders less precise.

The third method for the expression of MLC results involves the establishment of some reference value for a given responder cell population to which a given test response can be compared. This reference should reflect the inherent responsiveness of the test cell under consideration. There are two methods for obtaining a reference value, as follows. (i) The maximal response (in cpm) to a panel of stimulator cells when the responder cell is individually stimulated by cells from individual members of the panel can be determined. We have observed that a minimum of three, and preferably five, unrelated donors gives a reasonably precise median value. (ii) The response to a pool of unrelated donor cells can be determined. The theoretical basis for this approach is that pooled stimulating cells should contain all possible cellular antigens to which responding cells could respond and should thus stimulate to a maximum level of prolifer-

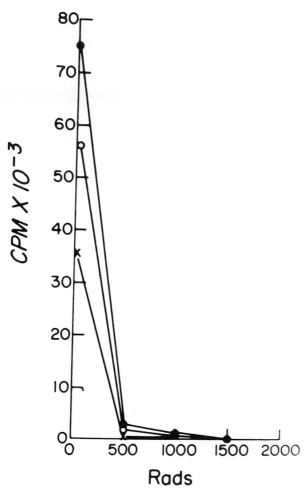

FIG. 3. Effects of various doses of radiation given to both responder and stimulator cells in three separate two-way MLC experiments (i.e., A_xB_x [O], B_xC_x [●], $C_x + A_x$ [×]). Results are expressed as the mean triplicate samples.

recipient. A typical example illustrating the basic MLC results and its interpretation is described below.

The HLA typing of the family is given in Tables 3 and 4. The mitogen response is shown in Table 4. The data are expressed as mean counts per minute RR, as described above in Presentation and treatment of MLC data. The family members include the patient, father (F), mother (M), and two siblings (both sisters; S_1 and S_2). In addition, three young, healthy, unrelated individuals were used as control responders and stimulators. The number of responder and stimulator cells was 5×10^4 cells of each per well, the X-ray dose to stimulator cells was 5,000 rads, and cells were cultured for 5 days. The MLC was pulsed with 1 μCi of [^{3}H]TdR for 6 h. All combinations of MLC were set up in triplicate. The mean cpm of the triplicate assays are shown in Table 2. In addition to raw mean cpm of triplicate values, the results are also expressed in terms of % RR, as defined above. Although the lymphocytes of the patient exhibited normal responses to PHA, concanavalin A, and pokeweed mitogen, they showed a significant response to autologous cells, and the RR was zero. Tests against self, S_1, and S_2 also showed no response. The patient is identical to S_1 at loci HLA-A, B, C, and DR (Table 3), and S_1S_2 combinations yield low RR values, whereas S_2S_1 has an RR value of >100 (Table 2). This asymmetric response suggests that S_2 has inherited genes which are homozygous at the D/DR locus. Indeed, DR typing shows that S_2 is homozygous at DR4, which is inherited from both parents. It is interesting to note that the lymphocytes of the patient exhibit normal responses to PHA, concanavalin A, and pokeweed mitogen (Table 4).

HLA-D TYPING

HLA-D typing is performed with the use of homozygous typing cells (5). These cells are identified among the offspring of marriages between first cousins or in families in which parents share HLA haplotypes. If one of the parents is homozygous, the probability of finding one of the offspring homozygous at HLA-D is increased. The offspring of unrelated individuals can also be homozygous if the parents share an HLA-D haplotype, but the frequency of this event is very low.

Like other HLA systems, the HLA-D region has been mapped with homozygous typing cells collected

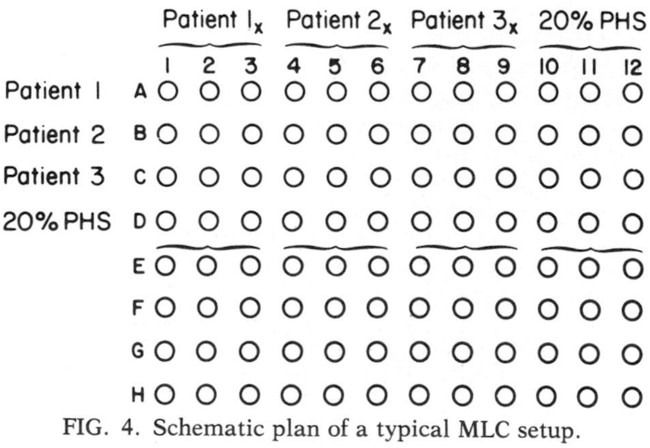

ation. The plateau value of stimulation can then be used to normalize the response. It has been suggested that pools consisting of 10 to 15 randomly selected donors approach such theoretical plateau values.

The general formula for relative response (RR) is as follows: % RR = {[(test cpm) − (autologous cpm)]/ [(median response cpm) − (autologous cpm)]} × 100.

Use of RR gives good correlation between repeat MLC assays on different occasions. A comparison of the coefficiencies of variance of the three basic methods described above shows that the RR has a smaller coefficient of variance and that the major portion of the variance in MLC data may be attributed to the biological variability rather than to technical error.

Clinical and genetic interpretations of MLC data

One of the major applications of the MLC assay is the identification of an appropriate transplant donor. Therefore, clinical MLC testing usually involves both patients and family members. A lack of response between the patient and potential donor may be a useful clue in choosing a favorable donor to the

FIG. 4. Schematic plan of a typical MLC setup.

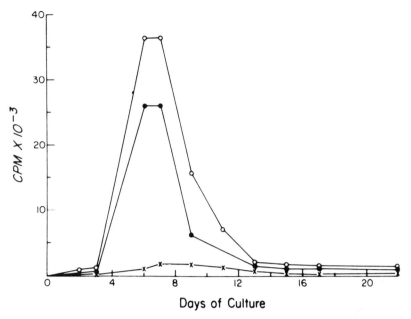

FIG. 5. Kinetics of MLC between cell A and autologous stimulator A_x (AA_x) (×), allogeneic stimulator B (AB_x) (○), and C_x (AC_x) (●), where cell A has phenotype Dw2,3, cell B has phenotype Dw3,5, and cell C has phenotype Dw2,–. Time represents total culture duration including the time of pulsing with [^{3}H]TdR. Results are expressed as mean of triplicate cultures.

worldwide during various international workshops. The testing laboratories had no prior knowledge of HLA-D typing of testing cells. Data thus collected were analyzed centrally, and it was found that some specificities were readily discriminated, while others were characterized with some difficulty. In particular, Dw1 and Dw2 are easiest to define, but all other specificities have been difficult to define clearly and uniquely. During the last international workshop, 19 HLA-D specificities were established. New designations and a complete listing of HLA-D phenotypes are given in chapter 130. Antigen frequencies may vary among ethnic groups or geographical locations. Thus

when the frequencies are compared it is important to know the ethnic background of donors.

Proliferative responses elicited by HLA-non-D antigens are a major contributory factor to poor discrimination in HLA-D typing. Also, low-level proliferative responses may result from the existence of some as yet

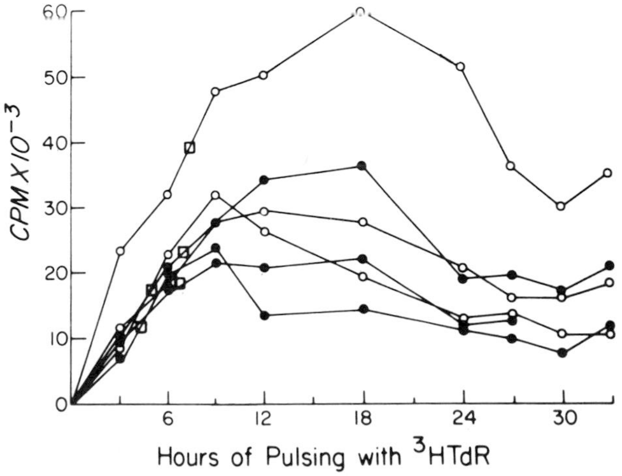

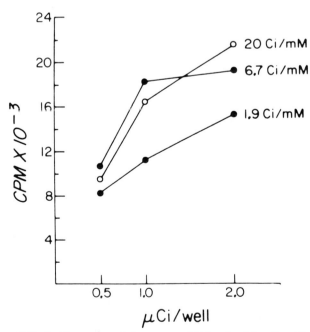

FIG. 6. Kinetics of [^{3}H]TdR uptake by six MLC. Six cultures (AB_x, BC_x, and AC_x, represented by open circles, and BA_x, CB_x, and CA_x, represented by closed circles) were labeled on day 6 for the indicated time. □, Value for each culture after an 18-h pulse on day 5.

FIG. 7. Mean cpm of six separate MLC pulsed for 6 h with [^{3}H]TdR of various specific activities (1.9, 6.7, and 20 μCi/mmol) and in various amounts (0.5, 1.0, and 2.0 μCi per well). The MLC assays were set up with responder and stimulator cells at 0.5×10^4 cells per well. Stimulator cells were inactivated with 5,000 rads.

TABLE 2. Five-member intrafamily MLC assay results

Patient	Patient		F		M		S_1		S_2		C_1		C_2		C_3	
	% RR	cpm	% RR	cpm	% RR	cpm	% RR	cpm	% RR	cpm	% RR	cpm	% RR	cpm	% RR	cpm
Auto$_x$[b]		2,128		1,135		1,117		427		409		1,122		574		1,745
Pool$_x$[c]		98,700		10,065		110,770		81,273		62,042		79.995		87,395		46,411
Patient	0.0	2,815	61.0	62,600	1.0	2,271	0.6	1,333	100.0	61,811	100.0	87,758	100.0	108,606	100.0	75,057
F	17.5	19,613	0.0	1,387	53.0	59,289	36.0	29,469	100.0	66,979	100.0	99,400	100.0	96,683	99.0	46,336
M	2.1	4,801	75.0	75,963	0.0	1,038	2.0	2,331	100.0	67,867	100.0	102,082	100.0	148,200	100.0	69,843
S_1	0.0	1,315	66.0	66,525	0.0	866	0.0	884	100.0	63,656	100.0	82,548	89.0	77,571	100.0	53,676
S_2	0.0	2,733	0.4	1,809	0.2	1,299	0.0	767	0.0	1,030	73.0	58,914	61,0	53,844	44.0	8,232
C_1	59.0	59,064	52.0	52,597	32.0	90,507	46.0	37,901	100.0	69,965	0.0	1,872	76.0	61,236	100.0	58,693
C_2		56,025	64.0	65,721	99.0	109,106	76.0	61,796	98.0	68,952	97.0	65,667	0.0	925	71.0	63,931
C_3	58.0	58,725	54.0	54,923	100.0	120,631	100.0	100,834	100.0	69,095	100.0	79,600	66.0	57,633	0.0	1,941
PHS (20%)		3,376		1,547		1,221		414		773		1,169		795		1,328

[a] C_1, C_2, and C_3 are healthy individuals unrelated to the patient, who were used as control responders and stimulators.
[b] Auto$_x$, Autologous control.
[c] Pool$_x$, Pooled-cell control.

unknown gene product in close linkage with the HLA-D genes.

Statistical analysis of HLA-D typing data

[^{3}H]TdR uptake data are expressed as RR for further statistical analysis. The basic criterion in deciding about the null (zero) response, thereby identifying the typing response, is whether two reactions are significantly different. This problem leads to the question of defining null response and positive response. Furthermore, the analysis should be independent of any assumption about the nature of the cellular reaction. This independence can be achieved by using analysis-of-variance, least-significant-difference, and multiple-range testing procedures. These tests make it possible to normalize data so that information from different experiments can be combined without introducing any statistical bias. Two major steps in data analysis are (i) defining clusters of like reactions and (ii) defining the range of responses attributable to a given HLA-D gene product.

A method of particular importance is the double-normalized-value method, in which responses are expressed in terms of a ratio of the 75th percentile of the range of responses for that responder, which is in turn expressed as a ratio of the 75th percentile of the range of reactions elicited by that particular stimulator. In this way an adjustment is made both for innate responsiveness of the responder cell and for innate stimulatory capacity of the stimulator cell. Cluster analysis is also used to identify groups. Responses are arranged into a predetermined number of groups by minimizing within-group variance and maximizing between-group variance.

Interpretation of HLA-D typing

Interpretation of HLA-D typing data is more complicated than interpretation of data from family MLC assays because of the difficulty in deciding objectively whether two reactions are significantly different. Clearly, to be useful as a typing cell, the homozygous cell should be able to stimulate a response in cells not possessing the determinant, but should produce no response in those cells which possess the same determinant (HLA-D type) as the typing cell. Figure 8 shows the results of two experiments with homozygous cells from donors Sc and JH. Each cell type was used to stimulate a random panel of responder cells. The RR to JH can be separated into two groups, i.e., 0 to 50 and 83 to 137% in one experiment and 0 to 49 and 64 to 114% in the other. The second experiment showed a clear separation at the 95% confidence level, but the first experiment showed two responses at the intermediate level, and the separation is not significant. The Sc cell type showed relative responses of 23 to 54 and 66 to 107% in the first experiment and 13 to 48 and 84 to 160% in the second. A complete separation at the 95% confidence level was observed in the second experiment, and some overlap was seen in the first.

For the JH cells, the 99% confidence interval for the high-responder group of the combined experiments gave an upper limit of 35% for typing response, whereas the lower value of the nontyping response for this group at the 99% confidence interval was 42%. The results of these experiments indicate that for RR values between 0 and 35%, we can be 99% sure that the response belongs to the low group, and this response can be called a typing response.

TABLE 3. HLA-A, B, C, and DR typing of a patient and members of his family

Relationship	Haplotype	Phenotype			
		HLA-A	HLA-B	HLA-C	HLA-DR
Patient	$\frac{a}{c}$	A2	B44	CW−	DR4
		A2	B35	CW4	DR1
F	$\frac{a}{b}$	A2	B44	CW−	DR4
		A32	B14	CW−	DR7
M	$\frac{c}{d}$	A2	B35	CW4	DR1
		A24	B35	CW4	DR4
S_1	$\frac{a}{c}$	A2	B44	CW−	DR4
		A2	B35	CW4	DR1
S_2	$\frac{a}{d}$	A2	B44	CW−	DR4
		A24	B35	CW4	DR4

TABLE 4. *Mitogenic response of lymphocytes from a patient and members of his family*[a]

Stimulator	Response of:											
	P		F		M		S_1		S_2		Control[b]	
	% RR[c]	cpm[d]	% RR	cpm	% RR	cpm	% RR	cpm	% RR	cpm	% RR	cpm
Mitogen												
PHA	100	243,371	100	208,263	100	173,630	34	58,696	86	147,191	100	171,470
ConA[e]	100	60,859	100	40,843	100	47,788	91	28,745	62	19,765	100	31,764
Pokeweed	82.3	30,362	100	42,361	100	48,662	100	52,670	65	24,087	100	36,893
Control medium only		325		1,039		228		81		240		274

[a] HLA typing of this family is shown in Table 3.

[b] A pool of cells from three unrelated individuals was used as a control.

[c] % RR = 100 × [(experimental cpm with mitogen − experimental cpm with medium alone)/(cpm of pooled cells with mitogen − cpm of pooled cells with medium alone)].

[d] [^{3}H]TdR values are the means of triplicate experiments.

[e] ConA, Concanavalin A.

It should be remembered that the significance of a moderate response among heterozygotes is not well understood. A moderate response may be related to the presence of a second locus contributing to MLC stimulation, as was recently observed with primed lymphocyte assays (see chapter 132).

CML

The ability to predict accurately the degree of immune response of the recipient to the donor, so that timely and proper donor selection can be made, is important in transplant medicine.

CML is of primary importance in allograft rejection. In this process, host (recipient) lymphocytes participate directly in the destruction of donor tissues by cell-cell interaction. In the first phase, the lymphocytes of the recipient come in contact with the lymphoid cells of the donor, which bear different histocompatibility antigens than those of the recipient. A small percentage of recipient lymphoid cells which have receptors for these foreign antigens respond by differentiation and proliferation. The sec-

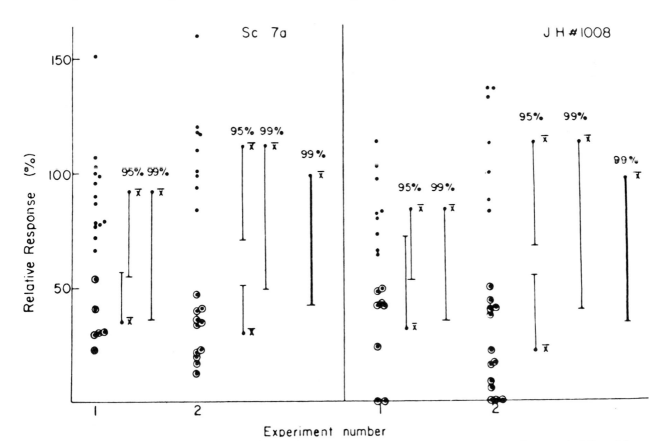

FIG. 8. Relative response of a responder cell panel to homozygous cells from donors JH and Sc. The 99 and 95% confidence intervals (one sided) have been denoted by vertical bars. Symbols: ●, experimental values; ⊙, typing response; x̄, mean values.

ond, or effector, phase involves destruction of the allograft by the sensitized lymphocytes. The in vitro procedure which mimics the destruction of the allograft is known as CML and is described in the following pages (6).

Generation of CTL in MLC

Fresh or previously frozen peripheral blood lymphocytes from the patient, members of the family, and unrelated individuals are used in appropriate combinations as responder or stimulator cells to generate CTL. Blood from patients is drawn into a heparinized syringe, transferred to sterile flasks, and diluted with RPMI 1640 medium as described above. Care must be taken to label blood samples correctly and to perform all procedures under sterile conditions. If cryopreserved cells are used, then the cells should be thawed by the procedures described above.

Cell counts, viability, and total recovery of lymphocytes from blood (if fresh blood is used) are determined by counting on a hemacytometer. Cell concentration is adjusted to 2×10^6 cells per ml. All stimulator cells are irradiated at 5,000 rads.

The MLC is set up in a Linbro plate with 24 2.0-ml, flat-bottom wells, each well containing 2×10^6 to 3×10^6 responder lymphocytes and an equal number of irradiated stimulator cells in culture medium. The culture medium contains 10 or 20% PHS. The cells are incubated at 37°C in a humidified atmosphere of 95% air and 5% CO_2 for 6 days. During this period, CTL are generated which specifically identify the stimulator cell.

Target cell preparation

A common procedure in preparing target cells is to activate nonirradiated stimulator cells with PHA (HA-16; Burroughs Wellcome Co., Research Triangle Park, N.C.). The lymphocytes are suspended in culture medium at a concentration of 2.0×10^6 and cultured in 2-ml wells in Linbro plates. These cells can be stimulated on day 3 with PHA (HA-16) at a final concentration of 1 µg/ml. On day 6, PHA-stimulated target cells are harvested and centrifuged ($200 \times g$) for 10 min. To the pellet, 100 µl of radioactive $^{51}Cr_2O_4$ is added. These cells are incubated for 1 h at 37°C and washed three times. The target cell concentration is then adjusted to 10^5 cells per ml.

CML test procedure

CML tests can be performed in round- or conical-bottomed 96-well microtiter plates (Linbro/Titertek; Flow Laboratories, Inc., McLean, Va.). Different dilutions of effector cells are prepared in culture medium and mixed with 100 µl of target cells (10×10^3 or 5×10^3 cells per well) to yield effector cell/target cell ratios of 100, 50, 25, 12.5, and 6.25. Triplicate wells are set up for each effector-target combination.

Prior to incubation, the plates are spun at $100 \times g$ for 3 min. After 4 h of incubation at 37°C, the plates are again centrifuged at $200 \times g$ for 3 min at 4°C, and a 125-µl sample of the supernatant is collected from each well. The amount of ^{51}Cr release determines the extent of lysis of the target cells. Spontaneous release is determined from ^{51}Cr release in the absence of effector cells, while the maximum release is determined by adding 1 N HCl or a detergent (Tween 20, 0.1%) to the appropriate wells.

Data analysis

Cytotoxicity data reduction and expression are critical to an understanding of the biological phenomenon involved. The presentations should clearly indicate lytic activity. The majority of investigators use tables or graphs in which cytotoxicity is expressed in terms of percent ^{51}Cr release at a single or several effector cell/target cell ratios. Alternatively, data can be expressed in lytic units (LU).

The cytotoxic activities of effector populations generated in MLC can be expressed in three different ways. The most common method is expression in terms of percent cytotoxicity, a quantity directly determined from the raw counts of ^{51}Cr release. The other two methods involve derived units, i.e., LU and cytotoxic units.

Percent cytotoxicity is calculated by the following formula (with all values in cpm): % cytotoxicity = 100 × {[(mean experimental value) − (mean spontaneous release)]/[(total releasable count) − (spontaneous release)]}, or, alternatively, % cytotoxicity = {[(experimental value) − (spontaneous release)]/(total count incorporated)} × 100.

The second method provides a conservative estimate of cytotoxicity.

The cytotoxicity can also be expressed as LU, which is defined as that number of effector cells required to kill a defined number of target cells, and is usually expressed as LU/10^7 cells, so that the value increases with increasing lytic activity.

Percent cytotoxicity plotted against the number of effector cells or the ratio of effector to target cells yields a sigmoid curve, suggesting a log-linear relationship between the number of killer cells and the amount of ^{51}Cr release. When plotted on a log-linear scale, this calculation yields a straight line. The best-fitted line by the least-squares method is employed to determine the number of effector cells capable of killing a defined number (e.g., 25%) of target cells.

Results and interpretation

In a typical CML test, results can be summarized as follows: when stimulator and responder cells differ with respect to HLA-A, B, and C determinants as well as HLA-D and DR determinants, there is (i) good proliferative response in the MLC phase and also good lysis of the specific (same as stimulator) target cells; (ii) lysis of any third-party target cell carrying the same haplotypes as the stimulator but absent on the responder cell; (iii) little or no lysis of third-party target cells carrying the HLA-D/DR determinant present on the stimulator cell and absent from the responder cell, but which carry the HLA-A, B, and C antigens of the responder cell; and (iv) significant lysis of third-party target cells which are stimulator but not responder cells, although HLA-D/DR antigens may be shared by the responder cells when stimulator and responders are identical for HLA-A, B, and C antigens but differ at HLA-D/DR determinants. In this case, good proliferation is observed, but there is no lysis of the specific target cell.

TABLE 5. Three-member intrafamily cell-mediated cytotoxicity test[a] results

Target cell	Response of effector cell[b]											
	P anti-P_x		P anti-M_x		P anti-F_x		P anti-PHL_x		M anti-PHL_x		F anti-PHL_x	
	% Cyt[c]	LU[d]	% Cyt	LU	% Cyt	LU	% Cyt	LU	% Cyt	LU	% Cyt	LU
Patient	15.9	3.2										
M			42.0	96.2	13.7	2.3						
F			32.2	55.6	2.3	3.6						
PHL							22.2	12.2	24.7	24.5	48.2	102.0

[a] Primary MLC combinations were established on day 0 with fresh peripheral blood lymphocytes from the patient and his family members and previously frozen pooled human lymphocytes.

[b] P, Patient; PHL, pooled human lymphocytes.

[c] % Cyt, Percent cytotoxicity at an effector cell/target cell ratio of 50.

[d] Per 10^7 cells.

Generally speaking, when third-party target cells carrying the HLA-D/DR determinants are present on the stimulator cell but absent from the responder cell, significant lysis of the target cell is observed. In stimulator-responder combinations which differ for HLA-A, B, and C but are identical for HLA-D/DR antigens, there is neither proliferative response in the MLC phase nor cytotoxic activity generated against the specific target cell. In other words, cells do not receive the signal to proliferate if the responder-stimulator combinations share HLA-D/DR antigens.

Thus, the following conclusions can be drawn: (i) to generate cytotoxic cells in the responder population, the stimulator cell should differ from the responder cell with respect to HLA-A, B, C, and D/DR antigens; and (ii) the lytic specificity of cytotoxic cells is not significantly controlled by HLA-DR antigen present on the stimulator but absent from the responder cell. Rather, this specificity depends primarily on HLA-A, B, and C antigens or antigens coded by genes very closely linked to the HLA-A, B, and C loci.

The results of a typical test of the family of a patient are presented in Table 5. The pooled human lymphocytes are a pool of cells from 10 unrelated normal individuals and were used as a target. Target cells were stimulated with PHA 3 days prior to testing, with PHA-stimulated targets. The effector cells generated in the MLC sometimes destroy targets in a nonspecific manner. Such self-killing may reflect autoimmune disease. To determine whether this is true, target cells autologous to the responder cells were used (Table 5). P anti-P_x was tested against P. The percent cytotoxicity was 15.9 at an effector cell/target cell ratio of 50, suggesting high autologous killing. However, P anti-M_x tested against M gave cytotoxic activity of 42.0%, and the corresponding lytic activity was 96.2 LU. In contrast, P anti-F_x did not show cytotoxic activity different from that of the autologous combination. When experiments are conducted to determine whether a patient can generate effector cell activity in CML, another control must be included. If a particular effector is unable to kill or destroy a control target, or PHL (Table 5), it may be due to lack of generation of effector cell resulting from a poor responder or stimulator cell preparation, i.e., a technical artifact. In testing functional ability, particularly for induction of proliferation and generation of a cytotoxic response, in the example cited the father (F) was found to be unable to generate CML activity against PHA blasts from the patient, whereas the mother, who also shares one haplotype with the patient, showed a strong cytotoxic activity against her own cells. Thus, we find that the patient was unable to generate a cytotoxic response against the father's cells. If we assume that PHA-activated T cells reflect the sensitivity of kidney cells to CTL, the CTL in the patient would not cause destruction of the donor kidney when the donor is the father. The father may thus be a good candidate for donating the kidney.

REAGENTS

PHS

PHS can be prepared in the laboratory or purchased from commercial sources. Serum from about 20 normal untransfused male donors is obtained. These sera are centrifuged at high speed (at least $5,000 \times g$) for about 30 min. Fat is removed from the top layer. Samples (1 ml) of serum from each individual sample are removed and tested for cytotoxicity, for the ability to support MLC, and for lymphocyte and background proliferation in autologous cultures. After being tested, equal volumes of individual sera are pooled. The PHS is divided into aliquots and frozen for future use. When PHS from commercial sources is obtained, the PHS should be tested for its ability to support cell proliferation and other functions.

Freezing medium

Although the basic ingredients of the freezing medium used in the cryopreservation of peripheral blood lymphocytes and cloned or MLC-activated T cells are the same, the relative proportions of these ingredients differ. To freeze peripheral blood lymphocytes, the freezing medium contains a cocktail of 60% RPMI 1640, 20% PHS, and 20% DMSO. Precooled DMSO is added drop by drop to the PHS-containing RPMI 1640 medium, and the mixture is kept on ice until used. The final concentration of DMSO after the cells have been added should be 5 to 10%. If T-cell clones, hybridoma clones, or MLC-activated cells are to be cryopreserved, the freezing medium is made of 40% PHS or fetal calf serum, 10% DMSO, and 50% RPMI 1640.

Medium for MLC and CML tests

For MLC and CML tests, RPMI 1640 is supplemented with 10% PHS; penicillin, 100 U/ml; streptomycin,

TABLE 1. HLA-DP gene frequencies in different ethnic groups (maximum-likelihood method of estimation)

Group	Gene frequency							χ^2	df
	DPw1	DPw2	DPw3	DPw4	DPw5	DPw6	"Blanks"		
Caucasians ($n = 533$)	0.067	0.129	0.074	0.430	0.017	0.014	0.269	17.76	15
Blacks ($n = 116$)	0.326	0.131	0.056	0.166	0.009	0.004	0.307	37.14	15
Chinese ($n = 17$)	0	0.158	0	0.031	0.457	0	0.355		

Six DP alleles have been described. Table 1 shows the gene frequency for DPw1 through DPw6 obtained at Georgetown University by F. M. Robbins for 533 Caucasian, 116 American black, and 17 Chinese donors. The frequencies for each allele vary widely both within racial groups and between racial groups. The gene frequencies obtained for Caucasians is consistent with the Hardy-Weinberg calculation for a single allelic system in equilibrium. However, the gene frequencies in the American black population fall outside the expected Hardy-Weinberg values ($P < 0.005$), suggesting the possibility of several genes playing a role in the response or nonequilibrium in the population sample studied.

Several monoclonal antibodies (ILR-1, B7/21, Tu39) produced in mice by immunizing with human antigens bind primarily to DP cell surface antigens, and recently several alloantisera which detect DP determinants have been identified by Johnson. The DP antigens are expressed on B cells and macrophages but not on resting T cells (6) and are found on the cell surface at about 1/10 the concentration of DR molecules. They also appear considerably more labile on the cell surface than DR does, rendering more difficult the task of typing these cells with complement-mediated cytotoxicity.

This low antigen density may also explain the observation that these antigens are weak stimulators in primary MLC. In PLT, DP antigens appear to stimulate primed cells to the same level as HLA-D/DR molecules. The reason for this relatively high stimulation by SB antigens in secondary leukocyte culture has not been determined. It may be due to properties unique to SB, to qualitative differences between primed and unprimed cells, or to the fact that an excess of stimulator cells is used in the secondary phase of PLT, masking quantitative antigenic differences.

To date, HLA-D, DR, and DP antigens have been demonstrated in PLT as allelic systems. More determinants, though, are clearly present. Primed reagents can be generated between cells from unrelated pairs of individuals who are HLA-D, DR, DQ, and DP identical. Using this priming method, Termijtelen has recently described an additional antigen called LBQ-1 which is encoded within the major histocompatibility complex.

Cloned PLT reagents

Although it is possible to generate populations of primed reagents with highly discrete specificity between two nearly identical cells, it is sometimes advantageous to isolate and expand single primed cells. Clones generated from PLs demonstrate remarkable specificity and diversity. Many of these allospecific clones recognize HLA-D and HLA-DR antigens. How-

ever, the reactivity detected by stimulating these cloned cells with panels of cells from 30 or more individuals rarely shows precise concordance with any classical HLA specificity such as D, DR, DP, or DQ (1). For example, many of the clones generated from a PL population recognizing DR1 will recognize cells from 90% of individuals serotyped as DR1 but fail to type the remaining 10%. The 10% of individuals missed by one clone from this PL population are generally not the same 10% missed by a second clone derived from the same PL population. Such discrepancies suggest at least two possible processes. First, these clones are recognizing distinct epitopes on a single DR1 molecule. Some of these epitopes may differ from one "DR1" molecule to another (microheterogeneity of DR1). Second, the epitopes responsible for the allospecificities that we call DR reside on several different molecules on a single cell, and some minor variation of one or more of these molecules does not significantly alter the serotyping pattern for DR, while radically altering the recognition by certain clonal reagents. The failure of the antisera to categorize individuals with minute differences may be because alloantisera contain many antibodies which recognize both several antigenic determinants on one molecule and determinants on several distinct molecules. Alloantisera which are used for HLA typing are selected on the basis of clustering broad groups, and it is likely that antisera which stray from classical definition tend to be considered variants and are not widely used.

Recombinant DNA methods reveal at least three distinct beta-chain genes and at least one alpha-chain gene in the HLA-DR subregion. Pairs of one alpha and one beta chain are expressed together on the cell surface, and at least two of the three possible DR subregion alpha-beta pairs are expressed (DR and BR-MT). The other two class II HLA subregions, DQ and DP, each contain at least two alpha- and two beta-chain genes. Thus, there are many potential molecules structurally similar to those known to be detectable in PLT (R. C. Giles and J. D. Capra, submitted for publication).

Polyclonal reagents, whether they are alloantisera, homozygous typing cells, or PLs, are likely to detect determinants on more than one of these molecules, whereas the cloned T cells each see unique epitopes. The analysis would be relatively simple at this point if these unique epitopes were not repeated on several different cell surface molecules. Fortunately, mutagenic and recombinant DNA techniques are being used to develop cells expressing single HLA class II molecules. The use of these unique cells together with cellular, serologic, and biochemical technologies should permit us to resolve the complexity of this system.

CLINICAL INDICATIONS

Cellular methods are not yet generally used to classify HLA-D region specificity in clinical settings, although MLC is performed routinely for confirming donor selection for both renal and bone marrow transplantation. Over the past 4 years HLA-DR serotyping has been adopted by nearly all HLA typing laboratories which support transplantation. Data suggest that matching is very important for successful long-term engraftment of related and cadaveric donor kidneys. DR typing, however, identifies only a limited number of the total HLA class II gene products from one individual; furthermore, the clinical role of the more recently identified class II antigens such as DP has not been addressed.

Two major reasons that cellular tests have not been used to define specificity are the scarcity of typing reagents and the difficulty of performing large-scale MLCs. For these reasons, the use of homozygous typing cells in primary MLC for routine typing is very unlikely. However, PLs can be generated and produced in quantity at a cost similar to that for procurement of HLA antisera. When high-quality reagents are used, PLT is at least as reliable as serotyping for HLA-D region antigens, as demonstrated in the Ninth International Histocompatibility Workshop (8). In this workshop, PLs were used to define HLA-DP specificities in 19 laboratories. In addition to producing large numbers of bulk PLs, it is also possible to produce on a large scale cloned cellular reagents which define HLA-D region molecules. These cloned reagents are extremely specific but are more difficult and costly to produce. Furthermore, great care must be taken in the selection of cloned reagents as some of these cells may recognize common epitopes on several different allospecific molecules, much the way that some monoclonal antibodies recognize common epitopes for several molecules. The power of cloned T cells is the ability to create reagents which define new epitopes and new cell surface structures. Careful screening of these cloned T cells against stimulator cells from donors with a wide range of HLA specificities can be used to select clones likely to identify unique determinants on single molecules. Thus, cloning and careful selection can eliminate the problem of defining multiple cell surface structures inherent in uncloned reagents such as bulk PLs and alloantisera.

It is now possible to use these PL methods in the clinical transplant setting. Once the reagents are provided, the test is reliable and relatively rapid (1 to 3 days). As there is no technical requirement of PLT that is not also a requirement of MLC (with the possible exception of the need for cryopreservation in PLT), any laboratory currently performing MLCs is capable of performing PLT.

Typing for DP antigens with high-quality PL reagents produces extraordinary specificity and reproducibility compared with primary MLC. The difference between "positive" and "negative" reactions is usually 10-fold or greater, making it possible to define the specificity of a test cell by quickly scanning the data visually. There are exceptions to this high-discrimination rule. In any large experiment (30 to 90 cells tested) a few cells will perform relatively poorly and require either datum normalization based on controls within the experiments to compensate for low responses of these poor cells or repeat testing. The likelihood of misclassification is further reduced by using two test reagents for each specificity. Using one test reagent for a specificity would result in an error rate for classification of approximately 10%, while using two reagents reduces this misclassification rate to approximately 1%. The importance of two reagents per specificity is further dramatized by the occasional occurrence of reactions in which one reagent which defines a DP specificity shows a strong positive response while the second reagent is clearly negative. This problem occurs most commonly in a discrepancy between the reagents originally described by Shaw et al. (6) as SB2A versus SB2B (DPw2) and SB5A versus SB5B (DPw5). In 10 to 15% of typings the 2B reagent produces a positive response when the 2A reagent is negative. In some cases, the discrepant cell is positive for both DPw6 reagents and is thus DPw6 positive and DPw2 negative. These reactions may be due to multiple epitopes on one molecule or to two distinct cell surface molecules. The likelihood of the presence of two molecules is increased by the fact that there are two alpha and two beta genes in the DP region as detected by recombinant DNA technology. The "problem" of the discrepancy between the two currently available DP2 reagents can be resolved by generating a new DPw2 bulk reagent or T-cell clone so that the second DPw2 reagent gives reactions identical to those of the SB2A reagent. Of equal importance is that the cause of the discrepancies must be resolved.

Several alternatives to PL generation are being developed concurrently. First, alloantisera which produce similar reaction patterns are being identified. Antisera producing reaction patterns closely correlated with DP typing by PLT have been described for the specificities DPw1, DPw3, and DPw5. Standard complement-mediated cytotoxicity has been used. This technique has several advantages over PLT. The complement-mediated test is performed in a large number of clinical laboratories, and the reagents, once developed, are much simpler to handle and distribute than are viable cryopreserved cells. However, it will require 3 to 5 years to acquire the necessary reagents. Second, it may be possible to develop monoclonal antibodies which define the same determinants. One allospecific monoclonal antibody, ILR-1, defines cells which express DPw2, DPw3, a subset of DPw4, and DR5. Groups of two to three monoclonal antibodies may better define the allospecificities of interest.

Two new approaches are evolving which may accelerate the development of allospecific monoclonal antibodies. First, the frequency of allospecific reagents against human determinants is likely to be much higher with human anti-human monoclonal antibodies than with mouse anti-human ones. Mice generally produce relatively broadly reactive antibodies reflecting the species differences. Second, as the amino acid sequence of human class II molecules is being defined, mice are being immunized with small peptides containing the amino acids of the allospecific portion of the molecule. This should reduce the problem of the mice producing primarily antispecies antibodies.

Another general approach uses recombinant DNA technology. It has been possible to identify a large number of class II genes in the HLA-D region of human chromosome 6 and to identify the coding sequence of some of these genes. Specific DNA probes which bind to portions of these HLA-D coding regions have been developed. The use of specific DNA probes along with restriction enzyme digests of DNA, followed by electrophoresis, provides an additional method of determining allospecificity. Since these recombinant DNA methods are very sensitive and reliable, they may become the method of choice for determining specificity. At present the recombinant methods require more time to complete than serotyping does but less time than PLT does. These DNA techniques may be modified to require far less time. However, 2 to 10 years may be required to produce optimal DNA probes and methods practical for the clinical laboratory. One word of caution is that this approach will retain many of the pitfalls of current serologic and cellular typing, such as cross-reactivity and molecular subtypes and supertypes.

Currently, therefore, the most rapid method of identifying new class II HLA determinants is PLT with T-cell cloning. In addition to the speed of development, the test is relatively rapid and reliable once standard reagents are produced. The primary drawback is the difficulty in handling and distributing cryopreserved viable cells. The increased availability of allospecific primed typing cells would permit the routine use of PLT for defining specificity for renal and bone marrow transplantation.

DATUM REDUCTION AND INTERPRETATION

To classify PLT responses objectively as positive or negative, the procedure of Shaw et al. (5) offers a good combination of ease of application and satisfactory results. They applied a clustering technique, developed by A. W. F. Edwards and L. L. Cavalli-Sforza, to divide responses of each PL reagent into a high and low cluster, using both untransformed data (arithmetic clustering) and log-transformed data (geometric clustering). The cutoff point between clusters may be either the same in both analyses or higher in the arithmetic clustering. Stimulators positive (i.e., in the high cluster) in both analyses are "positive," those positive by geometric clustering only are "ambiguous," and all others are "negative." A BASIC program to perform the cluster analysis is available from one of us (M.J.S.). Two reagents are used to define each antigen. To be labeled positive for the antigen, a stimulator must be definitely positive with one reagent and positive or ambiguous with the other; all other stimulators are considered negative for the antigen.

Although the technique of cluster analysis provides a useful method of scoring positive and negative reactions for most cells being tested, it can produce misleading results for a few cells (usually relatively poor stimulator cells). This can occur if the test cell has low viability or has few B cells or macrophages or both. Several methods can be used to identify these low stimulators. First, a nonirradiated aliquot of each stimulating cell can be stimulated by pokeweed mitogen. As pokeweed mitogen is a good B-cell mitogen, although it also stimulates other cell subsets, the magnitude of this response is related to the capacity of the cell population to stimulate a PL. Second, nonspecific PLs can be generated by stimulating peripheral blood leukocytes with a mitogen such as phytohemagglutinin (PHA) instead of allogeneic cells. These PHA-primed cells are restimulated by any cell which is not HLA-D identical to the primed cell.

The PHA-primed cells or pokeweed mitogen can be incorporated into the experimental design, and the results can be used to normalize the experimental counts per minute. The normalized values more accurately reflect the presence of the specificities being tested. Such values are analyzed by a clustering technique such as that described above or the Smirnov-Kolmagorov technique.

REAGENTS

PBS. Make 0.01 M solutions of monobasic (NaH_2PO_4) and dibasic (Na_2HPO_4) sodium phosphate salts in saline (0.85% NaCl) in double-glass-distilled water (solutions A and B, respectively). Mix 230 ml of solution A and 770 ml of solution B, check the pH, and adjust it to 7.3 if necessary. Filter sterilize and store the mixture at room temperature, or refrigerate it. Phosphate-buffered saline (PBS) can also be made as a 10× solution, which must be stored at room temperature. The pH should be adjusted after dilution to 1×.

Pooled human serum (PHS). Separate serum pools are prepared for use in cultures and for freezing and washing cells. Serum is obtained from clotted blood of approximately 20 untransfused male donors. One can substitute plasma with heparin (10 U/ml) but not with acid-citrate-glucose or similar anticoagulants. Sera are centrifuged at high speed (at least 3,000 rpm [2,500 × g] in a typical floor-model centrifuge), filtered (0.45-μm pore size), and frozen, keeping individual sera separate and reserving 1 ml of each for testing. Individual serum samples are tested in MLC, and those giving acceptable results (good cell proliferation in mixed cultures and low background proliferation in autologous cultures) are pooled for use in culture. Sera giving weak MLC or high background are pooled separately for use in wash and freezing media (see below).

Wash medium. Wash medium is PBS supplemented with 5% PHS (using PHS from the freezing-washing pool). Some laboratories prefer using 10% fetal calf serum with 10 U of heparin per ml to reduce problems with cell clumping.

Freezing medium. Freezing medium is 70% PBS, 20% PHS, and 10% dimethyl sulfoxide (DMSO). DMSO is added last, while swirling the 4°C PBS-PHS solution to avoid a high local DMSO concentration, and the solution is kept on ice until used. Tissue culture medium with 10 to 20% PHS can be used in place of PBS. Some laboratories use 15 to 20% DMSO followed by the addition of this solution to an equal volume of cells in tissue culture medium with 10% PHS. The final concentration of DMSO after adding the freezing medium to the cells should be 7.5 to 10%. If tissue culture medium is used in place of PBS, heparin (10 U/ml) should be added.

RPMI 1640. RPMI 1640 without HEPES (*N*-2-hydroxyethylpiperazine-*N'*-2-ethanesulfonic acid) buffer, bought as a liquid or powder, is used for priming cultures and maintaining clones (HEPES-buffered medium can be used, but it is more expensive). RPMI 1640 with 25 mM HEPES is used for PLT test cultures.

Medium for priming cultures. Medium for priming cultures is RPMI 1640, supplemented with 10% PHS.

Medium for PLT test cultures. Medium for PLT test cultures is HEPES-buffered RPMI 1640, supplemented with 5 to 10% PHS. Antibiotics such as penicillin (50 U/ml) plus streptomycin (50 μg/ml) or gentamicin (50 μg/ml) may be used if desired.

Clone medium. Clone medium includes the following: 10% PHS, 0.1% ITS (insulin, transfusion, selenium) Premix (Collaborative Research, Inc., Waltham, Mass.) (optional), IL-2-containing conditioned medium (CM; described below) at a concentration determined by testing (usually 10 to 40%), and RPMI 1640 to volume.

IL-2-containing CM. PBMC are gamma irradiated (1,000 rads from a cesium-137 irradiator) and adjusted to 10^6/ml in RPMI 1640 with 1% PHS and 1% (vol/vol) PHA-M or 0.08% PHA-P solution (Difco Laboratories, Detroit, Mich.). Cells are stimulated with the PHA at 37°C for 48 h, supernatants are harvested, and cells are removed by centrifugation and filtration. Some laboratories include Daudi lymphoblastoid cell lines (LCL; 5×10^5 cells per ml) or a costimulant. CM is tested in triplicate, in doubling dilutions from 80 to 0.625%, for maintenance of proliferation of at least one IL-2-dependent human T-cell clone or T-cell line. Test clones are plated at 10^4 per well in 96-well, flat-bottom culture plates in 0.2 ml of clone medium containing the various dilutions of CM. Thymidine incorporation is assessed by liquid scintillation counting as for PLT (described later). The CM concentration used for subsequent cultures is twice that needed to give maximal stimulation of the test clone(s).

All media can be filter sterilized (0.2-μm pore size), aliquoted into 100-ml bottles immediately after preparation, and stored at 4 or −20°C. After 1 month or more at 4°C, fresh L-glutamine (200 mM stock, stored frozen) is added (1%, vol/vol). If desired, the pH can be adjusted by sterile bubbling of CO_2 into the medium. Except as noted above, the various culture media and components are available from GIBCO Laboratories, Grand Island, N.Y., and Flow Laboratories, Inc., McLean, Va., as well as from other sources.

Ficoll-Hypaque solution. In a 1-liter graduated cylinder, dissolve 51.2 g of Ficoll 400 (Sigma Chemical Co., St. Louis, Mo.) in approximately 800 ml of double-glass-distilled H_2O, and then add 160 ml of 50% Hypaque (Winthrop Laboratories, Div. Sterling Drug, Inc., New York, N.Y.). While stirring, add double-glass-distilled H_2O to adjust the specific gravity to 1.077 (indicated by a hydrometer).

Trypan blue solution. Trypan blue solution is 0.25% (wt/vol) trypan blue in PBS, filter sterilized and stored at room temperature.

Scintillation cocktail. Scintillation cocktail is PPO (2,5-diphenyloxazole; 6.0 g/liter or 22.7 g/gal) and POPOP [1,4-bis(5-phenyloxazolyl)benzene; 10.0 mg/liter or 37.9 mg/gal] in toluene or pseudocoumene. Similar cocktails are available commercially.

LABORATORY PROCEDURES

Preparation of bulk PLs.

Cryopreserved PBMC from the chosen responder and stimulator are thawed by shaking frozen vials manually in a 37°C water bath until only a small ball of ice remains in each vial; vials are removed from the bath, shaken a few more seconds, and placed on ice. Contents of vials are immediately transferred to sterile centrifuge tubes, slowly diluted 10-fold with ice-cold wash medium (described earlier), centrifuged gently (120 $\times$ g, 5 min), and suspended in 1 to 2 ml of priming medium (described above). Some laboratories add 10 U of heparin to the suspension medium to reduce clumping of cells. Cells are then kept at room temperature until ready for culture.

Cell counts and viability are determined by counting on a hemacytometer after diluting to a convenient concentration for visual counting with trypan blue solution. Cells with less than about 80% viability dye exclusion probably should not be used. Dye exclusion tends to grossly overestimate functional viability. Cells are diluted to 2 $\times$ 10^6/ml with priming medium, and cells to be used as stimulators are gamma irradiated (2,000 rads). Responding and stimulating cells (5 ml of each) are placed in a 25-cm^2 tissue culture flask (e.g., Corning no. 25100, Falcon no. 30130, or Costar no. 3050). Flasks are incubated upright in a 37°C, humidified, 5% CO_2 incubator with the cap slightly loose (so that it can be wiggled up and down slightly) for 10 days. Usually no medium is added or changed during this time. However, an additional 5 to 10 ml of medium with 10% PHS may be added. If the culture becomes acidic, tissue culture medium may be exchanged with fresh medium, and if necessary the growing cells may be split into several flasks. The cells are now primed; i.e., a selection has been achieved such that, among the T cells of responder R, those with receptors for foreign antigens of stimulator S have proliferated, while those with receptors for other antigens have not or have even died. The primed cells can now be used as a reagent to type other individuals for the antigen(s) that R recognized on S; they can either be used immediately for PLT or be frozen for later use.

Significant variations on the priming protocol

1. If freshly isolated (i.e., never frozen) PBMC from the two donors are available, results will be better, but the culture volume should be increased to 20 ml per flask as the greater cell growth may deplete nutrients.

2. It is often necessary to prime cells twice when attempting to detect "weak" antigenic differences. When cells used in priming are DR matched, for example, one can prime first for 10 days and then for 6 days. For the second culture, 10-day-primed cells are centrifuged (120 $\times$ g, 5 min), counted, and suspended at 10^6/ml. The number of responding cells (already primed once) is 5×10^6, half the number used for the first culture, while the number of stimulating cells, 1 $\times$ 10^7, is the same as before. Some laboratories use 5 $\times$ 10^7 stimulating cells at this point.

3. If desired, cell numbers and culture volumes can be reduced fivefold, with a corresponding reduction in the number of primed cells, by using culture plates with 24 2-ml wells in place of the flasks described above. Such plates are made by Costar and Linbro, as well as by others.

Preparation of cloned PLs

Cells are primed in bulk as described above but are removed from culture after 6 days for cloning. Activated (blast) cells can be further enriched by density- or size-dependent separation, since they are larger and less dense than nonactivated lymphocytes. This is not necessary, however, if one uses an IL-2 preparation that is nonstimulatory for unactivated cells for the cloning procedure. If separation procedures are used, place the cells back in culture overnight, in clone medium (described above), before cloning. For some specificities it may be necessary to culture for up to 10 days or perform a secondary stimulation before cloning. This is particularly true with weak antigens or when there is a low frequency of potential responding clones in peripheral blood.

Special precautions during cloning include careful maintenance of the pH of cloning and dilution media, minimizing evaporation from the 10-μl cultures, and eliminating cell clumps. To maintain pH, media can be made slightly less than pH 7.3 (judged by color) with sterile CO_2, and tubes are left capped as much as possible. To minimize evaporation, PBS is used to cover the inside bottom of the Terasaki trays, excluding the wells themselves, before cloning begins (trays can be flooded, and PBS can be aspirated from the wells). Alternatively, trays are placed in a plastic container with moist paper towels in the bottom. The container is left open at one corner to allow the 5% CO_2 to enter. Cell clumps can be eliminated by pipetting the cell suspension, in 2 ml, at least 50 times with a Pasteur pipette immediately before dilution.

Gamma-irradiated (4,000 rads) lymphocytes from the stimulator (10^6/ml in clone medium) are used as a source of antigen and as feeder cells. Cells to be cloned are taken directly from culture, counted, pipetted as described above, and diluted (in two to three steps) to 30 cells per ml, the first dilution(s) being done with RPMI 1640 with at least 5% PHS and the final dilution being in the feeder cell suspension just described. The final cell suspension is plated into Terasaki trays at 10 to 20 μl per well. Final (average) cell numbers per well are 0.3 cell to be cloned and 10^4 feeder cells. The large excess of feeder to stimulator cells is the most important requirement at this stage.

On days 6 to 8 after cloning, clones at least two-thirds confluent are transferred to 0.2-ml, flat-bottom wells. On day 9, any remaining clones at least one-fourth confluent are transferred. When confluent in 0.2-ml wells, clones are transferred to 2-ml wells. All clone culture is in clone medium. Clones receive irradiated (4,000 rads) stimulator PBMC (10^6/ml) upon transfer to 0.2-ml wells and every 7 to 10 days thereafter. Upon reaching 4×10^6 cells (approximately when confluent in two 2-ml wells), clones are frozen in five vials each. Clones failing to reach this number within about 4 weeks of cloning are generally of little use and are discarded. If clones are to be frozen within

5 days after receiving feeder cells, one-fifth of the cells should be left in culture until 6 days post-feeder cells and frozen in a single vial. This last vial should be used for preliminary PLT testing as described below.

One aliquot of each clone is thawed and tested in PLT as described later for response to cells from the original responder R and stimulator S. A clone is potentially useful in PLT if the response to S (in counts per minute) is at least 10 times that to R.

Clones sufficiently reactive in PLT are expanded in culture to produce additional frozen vials; other clones are discarded. Clones are expanded in 2-ml wells or upright flasks as for bulk priming cultures, with 1×10^5 clone cells and 5×10^5 to 1×10^6 feeder cells per ml. When cells of the original stimulator are not available for use as feeders, one can substitute PBMC of any person whose cells have been found to be stimulatory for the clone in question.

Clones are grown for one or two 7- to 10-day cycles, splitting cultures when the cell density is approximately 2×10^6/ml, until one can freeze at least 10 vials of 2×10^6 cells each. Clones yielding fewer than 2×10^7 cells after two cycles are usually discarded. Cells from this second freeze are tested in PLT to determine whether their specificity makes them useful. If so, other vials of the second freeze can be thawed and clones can be expanded to obtain a working stock for large-scale testing. Clones can thus be expanded in stages as needed, so that the number of vials on hand at any time is not excessive. The extent to which clones can be expanded is controversial; some believe that there is a limit to the number of divisions a cell can undergo. There are three major reasons for the loss of clones in addition to the possibility of limited innate growth potential: (i) contamination, particularly with mycoplasma; (ii) IL-2 deficiency; and (iii) nutrient deficiency during rapid growth.

A modest variation from optimal culture conditions for a few hours can cause the rapid loss of the growing cells. At times the clones may become unreactive to the stimulation cells but continue to grow in IL-2. Specificity from one expansion may be lost, but a second cryopreserved aliquot may be expanded successfully. It is possible to obtain more than 10^{10} cloned cells if meticulous care is taken with the growth process.

Freezing of PLs

Primed cells are frozen by the same methods used for fresh cells. As for any cells to be frozen, it is very important to keep cells ice cold at all times when they are in the freezing solution. Cells are centrifuged and suspended in freezing solution. Alternatively, the cells are suspended at twice the final concentration in tissue culture medium with 10% PHS and heparin (10 U/ml), and an equal volume of freezing medium with twice the final concentration of DMSO is added slowly. Cells are aliquoted in desired amounts (5×10^5 to 1×10^8 per vial) in polypropylene or glass freezing vials (e.g., Nunc no. 1076, available from GIBCO), stored at $-80°C$ in a thin cardboard box or open container for 2 h or overnight or in a controlled-rate freezer ($-1°C$/min to $-80°C$), and transferred to liquid nitrogen-cooled storage.

PLT test procedure

PLT can be performed in round-bottom, 96-well microtiter trays (e.g., Linbro Titertek no. 76-014-05) in 0.15-ml cultures with 5×10^3 to 2×10^4 PLs per well. Stimulating cells can be nonirradiated PBMC (5×10^4 cells) or heavily gamma-irradiated LCL (12,000 rads, 5×10^3 cells per well). Triplicate cultures are incubated for 40 or 64 h or both with a [^{3}H]thymidine pulse (5 Ci/mmol, 1 µCi per culture) for the last 16 h. Cultures are stopped by cooling at 4°C (15 min to 1 week), and samples are harvested onto glass fiber filters for liquid scintillation counting.

1. Stimulator cells are thawed in groups that can be handled quickly. It is optimal to handle the cells of only one person at a time. Each group of vials should be thawed and slowly diluted in 10-fold medium with 10% PHS and heparin to avoid hypotonic shock (10% DMSO is hypertonic), centrifuged, and suspended in 1 ml of the HEPES-containing medium (described earlier) before the next group is thawed. Once suspended in culture medium, cells can be left at room temperature until put into culture. (If LCL are used as stimulators, they should be thawed and grown in bulk culture for at least 2 to 3 days before irradiating [12,000 rads] for PLT.) For large experiments (30 to 90 stimulators cells), the stimulator cells can be plated 12 to 24 h in advance of the PLs.

2. When all stimulators are in culture medium, determine viable cell counts and dilute each to 5×10^5 (PBMC) or 5×10^4 (LCL) per ml in the needed volume.

3. Using a Hamilton syringe (1002N) and repeating dispenser (PB600-1), dispense stimulators in triplicate (100 µl per well) in the microtiter trays. If possible, cells should be arranged so that each PL is contained within a single plate; i.e., stimulators, not PLs, should be split among several culture plates. Place microtiter trays, with stimulating cells, in the incubator.

4. Thaw bulk or cloned PLs as described for stimulating cells, and determine viable cell counts. (Once the technician is experienced, morphology will be better than dye exclusion as an indicator of viability, since many cells in poor condition do exclude dye. Only healthy looking cells are counted.)

5. Dilute PLs to the desired number of cells per milliliter (20 times the number needed per well). (Before doing an important test, one should test an aliquot of each PL at concentrations from 5×10^3 to 2×10^4 per well to determine the cell number needed for adequate discrimination between positive and negative stimulators.)

6. Dispense PLs into culture trays (50 µl per well). Wrap trays, individually or in groups, in Saran Wrap or other plastic wrap to minimize evaporation, and make a small hole in each wrapping.

7. Incubate for 24 h (approximately). Some laboratories incubate for 48 or 72 h.

8. Add 50 µl of [^{3}H]thymidine solution (5 Ci/mmol, diluted to 20 µCi/ml in RPMI 1640) to each well, and incubate overnight.

9. Stop cultures by cooling at 4°C for at least 15 min. They can be left for 1 week at this point if necessary.

10. Harvest cells onto glass fiber filter paper (Whatman no. 1827-866) with a multiple-sample harvester (available from Cambridge Technology, MA Bioproducts, Otto Hiller, and Skatron, as well as from others), washing wells 20 times with distilled water. Leaving the vacuum on, open the harvester and squirt water liberally over the entire filter strip to wash off any tritium label that may have leaked out around the O-rings of the harvester.

11. Let the filter strips dry thoroughly. If desired, drying can be hastened by heating in an oven or with heat lamps.

12. Place filter spots into numbered shell vials (1 dram, 15 by 45 mm), and add 0.5 ml of scintillation cocktail to each.

13. Verify that each filter spot is immersed in scintillation cocktail, and determine the counts per minute with a liquid scintillation counter.

14. Analyze the data as described above (Datum Reduction and Interpretation).

LITERATURE CITED

1. **Eckels, D. D., and R. J. Hartzman.** 1982. Characterization of human T-lymphocyte clones (TLC's) specific for HLA-region gene products. Immunogenetics **16**:117–133.

2. **Hartzman, R. J., F. Pappas, P. J. Romano, A. H. Johnson, and D. B. Amos.** 1978. Dissociation of HLA-D and HLA-DR using primed LD typing. Transplant. Proc. **10**:809–812.

3. **Mawas, C., D. Charmot, and M. Sasportes.** 1975. Secondary response of in vitro primed human lymphocytes to allogeneic cells. I. Role of HLA-antigens and mixed lymphocyte reactions stimulating determinants in secondary in vitro proliferative response. Immunogenetics **2**:449–463.

4. **Shaw, S., R. DeMars, S. F. Schlossman, P. L. Smith, L. A. Lampson, and L. A. Nadler.** 1982. Serologic identification of the human secondary B cell antigens: correlation between function, genetics and structure. J. Exp. Med. **156**:731–743.

5. **Shaw, S., R. Duquesnoy, and P. L. Smith.** 1981. Population studies of the HLA-linked SB antigens. Immunogenetics **14**:153–162.

6. **Shaw, S., A. H. Johnson, and G. M. Shearer.** 1980. Evidence for a new segregant series of B cell antigens that are encoded in the HLA-D region and that stimulate secondary allogeneic proliferative and cytotoxic responses. J. Exp. Med. **152**:565–580.

7. **Sheehy, M., P. Sondel, M. Bach, R. Wank, and F. Bach.** 1975. HLA typing: a rapid assay using primed lymphocytes. Science **188**:1308–1310.

8. **Wank, R., and D. J. Schendel.** 1985. Joint report: genetic analysis of HLA-D region products defined by primed lymphocyte typing, p. 289–300. In E. D. Albert and W. Mayr (ed.), Histocompatibility testing (1984). Munshgaard, Copenhagen.

9. **Wank, R., D. J. Schendel, J. A. Hansen, and B. Dupont.** 1978. The lymphocyte restimulation system: evaluation by intra-HLA-D groups priming. Immunogenetics **6**:107–115.

Chapter 133

Use of the Southern Blotting Procedure for the Detection of Restriction Fragment Length Polymorphisms

P. ANDREW BIRO AND DAVID GLASS

The detection of restriction fragment length polymorphisms (2) in eucaryotic DNAs by the Southern blotting procedure (9) is becoming an established technique that holds great promise in clinical research. It can be used for the prenatal diagnosis of inherited diseases, even those for which no other genetic markers are available. It is already being used in the study of hemoglobinopathies and may soon be available for the diagnosis of such diseases as Huntington's chorea (6). In the immune system it will be possible to tissue type for all classes of major histocompatibility gene products by this method, and the recent isolation of genes coding for components of the T-cell receptor may reveal further possible applications, for example in the study of immune deficiency syndromes.

The major advance that this technique represents results from the discovery of enzymes capable of recognizing and cleaving DNA molecules at short, defined sequences. These enzymes, known collectively as restriction enzymes, can be isolated from a great variety of microbial organisms and are commercially available from several suppliers.

A restriction fragment length polymorphism can be detected as a result of a change (usually a point mutation) in the primary sequence of the DNA such that a particular restriction enzyme recognition site is either created or deleted. Cleavage of total DNA by that enzyme will produce approximately 10^6 restriction fragments, including one or more polymorphic variants with altered electrophoretic mobilities which can be resolved on agarose gels. After electrophoresis the DNA is transferred to a solid support medium such as nitrocellulose and then probed by hybridization to a radioactively labeled RNA or DNA which is complementary to at least a part of one or more of the fragments. Such a probe is frequently either a cDNA clone of the mRNA from a particular gene or a relatively short section of cloned, single-copy genomic DNA. For the diagnosis of diseases which have no known genetic markers, such as Huntington's chorea, randomly isolated, polymorphic DNA probes, which can be mapped to their respective chromosomes by standard techniques, are being used in an attempt to demonstrate a genetic association between the disease and the DNA polymorphism.

It is important to remember that less than half of the DNA of any restriction fragment encompassing a gene is likely to code for a translated protein product. Most of the DNA is composed of flanking or intervening sequences or codes for the 3′ or 5′ untranslated regions of the mRNA. Consequently, a restriction fragment length polymorphism will not usually be associated with an equivalent protein polymorphism, nor is it likely to be the cause of the disease under study. It is simply a linked, although possibly very closely linked, genetic marker and, except in very rare instances, will not correlate absolutely either with the diseased state or with any other genetic marker. However, these limitations do not affect the validity or the potential usefulness of the technique which can be used to generate markers, at will, from any point in the genome.

PRINCIPLES OF THE METHOD

High-molecular-weight DNA is prepared from suitable tissue (most often whole blood), and a small amount, 5 to 20 μg, is cleaved by an appropriate restriction endonuclease. After the completeness of the digestion is verified, the individual restriction fragments are resolved on the basis of their lengths by electrophoresis through agarose, forming a relatively uniform smear of DNA. This is unlike the cleavage of a simple DNA such as a viral DNA which produces well-resolved, clearly distinguishable bands. However, the tandemly repeated sequences which are present in eucaryotic DNAs and have uniformly spaced cleavage sites do create a characteristic pattern of a few rather diffuse bands superimposed upon the DNA smear.

The gel can be stained with ethidium bromide to allow the DNA to be visualized under UV light and photographed. The DNA is then transferred to a suitable membrane support medium, either electrophoretically with a custom-designed apparatus or by the original capillary-action method of Southern (9, 10). In this procedure the DNA is first denatured by soaking the gel in dilute sodium hydroxide and then neutralized in a sodium acetate or Tris hydrochloride buffer. After the excess solution is rinsed off, the gel is placed on Whatman paper which is in contact with a large reservoir of 20× SSC (1× SSC is 0.15 M NaCl plus 0.015 M sodium citrate). A sheet of support medium such a nitrocellulose is placed over the surface of the gel and overlaid with paper towels or sponges. The DNA transfers to the nitrocellulose by capillary action over a period of several hours, after which the support medium is removed, rinsed in 2× SSC, dried, and baked.

The DNA on the membrane can now be hybridized to radioactively labeled probe in a small volume of solution under standard conditions. After a careful washing to remove the unhybridized probe, the membrane is subjected to autoradiography to detect the fragments complementary to the probe.

METHODS

Many of the techniques employed in Southern blotting are standard procedures in nucleic acid biochemistry, and more detailed descriptions can be found in handbooks such as *Molecular Cloning: A Laboratory Manual* (7) or selected volumes in the *Methods in Enzymology* series.

Preparation of DNA samples

DNA can be extracted from a wide variety of fresh and frozen tissues. Liver, spleen, and placenta are good sources of high-molecular-weight DNA from whole organs, and blood or, less commonly, sperm are the best sources of DNA from living donors. Lymphocytes from particularly valued donors can be transformed, for example by Epstein-Barr virus, to establish permanent cell lines which can provide an infinite amount of DNA.

The method of Blin and Stafford (1) gives the greatest yield and highest-molecular-weight DNA. Briefly, the tissue is cut into small pieces, frozen in liquid nitrogen, and pulverized in a Waring blender at the temperature of the liquid nitrogen. The still-frozen, powdered material is then sprinkled over the lysing buffer (see below, Reagents) and incubated at 37°C. Care must be taken in handling the liquid nitrogen, especially while using the blender. We have always pulverized the tissue in a metal container covered with cloth towels. It is not normally necessary to perform this step when extracting DNA from readily lyseable material such as cultured cells, sperm, or blood. However, for solid tissues such as liver or spleen it is the method of choice.

Whole blood is a common starting point, and DNA can be extracted from cells by one of several methods, including a buffy-coat preparation collected by sedimentation for 1 h through 6% dextran at 37°C (3). Alternatives to this method include the preparation of a pellet of nuclei by centrifugation of cells through a Triton X-100 sucrose density gradient. By either of these methods, 30 ml of whole blood should yield enough DNA for over 20 digests.

The DNA is incubated in the lysis buffer at 37°C or above (up to 55°C) for several hours until no further loss of turbidity is observed. The solution should be viscous and clear at this time. Denatured proteins are removed by extracting the DNA with an equal volume of phenol which has been equilibrated with lysis buffer lacking the proteinase K and sodium dodecyl sulfate (SDS). The extractions are carried out gently so as not to shear the DNA. The phases are separated by medium-speed centrifugation, e.g., in a Sorvall RC-5 apparatus. The aqueous phase containing the DNA is usually the upper layer, but in some circumstances, for example in high-salt solutions, a phase inversion may occur and the phenol phase becomes the upper layer. It is best not to discard either phase until its composition has been verified. If the DNA is very concentrated it may be hard to remove the aqueous layer without carrying over the interphase and some of the phenol. The use of a wide-mouthed pipette (for example a 10-ml plastic pipette with the tip cut off) is recommended. Alternatively, some of the aqueous layer can be left behind and then re-extracted with buffer to recover the rest of the DNA.

At the end of two or three cycles of phenol extraction, no interphase should remain and the solution should be clear. Residual phenol is removed from the aqueous layer by extraction with chloroform (again, the upper phase is the aqueous one). A phenol-chloroform-isoamyl alcohol mixture (24:24:1) may be used instead for the extractions.

Glass containers are recommended since many plastics are sensitive to organic reagents such as phenol and chloroform.

Residual SDS and the chloroform or phenol are removed either by dialysis or by ethanol precipitation. Dialysis is carried out first against a high-salt buffer (1 M NaCl in TE buffer) at room temperature to accelerate the removal of the phenol and SDS and subsequently against a low-salt buffer (TE) in the cold. Some expansion in volume occurs during this process, and the dialysis bag needs to be sufficiently large to accommodate the increase without bursting. Dialysis is continued until an organic smell can no longer be detected from the bag.

Alternatively, the DNA can be concentrated by ethanol precipitation. Sodium acetate (3 M, pH 7.0 to 8.0) is added to the DNA solution to a final concentration of 0.3 M, followed by 2 volumes of 95% ethanol. The solution is inverted until it is fully homogeneous. A stringy precipitate should form rapidly, although to ensure maximum recovery of DNA from dilute solutions, the precipitate should be cooled at 4°C for several hours, at −20°C for 2 h, or at −70°C for 15 min. The solution can be stored at this stage in the cold for long periods of time. Although the precipitate can often be sedimented by medium-speed centrifugation, occasionally it floats on the surface and can either be decanted into a microcentrifuge tube or collected by high-speed ultracentrifugation. The pellet is carefully rinsed with 70% ethanol, dried, and resuspended in sufficient TE buffer to give an approximate DNA concentration of 0.5 mg/ml. Resuspension is slow and may take many hours even at room temperature; occasional stirring accelerates the process.

Typical yields are about 1 mg of DNA per g of tissue. Although DNA prepared by this method is sufficiently clean to be digested by restriction enzymes, it still contains considerable quantities of RNA which prevent its quantitation by spectrophotometry. The RNA can be hydrolyzed by incubation with heat-treated RNase A. A 1-mg/ml solution of RNase A is placed in a boiling water bath for about 2 min to destroy DNases and then slowly cooled to room temperature to allow the RNase to renature. One microgram of RNase is sufficient to treat 20 μg of DNA. The RNase can be removed by treatment with proteinase K followed by phenol extraction, and the DNA can be freed from small oligoribonucleotides by dialysis. However, it is not normally necessary to inactivate the RNase, which does not interfere with the subsequent steps. The DNA concentration can now be measured by spectrophotometry: a DNA solution of 50 μg/ml has an optical denisty (OD) of 1.0 at 260 nm. For optimal results the DNA concentration should be adjusted to give OD readings between 0.2 and 1.0. The purity of the DNA can also be assessed at this time; an OD_{260}/OD_{280} ratio of 1.8 or higher indicates the DNA is free of protein.

When processing multiple samples, we normally omit the RNase treatment and estimate DNA concentrations by analzying small DNA samples, usually between 0.01 and 0.001 μg, on agarose and comparing their ethidium bromide-induced UV-fluorescence intensities with that of a previously calibrated standard DNA sample. This method, although crude, is sufficient for most purposes.

Restriction endonuclease digestion

Before the addition of restriction enzymes, each DNA sample should be tested to ensure that it is free of trace quantities of endogenous nucleases which have survived the preparation process. A few micrograms of each DNA are incubated in restriction enzyme buffer for several hours at 37°C before analysis on agarose. The DNA should have survived the treatment intact and should appear as a broad band near the origin of the gel; no forward migration of the DNA should be observed. Occasionally, a sample will contain endonucleolytic activity which will be stimulated by the magnesium in the restriction enzyme buffer and will degrade the DNA. The endonuclease can be inactivated by an additional cycle of treatment with proteinase K and phenol extraction.

Purified DNA solutions can usually be kept at 4°C for many weeks. However, for long-term storage the DNA should be maintained either at −20°C or below or as a precipitate in 70% ethanol.

Eucaryotic DNAs prepared by this method are sensitive to cleavage by nearly all restriction enzymes. The major exceptions are those enzymes which contain CpG dinucleotides as part of their recognition sequence. In eucaryotes, CpG palindromic doublets are extensively, but variably, methylated on one or both DNA strands. Methylation protects those sites from cleavage by most (but not all) restriction enzymes. There are some enzymes which generally recognize 4-base-pair (bp) sequences, such as *Taq*I (TCGA), which can cleave methylated DNA.

Different enzymes which share common recognition sequences are known as isoschizomers. Some enzymes are inhibited by methylation while their isoschizomers are not, and such enzyme pairs have been used to study the patterns of methylation in different tissues and the changes in methylation during periods of gene activity. However, a detailed description of the use of these enzymes is outside the scope of this chapter.

Many restriction enzymes are commercially available and nearly all of them are type II, in that they have defined recognition sequences and precise cleavage sites. Many recognition sequences are palindromes, and their enzymes cleave symmetrically about their axes of symmetry. There are exceptions; for example, *Mbo*II, which recognizes the sequence GAAGA and cleaves 8 bases downstream on the 5′→3′ strand and 7 bases downstream on the 3′→5′ strand. In such cases, the orientation of the sequence in the DNA will affect the position of cleavage. Type I enzymes, on the other hand, have defined recognition sequences but cleave at variable distances from them. (For a more detailed description of restriction enzymes and their properties, see one of the listings published periodically in *Nucleic Acids Research*.) Generally speaking, enzymes which recognize 6-bp sequences and cleave DNA approximately every 4,000 bp are more useful for these studies than those which cleave more frequently to produce shorter fragments, thereby creating additional technical difficulties.

The choice of which enzyme(s) to use must be left to the individual. There is no "best enzyme," and, when searching for a new polymorphism, it may be necessary to screen every readily available specificity. There is considerable variation both in the cost of different enzymes, presumably depending on their ease of preparation and yield, and in their activities, susceptibility to inhibition, stability, and purity. The researcher should consult the catalogs of the different suppliers for current information. We believe that the well-characterized enzymes, such as *Hin*dIII, *Eco*RI, *Bam*HI, and *Pst*I, which are relatively inexpensive and widely utilized, should be tried first.

The concentration of the DNA to be digested should be 0.1 to 1.0 μg/μl and may be adjusted with water if necessary. The appropriate restriction endonuclease buffer is added to the solution, most conveniently in 10× concentrated form. Sufficient enzyme is then added to digest the DNA, and the incubation is performed at the recommended temperature, usually 37°C, but it is important to remember that some enzymes, such as *Bcl*I, require elevated temperatures (see the manufacturer's data sheets). The amount of enzyme needed to ensure complete digestion is somewhat variable, and some enzymes are more robust than others. As a guide, at least 1 U of an enzyme should be used per μg of DNA until sufficient experience has been gained with that enzyme to know whether it can be stretched or whether more than 1 U/μg is needed. Some enzymes lose their activity more rapidly than others, and, again, the manufacturer's data sheets normally give some indication of the actual performance. Many researchers add an equal amount of phage lambda DNA to a parallel incubation and assess the completeness of digestion by visualizing the cleaved phage DNA bands over the smear of eucaryotic DNA. However, this method is imperfect since it only indicates the progress of the digest on the phage DNA and not directly on the human DNA. Differences in the purity of the DNAs and in the rates of cleavage of different sites may affect their relative extents of digestion.

After the samples are displayed on agarose, a relatively uniform smear of DNA should be observed, the top of which is slightly behind the 23-kilobase band of *Hin*dIII-cut phage lambda DNA. This DNA is frequently used as a size marker and is commercially available. The bottom of the smear almost extends to the gel front. The appearance of the characteristic pattern of bands produced by the repeated sequences serves as a useful indication of the integrity of the digestion (Fig. 1).

The cleaved DNA can be either stored frozen or concentrated by ethanol precipitation. It is not normally necessary to extract the spent restriction enzyme, although this is frequently done.

All restriction enzymes require a magnesium-containing buffer, usually Tris hydrochloride, magnesium chloride, and various amounts of NaCl. The chief differences among the buffers are in the recommended salt concentrations: low, medium, or high (10, 50, and 150 mM NaCl, respectively). Nearly all enzymes will work in one of the standard buffers (10 mM Tris hydrochloride [pH 7.5], 10 mM MgCl$_2$, and either 10 mM β-mercaptoethanol or 1 mM dithiothreitol plus either low, medium, or high salt). At least one supplier

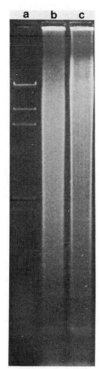

FIG. 1. Ethidium bromide-stained gel photographed under UV light. Lanes: a, *Hin*dIII-digested phage lambda DNA; b and c, *Eco*RI-digested total human DNA, showing characteristic pattern of repeated sequences.

(New England BioLabs, Inc.) publishes a list of salt requirements for different enzymes, and many have little or no preference for any particular salt concentration. Consequently, it is not necessary to prepare a unique buffer for each enzyme, and, when performing multiple digests on the same DNA, it is often possible to carry out simultaneous incubations with more than one enzyme or to adjust (increase) the salt concentration of the buffer between serial digests by enzymes with different salt requirements. However, some enzymes do have absolute requirements for particular components, for example for KCl in place of NaCl. In such cases the manufacturer's recommendations must be followed.

Preparation of agarose gels

The digested DNA is subjected to electrophoresis through agarose. Restriction enzymes which have 6-bp recognition sequences will produce DNA fragments that are on average between 4,000 and 6,000 bp long (assuming G+C content of about 40%) and resolve well on 0.7% agarose. Enzymes which cleave more frequently will require a stiffer gel: 1.0% up to about 1.5%, depending on the enzyme and on the known sizes of any particular fragments to be resolved. A 1.5% gel will separate fragments down to 300 bp or less, which is approximately the lower limit of this method since smaller fragments do not permanently bind to many of the support media and produce weak hybridization signals due to their short lengths.

Ordinary agarose (e.g., Sigma type I, low electroendoosmosis) is used for the gels; we have not found it necessary to use the highest-quality agarose, which is considerably more expensive than the reagent-grade material. Many suppliers also market high- and low-gelling-temperature varieties. These products are used for special purposes and should not be used for the studies described here. The agarose is added to the required volume of 1× TAE buffer and boiled gently. The flask is shaken occasionally to prevent burning the agarose, and some additional water should be included to compensate for losses by evaporation during boiling. When the agarose has completely dissolved, the solution is cooled to about 55°C, with some swirling to prevent localized gelling. The gel is now cast, and the desired slot-formers are inserted. When completely set, the slot-formers are removed and the gel is ready to be run. When using a flat-bed apparatus, the gel should be submerged in TAE buffer to prevent shinkage. The cooling process can be accelerated by placing the gel in the cold room.

A variety of gel apparatuses are commercially available or can be constructed by a plastics workshop. Vertical gels, which are cast between glass plates, can also be used, although endosmotic effects cause the DNA to smear during entry and produce diffuse bands. Horizontal gels, which are run completely submerged in buffer, give better results.

A minimum of 5 to 10 μg of DNA per lane is required for the detection of single-copy sequences. The width of the slot-former should be between 0.5 and 1.0 cm and the thickness between 0.1 and 0.2 cm. The maximum amount of eucaryotic DNA which can be routinely run on a gel without overloading is 0.5 μg/mm² of slot surface; hence 10 μg of DNA would require 20 mm² of slot surface and, if loaded into a 0.5-cm lane, would necessitate a slot height of 0.4 cm. Most slot-formers do not extend through to the base plate; instead, they create pockets in the gel. They also cause some distortion at the gel surface due to surface tension. Therefore, to compensate for these effects, the total height of the gel is increased to 0.6 cm. A small amount of tracking dye and either sucrose or glycerol are added to the DNA, and the volume of the sample is adjusted to completely fill the slot. On a 0.7% gel, xylene cyanol will migrate with DNA 5 to 7 kilobases in length and bromophenol blue with DNA about 0.4 to 0.7 kilobases in length. A size marker, such as *Hin*dIII-digested phage lambda DNA, is normally included in a separate lane to provide a molecular weight standard.

Electrophoresis is continued until the bromophenol blue is at least 8 cm from the origin, although longer runs will increase the separation of the DNA fragments. Optimal resolution is obtained with low-voltage gradients; gels are typically run overnight for up to 18 h. Some experimentation may be required to establish the correct voltage for such a run; we found about 0.25 V/cm to be sufficient. Unless very long runs are planned, it is not necessary to recirculate the running buffer.

On completion of the electrophoresis, the gel is carefully removed from the apparatus and soaked in dilute (0.5 μg/ml) ethidium bromide solution for about 30 min, and the DNA is visualized under UV light. Short-wavelength light can be used since it produces the highest fluorescence intensities, even though it is more destructive to the DNA than long-

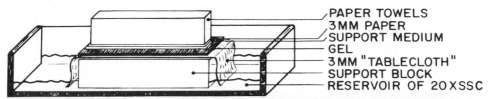

FIG. 2. Southern blotting apparatus.

wavelength UV light. The gel can be photographed through a red filter by using an appropriate camera mounted on a copy stand. Several UV and photographic systems are commercially available. A ruler should be placed alongside the gel for the calibration of the relative mobilities of the DNAs and the size marker. In addition, the positions of the phage lambda DNA bands can be marked in indelible ink on the gel and subsequently on the support membrane.

The DNA is denatured to form single strands by soaking the gel in 0.5 M NaOH–1 M NaCl for approximately 30 min with gentle periodic agitation. The single strands will bind to the support medium, whereas native, double-stranded DNA will not. When transferring samples from higher-percentage gels, it is sometimes necessary to cleave the DNA into smaller fragments to ensure complete transfer to the support medium. This is accomplished by depurinating the DNA by soaking the gel in dilute acid (0.2 M HCl works well) for 30 min before the denaturation treatment. However, we have not found this to be routinely necessary.

The NaOH is subsequently removed by immersing the gel either in 1 M Tris hydrochloride–3 M NaCl (pH 7.0) or in 3 M sodium acetate (pH 5.5 to 6.0) until completely neutralized. This is one of the most critical steps in the procedure, and it is slow relative to the denaturation process. It may take up to an hour, and it is easy to leave residual NaOH in the gel which can subsequently destroy the nitrocellulose. For this reason we prefer to use sodium acetate, which has a lower pH than Tris hydrochloride and neutralizes the alkali more efficiently.

The DNA is transferred to the support medium by placing the gel on one or more sheets of wet Whatman 3MM filter paper which dip into a large reservoir of 20× SSC (Fig. 2). A platform of glass plates is set up in a large baking dish or tray containing the SSC solution, and two sheets of 3MM paper are draped over the platform to form a "tablecloth." A sheet of support membrane is cut to size slightly smaller than the gel itself and wetted by flotation in 2× SSC. If air bubbles become trapped in the membrane during wetting, the membrane should be dried before being re-wet. The membrane is placed carefully on the gel surface, taking care to squeeze out any air bubbles. The support medium is overlaid by a slightly smaller sheet of wet 3MM paper, and many layers of absorbent material, such as paper towels, are stacked on top. A small weight such as a glass plate can be placed on the paper towels to aid the transfer process. It is important that neither the support medium nor any of the paper hangs over the side of the gel to make contact with the tablecloth since SSC will bypass the gel without transferring DNA. The tablecloth can be covered with a plastic wrap to prevent this. Transfer is

allowed to proceed for several hours, normally overnight, after which the positions of the slots at the origin of the gel are marked on the membrane with indelible ink to provide registration marks for the determination of the mobilities of the polymorphic fragments.

Several different kinds of support media are available, including nitrocellulose and chemically derivatized (diazotized) papers (8). The latter have some benefits for transferring RNAs and small DNA fragments but offer no significant advantages to these studies. Although nitrocellulose has been the traditional support medium, it is very brittle when dry and highly sensitive to residual alkali and overbaking (see below). For these reasons, we prefer the newer, nylon-based membranes, such as Pall-Biodyne, which are more durable than nitrocellulose and produce the same results. Both types of membrane are available in a variety of pore sizes; conventionally, 0.45-μm nitrocellulose and 1.2-μm nylon membranes are used for these experiments. Membranes with smaller pore sizes, such as 0.12-μm nitrocellulose, have been used for the transfer of small (<1,000 bp) DNA fragments.

Several companies manufacture electroblotting devices, which transfer the DNA to the support medium electrophoretically. These devices offer greater speed and require less handling of the gel. The researcher should consult manufacturers' catalogs for further details.

Finally, the membrane is carefully lifted from the gel and processed in accordance with the manufacturer's instructions. Nylon membranes are treated slightly differently from nitrocellulose, which is rinsed in 2× SSC, dried, and baked under vacuum at 80°C for 2 h. The temperature of the oven should not exceed 80°C since this will cause singing of the nitrocellulose. The gel can be restained with ethidium bromide to verify the completeness of the transfer.

Hybridization

Hybridization is carried out under one of several standard conditions (7): for example, in a solution containing 4× SCC, 1× Denhardt solution, 10% sodium dextran sulfate, boiled salmon sperm DNA (50 μg/ml) as carrier, and 0.5% SDS at 68°C for 12 to 18 h. Alternatively, hybridization can be carried out in a similar solution containing 50% formamide, usually at 42°C. By increasing the temperature (to as high as 56°C), a much greater degree of hybridization stringency will be achieved: only perfectly matched duplexes will be formed (4). Dextran sulfate increases the rate of hybridization and is not essential; however, we normally include it. For a more complete discussion of the effects of temperature and salt concentration on hybridization, see reference 9.

After baking, the membrane is wetted by flotation in 2× SSC at room temperature, ensuring that no air bubbles remain trapped underneath. If air pockets form, the membrane should be dried before being re-wetted. It is subsequently placed in an air-tight plastic bag such as a sandwich bag, and sufficient hybridization fluid is added to cover the membrane. As much air as possible is eliminated from the bag before it is sealed by heat and pressure and immersed in a water bath at the appropriate hybridization temperature for at least 1 h. This prehybridization process thoroughly saturates the filter with fluid and blocks any imperfections in the membrane which may bind the probe nonspecifically.

The radioactively labeled probe DNA is denatured by being heated in a boiling water bath for 2 min. The bag containing the filter is cut open at one corner, and the probe is carefully introduced through a Pasteur pipette. After the bag is resealed, the probe is spread uniformly throughout the bag, which is then placed flat in the water bath to maintain an even distribution of the probe. A shaking water bath can be used for this purpose. Several filters can be inserted in the same bag. Typically, a 20- by 15-cm filter requires about 40 ml of solution and additional filters an extra 5 ml each.

Hybridization is carried out for 12 to 20 h (usually overnight), after which the bag is cut open along one edge, and the filter(s) is quickly removed and immersed in a large (e.g., 500 ml) volume of 2× SSC–0.1% SDS. The spent hybridization fluid is disposed of as liquid radioactive waste. Alternatively, the bag can be opened under the SSC solution. The filters are rinsed with several changes of 1- to 2× SSC until no radioactivity can be detected in the wash. To remove the last traces of excess radioactivity, the later washes are carried out at high temperature. A final wash of 0.5× SSC at 67°C is often sufficient, but frequently more rigorous conditions (e.g., several changes of 0.2× SSC at 67°C) are required to obtain a completely clean filter. The use of lower SSC concentrations or higher temperatures will result in some loss of signal, especially from imperfectly matched duplexes, and this can be used to eliminate undesired signals from related genes, e.g., when probing for HLA-DR polymorphisms from HLA-DC or -SB genes. When scanned by a hand-held monitor, the filter should be silent. Some counts may be detected over areas of the filter whch bind DNA, but the edges should be silent. Continued washing may be successful in further reducing any remaining background, but occasionally air bubbles form during the hybridization and create local areas of extremely high radioactivity which cannot be removed by further washing.

The membrane is dried, placed between sheets of Saran wrap, and subjected to autoradiography using the fastest X-ray film available, currently Kodak XAR-5, together with an appropriate intensifying screen such as DuPont Lightning Plus. Bands should be visible after 1 to 2 days at −70°C, but longer exposures may be necessary to detect distantly related sequences or regions of short homology (Fig. 3). The mobilities of the polymorphic fragments can be measured by placing the developed X-ray film over the membrane and using the registration marks to indicate the origin of the gel. Their molecular weights can

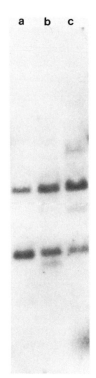

FIG. 3. Autoradiogram of Southern blot. Human DNA samples were digested by PstI and hybridized to an HLA-DR β-chain-specific probe to demonstrate HLA-D region polymorphisms. Lanes: a, DNA from the LB (DR 6,6) cell line; b, DNA from the JY (DR 4,6) cell line; c, DNA from the Priess (DR 4,4) cell line.

be determined by comparing their mobilities with the bands of the size marker.

If the filter is still damp when placed at −70°C, it is often possible to continue washing it after a first exposure to eliminate cross-hybridizing sequences. Previously hybridized probe may be removed by soaking the filter in dilute NaOH (5 to 20 mM) for a few minutes at room temperature before being neutralized by Tris hydrochloride. Membranes can usually be reused a few times although, we have found, with some successive reduction of signal.

Labeling of probe

Although the growth and preparation of recombinant DNA clones is outside the scope of this chapter, several methods for labeling DNA to high specific activity (>10⁸ cpm/μg) have been described. The most commonly used method is nick translation, which is outlined briefly below.

The sample to be labeled is treated with trace amounts of DNase I, which produces random single-stranded nicks in the DNA. DNA polymerase I (Kornberg polymerase) has exonuclease activity and will sequentially degrade the broken strand in a 5′→3′ direction starting at a nick and creating a gap in that strand. A second molecule of the polymerase will repair the gap, proceeding in the same direction as the exonuclease and using the 3′ end of the nicked strand as the primer and the exposed strand as the template. α-³²P-labeled deoxynucleoside triphosphates (dNTPs) can be incorporated into the resynthesized strand. Using one or more commercially available radioactive dNTPs with a specific activity greater than 2,000 to 3,000 Ci/mmol, small amounts of DNA can be labeled to an activity of $>10^9$ cpm/μg.

The synthesis of a probe with the highest possible specific activity is essential for the detection of single-copy sequences. A small amount of DNA (about 0.01 μg) is resuspended in 10 to 20 μl of nick translation buffer (10 mM Tris hydrochloride [pH 7.5], 10 mM MgCl$_2$, 10 mM NaCl) containing about 50 μCi of each of one or more radioactive dNTPs (specific activity, >2,000 Ci/mmol). The concentrations of the other, unlabeled dNTPs should be about 50 μM each. A trace amount of DNase I is added to the solution, together with 0.25 μl (1 to 2 U) of DNA polymerase I (whole enzyme), and incubated for about 30 min. We have found it convenient to perform the incubation at room temperature, although other investigators prefer a lower temperature (often 16°C). Excess, unincorporated dNTPs are removed by chromatography through a small (1-ml) Sephadex G-50 column (or the equivalent). Up to 30 to 50% of the labeled dNTPs should have been incorporated into the DNA. It may be convenient to monitor the progress of the reaction by passing samples (0.5 μl) of the incubation mix through the column at 10-min intervals and terminating the reaction when 30% of the radioactivity is excluded by incorporation into the DNA. Spin columns may be used for this process (7). Blue dextran is used as a marker for the excluded volume, and the column is developed with a low-salt buffer such as 10 mM Tris hydrochloride (pH 7.5) containing 5 mM EDTA to inactivate the enzymes.

The amount of DNase I to be added must be determined empirically since preparations differ in their activities. A series of 10× dilutions of the enzyme in storage buffer is prepared to cover the range from 10 ng down to 10 pg of enzyme per μl of solution. Samples (0.01 μg) of DNA are incubated with 1 μl of each of the enzymes dilutions for 30 min at room temperature and immediately analyzed on a 0.7% agarose gel. Samples which have received excess enzyme will be degraded and may not be visible; samples which have received insufficient enzyme will remain intact, whereas samples receiving the correct amount of enzyme will show a limited amount of degradation, detectable by some forward migration of the DNA in the gel. A stock solution of DNase I can be prepared in 50% glycerol–1 mM EDTA–10 mM Tris hydrochloride [pH 7.5]–1% bovine serum albumin and is relatively stable at −20°C.

The novice is urged to purchase one of the commercially available kits for carrying out this reaction because it is a critical step in the detection of single-copy sequences.

A 0.01-μg portion of labeled probe is sufficient for 100 ml of hybridization solution. We have found that such highly labeled probe is subject to rapid radiolytic decomposition and cannot be stored for more than 2 or 3 days at −20°C.

A variety of other methods, such as the SP6 transcription system (5), are available for preparing radioactively labeled probes, and the appropriate references or suppliers' catalogs should be consulted. The nick translation system is the most universal and can be used to label any type of double-stranded DNA, e.g., fragment, or whole DNA in linear or circular form.

REAGENTS

TE buffer (10 mM Tris hydrochloride [pH 7.5], 1 mM EDTA)

TAE buffer (0.04 M Tris acetate [pH 7.9], 0.002 M EDTA)

DNA lysis buffer (10 mM Tris [pH 7.5], 10 mM EDTA, 100 mM NaCl, 1% SDS, proteinase K [20 μg/μl])

3 M Sodium acetate (pH 5.2 to 5.5) (408 g of sodium acetate · 3H$_2$O in 800 ml of water; adjust to pH 5.2 to 5.5 with glacial acetic acid; add water to 1,000 ml)

SUPPLIERS

Restriction enzymes and DNA modification enzymes (New England BioLabs, Inc., Beverly, Mass.; Bethesda Research Laboratories [BRL], Inc., Gaithersburg, Md.; Boehringer Mannheim Biochemicals, Indianapolis, Ind.; International Biotechnologies, Inc., New Haven, Conn.; plus many other smaller companies)

Proteinase K (Sigma Chemical Co., St. Louis, Mo.; Boehringer Mannheim)

DNase I (Worthington Diagnostics, Freehold, N.J.)

Support media

  Nitrocellulose (Schleicher & Schuell, Inc., Keene, N.H.; Millipore Corp., Bedford, Mass.; Whatman Ltd., Maidstone, England)

  Nylon membranes (Bio-Rad Laboratories, Richmond, Calif.; Pall-Biodyne, ICN Pharmaceuticals, Irvine, Calif.; New England Nuclear Corp., Boston, Mass.)

Agarose (Sigma)

Electrophoretic apparatus, (Bio-Rad Laboratories; BRL; Hoeffer Scientific Instruments, San Francisco, Calif.)

Sodium dextran sulfate (Sigma; Pharmacia Fine Chemicals, Piscataway, N.J.)

This work was supported in part by the Easter Seals Foundation, the Gebbie Foundation, the Lions Club of Massachusetts, the New England Peabody Home for Crippled Children, Public Health Service grants AM30486 and AM05577 from National Institutes of Health, and the Multipurpose Arthritis Center (AM205860 P16).

LITERATURE CITED

1. **Blin, N., and D. W. Stafford.** 1976. Isolation of high-molecular-weight DNA. Nucleic Acids Res. **3**:2303–2308.
2. **Botstein, D., R. L. White, M. Skolnick, and R. W. Davis.** 1980. Construction of a genetic linkage map in man using restriction fragment length polymorphisms. Am. J. Hum. Genet. **32**:314–331.
3. **Boyum, A.** 1976. Isolation of lymphocytes, granulocytes and macrophages. Scand. J. Immunol. **5**(Suppl. 5):9–15.
4. **Fisher, J. H., J. F. Gusella, and C. H. Scoggin.** 1984. Molecular hybridization under high stringency permits cloned DNA segments containing reiterated DNA sequences to be assigned to specific chromosomal locations. Proc. Natl. Acad. Sci. U.S.A. **81**:520–524.
5. **Green, M. R., T. Maniatis, and D. A. Melton.** 1983. Human β-globin pre-mRNA synthesised in vitro is accurate-

ly spliced in *Xenopus* oocyte nuclei. Cell **32**:681–694.

6. **Gusella, J. F., R. E. Tanzi, M. H. Anderson, W. Hobbs, K. Gibbons, R. Raschtchian, T. C. Gilliam, M. R. Wallace, N. S. Wexler, and P. M. Conneally.** 1984. DNA markers for nervous system diseases. Science **225**:1320–1326.

7. **Maniatis, T., E. F. Fritsch, and J. Sambrook.** 1982. Molecular cloning: a laboratory manual. Cold Spring Harbor Laboratory, Cold Spring Harbor, N.Y.

8. **Seed, B.** 1982. Diazotizable arylamine cellulose papers for the coupling and hybridization of nucleic acids. Nucleic Acids Res. **10**:1799–1810.

9. **Southern, E. M.** 1975. Detection of specific sequences among DNA fragments separated by gel electrophoresis. J. Mol. Biol. **98**:053–517.

10. **Southern, E. M.** 1979. Gel electrophoresis of restriction fragments. Methods Enzymol. **68**:152–176.

TABLE 3. Limited repertoire of useful genetic systems

System	Whites		Blacks	
	P_e	P_{cum}	P_e	P_{cum}
ABO	0.1537	0.1537	0.1916	0.1916
Rh	0.2258	0.3448	0.1827	0.3393
MNSs	0.2408	0.5025	0.2506	0.5049
Kell	0.0400	0.5224	0.0083	0.5090
Duffy	0.1854	0.6109	0.1534	0.5843
Kidd	0.2868	0.6836	0.1558	0.6491
HLA-A,B	0.96	0.9873	0.95	0.9825

confidence by limited testing if HLA is included. The repertoire of markers commonly employed is shown in Table 3. This series of markers will exclude 99% of falsely accused white men and 98% of falsely accused black men, provided that the HLA antiserum panel can identify all the HLA-A and -B alleles defined by the Ninth International Histocompatibility Testing Workshop (Table 4). If antisera for only the basic, or broad, specificities are used, the P_{cum} is reduced to approximately 97% for whites and 95% for blacks.

Exclusions

There are two types of exclusions. (i) The child possesses a gene not present in either parent. (ii) The child fails to inherit either allele present in the alleged father.

Given its power, the HLA system will exclude most falsely accused men. Further, in tests using a limited number of other systems, most often the exclusion will be found only with HLA. HLA exclusions will usually be of both type 1 and type 2. A falsely accused man who carries common antigens may not be excluded by HLA but may be excluded by one or more other systems. These exclusions will usually be of only type 1 or type 2. Exclusions by only a single system, other than HLA, should induce caution and lead the investigator to repeat the typing of the excluding system, using different reagents or fresh blood samples, if possible. Laboratory irregularity is suspected especially in cases in which the likelihood of paternity based on the nonexcluding systems is high. The cautious investigator will, of course, carry out additional tests to seek other excluding systems.

Nonexclusions

The next section details with the application of statistical methods to the genetic profiles of the individuals involved in cases of disputed paternity. The need for an understanding of Mendelian principles of heredity, the genetics of each marker system, and biostatistics has already been discussed. The statistical analysis of nonexclusionary results is based on the principle of Hardy-Weinberg equilibrium and probability theory. There is sufficient space here for only a brief review of the fundamental concepts.

STATISTICAL ANALYSIS

Laws of probability

The multiplication law of probability states that the probability of two or more independent events occur-

ring is equal to the product of the probabilities of the individual events.

For example, if the probability of drawing an O allele (ABO system) from the population is r, the probability of drawing two such alleles is $r \times r = r^2$.

The addition law of probability states that the probability that one of two or more mutually exclusive events will occur is equal to the sum of the probabilities of the individual events.

For example, if the population frequencies of the O and A alleles of the ABO system are r and p, the probability of drawing either of these alleles from the population is given by $r + p$.

Hardy-Weinberg equilibrium

A population in which two alleles, A and B, occur with the frequencies p and q will consist, after one generation of random mating, of three genotypes in the equilibrium proportion $p^2:2pq:q^2$ (AA:AB:BB).

For an individual drawn from a population in Hardy-Weinberg equilibrium, the probability of the genotype can be determined using probability laws. The genotype requires two independent events, i.e., drawing two alleles; thus, the probability of the genotype is governed by the multiplication law. The probability of an OO genotype is r^2, while that of the AO genotype is $2pr$ rather than just pr since that genotype can occur two different ways: maternal gene A and paternal gene O or the converse.

Some phenotypes may consist of more than one genotype. Their probabilities involve the addition law of probability. For example, an ABO type A phenotype will occur with either an AA or an AO genotype; therefore, the probability of the type A phenotype, $P(A)$, is given by:

$$P(A) = P(AA) + P(AO)$$
$$= p^2 + 2pr$$

Conditional probability

Conditional probability is the probability of one event conditional upon another event or condition. The effect is that the universe in which we are working is reduced. The genotype probabilities given above are absolute probabilities. However, we may wish to know the probability of a genotype conditional upon the phenotype. If we ask what is the probability of an AA genotype given that the phenotype is A, intuitively we can see that this conditional probability will be different from the absolute probability since the universe has been reduced to only those individuals with either of two genotypes, AA or AO. This probability is given by:

$$P(AA|A) = \frac{P(AA)}{P(AA) + P(AO)}$$
$$= \frac{p^2}{p^2 + 2pr} = \frac{p}{p + 2r}$$

In addition to genotype probabilities which are conditional upon the phenotype, they may also be conditional upon certain genetic relationships. A child's genotype (and thus phenotype) is conditional

TABLE 4. P(phenotypes|hypothesis)

Genotypes		Probabilities[a]					
M	AF	P(M)	P(AF)	P(C|M,AF)	P(C|M)	P(M,AF,C|M,AF)	P(M,AF,C|M)
				Condition 1: M:A, AF:A, C:O			
AO	AA	$2pr$	p^2	$\emptyset$	$(1/2)r$	$\emptyset$	p^3r^2
AO	AO	$2pr$	$2pr$	$1/4$	$(1/2)r$	$\dfrac{p^2r^2}{X_1{}^b}$	$\dfrac{2p^2r^3}{Y_1{}^c}$
				Condition 2: M:A, AF:A, C:A			
AA	AA	p^2	p^2	1	$p+r$	p^4	$p^4(p+r)$
AA	AO	p^2	$2pr$	1	$p+r$	$2p^3r$	$2p^3r(p+r)$
AO	AA	$2pr$	p^2	1	$p+(1/2)r$	$2p^3r$	$2p^3r[p+(1/2)r]$
AO	AO	$2pr$	$2pr$	$3/4$	$p+(1/2)r$	$\dfrac{3p^2r^2}{X_2{}^d}$	$\dfrac{4p^2r^2[p+(1/2)r]}{Y_2{}^e}$

[a] Frequencies of the A and O alleles are designated p and r, respectively. See the text for explanations of column headings.
[b] $X_1 = p^2r^2$.
[c] $X_2 = p^4 + 4p^3r + 3p^2r^2 = p^2(p + 3r)(p + r)$.
[d] $Y_1 = p^2r^2(p + 2r)$.
[d] $Y_2 = (p^4 + 2p^3r)(p + r) + 2p^2r(p + 2r)[p + (1/2)r] = p^2(p + 2r)(p^2 + 3pr + r^2)$.

upon its parents' genotypes. Therefore, when a mother and father have the genotypes AO and OO, the probability of their child having an AO genotype is not $2pr$ as in the previous example above but $1/2$: $P(C_{AO}|M_{AO},F_{OO}) = P(A_M$ and $O_F) = (1/2) \times 1 = 1/2$, where C_{AO}, M_{AO}, and F_{OO} are the genotypes of the child, mother, and father, and M_A and F_O are the maternal and paternal genes contributed to the child.

If only one parent is known, the probability of a child is determined from the probabilities of drawing one gene from that parent and the other from the random population (RP). For example, the probability of an AO child given an AO mother is:

$$P(C_{AO}|M_{AO}) = P(M_A)P(RP_O) + P(M_O)P(RP_A)$$
$$= (1/2)r + (1/2)p$$

In paternity cases, the genotypes are often not known. For example, in the situation described above, we would recognize only that the phenotypes are A. This complicates the calculations further, as shown in examples below.

P(observations|hypotheses)

There are two components in the statistical analysis of paternity cases: (i) the observations or events and (ii) the hypotheses or conditions. The observations are the test results. The hypotheses include the various conditions which can explain the observations. In the standard three-party case (mother, child, alleged father), maternity is assumed, and if genetic tests do not exclude paternity, there are two mutually exclusive hypotheses: (i) the alleged father is the biological father or (ii) the alleged father is not the biological father, but possesses genes that the child could only have inherited from his or her true father.

The initial values to be obtained are the conditional probabilities of the observations given the hypothesis P(observations|hypothesis). Many laboratories, in the standard three-party case, have designated as X the

conditional probability obtained under the hypothesis of paternity and as Y the conditional probability obtained under the hypothesis of nonpaternity. To determine P(observations|hypothesis), two different questions may be asked. (i) What is the probability of observing the phenotypes of the individuals tested given either that they are a mother, child, and father (paternity) or given that they are a mother, child, and a falsely accused man (nonpaternity)? (ii) What is the probability that a child of this phenotype would result from a union of gametes either from this woman and this man (paternity) or from this woman and someone other than this man (nonpaternity)? Depending on which question is asked, different calculations are performed and different X and Y values are obtained. However, the X/Y ratio (commonly called the paternity index) will be the same for both approaches. Since the X/Y ratio determines the final outcome of the analysis, either approach may be used and both will be demonstrated here.

P(phenotype|hypothesis)

Two examples of these calculations are provided in Table 4 as a format for this discussion. These examples assume that the mother and biological father are unrelated. First, the genotype combinations possible for the phenotypes of the mother (M) and alleged father (AF) are listed. Because maternity is assumed, it is necessary to list only those genotypes of the mother that are compatible with those of her child, as shown for condition 1. In practice, it is better to list all of the genotypes possible for the mother's phenotype and then to eliminate those that are incompatible with the child's phenotype. Although more time-consuming, this practice reduces appreciably the chance of mistakenly omitting a genotype. All possible genotypes are listed for the alleged father since, under the hypothesis of nonpaternity, his genotype is not restricted by that of the child. Next, the probabilities for each of the genotypes, designated P(M) and P(AF), are determined. If these individuals are drawn from a population in Hardy-Weinberg equilibrium, their genotype probabilities can be determined using the multiplication law of probability, as discussed above. Allele frequencies from an appropriate sample are used for the allele probabilities. An appropriate sample is one that is large enough to reduce sampling error and that has been drawn from the same racial group as that of the subject under consideration.

It was noted above that the probability of the child's phenotype is conditional upon the genotypes of the parents. Under the hypothesis of paternity, both parents are known; therefore, for each genotype combination of the mother and alleged father, we determine the conditional probability (X) of the child, denoted $P(C|M,AF)$. Under the hypothesis of nonpaternity, we are given only one parent, the mother, and we determine the conditional probability (Y) of the phenotype of the child given the mother, i.e., $P(C|M)$.

It has been noted that when both the child and the mother have the AO genotype, $P(C_{AO}|M_{AO}) = (1/2)(r + p)$. However, in Table 4 (condition 2) $P(C_A|M_{AO}) = p + (1/2)r$.

This occurs because, knowing only that the child is phenotype A, we must consider two possible genotypes, AA and AO. When the mother's genotype is AO, the combinations of gametes which result in a type A child are as follows. If the maternal gamete is A $(P = 1/2)$ and the paternal gamete is A or O $(P = p + r)$, then the probability that the child is A is $(1/2)(p + r)$. Alternatively, if the maternal gamete is O $(P = 1/2)$ and the paternal gamete is A $(P = p)$, then the probability that the child is A is $(1/2)p/[p + (1/2)r]$.

The probabilities of observing all three individuals for any single genotype combination within a system are:

$$X = P(M,AF,C|M,AF) = P(M) \times P(AF) \times P(C|M,AF)$$

and

$$Y = (M,AF,C|M) = P(M) \times P(AF) \times P(C|M)$$

under the hypotheses of paternity and nonpaternity, respectively. As shown in Table 4, when more than one genotype is possible for either parent, the total $P(\text{observations}|\text{hypothesis})$ is given by the sum of the values obtained for each genotype combination. Then, $X = \Sigma\Sigma P(M,AF,C|M,AF)$, which is $X = \Sigma\Sigma[P(M) \times P(AF) \times P(C|M,AF)]$. Similarly, $Y = \Sigma\Sigma P(M,AF,C|M)$, which is $Y = \Sigma\Sigma[P(M) \times P(AF) \times P(C|M)]$ when M and AF are unrelated.

P(gametes|hypothesis)

In the method described above, we listed various genotype combinations for the mother and the alleged father and determined, for each combination, the probability of a child of a given phenotype deriving from one or both of those parental genotypes. In this second approach, we determine the various gamete combinations which would result in the child's phenotype and calculate the probability of those gametes being drawn from the mother and alleged father (paternity) or from the mother and an unknown, unrelated man (nonpaternity). (Analysis of condition 2 of Table 4 by this method is shown in Table 5).

TABLE 5. $P(\text{gametes}|\text{hypothesis})^a$

Gametes		Probabilities				
MG	PG	$P(MG)$	$P(AFG)$	$P(RPG)$	$P(MG,AFG)$	$P(MG,RPG)$
A	A	$\dfrac{p + r}{p + 2r}$	$\dfrac{p + r}{p + 2r}$	p	$\dfrac{(p + r)^2}{(p + 2r)^2}$	$\dfrac{(p + r)p}{p + 2r}$
A	O	$\dfrac{p + r}{p + 2r}$	$\dfrac{r}{p + 2r}$	r	$\dfrac{(p + r)r}{(p + 2r)^2}$	$\dfrac{(p + r)r}{p + 2r}$
O	A	$\dfrac{r}{p + 2r}$	$\dfrac{p + r}{p + 2r}$	p	$\dfrac{(p + r)r}{(p + 2r)^2}$	$\dfrac{pr}{p + 2r}$
					X	Y

^{a} See the text for explanations of column headings. $X = [(p + r)^2 + 2(p + r)r]/(p + 2r)^2$ and $Y = [(p + r)^2 + pr]/(p + 2r)$.

The gamete probabilities of the mother and alleged father, $P(MG)$ and $P(AFG)$, are conditional upon their genotypes, which are, in turn, conditional upon their phenotypes. These probabilities are determined as follows:

$$\sum_{i=1}^{n}[P(\text{gamete}|\text{phenotype}) = P(\text{gamete}|\text{genotype}_i) \times P(\text{genotype}_i|\text{phenotype})]$$

For example, the probability of an A individual producing an A gamete is 1 if that individual is homozygous AA and 1/2 if heterozygous AO. As shown earlier, the conditional probabilities of the two genotypes are given by:

$$P(AA|A) = \frac{p^2}{p^2 + 2pr} = \frac{p}{p + 2r}$$

$$P(AO|A) = \frac{2pr}{p^2 + 2pr} = \frac{2r}{p + 2r}$$

Then,

$P(A \text{ gamete}|A \text{ phenotype})$

$$= 1\left(\frac{p}{p + 2r}\right) + 1/2\left(\frac{2r}{p + 2r}\right) = \frac{p + r}{p + 2r}.$$

The probability of drawing the paternal gamete from the random population, $P(RPG)$, is simply the frequency of that allele in the population.

The X and Y values are, then, the probability of drawing any of the appropriate gamete combinations from the mother and the alleged father or from the mother and the random population as follows:

$$X = \Sigma\Sigma P(MG,AFG) = \Sigma\Sigma P(MG)P(AFG)$$

$$Y = \Sigma\Sigma P(MG,RPG) = \Sigma\Sigma P(MG)P(RPG)$$

Choice of method

For the standard three-party case, the second method is probably less cumbersome because it uses numbers which are larger, easier to manage, and less subject to rounding errors. However, when modifications are necessary to accommodate special circum-

TABLE 6. Probability of paternity

Method	Posterior probability $\left(\dfrac{X}{X + Y}\right)$
1	$\dfrac{X}{X + Y} - p^2(p + 3r)(p + r) \dfrac{X}{p^2(p + 3r)(p + r) + p^2(p + 2r)(p^2 + 3pr + r^2)}$
	$= \dfrac{(p + 3r)(p + r)}{(p + 3r)(p + r) + (p + 2r)(p^2 + 3pr + r^2)}$
2	$\dfrac{X}{X + Y} = \dfrac{(p + r)^2 + 2(p + r)r}{(p + r)^2 + 2(p + r)r + (p + r)^2(p + 2r) + pr(p + 2r)}$
	$= \dfrac{(p + r)(p + r + 2r)}{(p + r)(p + r + 2r) + (p + 2r)(p^2 + 2pr + r^2 + pr)}$
	$= \dfrac{(p + 3r)(p + r)}{(p + 3r)(p + r) + (p + 2r)(p^2 + 3pr + r^2)}$

stances such as consanguinity or multiple children, the logic of the first method is easier to follow.

Cumulative P(observations|hypotheses)

As discussed above, it is desirable to utilize multiple genetic systems to resolve cases of disputed parentage. The X and Y values must be calculated for each independently inherited system. Cumulative conditional probabilities are then calculated using the multiplication rule, as follows:

$$X_c = \prod_{i=1}^{n} X_i \quad \text{and} \quad Y_c = \prod_{i=1}^{n} Y_i,$$

where X_c (or Y_c) is the cumulative probability for n systems and X_i (or Y_i) represents the probability of an individual system.

The X/Y ratios determined from the values obtained under each of the two approaches are given in Table 6 for condition 2 of Table 4. It should be noted that although different X and Y values are obtained by the two approaches, the X/Y ratios are identical. Thus, in the ordinary three-person case, the outcome is the same.

Problem. Table 7 shows the application of method 1 to a real case utilizing the genetic systems listed in Table 1.

EVALUATING THE HYPOTHESES

Probability of Paternity

There is universal agreement that the preferred statistical analysis is Bayesian. Bayes' Theorem uses the a priori probabilities of the hypotheses and the conditional probabilities of the observations given the hypotheses to determine the final or posterior probability of a hypothesis given the observations. Let $P(A_i)$ = the prior probability of hypothesis A_i.

Since the hypotheses must account for all the conditions under which the observations can occur, the sum of the prior probability values must equal 1, i.e.,

$$\sum_{i=1}^{n} P(A_i) = 1,$$

where $P(Z|A_i)$ is the conditional probability of the observations given, the hypotheses A_i (in the standard three-party case, these are the X and Y values) and $P(A_i|Z)$ is the posterior probability of the hypothesis A_i, given the observations Z. Then,

$$P(A_i|Z) = \frac{P(A_i)P(Z|A_i)}{\sum_i P(A_i)P(Z|A_i)}.$$

In the standard three-party case, if the hypotheses of paternity and nonpaternity are represented by A_x and A_y, respectively, the probability of paternity is given by:

$$(A_x|M,C,AF) = \frac{P(A_x)X}{P(A_x)X + P(A_y)Y}.$$

Prior probability

Selection of an appropriate value for the prior probability is a matter of some concern to geneticists and biostatisticians. To illustrate the problem, our individual points of view are set forth. Several approaches to constructing prior probabilities have been proposed, each with both good and bad points. We mention here only a brief review of some of the more popular methods along with some comments. As noted by Hummel et al. (10), the concern over an appropriate value for prior probability may be reduced as the number of discriminating test systems increases, since the effect of prior probability diminishes as the ratio of X to Y increases.

If accurate information were available, the number of potential fathers and the relative frequency of encounters with the mother during her fertile period relative to conception of the child could be used to establish a valid prior probability. As pointed out by Ellman and Kaye, this information is rarely reliable (7). Nevertheless, if this number were known, and only

TABLE 7. Likelihood of paternity[a]

System	Trio tested			Likelihoods		
	AF	M	C	X	Y	X/Y
ABO	O	A	O	0.4130	0.2932	1.4085
Rh	CcDee	ccDee	ccDee	0.4490	0.6403	0.7013
MNSs	NNss	NNSS	NNSs	1.0000	0.3800	2.6316
Kell	kk	kk	kk	1.0000	0.9962	1.0038
Jk	aa	aa	aa	1.0000	0.7315	1.3671
Fy	b	ab	b	0.5000	0.4375	1.1429
Lu	ab	bb	ab	0.5000	0.0200	25.0000
P_1	0	0	0	1.0000	0.1292	7.7399
Le	0	0	0	1.0000	0.4303	2.3240
ADA	1-1	1-1	1-1	1.0000	0.9785	1.0220
AK	1-1	1-1	1-1	1.0000	0.9901	1.0100
EAP	BB	BB	BB	1.0000	0.8308	1.2037
PGM_1	1-1	1-1	1-1	1.0000	0.7673	1.3033
6PGD	AA	AA	AA	1.0000	0.9645	1.0368
Hp	1-1	2-1	1-1	0.5000	0.2934	1.7044
Tf	CC	CC	CC	1.0000	0.9444	1.0589
Gc	1-1	1-1	1-1	1.0000	0.8924	1.1206
CA II	1-1	1-1	1-1	1.0000	0.8986	1.1128
Js	bb	bb	bb	1.0000	0.9100	1.0989
GPT	2-1	2-1	2-1	0.5000	0.5000	1.0000
HLA	A2,B35,A3,B45	A26,B57,A1,B8	A2,B35,A26,B57	0.0316	0.0097	3.2606
Cumulative likelihoods				$X_{cum} =$ 0.0004434	$Y_{cum} =$ 0.00000001789	$X_{cum}/Y_{cum} =$ 24,788

$X_{cum}/(X_{cum} + Y_{cum})] \times 100 = 99.996\%$

[a] See the text for an explanation of column heads.

one possible father could be tested, a rational prior probability could be constructed by assigning an equal prior probability of conception to each separate encounter. The prior probability of paternity for each man would be the proportion of the total number of encounters in which he was the partner.

A prior probability currently in vogue is based on the reasoning of Essen-Möller and Quensel, who proposed that, in the absence of reliable information on which to base the assignment of prior probability values, the prior probability should not favor either hypothesis (8). The use of the so-called uniform priors is defended on the grounds that it maintains the symmetry of the Bayesian analysis. The result, however, is to convert a perfectly sound likelihood into a dubious posterior probability. This approach may have gained popularity not so much because of its philosophy but because it simplifies the calculation, since the posterior probability reduces to $X/(X + Y)$, designated W by Essen-Möller.

This approach is equivalent to assuming that, for each case, there are two men who are equally likely to be the father. Were this true, when a test system with a high probability of excluding a falsely accused man is used, the observed exclusion rate should be near 50%. However, this is not the case, probably because mothers tend to identify true fathers and because they are informed by their counsels that current test procedures have a high probability of excluding falsely accused men. The observed exclusion rate in the laboratory of one of the authors of this chapter (A.A.Z.) is about 20%, whereas the exclusion rate in the laboratory of the other (W.B.B.) is about 10%.

Noting that the exclusion rate in his laboratory is also about 20%, Hummel has suggested that the fre-

quency with which true biological fathers are correctly identified should be used as the probability that a woman has, a priori, correctly identified the true father (10). A.A.Z. had independently arrived at this opinion based on the idea that, when this approach is limited to cases in which a woman seeks to prove the identity of the true father, she utilizes information available only to her. The defense of this approach rests on its comparison to other applications of probabilities as applied to individual situations such as population gene frequencies. For example, given a phenotype, an individual is not 60% homozygous and 40% heterozygous; the individual is either a homozygote or a heterozygote.

W.B.B., however, is opposed to this approach. Her argument is that no laboratory's exclusion rate represents the true rate of nonpaternity in the population, viz., the different rates in our two laboratories. W.B.B. suggests that to assign a prior probability of 0.80 or 0.90 to the alleged father and 0.20 or 0.10 to the "random man" is incompatible with both scientific impartiality and legal justice (6). Furthermore, a laboratory's exclusion rate may be 20% one year but may drop to 10% the next, requiring constant changes of the prior probability. It would be difficult under such circumstances to guarantee that a valid prior probability was used in a given case. W.B.B. also rejects the argument that a prior probability of paternity based on the rate of exclusion is comparable to the a priori probability of heterozygosity based on gene frequencies. The latter are based on population samples which asymptotically approach true frequencies. Given the phenotype of an individual of unknown genotype, the likelihoods of possible genotypes are estimated based on prior data, i.e., population fre-

TABLE 8. Influence of prior probability on the probability of paternity (posterior probability)

Prior probability	Posterior probability in:	
	Limited systems (CP[a] = 0.9250)	All systems (CP = 0.99996)
0.01	0.1108	0.99605
0.05	0.3936	0.99924
0.10	0.5781	0.99964
0.20	0.7551	0.99984
0.30	0.8406	0.99991
0.40	0.8916	0.99994
0.50	0.9250	0.99996
0.60	0.9487	0.99997
0.70	0.9664	0.99998
0.80	0.9801	0.99999
0.90	0.9911	0.99999
0.95	0.9957	0.99999
0.99	0.9992	0.99999

[a] CP, Conditional probability.

quencies. The objective probability is, of course, 1 or 0, and if pertinent data were available, such as typing of parents or offspring, the outcome would be certain. The indeterminacy inherent in paternity cases, however, is not susceptible to this objective kind of resolution.

Ellman and Kaye (7) have suggested a chart approach to show the various posterior probabilities possible using different prior probabilities. On the one hand, while this method is impartial and also maintains the symmetry of Bayesian analysis, it places on jurists the burden of numerically weighting nonparametric data. On the other hand, this approach can be defended because it clearly illustrates the impact a valid prior probability would have on the final probability in the case in question. For those cases with a low likelihood ratio (conditional probability), the effect of a high prior probability would be great, while it would be trivial on those with high ratios. This is illustrated in Table 8 by utilizing the data in Table 7. In the first calculation the limited list of genetic markers shown in Table 3 was used, while in the second calculation all of the systems listed in Table 7 were included. These outcomes should instruct the jurists that the nonbiological evidence must be carefully considered in the cases with relatively low likelihood ratios. The likelihood (conditional probability) using the limited markers was 92.5%, a level considered convincing by many judges; yet a modest decrease in the prior probability, from 0.5 to 0.4, is sufficient to cast real doubt on the hypothesis of paternity.

To avoid the controversy over prior probabilities, some individuals omit prior probabilities. When this is done, one must take great care to interpret the results accurately since, in the absence of a prior probability, $X/(X + Y)$ is no longer the probability of paternity but rather the relative probability, or likelihood, of making the observations when the man is the father. To interpret $X/(X + Y)$ as the probability of paternity implies prior probability values of 0.5 for both hypotheses.

In the summary of the Airlie Conference on Inclusion Probabilities in Parentage Testing it is noted that the majority of conference participants felt that the "assignment of a prior probability is not usually the province of the laboratory scientist" (p. xiii, reference

6). As noted above, the probability of paternity, a statistic usually requested by the court, cannot be determined without inclusion of a prior probability. Therefore, if a probability of paternity is calculated, the scientist should always state in the report what prior probability values were used and why. Then, by using one of the simple algebraic equations shown below, the recipient of this information can incorporate any other prior probability values.

$$PP_n = \frac{b(1 - a)PP_o}{b(1 - a)PP_o + a(1 - b)(1 - PP_o)}$$

where PP_n is the new probability of paternity, PP_o is the original probability of paternity, a is the original prior probability used to calculate PP_o, and b is the new prior probability. When $a = 1 - a = 0.5$,

$$PP_n = \frac{bPP_o}{bPP_o + (a - 1)(1 - PP_o)}$$

SPECIAL CONSIDERATIONS

The procedures described above are applicable to the standard three-party case when there is no consanguinity and the genetic systems are all inherited independently. Although this type of case occurs most often, there are exceptions which require modifications in the calculations. A complete discussion of the mathematical treatment is too exhaustive for this chapter; however, a brief review of some of the special circumstances is included so that the reader will recognize situations for which the standard calculations described here are inappropriate.

Linked loci

Several systems in use, including the MNS, Gm, HLA, and possibly Rh systems, are controlled by linked loci. All of these systems exhibit linkage disequilibrium, i.e., nonrandom association of the alleles of linked loci. Consequently, haplotype frequencies which take linkage disequilibrium into account must be used. In the MNS, Gm, and Rh systems, recombination is either extremely rare or unknown and may be ignored in the calculations. However, in the HLA system, the recombination frequency, Θ, between the HLA-A and -B loci which are most commonly tested in parentage cases is nearly 1% ($\Theta \cong 0.008$). This will have an effect on the likelihood of paternity in cases where the X value begins to approach the recombination rate. The magnitude of this effect is shown for some theoretical values of X and Y in Table 9. In practice, while the extreme differences seen for cases in which $X < Y$ may not occur, an appreciable effect is possible. This is shown by the following example using haplotypes with extreme differences in relative genotype probabilities. The phenotypes are mother, HLA-A2,A3,B7,B44; alleged father, A1,A30,B8,B13; and child, A2,A30,B8,B44. Using HLA haplotype frequencies for Caucasoids assuming $P (A_x) = P(A_y)$ and ignoring Θ, the posterior probability of paternity is 61.49%. When recombination is included in the calculation ($\Theta = 0.008$), the posterior probability is 87.02%.

TABLE 9. The effect of recombination on the probability of paternity[a]

X	Y			
	0.005		0.001	
	NR	R	NR	R
0.4999	99.01	99.00	99.80	99.80
0.4995	99.01	99.00	99.80	99.80
0.4990	99.01	99.00	99.80	99.80
0.4950	99.00	98.99	99.80	99.80
0.4900	98.99	98.98	99.80	99.79
0.4750	98.96	98.95	99.79	99.79
0.4500	98.90	98.89	99.78	99.78
0.4000	98.77	98.76	99.75	99.75
0.1000	95.24	95.34	99.05	99.03
0.0500	90.91	91.41	98.04	98.15
0.0250	83.33	85.12	96.15	96.62
0.0100	66.67	73.46	90.91	93.26
0.0050	50.00	64.08	83.33	89.92
0.0010	16.67	49.92	50.00	83.29
0.0005	9.09	47.32	33.33	81.79
0.0001	1.96	45.05	9.09	80.39

[a] Posterior probabilities were calculated with equal prior probabilities. For each value of Y, a posterior probability was calculated, first ignoring recombination (NR) and then allowing for recombination (R) at a frequency of $\Theta = 0.008$.

Consanguinity

In the discussion of the calculations of X and Y, it was noted that when the mother and the alleged father are drawn from populations in Hardy-Weinberg equilibrium, their genotype probabilities can be determined by applying probability theory and that the probability of observing these two individuals is $P(M)P(AF)$. However, when these individuals are related, their genotypes are not independent since they may share an allele identical by descent. In cases in which the genotypes of the mother or the alleged father, or both, are ambiguous, the effect of that relationship on genotype probabilities must be accounted for in the calculations.

In cases in which the mother claims that two or more possible fathers are related to each other, the calculation of Y cannot be based on population data. In such cases, the likelihood of all possible genotypes of the alleged father and other possible fathers (not tested) must be calculated given the degree of relationships, i.e., whether the alleged father is a first-degree relative, such as mother's father or brother, or a second-degree relative, such as first cousin or grandfather.

This is especially relevant to the assignment of rare genotypes. Returning to the example given above, based on population haplotype frequency, it is almost 400 times more likely that the alleged father's genotype is A1,B8/A30,B13 rather than A30,B8/A1,B13. If we add the information that a first- or second-degree relative of the alleged father has an A30,B8 haplotype, we can intuitively see that the A30,B8/A1,B13 genotype becomes less unlikely for the alleged father.

Deficient information

In cases in which the mother is unavailable for testing, likelihoods may still be calculated for nonexclusions. These ratios will be reduced commensurate with the missing data. Some compensation for missing data is possible if maternal relatives can be tested. The degree of compensation is proportionate to the closeness of the relationships. Maternal grandparents and sibs are particularly useful.

Extended families

In cases in which there is more than one child, all of the individuals tested should be evaluated as a unit. For example, in two-child cases, four hypotheses should be evaluated, i.e., that the alleged father is (i) the father of both children, (ii) the father of the first but not the second child, (iii) the father of the second but not the first child, and (iv) the father of neither child. If the children are evaluated separately, as if this were a series of one-child cases, it is possible to miss exceptional circumstances which could drastically affect the probability, or even eliminate the possibility, of paternity for both children. For example, in a case in which the individuals have the following ABO phenotypes: mother (O), child 1 (A_2), child 2 (O), and alleged father (A_1), we can see that if the children were considered individually, the alleged father would be excluded in neither case. However, if we consider the children simultaneously, we can see that the man cannot be the father of both children. Perhaps the most meaningful probability in this case is the probability that the man is the father of one child, not specifying which one.

Racial admixture

It was noted above that the gene frequencies used should be appropriate for the race of the individuals. This is not possible when the mother or the alleged father, or both, are of mixed racial ancestry. Mickey et al. (11) have dealt with the problem of determining genotype probabilities for such individuals. The question remains concerning what population frequencies to use for the alternative hypothesis. For example, a recent case in one of our laboratories involved a mother whose background was Chinese, Caucasoid, Black, and West Indian. The alleged father was Caucasoid. Because the mother might have chosen another partner from more than one population, three separate calculations of Y were carried out using the frequencies of the White, Black, and Chinese populations. The West Indian Y value could not be calculated because of insufficient gene frequency data from that population.

APPLICATIONS AND LIMITATIONS

By 1983, 33 of the 50 United States had passed legislation permitting the admission into court proceedings of inclusionary as well as exclusionary evidence in cases of disputed parentage. The increased use of this information is encouraging. However, the fact that one-third of the states choose to ignore the usefulness of genetic information is discouraging. Controversy over the admissibility of inclusionary evidence is due, in part, to a lack of understanding by both the public and members of the legal system. For example, in 1982, Page-Bright referred to "recent advances in genetic research" (13), apparently unaware that typing has been available for the markers listed in Table 1 since 1970 and that Bayes' Theorem dates from 1763 (5). Statutes of various states and statements in law journals (reviewed by Ellman and Kaye [7] and Page-Bright [13]) often imply that HLA is something other than a blood test. This reflects, more than anything, a lack of appreciation that the focal point of analysis is the genome and not the blood. Finally, there is the valid concern that a jury will be overwhelmed or "mesmerized" by sheer numbers. Yet, as scientists, we can see that to disregard the genetic and statistical information, or to utilize only part of it, is equally inappropriate. Therefore, if the application of science to questions of paternity is to be properly evaluated, scientists performing such analyses must have sufficient understanding of the principles involved not only to carry out the analyses but also to interpret their meaning to those untrained in genetics and statistics. The probability or odds stated by the scientist are based only on the results of the genetic marker tests performed on blood specimens from the individuals. It is a numerical value used to accept or reject a hypothesis. Those responsible for adjudicating the issue of paternity, and not the scientist, should determine the relative weight to be given to this information. It is incumbent on them to evaluate all evidence in making this determination. Nonetheless, it is the scientist's responsibility not to allow the significance of the data to be diminished by taking less than the utmost care to perform accurate and valid analyses, which include clear communication with nonscientists, i.e., the litigants, their legal counsels, and the jurists.

LITERATURE CITED

1. **American Association for Clinical Histocompatibility Testing.** 1981. Laboratory manual. American Association for Clinical Histocompatibility Testing, New York.
2. **American Association of Blood Banks.** 1977. Technical manual. J. B. Lippincott Co., Philadelphia.
3. **Baur, M. P., and J. A. Danilovs.** 1980. Population analysis of HLA-A,B,C,DR, and other genetic markers, p. 955–993. *In* P. I. Terasaki (ed.), Histocompatibility testing 1980. University of California Tissue Typing Laboratory, Los Angeles.
4. **Baur, M. P., and J. A. Danilovs.** 1980. Reference tables of two- and three-locus haplotype frequencies for HLA-A,B,C,DR,Bf, and GLO, p. 994–1210. *In* P. I. Terasaki (ed.), Histocompatibility testing 1980. University of California Tissue Typing Laboratory, Los Angeles.
5. **Bayes, T.** 1763. An essay towards solving a problem in the doctrine of chances. Phil. Trans. R. Soc. Lond. **53:**370–418.
6. **Bias, W. B., D. A. Meyers, and E. A. Murphy.** 1983. Theoretical underpinnings of paternity testing, p. 51–62. *In* R. H. Walker (ed.), Inclusion probabilities in parentage testing. American Association of Blood Banks, Arlington, Va.
7. **Ellman, I. M., and D. Kaye.** 1979. Probabilities and proof: can HLA and blood group testing prove paternity? N.Y.U. Law Rev. **54:**1131–1162.
8. **Essen-Möller, E., and C.-E. Quensel.** 1939. Zur Theorie das Vaterschaftsnachweises aufgrund von Ähnlichkeitsbefunden. Z. Ges. Gerichtl. Med. **31:**70–96.
9. **Harris, H., and D. A. Hopkinson.** 1976. Handbook of enzyme electrophoresis in human genetics. North-Holland Publishing Co., Amsterdam.
10. **Hummel, K., J. Conradt, and I. Kundinger.** 1981. The realistic prior probability from blood group findings for cases involving one or more men, p. 73–79. *In* K. Hummel and J. Gerchow (ed.), Biomathematical evidence of paternity. Springer-Verlag, New York.
11. **Mickey, M. R., J. Tiwari, J. Bond, D. Gjertson, and P. I. Terasaki.** 1983. Paternity probability calculations for mixed races, p. 325–347. *In* R. H. Walker (ed.), Inclusion probabilities in parentage testing. American Association of Blood Banks, Arlington, Va.
12. **Mourant, A. E., A. C. Kopec, and K. Domaniewska-Sobczak.** 1976. The distribution of the human blood groups and other polymorphisms. Oxford University Press, New York.
13. **Page-Bright, B.** 1982. Proving paternity—human leukocyte antigen test. J. Forensic Sci. **27:**135–153.
14. **Steinberg, A. G., and C. E. Cook.** 1981. The distribution of the human immunoglobulin allotypes. Oxford University Press, New York.

Chapter 139

HLA and Disease

ARNE SVEJGAARD

A variety of human diseases have been found to arise more often in individuals carrying certain HLA antigens than in those lacking them. The associations between HLA and disease have been the subject of several recent reviews (3, 6, 8), and in general they are much stronger than those which have been found between various other blood groups and diseases. This new field of immunogenetic research is likely to be fruitfully continued for some time because new HLA markers are still being discovered and because the existence of such associations may provide insight into not only the genetics but also the etiology of the HLA-associated disorders.

The purpose of this chapter is to outline how such studies may be performed so that the clinical immunologist can plan and perform them and evaluate critically the data reported by other investigators.

It should be stressed that the list of references primarily includes surveys which should be consulted for further detail in case detailed data are needed.

METHODS

Since a simple survey of the HLA system has recently appeared (7) and the techniques for HLA typing have been discussed elsewhere in this manual, only the problems related to the study of HLA in disease are discussed here. In particular, the methodology and the pitfalls inherent in such studies are stressed.

Population studies or family studies, or both, may be used when attempting to establish whether or not the HLA system is involved in the susceptibility or resistance to a disease. In general, population studies are easier to perform, but in some cases a relationship can only be established by family studies. In addition, family studies may help to clarify the genetics of disorders already known to be HLA associated.

Population studies

Population studies require a group of unrelated patients and a group of unrelated healthy control individuals. The selection of these individuals, the sources of typing errors, and the statistical treatment of the results are discussed below.

Selection of patients and controls. Although it may not be of great importance in a preliminary study, it is worth noting that the patients who are HLA typed often represent selected groups; in most cases, these are patients who attend or have attended hospital clinics, and such patients tend to be more severely affected than those who have never been admitted to a hospital. Moreover, the patients who are most troubled by their disease are more likely to cooperate. Thus, the psoriatic patients who have been HLA typed so far are probably biased towards being more severely affected. This is less of a problem for diseases which are inevitably treated in hospitals, but here another

source of bias may arise: in retrospective studies of lethal diseases, patients who die early in the course of the disease obviously "escape" HLA typing, and, accordingly, there is a bias towards too many long-term survivors in the group of patients who are HLA typed. If an HLA antigen is more frequent in such patients than in controls, the possibility should be kept in mind that this HLA antigen confers resistance to death rather than susceptibility to the disease. Such a relationship can only be unraveled by a prospective study of all newly diagnosed patients.

With regard to "unrelatedness" of the patients, it is usually sufficient to ask patients whether they have affected relatives and then to make sure that these are not included in the study. However, for very rare recessive disorders, it is striking how often individuals do not know that they are related. In this context, it should be remembered that patients with such rare recessive disorders often are inbred (e.g., offspring of first cousins or even of incest) and thus homozygous on more loci (including HLA) than outbred individuals. Obviously, patients belonging to the same isolate group often share many genes (e.g., HLA genes and disease genes not linked to HLA), which may cause spurious associations between HLA and a disease.

Special problems arise when studying mixed populations which have not yet reached equilibrium (stratification), and it may be difficult to find good control groups for such patients. For example, it is well known that the degree of Caucasian admixture varies among American Blacks, and American Blacks who develop a "Caucasian" disease are more likely to have more "Caucasian" genes (including HLA) than other Blacks. This may lead to a spurious association between "Caucasian" HLA antigens and a "Caucasian" disease in these patients. On the other hand, an association, for example, between a "Caucasian" disease and an "African" HLA antigen, may be meaningful.

Thus, the selection of a control group may be difficult, and it is worth mentioning that HLA antigen frequencies also vary considerably within the same racial group. However, large amounts of normal materials are now available from different countries (5), and it may be useful to compare the control groups with some of these.

The control groups often consist predominantly of blood donors, and so far it has not been possible to show that these differ from the normal population; if there are differences, they are apparently small. Moreover, the HLA antigen frequencies do not seem to differ between different age groups or between sexes. Accordingly, blood donors constitute in general a satisfying control group, provided ethnic differences are taken into account. Unrelated individuals involved in paternity testing and other healthy randomly selected individuals may also be included.

Serological pitfalls. Serological pitfalls are discussed elsewhere in this manual, but it is worth

TABLE 1. The 2 × 2 table[a]

| Group | No. of individuals: | | Total |
	With antigen	Without antigen	
Patients	a	b	$a + b$
Controls	c	d	$c + d$
Total	$a + c$	$b + d$	$N = a + b + c + d$

[a] Frequency of antigen in patients (hp): $hp = a/(a + b)$. Frequency of antigen in controls (hc): $hc = c/(c + d)$. Relative risk (RR):

$$\text{Woolf's } RR = \frac{ad}{bc} = \frac{hp(1 - hc)}{hc(1 - hp)} \text{ and}$$

$$\text{Haldane's } RR = \frac{(a + \frac{1}{2})(d + \frac{1}{2})}{(b + \frac{1}{2})(c + \frac{1}{2})}.$$

Etiologic fraction (EF):

$$EF = \left(\frac{RR - 1}{RR}\right) hp \text{ for } RR > 1.$$

Preventive fraction (PF):

$$PF = \frac{(1 - RR)hp}{RR(1 - hp) + hp} \text{ for } RR < 1.$$

Chi square (1 degree of freedom [df]):

$$\chi^2 = \frac{(ad - bc)^2 N}{(a + b)(c + d)(a + c)(b + d)}$$

and with Yate's correction

$$\chi^2 = \frac{([ad - bc] - N/2)^2 N}{(a + b)(c + d)(a + c)(b + d)}.$$

For example, in comparing diabetic patients to controls for HLA-DR3 or -DR4, or both, where $a = 120$, $b = 11$, $c = 389$, and $d = 315$ ($N = 835$), the following values are obtained: $hp = 120/131 = 0.916$ (91.6%); $hc = 389/704 = 0.553$ (55.3%); Woolf's $RR = (120 \times 315)/(11 \times 389) = 8.8 = [0.916(1 - 0.553)]/[0.553(1 - 0.916)]$; Haldane's $RR = [(120 + \frac{1}{2})(315 + \frac{1}{2})]/[(11 + \frac{1}{2})(389 + \frac{1}{2})] = 8.5$; $EF [(8.8 - 1)/8.8]0.916 = 0.81$; $\chi^2 = [(120 \times 315 - 11 \times 389)^2 835]/(131 \times 704 \times 509 \times 326) = 61.3$, which for 1 df gives $P \ll 10^{-10}$; Fisher's exact test gives $P = 2 \times 10^{-17}$.

mentioning that in some disorders, e.g., systemic lupus erythematosus, the lymphocytes are more susceptible to the action of antibody and complement, which may cause false-positive reactions due to weak unknown extra antibodies in the typing sera. Chronic lymphocytic leukemia is a special case because most of the circulating leukocytes are B lymphocytes which may react with unknown anti-DR antibodies in the anti-HLA-ABC typing sera.

On the other hand, it has also been found that the treatment of patients with chloramphenicol may cause a disappearance of detectable HLA antigens on lymphocytes, and it is not known whether other drugs have similar properties.

The best way to exclude such typing errors is to type the healthy relatives and determine whether the HLA antigens of the patients are inherited.

Statistical treatment of the results. The comparison between patients and controls is usually done by using a 2 × 2 table (Table 1) for each of the antigens studied. Distinction should be made between the strength of an association and its statistical significance.

The strength is usually estimated by either the relative risk (10) or the etiologic fraction (1, 2). The relative risk is simply the cross-product ratio (equal to the odds ratio) of the four entries in the 2 × 2 table (Table 1). This risk indicates how many times more often the disease occurs in individuals with the antigen compared to those without it. A relative risk greater than one is seen when the antigen is more frequent in patients than in controls and indicates increased risk, whereas decreased frequency of an antigen in the patient group gives a risk less than one, i.e., a decreased risk. When there is no difference between patients and controls, the risk is one. For example, it appears from Table 1 that individuals who are HLA-DR3 or -DR4 positive, or both, have about eight to nine times greater risk of diabetes than individuals who do not carry any of these antigens. The absolute number of patients and controls in the 2 × 2 table is not necessary to estimate the relative risk, as it can also be determined from the frequencies of the antigens in patients and in controls as shown in Table 1, but these numbers (or the total numbers of patients and controls) should always be given, because they are needed for significance testing and for combining various data sources (cf. below).

If an antigen is present or absent in all patients, the relative risk is indefinite or zero, respectively. This is inconvenient for several reasons, and in these cases Haldane's modification (Table 1) can be used.

The etiologic fraction can be estimated when the relative risk is greater than one and is also called the attributable risk at the population level (2) or the delta (1) value. Roughly speaking, this value indicates how much the factor(s) under study contributes to the disease at the population level. It is easily computed from the relative-risk value and the frequency of the antigen in patients, as shown in Table 1. For example, HLA-DR3 and -DR4 together "contribute" about 81% to the susceptibility to insulin-dependent diabetes. It should be noted that the etiologic fractions for different antigens are not additive. Under certain strict conditions, which are rarely fulfilled, the etiologic fraction may give information on the degree of linkage disequilibrium between the markers under study and a hypothetical disease-disposing gene (1).

When the relative risk is less than one, the preventive fraction must be used instead of the etiologic fraction (Table 1). Both of these fractions vary between 0 (no association) and 1.0 (maximal association).

Both the relative risk and the etiologic (preventive) fraction tell something of the biological importance of an association, but these estimates of the strength of an association have rather different meanings: while the relative risk refers to the risk of a single individual, the etiologic fraction refers to the "involvement" of the HLA factor in question in the entire population.

The statistical significance of an association can be evaluated by Fisher's exact test or by various approximate tests, e.g., a chi-square test. Fisher's exact test gives the exact probability (P) of finding differences as extreme as or more extreme than that observed. This is the only reliable test when one or more of the expected numbers in the 2 × 2 table is less than five, but it can also be applied to large samples by using computers. It is a one-sided test, and thus as a crude rule the P value should be multiplied by two if there is no a priori assumption that an antigen has either decreased or increased frequency. When the expected numbers in the 2×2 table are greater than five, the approximation of the chi-square test to the exact test is usually good, and this value is easier to compute (Table 1). Occasionally, Yate's correction for discontinuity is used, but it should be noted that this correction is not a correction for small numbers. When several chi-square values are to be added, Yate's correction must not be used. In addition to the classical chi-square test shown in Table 1, an extension of the relative risks may also be used to create chi-square values (see Table 4).

The main reason to stress the distinction between the strength and the statistical significance is that a relative risk may well be high but insignificant (when the number of patients or controls, or both, is low), and, conversely, a risk differing only slightly from unity may do so in a statistically highly significant way when large numbers of individuals have been studied.

The level of significance is somewhat complicated in these studies because numerous antigen frequencies are usually compared between patients and controls. Usually, 20 or more antigens are studied, and on an average one of these will differ significantly at the 5% probability level by chance alone, i.e., if there is no true difference. This phenomenon (type I or alpha error) may be taken into account by multiplying the P values by the number of antigens studied. Moreover, if additional comparisons are made (e.g., of various subgroups of patients or of various phenotypic combinations), correction should be done for all comparisons. For example, if 30 antigens are compared between three subgroups of patients, each two-sided P value should be multiplied by $3 \times 30 = 90$. Although this correction yields a conservative measure, I would still recommend that the P values after multiplication be evaluated by the following scheme: $0.05 > P > 0.01$ is probably significant; $0.01 > P > 0.001$ is significant; and $P < 0.001$ is highly significant. A P value of 0.05 indicates that the observed difference will be found in 1 of 20 random investigations if there is no difference, and "1-in-20" is not a rare occurrence. Obviously, multiplication times the number of comparisons made is not necessary in a second study showing deviation of the same antigen in the same disease. In fact, such subsequent studies are the best way to prove or disprove an association.

It is sometimes assumed that the number of controls should equal the number of patients. This is a misunderstanding, but it derives from the fact that, if a difference is to be established by investigating the smallest possible number of individuals (patients plus controls), this is done by investigating equal numbers in the two groups. If possible, however, it is convenient to have a large control group, because this gives more accurate estimates of the antigen frequencies and the risk and because it increases the statistical significance of an association. In this relation, it is worth noting that even with a large amount of control material it is more difficult to establish a decreased than an increased frequency of an antigen with a

TABLE 2. Associations detectable as significant in various sample sizes

Frequency (%) of character in controls	Lower/upper limits of frequencies (%) of character in patients with a patient (no.):control (no.) sample size of [a]:			
	20:10	20:20	50:50	100:100
0	/10	/50	/24	/12
10	/45	/70	/42	/31
20	/60	/80	/58	3/44
30	/75	/90	2/68	9/56
40	0/85	/95	8/76	16/66
50	10/90	0/100	14/86	25/75
60	15/100	5/	24/92	34/84
70	25/	10/	32/98	44/91
80	40/	20/	44/	56/97
90	55/	30/	58/	69/
100	90/	50/	76/	88/

[a] Limits detectable as significant (one-sided, noncorrected $P = 0.00025$). The minimal and maximal relative-risk values for increased and decreased risks, respectively, were as follows for the four groups: 20:10, 0.17–6.0; 20:20, 0.06–16.0; 50:50, 0.21–4.8; 100:100, 0.33–3.0.

frequency below 50% in controls. In the former case, more patients should be studied.

Table 2 gives the lower and upper limits of the antigen frequencies in patients which can be shown to be significantly different in various sample sizes of patients and controls. The significance level, one-sided $P = 0.00025$, corresponds to a borderline significance level ($P_c = 0.05$) when correction is made for one-sidedness and 100 comparisons are made, which may easily be the case when polymorphic DNA markers are included. Indeed, the study of DNA markers has just begun, and therefore the number of controls will be limited for some time; this is why we used equal numbers of patients and controls in three of the examples. It appears that when only 20 patients and 20 controls are studied, only very strong association can be demonstrated (risks outside the range 0.06 to 16.0), whereas studies of 50 patients and 50 controls are about as powerful as studies of 20 patients and 10,000 controls. It may be concluded that even when resources are limited, more than 20 patients and 20 controls should be studied. If attempts are made to establish which markers show the strongest association (cf. below), even 50 patients and 50 controls are low numbers.

Table 3 shows an analysis of the HLA-A and -B antigen frequencies in an early study of 85 patients with insulin-dependent diabetes compared with 1,967 controls. It appears that only the P values for HLA-B7 and -B8 can stand the test of being multiplied times 2 (for one-sidedness) and 23 (for the number of antigens investigated). The increase of HLA-B15 remains probably significant after this procedure, whereas all other P values are insignificant. It is now clearly established that the positive associations for HLA-B8 and -B15 in this disease are due to linkage disequilibrium between these markers and HLA-DR3 and -DR4, respectively, which show stronger associations than do HLA-B8 and -B15, and that the decreased frequency of HLA-B7 is secondary to an almost entire absence of HLA-DR2 (cf. below).

Combination of data from various sources cannot be done by simply adding the entries in the 2×2 tables,

TABLE 3. HLA antigen frequencies (%) in juvenile diabetes and controls

Antigen	Controls (N = 1,967)	Patients (N = 85)	Relative risk	Fisher's P	P × 2 × 23
HLA-A1	31.1	32.9	1.09	0.40	
HLA-A2	53.6	64.7	1.58	0.03	1.4
HLA-A3	26.9	25.9	0.95	0.47	
HLA-A9	17.3	27.1	1.78	0.02	0.92
HLA-A10	9.6	5.9	0.59	0.17	
HLA-A11	10.1	7.1	0.68	0.24	
HLA-A28	10.0	7.1	0.69	0.25	
HLA-Aw19	17.8	7.1	0.35	0.004	0.18
HLA-B5	10.6	7.1	0.64	0.19	
HLA-B7	26.8	10.6	0.32	0.0003	0.01
HLA-B8	23.7	44.7	2.60	0.00003	0.001
HLA-B12	25.2	16.5	0.57	0.03	1.4
HLA-B13	4.3	4.5	1.06	0.54	
HLA-B14	4.5	0.0	0.00	0.02	0.92
HLA-B15	17.9	32.9	2.25	0.0008	0.04
HLA-B16	5.4	10.6	2.08	0.04	1.84
HLA-B17	7.7	4.7	0.59	0.22	
HLA-B18	7.1	9.4	1.36	0.26	
HLA-B21	3.5	2.4	0.68	0.44	
HLA-B22	3.8	2.4	0.61	0.37	
HLA-B27	8.6	14.1	1.74	0.07	
HLA-B35	13.1	10.6	0.79	0.32	
HLA-B40	17.9	18.8	1.06	0.47	

as this may give spurious values for both the risk and the significance. A procedure which can be used was developed by Woolf (10), and a worked-out example is shown in Table 4 for HLA-B8 in immunoglobulin A (IgA) deficiency in blood donors. The relative risk varies considerably (from 2.4 to 8.4) between the three different studies, but the calculations show that there is no significant heterogeneity between the three risks, and, accordingly, the combined estimate of the relative risk (3.0) gives the best picture of the situation. In addition, the deviation of this estimate is extremely significant. On the basis of the combined estimate, it is possible to calculate the most likely frequency of HLA-B8 in a given population by means of the formula: $hp = X \times hc/(1 - hc + X \times hc)$, where hp and hc are the frequencies of B8 in patients and controls, respectively, and X is the relative risk. For example, in the third population the control frequency of B8 is $hc = 812/(812 + 2489) = 0.246$, and the best estimate of hp in this population now is $hp = 3.0 \times 0.246/(1 - 0.246$

$+ 3.0 \times 0.246) = 0.495$ or 49.5%. Incidentally, the increased frequency of B8 in this condition has subsequently been shown to be due to a stronger increase of DR3.

Which markers are most strongly associated? The question of which markers are primarily involved is, of course, difficult to answer as long as we do not know all HLA markers and their functions. However, it is possible to investigate which markers from the different segregant series show the strongest association. The magnitude of the relative risk or the etiologic fraction may give some indications in this direction, but it is often difficult to obtain significant differences between the relative risks for two different factors known to be in linkage disequilibrium with each other in the general population. When the associations of two factors from two different series are compared, it is useful to test whether one of them shows an association both in individuals carrying and in those lacking the other factor. This procedure is exemplified in Table 5, where we first compared the frequency of DR3 in B8-positive patients with insulin-dependent diabetes with that in a corresponding group of controls. It appears that DR3 is significantly ($P = 0.027$) increased in this subgroup with an odds ratio of 7.2. It also appears that DR3 is significantly increased in B8-negative patients as compared to B8-negative controls. Accordingly, DR3 is increased in both B8-positive and B8-negative patients. In contrast, when making the opposite comparisons, it appears that B8 is not increased in either DR3-positive or DR3-negative patients. Thus, we conclude that the B8 association in insulin-dependent diabetes is entirely secondary to a stronger association with DR3 and is solely due to the well-known linkage disequilibrium between B8 and DR3. However, it is as yet unknown whether the primary (causative) association is with the DR3 determinant itself or with another still unknown HLA factor associated with this determinant.

The analysis illustrated in Table 5 does not always give such clear-cut results; sometimes it is difficult to decide whether the association involves just one or both factors. This may be the case when there are few data, when both factors are indeed associated, or when the association primarily involves a factor controlled by a gene located between those controlling the two factors investigated. It is sometimes assumed that an entire haplotype (e.g., *HLA-A1,B8,DR3*) is associated. In general, this is difficult to test when

TABLE 4. Calculation of combined relative risk of IgA deficiency in HLA-B8-positive individuals[a]

Study no.	No. of patients B8+ (a)	No. of patients B8− (b)	No. of controls B8+ (c)	No. of controls B8− (d)	Relative risk (x = ad/bc)	y = ln x	Variance of y (V = 1/a + 1/b + 1/c + 1/d)	Weight (w = 1/V)	yw	χ² = Y²w
1	27	35	137	471	2.65	0.975	0.0750	13.33	13.00	12.68
2	14	5	68	204	8.40	2.128	0.2910	3.44	7.32	15.58
3	14	18	812	2,489	2.38	0.867	0.1286	7.78	6.75	5.85
Total								24.55	27.07	34.11

[a] Combined estimate, $Y = \Sigma wy/\Sigma w = 27.07/24.55 = 1.1026$; combined estimate of relative risk, $X = \text{antilog}_e Y = 3.01$; standard deviation of $Y = 1/\sqrt{\Sigma w} = 1/\sqrt{24.55} = 0.2018$; 95% limits of $Y = 1.1026 \pm 1.96 \times 0.2018 = 0.7071$ and 1.4981; 95% limits of $X = \text{antilog}_e 0.7071$ and $\text{antilog}_e 1.4981 = 2.03$ and 4.47; significance test for relative risk differing from 1.0 = $\chi^2_{signif.} = Y^2\Sigma w = (1.1026)^2 \times 24.55 = 29.85$, which for 1 degree of freedom (df) gives $P = 10^{-8}$; test for heterogeneity between the three sets of data: $\chi^2_{het.} = \chi^2_{total} - \chi^2_{signif.} = 34.11 - 29.85 = 4.26$, which for 2 df (number of studies minus one) gives $P = 0.12$. Data obtained from reference 8.

TABLE 5. Testing which factor is most strongly associated[a]

Group and population	No. of individuals in which factor[b] is:		Odds ratio[c]	P
	Present	Absent		
HLA-B8[+]				
Diabetics	35	1	7.2	0.027
Controls	58	12		
HLA-B8[-]				
Diabetics	15	42	3.7	0.001
Controls	17	174		
HLA-DR3[+]				
Diabetics	35	15	0.72	0.28
Controls	58	18		
HLA-DR3[-]				
Diabetics	1	42	0.32	0.22
Controls	13	172		

[a] Data obtained from reference 4.
[b] Factor: DR3 for HLA-B8[+] and -B8[-] populations, B8 for HLA-DR3[+] and -DR3[-] populations.
[c] The odds ratio corresponds to the relative risk.

dealing with common haplotypes. The results in Table 5 argue against this possibility for the *HLA-B8,DR3* haplotype in insulin-dependent diabetes.

The problems of defining the strongest association become increasingly more difficult the stronger the linkage disequilibrium between the factors under examination, i.e., the closer the corresponding genes are located on the chromosome. Thus, it may be anticipated that it will be difficult to decide between various possibilities when DNA markers are also included in these studies.

Family studies

When an association has been established in unrelated individuals, it is usually worthwhile to perform family studies to obtain further insight into the genetics of the disorder. On the other hand, diseases not associated with known HLA factors may still be controlled by unknown HLA factors not strongly associated with known ones. This relationship can only be clarified by family studies.

The simplest form of family study consists of questioning the propositi of a possible family history, keeping in mind that the patients are not always informed on whether their relatives are affected or not. The relevant figure concerns the frequency of the disease among first-degree relatives: parents, siblings, and children. These groups should be treated separately until it is seen that there are no differences between them; e.g., the incidence in children is usually lower than in parents and siblings if the disease does not have an early onset. It is not sufficient to know that there are one or two affected siblings or children; the total numbers of siblings and children must be known. By comparing the frequency of the disease in first-degree relatives of patients carrying the disease-associated HLA factor with the corresponding frequency for the remaining patients, it may, for example, be found that the former patients have more affected relatives, which indicates that if other HLA factors are involved then they are not as important.

A more laborious kind of family study is the typing of kindreds with more than one affected member to see whether the disease is always inherited together with the disease-associated HLA antigen. One important pitfall in such family studies is the biased ascertainment of the families, as they are selected because they contain two or more affected members. Accordingly, they are likely to possess more disease liability genes than families with isolated cases.

Perhaps the worst difficulty in family studies derives from the fact that most diseases have varying degrees of penetrance and varying age at onset because environment plays a role in their manifestations (i.e., they are multifactorial). Hence, the absence of psoriasis in a Cw6-positive relative of a Cw6-positive psoriatic is not informative, since the disease may become manifest at a later time. Phrased more directly: only affected relatives are really informative. Nevertheless, when the ages are taken into account, such family studies may provide important information regarding the risk of developing the disease for relatives with various HLA phenotypes.

In several cases, important information may be obtained by typing affected sibling pairs (sib pairs), or triplets, and investigating the proportions of sib pairs sharing both, one, or no parental haplotypes (9). It is worth noting that two siblings with the phenotypes of, say, HLA-A1,2;B7,8 and HLA-A1,9;B8,12 need not share the same parental *HLA-A1;B8* haplotype; the parents should also be typed if possible to clarify the situation.

If the HLA system is not involved in the development of a disease, affected sib pairs will share HLA haplotypes with the same frequencies as seen in healthy sib pairs from normal families: one-fourth of the pairs will share both, one-half will share one, and the remaining one-fourth will share none of the parental haplotypes. Accordingly, if the proportion of haplotype sharing differs from this expectation (1:2:1), it has been established that the HLA system is involved in the disease in question and that this is true whether or not the disease shows HLA association(s) at the population level. Indeed, for diseases without associations with known HLA factors, sib-pair studies are useful in determining whether the HLA system plays a role for that disease. Moreover, even for HLA-associated disorders, the sib-pair method provides additional useful information.

The degree of haplotype sharing depends on the mode of inheritance and the frequency of the disease susceptibility gene. If the susceptibility is simple recessive (with or without complete penetrance) and the frequency of the susceptibility gene is low (e.g., 0.01), virtually all affected sib pairs will be HLA identical; in such cases, only four affected sib pairs are needed to demonstrate the association ($[1/4]^4 = 0.004$). If the susceptibility is dominant and the gene is rare, almost all affected sib pairs will share one or both haplotypes, and at least 16 pairs are needed to obtain significance at the 1% probability level ($[3/4]^{16} = 0.01$). However, if the gene is more frequent, these clear-cut pictures will not be seen; but even here the actual distribution of haplotype sharing among affected sib pairs may be used to test various genetic models.

TABLE 6. HLA haplotype sharing in sib pairs affected with insulin-dependent diabetes or rheumatoid arthritis[a]

No. of haplotypes shared (expected frequency)	Diabetes				Rheumatoid arthritis			
	No. of sib pairs observed	Frequency (%)	No. expected	χ^2	No. of sib pairs observed	Frequency (%)	No. expected	χ^2
2 (25%)	154	58.6	65.8	118.2	10	20	12.3	0.43
1 (50%)	97	36.9	131.5	9.1	28	57	24.5	0.50
0 (25%)	12	4.6	65.8	44.0	11	22	12.3	0.14

[a] Data was obtained from reference 4 and from the 9th International Histocompatibility Workshop. χ^2 = (no. of sib pairs observed − no. expected)^2/no. of sib pairs expected. Total χ^2 values are 171.3 ($P = 10^{-37}$ for 2 degrees of freedom [df]) and 1.07 ($P = 0.59$ for 2 df) for diabetes and rheumatoid arthritis, respectively.

Table 6 shows the degree of haplotype sharing observed in sib pairs affected with insulin-dependent diabetes or rheumatoid arthritis. For insulin-dependent diabetes, the distribution is highly significantly different from that expected. This observed distribution has been used directly to rule out a dominant model for all possible frequencies of the hypothetical diabetes susceptibility gene and indirectly to exclude a recessive model because this would only be compatible with the observations for gene frequencies which are so high that they do not fit population and family frequencies for this disease. In contrast, the sib-pair data on rheumatoid arthritis do not differ from expectations despite the well-established association between this disease and HLA-DR4. This observation may be explained by the possibility that the frequency of the rheumatoid-arthritis susceptibility gene is common and that the penetrance is low. This example illustrates that family studies may not always reveal a relationship between HLA and a disease.

For diseases (or conditions) inherited in a simple Mendelian way (autosomal dominant or recessive), the HLA system is very powerful in classical linkage studies. In the case of recessivity, even families with just one affected child give information provided there is one or more healthy siblings to the propositus. Special computer programs have been developed for linkage studies, and some can even take into account incomplete penetrance and various age-at-onset values. Classical linkage studies showed, for example, that C2 deficiency and congenital adrenal hyperplasia are closely linked to HLA.

ASSOCIATIONS

Table 7 lists the most important associations which have so far been established between various HLA factors and certain diseases. Only the antigens showing the supposedly strongest associations are indicated. It appears clearly that most of the associations primarily involve HLA-DR antigens, but it should be noted that HLA-DP and -DQ antigens and complement variants have generally only been studied to a limited degree or not at all. The strength of the various associations varies considerably both when expressed as the relative risk and as the etiologic fraction. For example, the two malignant disorders, Hodgkin's disease and acute lymphatic leukemia, show very weak associations whereas most of the remaining associations are strong. It should be stressed that the strength of an association at the population level may not reflect the true involvement of HLA in the disease in question. This is exemplified

by the fact that the entire genetic background of congenital adrenal hyperplasia is located in the HLA region, but the association between this disorder and HLA-B47 is far from absolute.

IMPLICATIONS

The associations, at the population level or in families, between HLA and disease have both scientific implications and more theoretical and practical clinical implications because these associations may be relevant in relation to the subdivision, genetics, etiology and pathogenesis, diagnosis, prophylaxis, and prognosis of various diseases.

Disease heterogeneity

In several cases, HLA studies have substantiated and extended earlier clinical assumptions that certain diseases are heterogeneous, i.e., that they consist of various entities. Perhaps the most marked example is diabetes, which was previously divided on the basis of age at onset in a juvenile form also characterized by occurrence in nonobese individuals requiring insulin. However, many endocrinologists and geneticists still held that the two forms represented different presentations of the same underlying disorder. Now, HLA studies have clearly shown that it is only the insulin-dependent form which is associated with HLA irrespective of the age at onset, whereas the non-insulin-dependent form is not HLA associated. This subdivision is obviously of great importance both because it shows that the two forms must have different pathogenetic mechanisms and because distinction between the two forms must also be made in analyses of their genetic backgrounds. Even within insulin-dependent diabetes, it has been hoped that the associations with DR3 on the one hand and DR4 on the other might help to distinguish two different subtypes of this disease, but so far attempts to demonstrate this have given equivocal results.

Some associations may also be used to tie various diseases together. For example, the HLA-B27 associations for ankylosing spondylitis, Reiter's disease, reactive arthropathy, and acute anterior uveitis indicate that these disorders may have a pathogenetic pathway in common.

Genetics

Two of the diseases in Table 7 were known in advance to have a clear-cut autosomal recessive mode of inheritance: congenital adrenal hyperplasia and

TABLE 7. Associations between HLA and some diseases[a]

Condition	HLA	Frequency (%) in:		RR	EF
		Patients	Controls		
Hodgkin's disease	A1	40	32.0	1.4	0.12
Acute lymphatic leukemia	A2	62	53.3	1.4	0.18
Idiopathic hemochromatosis	A3	76	28.2	8.2	0.67
	B14	16	3.8	4.7	0.13
Behcet's disease	B5	41	10.1	6.3	0.34
Congenital adrenal hyperplasia	B47	9	0.6	15.4	0.08
Ankylosing spondylitis	B27	90	9.4	87.4	0.89
Reiter's disease	B27	79	9.4	37.0	0.77
Acute anterior uveitis	B27	52	9.4	10.4	0.47
Subacute thyroiditis	B35	70	14.6	13.7	0.65
Psoriasis vulgaris	Cw6	87	33.1	13.3	0.81
Dermatitis herpetiformis	DR3	85	26.3	15.4	0.80
Celiac disease	DR3[b]	79	26.3	10.8	0.72
IgA deficiency in blood donors	DR3[b]	64	26.3	5.0	0.51
Sicca syndrome	DR3	78	26.3	9.7	0.70
Idiopathic Addison's disease	DR3	69	26.3	6.3	0.58
Graves' disease	DR3	56	26.3	3.7	0.42
Insulin-dependent diabetes	DR3, 4, or both	91	57.3	7.9	0.80
	DR2	10	30.5	0.2	—
Myasthenia gravis	DR3	47	26.3	2.5	0.28
SLE	DR3	67	26.3	5.8	0.55
Idiopathic membraneous nephropathy	DR3	75	20.0	12.0	0.69
Zw[a]-immunized mothers[c]	DR3	95	15	113	0.94
Narcolepsy	DR2	100	25.8	—	1.00
Multiple sclerosis	DR2	59	25.8	4.1	0.45
Optic neuritis	DR2	46	25.8	2.4	0.27
Goodpasture's syndrome	DR2	88	32.0	15.9	0.82
Rheumatoid arthritis	DR4	69	32.1	4.7	0.54
Pemphigus	DR4	87	32.1	14.4	0.81
IgA nephropathy	DR4	49	19.5	4.0	0.37
Hydralazine-induced SLE	DR4	73	32.7	5.6	0.60
Postpartum thyroiditis	DR4	72	32.2	5.3	0.58
Hashimota's thyroiditis	DR5	19	6.9	3.2	0.13
Pernicious anemia	DR5	25	5.8	5.4	0.20
Juvenile rheumatoid arthritis	DRw8	23	7.5	3.6	0.17
	B27	25	9.4	3.2	0.17
Primary glomerulonephritis	C4B* 2.9[d]	25	1.5	22.0	0.24

[a] These data derive from many different sources (6, 8). Most of the antigen frequencies refer to a Danish population, but when just one study has been reported, the frequencies given in that population are used. All data refer to Caucasoids. *RR*, Relative risk; *EF*, etiologic factor; SLE, systemic lupus erythematosus. In the case of C2 deficiency, the *A25,B18,DR2* haplotype increased.

[b] DR7 also increased.

[c] Zw[a] is a platelet-specific alloantigen.

[d] C4B* 2.9 is a rare variant of complement factor C4B.

complement factor C2 deficiency. Both of these were easily shown to be closely linked to the HLA system, and subsequent studies have shown that the genes responsible for these conditions are located between the HLA-B and -DR loci. These two conditions are both present at birth and have complete penetrance (i.e., they are always expressed in individuals with the genetic background), which is in contrast to the remaining disorders in Table 7, all of which are characterized by varying age at onset and, in most cases, incomplete penetrance, making genetic analyses more difficult. The penetrance of a disease can be established by twin studies: if it is complete, monozygotic twins will always be concordant for the disease.

HLA studies made it clear that idiopathic hemochromatosis is also an autosomal recessive disease with an almost complete penetrance, but here the age at onset is variable, and it rarely manifests itself until after the age of 20 years.

HLA studies also revealed that the genetic susceptibility to ankylosing spondylitis is largely due to an HLA gene with dominant action. This gene may be either *HLA-B27* itself or an as yet unknown HLA gene closely associated with *B27*. However, the penetrance is not complete. The disease is not purely genetic, and the same is true of virtually all of the other diseases listed in Table 7 (except the autosomal recessive ones just mentioned): they are not inherited as such; it is the susceptibility to these diseases which is inherited. The HLA associations show that at least part of this genetic susceptibility is due to one or more genes in the HLA region.

One of the diseases which has been the subject of the most intensive genetic studies, including HLA, is insulin-dependent diabetes, but as yet no final conclusions have been reached concerning how the susceptibility is inherited. Although, as mentioned above, both dominant and recessive models (with or without complete penetrance) have been ruled out, a model intermediate between dominance and recessivity is still possible. However, we favor the possibility that there is more than one HLA gene which causes susceptibility to insulin-dependent diabetes, each by its own mechanism.

Mechanisms which can explain the association

It is beyond the scope of this chapter to go into the details of the mechanisms which can explain the associations, but some of those which have been suggested most often are summarized below with reference to our present knowledge of the biological function of the HLA system.

It is now generally accepted that the class II molecules (e.g., HLA-DR, -DP, and -DQ) are the immune response (Ir) determinants in humans which are involved in the presentation of antigen in the early phase of the thymus-dependent immune response. There is also increasing evidence that the HLA-D region may control immune suppression (Is) determinants. Accordingly, it seems that most of the HLA-DR associations listed in Table 7 are due to the action of the Ir or Is determinants, or both. Perhaps the best candidate of an Ir gene involvement is the maternal immunization against the fetal, platelet-specific Zw^a antigen. Other likely candidates are dermatitis herpetiformis and celiac disease, which both seem to involve hypersensitivity to a component in gluten. Most of the other DR-associated disorders are characterized by various degrees of autoimmunity, which again supports the assumption of Ir or Is gene involvement, but the specificities of the corresponding determinants are unknown.

Class I, i.e., HLA-ABC molecules are also involved in thymus-dependent immune responses, but they play their role at a later stage, i.e., in the lysis of virus-infected or hapten-conjugated target cells by cytotoxic killer T lymphocytes. However, at present it is entirely unknown whether this mechanism is the basis for some of the HLA-ABC associations. Indeed, in congenital adrenal hyperplasia and idiopathic hemochromatosis, thymus-dependent immunity is not involved: the former seems to be due to the absence of a gene controlling 21-hydroxylase in the adrenal cortex, and the latter to the absence of a gene controlling absorption of iron from the gut. These two examples illustrate that caution is needed when conclusions are drawn from a mere HLA association to the pathogenesis of a disease.

The class III (complement) molecules are involved in the elimination of certain bacteria and in the handling of immune complexes, which agrees with the observation that C2 and in particular C4 deficiencies are characterized by increased susceptibility to certain infections and to lupuslike syndromes. It is conceivable that less severe quantitative deficiencies and perhaps qualitative differences between variants may also predispose to certain diseases, in particular when immune complexes are involved, e.g., glomerulonephritis.

Finally, as mentioned above, the HLA system also controls some nonimmune functions. For example, there is evidence that class I molecules are involved in the interactions between certain ligands (e.g., hormones) and their receptors on the cell surface. Thus, there is ample room for speculations concerning the mechanisms behind the HLA associations.

CLINICAL APPLICATIONS

Diagnosis

Typing for HLA-B27 has become a diagnostic tool in doubtful cases of ankylosing spondylitis or Reiter's disease because it can be considered a diagnostic test with about 8.5% false-positive results (the average frequency in Caucasoids of European ancestry) and about 10 and 23% false-negative results (the frequencies of B27-negative patients with ankylosing spondylitis and Reiter's disease, respectively). As illustrated in Table 8, the power of this test depends strongly on the a priori probability of the disease in question. For example, if the a priori probability of ankylosing spondylitis is 50%, then the a posteriori probabilities of the disease are $(1 - 0.1) \times 0.5/[(1 - 0.1) \times 0.5 + 0.085 (1 - 0.5)] = 0.91$ or 91% if the patient is B27 positive but only $0.1 \times 0.5/[0.1 \times 0.5 + (1 - 0.085)(1 - 0.5)] = 0.10$ or 10% if the patient is B27 negative. It should be noted that when the a priori probability is high (say 70% or more), the a posteriori probabilities are still high even in B27-negative patients, indicating that HLA typing is of limited value for routine purposes in such cases.

Apart from these two conditions, diagnostic use of HLA typing for routine purposes would only be indicated in very rare cases at the present time. However, this situation may change, for example, if better markers become available for a given disease (e.g., multiple sclerosis). Moreover, HLA typing may also be indicated for scientific purposes in certain clinical research projects.

A special case of diagnostic use of HLA typing arises when a couple has given birth to a child with congenital adrenal hyperplasia due to 21-hydroxylase deficiency (11- and 17-hydroxylase deficiencies are not linked to HLA). In subsequent pregnancies, it is possible to determine the affection status of the expected

TABLE 8. Diagnostic value of HLA typing: dependency of a posteriori probabilities of disease (after HLA typing) on the a priori probabilities[a]

A priori probability (%)	A posteriori probability (%) for subjects with (+) and without (−) antigen HLA-B27 in:			
	Ankylosing spondylitis		Reiter's disease	
	+	−	+	−
10	54	1	50	3
20	73	3	69	6
30	82	5	80	10
40	88	7	86	14
50	91	10	90	20
60	94	14	93	27
70	96	20	95	37
80	98	30	97	50
90	99	50	99	69

[a] Frequencies of HLA-B27 were 8.5 in controls and 90 and 77% in ankylosing spondylitis and Reiter's disease, respectively.

child by HLA typing the patients, the parents, and fetal cells. If the latter are HLA genotypically identical to those of the patient, the expected child is also affected, and the parents may be offered an abortion. HLA typing of fetal cells is not always easy, but it may be anticipated that such prenatal diagnosis becomes easier when the DNA technology is refined.

Prophylaxis

The above prenatal diagnostic use of HLA typing may also be considered prophylactic. Another case for the application of HLA typing in prophylaxis is idiopathic hemachromatosis. By typing the proband, the parents, and the siblings, it can be established which of the latter has the genetic background of this disease, i.e., those who are HLA genotypically identical to the proband. The iron status of such siblings should be followed so that depletion of excessive iron stores can be instituted before irreversible organ damage develops.

Prognosis

In certain cases, the prognosis of an HLA-associated disease is related to the HLA type of the patient. For example, Reiter's disease and reactive arthropathy runs a more severe and prolonged course in B27-positive than in B27-negative patients. Multiple sclerosis progresses more rapidly in DR2-positive than in DR2-negative patients, and Graves' disease relapses more frequently after medical treatment in DR3-positive than in DR3-negative patients. However, the practical, clinical value of these relationships is limited.

This study was aided by grants from the Medical Research Councils of Denmark and the European Economic Community.

The expert secretarial assistance of Christina Dam-Sørensen is gratefully acknowledged.

LITERATURE CITED

1. **Bengtsson, B. O., and G. Thomson.** 1981. Measuring the strength of associations between HLA antigens and diseases. Tissue Antigens **17:**356–363.
2. **Green, A.** 1982. The epidemiologic approach to studies of association between HLA and disease. II. Estimation of absolute risks, etiologic and preventive fraction. Tissue Antigens **19:**259–268.
3. **Möller, G. (ed.).** 1983. HLA and disease susceptibility. Immunol. Rev. **70:**1–218.
4. **Platz, P., B. K. Jakobsen, N. Morling, L. P. Ryder, A. Svejgaard, M. Thomsen, M. Christy, H. Kromann, J. Benn, J. Nerup, A. Green, and M. Hauge.** 1981. HLA-D and -DR antigens in genetical analysis of insulin-dependent diabetes mellitus. Diabetologia **21:**108–115.
5. **Ryder, L. P., E. Andersen, and A. Svejgaard (ed.).** 1978. An HLA map of Europe. Hum. Hered. **28:**171–210.
6. **Ryder, L. P., E. Andersen, and A. Svejgaard (ed.).** 1979. HLA and Disease Registry, 3rd report. Munksgaard, Copenhagen.
7. **Svejgaard, A., M. Hauge, C. Jersild, P. Platz, L. P. Ryder, L. Staub Nielsen, and M. Thomsen.** 1979. The HLA system: an introductory survey, 2nd revised ed. S. Karger, Basel.
8. **Svejgaard, A., P. Platz, and L. P. Ryder.** 1983. HLA and disease 1982—a survey. Immunol. Rev. **70:**193–218.
9. **Suarez, B., D. O'Rourke, and P. van Eerdewegh.** 1982. Power of the affected-sib-pair method to detect disease susceptibility loci of small effect: an application to multiple sclerosis. Am. J. Med. Genet. **12:**309–326.
10. **Woolf, B.** 1955. On estimating the relation between blood group and disease. Ann. Hum. Genet. **19:**251–253.

Chapter 140

Section O. Immunopathology and Immunohistology

Introduction

DAVID T. ROWLANDS, JR.

Tissue methods are assuming increasing significance in clinical and laboratory immunology. The fundamental technology of these methods has long been the central armamentarium of pathologists, in that special stains on appropriately prepared specimens have been available for much of this century and immunologic methods have been applied to tissue sections for several decades. The recent development of improved methods for localizing antibodies in tissues and the nearly concurrent development of monoclonal antibody technology have significantly enlarged the repertoire of methods for identifying tissue antigens, including those of neoplasms.

Because of the obvious implications of these methods in the field of immunologic diagnosis, it was considered appropriate to include basic information relative to these methods in this manual. The first chapter deals with the use of immunofluorescence in tissues. The second chapter is concerned with the use of immunohistochemistry to better define undifferentiated malignant tumors. The third presentation introduces the methodology used in now-conventional electron microscopy. The fourth paper outlines the state of the art in immunologic diagnoses that make use of lymphocytes in solid tissues. The final presentation is a more detailed view of nonlymphocyte tumor markers.

With the exception of electron microscopy, the required instrumentation is relatively simple. An abundance of suitable reagent kits is becoming available commercially, so variability in reagent quality can now be generally avoided. However, as will become clear in the various presentations, it is necessary to observe and apply care and attention to technical details to avoid significant interpretive errors.

Many of the methods demand the use of fresh, quick-frozen tissues, but the methods at hand are being constantly adapted to use paraffin sections. This state of the art means that many studies can be done only on surgically removed tissues. These constraints are most critical in the case of fluorescence and electron microscopic studies. Enzyme-linked assays are perhaps more generally applicable to paraffin-embedded tissues than are methods which use fluorescent tags. The tissue fixative is an obvious corollary to these concerns for morphologic and antigen preservation. The appropriate fixative varies with the assay to be employed. The tissues themselves are of lesser importance. Among the blood-forming organs likely to be important to immunologists, the spleen holds a special place in that its sections must be exceedingly thin (1 to 2 mm) if proper penetration of the fixative is to occur. The preparation of tissues for staining and evaluation is equally important. The ultimate objective is to maintain tissue and cell structures along with antigenicity. The methods used for fixation and preparation are the main determinants of how rapidly the tissues must be used and the conditions necessary for storage. For example, frozen sections will, in some cases, provide optimum preservation of antigens but will preserve structure less well. Tissues preserved as frozen sections require special care, with facilities for storage at −70°C being needed in most instances. Even under these austere conditions, the degree of preservation will vary with the antigen in question. Little is available in the way of general principles as to which antigens are well preserved under these conditions, so trial and error is required when new systems are under study.

Certain studies will require that cells be prepared as single cell suspensions or be treated with enzymes or both. The single cell suspension of lymphoid cells is done by gently teasing the tissues into small fragments and passing the cells through a wire mesh. Enzymes, such as trypsin, may be needed to separate these cells. Such treatment causes little cellular injury. Instead, the reactivity of antigens on the cell surfaces appears enhanced. This enhanced activity may be due to the removal of interfering substances. A second method for the removal of surface contaminants is the overnight incubation of cells in appropriate medium. Care must be taken to ensure that the cells remain viable during this incubation and that there is no selective loss of cell populations. This precaution is especially important in populations of abnormal cells. Estimations of viability can be made by direct observations of the cells or, better, by the ability of these cells to exclude vital dyes.

The staining methods alluded to will provide the means for localization of antigens. It will still be essential to be able to evaluate the structures of the cells and tissues involved. In some cases, this evaluation will be made directly, without staining, whereas in other cases, staining will be required to classify the cells by conventional criteria and to evaluate tissue damage. The stains used are those available in conventional histology laboratories. Since the quality of these stains and tissue preparations varies with the conditions of fixation and processing, it may be necessary, on occasion, to compromise the quality of the morphologic detail or the quality of the immunologic reaction. Experimentation to achieve optimal results is necessary when these concerns arise.

Despite the plethora of advanced techniques at our disposal, precise conventional morphology is not yet replaceable. Without the expertise of a knowledgable morphologist, errors are likely to occur even in those neoplasms with available immunologic markers. This point will become especially clear when the immuno-logic methods for evaluating solid tumors are consid-ered. The selection of appropriate staining methods requires a clear idea of the diagnostic possibilities.

The incorporation of histologic methods into the armamentarium of the clinical immunologist already has had considerable impact. It is hoped that these presentations will add appropriate emphasis to the utility of these methods and will alert users to the care necessary to avoid critical pitfalls.

Chapter 141

Tissue Immunofluorescence

RAFAEL VALENZUELA AND SHARAD D. DEODHAR

Immunofluorescence is a reliable, simple, rapid, and relatively inexpensive immunohistological technique used extensively in the clinical laboratory. Originally developed by Coons et al. in 1942 for the demonstration of microbial antigens in tissues (2, 3), it is now used to demonstrate many other cell and tissue antigens in numerous clinical conditions, principally in immunologic renal and skin diseases.

It is generally accepted that a complete evaluation of kidney and skin biopsy specimens, such as in cases of glomerular and tubulointerstitial disorders, connective tissue diseases, bullous dermatoses, and other disorders, must include direct immunofluorescence examination for the demonstration of tissue-bound immunoglobulins, complement components, fibrin-related products, and other immunoreactants. It is also important that in some of these conditions (e.g., anti-glomerular basement membrane disease, pemphigus, and pemphigoid diseases) the patient's serum be analyzed by indirect immunofluorescence for appropriate circulating autoantibodies. Immunoperoxidase has also been used as an alternative technique for the study of kidney and skin biopsies. However, most of the clinical experience to date relates to immunofluorescence.

This chapter deals with the direct immunofluorescence technique as performed routinely in the clinical laboratory with well-characterized commercial fluorescein isothiocyanate (FITC)-labeled antisera. Additional information about the basic principles of fluorescence microscopy and immunochemical aspects of labeled antibodies can be found in various monographs (1, 4, 6).

DIRECT IMMUNOFLUORESCENCE

Principle

In the direct immunofluorescence technique, the tissue sections are incubated with fluorescent antibodies under conditions which allow the binding of such antibodies to specific tissue antigens. The unbound antibodies are then washed off the sections, and the bound antibodies are visualized with a fluorescence microscope.

Specimens

The biopsy material (i.e., from kidney, skin, etc.) should be received in the fresh state without any fixative. To avoid dehydration, the specimen must be carried in saline-soaked cotton gauze. Ideally, the tissue should be snap-frozen in liquid nitrogen as soon after removal as possible. If the tissue cannot be frozen immediately, it is best stored at 4°C, wrapped in saline-soaked cotton gauze, for no longer than 24 h. Alternatively, acceptable results can be obtained by preserving the biopsy specimens in Michel transport medium (solution of ammonium sulfate in a neutral buffer) for as long as 2 weeks (4). After being removed from this medium, the specimen must be washed three times, for 10 min each time, in neutral buffer. Fixed, paraffin-embedded tissue is not satisfactory.

Procedure

There are several modifications of the original method. In our experience, excellent results are obtained with the following procedure.

1. Precool cryostat chuck in liquid nitrogen for about 1 min.

2. Immobilize the biopsy specimen on top of the precooled cryostat chuck by using a few drops of water. As the water begins to freeze, the chuck should be inverted to eliminate excess water.

3. Place the chuck in liquid nitrogen to snap-freeze the tissue. As a rule, the tissue can be considered adequately frozen when the liquid nitrogen stops bubbling. At this stage, the frozen specimen can be stored at −70°C for as long as necessary.

4. Cut 6-μm sections of frozen biopsy specimen on a tissue cryostat at −20°C. The number of sections depends on the number of fluorescent antisera required. Additional sections should be used as negative controls.

5. Place six sections on each standard histologic slide. Separate the sections from each other by liquid embroidery fluid lines. These lines will prevent intermixing of the fluorescent antisera as the antisera are applied to each of the tissue sections.

6. Allow the slides to air dry for at least 10 min. Inadequate drying of the sections may cause them to detach from the slide during the washing procedure.

7. Overlay each tissue section with the appropriate fluorescent antiserum. Verify that the whole section area is covered by antiserum.

8. Incubate the slides for 20 min in a closed humidity chamber at room temperature.

9. Wash the unreacted antiserum off the sections by dipping the slides sequentially into three jars of 0.01 M phosphate-buffered saline (PBS), pH 7.2. After the three rinses, the slides are immersed in a fourth jar of PBS for 15 min.

10. Drain the slides, and wipe excess buffer from around the sections with cotton gauze. Put cover slips on the slides, with a drop of buffered glycerol (90% glycerol) as the mounting medium.

11. Examine the slides with a fluorescence microscope. The ideal combination of excitation and barrier filters should be determined by the absorption and emission spectra of the fluorochrome. The absorption peak of FITC is about 490 nm (blue), and the emission peak is 520 nm (green).

Quality control

1. It is advisable to test new lots of fluorescent antisera for specificity by appropriate immunologic

procedures such as immunoelectrophoresis or Ouchterlony gel diffusion analysis or both.

2. Determine the appropriate working dilutions of new batches of fluorescent antisera by testing various dilutions (1:10, 1:20, 1:30, 1:40, and 1:80) on a known positive tissue. Select the dilution that gives maximal antigen-specific fluorescence with minimal background fluorescence.

3. For kidney biopsies, stain additional sections with toluidine blue. Verify by light microscopy that the sections contain glomeruli. If none is present, try a deeper cut into the tissue. For skin biopsies, verify that the sections contain epidermis.

4. Include known positive and negative tissue samples with each direct immunofluorescence run. Stain the samples with each of the fluorescent antisera used. This staining will monitor the immunoreactivity of the antisera.

5. Include additional sections for each tissue specimen studied. Ideally, these sections should be incubated with the appropriate fluorescent nonimmune sera (goat, rabbit, etc.) and washed in PBS. A simple wash in PBS should be sufficient if the desired nonimmune sera are not available. These sections should be used to evaluate tissue autofluorescence and nonspecific fluorescence.

6. Occasionally, it may become necessary to verify the specificity of a given positive immunofluorescent reaction. Verification is usually accomplished by blocking the tissue fluorescent reaction, either by preincubating the tissue section with saturating amounts of unlabeled antiserum or by preabsorbing the fluorescent antiserum with the involved antigen.

REAGENTS AND MATERIALS

1. FITC-labeled antisera to human proteins. Satisfactory preparations with well-defined protein/fluorescein ratios are now available from many commercial sources for the following antisera: immunoglobulin G (IgG), IgA, IgM, kappa, lambda, C3, C4, C1q, and fibrinogen.
2. Glycerol (reagent grade)
3. PBS (0.01 M phosphate, 0.15 M NaCl), pH 7.2
4. Pasteur pipette (5¾ in. [ca. 14.6 cm] long)
5. Histologic glass slides (with frosted edges)
6. Coplin jars, staining rack, and staining dish
7. Large plastic container with cover
8. Tissue cryostat
9. Fluorescence microscope with appropriate combination of excitation and barrier filters
10. Freezer (−70°C)

INTERPRETATION

For the proper evaluation of kidney and skin biopsy specimens, specific fluorescence must be distinguished from nonspecific fluorescence and autofluorescence. Specific fluorescence should be evaluated by specific criteria.

Autofluorescence and nonspecific fluorescence

The elastic fibers, cytoplasmic granules of the sweat glands and renal tubular epithelium, and certain cytoplasmic lipoproteins autofluoresce yellow, green-

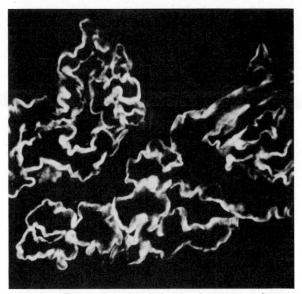

FIG. 1. Diffuse, generalized, linear deposition of IgG in the glomerular basement membrane. Goodpasture syndrome. FITC-labeled goat anti-human IgG. ×1,400. Reprinted by permission from reference 9.

ish yellow, or brownish yellow when the regular filter combination recommended for FITC is used (7–9).

Various patterns of nonspecific green fluorescence

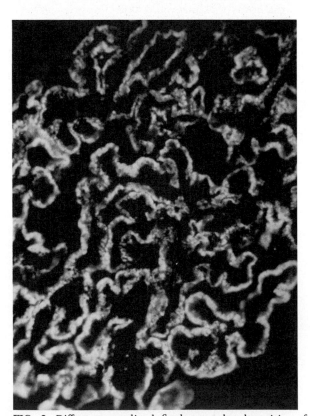

FIG. 2. Diffuse, generalized, finely granular deposition of IgG in the glomerular basement membrane, with preservation of its normal silhouette. Idiopathic membranous glomerulonephritis. FITC-labeled goat anti-human IgG. ×1,414. Reprinted by permission from reference 9.

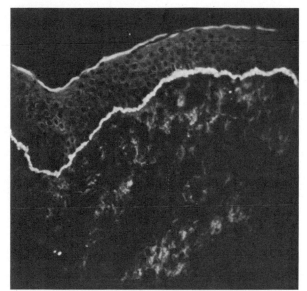

FIG. 3. Diffuse, linear deposition of IgG along the dermal-epidermal junction (basement membrane zone). Bullous pemphigoid. FITC-labeled goat anti-human IgG. ×350. Reprinted by permission from reference 7.

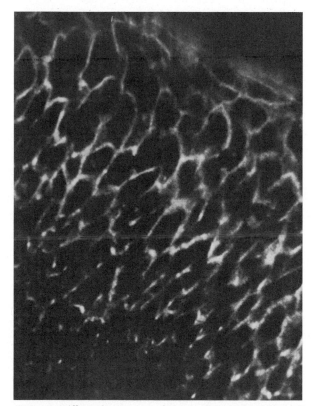

FIG. 4. Diffuse deposition of IgG in the intercellular substance of the epidermal cells. Pemphigus vulgaris. FITC-labeled goat anti-human IgG. ×1,414. Reprinted by permission from reference 7.

can be observed as a result of using either antisera with very high fluorescein/protein ratios or suboptimally diluted fluorescent antisera. Other factors responsible for nonspecific fluorescence include the presence of large protein aggregates or heterophilic antibodies in the antisera, nonspecific binding of the fluorochrome to certain tissue proteins, and accumulation of serum proteins in the tissue as a consequence of proteinuria or vascular leakage (7–9).

Specific fluorescence

The criteria that should be considered in describing the different immunofluorescence patterns observed in kidney and skin diseases are as follows: (1) the exact histologic location of the deposits (e.g., glomerular basement membrane, mesangial area, dermal-epidermal junction, intercellular substance of the epidermal cells, vessel walls, etc.); (ii) the distribution (focal, diffuse, etc.) and morphology (linear, finely granular, coarsely granular, globular, etc.) of the fluorescent deposits; and (iii) the protein content of the deposits (IgG, C3, etc.). Specific immunofluorescence patterns can be described consistently by these criteria (Fig. 1 through 4). In turn, these patterns can be correlated with histopathologic and ultrastructural findings as well as with the clinical aspects of each disease. Illustrations of the various immunofluorescence patterns associated with renal and skin diseases and their detailed interpretation for differential diagnoses are beyond the scope of this chapter. Comprehensive monographs on this particular subject are available (7–9).

LITERATURE CITED

1. **Beutner, E. H., R. S. Nisengard, and B. Albini (ed.).** 1983. Defined immunofluorescence and related cytochemical methods. Ann. N.Y. Acad. Sci. **420.**
2. **Coons, A. H., H. J. Creech, R. N. Jones, and E. Berliner.** 1942. Demonstration of pneumococcal antigen in tissues by use of fluorescent antibody. J. Immunol. **45:**159–170.
3. **Coons, A. H., and M. H. Kaplan.** 1950. Localization of antigen in tissue cells. II. Improvements in a method for the detection of antigen by means of fluorescent antibody. J. Exp. Med. **91:**1–13.
4. **Kawamura, A., Jr. (ed.).** 1977. Fluorescent antibody techniques, 2nd ed. University Park Press, Baltimore.
5. **Michel, B., Y. Milner, and K. David.** 1973. Preservation of tissue-fixed immunoglobulins in skin biopsies of patients with lupus erythematosus and bullous diseases—preliminary report. J. Invest. Dermatol. **59:**449–452.
6. **Nairn, R. C.** 1976. Fluorescent protein tracing, 4th ed. Churchill Livingstone, Edinburgh.
7. **Valenzuela, R., W. F. Bergfeld, and S. D. Deodhar.** 1984. Interpretation of immunofluorescent patterns in skin diseases. American Society of Clinical Pathologists Press, Chicago.
8. **Valenzuela, R., and S. D. Deodhar.** 1980. Interpretation of immunofluorescent patterns in renal diseases. Pathobiol. Annu. **10:**183–221.
9. **Valenzuela, R., and S. D. Deodhar.** 1981. Interpretation of immunofluorescent patterns in renal diseases. American Society of Clinical Pathologists Press, Chicago.

Chapter 142

Diagnostic Immunohistochemistry and Electron Microscopy of "Undifferentiated" Malignant Tumors

HENRY A. AZAR AND CARMEN G. ESPINOZA

The recent introduction of immunoperoxidase techniques, including the highly sensitive avidin-biotin complex (ABC) method currently favored in our laboratory, and the availability of an increasing number of commercially produced polyclonal and monoclonal antibodies against a variety of cellular markers have contributed significantly to the definitive histopathologic diagnosis of seemingly undifferentiated or anaplastic tumors and of tumors of uncertain histogenesis (2, 4, 5, 8, 9). Most immunoperoxidase methods are used in staining Formalin-fixed, deparaffinized tissue sections, as in the demonstration of relatively stable cell constituents such as cytoskeletal intermediate filaments (3, 7), S-100 protein (6) (initially isolated from a bovine brain extract and thought to be a nerve tissue-specific protein), and a variety of hormones, enzymes, and tissue-specific antigens. Other methods require frozen sections or fresh touch preparations, as in the demonstration of immunologic phenotypes of lymphoid cells with monoclonal antibodies (10).

Whereas it is often desirable or inevitable, because of sampling problems and cost effectiveness, to resort solely to immunohistochemical methods in the study of "undifferentiated" tumors, transmission electron microscopy done alongside immunohistochemistry serves to further narrow the differential diagnosis of these tumors and helps in determining their precise diagnosis (1).

CLINICAL INDICATIONS

The indications for applying immunohistochemical methods with or without parallel transmission electron microscopy are principally in the study of undifferentiated or "anaplastic" malignant tumors, which are often difficult or impossible to classify by means of light microscopy, including the use of traditional histochemical special stains. In adults, nondescript large-cell malignancies generally include anaplastic carcinomas, amelanotic malignant melanomas, and non-Hodgkin's malignant lymphomas of large-cell type (histiocytic malignant lymphomas in the Rappaport classification). In children, the precise diagnosis of small-cell malignancies often presents problems, and the distinction between Ewing's sarcoma, other primitive mesenchymal tumors, neuroblastomas, and malignant lymphomas is often based on rather tenuous light microscopic criteria.

In addition to these situations, immunohistochemistry and electron microscopy may be applied to the diagnosis of tumors of uncertain histogenesis, for example, spindle cell tumors in which the differential diagnosis includes a sarcomatoid form of squamous cell carcinoma, a true sarcoma, and a spindle cell variant of malignant melanoma. In a disseminated malignancy such as a metastatic adenocarcinoma in lymph nodes or

in the skeleton, it may be desirable to identify a possible primary site of origin such as the prostate or the breast. This identification can usually be accomplished by using primary antisera against prostate-specific antigen or against alpha lactalbumin or lactoferrin.

Immunohistochemistry and electron microscopy do not generally establish whether or not a lesion is malignant; criteria of malignancy are best based on cytological and architectural features observed by light microscopy. These ancillary methods do help in classifying tumors by revealing immunohistochemical or ultrastructural features of differentiation. We are encouraged to speculate that no matter how undifferentiated or anaplastic tumor cells are, they share with their ancestral embryonal or reserve cells certain functional or structural characteristics that are expressions of cell differentiation.

Because tissue specimens are often sent to consultants or specialized surgical pathology laboratories with little or no clinical information and no accompanying tissue sections or paraffin tissue blocks, it is important to outline the following specimen requirements.

(i) Tissue examination or consultation request form on which are entered pertinent clinical and laboratory data, including age and sex of the patient, precise site of biopsy, differential diagnosis or indication for special studies, and previous biopsies, if done

(ii) A representative histologic section

(iii) Paraffin tissue block(s) and, from lesions suspected of representing non-Hodgkin's lymphoma, several fresh, small fragments (0.4 by 0.3 by 0.2 mm) of tissue placed in Michel transport medium (obtained as 10-ml vials from Zeus Scientific, Inc., Raritan, N.J.)

(iv) Fine fragments (1 to 2 mm^3) of representative tumor tissue fixed immediately in 2.5% buffered glutaraldehyde for possible electron microscopic study

The best time to save tissue for possible immunohistochemical or electron microscopic studies is during operating room consultations or immediately after frozen sections are made, when the pathologist has access to fresh, unfixed specimens. Frozen sections or thick, untrimmed, Formalin-fixed tissue blocks are far less suitable for electron microscopy than are small fragments of fresh tissue immediately fixed in glutaraldehyde. Necrotic, hemorrhagic, or crushed areas should be avoided. For immunocytochemistry, buffered-Formalin fixation seems to be adequate for most cell markers, except for T-lymphocyte panels, which require frozen sections. B5 or Zenker solution is favored for the preservation of immunoglobulins.

PRIMARY ANTISERA AND REAGENTS FOR IMMUNOHISTOCHEMISTRY

Primary antisera are commercially available as polyclonal antisera raised in rabbits immunized with

TABLE 1. Cell markers in tumors most commonly tested for in paraffin-embedded tissues[a]

Cell tumor marker	Type of tumor[b] frequently demonstrating marker
Intermediate filaments	
Keratins	Most epithelial tumors, including most carcinomas, thymoma, mesothelioma, and synovial sarcoma
Glial fibrillary acidic protein	Most gliomas, including glioblastoma multiforme
Desmin (monoclonal antibody)	Muscle tumors
Vimentin (monoclonal antibody)	Most mesenchymal tumors, principally nonmuscle sarcomas, but also some epithelial and neuroectodermal tumors
Oncofetal proteins	
Carcinoembryonic antigen	Most epithelial tumors, particularly adenocarcinomas, and embryonal carcinoma
Alpha fetoprotein	Yolk sac tumor or entodermal sinus tumor and hepatocellular carcinoma
"Specific" cell products or tissue-specific proteins	
Kappa or lambda light chains	Multiple myeloma and some differentiated B-cell lymphomas
S-100 protein[c]	Melanocytic tumors, particularly amelanotic melanomas, neurofibroma, and neurilemmoma; salivary gland tumors; chondroid tumors; histiocytosis X (Langerhans cells)
Factor VIII antigen	Hemangiomas and Kaposi's sarcoma
Prostate-specific antigen	Adenocarcinoma of prostate
Alpha lactalbumin	Adenocarcinoma of breast
Lactoferrin	Adenocarcinoma of breast
Surfactant (not commercially available)	Some bronchiolo-alveolar carcinomas
Epithelial membrane antigen (monoclonal antibody)	Most epithelial tumors
Leukocyte common antigen (monoclonal antibody	Most lymphomas and hemopoietic neoplasms
Hormones	
Calcitonin	Medullary carcinoma of thyroid
Thyroglobulin	Adenocarcinoma of thyroid
Human chorionic gonadotropin	Choriocarcinoma, embryonal carcinoma, and miscellaneous carcinomas (lung, breast)
Enzymes	
Prostatic acid phosphatase	Adenocarcinoma of prostate
Lysozyme (muramidase)	Chloromas
Neuron-specific enolase	Neuroectodermal tumors; many nonspecific reactions

[a] All primary antisera are polyclonal antibodies except when otherwise indicated.

[b] The primary antiserum also decorates histogenetically related normal or reactive cells. In other words, the marker is not a tumor-specific antigen.

[c] S-100 protein, although a useful marker for a variety of neuroectodermal tissues, is an antigen also found in certain epithelial and mesenchymal cells.

human cell antigens and as monoclonal antibodies obtained from stable hybridomas grown in tissue culture. The production of clinically useful monoclonal antibodies is steadily increasing, but, currently, most laboratories (including our own) favor the use of cheaper and more readily available polyclonal antisera.

Antisera used in tumor diagnosis are grouped according to the types of cellular antigens they react with. The commonest cell markers tested for in the immunohistochemistry of tumors are listed in Table 1. Antisera and other reagents (secondary or binding antibodies, peroxidase complexes, chromagens, etc.) are supplied by Dako Corp., Santa Barbara, Calif., and Immunolok, Carpenteria, Calif., and are available at suppliers of primary antisera used in radioimmunoassays. Kits for ABC immunohistochemical staining are supplied by Vector Laboratories, Burlingame, Calif. As affinity-purified polyclonal antibodies become commercially available, these will gradually replace the currently popularized antisera.

For monoclonal antibodies to leukocytes (including T-lymphocyte subset) antigens, we have used products from Ortho Diagnostic Systems, Westwood, Mass., and from Becton Dickinson Monoclonal Center, Mountain View, Calif. Monoclonal antibodies to vimentin and other intermediate filaments are supplied by Labsystems, Chicago, Ill.

PROCEDURES

ABC immunoperoxidase procedure

Principle. The ABC method (4) is an indirect immunoperoxidase procedure similar to the peroxidase-antiperoxidase technique and applicable to Formalin-fixed, deparaffinized tissue sections. This highly sensitive method is based on the ability of the egg white glycoprotein avidin to bind non-immunologically four molecules of the vitamin biotin. As in the peroxidase-antiperoxidase technique, three reagents are used: (i) a primary antiserum specific for the tissue antigen to be localized in tissue sections; (ii) a secondary biotinylated antibody capable of binding to the primary antibody; and (iii) the avidin-biotin-peroxidase complex.

By its indirect binding to the tissue antigen, the peroxidase enzyme helps locate the antigen by reacting with a chromagen in the presence of a source of oxygen. Because the secondary biotinylated antibody has numerous binding sites for the tertiary reagent complex, the resultant peroxidase reaction is greatly amplified. Thus, the ABC procedure allows a greater dilution of the primary antibody, reduced background staining, and shorter incubation periods.

Staining procedure. The staining procedure recommended for the use of the ABC kit supplied by Vector Laboratories has been modified by Sudha Pillarisetti and Sandra K. Livingstone of our laboratory to include trypsinization.

ABC staining procedure for polyclonal antibodies

1. Cut paraffin sections at 4 to 5 μm, and attach them to slides with an appropriate glue.

2. Dry in the oven (not to exceed 60°C) for at least 1 h.

3. Deparaffinize the sections, and remove the mercury pigment if needed. Place in phosphate-buffered saline (PBS; 0.01 M, pH 7.6) for 5 min.

4. Block endogenous peroxidase with 3% hydrogen peroxide in distilled water for 10 to 30 min. Wash in PBS for 5 min.

5. Trypsinize with 0.15% trypsin in 0.4% calcium chloride (anhydrous) in distilled water, pH 7.6 (adjust with 0.1 N sodium hydroxide), for 45 min.

6. Wash in running tap water for 10 min. Rinse in distilled water. Wash in PBS for 5 min.

7. Block nonspecific binding with normal goat serum (1:100) in a moisture chamber for 20 min.

8. Drain the slides, and incubate them with primary rabbit antiserum for 1 h in a moisture chamber. Rinse the slides individually, and place them in PBS for 5 min.

9. Incubate the sections with biotinylated secondary goat antibody to rabbit immunoglobulin (1:100) in a moisture chamber for 20 min. Rinse the slides individually, and place them in PBS for 5 min.

10. Incubate with ABC (avidin-biotin-PBS, 1:1:100) in a moisture chamber for 20 min. Rinse the slides individually, and place them in PBS for 5 min.

11. Develop the reaction with 3,3-diaminobenzidine tetrahydrochloride (6 mg/10 ml of Tris hydrochloride buffer, pH 7.6, plus 2 drops of 3% hydrogen peroxide) for 5 min or less.

12. Stop the reaction by rinsing the slide with distilled or tap water. Wash in running tap water for 10 min.

13. Counterstain with Mayer hematoxylin, with 3 to 5 quick dips. Wash in running tap water for 10 min.

14. Dehydrate, clear, and mount with resinous mounting medium.

ABC staining procedure for monoclonal antibodies. For paraffin sections, the steps for staining are essentially the same as for polyclonal antisera, except that a primary mouse monoclonal antibody and a biotinylated horse antibody to mouse immunoglobulin are used. For frozen sections, trypsinization is omitted. Because of its bubbling effect, hydrogen peroxide should not be used in cryostat sections embedded in OCT compound (Miles Scientific, Naperville, Ill).

The optimal dilution of the primary antibody is determined for each antigen by using a wide range of dilutions. Excess antibody could cause a prozone effect and should be avoided. When results are interpreted, an excellent positive preparation should show an intense brown staining in cells containing the antigen, negative staining in the negative control section or in the section in which a nonimmune serum is used, and no background staining.

Controls. Three types of controls are run along the unknown section and under the same conditions: (i) a positive control section containing the antigen to be tested; (ii) a negative control section lacking the antigen to be tested; and (iii) a control section containing the antigen to be tested but in which the primary specific antibody has been substituted for by another primary antibody or by a nonimmune serum of the same species.

In addition to the above controls, the unknown section may contain built-in positive and negative controls. For example, in an antikeratin reaction, the unknown section may contain areas of normal squamous or respiratory epithelium, which should give a positive keratin reaction, and areas of smooth or skeletal muscle, which should react negatively.

Pitfalls and need for standardization in immunohistochemistry

It is now recognized that immunohistochemical methods are fraught with many pitfalls due to poor technique, nonspecific binding of primary antisera, and variability of expression of antigens in fixed tissues (2). There is much to be learned about the presumed specificity of antibody reactions and their reproducibility under different conditions of tissue fixation and processing.

In addition to the necessity for controls, there is a dire need for standardization of immunohistochemical procedures by providing users with sets of tumor sections tested with antisera panels of specified commercial origin. The dissemination of these "standards" could be done by a professional organization that would monitor the accuracy and reproducibility of specific immunohistochemical reactions in such tumor samples. Serially transplantable human tumor xenografts in athymic (nude) mice maintained in our laboratory serve as a "living tumor bank" and provide an excellent source of 20 different types of tumor.

Electron microscopic methods

Fine tissue fragments are promptly fixed in 2.5% buffered glutaraldehyde, postfixed in 1% osmium tetroxide, and embedded in Epon. Sections 1 μm thick are examined for orientation, and representative tumor areas are selected for ultrathin sectioning. The thin sections are stained with uranyl acetate and lead citrate and viewed under a transmission electron microscope.

INTERPRETATION

The pathologist should always interpret immunohistochemical preparations with appropriate positive and negative controls. Crushed and necrotic tissues,

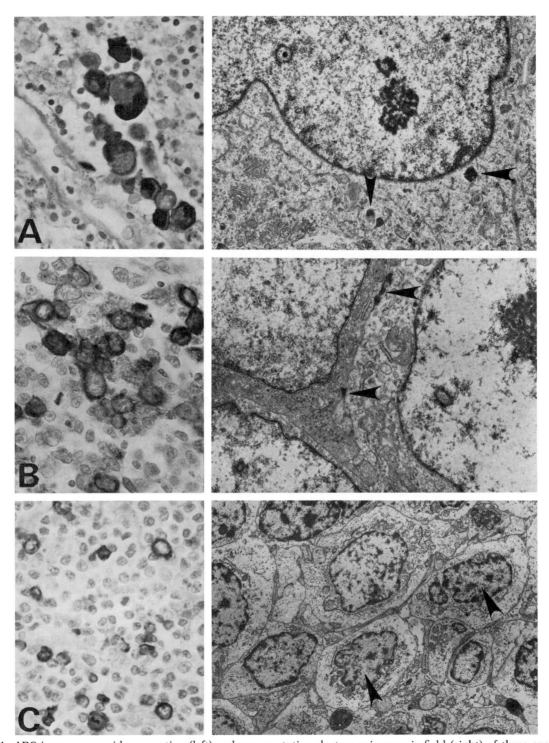

FIG. 1. ABC immunoperoxidase reaction (left) and representative electron microscopic field (right) of three examples of undifferentiated malignant tumors. (A) Amelanotic malignant melanoma. Positive immunostaining for S-100 protein (×1,000) and electron micrograph showing premelanosomes at arrows (×9,100). (B) Anaplastic carcinoma. Positive immunostaining for keratin (×1,000) and electron micrograph showing well-developed desmosomes at arrows (×11,000). (C) Malignant lymphoma, large-cell type. Positive immunostaining for lambda light chain (×1,000) and electron micrograph showing large cleaved nuclei at arrows (×2,500).

entrapped normal or hyperplastic cells masquerading as tumor cells, macrophages engulfing cell antigens or nonspecifically binding antibodies, and residual endogenous peroxidase activity in a variety of leuko-

cytes can all give false-positive reactions. False-negative reactions can be minimized by running positive controls under the same conditions as those applied to unknown sections and by including, whenever possi-

tures of paraformaldehyde and glutaraldehyde (3) or formaldehyde and glutaraldehyde (8). By a process of trial and success, an investigator with a given investigative problem may manipulate the combinations and concentrations of these fixatives to achieve an optimal outcome.

In processing human tissues for diagnostic microscopy we have found an aqueous solution of 4% glutaraldehyde buffered in 0.1 M sodium cacodylate to be appropriate. The 1-mm fragments of tissue are placed in a glass vial containing 5 ml of the buffered fixative and kept for 4 to 6 h in a refrigerator. After fixation, the specimens are rinsed for 10 to 15 h in one to three changes of an aqueous, 0.1 M cacodylate-buffered, 7.5% solution of sucrose. At this point the fixed specimen may be sent in the mail, stored for several days (preferably in the refrigerator), or secondarily "fixed" with osmium tetroxide if enhancement of the ultimate image contrast is desired. Such secondary postfixation is achieved by placing the glutaraldehyde-fixed, sucrose-washed specimens in 5 ml of aqueous 1% osmium tetroxide buffered with 0.1 M S-collidine. Osmium tetroxide should be handled within a fume hood to avoid inhalation of or skin contact with toxic fumes.

At this point, en bloc staining with uranyl acetate is optional, since sections of the tissue will be stained later with uranyl acetate and other heavy-metal stains. If desired, the tissue blocks may be placed for 1 h in aqueous 0.5% uranyl acetate in Veronal hydrochloride buffer.

The choice of appropriate buffers to be used with these fixatives is discretionary (7). The use of phosphate and cacodylate buffers runs a risk of generating heavy-metal precipitates during later staining with uranyl compounds. For this reason, some circumstances call for Veronal hydrochloride buffer.

EMBEDDING

The purpose of embedding fixed cell suspensions or blocks of tissue is to replace the water compartment with a matrix material sufficiently rigid to maintain tissue and cell structures, smoothly penetrable by a sectioning device, and resistant to the physical trauma generated by the electron beam of the microscope. After fixation and washing (and en bloc staining), specimens are dehydrated in a series of 35, 70, 95, and 100% (absolute) ethyl alcohol. Each alcohol rinse should be for 15 min, except with the absolute alcohol, there should be two rinses for 15 min each. Finally, the dehydrated tissues should be penetrated by propylene oxide solvent twice for 15 min each time.

Of several plastic resins available for tissue embedding, those most suitable and frequently utilized are Epon 812 (7) and Spurr ERL 4206 (6). We have had success with each, but we will describe the embedding procedure with Epon. The dehydrated specimens are placed in a 1:1 mixture of propylene oxide and Epon, with gentle stirring for 1 h. The Epon-infiltrated specimens are then placed in a 3:7 mixture of propylene oxide and Epon for further infiltration at room temperature. Each Epon-infiltrated block of tissue is then placed into a gelatin or polyethylene capsule of liquid Epon and encouraged to settle to the bottom or apex of the capsule. Capsules are labeled

(by a strip of labeled paper placed within the Epon at the rim of the capsule) and placed in a 60°C oven (for up to 2 days if necessary) to achieve polymerization of the Epon resin. Tissue identity, origin, and block number should be recorded in a log book, and polymerized blocks may be stored in properly labeled slide-type pillboxes.

SECTIONING

The sectioning of embedded specimens is a two-step procedure. First, sections approximating 0.5 μm in thickness are made with a glass knife mounted in an ultramicrotome and stained with alcaline toluidine blue for screening examination by a regular light microscope (7). Sections and areas containing structures desired for electron microscopic study are thereby identified; the corresponding blocks are trimmed appropriately and remounted in the ultramicrotome, which is fitted with either a high-quality glass knife or a suitable diamond knife. Ultrathin sections (around 50 nm thick) which appear silvery or gray-white rather than yellow or violet are cut, floated on a water bath fitted to the edge of the microtome knife, and picked up from the bath onto a copper grid disk coated with collodion-carbon. Skilled technicians can prepare ribbons of sections spread across the center of the copper grid so that serial sections can be examined.

STAINING

Single- or double-staining procedures may be performed, depending on the degree of image contrast desired (2, 4). We prefer relatively high-contrast specimens; hence, a double-staining procedure incorporating aqueous uranyl magnesium acetate (7.5%) and lead citrate (0.1%) will be described. A grid with adherent tissue sections is floated upside down on the surface of a drop of uranyl magnesium acetate which is on a wax platform in the center of a coverable plastic dish. After 15 min of exposure to the stain, the grid is rinsed by dipping it with forceps in distilled water, and it is dried on the surface of absorbent filter paper. Dried grids are then stained with lead citrate in a manner similar to that described for uranyl staining except that a few pellets of NaOH are placed in the covered plastic staining dish to absorb carbon dioxide gas and thereby avoid heavy-metal carbonate precipitates. The doubly stained grids are then again rinsed in carbon dioxide-free distilled water, dried as before, and placed on a piece of filter paper in a covered petri dish or into a compartment of a grid storage slide box. The grid containers may be stored in a desiccator to maintain a dehydrated condition until examination in the electron microscope.

ELECTRON MICROSCOPIC EXAMINATION AND PHOTOMICROGRAPHY

Knowledge about and attention to the details of operation of an electron microscope will result in better performance and a higher-quality photomicrographic product (7). The information required to achieve competence in operating an electron microscope is beyond the scope or intention of this presentation; however, certain fundamental principles are useful for the curious or beginning user. There are essential similarities as well as important differences between an electron microscope and a light microscope. The illuminating source in an electron microscope is a beam of high-velocity electrons, rather than light, accelerated into a sealed microscope column under vacuum. The functions of an electronic electron accelerator, pinhole diaphragm, and electromagnetic condenser lens are analogous to the functions of the light source, diaphragm, and glass condenser, respectively, in the light microscope. Instead of several insertable objective lenses, the electron microscope possesses only a single objective lens, the magnifying capacity of which is modified electromagnetically by the operator. A projector lens in the electron microscope projects the object image onto a phosphorescent screen which may be mechanically removed to further project the specimen image onto photographic film. The entire electron microscope column, from electron gun filament through lenses and specimen to phosphorescent screen and film, is maintained under vacuum. Photography is essential to generate a permanent record of electron microscopic observations and to achieve photographic resolution of finer ultrastructural details. In light microscopy, the human retina or photographic film detects light of various colors, transilluminated through the stained specimen. In electron microscopy, a phosphorescent screen or black-and-white photographic film detects contrast "shadows" of components of the specimen. These shadows are created by the various degrees of electron opacity generated by the differential uptake of osmium and other heavy-metal stains by different structural components of the specimen.

Ideally, grid specimens and film should be dehydrated before being introduced into the electron microscope column. This dehydration reduces both pump-down time and contamination of the column with moisture. Although earlier electron microscopes utilized plate glass negatives for photomicroscopy, now lightweight, thin, flexible sheet film or 35-mm roll film is used, depending on the make of electron microscope and the photographic mechanism. Many models of electron microscopes are now made to suit medical diagnostic or high-resolution research laboratory needs. These and other major instruments and supplies required to operate a complete electron microscopy laboratory are quite costly. A good darkroom or access to a professional darkroom facility equipped to develop negatives and prepare high-fidelity photographic enlargements of negatives is essential for complete ultrastructural analyses of electron microscope-generated images, for maintenance of permanent visual records, and for possible later presentation or publication of observations. The consistent acquisition of precipitate-free images, chatter-free

sections, well-fixed and optimally stained specimens, and crisp, well-focused photographic images is a high-cost technical skill and an art requiring well-trained and highly motivated personnel; good, well-serviced equipment; and persevering diligence. The professional using electron microscopy should devote ample time to the actual examination of specimens and to the review and analysis of enlarged electron photomicrographs.

SUMMARY

Electron microscopy can serve independently or in conjunction with other modalities of microscopy to evaluate the normal and abnormal structures of biological specimens and to render pathologic diagnoses in medicine. An electron microscopy laboratory is costly, it is instrumentation and skill intensive, and it requires fastidious attention to technical details. Investigator interest and commitment as well as the availability of financial resources will determine whether users establish their own laboratory or consider joining an existing laboratory as collaborators or fee-for-service users.

A variety of highly specialized techniques of specimen preparation and electron microscopic instrumentation are available for unique application to specific project and study requirements. These techniques include immunoelectron microscopy, high-resolution radioelectron microscopy, negative imaging, shadowcasting and scanning electron microscopy, elemental and diffraction analysis, and freeze fracturing, to name a few. Any reader with curiosity about or interest in these modalities of ultrastructural analysis should refer to special readings on these topics.

LITERATURE CITED

1. **Farquhar, M. G., R. L. Vernier, and R. A. Good.** 1957. An electron microscopy study of the glomerulus in nephrosis, glomerulonephritis and lupus erythematosus. J. Exp. Med. **106:**649–660.
2. **Hayat, M. A.** 1981. Principles and techniques of electron microscopy, vol. 1. Biological applications, p. 301–340. University Park Press, Baltimore.
3. **Karnovsky, M. J.** 1965. A formaldehyde-glutaraldehyde fixative of high osmolality for use in electron microscopy. J. Cell. Biol. **27**(Suppl.):137–138.
4. **Pease, D. C.** 1964. Histological techniques for electron microscopy, 2nd ed. Academic Press, Inc., New York.
5. **Pease, D. C., and R. F. Baker.** 1950. Electron microscopy of the kidney. Am. J. Anat. **87:**349–389.
6. **Spurr, A. R.** 1969. A low viscosity epoxy resin embedding medium for electron microscopy. J. Ultrastruct. Res. **26:**31–43.
7. **Trump, B. F., and R. T. Jones.** 1978. Diagnostic electron microscopy, vol. 1. John Wiley & Sons, Inc., New York.
8. **Yanoff, M.** 1973. Formaldehyde-glutaraldehyde fixation. Am. J. Ophthalmol. **76:**303–304.

Chapter 144

Lymphocyte Markers in Solid Tissues

RAYMOND R. TUBBS

Malignant lymphomas have come to be recognized as neoplasms of the immune system. These neoplasms display the antigenic properties, and in some instances the functional characteristics, of corresponding normal mononuclear cell populations. Tissue immunotyping is designed to profile the antigenic expression of immunoglobulin and non-immunoglobulin surface and cytoplasmic molecules peculiar to individual stages of T- and B-lymphocyte and monocyte-macrophage maturation. The derived immunotype is used as a corroborative tool, confirming and reinforcing histopathologic interpretation. Independent clinical relevance has been well established for immunologic subtypes of acute lymphocytic leukemia. Generally, with rare exceptions, such independent prognostic information has not been confirmed for non-Hodgkin's lymphomas in solid tissue (4, 5).

Diagnostic applications of tissue immunotyping include the classification of undifferentiated large-cell neoplasms, profiling of immunoglobulin light-chain expression as an index of clonality, differentiation of reactive hyperplasias from malignant lymphomas, and corroboration of histopathologic diagnoses by formulation of B- and T-cell subphenotypes (1). The technology and applications are of relatively recent vintage, and much work still needs to be done.

A variety of methods can be used to study tissue antigens. Space limitations preclude an in-depth review, and the reader is referred to one of several review articles on the subject (2). For an analysis of surface immunoglobulin and non-immunoglobulin surface antigens for flow cytometry or manual immunofluorescence, either the direct or indirect immunofluorescence procedure is utilized (1). Cytocentrifuge preparations (CCP) made from the derived fresh-cell suspension can be processed and immunostained in the same manner as frozen tissue sections (FSIP; 3). Two basic techniques are recommended for the study of FSIP and CCP (3, 6–9). For immunoglobulin immunotypes, the direct immunoperoxidase procedure is preferred, with multiple dilutions with and without hematoxylin counterstain for morphologic correlation. For non-immunoglobulin differentiation antigens, either an indirect immunoperoxidase or avidin-biotinylated peroxidase complex (ABC) procedure is preferred.

CLINICAL INDICATIONS

Since the question of independent clinical relevance for immunotyping is still unanswered (4, 5), the principal indication for the procedure is as an adjunct to conventional histopathologic interpretation.

At the present time, a multiparameter approach is preferred, using both cell suspension and immunohistologic methods. If a choice between methods must be made, a combination of FSIP immunohistology with immunoperoxidase-stained CCP is preferred over manual immunofluorescence or flow cytometric analysis of a cell suspension. Although quantitation is somewhat difficult by immunohistologic and immunocytologic procedures, this disadvantage is outweighed by the ability to perform morphologic correlations. Furthermore, image analysis-derived quantitation of immunocytologic and immunohistologic preparations may soon become routine. Concordance for immunotyping has been documented for FSIP as compared with flow cytometry and manual immunofluorescence of derived cell suspensions (2). A variety of immunotyping methods exist among laboratories, and further standardization needs to be developed.

The pitfalls of lymphoma immunotyping include the sampling error sometimes accorded a derived cell suspension, the erroneous use of paraffin sections for typing, and the potential for misinterpretation of immunoglobulin types as a consequence of interstitial immunoglobulin adherent to collagen and vascular endothelium in desmoplastic and richly vascularized neoplasms. Most of these problems can be identified and circumvented by the use of the multiparameter approach as outlined above, with CCP, FSIP, flow cytometry, and manual immunofluorescence.

INTERPRETATION

The interpretation of immunotyping results is qualitative and semiquantitative for FSIP and CCP and quantitative for flow cytometry and manual immunofluorescence. At this time, the ability to generate quantitative information from immunohistologic and immunocytologic preparations is just being developed. Since the FSIP and CCP give generally excellent morphologic correlation, the ability to qualitatively identify antigen expression for a certain morphologic subpopulation is very useful, and quantitative information may add little to the exercise.

Physiologic hyperplasias are generally characterized by an exaggeration of the functional compartments of non-immunoglobulin antigens of the human lymph node or spleen (2, 3, 8). Follicular hyperplasias are characterized by polyclonal immunoglobulin light-chain expression, defined as both κ and λ light chains in the same follicle, with a ratio of approximately 1.5 (2, 3, 8).

Two general patterns of immunohistologic staining are observed in non-Hodgkin's lymphomas. These patterns reproduce the follicular and diffuse lymphomatous architectural growth patterns of non-Hodgkin's lymphoma. Immunoglobulin D (IgD)-positive mantle zones are usually absent. Individual neoplastic follicles show clonal excess (only κ or only λ) staining. Heavy-chain isotype expression in follicular lymphomas may be IgM, IgD, or IgG, but most commonly is IgM. Variable numbers of T cells are identified within neoplastic follicles, but the cells are

TABLE 1. Values for antigenic markers in cell suspensions[a] derived from benign solid tissues[b]

Antigenic marker	Mean (range) (%) for tissues from:	
	Spleen	Benign hyperplastic lymph nodes
Immunoglobulins[c]		
Total	52.8 (29.5–63.9)	49.7 (40.9–62.1)
IgM	26.1 (13.7–37.8)	32.9 (16.9–52.7)
IgD	24.8 (11–40.6)	33.9 (15.0–51.0)
IgG	17.5 (9.7–24.2)	10.1 (5.1–12.0)
IgA	5.1 (4.0–6.9)	8.3 (3.2–11.9)
κ	31.1 (15.7–41.9)	32.0 (17.1–49.1)
λ	20.4 (10.6–34.4)	19.2 (11.9–29.8)
κ/λ ratio	1.6 (1.2–1.7)	1.8 (1.3–2.3)
Non-immunoglobulin differentiation antigens		
Leu10	24 (17.8–29.1)	44.7 (30.1–66.3)
Ca11a	0.8 (0–1.7)	0.5 (0–1.5)
Leu1	36.8 (19.8–60.4)	39.1 (30.9–45.2)
Leu2a	13.5 (9.0–18.4)	9.3 (3.0–25.2)
Leu3a and b[a]	20.8 (10.7–31.1)	27.9 (17.3–54.2)
HLA-DR[a]	41.7 (18.6–60.0)	44.7 (27.4–67.1)
Leu3/Leu2 ratio[a]	1.3 (0.6–1.9)	6.3 (2.3–11.6)

[a] Suspensions not macrophage depleted. Leu3 is expressed on macrophage subpopulations.
[b] These tissues represent cases without malignant histopathologic changes, and the values cannot be considered normal reference values. The grossly "normal" tissues were obtained from ill patients undergoing laparotomy or other apparently unrelated surgical procedures and showed diverse benign histopathology including follicular hyperplasia and sinus histiocytosis.
[c] With FITC-F(ab′)$_2$ conjugates.

confined principally to the interfollicular zone. Diffuse lymphomas are characterized by a diffuse immunostaining pattern. In most diffuse non-Hodgkin's lymphomas, a definition of immunotype can usually be made with ease. However, in diffuse lymphomas of mixed histology, it may be difficult to determine the precise immunotype from FSIP alone, and additional information from the CCP and paraffin sections stained with the LN monoclonal antibody series can be helpful in this setting (8). Usually, a large, atypical LN-2-positive large-cell population with immunoglobulin clonal excess is identified in diffuse mixed lymphoma; smaller lymphocytes are T11 positive, and numerous macrophages are identified. CCP reflect the predominance of one immunoglobulin light-chain type and can be selectively assessed for marker expression by the large atypical cells.

In CCP from small lymphocytic lymphoma, only semiquantitative assessments can be made. In follicular and diffuse, small, cleaved-cell types and in large-cell lymphomas, the cytologically atypical population can be correlated with the expression of the immunoglobulin or differentiation antigen immunotype, contrasted with the usual minor contaminating subpopulation of T cells in CCP.

Ranges for derived cell suspensions from benign spleens and hyperplastic lymph nodes are summarized in Table 1. It is emphasized that these values cannot be considered "normal" reference values. The tissues from which the suspensions were derived showed a spectrum of physiologic benign changes, including follicular hyperplasia, sinus histiocytosis, and splenic sinusoidal congestion. All tissues were of necessity derived from ill patients. Immunoglobulin clonal excess for a population in the suspension is defined for cell suspensions having a κ/λ ratio of >3 or <1. The quantitative data should be interpreted in conjunction with the FSIP and CCP, since the derived cell suspension reflects a heterogeneous mixture of neoplastic and nonneoplastic cells for which few morphologic correlations can be made in the absence of cell sorting or panning procedures.

REAGENTS AND TEST PROCEDURES

Immunohistochemistry for Lymphoproliferative Disorders: Initial Screen for Surface-Cytoplasmic Immunoglobulins

Reagents

3-Amino-9-ethylcarbazole (AEC; Sigma Chemical Co., IsoPac), 25 mg
Poly-L-lysine (Sigma, no. P1524)
Acetic acid-sodium acetate buffer, 0.02 M, pH 5.2
N,N-Dimethylformamide (J. T. Baker Chemical Co., no. 9221-1)
30% Hydrogen peroxide (Fisher Scientific Co., no. H325)
Modified phosphate-buffered saline (PBS) buffer
Stock solution. Dissolve in distilled water; dilute up to 1 liter; add K_2HPO_4 first, and stir it in, with heat if necessary.

NaCl . . . . 180 g
NaH_2PO_4 . . . . 33 g
K_2HPO_4 . . . . 188 g

Working solution. Use 40 ml of stock PBS in 960 ml of distilled H_2O and 20 mg of Merthiolate.
Affinity-purified antibody conjugates
Peroxidase-conjugated anti-kappa Fab (HPO-aκ) (Tago, Inc.; no. 2396), 1:100 and 1:300 in modified PBS

Peroxidase-conjugated anti-lambda Fab (HPO-aλ) (Tago, no. 2398), 1:100 and 1:300 in modified PBS

Peroxidase-conjugated chrompure goat IgG (negative control, HPO-C) (Jackson Immunoresearch Laboratory, no. 005-3004), 1:100 and 1:300 in modified PBS

Procedure

Cut 8-μm cryostat-frozen sections onto slides coated with poly-L-lysine (0.1% in distilled water) as soon as tissue is received. Cut three slides with three sections; two sections on each slide will be immunostained, and one section will serve as a negative control. Air dry overnight at room temperature.

Fix the frozen sections, tonsil control, and three cytospins (see below) for 10 min in fresh reagent grade acetone. Air dry.

Wash with modified PBS for 5 min, and wipe around the sections.

Apply the antibodies as follows.

    (i) To the first slide and the tonsil control slide, apply HPO-aκ (1:300) to the left section, HPO-aλ (1:300) to the section on the right, and HPO-C to the third section.

    (ii) To the second slide, apply antibody (1:100) in the same format as above.

    (iii) To the third set of slides, apply HPO-aκ (1:100) to the left tissue section and one cytospin. To the right-hand tissue section and one cytospin, apply HPO-aλ (1:100). To the middle section and the third cytospin, apply HPO-C (1:100). This set of slides will be counterstained after AEC is added.

    (iv) Incubate for only 10 min at room temperature in a humidified chamber.

Wash with modified PBS, with multiple changes over 5 min.

Develop the AEC color reaction product for 10 min as follows. Dissolve 25 mg of AEC (Sigma Isopac) in 10 ml of dimethylformamide. Add 100 ml of 0.02 M acetate buffer, pH 5.2. Add 40 μl of 30% hydrogen peroxide. Stain the slides for 10 min.

Observe the usual AEC precautions. Use gloves, and do all AEC reactions under a hood. Discard the AEC solution and the first PBS wash into a proper container.

Wash in PBS for 5 min, with multiple changes.

Counterstain the cytospins and three frozen section slides with fresh hematoxylin (no alcohol).

Add cover slips with Aquamount (Lerner Labs). Do not dehydrate in alcohols. Seal the edges of the cover slips with nail polish, and label the slides.

Lymphocyte Differentiation Antigens: Initial Screen for ABC Method (with Indirect Option)

Required reagents

Poly-L-lysine (Sigma, no. P1524)
AEC (Sigma Isopac), 25 mg
Modified PBS buffer (see immunoglobulin procedure above)
Acetate buffer, 0.02 M, pH 5.2
30% Hydrogen peroxide (Fisher, no. 4325)
N,N-Dimethylformamide (Baker, no. 9221-1)

Reagent grade acetone
Mouse ABC kit (Vector, no. PK-4002)
HPO–anti-mouse IgG (Dako, no. P-260; optional for indirect modification)
Monoclonal antibodies
T11 (Coulter, no. 6602137), 1:40
Leu1 (Becton Dickinson, no. 7300), 1:15
Leu14 (Becton Dickinson, no. 7510), neat
J5 (Coulter, no. 6602143), 1:40
B1 (Coulter, no. 6602140), 1:5
B2 (Coulter, no. 6602146), 1:5
Mouse IgG control (Jackson, no. 015-003), 0.1 mg/ml

Procedure

Air dry 8-μm cryostat-frozen sections overnight at room temperature on slides coated with poly-L-lysine (0.1% in distilled water). Fix with reagent grade acetone for 10 min, and allow to air dry.

Preform the ABC at this time. (See below.)

Use a modified PBS wash, with three changes over 5 min.

Apply mouse monoclonal antibodies and mouse IgG control to the sections, and incubate them in a humidified chamber at room temperature for 15 min.

Use a modified PBS wash, with three changes over 5 min.

(For tissues rich in endogenous biotin, a simple indirect immunoperoxidase procedure can be used instead of the ABC method. At this point, substitute HPO–anti-mouse IgG (Dako P-260; 1:60) for 15 min, wash, and develop the reaction product in AEC as described above.)

Apply biotinylated affinity-purified horse anti-mouse immunoglobulin (1:200) in modified PBS (15 min, room temperature).

Use a modified PBS wash, with three changes over 5 min.

Apply preformed ABC for 15 min in a humidified chamber at room temperature. ABC contains the following:

20 μl of reagent A-avidin DH
20 μl of reagent B-biotinylated horseradish peroxidase
1.6 ml of modified PBS (preform and leave at room temperature for at least 30 min before use)

Use a modified PBS wash, with three changes over 5 min.

Develop the AEC color reaction product for 10 min at room temperature (see immunoglobulin procedure above).

Wash in PBS for 5 min, with multiple changes. Counterstain with hematoxylin, and mount the cover slip with Aquamount. Do not dehydrate in alcohols.

Seal the edges of the cover slips with nail polish, and label the slides.

Cell Suspension Immunofluorescence: Direct Technique

Reagents

Modified RPMI (GIBCO Laboratories, no. 320-1875, with 5% heat-inactivated newborn calf serum

[GIBCO, no. 230–6010], 25 mM HEPES [*N*-2-hydroxyethylpiperazine-*N'*-2-ethanesulfonic acid], and 0.5% garamycin), 4% paraformaldehyde, clear Hanks solution (GIBCO, no. 310-4025)
Trypan blue (Sigma, no. T9520), 0.2% in cell suspension
Controls
1. Fluorescein isothiocyanate (FITC)-goat IgG control (Jackson, no. 005-1006)
2. FITC-mouse IgG control (Becton Dickinson, no. 9041)
Antibodies
3. FITC–anti-total Ig (Tago, no. 4203)
4. FITC–anti-IgM (Tago, no. 4202)
5. FITC–anti-IgD (Kallstead, no. 2093)
6. FITC–anti-IgG (Tago, no. 4200)
7. FITC–anti-IgA (Tago, no. 4201)
8. FITC–anti-κ (Tago, no. 4206)
9. FITC–anti-λ (Tago, no. 4208)
10. FITC–Leu10 (Becton Dickinson, no. 7453)
11. FITC–Calla (Becton Dickinson, no. 7503)
12. FITC–Leu1 (Becton Dickinson, no. 7303)
13. FITC–T11 (Coulter, no. 4235259)
14. FITC–Leu9 (Becton Dickinson, no. 7484)
15. FITC–Leu2a (Becton Dickinson, no. 7313)
16. FITC–Leu3a and b (Becton Dickinson, no. 7413)
17. FITC–HLA-Dr (Becton Dickinson, no. 7363)
Reagents 1 and 3 through 9 are F(ab')$_2$ immunoglobulin fragments.

Procedure

1. Make a single-cell suspension as follows.
   (i) Force thin slices of tissue through a 20-mesh brass screen (Fisher, no. 14-295B).
   (ii) Dislodge the remaining tissue from the front and back of the screen with modified RPMI (use a 3-ml plastic syringe with an 18-gauge needle).
   (iii) Remove the needle from the syringe, and forcefully aspirate small tissue fragments in modified RPMI into the syringe.
   (iv) Pass the crude suspension through Fisher Spectra Mesh (41-μm mesh, nylon, no. 08-670-202), purify over a density gradient (Ficoll), wash, count, and assess the viability with trypan blue. (The Ficoll step is optional, but preferred.)
   (v) Prepare 12 cytospins for immunoperoxidase staining from a sample of the suspension (2 × 10^6 cells in 1 ml of modified RPMI). Air dry briefly, and then dip the cytospin slide in and out of acetone for a total of 5 s. Air dry overnight at room temperature.
2. Place 10^6 washed cells of ≥95% viability in each of 17 labeled incubation tubes.
3. Centrifuge the tubes at 1,700 rpm at 4°C for 5 min. Pour off the supernatant, vortex, and add 100 μl of cold modified RPMI. Vortex and put on ice.

4. If Fc receptor binding is a problem, preincubate at this point with goat IgG (tube 1 and tubes 3 through 9; Jackson, no. 005-0004) and mouse IgG (tube 2 and tubes 10 through 17; Jackson, no. 015-0003) for 5 min.
5. Add 5 μl of each primary antibody to the corresponding labeled tube; be certain that antibody is delivered to the suspension. Keep antibodies, buffers, and cells at 4°C at all times. Use a pipette tip only once: failure to do so will cross-contaminate monoclonal antibodies.
6. Incubate on ice for 30 min. After the 30-min incubation, add 4 ml of cold modified RPMI to each tube by using a dispenser jar.
7. Centrifuge the tubes at 1,700 rpm for 5 min at 4°C.
8. Pour off the supernatant, vortex the tubes, and resuspend the cells in 4 ml of cold modified RPMI.
9. Centrifuge the tubes at 1,700 rpm at 4°C for 5 min. Pour off the supernatant, and vortex the tubes. Add 200 μl of 0.5% paraformaldehyde to the vortexed cells if analysis is to be delayed, or suspend the cells in clear Hanks solution (4°C) for immediate manual or flow cytometric analysis.

LITERATURE CITED

1. **Aisenberg, A. C.** 1979. Current concepts in immunology: cell-surface markers in lymphoproliferative disease. N. Engl. J. Med. **301**:512–518.
2. **Falini, B., and C. R. Taylor.** 1983. New developments in immunoperoxidase techniques and their application. Arch. Pathol. Lab. Med. **107**:105–117.
3. **Fishleder, A., R. R. Tubbs, J. Valenzuela, and D. Norris.** 1984. Immunophenotypic characterization of acute leukemia by immunocytology. Am. J. Clin. Pathol. **81**:611–617.
4. **Gold, E. J., R. H. Mertelsman, D. A. Filippa, T. H. Szatrowski, B. Koziner, and B. Clarkson.** 1983. Prognostic significance of receptors for the third component of complement and heavy chain phenotype in diffuse B cell lymphoma. Blood **62**:107–111.
5. **Horning, S. J., R. S. Doggett, R. A. Warnke, R. F. R. Dorfman, R. S. Cox, and R. Levy.** 1984. Clinical relevance of immunologic phenotype in diffuse large cell lymphoma. Blood **63**:1209–1215.
6. **Tubbs, R. R., A. Fishleder, R. A. Weiss, R. A. Savage, B. A. Sebek, and J. K. Weick.** 1983. Immunohistologic cellular phenotypes of lymphoproliferative disorders. Comprehensive evaluation of 564 cases including 257 non-Hodgkin's lymphomas classified by the International Working Formulation. Am. J. Pathol. **113**:207–221.
7. **Tubbs, R. R., and K. Sheibani.** 1984. Immunohistology of lymphoproliferative disorders. Sem. Diagn. Pathol. **1**:272–286.
8. **Tubbs, R. R., K. Sheibani, R. A. Weiss, R. A. Sebek, and S. D. Deodhar.** 1981. Tissue immunomicroscopic evaluation of monoclonality of B-cell lymphomas: comparison with cell suspension studies. Am. J. Clin. Pathol. **76**:24–28.
9. **Warnke, R., and R. Levy.** 1980. Detection of T and B cell antigens with hybridoma monoclonal antibodies: a biotin-avidin-horseradish peroxidase method. J. Histochem. Cytochem. **28**:771–776.

Chapter 145

Nonlymphocyte Tumor Markers in Tissues

A. E. SHERROD AND CLIVE R. TAYLOR

The practice of surgical pathology involves the examination of tissue sections and ultimately the offering of an opinion based on established histologic criteria. Subjective as this opinion may be, it often is nonetheless translated into a diagnosis on which therapy may be based. This form of histologic diagnosis has proven relatively successful over the past century, and numerous new histologic entities are being added to the literature. It has not been possible, however, to develop for histology the objective criteria offered by many other laboratory tests.

Histochemical methods were introduced in the latter part of the 19th century by pathologists searching for more objective methods, aside from the examination of morphologic features, for cellular recognition and diagnosis. Histochemical techniques revealed differences in staining patterns and intensities based on variations in the microchemical computation of cells in the reactivity of various cellular substrates with their corresponding enzymes. Most such methods, however, have limited specificity, since generally the chemical compositions of different cells show more similarities than differences.

Immunoperoxidase methods may be viewed as additional "special stains" to be used in conjunction with both histochemistry and morphology, but having a higher order of specificity. The rapid acceptance of immunoperoxidase methods may be attributed to the fact that they are not new techniques, but rather amalgamations of two established, well-tested techniques. The demonstration of peroxidase enzymatic activity is an exploitation of histochemical methods, whereas the theoretical basis of immunoperoxidase is related to the specificity of the antigen-antibody reaction, the utility of which was established in earlier immunofluorescence methods.

The immunofluorescence method for recognizing antigens in tissue sections was introduced by Coons and his associates. However, this method was generally applied to frozen sections and was considered unreliable on conventionally processed surgical specimens. Furthermore, the suboptimal morphologic detail of fresh cryostat sections, as well as the dark background resulting from use of light in the UV wavelength, limited surgical pathologists in the use of orthodox histology, a discipline to which they may have committed years in training. The conjugation of antibody to horseradish peroxidase in place of fluorescein isothiocyanate represented the initial step in the development of immunoperoxidase as a viable alternative to proven immunofluorescence methods. Peroxidase-labeled antibodies allowed the examination of labeled-antibody preparations by light microscopy; although initially this labeling was restricted predominantly to frozen sections, which, as with immunofluorescence, gave less than satisfactory morphology, some antigens were identified in routinely processed Formalin-fixed, paraffin-embedded tissues.

This procedure finally gave the surgical pathologist the desired histologic detail as well as the added benefit of being able to evaluate tissues long since stored as paraffin blocks. Although the early era of immunoperoxidase methodology was restricted to the demonstration of only a few antigens in paraffin-embedded tissues, the list has now grown considerably, from a small handful in 1974 to well over a hundred at the present time (Table 1).

Variations on the immunoperoxidase theme have been explored to examine alternatives to the use of directly conjugated antibodies. This work has led to the development of unlabeled-antibody methods with their peculiar advantages and disadvantages.

It is apparent that some methods are better than others for routine pathology laboratory use (see below). Also, although not all the antigens thus far described in paraffin sections have proven useful for diagnostic purposes, some have been shown to be of diagnostic utility. Presumably others remain to be discovered; the recent development of antibodies against the different intermediate filaments that characterize distinct basic cell types appears especially promising.

VARIATIONS OF THE IMMUNOPEROXIDASE TECHNIQUE

As with earlier immunofluorescence techniques, initial immunoperoxidase studies utilized direct or indirect conjugate methods. These techniques are illustrated in Fig. 1. The peroxidase-antiperoxidase (PAP) method (Fig. 1) was developed to avoid some of the problems associated with conjugated antibodies, including the reputed difficulty in the preparation of high-quality conjugates in which neither free label nor free antibody remained. First used for the demonstration of antitreponemal antibodies (9), the PAP method gained wide acceptance largely because of its increased sensitivity compared with that of other techniques. The PAP method is based upon linkage of the substrate to the antigen under investigation solely by immunologic binding and not through chemical reactions.

Other techniques have since been developed. These techniques include the use of staphylococcal protein A, either as a peroxidase conjugate or as a linking reagent in the PAP system; the use of hapten-linked antibody; and the various avidin-biotin systems, which exploit the high binding affinity these two substances have for one another. In the basic avidin-biotin technique, the localization of biotinylated antibody in the tissue is revealed by the addition of an avidin-peroxidase conjugate. Another variation using this technique was developed by Hsu and colleagues, in which a conjugate of avidin, biotin, and peroxidase is formed before the conjugate is added to the tissue section (5). This avidin-biotin conjugate (ABC) proce-

TABLE 1. Antigens demonstrable in "routinely" processed paraffin sections

Antigen class	Antigen[a]
Hormones	ACTH, GH, LH, LTH, FSH, TSH, parathormone, calcitonin, thyroxine, thyroglobulin, hCG, βhCG, testosterone, estradiol, progesterone, insulin, glucagon, somatostatin, VIP, gastrin, secretin, motilin, neurotensin, cholecystokinin, renin, vasopressin, oxytocin, neurophysin
Receptors	Transferrin receptor protein, estrogen receptor protein
Other tissue components	Laminin, fibronectin, collagens, amyloid A protein
Other cellular components	Lysozyme (muramidase), lactoferrin, transferrin, ferritin, hemoglobin A, hemoglobin F, myoglobin, actin, myosin, keratin, α-1-antitrypsin, α-1-chymotrypsin, α-fetoprotein, CEA, mammary epithelial membrane Ag, hepatorenal Ag, pancreatic Ag, melanoma Ag, PAP, PSA, GFAP, tyrosine hydroxylase, myelin basic protein, enkephalin(-like) Ag, substance P, enolases, adenosine desminase, terminal transferase, carbonic anhydrase, cathepsin D, converting enzyme, factor VIII-related Ag, creatine kinase, intestinal mucin Ags, HLA Ags, blood group Ags, surfactant apoprotein, S-100 Ag, neurofilament, vimentin, desmin
Infectious agents	Herpes I and II, hepatitis B surface Ag, mouse mammary tumor virus Ag, rubella, baboon endogenous virus, measles Ag, respiratory syncytial virus, buffalo pox, *Legionella* spp., *Klebsiella* spp., group B streptococcus, influenza, polio, varicella-zoster, cytomegalovirus, parainfluenza, lymphocytic choriomeningitis virus, Moloney virus, Friend virus, Shope fibroma virus, simian virus 40, human papilloma virus, distemper virus, rotavirus, polyoma virus, *Chlamydia* spp., *Mycoplasma* spp., *Trichomonas* spp., *Toxoplasma* spp., *Trichophyton* spp.
Immunoglobulin components	κ and λ light chains; γ, α, μ, δ, and ε heavy chains; J chain; secretor piece
Complement components	C1, C3

[a] For abbreviations, see legend to Fig. 2. Ag, Antigen.

dure (Fig. 1) has a sensitivity comparable to that of the PAP method.

Of these techniques, the PAP and ABC methods have gained the greatest popularity. Immunostaining kits are available which incorporate one or the other of these methods and include all of the necessary reagents. A pathologist anticipating a limited number of cases for evaluation with a particular antibody may be well advised to utilize the kit form, as the titers of the reagents have been properly determined for optimal specificity with a low level of background staining. However, it may be more economical, when dealing with large numbers of tissue sections, to purchase the reagents separately and establish one's own in-house procedure. This choice requires determining the optimal dilutions for each immunologic reagent by a checkerboard titration in which each of the reagents is used in serial dilutions with each of the other reagents (4).

CONTROLS

Proper controls are necessary for the validation of any immunohistologic stain. In practice, these controls consist of tissue known to contain the antigen in question; ideally, the tissue should be processed in the same manner as sections that are being evaluated for diagnostic or investigative purposes. The presence of specific staining in a positive control ensures not only that the immunoperoxidase system is working, but also that the method of tissue processing is satisfactory for that antigen. If no staining is seen in the positive control, it may be necessary to use frozen sections to determine whether the failure is in the staining procedure or the mode of tissue processing.

A negative control is often useful in the evaluation of the validity of an immunostain, especially when there is a high degree of background reactivity. The usual negative control is represented by an additional tissue section treated in a manner identical to the test section, except that the primary antibody is omitted and replaced by serum from the species in which the primary antibody was raised. In certain instances, a parallel tissue section exposed to substrate reagent alone may prove useful in the evaluation of endogenous peroxidase activity (4).

FIXATION

A growing list of antigens has been demonstrated in fixed tissues. On the other hand, it is apparent that many other antigens are either destroyed or sufficiently altered by fixation that they are unrecognizable by their corresponding antibodies. Although it is not clear exactly how most fixatives affect individual antigens, it is apparent that different antigens respond differently to different fixatives. There are some general guidelines. As an example, if Formalin is used, it should be freshly made and buffered. Fixation, whatever the fixative, should be allowed to proceed for as short a time as possible, which necessitates proper trimming of tissue to allow for even and rapid fixation. Once the tissue is properly fixed, it should not be stored in Formalin, but rather transferred to 70% ethanol until the processing procedure can be continued. Prolonged exposure to Formalin (or other fixa-

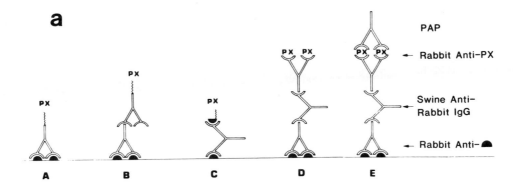

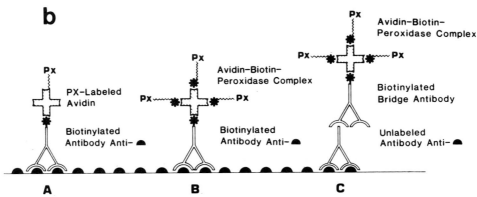

FIG. 1. (a) Immunoperoxidase procedures. A, Peroxidase-antibody conjugate, direct method; B, peroxidase-antibody conjugate, indirect method; C, labeled-antigen method; D, enzyme bridge method; E, PAP immune complex method. (b) Biotin-avidin immunoenzymatic procedures. A, Labeled avidin-biotin method; B, direct biotinylated method; C, indirect biotinylated ABC method. Symbols: PX, peroxidase; ✱, biotin; ⊹, avidin; ▲, antigen.

tives) results in progressive loss of antigenicity. During embedding, the paraffin bath should be held at less than 60°C; this limit also applies to oven temperature if a period of incubation is used to promote adherence of sections to the slides. Other fixatives, such as Bouin, Zenker, Carnoy, and B-5, have been used with varied success. Experience shows that certain antigens will be found to tolerate certain of these fixatives better than others. An extensive literature has developed concerning fixation (1); there is no universally satisfactory fixative for immunostaining, but for many antigens, Carnoy is preferable to Formalin.

USE OF PROTEOLYTIC ENZYMES

When working with Formalin-fixed, paraffin-embedded tissue, better immunostaining results may be achieved through the use of proteolytic enzymes. In many instances, not only will partial digestion of the tissues reduce background staining, but it will also enhance the staining of certain antigens. Several postulates have been advanced to explain this observation. It has been suggested that, after enzyme treatment, better penetration of sections by antisera occurs in tissues which were initially rendered impermeable because of fixation. Digestion may alter the electrostatic charge of the tissue, resulting in improved

bonding of antibody to antigen. It has also been proposed that enzymatic treatment may unmask immunoreactive sites facilitating antigen-antibody interaction. "Predigestion" of tissue may thus be indicated in certain instances, but as a general rule does not apply to tissues processed in fixatives other than Formalin; also, with some antigens, predigestion may do more harm than good, resulting in antigen destruction. In addition to different components of complement and immunoglobulins, enhanced staining has been seen for factor VIII antigen and the cellular intermediate filaments (cytokeratin and vimentin). Accumulated experience in the use of proteolytic enzymes will almost certainly reveal other antigens which will show enhanced staining by this technique.

A wide variety of proteolytic enzymes is available. The most reliable and useful have been trypsin, protease, and pronase. Enzymatic activity varies not only with the type of enzyme, but also from one lot to the next of the same enzyme. It is therefore necessary to evaluate each enzyme for optimal concentration and length of time necessary to allow for tissue digestion. With either trypsin or protease, working concentrations usually remain between 0.1 and 0.05%, with the time of enzymatic treatment of tissues ranging from 5 to 25 min. Controls must be employed simultaneously and treated in a manner identical to that used to treat the tissue under evaluation.

IMMUNOHISTOLOGIC APPROACH TO TUMOR DIAGNOSIS

Not infrequently the pathologist may encounter a tumor which is so "poorly differentiated" that classification by morphologic features alone is not possible. Electron microscopy may be helpful in providing ultrastructural evidence of squamous, muscle cell, or glandular differentiation, but, more often than not, the actual origin of the neoplasm cannot be determined; also, the pathologist frequently does not have material available for electron microscopic studies. Histochemical stains may also be of some value, such as the presence of periodic acid-Schiff-positive material or mucins in adenocarcinomas, but these types of stains are not specific with regard to the identification of particular cell or tumor types.

Immunohistochemistry offers the advantage of precise identification of cell types. At present, the number of antibodies available for this purpose is limited, but new antibodies are being constantly introduced.

Figure 2 provides an approach to the use of immunohistochemical methods in facilitating the diagnosis of unknown tumors. The antigens listed are those for which there is reasonable evidence in the literature for their general utility and reproducibility of staining. A number of other antibodies of equal or greater potential value have been described (i.e., anti-pancreatic cancer antigen, anti-lung cancer antigens), but data relating to their usefulness are either nonexistent, limited, or subject to such controversy that no recommendation can at present be given.

One approach is to screen tumors of unknown origin with antibodies against carcinoembryonic antigen (CEA) and keratin. The great majority of carcinomas have been shown to display some degree of reactivity with one or both of these antibodies in at least some of the carcinoma cells. Squamous carcinomas generally show more extensive positivity with antikeratin antibody, whereas adenocarcinomas are often positive with anti-CEA. However, the observation of some overlap of reactivity with these two antibodies precludes an absolute diagnosis. Part of the difficulty stems from the antibodies themselves. Not all anti-CEA antibodies are identical; some contain activity against nonspecific cancer antigen in addition to activity against CEA. Antibodies with significant nonspecific cancer antigen activity, in addition to CEA specificity, show a wider spectrum of positivity than highly purified CEA antibodies or monoclonal antibodies to CEA. Even with the use of monoclonal antibodies to CEA, reactivity may be observed in many different neoplasms. Colonic carcinoma typically shows some degree of reactivity for CEA (Fig. 3), but positivity has also been found in a variety of other adenocarcinomas of endodermal derivation, including carcinomas of the pancreas, stomach, and lung. Breast carcinoma has also been shown to be positive in 30 to 50% of cases. Tumors with definite squamous differentiation are less often CEA positive, but scattered CEA-positive cells have been identified in squamous carcinomas from the cervix and lung.

Likewise, antibodies against keratin derived from different sources have not always shown a uniform pattern of positivity. Some antibodies (antisera) seem mainly to identify cross-linked or high-molecular-weight keratin, such as is found in keratinizing squamous epithelium, while other antibodies more readily detect the nonlinked or low-molecular-weight keratin that exists as part of the cytoskeleton of diverse epithelial cell types. Mesothelial tumors and adenocarcinomas have shown various degrees of positivity with such antibodies.

These differences of immunostaining against keratins of different molecular weights can be largely explained by more basic research centered on identifying components of the cytoskeleton (intermediate filaments) found in almost all vertebrate cells (8). The diameter of intermediate filaments varies from 7 to 11 nm; these filaments are therefore considered intermediate between microfilaments (6 nm) and microtubules (25 nm). Different intermediate filaments can be identified by immunologic techniques. The filaments have been found to consist of polymers in which the major polypeptides vary in molecular weight from approximately 40 to 70,000; constituents with even higher molecular weights have been identified in neurofilaments. According to most investigators, there are five distinct subgroups of intermediate filaments: (i) cytokeratins found in true epithelia, (ii) neurofilaments found in many but not all neurons, (iii) glial fibrilliary acidic protein (GFAP) filaments found in various glial cells such as astrocytes and Bergmann glial cells, (iv) desmin filaments found in most myogenic cells, and (v) vimentin filaments found in various nonepithelial cells of so-called mesenchymal origin. It should also be noted that a limited number of cell types appear to lack intermediate filaments, forming a sixth subgroup.

The majority of major cell types contain only one type of intermediate filament. Both keratinizing and nonkeratinizing types of epithelial cells—not just squamous epithelium, but also the glandular, ductal, or lining epithelia of the liver, pancreas, intestine, lung, urinary bladder, and endometrium—react with antibodies against cytokeratin. Thymus reticular epithelium is also positive for cytokeratin. Vimentin intermediate filaments are associated with endothelial cells, fibroblasts, macrophages, chondrocytes, lymphocytes, and other cells of mesenchymal origin. Desmin is characteristic of most myogenic cells, including cells of cardiac, skeletal, and visceral smooth muscles. Interestingly, this intermediate filament is found in some but not all vascular smooth muscle cells. GFAP is present in many glial cell types, such as astrocytes, Bergmann glia, and cells of the glia limitans, whereas neurofilaments are found in most but not all neurons.

Some cells contain two intermediate filaments simultaneously. Such cells are certain astrocytes, which demonstrate both vimentin and GFAP, and some vascular smooth muscle cell types, which have both desmin and vimentin. The presence of cytokeratin and vimentin within the same cell is rarely seen, but it has been described in certain instances, such as in some cells of the parotid gland and in pleomorphic adenomas. At present, no cell has been found to express two types of intermediate filament without vimentin as one of the constituents. It is not certain whether three intermediate-filament types can exist in the same cell. As previously mentioned, certain types of cells contain no intermediate fila-

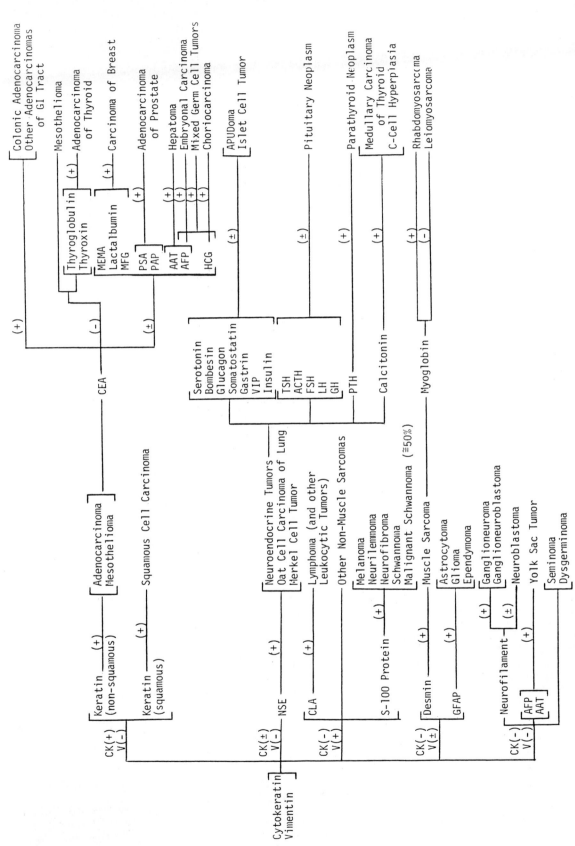

FIG. 2. Diagnostic algorithm for immunohistochemical diagnosis of tumors. The immunohistochemical reactivity of some tissues listed (particularly those indicated by ±) remains controversial, with differences in immunostaining being observed in different laboratories. These differences may be attributed to variations in antibody specificity, tissue fixation, tissue processing, staining techniques, and newly developed antibodies that have not been fully evaluated. CK, Cytokeratin; V, vimentin; MEMA, mammary epithelial membrane antigen; MFG, milk fat globule; PSA, prostate-specific antigen; PAP, prostatic acid phosphatase; AAT, alpha-1-antitrypsin; AFP, alpha-fetoprotein; HCG, human chorionic gonadotropin; NSE, neuron-specific enolase; VIP, vasoactive intestinal polypeptide; TSH, thyroid-stimulating hormone; ACTH, adrenocorticotropic hormone; FSH, follicle-stimulating hormone; LH, leutinizing hormone; GH, growth hormone; CLA, common leukocyte antigen; PTH, parathormone.

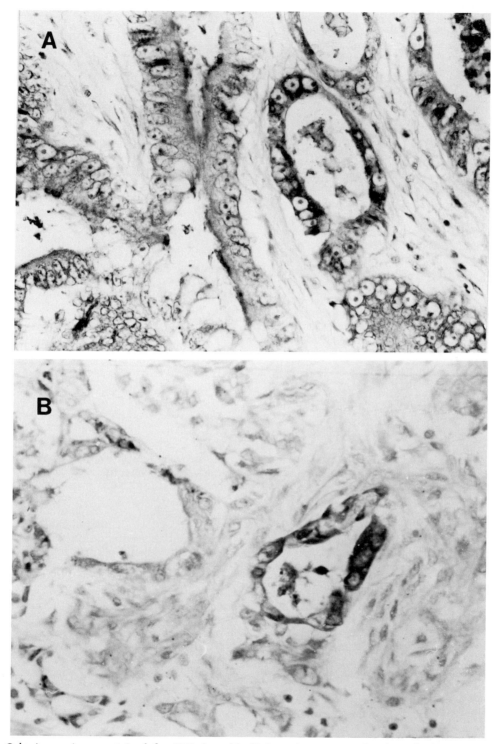

FIG. 3. (A) Colonic carcinoma stained for CEA (gray-black) by using a monoclonal antibody and the PAP method. Hematoxylin counterstain (400× objective). (B) Yolk sac carcinoma (endodermal sinus tumor) stained for alpha-fetoprotein (gray-black) by using a conventional antiserum and the PAP method. Hematoxylin counterstain (400× objective).

ments; this fact has been found to be true of germ cells.

With regard to the classification of neoplasms, it has been shown that essentially all carcinomas (i.e., epithelium-derived tumors), regardless of the site of the tumor or the degree of differentiation, stain positively for cytokeratin. But different tumors show differing amounts and arrangements of cytokeratin filaments. It now appears that there are some 19 distinct components of cytokeratin which differ in molecular weight and isoelectric point. These components are responsible for complex cytokeratin patterns which vary in different epithelia and to some extent may be more characteristic of certain epithelia than others. For example, epithelial cells found in colon and small intestine contain cytokeratin consisting of components 8 and 18, whereas high-molecular-weight components 1 and 2 are restricted to keratinizing epidermis and the epithelium of the anal canal and ectocervix.

It would seem reasonable, then, that in situations where the question involves an undifferentiated carcinoma versus some other type of neoplasm, a cytokeratin antibody of broad specificity is indicated. Once the carcinomatous nature of a neoplasm has been confirmed, then antibody with more limited specificity may be utilized to classify the tumor (e.g., components 8 and 18 for hepatocellular carcinoma). Likewise, antibodies to desmin and vimentin can be useful in identifying soft-tissue sarcomas. Antibodies to desmin distinguish sarcomas of muscle cell origin, including leiomyosarcoma and rhabdomyosarcoma, from other sarcomas which contain vimentin only. Rhabdomyosarcoma and leiomyosarcoma cannot be distinguished with antibody to desmin, since both tumors are desmin positive. Although vimentin has been found in some muscle sarcomas, nonmuscle sarcomas thus far examined have contained vimentin but not desmin. Tumors as diverse as liposarcoma and lymphoma have been shown to be vimentin positive and desmin negative.

Essentially all soft-tissue tumors have been shown to be negative for cytokeratin, so that antibodies to cytokeratin, vimentin, and desmin appear to be capable of distinguishing among carcinomas, nonmuscle sarcomas, and muscle sarcomas.

GFAP is considered the most specific marker for gliomas. If a tumor stains positively for GFAP, then the tumor is probably glial in origin. However, negative results have been found in some undifferentiated tumors thought to be of glial origin. Also, the small round cells in glioblastoma multiforme have shown little or no staining, whereas the large atypical multinucleated cells stained strongly. GFAP is also found in ependymomas.

Neurofilaments have been found in ganglioneuroblastoma and pheochromocytoma in relatively large amounts; however, staining in neuroblastomas is still controversial, discrepancies being found when negative paraffin-embedded material is compared with frozen tissue.

Although metastases from solid tumors seem to retain the intermediate filament of the primary neoplasm and generally do not acquire additional intermediate filaments, there are some reports of tumor cells within body fluids (i.e., ascites or plural effusions) which may be positive for both cytokeratin and vimentin.

The antibodies to intermediate filaments can be used not only to identify basic tumor types but also in some instances to subclassify tumors by using antibodies with narrower ranges of specificity (e.g., cytokeratins of various molecular weights). A battery of second-stage immunostains may then be utilized in an attempt to define more precisely the tumor under investigation. Again the range of antibodies available for the precise definition of tumors is limited, but growing rapidly.

PRESUMPTIVE CARCINOMAS AND ENDOCRINE TUMORS

Thyroglobulin and thyroxine

The follicular epithelial cells of the thyroid gland show various degrees of staining in paraffin sections treated with antibody against thyroglobulin, thyroxin, or triiodothyronine. The intensity of staining varies from cell to cell and follicle to follicle. Staining is usually more intense within the follicular cell cytoplasm than within the colloid stored within follicles, which characteristically shows a faint blush of reactivity. To date, the most commonly reported use of antithyroglobulin or antithyroxine antibody has been in the differential diagnosis of metastatic tumors derived from the thyroid. The majority of lesions metastatic from the thyroid follicular epithelium appear to contain some detectable thyroglobulin or thyroxine, though often the proportion of cells that show a positive reaction is very low. Clearly, however, the possibility does exist that poorly differentiated metastases may be poorly differentiated not only in a morphologic sense, but also in a functional sense and may contain no detectable thyroglobulin or thyroxine.

Calcitonin

Medullary C-cell carcinoma of the thyroid is derived from the so-called parafollicular C cells that produce calcitonin. The cells that form medullary C-cell carcinoma commonly produce calcitonin, often in sufficiently large amounts for physiologic effects to be seen within the patient, and calcitonin may be demonstrated within the cells of medullary C-cell carcinoma by immunoperoxidase techniques in paraffin sections. The intensity of staining varies from cell to cell, and the proportion of cells showing detectable staining varies from tumor to tumor. DeLellis (2) has described a particularly exciting practical use of calcitonin staining with reference to the diagnosis of medullary C-cell carcinoma, which may occur in either familial or sporadic form. Familial cases of C-cell carcinoma typically show an associated C-cell hyperplasia in the residual uninvolved thyroid; sporadic cases show normal numbers of C cells. Thus, examination of the residual thyroid for the number of C cells will effectively distinguish a familial from a sporadic case. Of even greater importance, in a clinical context, is that it has become apparent that only those family members showing C-cell hyperplasia are at risk. Thus, an approach advocated by DeLellis and colleagues is biopsy of the thyroids of family members of a familial case of medullary C-cell carcinomas, with consideration of thyroidectomy in those individuals showing C-cell hyperplasia.

Immunohistologic studies have also cast light on the microanatomy of the thyroid, revealing that "parafollicular C cells" are not truly parafollicular, but are situated within the confines of the basement membrane of adjacent follicles. These cells occupy a position in relation to the thyroid follicular epithelium somewhat analogous to that occupied by the diffuse neuroendocrine cells of the gut.

Parathormone

Parathormone can be successfully stained in paraffin sections and may be used for the identification of normal parathyroid tissue or parathyroid carcinoma, particularly when the carcinoma occurs as a metastasis. It is worth pointing out, however, that ectopic hormone production by tumors does occur, and parathormone, in particular, may be produced by tumors that are not of parathyroid origin. Immunostaining for parathormone may thus be attempted in tumors resected from patients with clinical evidence of parathormone hyperactivity in an effort to establish that the resected tumor is indeed responsible for the increased levels of parathormone. Another indication for carrying out a stain for parathormone would be in thoracic surgery, during parathyroidectomy, to confirm that tissue removed is parathyroid. A rapid-frozen section can readily be stained for the presence of the hormone. Such a stain carried out at 37°C may take only half an hour, which is consistent with the needs of the surgeon.

Pituitary hormones

Pituitary hormones were among the first antigens shown to be demonstrable within paraffin sections. Subsequently, the pituitary has proved to be a fertile area for investigation. Numerous papers have been published, to the extent that the standard pathology texts relating to the pituitary gland are largely obsolete. It is no longer sufficient simply to stain with orange G, tetrachrome, or periodic acid-Schiff in an attempt to assess hormonal activity of normal pituitary tissue or pituitary adenoma. It has become clear that the only accurate, reliable method of determining the function of excised pituitary tissue is to perform an immunostain. All of the major pituitary hormones have been successfully stained by immunoperoxidase techniques in paraffin sections; the pattern of staining can be utilized to distinguish normal pituitary tissue from hyperplastic pituitary tissue from pituitary adenoma. In normal pituitary tissue, cells containing an individual hormone occur in clusters of 3 to 5 cells; in hyperplasia, the cell clusters are generally larger, numbering 10 or more cells; in pituitary adenoma, complete fields are encountered that consist of a single cell type, usually containing only a single hormone. It has also become apparent that one other basic rule, i.e., that individual pituitary cells produce only one hormone, does not hold true, though the extent of double production of hormones has not been fully established.

Islet cell hormones

The nature and pattern of hormone production by islet cell tumors of the pancreas may also be accurately determined by immunostaining for insulin, glucagon, somatostatin, vasointestinal polypeptide, and gastrin. This staining is particularly useful in determining whether a particular tumor is responsible for an observed clinical effect (e.g., the demonstration of gastrin in relation to recurrent peptic ulceration).

Neuron-specific enolase

Normally, neuron-specific enolase is found in neurons and cells of the amine precursor uptake and decarboxylation (APUD) system. Although this protein enzyme may be used to mark tumors arising from these two cell types, it is not as specific as originally claimed, being found in variety of other tumors. Its usefulness is restricted largely to identification of APUDOMAS and tumors of the diffuse neuroendocrine system, as well as oat cell carcinomas of the lung.

Alpha-1-antitrypsin and alpha-fetoprotein

Both alpha-1-antitrypsin and alpha-fetoprotein are alpha-1-globulins; although both are produced in the fetal liver, only alpha-1-antitrypsin is normally produced in the adult. Both of these proteins are found in hepatocellular carcinoma and endodermal sinus (yolk sac) tumor (Fig. 3), generally as intracellular inclusions. Alpha-fetoprotein has also been found within other germ cell tumors that lack overt yolk sac differentiation, particularly within embryonal carcinomas.

Sex hormones

In the past, specific hormone production was generally assigned to specific cell types. Theca cells were thought to produce estrogen, and Leydig cells were responsible for the production of testosterone. Granulosa and Sertoli cells were generally regarded as inactive. By using specific antibodies to testosterone, estradiol, and progesterone, it has now been shown that all these cells may be functionally active and have the capacity to synthesize both estrogen and androgens. This observation has proved of value in the identification of hormone-producing gonadal stromal tumors (6).

PROSTATIC ACID PHOSPHATASE AND PROSTATE-SPECIFIC ANTIGEN

The detection of elevated levels of prostatic acid phosphatase (PAP) in serum has value in detecting the presence of extensive prostatic carcinoma. The PAP is released by the tumor cells. Benign normal prostate cells also contain PAP, detectable by immunoperoxidase methods in paraffin sections; indeed, on a cell-to-cell basis, normal prostatic epithelial cells stain more intensely than do prostate cancer cells. The value of staining tissue for PAP is not in distinguishing benign prostate from malignant prostate cells, but in identifying a poorly differentiated carcinoma of unknown origin as prostatic carcinoma. In our experience, PAP is present in almost all prostatic cancers, primary or secondary, and has not been observed in other cancers. Prostate-specific antigen, prepared from semen, has a similar distribution, and the antibody may be used in a similar manner. Our experiences parallel those of other investigators.

BREAST-RELATED ANTIGENS

Breast cancer has been the subject of extensive immunohistologic research. Some monoclonal antibodies exist which in some cases are able to distin-

TABLE 2. Commercial immunostaining kits and reagents

Company and location	Materials available
Vector, Burlingame, Calif.	ABC kits
Biogenex, Dublin, Calif.	Approx 40 immunohistology kits
Labsystems Inc., Chicago, Ill.	Antibodies to intermediate filaments
Ortho, Carpenteria, Calif.	Broadest range of kits, including monoclonal antibodies to T and B cells
Becton Dickinson Monoclonal Antibody Unit, Mountain View, Calif.	B- and T-cell kits
Biomeda, Foster City, Calif.	Approx 20 immunohistology kits
Miles Laboratories, Naperville, Ill.	Approx 50 immunohistology kits
Dako, Santa Barbara, Calif.	Approx 40 immunohistology kits
Hybritech, San Diego, Calif.	Monoclonal antibodies to CEA, etc.
Techniclone, Costa Mesa, Calif.	LN antibodies, reactive with lymphocytes in paraffin sections

guish breast cancer from normal breast tissue. There have been claims that antibody against transferrin or transferrin receptor may serve the same purpose, whereas lactoferrin is detected both in benign breast epithelial cells and in some carcinomas. Other antibodies (e.g., versus mammary epithelial membrane antigen, milk fat globule antigen, and lactalbumin) facilitate the distinction of breast tissue (normal or malignant) from other tissues.

PRESUMPTIVE SARCOMAS: KERATIN NEGATIVE, VIMENTIN POSITIVE

S-100 protein

S-100 protein is an acidic protein first isolated from bovine brain extract. It has been shown to be widely distributed within the supporting cells of central and peripheral nervous systems (astrocytes, oligodendrocytes, and Schwann cells) and their respective tumors. It is not, however, restricted to the nervous system, as it has been found in other cells, including chondrocytes, some histiocytes, interdigitating reticulum cells, and nevi, with rare reports of reactivity in some carcinomas. Antibody to this protein has been found useful in the identification of benign nerve sheath lemmoma tumors (neurofibroma, neurilemmoma, and granular cell tumor). S-100 protein is less helpful in the identification of malignant Schwannomas, as less than half of these tumors have been shown to mark with this protein. The vast majority of malignant melanomas, including amelanotic forms, contain S-100 protein, making it a useful marker for the differentiation of malignant melanomas from many carcinomas. Tumors suspected of melanoma may be more reliably identified by using monoclonal antibodies against melanoma-related antigens; these antibodies are particularly effective in frozen sections, but some have been reported to be effective in paraffin sections.

Myoglobin

An oxygen-binding heme protein, myoglobin is present in striated muscle tissues and has been demonstrated by immunohistochemical methods in normal and neoplastic skeletal muscle cells. It is generally considered a specific marker for skeletal muscle neoplasms, being useful for the diagnosis of rhabdomyo-sarcoma. It is best used in conjunction with antidesmin antibody.

Factor VIII-associated antigen

Kaposi's sarcoma is of great current interest due to a high frequency of occurrence in the so-called homosexual-related immunodeficiency syndrome. The sarcomatous cells are believed to be derived from endothelium, an observation supported by the frequent occurrence of factor VIII-associated antigen within the tumor cells when they are stained by immunohistologic techniques. The fact that Kaposi's sarcoma does stain for factor VIII-associated antigen has been used in the differential diagnosis of this lesion from undifferentiated sarcomatous proliferations.

Common leukocyte antigen and lymphocyte-related antigens

There are numerous monoclonal antibodies against leukocyte surface antigens that distinguish among T cells, B cells, monocytes, granulocytes, and various differentiation subsets. These antibodies can be used to recognize leukocytes and the corresponding neoplasms in frozen sections. Unfortunately, the great majority of these antibodies will not detect the corresponding antigens in fixed paraffin sections. However, a few antibodies effective in paraffin sections have become available.

One such antibody reacts with common leukocyte antigen reliably in sections fixed with Formalin and in sections optimally fixed with B-5; the antibody reacts less well if Formalin fixation is too short. Applied to an undifferentiated neoplasm, positive cell membrane staining is evidence in favor of a lymphoma (or, less often, of granulocytic sarcoma or a histiocytic tumor) (10).

Three other monoclonal antibodies, designated LN-1, LN-2, and LN-3, also are effective in fixed paraffin sections, B-5 being preferable to Formalin. LN-1 reacts, among lymphoid cells, only with follicular center B cells and follicular center cell lymphomas; LN-2 reacts with most B-cell lymphomas and some normal and neoplastic histiocytes (but not T-cell lymphomas; all nonlymphomas are nonreactive); LN-3 has anti-Ia activity and reacts with B cells and histiocytes.

Clearly, the reagents may be forerunners of panels of highly discriminatory antibodies.

CONCLUSION

Immunohistochemistry has provided a new and more scientific approach to diagnostic pathology, offering an alternative to diagnosis by morphology alone. The techniques involved are simple and practical, allowing identification of many tissue antigens in paraffin-embedded tissues. Areas of uncertainty still remain, but with further investigation and research, the role of specific antibodies will be more completely defined for diagnostic as well as therapeutic use. Some commercial (kit) sources are listed in Table 2.

LITERATURE CITED

1. **Banks, P. M.** 1979. Diagnostic applications of an immunoperoxidase method in hematopathology. J. Histochem. Cytochem. **27**:1192–1194.
2. **DeLellis, R. A. (ed.).** 1981. Monographs in diagnostic pathology: diagnostic immunohistochemistry. Masson Publishing U.S.A., Inc., New York.
3. **Epstein, A. L., R. J. Marder, J. N. Winter, and R. I. Fox.** 1984. Two new monoclonal antibodies (LN-1, LN-2) reactive in B-5 Formalin-fixed paraffin-embedded tissues with follicular center and mantle zone human B lymphocytes and derived tumors. J. Immunol. **133**:1028–1036.
4. **Falini, B., and C. R. Taylor.** 1983. New developments in immunoperoxidase techniques and their applications. Arch. Pathol. Lab. Med. **107**:105–117.
5. **Hsu, S. M., L. Raine, and H. Fanger.** 1981. Use of avidin-biotin peroxidase complex (ABC) in immunoperoxidase techniques: a comparison of ABC and unlabelled antibody (PAP) procedures. J. Histochem. Cytochem. **29**:577–580.
6. **Kurman, R. J., C. R. Taylor, and U. Goebelsmann.** 1981. Immunocytochemistry diagnosis and classification of ovarian and testicular neoplasms, p. 137–148. *In* R. A. DeLellis (ed.), Monographs in diagnostic pathology: diagnostic immunohistochemistry. Masson Publishing U.S.A., Inc., New York.
7. **Nadji, M., A. R. Morales, J. Ziegles-Weissman, and N. S. Penneys.** 1981. Kaposi's sarcoma: immunohistologic evidence for an endothelial origin. Arch. Pathol. Lab. Med. **105**:274–275.
8. **Osborn, M., and K. Weber.** 1983. Biology of disease. Tumor diagnosis by intermediate filament typing: a novel tool for surgical pathology. Lab. Invest. **48**:372–394.
9. **Sternberger, L. A.** 1978. Immunocytochemistry, 2nd ed. John Wiley & Sons, Inc., New York.
10. **Warnke, R. A., K. C. Gatter, and B. Fallini.** 1983. Diagnosis of human lymphoma with monoclonal antileukocyte antibodies. N. Engl. J. Med. **309**:1275–1281.

Chapter 146

Section P. Laboratory Management and Administration

Organization of the Clinical Immunology Laboratory

SHARAD D. DEODHAR

There has been rapid progress in the field of immunology during the past 2 decades, and significant advances have been made not only in our understanding of the basic mechanisms of the immune response, but also in the clinical applications of these mechanisms on a practical level. Historically, the applications of immunology to laboratory medicine were primarily in the areas of infectious disease serology and, later, blood banking. In recent years, the scope of immunology has widened greatly, and its practical applications now extend to various clinical areas such as rheumatology, dermatology, nephrology, allergy and hypersensitivity diseases, cardiology, neurology, pediatrics, gastroenterology, and two other major areas, namely, transplantation and cancer immunology. A plethora of laboratory tests involving immunologic techniques or designed to evaluate various components of the immune system have now become available, and clinical laboratories are faced with the problem of providing service in many or all of the areas mentioned. Recent legislative changes such as introduction of the concept of diagnosis-related groupings have made it necessary that these services be provided in an efficient and cost-effective fashion. An attempt will be made here to present some approaches to organizing a clinical immunology laboratory that would provide most of the immunologic services needed in a large community hospital while at the same time emphasizing quality assurance, efficiency, and cost control.

PROPOSED ORGANIZATION

In the past, different immunologic test procedures were carried out in different clinical laboratories, such as laboratories for microbiology, serology, blood banking, and other services. There is, however, a distinct trend now among large medical centers to create a specific, well-defined clinical immunology laboratory so that appropriate service to the various clinical departments can be provided in a well-coordinated fashion. The tests or procedures generally considered in the realm of the clinical immunology laboratory may include immunomicroscopy, agglutination techniques, various techniques involving immunoprecipitation, nephelometry for the measurement of various serum or other body fluid components, evaluation of complement components, histocompatibility testing or tissue typing, various tests involving cell-mediated immune function, quantitation of lymphocyte subsets by flow cytometry, radioimmunoassays (RIAs), enzyme-labeled immunoassays (EIAs), and others. Admittedly, there always has been and always will be a great deal of overlap between the activities of

such a unit and those of other clinical laboratories in any given large health care institution. However, organization of the laboratories, based on the concept of centralization of special techniques, can avoid the costly duplication of space, equipment, and skilled technical personnel. The recent focus on cost containment in various segments of the health industry makes it essential that the concept of centralization be applied as widely as possible, particularly in those situations involving the use of highly expensive instruments or highly skilled technical personnel.

The laboratory components of a typical clinical immunology unit may be divided as follows: (i) general immunology laboratory, (ii) cellular immunology laboratory, (iii) histocompatibility-testing or tissue-typing laboratory, and (iv) RIA, EIA, or tumor marker laboratory. The test activities in each of these subunits must be based on the usual quality control considerations, such as procedural selection for a given test, quality of reagents, proper instruments, specimen collection and storage, safety procedures, appropriate standards and positive and negative control specimens, data processing, interpretation and reporting, and appropriate cost accounting of each test procedure. An excellent discussion of these quality assurance practices as related to the clinical immunology laboratory has been provided in two recent monographs (1, 2).

GENERAL IMMUNOLOGY LABORATORY

The general immunology laboratory should be able to perform tests such as various immunoprecipitation techniques, immunomicroscopy involving fluorescence- and enzyme-labeled reagents, analysis of various complement components, agglutination tests, serum protein analyses, including those performed by the nephelometric techniques, and other procedures. The space, equipment, and personnel for such a unit should be arranged to suit the appropriate clinical needs of a given institution. Specific guidelines for the design of laboratories can be obtained from the American Public Health Association (1).

Various serologic tests for the evaluation of infectious diseases can also be performed in the general immunology laboratory. The most frequently performed tests in this laboratory are usually those related to the detection of circulating autoantibodies in various autoimmune diseases. The popular indirect immunofluorescence tests include those for various antinuclear antibodies, mitochondrial antibodies, smooth-muscle antibodies, antibodies localizing in the intercellular region and in the basement membrane of the skin, antibodies to cytoplasmic components of parietal cells, adrenal cortical cells, thyroid epithelial cells, and many others. Of these, the test for antinuclear antibody is probably the most commonly requested, since it is thought to be the best screening test for all diseases in the systemic lupus erythematosus and related connective tissue disease categories. The direct immunofluorescence test, as performed on tissue biopsy specimens such as those of renal, skin, muscle, liver, and other tissues, is also clinically important. The measurement of serum proteins, including various immunoglobulins, complement components, C-reactive protein, and many others, is now carried out by automated nephelometry in most laboratories. The nephelometric technique has certain distinct advantages over the previously used agar diffusion techniques for the measurement of these serum components. Immunoelectrophoretic procedures are performed primarily for the characterization of monoclonal gammopathies. The agglutination techniques are particularly useful in the measurement of thyroglobulin antibodies and microsomal antibodies in the study of patients with autoimmune or Hashimoto's thyroiditis. Also, latex agglutination still enjoys a great deal of popularity for the measurement of rheumatoid factor, although nephelometric techniques have been introduced in this situation also.

CELLULAR IMMUNOLOGY LABORATORY

The cellular immunology laboratory can be designed to perform those tests dealing with the evaluation of cell-mediated immunity and the study of lymphocyte subsets in general. The procedures may include a lymphocyte blast transformation test with various mitogens such as phytohemagglutinin, concanavalin A, and pokeweed mitogen; the study of proliferative responses to specific antigens; lymphocyte cytotoxicity tests against various target cells, including tumor cells and others; tests for monocyte function; quantitation of T- and B-cell subsets; and various other procedures as needed. Since many of the procedures performed in this unit involve cell culture techniques, this laboratory must meet the usual rigid, sterile requirements for the actual cell culture part of the work. To minimize the danger of contamination, this laboratory should be properly enclosed, and it should be designed to minimize traffic flow. It should also be equipped with certain special devices such as overhead UV light and a positive air pressure system equipped with appropriate filters and laminar-flow hoods. In addition, this laboratory should also have appropriate cell culture incubators, a phase microscope for studying cell cultures, and other standard equipment for such operations. Ideally, the cell culture laboratory should be divided into two parts, i.e., one for the rigid, sterile work necessary for long-term cultures and the other for work with short-term cultures, preparation of reagents, processing of specimens for final evaluations, and other such procedures that do not require absolute sterility.

In most clinical laboratories, the quantitation of T- and B-cell subsets is still carried out by rosetting techniques involving sheep erythrocytes and other appropriate reagents. However, the introduction of flow cytometry and the availability of automated instruments have provided a major advance in the area of T- and B-cell quantitation and the study of the various lymphocyte subsets. Measurements of T-cell subsets, particularly the ratio of T-helper to T-suppressor cells, has proved to be extremely helpful in the study of patients with acquired immune deficiency syndrome (AIDS) and a wide variety of autoimmune diseases, including systemic lupus erythematosus and others; in the monitoring of renal and other transplant patients; and in the study of patients with immunodeficiency and lymphoproliferative diseases. Although flow cytometry is still limited to a few large institutions in this country, the increasing availability of simpler, less expensive instruments promises to make this approach far more popular in the near future.

HISTOCOMPATIBILITY-TESTING OR TISSUE-TYPING UNIT

Histocompatibility testing is a specialized type of service which is essential if a given institution is involved in clinical transplant programs. In most parts of the country, such units provide regional service in that they perform histocompatibility testing for all transplants done in a given geographic area. Thus, the histocompatibility laboratory at Cleveland Clinic Foundation performs all tissue-typing procedures on donors and recipients in the transplant programs in northeastern Ohio. Another important area of activity for this laboratory is the study of various disease associations, particularly with respect to HLA-DR antigens. Another important application of the histocompatibility antigen determinations has been in the area of paternity testing. The data derived from HLA testing are being used increasingly in this regard.

RIA-EIA TUMOR MARKER LABORATORY

The RIA-EIA tumor marker laboratory can perform various hormonal determinations, drug level studies, measurements of tumor markers such as carcinoembryonic antigen and alpha-fetoprotein, and many other tests. In many institutions around the country, these techniques are performed by various clinical laboratory departments, including endocrinology, clinical chemistry, and radiology. However, the techniques are essentially immunologic, involving antigen-antibody reactions, and therefore one can consider them another integral part of the clinical immunology laboratory activities. The current trend is toward automation of various RIA and EIA procedures, and automated equipment is available for the performance of many of these procedures. Automation is particularly helpful for high-volume tests such as those for T3, T4, digoxins, etc. One major advantage in performing all such analyses in one laboratory unit is that efficient service can be offered with respect to time, effort, and cost.

PROFICIENCY TESTING

Every clinical immunology laboratory must, at any time, be ready to demonstrate and document its competence in performing any of the procedures that are carried out as part of its routine clinical service.

In-house quality control programs are very important in this regard, and it is suggested that approximately 20 to 25% of the total laboratory effort be directed to the performance of tests on quality control specimens such as various standards, positive and negative controls, and appropriate unknowns as provided by various national proficiency testing programs. Participation in such programs is strongly recommended, and at the present time such programs are offered by the Centers for Disease Control in Atlanta, Ga., and the College of American Pathologists. At present, both of these programs are voluntary for those laboratories that do not participate in interstate mailing of specimens. For those laboratories that do receive specimens from out of state, participation in one of these programs is required. Participation in these programs involves performing various tests on certain unknown specimens, and the results of all participating laboratories are then compared with those of the referee laboratories. The performance of each laboratory is then graded as acceptable or unacceptable. The results are also analyzed on the basis of the particular technique employed for a given test, the source of the reagents used, and, in some cases, the specific instrument being used. The data derived from these programs have been extremely helpful in comparing the performances of different sets of reagents, kits, etc., and in studying interlaboratory variations of the various test results.

LICENSURE AND CERTIFICATION OF PERSONNEL

In any clinical service laboratory, the technical personnel represent the single most important item for maintaining high-quality performance. For the various types of immunologic procedures described here, the individual in a technical position should have, as background education, either a bachelor's degree in one of the biological sciences or a medical technologist certification such as that given by the Board of Registry of the American Society of Clinical Pathologists or by the American Society of Medical Technology. Previous experience in an immunology laboratory is very helpful, but not essential, for employment in a clinical immunology laboratory. Special certification in clinical laboratory immunology is now available through the Board of Registry of the American Society of Clinical Pathologists, at both the categorical and the specialist levels. Both of these certifications require certain periods of practical experience in a clinical setting as well as a formal educational background. These examinations are given annually, and specific details can be obtained by writing to the Board of Registry office in Chicago, Ill. For individuals with a doctoral degree (Ph.D. or M.D.) and 6 years of experience in a clinical setting, the American Society for Microbiology, through its Board of Medical Laboratory Immunology, offers a certification examination, also given annually. For pathologists, anatomic or clinical, the American Board of Pathology offers a special certification in immunopathology, and the appropriate written and practical examinations are also given annually. Thus, it is now possible for all the personnel in a given clinical immunology laboratory, at both the technical and professional levels, to acquire appropriate certification from one or more of the agencies mentioned. It is essential that the professional director of the laboratory have appropriate certification, and it is strongly recommended that as many of the technical personnel as possible acquire certification. These certification programs make it possible to recognize the experience and talents of individuals working in clinical immunology laboratories, and the programs help to maintain the level of excellence expected of these laboratories.

CONCLUSION

The recent expansion and progress in clinical immunology has resulted in a dramatic increase in the number of immunologic diagnostic tests performed in clinical laboratories. To achieve maximum efficiency and cost containment, it is recommended that the various laboratory activities be centralized as much as possible, and in certain highly specialized situations, the facilities may even be shared among different institutions in a given geographic region. The various component laboratories described above need not be physically separate or distinct; rather, they can be considered separate in an administrative sense. In the final analysis, each institution must arrive at its own organization to meet its own needs.

LITERATURE CITED

1. Deodhar, S. D., W. E. Braun, L. P. Cawley, P. W. Keitges, R. M. Nakamura, G. M. Penn, G. Reynoso, and E. S. Tucker. 1978. Immunology, p. 745–786. *In* S. L. Inhorn (ed.), Quality assurance practices for health laboratories. American Public Health Association, Washington, D.C.
2. Rippey, J. H., and R. M. Nakamura. 1983. Diagnostic immunology: technology assessment and quality assurance. College of American Pathologists, Skokie, Ill.

Chapter 147

Quality Control in Immunoserology

ROGER N. TAYLOR

The purpose of this chapter is to present concepts of quality control that are peculiar to immunologic test results, especially those from serologic titrations. Since extensive literature addresses the general principles and formulas used for quality control, they will not be repeated here (1, 2, 5–8, 15). Although the following discussion will be limited to internal quality control, the same principles could be applied to proficiency testing (external quality control).

Two of the most common problems related to the quality control of immunologic test results are ignoring the need to measure actual variation and disregarding the fact that the results frequently have a log-Gaussian distribution rather than a Gaussian distribution. It is commonly held dogma that serologic test results vary by plus or minus one dilution and that, therefore, a fourfold difference is significantly different. These ideas are still used for quality control of serologic test results despite the facts that the assertions are vague and undocumented and that there is evidence that these ideas are usually not true (9).

For some immunologic tests, Gaussian-based statistical calculations are improperly used when it is known that the results more nearly approximate a log-normal distribution; e.g., with immunoglobulins. More appropriate methods of measuring variation in immunoserology will be the primary emphasis of this chapter.

DESIRABLE CHARACTERISTICS OF A MEASUREMENT SYSTEM

An ideal system for measuring variation in immunologic tests would include the following desirable features.

1. The system should be easy to use.
2. It should be a sensitive indicator of performance problems.
3. It should be capable of being related to clinical requirements.
4. It should be compatible with the other systems used in the laboratory.
5. It should be easily automated.
6. It should permit the establishment of quality control charts.
7. It should permit the measurement of precision as well as accuracy.
8. It should permit the use of standard statistical tests.
9. It should permit the derivation of probability values.
10. It should be useful for making interlaboratory, intermethod, or intertechnologist comparisons.
11. It should not be biased toward any specific measurement system.
12. It should permit the reporting of continuous (as opposed to discrete) results such as those that can be

obtained from nephelometry, fluoroimmunoassay, enzyme immunoassay, and radioimmunoassay.

13. It should permit the reporting of central values that are not restricted to the discrete values in a particular system of measurement and should take into consideration the fact that the best estimate of central tendency (analyte concentration) may not be a possible result in any particular assay system.
14. The estimate of variation should not change appreciably when samples with slightly different mean values are tested.
15. It should be applicable to measurement systems that produce irregular (not uniformly spaced) results, such as the Rantz and Randal system used for anti-streptolysin O.

VARIATION IN SEROLOGIC TESTS

Do serologic test results vary by plus or minus one dilution and is a fourfold difference significant?

Even though these ideas are commonly accepted, little thought seems to have been given to what they actually mean or what the implications of their acceptance are. In most cases, the plus-or-minus-one-tube rule has been taken to mean that as long as none of the results differ by more than one tube from the central result, the variation is acceptable. In some cases, the rule is interpreted to mean that variation is acceptable as long as replicate titers remain within a twofold range. Sometimes the plus-or-minus-one-tube rule is used when dilution schemes other than twofold are used or when irregular dilution schemes are used.

These interpretations do not take into account the fact that frequently the true result may be between two tubes; i.e., the true result may not be one of the possible discrete values in a particular assay system. They also ignore the fact that within these limits there can be great differences in the percentage of results that are identical when the same specimen is repeatedly measured (9). The implicit assumption underlying this rule and these interpretations is that the variation in all serologic tests, in all laboratories, and under all conditions is the same.

The problem of measuring variation in serologic test results has been investigated by others at the Centers for Disease Control, and various methods of measuring variation have been proposed (3, 14), but we prefer the simpler method that has been in use in proficiency testing since 1972 (9–13; R. N. Taylor, Ph.D. thesis, University of Utah, Salt Lake City, 1974). Our method consists simply of converting the results to logarithms (to any convenient base), calculating the mean and standard deviation by the commonly used formulas, and converting back to the original form (antilogarithm).

The simplicity of the calculation is demonstrated in the following example.

Result	Log$_2$	(Log$_2$)^2
1	0	0
2	1	1
4	2	4
$n = 3$	$\Sigma X = 3$	$\Sigma X^2 = 5$

Geometric mean

$$\overline{X}_G = \text{antilog } \overline{X}_{\log}$$

$$\overline{X}_{\log} = \frac{\Sigma X}{n}$$

$$\overline{X}_{\log} = \frac{3}{3}$$

$$\overline{X}_{\log} = 1$$

$$\overline{X}_G = 2$$

Geometric standard deviation

$$S_G = \text{antilog } S_{\log}$$

$$S_{\log} = \sqrt{\frac{\Sigma X^2 - \frac{(\Sigma X)^2}{n}}{n - 1}}$$

$$S_{\log} = \sqrt{\frac{5 - \frac{(3)^2}{3}}{3 - 1}}$$

$$S_{\log} = 1$$

$$S_G = 2$$

The results 1, 2, and 4 have corresponding logs to the base 2 of 0, 1, and 2, respectively, and logs squared of 0, 1, and 4, respectively. There are three values with the sum of their logs equal to 3 and the sum of their logs squared equal to 5. By substituting the values into the formula for the mean, we get a value of 1 as the mean of the log results. The antilog of 1 is 2; therefore, the geometric mean of the results 1, 2, and 4 is 2. By substituting the appropriate values into the formula for the standard deviation and solving the equation, we get a standard deviation of the log values of 1. The antilog of 1 is 2, so the geometric standard deviation of the results is also 2.

This method is a simple adaptation (log conversion) of the method that is commonly used in other clinical laboratory disciplines and defines variation in terms of standard deviations (geometric). It avoids the confusion that has resulted from conflicting definitions of repeatability, replicability, and reproducibility that are used in serology (4, 5, 7). Variation can be measured within or among samples, technologists, tests, or laboratories.

This method of measuring variation in serologic test results is similar to the method used in other laboratory disciplines, but the results must first be log transformed because most, if not all, serologic test results and many other test results are approximately log-normally distributed. It is convenient to describe variation in measurements by reference to the normal curve for a number of reasons: (i) the mean value is the best estimate of the true value, (ii) the calculation of two simple parameters (mean and standard deviation) completely describes the distribution and will therefore permit calculations of the percentage of results that will be within any defined limits of the curve, and (iii) many common statistical tests are based on the normal curve or modifications of it. Therefore, comparison between or among items can be made, and the probability of significant differences can be estimated.

FREQUENCY DISTRIBUTION

One of the first things that must be done in analyzing data for quality control is to determine the shape of the frequency distribution. Control sera that represent the range of values to be expected when assays on patient samples are performed should be selected with emphasis on the critical or borderline levels or titers. After the results of at least 30 assays on each of the control sera have been collected, the data can be examined to see if the distribution fits the normal or log-normal curve. Statistical tests (chi-square test and Kolmogorov-Smirnov test) are available to determine if a set of results differs significantly from a specific theoretical distribution (13), but in many cases rough approximations are satisfactory. Preparation of a simple frequency distribution histogram is a good first step. Use bars of equal size that have increments characterized by a common difference, i.e., 1, 2, 3, 4, 5, etc., to check for a normal distribution; use bars of equal size that have increments with a common ratio, i.e., 1, 2, 4, 8, 16, etc., to check for a log-normal distribution. If the distribution does not fit the expected curve at all, it will be apparent from the histogram and will eliminate the need for further evaluation. If the histogram is symmetrical and looks like the Gaussian curve, other quick tests can be applied.

The next step is to calculate the means and standard deviations to see if those statistics look acceptable. Calculate arithmetic means and standard deviations for the normal distribution and geometric means and standard deviations for log-normal distributions (see the formulas above). If the differences between the mean and the median and the mean and the mode are small, if approximately 68% of the results are within 1 standard deviation of the mean, and if approximately 95% of the results are within 2 standard deviation limits, the results are probably close enough to normal or log-normal to justify using parametric statistical tests.

When the variation is small, it may not make much difference whether arithmetic or geometric parameters are used. Table 1 shows some examples of the relationship between arithmetic and geometric parameters calculated from a log-normal distribution. When the geometric standard deviations are small, the 95% limits are about the same with either assumption (normal or log-normal). In addition, there is a good correlation between the geometric standard de-

TABLE 1. Relationship between arithmetic and geometric parameters calculated from a log-normal distribution.

Actual geometric parameters			Calculated arithmetic parameters			
Mean	SD	95% limits	Mean	SD	CV[a] (%)	95% limits
100	2.00	25–400	127	100	79	−73–327
100	1.41	50–200	106	38	36	31–182
100	1.19	71–141	102	18	18	66–137
100	1.09	84–119	100	9	9	83–117
100	1.04	92–109	100	4	4	92–108
100	1.02	96–104	100	2	2	96–104
100	1.01	98–102	100	1	1	98–102
100	1.00	100–100	100	0	0	100–100

[a] CV, Coefficient of variation.

viation and the arithmetic standard deviation, i.e., 1.01 versus 1, 1.02 versus 2, 1.04 versus 4, etc. When variation is large, it is critical that the appropriate distribution assumption be used. For example, the calculated mean, standard deviation, and 95% limits are substantially different from the geometric counterparts when the geometric standard deviation is 2.00 (mean, 100 versus 127; standard deviation, 2.00 versus 100; 95% limits, 25 to 400 versus −73 to 327).

QUALITY CONTROL CHARTS

Measurements are subject to two kinds of errors, i.e., random and systematic. Systematic errors (accuracy errors) appear as bias; i.e., results are consistently either higher or lower than the true value. Random errors (precision errors) are indicated by the inability to repeatedly reproduce the same result or relationship.

Systematic error in a test procedure commonly arises from those errors inherent in the test equipment, reagents, or calibrations. This error is usually reasonably constant from day to day. A temporary systematic error would result from a shift in the calibration of an instrument, from a change in reagents, or from the use of a standard that had deteriorated. This error would be quite constant until the problem was recognized and corrected.

When multiple determinations are run on the same material, the mean is usually considered the best estimate of the true value, but without some standardization, the true value is open to question. It is important, therefore, that certified reference samples with defined or established reference values be available to check the closeness of the observed values to the reference values that are considered the true values. The determination of the accuracy of a result is impossible when there is no definitive standard for the substance being measured and especially if different procedures give different values for the same material. For many tests, standard materials or standard methods or both are available.

"Precision" refers to the ability of a test to give essentially the same value in repeated applications on the same or similar material and is a measure of random error. Many sources of error are controlled for samples tested in replicate on the same day, in the same run, by the same technologist, and with the same method, standards, and reagents. In this case, the systematic errors are constant (because they were consistently applied) and do not enter into the precision measurement. The resulting error is the random error of the assay.

Youden and Steiner have shown that precision can be measured without the necessity of making any repeat determinations, even duplicates (15). Measuring precision on samples that are not duplicates has the benefit of providing more estimates of systematic error with no additional work, and it is less subject to censorship. If it is known that samples are duplicates, the results are more susceptible to compromise.

The best way to estimate precision is to perform single determinations on each of two similar materials. Each measurement contains both systematic and random error, but when the differences are obtained, the systematic error in one is subtracted from the systematic error in the other, and the variation in the remainder is an estimate of twice the random error. The standard deviation of the results from a single material can be estimated by dividing the standard deviation of the difference by the square root of 2. If duplicate measurements are made on a single sample or if single measurements are made on duplicate samples, variation can be used to estimate precision. When the samples are not duplicates, the variation in the difference can also be used to measure precision.

This method of analysis can be modified to be applicable to log-normal data by converting the test results to logarithms. Because serologic dilutions are based on twofold dilutions, logarithms to the base 2 are convenient for this example. For the dilutions 1:1 (undiluted), 1:2, 1:4, 1:8, 1:16, etc., the corresponding titers (reciprocal dilutions) are 1, 2, 4, 8, 16, etc., and the corresponding logarithms to the base 2 are 0, 1, 2, 3, 4, etc.

Measuring the difference between the two samples in logarithms is equivalent to measuring the ratio of two samples. If one sample has a titer of 8 and another has a titer of 4, their corresponding log values are 3 and 2. The difference between samples is one twofold dilution, which is the same as a ratio of 2. The titer 8 divided by 4 is also a ratio of 2.

The variability in immunologic tests can and should be monitored with the same methods applicable to other quantitative tests. The results of repeated testing of control sera should be accumulated until there are enough values (generally at least 30 results) to allow reasonably reliable calculations of the geometric mean and standard deviation. Control sera should be available in sufficient quantity to last 6 months or more, if possible, to provide continuous monitoring as reagents or kits change. The results obtained for each control serum (high titer or concentration, low titer or concentration, and negative or normal) should then be used to construct quality control charts similar to those recommended for other areas of the laboratory.

The charts should indicate the mean and the upper and lower acceptability limits and should provide for the routine plotting of control results so that shifts, trends, and "out of control" results can be readily detected. Separate charts should be prepared for accuracy and precision.

The control limits can be calculated in a way similar to the way arithmetic limits are calculated. The range of 1 geometric standard deviation is expressed as the geometric mean multiplied or divided by 1 geometric standard deviation rather than ±1 arithmetic standard deviation. The range for 1 geometric standard deviation includes all values between the geometric mean divided by the geometric standard deviation and the geometric mean multiplied by the geometric standard deviation. The range for 1 geometric standard deviation for a group of values with a geometric mean of 80 and a geometric standard deviation of 2 would be from 40 (80 divided by 2) to 160 (80 multiplied by 2). To calculate ranges other than that for 1 geometric standard deviation, the geometric standard deviation is raised to the power of the number of geometric standard deviations desired. For example, the range for 2 geometric standard deviations is the geometric mean multiplied and divided by the geometric standard deviation squared, and the range for 3 geometric standard deviations is the geometric mean multiplied and divided by the geometric standard deviation cubed. From the example above, the range for 2 geometric standard deviations would be from 20 (80 divided by 2^2) to 320 (80 multiplied by 2^2), and the range for 3 standard deviations would be from 10 (80 divided by 2^3) to 640 (80 multiplied by 2^3). It is not necessary that any of the values be whole numbers. The limits for 1.41 geometric standard deviations for the same example would be from 30 (80 divided by $2^{1.41}$ [2.66]) to 213 (80 multiplied by $2^{1.41}$). In some cases it is easier to use the traditional formulas on the log-transformed data and then convert the results back to the original form after the limits have been calculated.

Ideally, the calculated control limits should be compared with the clinical requirements for a particular analyte before a test is used for reporting patient test results. If the accuracy, precision, and other parameters do not meet the clinical requirements, the methodology should be reviewed for possible ways of improving performance, or other methods should be considered. At present, it is difficult to comply with this ideal because consensus clinical requirements do not exist. The tentative recommendations that have been proposed should be used with caution until they have been extensively examined by the clinical laboratory community (10).

For more in-depth discussion of these procedures and for examples of quality control charts prepared by this method, refer to the Centers for Disease Control publication *Quality Control for Immunologic Tests* (13). Appendices A through C are examples of computer programs that can be used to perform the calculations described and prepare quality control charts.

STATISTICAL SIGNIFICANCE

In addition to accepting the idea that serologic tests have a variation of plus or minus one tube, serologists have also accepted the idea that a fourfold rise in titer constitutes a significant change. The idea that a fourfold titer difference constitutes a statistically significant change disregards the fact that variations in serologic test results are not the same in all tests or for all procedures. In practice, such change may or may not be significantly different (9). Table 2 shows the

ratio of results required between two serologic test results for the differences to be statistically significant for selected geometric standard deviations. This table can be used to determine the significance of differences between results at given geometric standard deviations. For example, if the geometric standard deviation is less than 1.284, then a twofold difference is significant at the 0.05 probability level. If each laboratory measured the intralaboratory precision for each test, it could very easily report to the physician not only titers on paired sera, but also the probability that the differences were statistically significant. On single samples, the laboratory could provide titers and confidence intervals. The estimates of intralaboratory precision would come directly from the statistical calculations used to set up the quality control charts and would require little additional effort.

CONCLUSION

The system used by the Centers for Disease Control has all the characteristics mentioned above that are desirable in an ideal measurement system, and it is strongly recommended that others use this or a similar system. By using the methods described, laboratorians can perform multiple tests on quality control samples, calculate the actual variation, and establish quality control charts. These charts can then be used to more accurately determine when the test is out of control, because the charts are based on actual, measured variation and calculated limits.

The methods can also be used to fill other needs for estimates of variation and significance, such as a difference in results between or among tests, laboratories, procedures, or technologists; for the measurement of variation in analyte levels in populations; and for the measurement of the statistical significance of differences between samples.

We recommend that serologists measure the actual variation in the tests they perform, that they establish controls with calculated acceptable limits, and that the significance of differences in results be calculated.

APPENDIX 1

The following is a BASIC program for the IBM-PC which calculates geometric quality control statistics from a series of quality control test results. The program is written to use double precision values, but the values may only be single precision in interpretive BASIC. The program should be compiled to take advantage of the double precision. It may require slight modification to run on other computers.

TABLE 2. Ratio of results required between two serologic test results for differences to be statistically significant for selected geometric standard deviations.

Precision	Ratio of results required for significant difference		
	$P < 0.05$	$P < 0.01$	$P < 0.001$
1.000	1.000	1.000	1.000
1.077	1.228	1.310	1.414[a]
1.100	1.302	1.414[a]	1.560
1.133	1.414[a]	1.575	1.792
1.160	1.509	1.716	2.000[a]
1.210	1.697	2.000[a]	2.435
1.284	2.000[a]	2.482	3.212
1.346	2.278	2.944	4.000[a]
1.464	2.878	4.000[a]	5.930
1.649	4.000[a]	6.158	10.320

[a] Ratio occurring in common dilution schemes.

```
10 PRINT "Enter values of X (-1 to Quit)"
20 INPUT "X = ",X#
30 IF X# = -1 THEN 80
40 N=N+1
50 SUM#=SUM#+LOG(X#)
60 SUM2#=SUM2#+LOG(X#)∧2
70 GOTO 20
80 PRINT "                N = ";N
90 MEAN#=EXP(SUM#/N)
100 SD#=EXP(SQR((SUM2#-SUM#∧2/N)/(N-1)))
110 PRINT "            Mean = ";MEAN#
```

```
120 PRINT "Standard Deviation = ";SD#
130 PRINT "1 SD Limits     =
        ";MEAN#/SD#;" to ";MEAN#*SD#
140 PRINT "2 SD Limits     =
        ";MEAN#/SD#/\2;" to ";MEAN#*SD#/\2
150 PRINT "3 SD Limits     =
        ";MEAN#/SD#/\3;" to ";MEAN#*SD#/\3
160 END
```

If you would like to have the values printed as they are entered, add the following line:

```
35 PRINT X#
```

If you would like to be able to calculate limits other than those listed, add the following lines.

```
151 INPUT "Enter number of standard deviations (−1
        to Quit)",ND
152 IF ND = −1 THEN 160
153 PRINT ND;" SD Limits = ";MEAN#/SD#/\ND;"
        to ";MEAN#*SD#/\ND
154 GOTO 151
```

APPENDIX 2

The programs below permit the entry of values into a dBase II file or the use of an existing dBase II file to calculate geometric statistical parameter estimates. (dBase III permits calculation of these estimates within the system.) It is assumed that the dBase and BASICA programs are on the same subdirectory or disk. If they are not, "Change Directory" commands can be entered into the DBMEAN.BAT file.

Before running the program, a DBF file called DBMEAN.DBF must be created. This file contains at least a numeric field, called VALUE, that is large enough and has enough decimal places to accept the entries. A suggested definition is: VALUE,N,10,4. From DOS, issue the command DBMEAN to run the program.

The first file is a systems batch file that controls the running of the other programs.

DBMEAN.BAT

```
ECHO OFF
DBASE DBMEAN.CMD
BASICA DBMEAN
DBASE DBDISP.CMD
ERASE DBMEAN.TXT
```

The next file is a dBase command file that permits the entry of values into the DBF file called DBMEAN.DBF. If the DBMEAN.DBF file already has entries in it, this file is not needed, and the command that calls this file (DBASE DBMEAN.CMD) should be removed from the batch file.

DBMEAN.CMD

```
SET ECHO OFF
SET TALK OFF
USE DBMEAN
DELETE ALL
```

```
PACK
?
? 'ENTER OBSERVATIONS (0 TO END)'
?
STORE T TO RUNNING
STORE 1 TO COUNT
DO WHILE RUNNING
    STORE STR(COUNT,3) TO I
    INPUT 'OBS #&I ' TO INVAL
    IF INVAL = 0
        STORE F TO RUNNING
    ELSE
        APPEND BLANK
        REPLACE VALUE WITH INVAL
        STORE COUNT+1 TO COUNT
    ENDIF
ENDDO
COPY TO DBMEAN SDF
QUIT
```

Because dBase II does not permit logarithmic conversion, it is necessary to exit to BASICA to transform the values. The following is the BASICA program, which converts the values and makes the statistical calculations.

DBMEAN.BAS

```
10 OPEN "DBMEAN.TXT" FOR INPUT AS #1
20 IF EOF(1) THEN 80
30 INPUT #1,X#
40 N=N+1
50 SUM#=SUM#+LOG(X#)
60 SUM2#=SUM2#+LOG(X#)/\2
70 GOTO 20
80 CLOSE #1
90 MEAN#=EXP(SUM#/N)
100 SD#=EXP(SQR((SUM2#−SUM#/\2/N)/N−1)))
110 L1#=MEAN#/SD#: U1#=MEAN#*SD#
120 L2#=MEAN#/SD#/\2: U2#=MEAN#*SD#/\2
130 OPEN "DBMEAN.TXT" FOR OUTPUT AS #1
140 PRINT #1,N: PRINT #1,MEAN#: PRINT #1,SD#
150 PRINT #1, L1#: PRINT #1, U1#: PRINT #1, L2#:
        PRINT #1, U2#
160 SYSTEM
```

The last file is a dBase command file, which reads the DBMEAN.DBF file and displays the results of the statistical calculations.

DBDISP.CMD

```
SET ECHO OFF
SET TALK OFF
USE DBMEAN
DELETE ALL
PACK
APPEND FROM DBMEAN.TXT SDF
GOTO TOP
?
?
?
? 'NUMBER OF VALUES =             ',VALUE
SKIP
? 'GEOMETRIC MEAN =             ',VALUE
SKIP
```

```
? 'STANDARD DEVIATION =              ',VALUE
SKIP
? '1 GEOMETRIC SD LIMITS:'
? '       LOWER                       ',VALUE
SKIP
? '       UPPER                       ',VALUE
SKIP
? '2 GEOMETRIC SD LIMITS:'
? '       LOWER                       ',VALUE
SKIP
? '       UPPER                       ',VALUE
?
?
?
QUIT
```

APPENDIX 3

The following is a listing of cell entries to set up quality control calculations on Lotus 1-2-3. The column on the left is the cell number, and the entries to the right of the cell numbers are the data to be entered in that cell.

```
B1: 'Geometric Statistical Calculations
B2: '         for Quality Control
B4: 'Result
C5: @IF(B5<>0,@LN(B5),B5)
D5: 'N
E5: @COUNT(RESULT)
D6: 'Geo. Mean
E6: @EXP(@SUM(LN−RESULT)/@COUNT
     (RESULT))
D7: 'Geo. SD
E7: @EXP(@SQRT((@COUNT(RESULT)/(@COUNT
     (RESULT)−1))*@VAR(LN−RESULT)))
E9: '1 S Limit
D10: 'Lower
E10: +E6/E7
D11: 'Upper
E11: +E6*E7
E12: '2 S Limit
D13: 'Lower
E13: +E6/E7/\2
D14: 'Upper
E14: +E6*E7/\2
```

Enter 1 through 10 in cells A5 through A14, and then copy the formula in C5 to C6 through C14 (with relative addresses). Use the /Range Name Create commands to name the ranges RESULT, B5 ... B14, and LN−RESULT, C5 ... C14.

To expand the system to permit more results, simply copy the formula in C5 into the expanded range of the C column, expand the definition of the RESULT and LN−RESULT range names, and enter the additional results in column B.

To calculate ranges other than for 1 and 2 standard deviations, copy the formulas in cells E13 and E14 into vacant cells, but change the 2 at the end of the formula to the desired number of standard deviations (the values need not be whole numbers). If you would like to experiment with different numbers of standard deviations, a cell could be used to accept the desired number, e.g., F10, and the formulas could then be modified to respond to changes in that value. In that case, the two formulas would be +E6/E7/\F10 for the lower limit and +E6*E7/\F10 for the upper limit.

LITERATURE CITED

1. **Barnett, R. N.** 1974. Clinical laboratory statistics. Little, Brown & Co., Boston.
2. **Freund, J. E.** 1976. Statistics: a first course, 2nd ed. Prentice-Hall, Inc., Englewood Cliffs, N.J.
3. **Hall, E. C., and M. B. Felker.** 1970. Reproducibility in the serological laboratory. Health Lab. Sci. **7:**63–68.
4. **Mandel, J.** 1971. Repeatability and reproducibility. Mater. Res. Stand. **11:**8–16.
5. **Mandel, J., and L. F. Nanni.** 1979. Measurement evaluation, p. 209–272. In S. L. Inhorn (ed.), Quality assurance practices for health laboratories. American Public Health Association, Washington, D.C.
6. **Natrella, M. G.** 1963. Experimental statistics. National Bureau of Standards handbook 91. National Bureau of Standards, Department of Commerce, Washington, D.C.
7. **Palmer, D. F., and J. J. Cavallaro.** 1980. Some concepts of quality control in immunoserology, p. 1078–1082. In N. R. Rose and H. Friedman (ed.), Manual of clinical immunology, 2nd ed. American Society for Microbiology, Washington, D.C.
8. **Snedecor, G. W., and W. G. Cochran.** 1967. Statistical methods, 6th ed. Iowa State University Press, Ames.
9. **Taylor, R. N.** 1983. Measurement of variation and significance in serologic tests. Ann. N.Y. Acad. Sci. **420:**13–21.
10. **Taylor, R. N.** 1984. Standards and quality assurance for immunologic tests: Centers for Disease Control survey program and problems of quality assurance, p. 115–127. In J. H. Rippey and R. M. Nakamura (ed.), Diagnostic immunology: technology assessment and quality assurance. College of American Pathologists, Skokie, Ill.
11. **Taylor, R. N., and K. M. Fulford.** 1981. Theory and application of the CDC diagnostic immunology proficiency testing program. Centers for Disease Control, Atlanta.
12. **Taylor, R. N., A. Y. Huong, and K. M. Fulford.** 1975. Measurement of variation in serologic tests. Center for Disease Control, Atlanta.
13. **Taylor, R. N., A. Y. Huong, K. M. Fulford, V. A. Przybyszewski, and T. L. Hearn.** 1979. Quality control for immunologic tests. Department of Health and Human Services publication no. (CDC) 82-8376. Center for Disease Control, Atlanta.
14. **Wood, R. J., and T. M. Durham.** 1980. Reproducibility of serological titers. J. Clin. Microbiol. **11:**541–545.
15. **Youden, W. J., and E. H. Steiner.** 1975. Statistical manual of the AOAC. Association of Official Analytical Chemists, Washington, D.C.

Chapter 148

Standardization of Reagents and Methodology in Immunology

IRENE BATTY

In recent years, there has been increasing emphasis on the importance of standardization of the reagents used in the clinical immunology laboratory (19). The primary aims of such standardization are to improve the quality of laboratory results and to provide a means to ensure uniformity in the designation of the concentration of clinically important substances in body fluids which cannot be adequately characterized by chemical and physical means.

Although immunology is a relatively young discipline, the time has long since passed, at least in the major areas, when comparability and uniformity of results could be ensured by the interchange of materials among interested workers. It is also no longer the case that most of the test systems and techniques are controlled by competent, involved laboratory immunologists; many tests are in routine use and are performed by technicians who, although technically competent, have little intimate knowledge of the immunological basis of the tests.

It might be thought that reagents which are used by scientists for in vitro tests in the laboratory, where expense, time and inclination are virtually the only factors which determine how well the reagents and the performance of the test are controlled, make up the area least in need of standardization. This situation might be true if each test result could be regarded in isolation and if there were no need to communicate results to others or to compare results obtained in different laboratories or even in one laboratory at different times.

EARLY WORK ON STANDARDIZATION

This point becomes clearer if we consider the history of biological standardization, which started in the late 1880s after Roux and Yersin and Behring and Kitasato had shown that certain bacterial species produce toxins and that animals receiving repeated doses of such toxins produce substances which specifically neutralize these toxins. It almost immediately became clear to these early workers that, if these phenomena were to be studied in anything more than the most superficial manner and have any practical application, it was necessary to quantify the interaction of these substances. By 1897, therefore, Ehrlich had produced his classical work on the standardization of diphtheria toxin, and Kraus had shown that when homologous antiserum and soluble antigen meet, a visible precipitate is produced; that is, the foundation of immunological standardization was laid.

ELEMENTS OF STANDARDIZATION

Units

The first stage in any attempt at quantification is the definition of units by which activity is to be measured. Units in the immunological context are analogous to the international and national physical units of length and mass in that the units are defined by reference to the activity of a given weight or, more rarely, a given volume of an arbitrarily designated standard preparation.

Originally, Ehrlich measured the potency of diphtheria toxin in terms of the least volume which, when injected by a stated route, would kill an animal of a designated species and weight within a certain time, that is, in terms of its minimal lethal dose. This parameter measures the toxicity of a toxin, and although it is independent of the ability of the toxin to combine with antitoxin, it has the grave disadvantage that such measurements are particularly sensitive to changes in the indicator systems. The apparent toxicity of a toxin has been found to vary with the diet of the indicator animal and even with the season of the year, as this affects the susceptibility of the animal. Such tests show poor reproducibility either within a single laboratory at different times or among laboratories at the same time. A further problem was that toxins were also found to lose toxicity both on storage and after treatment with a variety of chemical reagents, without any diminution in the ability to combine with antitoxin. Therefore, although Ehrlich originally defined the unit of antitoxin as the smallest amount of antiserum which would neutralize 100 minimal lethal doses of toxin, a unit of antiserum is now defined as that amount of an antiserum which has the same ability to combine with a volume of toxin, some of which may be toxoid, as had the arbitrary unit of antitoxin in the original serum laid down by Ehrlich, that is, as a certain weight of his dried standard preparation of antitoxin. In this example, 1 IU of diphtheria antitoxin has the same combining, neutralizing activity as 0.0628 mg of the present international standard.

Size of units. Although the weight of the standard preparation to which unit activity is assigned may have been related originally to a particular degree of biological activity, the weight is not necessarily related to other activities of the antibody. It happens, therefore, that some units appear small for certain purposes and large by other criteria. For instance, a therapeutic dose of tetanus antitoxin contains thousands of units, whereas a reasonable level of circulating tetanus antitoxin in an immune animal is only a fraction of a unit.

Comparability of units. There is no relationship between the unit of one specific antibody and the unit of a different antibody; for example, a unit of immunoglobulin G (IgG) will not precipitate the same mass of specific immunoglobulin as a unit of IgE. In the early days of standardization, antibodies were almost always used as the standard materials because they tended to be more stable. Nowadays, it is the custom to choose a standard on the basis of the precision with which it can be characterized and the ease with which a sufficiently large homogeneous batch of material can be accurately divided into small portions and lyophilized.

Continuity of units. Great care is taken to ensure that the international unit of any specific substance represents the same amount of activity when it becomes necessary to change standards by comparing the old with the new in an international collaborative assay. The unitage is then assigned to the new standard in terms of the old so that the activity per unit remains the same, although the weight of dried material which contains the activity is likely to be different.

Reagents under consideration

A very high proportion of tests used in diagnostic laboratories, particularly in the fields of microbiology and hematology, depends on reactions between antigens and antibodies; i.e., the tests are immunologically based. However, many reagents used in such tests, for example, blood-grouping antisera and agglutinating sera, are properly outside the scope of this chapter. The discussion will be confined to those reagents which are used for detection and quantitation in an immunological context.

The problem of standardizing the reagents for and methods of immunological tests has two other major facets which govern attempts at achieving a solution to the problem.

Complexity

The first problem is the complexity of the materials being considered. It is now possible to obtain many of the antigens under consideration in a relatively pure form, but, however pure the antigen, the antibodies raised against it will be heterologous, differing at least in specificity, class, and avidity. The choice of materials for an antibody standard is therefore extremely difficult. When monoclonal antibodies (Mabs) were first produced, it was hoped that their epitope specificity would make the problem of choosing an antibody standard much simpler. This hope has not yet

proved to be the case, although Mabs have played a most useful part in identifying the antigens and thus, eventually, the nature of the antibodies being measured. However, for the most commonly used tests in the immunological laboratory, polyclonal antibody standards are still the most commonly used and will be until it is determined whether the Mab is capable of reacting with all molecules of the designated type and has the requisite stability.

Many of the antigens used in clinical immunology are still complex; for example, the crude extract of *Candida albicans* used to detect immune deficiencies may have at least 70 antigenic components, all capable of eliciting antibody responses. If such antigens are purified, the result is commonly an unstable material unsuitable for use as a standard.

Functional activity

The second problem is the importance to the user of functional activity. The problem would be slightly simpler if it were sufficient to quantitate the number of molecules of the designated substance present in the biological fluid, but it is sometimes more important to estimate the functional activity of the material present. In complement, for example, it may be desirable to know both the hemolytic and chemotactic properties. For certain antigens it may be necessary to estimate both the antibody-binding and immunogenic capacities.

Standard reference materials

For a list of international standards/reference preparations and useful reference preparations available from the World Health Organization (WHO), see Tables 1 and 2. The first step in producing standard reference materials is the writing of the specification, which should result from the combined effort of a group of experts in the field drawn from all countries where clinical immunology backed by laboratory work of a high standard is practiced on a large scale. It is likely that such a group can write a reasonably unequivocal specification for a standard material which will be satisfactory when used under many different circumstances. Such a group of experts is best sponsored by the appropriate international sci-

TABLE 1. International standards/reference preparations available for immunological use (WHO)

Prepn	Quantity/ampoule (IU)	Yr of establishment	Wt containing 1 IU (mg)
Rheumatoid arthritis serum	100	1965	0.171
ANF serum (homogeneous)	100	1970	0.186
Human serum IgG, IgM, and IgA	100	1970	0.1847
Human serum IgD[a]	100	1971	0.81
Human serum IgE	11,500	1973	0.06562
Alpha-fetoprotein, human	100,000	1975	0.001399
Carcinoembryonic antigen, human	100	1975	0.0236
FITC-conjugated sheep anti-human immunoglobulin	100	1976	0.0594
FITC-conjugated sheep anti-human IgM (μ chain)	100	1978	0.0447
Serum proteins (albumin, alpha$_1$-antitrypsin, alpha$_2$-immunoglobulin, C3 ceruloplasmin, transferrin)	100	1978	1.114
Human complement components C4, C5, C1q, and factor B	100	1980	1.107
FITC-conjugated sheep anti-human IgG (γ chain)	100	1981	0.0923
Peroxidase-conjugated sheep anti-human immunoglobulin	100	1982	0.3126

[a] British standard.

TABLE 2. Useful reference preparations available for immunological use (WHO)

Prepn	Yr of establishment
Myeloma serum HL high titer of IgM antinuclear activity	1978
Nuclear ribonucleoprotein antibody	1983
Smooth muscle (antiactin) antibody	1983
Mitochondrial antibody	1983

entific society, for example, the International Union of Immunological Societies (IUIS), working in conjunction with WHO. Appendix 1 gives the specification of an anti-human IgM conjugate prepared in such a way.

WHO, which has many years of experience in the standardization of biological substances, in particular of vaccines and antisera for prophylactic and therapeutic use, has written the specifications for freeze-drying (lyophilizing) such materials (20). These methods have not been superseded, although such methods should always be considered critically whenever the standardization of a different antigen or antibody or of an antigen or antibody for use in a different situation is being undertaken. It is conceivable that changes take place during freeze-drying that, without necessarily affecting potency, do affect suitability for a particular purpose. An instance of such a change is the present international standard for IgG, IgM, and IgA, which, though highly satisfactory for radial immunodiffusion, reconstitutes to give a slightly turbid solution unsatisfactory for nephelometric measurement by automated techniques, as it gives too high a blank reading.

The second step is the procurement of material to meet the specifications. This material may come from a hospital or research laboratory or from a commercial undertaking. It is important to prepare a large batch, sufficient for at least 4,000 ampoules, as replacement necessitates a further collaborative comparative assay and is time and labor consuming.

The third step is the international collaborative assay of the material. Again, this assay is undertaken by acknowledged experts drawn from as many countries as possible, so that the material is tested under many different conditions. The design of the protocol of such a collaborative assay is best done in consultation with a statistician.

Stability. It is essential that any material used as an international standard retain its activity undiminished throughout its life-span as a standard and suffer no loss of activity under the conditions to which it might reasonably be subjected during distribution. To ensure that it retains its activity, several ampoules of the material are subjected to accelerated degradation tests by storing them at three or more different temperatures, for example, at -30, 4, 25, 37, and 56°C, for at least 2 months, testing the activity by the most precise method available, and constructing Arrhenius plots (4).

It is of course essential that degradation has been shown to be a first-order reaction before such methods are used. Kirkwood and Tydeman have recently published useful studies of the statistical facets of stability testing of biological standards, including the principles of design of the tests (6).

Methods

It should be appreciated that it is counterproductive to insist that a standard methodology be used in all clinical immunology laboratories, even if any regulatory authority were in a position to insist on it. It is generally agreed that what is required is a reference method which, if followed closely, should give the correct value within the agreed limits to the standard material and by inference to other similar materials. Given such a method, users can both control their own methods and set up their own laboratory standards for day-to-day use. It is implied by this idea that any reference method correctly applied will enable the users to obtain results which they can confidently state are inside or outside the agreed reference ranges for the population under consideration. That being said, studies (1) have shown that more consistent estimates of potency are sometimes made with the local method than with the reference method. Familiarity with an imperfect technique compensates for its inadequacies, whereas lack of familiarity with the reference technique may result in both less precision and less accuracy. Readers are recommended to consult a joint IUIS-WHO Working Group report on the use and abuse of laboratory tests in clinical immunology ("Use and Abuse of Laboratory Tests: Critical Considerations of Eight Widely Used Diagnostic Procedures," WHO unpublished document, 1981).

IMMUNOGLOBULINS

Methods of the test

The most commonly used methods for measuring the immunoglobulins are radial immunodiffusion (10), electroimmunoassay (9), automated immunoprecipitation (8), radioimmunoassay (3), enzyme-linked immunosorbent assay (16), and the radioallergosorbent test (RAST) for IgE (5, 18).

Whicher et al. have published a very good review of immunochemical assays for immunoglobulins, which should be referred to if greater detail is required on principles, methods, and calculations (17).

Radial immunodiffusion. Of the methods listed, radial immunodiffusion (10) has the longest history and the most complete documentation. The method is given in more or less detail in most recent textbooks of immunological methods, and the Association of Clinical Pathologists has issued a methods broadsheet which sets out the method in great detail. The points in the method which are critical if results are to be precise (i.e., reproducible) and accurate (i.e., in the case of the standard, close to the agreed value) are emphasized. Examples of such critical points are the importance of the uniformity of depth of the agar, the need for wells freshly cut and with precise dimensions neither distorted by contraction nor rounded by time, and the accuracy with which the wells should be filled. The sensitivity of the method (12), which depends on the ability to visually detect antigen-antibody precipitates in gels, can be increased if, after the reaction has been allowed to run to completion, the plate is washed and then treated by applying a second antiserum which contains radioactive antibody to the antibody immunoglobulin in the precipitate; e.g., if goat serum was used in the plate, then a radioactive antibody to goat immunoglobulin would be used. The area of the ring shows a linear relationship to the initial concentration of antigen in the well.

Electroimmunoassay (rocket immunoassay). Electroimmunoassay (9) is increasingly being used where radial immunodiffusion would previously have been used. Electroimmunoassay has a slight advantage over the radial immunodiffusion technique because it is easier to accurately measure a peak height than to measure the area of a circle, and such a measurement can give a result in less time. For a given antibody concentration, the relationship between the distance traveled by the precipitate and the antigen concentration is linear. In both methods, the use of a standard antigen of known potency is virtually obligatory. For immunoglobulins there are international reference preparations for IgG, IgM, and IgA (13) and research standards for IgD (14) and IgE (15) against which laboratory standards (pools of healthy adult sera held in small portions at −70°C or lower) should be calibrated.

Automated immunoprecipitation. Automated immunoprecipitation is based on a nephelometric approach (8) to antigen-antibody combinations. An admixture of suitably diluted monospecific antiserum with a microvolume of the sample is passed through delay and mixing coils. The binding of antigen to soluble antibody is observed by the increase in light scattering of a beam of incident light. The intensity of light scattered is proportional to the molecular weight and concentration of the particles. This method has the advantages that it has been automated and that as many as 50 to 100 determinations can be made in 1 h, but it is important that the samples and standards tested have minimal initial turbidity, and the quality of the results depends to a large extent on the quality of the antibodies used.

Radioimmunoassay. Although it is more cumbersome and needs a higher degree of skill and more expensive equipment than the methods already discussed, radioimmunoassay (3) as a method of quantitating proteins has the advantage of being a relatively simple way to measure picogram amounts of specific protein. There are several methods available for separating bound and free antigens, with the double-antibody and solid-phase methods being the most common. Which method is used is less important than that it be controlled by the use of appropriate standards, although it is important to determine that the efficiency of the separation is such that no labeled antigen is found in the "bound" fraction in the absence of antibody and that all the labeled antigen is found in the "bound" fraction in the presence of excess antibody.

Enzyme immunoassay. Enzyme immunoassay (16) has proved to be as sensitive as radioimmunoassay, but except for the measurement of IgE and IgD, such sensitivity is not essential.

Other assays of this type have recently been used for the quantitation of immunoglobulins; for example, both immunofluorometric and immunoradiometric assays have considerable sensitivity, and the former can be used with most laboratory fluorimeters.

RAST. The RAST (18) is virtually limited in its use to allergologists, as it is used to measure IgE reagins which appear to react as functionally monovalent molecules. The allergen is conjugated with an insoluble substrate and added to the serum under test. After time is allowed for the allergen-specific antibodies to react, the insoluble complex is washed, and radioactively labeled anti-IgE antibodies are added. After further washes of the complex, the concentration of label is determined by counting, and the IgE reagin content of the serum is thus established. The problems of standardization in this test system are mainly dependent on the resolution of the problems of standardizing the allergen preparations used. The IUIS and the International Union of Allergologists are currently working on the standardization of the RAST technique, and international reference preparations of three of the most commonly occurring allergens, i.e., short ragweed (*Ambrosia elatior*) pollen extract, timothy (*Phleum pratense*) pollen allergenic extract, and house dust mite (*Dermatophagoides pteronyssinus*) extract, are now available from WHO.

Serum proteins

The methods given for measuring immunoglobulin (other than RAST) have also in recent years been used for the measurement of other serum proteins, and as with the immunoglobulins, the quality of the results obtained depends largely on the quality of the antibodies used in the test system. The most important qualities of these antisera are that they be monospecific, at least so far as the sensitivity of the test system is capable of detecting any contaminating antibodies, and of high avidity, so that antigen binding is firm and does not readily dissociate. An international standard for six serum proteins is now available from WHO (see Appendix 2). This standard is also calibrated against the first international standard for IgG, IgM, and IgA and reconstitutes to a crystal-clear solution; thus it is suitable for nephelometric measurements.

AUTOANTIBODIES

Methods of the test

The following tests are the most commonly used: immunofluorescence, enzyme-labeled antibody, and hemagglutination tests.

Immunofluorescence. With the immunofluorescence technique, one is faced not only with the inherent variability of the immunological reagents because of the inhomogeneity of antibodies, but also with differences in labeling efficiencies, substrates, and optical systems, including the light sources and type of illumination used.

However, that being said, there is no doubt as to the crucial importance of the conjugate in any attempt to obtain reproducible results both within and between laboratories. To have a conjugate which in the quantitation of autoantibodies gives good strong specific staining at the recommended working dilution without any nonspecific or unwanted staining of the substrate, so that a sharp endpoint is achieved, it is essential to start with a high-titered anti-human globulin serum. Ideally, such a serum is best raised by using as antigen purified immunoglobulin from a pool composed of bleedings from a large number of donors, so that the reagent will recognize all classes of immunoglobulins equally. When monospecific conjugates are required, it is not sufficient to show that the starting serum is monospecific by gel diffusion techniques or, even after conjugation of the globulins, by its ability to stain or not stain monoclonal bone marrow smears. Rather, the serum should be shown to be monospecific by an indirect immunofluorescence test in which one uses in the sandwich patient's sera of known reactivity of particular class specificities against the substrate. That is, the monospecificity of the conjugate must be established by using the most sensitive test system in which it may be used.

It has also been found that the fluorochrome used can adversely affect the performance of the conjugate. Fluorescein isothiocyanate (FITC) has the highest emission intensity of those fluorochromes commonly used, but even with FITC, it is essential to use preparations of the highest purity. Impurities give rise to variability in performance and invalidate the calculation of the fluorochrome/protein ratio, on which the sensitivity of the test depends. Impurities are a common cause of nonspecific staining. A standard test for the labeling efficiency of FITC has been promulgated by the U.S. National Committee for Clinical Laboratory Standards, and a document outlining the parameters which govern the production of good conjugates has been issued by the Medical Research Council of Great Britain's working party on the use of antisera to immunoglobulins (11). Mabs have been shown to make good conjugates, but their universality is not yet proven.

Standardization of immunofluorescence materials and techniques is still far from perfect, but the report of a joint IUIS-WHO consultation produced recommended methods for the fluorescent-antibody test for antinuclear factor (ANF), *Treponema pallidum* antibodies (FTA-ABS), and *Toxoplasma* antibodies (Appendix 3). A group under the auspices of WHO, the New York Academy of Sciences, IUIS, and other interested parties has now met six times, and a study of the reports of these meetings will give the reader a deeper insight into the problems involved (2, 7).

Enzyme (e.g., peroxidase)-labeled antibody tests and hemagglutination tests. The enzyme-labeled antibody and hemagglutination test systems for quantitating autoantibodies have only recently been the subject of much study from the point of view of their standardization. Workers in the field have relied on the use of WHO-designated expert reference centers to help them resolve problems of method and confirm comparability of results. There is now available from WHO an international reference preparation of horseradish peroxidase anti-human immunoglobulin suitable for use in immunohistochemistry.

Detection of immune complexes. Since 1972, a multitude of methods have been devised for the measurement of immune complexes. Of these methods based on different principles, 18 were initially assessed by the IUIS subcommittee on standardization for immune complexes on 24 preparations; this number was whittled down to 10 preparations and 8 methods at the next stage. The most favored methods at present are C1q solid-phase or fluid-phase binding tests, conglutinin assays, monoclonal rheumatoid factor inhibition, and the Raji cell assay. All have their pitfalls ameliorated to some extent by the use of standards.

Reference preparations of aggregated IgG and of preformed immune complexes (tetanus toxoid antigen-antibody complexes) are available on request from V. Nydegger, Service de Transfusion CRS, Laboratoire Central, Berne 22, Switzerland.

B- and T-cell determinations

There are two methods most commonly used for T-cell markers, i.e., sheep erythrocyte rosettes and Mabs appropriately labeled, usually with fluorochromes; the second method appears to give the most consistent results.

Surface membrane immunoglobulin is probably the most reliable marker for B cells. The immunoglobulin reacts with fluorochrome-labeled antibody to Fab or a mixture of anti-kappa anti-lambda light chains. Mabs reacting specifically with all B cells do exist, as do Mabs to subsets.

The necessity for standardization and quality control is not as readily appreciated with immunological reagents as it is with drugs. In the past, methods used in the diagnosis of pathological conditions were relatively insensitive, and it was comparatively easy to distinguish between normal and abnormal states, but the highly sensitive techniques now used have shown that in most circumstances these differences in level are quantitative rather than qualitative. It is clear, therefore, that the precision and accuracy of test methods and the standardization and quality control of reagents should no longer be neglected.

APPENDIX 1

Anti-IgM Conjugate Specification

Specificity

1. The anti-IgM conjugate must be class specific for human IgM in the definitive fluorescent-labeled antibody tests for syphilis, toxoplasma, rubella, etc.
2. The conjugate must not react with other immunoglobulin classes, light chains, or complement components or exhibit other inappropriate reactions in the definitive fluorescent-labeled antibody test systems.
3. The conjugate must be free from immune complexes and all other human serum components.
4. Insolubilized absorbents should be used.

Potency

1. The conjugate must have a plateau titer of at least 1:8 in a congenital syphilis system.
2. The conjugate must not show nonspecific staining at a concentration of less than four times the endpoint titer.

Immunogen

As immunogen, use purified IgM from a pool of monoclonal sera or from normal human sera.

Filling and freeze-drying

Filling and freeze-drying should be done according to the recommendations in reference 20, p. 111–114.

Stability data

Adequate stability data must be provided.

Necessary information

Information on the material as laid down at the 1968 London meeting on standardization of immunofluorescence and by the Medical Research Council working party (11) should be provided as follows.

1. Name and address of the manufacturer
2. Proper name of the product and its batch or lot number
3. Manufacturer's recommended expiration date
4. Type of fluorochrome used to label the antibodies
5. (a) If a standard is available, give the potency in relation to the standard, or (b) if a standard is not available, give the intended working dilution (with range) as found in a specified test.
6. Ratio of optical densities before the addition of any stabilizers
7. Any special information about processing, including additions and absorptions
8. Any known cross-reactivity, especially to immunoglobulin of other species
9. Type and concentration of preservative present, if any

APPENDIX 2

List of Substances to be Estimated

Immunoglobulins: IgG, IgM, IgA, IgD, IgE

Other serum proteins: in particular, prealbumin, albumin, alpha$_2$-macroglobulin, alpha$_1$-glycoprotein, hemopexin, transferrin, haptoglobin, ceruloplasmin, alpha$_1$-antitrypsin, beta-lipoprotein

Autoantibodies: against adrenal gland, gastric parietal mucosa, glomerular basement membrane, intrinsic factor, mitochondria, parathyroid gland, parotic duct cells, skin, smooth muscle, striated muscle, sperm, thyroglobulin, thyroid microsomes, and single- and double-stranded DNA
Complement
Immune complexes
B and T cells

APPENDIX 3

Provisional Recommended Methods of Test

ANF test

Reagents, minimum
1. Fluorescein-labeled anti-human IgG
2. Phosphate-buffered saline (PBS), pH 7.6

NaCl	8.5	g
Na$_2$HPO$_4$	1.28	g
NaH$_2$PO$_4 \cdot$ 2H$_2$O	0.156	g
Distilled water to	1	liter

3. Mounting fluid, pH 9 (buffered glycerol)

NaHCO$_3$	0.0715	g
Na$_2$CO$_3$	0.016	g
Distilled water to	10	ml
Glycerol to	100	ml

4. Cryostat sections of rat liver
5. WHO international standard human ANF serum

Method, commonly accepted
1. All dilutions should be made in PBS.
2. Standard ANF serum is allowed to react with the substrate for 30 min at room temperature (20 to 25°C) in a humid chamber.
3. Wash for 30 min in at least two changes of PBS, with gentle agitation.
4. Drain, and remove the excess moisture from around the edges with lint-free absorbent.
5. Dilutions of conjugate in PBS are allowed to react for 30 min at room temperature in a humid chamber.
6. Wash for 30 min in at least three changes of PBS.
7. Drain the slides, rinse them in distilled water, drain them, and mount them in the mounting fluid given above.

Results
Plateau of ANF = ANF titer obtained with at least three twofold-titer steps of conjugate
Plateau endpoint = last dilution of conjugate giving the ANF plateau
When possible, the emission should be measured.

Toxoplasma sp. test

Reagents, minimum
1. Fluorescein-labeled anti-human IgG
2. PBS, pH 7.6, as described above under ANF test
3. Mounting fluid, pH 9 (buffered glycerol), as described above under ANF test
4. *Toxoplasma gondii* RH strain
5. Methyl alcohol (absolute) or dry acetone
6. WHO international standard *Toxoplasma* serum
7. Evans blue, 0.5 g in 50 ml of PBS

Method, commonly accepted
1. Air dry the antigen smear, and fix it for 10 min in absolute alcohol or dry acetone.
2. Wash the slides for 5 min in PBS.
3. Allow the serum to react with antigen for 30 min at room temperature (20 to 25°C) in a humid chamber.
4. Wash the slides for 30 min with at least three changes of PBS, with gentle agitation.
5. Allow dilutions of the conjugate to react with the preparation for 30 min at room temperature in a humid chamber.
6. Wash the slides for 1 h in at least four changes of PBS.
7. Rinse with distilled water, blot, and mount in mounting fluid as given above.
8. All conjugate dilutions should be made so that a final concentration of 0.2% Evans blue is attained.

Note: The use of Evans blue reduces the sensitivity of the test.

Results
Plateau of *Toxoplasma* = *Toxoplasma* titer obtained with at least three twofold-titer steps of conjugate
Plateau endpoint = last dilution of conjugate giving the *Toxoplasma* plateau
Where possible, the emission should be measured.

FTA-ABS test

Reagents, minimum
1. Fluorescein-labeled anti-IgG
2. PBS, pH 7.6, as described above under ANF test
3. Mounting fluid, pH 9 (buffered glycerol), as described above under ANF test
4. *Treponema pallidum*, well washed
5. WHO international standard positive syphilitic serum
6. Sorbent
7. Dry acetone

Method, commonly accepted
1. All dilutions are to be made in PBS.
2. Ensure the even distribution of treponemes; if necessary, break up clumps by repeated aspiration into a syringe with a 25-gauge needle.
3. Fix in dry acetone for 10 min.
4. Inactivate the serum at 56°C for 30 min.
5. Prepare serum-sorbent mixtures not more than 30 min before they are used.
6. Allow the serum to react with the treponemes on the slide for 30 min at 37°C in a humid chamber.
7. Wash the slide in four changes of PBS for 20 min at room temperature.
8. Allow the conjugate to react with the preparation for 30 min at 37°C in a humid chamber.
9. Wash the slides in four changes of PBS for 20 min, rinse in distilled water, and blot gently.
10. Mount in mounting fluid as given above.

Results
Plateau of FTA-ABS = FTA-ABS titer obtained with at least three twofold-titer steps of conjugate

Plateau endpoint = last dilution of conjugate giving the FTA-ABS plateau

Where possible, the emission should be measured.

LITERATURE CITED

1. **Anderson, S. G., M. W. Bentzon, V. Huba, and P. Krag.** 1970. International reference preparation rheumatoid arthritis serum. Bull. W.H.O. **42**:311–315.
2. **Hijmans, W., and M. Schaeffer.** 1975. The 5th International Conference on Immunofluorescence and the Related Staining Techniques. Ann. N.Y. Acad. Sci. **254**:21–172.
3. **International Atomic Energy Agency.** 1974. Radioimmunoassay and related procedures. Standardization and control of reagents and procedures. Medicine **1**:3–87.
4. **Jerne, N. K., and W. L. M. Perry.** 1956. The stability of biological standards. Bull. W.H.O. **14**:167–182.
5. **Johansson, S. G. O., H. Bennich, and T. Berg.** 1971. In vitro diagnosis of atopic allergy. III. Quantitative estimation of circulating IgE antibodies by the radio allergosorbent test. Int. Arch. Allergy **41**:443–451.
6. **Kirkwood, T. B. L.** 1984. Design and analysis of accelerated degradation tests for the stability of biological standards. II. Principles of design. J. Biol. Stand. **12**:215–224.
7. **Knapp, W., K. Holubar, and J. Wick (ed.).** 1978. Immunofluorescence and related staining techniques. Proceedings of the VIth International Conference on Immunofluorescence and Related Staining Techniques, Vienna, Austria, 1978. Elsevier/North-Holland Biomedical Press, Amsterdam.
8. **Larson, C., P. Orenstein, and R. F. Ritchie.** 1971. Automated nephelometric determination of antigen antibody interaction: theory and application, p. 101. *In* Advances in automated analysis. Mediad Inc., Tarrytown, N.Y.
9. **Laurell, C. B.** 1966. Quantitative estimation of proteins by electrophoresis in agarose gel containing antibodies. Anal. Biochem. **15**:45–52.
10. **Mancini, G., A. O. Carbonara, and J. F. Heremans.** 1965. Immunochemical quantitation of antigens by single radial immunodiffusion. Immunochemistry **2**:235–254.
11. **Medical Research Council Working Party.** 1971. Recommendations on the characterization of antisera as reagents. Immunology **20**:1–10.
12. **Rowe, D. S.** 1969. Radioactive single radial diffusion. A method of increasing the sensitivity of immunochemical quantification of proteins in agar gel. Bull. W.H.O. **40**:613–616.
13. **Rowe, D. S., S. G. Anderson, and B. Grab.** 1970. A research standard for human serum immunoglobulins IgG, IgA and IgM. Bull. W.H.O. **43**:535–552.
14. **Rowe, D. S., S. G. Anderson, and L. Tackett.** 1970. A research standard for human serum immunoglobulin D. Bull. W.H.O. **43**:607–609.
15. **Rowe, D. S., L. Tackett, H. Bennich, K. Ishizaka, S. G. O. Johansson, and S. G. Anderson.** 1970. A research standard for human serum immunoglobulin E. Bull. W.H.O. **43**:609–611.
16. **van Weeman, B. K., and A. H. W. M. Schuurs.** 1971. Immunoassay using antigen-enzyme conjugates. FEBS Lett. **15**:232.
17. **Whicher, J. T., C. Warren, and R. E. Chambers.** 1984. Immunochemical assays for immunoglobulins. Ann. Clin. Biochem. **21**:78–91.
18. **Wide, L., H. Bennich, and S. G. O. Johansson.** 1967. Diagnosis of allergy by an in vitro test for allergen antibodies. Lancet **ii**:1105–1107.
19. **World Health Organization.** 1972. 24th report of the WHO Expert Committee on Biological Standardization, p. 7. World Health Organization technical report series no. 486. World Health Organization, Geneva.
20. **World Health Organization.** 1978. Guidelines for the preparation and establishment of reference materials for biological substances. WHO/BS/626/78. World Health Organization, Geneva.

Chapter 149

Proficiency Testing and Clinical Laboratory Immunology

JOHN H. RIPPEY

Interlaboratory comparisons, external quality control, proficiency testing, and surveys are essentially synonymous terms. Which term is utilized depends on whether one is placing emphasis on similarities and differences, accuracy, regulatory requirement, or state-of-art monitoring. Regardless of emphasis, such programs compare the results from different laboratories on common specimens. Most commonly, the samples are sent to the participant laboratories on a quarterly basis, with subsequent centralized tabulation of the results from each participant's worksheet forms.

The first laboratory comparison program was a syphilis serology program, launched by the U.S. Public Health Service in 1935 (4). F. William Sunderland developed a chemistry survey program in 1945 under the auspices of the Philadelphia County Medical Society (2). The College of American Pathologists began their first survey efforts in 1948, but they did not initiate their Diagnostic Immunology Surveys until 1968. More recently, immunology and immunochemistry proficiency testing programs on a nationwide scale have been sponsored by the Centers for Disease Control, the American Association of Bioanalysts, and the American Association of Clinical Chemists.

The earliest interest in interlaboratory comparisons was centered on state-of-the-art monitoring. The marked growth of these comparison programs during the past 15 years has been predominantly due to state and national regulatory requirements. Currently, laboratory utilization of such programs is being enhanced by reagent method tabulations and educational components.

SURVEY DESIGN

Survey program design involves analyte selection, number of challenges per analyte number of mailings per year, and sample preparation. Survey challenges are generally available for most routine qualitative immunology tests, as well as for the more common titration procedures and for most quantitative fluorescent, enzymatic, and isotopic immunoassays. Flow cytometry and immunologic cell marker challenges, although needed, are not yet available. However, such challenges are presently being developed.

The challenges that are currently available are usually offered in sets of related tests or test procedures. The ideal situation would make it possible for each individual laboratory to purchase analyte challenges for only those tests it regularly performs. This ideal has been more closely approximated with the introduction of minimodule surveys, but true single-test menu ordering has not yet been perfected.

The number of challenges per analyte and the number of mailings per year have been, to date, largely dictated by regulatory requirement. As a general observation, most regulatory agencies have decreased the required number of challenges for well-standardized procedures such as syphilis serology tests. In contrast, some current regulatory proposals for alpha-fetoprotein testing suggest a relatively large number of challenges.

Sample preparation represents a continuous potential problem for immunology surveys, due to ever-changing instrumentation and methodology. The preferred sample is a stabilized liquid serum, mixed serum, or spiked serum. Spiked saline and albumin samples are definitely suboptimal. Antibody integrity is sometimes compromised by the lyophilization process. On the other hand, complement samples must be lyophilized for stability. Serum samples spiked with more than one antibody, such as rheumatoid factor plus rubella antibody, are distinctly inferior to singly spiked samples, giving a much broader spectrum of variability in interlaboratory results (7).

RESULT TABULATIONS

Appropriate result tabulations are contingent on understandable worksheets, clear instructions, current computer programing, and accurate data entry. Complicated worksheets for results and imprecise instructions reduce a survey to an evaluation of "formsmanship," rather than laboratory proficiency. Laboratorians are usually subjected to survey worksheets only four times a year. Consequently, their accuracy in the use of these forms is in no way analogous to their accuracy in the use of their routine laboratory forms every day at work.

For immunology surveys, it is preferable for the tabulation format to list analyte results by groupings that specify both method and commercial reagent. There is a relative unavailability of widely accepted reference standards for many immunology tests and procedures. Due to this lack of standardization, different reagents and methods often do not yield comparable results. By employing reagent-method groupings for survey result tabulations, individual laboratory evaluations are more meaningful, and useful reagent method performance data are provided to the survey participants.

EVALUATION FORMATS

Numerous approaches can be taken in regard to participant result evaluation. The three most prevalent mechanisms are fixed-criterion formulas, referee laboratory results, and participant consensus results. The fixed-criterion approach lends itself best to procedures with accepted, available reference standards and to procedures for which analytical goals based on medical utility can be relatively well defined. Generally, immunology testing is not characterized by either of these features.

Participant evaluations based on referee laboratory results have the potential disadvantage that the referee laboratory group may be composed of a relatively small number of elite testers, many using the same reagent and method. Evaluations referenced to the results of a few single-reagent-method laboratories are not comparable to results in the working world, where there are many methods and numerous reagents. This type of evaluation becomes even less meaningful when it involves an analyte challenge lacking available reference standards. In addition, this type of evaluation, if fully backed with regulatory impact, could possibly stifle the development of superior emerging methodology.

Evaluations based on participant consensus by reagent-method groupings circumvent many of the problems inherent in immunology proficiency testing. As usually instituted, qualitative challenge results are tabulated by reagent and method, and the result achieved by 80% or more of the reagent-method participants is designated the acceptable result (7). Similarly, quantitative challenge results are tabulated by reagent and method, the reagent-method mean is calculated, and reagent-method participants achieving results within ±2 standard deviations are evaluated as acceptable. This type of format allows evaluations to be made within the framework of current capability and makes use of statistical data that working laboratorians can use and understand. While there are definite arguments for transforming participant results to geometric data and constructing fairly intricate arithmetic formulas and ratios for evaluation purposes (9), such numerical manipulations tend to be difficult to understand, decrease the useful informational feedback to participants, and could possibly reduce the use of surveys to solely a regulatory vehicle.

OBJECTIVES

Surveys with adequate specimen integrity, accurate result tabulations, and understandable informational feedback to participants not only fulfill regulatory requirements, but also provide an excellent vehicle for interlaboratory, methodology, and reagent comparisons. This is particularly true for the many relatively inexact procedures performed in the diagnostic immunology laboratory. Whether this mechanism has actually succeeded in educating laboratorians and improving laboratory performance has been questioned (8).

Due to the infrequency of mailings (usually quarterly), surveys have never been intended to function as a laboratory's sole quality control program. To some degree, external quality control is a parameter of accuracy, and internal quality control is a parameter of precision (6). There has long been interest in attempting to combine many of the features of both external and internal quality controls into a single program, but such a program has not yet been realized.

Proficiency testing programs are not in themselves reliable indicators of adequate or inadequate laboratory performance (1). Functioning, daily, internal quality control formats, accepted available reference standards, and periodic accreditational inspections are equally important in producing quality laboratory results (3, 5). Laboratorians, sponsors of survey programs, regulatory agency personnel, and reference standard manufacturers all need to maintain an awareness of the appropriate balances between these interrelated features of laboratory quality control.

LITERATURE CITED

1. **Batsakis, J. G.** 1982. Response to report of the Office of Inspector General to Assistant Secretary of Health on proficiency testing, p. 14–15. College of American Pathologists, Skokie, Ill.
2. **Belk, W. P., and F. W. Sunderman.** 1947. A survey of the accuracy of chemical analyses in clinical laboratories. Am. J. Clin. Pathol. **17:**853–861.
3. **Boutwell, J. H.** 1975. The perspective of Center for Disease Control, p. 17. *In* M. Davis (ed.), Proceedings of Second National Conference on Proficiency Testing. Informational Services Inc., Bethesda, Md.
4. **Cumming, H. S., H. H. Hazen, A. H. Sanford, F. E. Senear, W. M. Simpson, and R. A. Vonderlehr.** 1935. Evaluation of serodiagnostic tests for syphilis in the United States: report of results. Vener. Dis. Inf. **16:**189–201.
5. **LaMotte, L. C.** 1975. The perspective of Center for Disease Control, p. 33–35. *In* M. Davis (ed.), Proceedings of Second National Conference on Proficiency Testing. Informational Services Inc., Bethesda, Md.
6. **Rippey, J. H.** 1983. Quality control in the diagnostic immunology laboratory. Pathologist **37:**252–253.
7. **Rippey, J. H.** 1983. The CAP surveys program and problems of quality assurance, p. 111–114. *In* J. H. Rippey and R. M. Nakamura (ed.), Diagnostic immunology: technology assessment and quality assurance. College of American Pathologists, Skokie, Ill.
8. **Taylor, R. N.** 1983. Standards and quality assurance for immunologic tests: Centers for Disease Control survey program and problems of quality assurance, p. 115–123. *In* J. H. Rippey and R. M. Nakamura (ed.), Diagnostic immunology: technology assessment and quality assurance. College of American Pathologists, Skokie, Ill.
9. **Taylor, R. N., A. Y. Huong, K. M. Fulford, V. A. Przybyszewski, and T. L. Hearn.** 1979. Quality control for immunologic tests. U.S. Department of Health and Human Services publication no. (CDC) 82-8376, p. 55–63. Public Health Service, Center for Disease Control, Atlanta.

Chapter 150

Use of Predictive Value Theory in Clinical Immunology

ROBERT S. GALEN

The predictive value model has been applied by a number of investigators for evaluating the clinical performance and effectiveness of clinical laboratory tests. In evaluating diagnostic procedures, the model facilitates selection of the best test. For a particular test, the model facilitates selection of the best methodology. Furthermore, the predictive value model can be expanded to deal with multiple tests. It has proven to be an expedient empirical tool for optimizing laboratory test selection, strategies, and interpretation.

PREDICTIVE VALUE OF LABORATORY DIAGNOSIS

Sensitivity, specificity, predictive value, and efficiency define the diagnostic accuracy of a laboratory test (5). Sensitivity, expressed as a percentage, indicates the frequency of positive test results in patients with a particular disease [TP/(TP + FN) × 100, where TP is true-positive and FN is false-negative], whereas specificity indicates the frequency of negative test results in patients without that disease [TN/(FP + TN) × 100, where TN is true-negative and FP is false-positive]. The predictive value of a positive test result indicates the frequency of diseased patients in all patients with positive test results [TP/(TP + FP) × 100]. The predictive value of a negative test result indicates the frequency of nondiseased patients in all patients with negative test results [TN/(TN + FN) × 100]. The efficiency of a test indicates the percentage of patients correctly classified (disease and non-diseased) by the test [(TP + TN)/(TP + FP + FN + TN) × 100].

A true-positive is a diseased patient correctly classified by the test. A false-positive is a nondiseased patient misclassified by the test. A false-negative is a diseased patient misclassified by the test. A true-negative is a nondiseased patient correctly classified by the test.

In screening for disease, the predictive value of the positive result is of the utmost importance. In the discussion that follows, predictive value will be used to refer to the predictive value of the positive test result. A marked change in predictive value occurs when there is a change in the prevalence of the disease in the population under study. For example, a laboratory test that was positive in 95% of diseased patients and negative in 95% of nondiseased patients is evaluated in Table 1. Note the change in predictive value that occurs for this test with changing prevalence of disease. It can readily be seen that a particular test has a higher predictive value when the disease occurs with a higher prevalence. This fact explains why a good diagnostic test frequently fails as a screening test when the drop in prevalence is quite marked. When clinical judgment is used in ordering laboratory tests,

the patient suspected of having a particular disease is placed in a new population with a higher prevalence or probability of disease. Therefore, the test performs much better.

Although predictive value theory has only recently found its way into the literature of laboratory medicine, the formula and concept are not at all new. The formula for calculating predictive value is frequently referred to as Bayes' formula and was published posthumously in 1763 (1). It is clear from the current medical literature that Bayes' equation is becoming increasingly popular. The formula may be presented in several variations, and it is important to recognize these variations as the following equation: predictive value = (prevalence)(sensitivity)/[(prevalence)(sensitivity) + (1 − prevalence)(1 − specificity)].

There has been considerable confusion in the literature concerning the meaning of the term "false-positive rate." In evaluating the statistical skills of physicians, Berwick and associates expected their subjects to know that the false-positive rate was equal to the number of false-positives divided by the number of true-negatives plus false-positives, or 1 minus specificity. They considered incorrect an answer in which the number of false-positives was divided by the total number of subjects studied, as well as an answer in which the number of false-positives was divided by the total number of positive results, or 1 minus predictive value (2).

Unfortunately, theirs is an inappropriate and misleading definition. It is inappropriate because a rate, in scientific parlance, usually refers to a quantity per unit of time. It is also misleading because there are, in fact, four useful false-positive ratios or proportions, not just one.

One false-positive ratio is defined by the proportion of results that are falsely positive for a particular disease when the test is employed in the study of a population in which that disease is totally absent, i.e., FP/(TN + FP). This proportion equals 1 minus specificity.

A second false-positive ratio is defined by the proportion of all results, both positive and negative, that are falsely positive for disease when the test is employed in the study of a population in which a particular disease is both present and absent, i.e., FP/(TN + FP + TP + FN).

A third false-positive ratio is defined by the proportion of all positive results that are falsely positive for disease when the test is employed in the study of a population in which a particular disease is both present and absent, i.e., FP/(TP + FP). This proportion equals 1 minus the predictive value of a positive result.

A fourth and final false-positive ratio is defined by the proportion of all false results that are falsely

TABLE 1. Predictive value as a function of disease prevalence[a]

Prevalence of disease (%)	Predictive value of test (%)
1	16.1
2	27.9
5	50.0
10	67.9
15	77.0
20	82.6
25	86.4
50	95.0

[a] For a laboratory test with 95% sensitivity and 95% specificity.

positive when the test is employed in the study of a population in which a particular disease is both present and absent, i.e., FP/(FP + FN).

Therefore, the term false-positive rate should be abandoned. There are at least four false-positive proportions, and each must be clearly defined to avoid confusion (6).

APPLICATION OF THE MODEL

In 1977, Foti and co-workers reported on a radio-immunoassay (RIA) procedure for prostatic acid phosphatase (PAP) (4). Table 2 summarizes their findings. The study by Foti et al. and the editorial by Gittes that followed resurrected acid phosphatase not only as a tumor marker, but as a cancer screening test: "The finding of an elevated prostatic acid phosphatase may soon no longer mean that cure is out of the question and that only palliative therapy may be used. A new excitement over this oldest of 'tumor markers' is in the air" (7). Gittes also writes that "the grim finding has been that overall, 90% of cases are first detected when they have already metastasized. The clear implication of the accompanying report is that mass screening on the basis of a blood test alone can reverse this gloomy experience" (7).

Both Foti et al. and Gittes committed the cardinal sin of ignoring disease prevalence and incidence. Is the test described by Foti et al. suitable for mass screening? It is quite simple to evaluate the usefulness of this test by using the predictive value model (3).

Foti and co-workers determined the sensitivity of RIA (based on current clinical staging criteria) to be 33, 79, 71, and 92% in stages I, II, III, and IV, respectively. The specificity of RIA has been measured in specific subgroups, but it is not available for the at-risk population as a whole. However, on the basis of specificity of 100% in normal subjects, 94% in benign prostatic hypertrophy, and 89% in patients with other carcinomas, a reasonable estimate of specificity would be 95%. The third factor, prevalence, is a function of age and the method of diagnosis. Estimates from autopsy series with step sections yield the highest rates, and clinical series yield the lowest rates. An overall estimate of prevalence of 25% for men over age 60 seems more than reasonable.

Finally, the cases must be staged. Clinical data, probably biased toward later stages, and autopsy data were combined to form an estimate that 15, 25, 35, and 25% of the patients with carcinoma would fall

into stages I, II, III, and IV, respectively (3). Figure 1 demonstrates how this test can be evaluated by using the predictive value model. On the basis of these estimates, the predictive value of RIA can be calculated to be 83%, with an overall sensitivity of 73%.

These calculations are representative of an unscreened population. If the population had been previously screened for prostatic carcinoma, the test would be detecting the incident, rather than the prevalent, cases. An incidence rate of 5% per year (5 to 10 times the maximal reported clinical incidence rate) is more than adequate to explain the rise in prevalence with age seen in autopsy populations. This rate yields a predictive value for a positive test of 43%. Therefore, 57% of the follow-up work would be unnecessary. With this rate, it would be neither medically prudent nor cost effective to use this test for screening purposes. With a lower incidence, the test would perform even more poorly. With a 1% incidence, the predictive value would be only 13%. Table 3 demonstrates the effect of prevalence on the predictive value of this test.

More recently, Watson and Tang, writing in *The New England Journal of Medicine* (the source of the first study and exuberant editorial), tried to answer some very fundamental and reasonable questions about the RIA. They calculated that the predictive value of a positive screening test in a randomly selected man was 0.41%. Therefore, only 1 of every 244 subjects (0.41/100) with a positive test would have carcinoma of the prostate. They write: "These calculations by themselves are persuasive evidence against the utility of the RIA-PAP [RIA for PAP] as a primary screening examination for prostatic carcinoma in the general male population and particularly in males whose prostate is normal according to rectal examination" (11). What about screening high-risk populations? "Even in the older age groups in which the prevalence is greatest, the RIA-PAP would have limited value as a screening test. Considering the high prevalence of latent histologic carcinoma in this age group (over 75), we predict a far superior rate of detection from 'blind' biopsies of the prostate than from the RIA-PAP" (11).

Other authors, writing in the same issue of *The New England Journal of Medicine*, evaluated 10 tests or

TABLE 2. Sensitivity and specificity of RIA for PAP[a]

Group	No. of patients	Sensitivity (%)	Specificity (%)
Patients with prostatic cancer	113	70	
Stage I	24	33	
Stage II	33	79	
Stage III	31	71	
Stage IV	25	92	
Patients without prostatic cancer	217		94
Normal controls	50		100
Benign prostatic hyperplasia	36		94
Total prostatectomy	28		96
Other cancers	83		89
Gastrointestinal disorders	20		95

[a] Data summarized from Foti et al. (4).

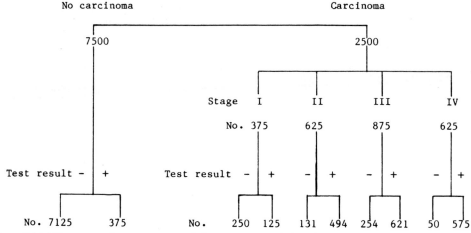

FIG. 1. Testing of 10,000 persons for carcinoma of the prostate and distribution of results in a hypothetical unscreened population. Prevalence, 25%; specificity, 95%; sensitivity, 73%; predictive value of positive results, 83%; predictive value of negative results, 91%; efficiency, 89%.

procedures in 300 symptomatic elderly men to determine which test is most accurate in the detection of prostate cancer. The conclusion was "that a skillful rectal examination is still the most accurate office test for the detection of prostatic carcinoma" (9).

Of the 10 tests or procedures, the least efficient test was the acid phosphatase by RIA. In fact, both the counterimmunoelectrophoresis and the Roy method for acid phosphatase performed better than RIA in their study. At the present time, I cannot help but agree with Watson and Tang, who say that "with regard to the initial detection of prostatic carcinoma it seems that the most economical and most reliable probe for detection remains not a needle in the patient's arm, but the gloved finger of the physician" (11).

Obviously, the introduction of an RIA for PAP generated some controversy in the medical literature. More assays were developed, clinical trials were conducted, and Gittes wrote another editorial on the subject: "Six years later, it is now clear that the radioimmunoassay did not and indeed could not live up to that hope . . . the specificity of only 94 percent undermined the potential of the test for screening purposes" (8). "Subsequent reports that the level of prostatic acid phosphatase was elevated in at least 6 percent of patients with benign prostatic hypertrophy strengthened the prediction that such an elevation was likely by overwhelming odds to be due to benign prostatic hypertrophy rather than prostatic cancer. The intervening years confirmed the futility of measuring prostatic acid phosphatase as a screening test" (8). "A marker specific for prostatic cancer may yet be found, which can overcome the mathematical advantage of the overwhelming incidence of benign prostatic hypertrophy. But for now the only reliable probe for detection of prostatic cancer is the examining finger of a physician performing a thorough examination" (8).

The predictive value of an RIA should and must be a criterion of the assay's evaluation. The fiasco with the RIA for PAP demonstrates what is likely to happen if the predictive value model is not used to evaluate new laboratory procedures before their introduction.

It is somewhat interesting to note that not only did Foti and co-workers in their original study and Gittes in his original editorial overlook the predictive value of the RIA under evaluation, but the reviewers of these articles in *The New England Journal of Medicine* also overlooked it. This fact is particularly interesting in light of the "mixed reviews" received by *Beyond Normality* when it was published in 1975 (5). *The New England Journal of Medicine* reported: "This book is a brief, somewhat chatty exposition of a general mathematical relation developed nearly two centuries ago by the Reverend Thomas Bayes" (10). This very same simple mathematical relation seems to have been lost upon many otherwise competent investigators, writers, and editors, including some in New England!

In summary, three relationships are possible between sensitivity and specificity for any test: the sensitivity may be greater than the specificity, the sensitivity may be equal to the specificity, or the sensitivity may be less than the specificity. Let us review what happens to the predictive value and efficiency under each of these circumstances in the face of fixed, as well as increasing, disease prevalence.

At a given prevalence, an incremental increase in specificity results in a greater increase in the predictive value of a negative test than does the same

TABLE 3. Effect of prevalence on predictive value of RIA for PAP

Prevalence (%)	Predictive value (%)[a]		Efficiency (%)
	+	−	
1	12.8	99.7	94.8
2	22.9	99.4	94.6
5	43.3	98.5	93.9
10	61.7	96.9	92.8
15	71.9	95.2	91.6
20	78.4	93.3	90.5
25	82.9	91.2	89.4
50	93.6	77.6	83.8

[a] +, Tests with positive results; −, tests with negative results.

incremental increase in sensitivity. As prevalence increases, the predictive value of a positive test increases, regardless of the relationship between sensitivity and specificity.

At a given prevalence, an incremental increase in sensitivity results in a greater increase in the predictive value of a negative test than does the same incremental increase in specificity. As prevalence increases, the predictive value of a negative test decreases, regardless of the relationship between sensitivity and specificity.

At a given prevalence (up to 50%), an incremental increase in specificity results in a greater increase in the efficiency of a test than does the same incremental increase in sensitivity. As prevalence increases, the efficiency of a test increases only if sensitivity is greater than specificity. When sensitivity is less than specificity, the efficiency of a test decreases with increasing prevalence. When sensitivity equals specificity, test efficiency is independent of prevalence and equal to sensitivity (or specificity). The value of test efficiency in all other cases falls between the values of test sensitivity and specificity, regardless of the relationship among sensitivity, specificity, and prevalence.

COMBINATION TESTING

Although it is quite simple to apply the predictive value model to the evaluation of a single test, the model can similarly be used to evaluate more than one test. In reality, it is rare to use the result of a single test as the final arbiter of a medical decision. But if we decide to use more than one test, a number of questions need to be answered. Which tests should we use? In what sequence should they be performed? How many tests are enough in a profile or battery of tests? How should the results be interpreted?

To see how the predictive value model can be used to answer these questions, let us consider situations where we use two tests, such as the Veneral Disease Research Laboratory and the fluorescent treponemal antibody tests, metanephrines and VMA tests, or the CPK and LDH isoenzyme tests. Two independent tests in a screening or diagnostic situation can be used in three different ways. (i) Test A is applied first, and all patients with a positive result are retested with test B (series approach: [++] = +). (ii) Test B is applied first, and all patients with a positive result are retested with test A (series approach: [++] = +). (iii) Tests A and B are used together, and all patients with positive results for either or both tests are considered positive (parallel approach: [+−] = +; [++] = +; [−+] = +).

Which approach or sequence is best? This depends on the testing situation and the sensitivity and specificity of the individual tests and their combinations.

TABLE 4. Multiple testing: hypothetical data for two tests (A and B)

Type of patient	No. of patients with test results of:			
	A+,B−	A−,B+	A+,B+	A−,B−
Diseased	190	40	760	10
Nondiseased	9,800	4,850	100	84,250

TABLE 5. Combination testing for hypothetical data

Test	Sensitivity (%)	Specificity (%)
Single (test A)	95.0	90.0
Single (test B)	80.0	95.0
Series (tests A and B)	76.0	99.9
Parallel (test A or B)	99.0	85.1

For the sake of the discussion, we will examine the hypothetical data presented in Table 4.

The sensitivity of test A is (190 + 760)/1,000, or 95%. The sensitivity of test B is (40 + 760)/1,000, or 80%. The sensitivity of the series combination (A and B positive [A+,B+]) is 760/1,000, or 76%, but the sensitivity of the parallel combination (A or B positive) is (190 + 40 + 760)/1,000, or 99%. With parallel testing, the combined sensitivity is greater than the individual sensitivities of the contributing tests.

The specificity of test A is (4,850 + 84,250)/99,000, or 90%. The specificity of test B is (9,800 + 84,250)/99,000, or 95%. The specificity of the series combination, however, is (9,800 + 4,850 + 84,250)/99,000, or 99.9%, since A+,B−; A−,B+; and A−,B− are all interpreted as negative results in series testing. The specificity of the parallel combination is 84,250/99,000, or 85.1%, since only A−,B− is considered a negative response.

Parallel testing results in the highest sensitivity but the lowest specificity, whereas series testing results in the lowest sensitivity but the highest specificity. Table 5 summarizes these findings. For tests run in parallel (A and B determined simultaneously) but considered positive if either component is positive and negative only if both are negative, the sensitivity is higher and the specificity is lower than in comparable series testing. The sensitivity is increased because some diseased patients are positive by one test, but not by the other. Similarly, there are more false-positive results in nondiseased patients. Of all the approaches, the parallel approach requires the most laboratory work, since both tests are performed on all patients in the population.

In evaluating clinical laboratory tests, it is essential that the laboratory have at its disposal simple ways of analyzing data sets. The predictive value model has proven to be effective in designing test strategies and evaluating the usefulness of laboratory tests. The widespread use of computers in laboratory medicine should permit this approach to data analysis to become routine in the next few years.

LITERATURE CITED

1. **Bayes, T.** 1763. An assay toward solving a problem in the doctrine of chance. Philos. Trans. R. Soc. London **53**:370–418.
2. **Berwick, D. M., H. V. Fineberg, and M. C. Weinstein.** 1981. When doctors meet numbers. Am. J. Med. **71**:991–998.
3. **Fink, D. J., and R. S. Galen.** 1978. Immunologic detection of prostatic acid phosphatase: critique II. Hum. Pathol. **9**:621–623.
4. **Foti, A. G., J. F. Cooper, H. Herschman, and R. R. Malvaez.** 1977. Detection of prostatic cancer by solid-phase radioimmunoassay of serum prostatic acid phosphatase. N. Engl. J. Med. **297**:1357–1361.

5. **Galen, R. S., and S. R. Gambino.** 1975. Beyond normality: the predictive value and efficiency of medical diagnoses. John Wiley & Sons, Inc., New York.

6. **Gambino, S. R., and R. S. Galen.** 1983. One man's rate is another man's ratio. Am. J. Clin. Pathol. **80:**127–128.

7. **Gittes, R.** 1977. Acid phosphatase reappraised. N. Engl. J. Med. **297:**1398–1399.

8. **Gittes, R. F.** 1983. Serum acid phosphatase and screening for carcinoma of the prostate. N. Engl. J. Med. **309:**852–853.

9. **Guinan, P., I. Bush, V. Ray, R. Vieth, R. Rao, and R. Bhatti.** 1980. The accuracy of the rectal examination in the diagnosis of prostate carcinoma. N. Engl. J. Med. **303:**499–503.

10. **McNeil, B. J.** 1976. Beyond normality: the predictive value and efficiency of medical diagnoses—book review. N. Engl. J. Med. **294:**1016.

11. **Watson, R. A., and D. B. Tang.** 1980. The predictive value of prostatic acid phosphatase as a screening test for prostatic cancer. N. Engl. J. Med. **303:**497–499.

AUTHOR INDEX

SUBJECT INDEX